FOR INSTRUCTORS

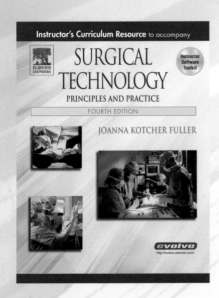

INSTRUCTOR'S CURRICULUM RESOURCE WITH CD-ROM
0-7216-9694-5

Available in both print and electronic formats, this helpful instructor's package provides all of the tools needed to quickly and consistently prepare for class. Key components include:
- Lecture Outline for every chapter
- Answers to all workbook exercises and case studies
- A comprehensive test bank in both print and CD-ROM formats in the ExamView test-generator platform
- PowerPoint lecture slides on the CD-ROM
- A correlation grid that compares text learning objectives with both the CAAHEP and ABHES required curriculum competencies

LESSON PLAN MANUAL
0-4160-2414-X

The Lesson Plan Manual is a compelling and practical tool designed to assist instructors in producing maximal student learning and growth while minimizing the time needed to develop lesson plans. The Lesson Plan Manual contains customizable chapter lesson plans that save time by already having assembled all of the teaching and learning components needed for classroom planning and preparation into one easy-to-use reference. Each lesson plan includes:
- Content competencies covered by the chapter
- Teaching Focus—a summary of what the student should learn in the lesson
- Material and resource lists
- Lesson preparation checklists to help instructors stay focused
- Key terms with page references
- Teaching modalities that are aligned with chapter learning objectives and chapter content in an at-a-glance grid format
- PowerPoint slides printed with embedded lecture notes that follow the text content

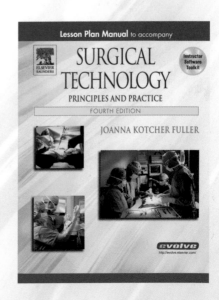

EVOLVE COURSE MANAGEMENT SYSTEM

http://evolve.elsevier.com/Fuller/surgical/

Evolve is an interactive learning environment that works in coordination with *Surgical Technology: Principles and Practice, 4th Edition,* providing Internet-based course content that reinforces and expands on the concepts that instructors deliver in class. In addition to the resources available to students, instructors are able to access all of the components of the *Instructor's Curriculum Resource,* including the computerized test bank, correlation grid, and PowerPoint slides. Instructors can also use Evolve to:
- Publish class syllabi, outline, and lecture notes
- Set up "virtual office hours" and email communication
- Share important dates and information through the online class *Calendar*
- Encourage student participation through *Chat Rooms* and *Discussion Boards*

Instructors are encouraged to contact their sales representative for more information about integrating Evolve into their curricula.

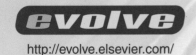

http://evolve.elsevier.com/

CONTENTS

Unit 1
THEORY AND TECHNIQUES IN SURGERY

Unit 2
SURGICAL PROCEDURES

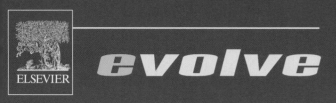

ELSEVIER

evolve

To access your Student Resources, visit the web address below:

http://evolve.elsevier.com/Fuller/surgical

- **Content updates**
  Updated with the most current information for surgical technology practice

- **Scored chapter quizzes**
  With answers and rationales, along with text page numbers, for review of concepts

- **Internet research activities**
  To challenge and intrigue while broadening comprehension

- **WebLinks**
  Links to hundreds of websites carefully chosen to supplement the content of each chapter of the textbook; regularly updated, with new links added as they develop

SURGICAL TECHNOLOGY
PRINCIPLES AND PRACTICE
FOURTH EDITION

JOANNA KOTCHER FULLER, CST, BA, BSN, MPH

University Hospitals Lothian Trust
Edinburgh, Scotland

Contributing Editor:

ELIZABETH NESS, BA, CST

Program Coordinator, Surgical Technology
Macomb Community College
Clinton Township, Michigan

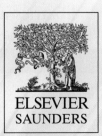

ELSEVIER
SAUNDERS

ELSEVIER
SAUNDERS

11830 Westline Industrial Drive
St. Louis, Missouri 63146

SURGICAL TECHNOLOGY: PRINCIPLES AND PRACTICE, FOURTH EDITION
Copyright © 2005 by Elsevier Inc.

NOTICE

Surgical technology is an ever-changing field. Standard safety precautions must be followed, but as new research and clinical experience broaden our knowledge, changes in treatment and drug therapy may become necessary or appropriate. Readers are advised to check the most current product information provided by the manufacturer of each drug to be administered to verify the recommended dose, the method and duration of administration, and contraindications. It is the responsibility of the licensed prescriber, relying on experience and knowledge of the patient, to determine dosages and the best treatment for each individual patient. Neither the publisher nor the author assumes any liability for any injury and/or damage to persons or property arising from this publication.

Previous editions copyrighted 1994, 1986, 1981

ISBN-13:   978-0-7216-9693-5
ISBN-10:   0-7216-9693-7

Publisher: Michael S. Ledbetter
Senior Developmental Editors: Laurie K. Gower, Lisa P. Newton
Publishing Services Manager: Pat Joiner
Project Manager: Gena Magouirk
Senior Design Project Manager: Bill Drone

Printed in the United States of America

Last digit is the print number: 9   8   7   6   5   4   3   2

Contributors

We extend a special acknowledgment to the following people who brought their expertise to bear by contributing content and valuable editorial input:

CHRISTINA L. BAUMER, PHD, RN, MED, CNOR, CHES
Division Chair, Continuing Education;
Program Director, Surgical Technology,
Lancaster General College of Nursing and Health Sciences,
Lancaster, Pennsylvania

RONALD W. BUTTS, CST, CFA, CSA
Senior Surgical Technologist/Surgical Assistant,
Munson Medical Center,
Traverse City, Michigan

ROBERT DOHENY, CST
Surgical Services,
William Beaumont Hospital,
Troy, Michigan

REBECCA CARR FERGUSON, RN, BSN, CNOR
Southeast Alabama Medical Center,
Dothan, Alabama

MARY GRACE HENSEL, RN, BSN, CNOR
Allegheny General Hospital,
Pittsburgh, Pennsylvania

JANET ANNE MILLIGAN, RN, CNOR
Surgical Technology Program,
College of Southern Idaho,
Twin Falls, Idaho

MARGARET MULCRONE, RN, MSN, CNOR
Staff Development Coordinator, Surgical Services,
St. Joseph Mercy—Macomb,
Clinton Township, Michigan

PATRICIA C. SEIFERT, RN, MSN, CRNFA, CNOR, FAAN
Perioperative Cardiac Care Coordinator, CVOR,
Inova Fairfax Hospital,
Falls Church, Virginia

KEN WARNOCK, CST
Surgical Technology Faculty,
Macomb Community College,
Clinton Township, Michigan

Reviewers

To ensure the accuracy of the material presented throughout this textbook, an extensive review and development process was used. This included several phases of evaluation by a variety of surgical technology instructors and experts in the various medical and surgical specialties. We are deeply grateful to the numerous people who have shared their comments and suggestions. Reviewing a book or supplement takes an incredible amount of energy and attention, and we are glad so many colleagues were able to take time out of their busy schedules to help ensure the validity and appropriateness of content in this textbook. The reviewers provided us with additional viewpoints and opinions that combine to make this text an incredible learning tool. We wish to thank the following editorial review team:

KAREN ALDRIDGE, CST
Central Carolina Technical College,
Sumter, South Carolina

MARYPAT ANNABLE, RN, CNOR, MSN
Surgical Technology Chair,
Onondaga Community College,
Syracuse, New York

PAMELA S. APPLETON, RN, BS, CNOR
Southern Illinois Collegiate Common Market,
Herrin, Illinois

MARGARET M. BANGERT, RN, BSN, MSED, CNOR
Ulster County Board of Cooperative Education,
Port Ewin, New York

CHRISTINA L. BAUMER, PHD, RN, MED, CNOR, CHES
Division Chair, Continuing Education;
Program Director, Surgical Technology,
Lancaster General College of Nursing and Health Sciences,
Lancaster, Pennsylvania

RICHARD H. BELL, PHD
Professor of Biology/Microbiology,
Macomb Community College,
Clinton Township, Michigan

CAMILLE L. CHURCH, CST
Olympia College,
Merrillville, Indiana

LORI CLIFTON, RN, BSN, CNOR
Clinton Township, Michigan

LYNDA CUSTER, CST, MA
Program Coordinator, Surgical Technology Program,
Baker College,
Clinton Township, Michigan

DIONA DAVIS, CST, CFA
College of Technology,
Montana State University,
Great Falls, Montana

IVONNE DELEON, ST, RN, CNOR
Central Carolina Technical College,
Sumter, South Carolina

CAROL DOLLAR, RN, BSN
Surgical Technology Program Coordinator,
Tulsa Technology Center,
Tulsa, Oklahoma

MICHAEL DORICH, B.ED, CAHI
Western School,
Monroeville, Pennsylvania

GITTHALINE A. GAGNE, CST, CRCST, MS
Connelley Technical Institute,
Pittsburgh, Pennsylvania

LINDA GROAH, RN, MS, CNOR
Tiburon, California

REBECCA NADINE KNIGHT, RN, BS, CNOR
Loma Linda University,
Loma Linda, California

WANDA KORZOWSKI, CSPDS

Manager, Sterile Processing,
St. John Providence Hospital & Medical Center,
Southfield, Michigan

MAUREEN LANGE, RNC, CNOR, MS

Elgin Community College,
Elgin, Illinois

KATHERINE B. LEE, CST, MS

Associate Professor;
Surgical Technology Program Director,
Richland Community College,
Decatur, Illinois

RUTH A. LETEXIER, BSN, CST, PHN

Surgical Technology Department,
Northwest Technical College,
East Grand Forks, Minnesota

JAYNE MACPHERSON, CST, BS

Bunker Hill Community College,
Chelsea, Massachusetts

MARY JANE MCCLAIN, MSN, RN, CNOR

Fresno City College,
Fresno, California

MARIETTA MCDUFFY, CST, BS

Surgical Technology Program,
Malcolm X College,
Chicago, Illinois

MARY E. MCNARON, CST, CNOR, RN, BSN, MS

Coordinator, Surgical Technology,
Gulf Coast Community College,
Panama City, Florida

KEVIN NEFF, MD

Assistant Clinical Professor, Department of Anesthesia,
Wayne State University School of Medicine,
Detroit, Michigan

ANNE E. REHM, RN, MSN, CNOR

Gwinnett Technical College,
Lawrenceville, Georgia

CLIFFORD SMITH, RN, CNOR, CRNFA, BSN

Director, Surgical Technology Program,
Mt. Aloysius College,
Cresson, Pennsylvania

KATHLEEN JEAN URIBE, CST, BSN, MA

Program Chair, Surgical Technology,
Southeast Community College,
Lincoln, Nebraska

KEN WARNOCK, CST

Surgical Technology Faculty,
Macomb Community College,
Clinton Township, Michigan

JOYCE ANNE TALLMAN WESTER, RN, BA, MA, CNOR

Pinellas Technical Education Center—Clearwater Campus,
Clearwater, Florida

TRACY L. WOODSWORTH, BSN

Instructor, Surgical Technology,
Mt. Hood Community College,
Gresham, Oregon

NANCY WRIGHT, RN, BS, CNOR

Surgical Technology Program Manager,
VA College,
Birmingham, Alabama

There are many individuals who have contributed to our lives in certain ways, providing something unique to us, from whom we gain valuable life experience and knowledge. Some of these experiences create who we are, how we think, and how we deliver these valuable messages to others. There are many people who have influenced who I am, and I would like to dedicate this textbook to the following people:

To all of my students past, present, and future, who have been my inspirations to write this textbook;

Beatrice Franklin, CST, MEd, my mentor as an instructor in the field of surgical technology. Bea's mentoring challenged me to "think outside the box" and deliver education in nontraditional meaningful ways;

Anne Marie Kaminski, RN, MSHA, who provided me valuable firsthand experience and instilled the work ethic that we are the patient advocates, always keeping in mind "the patient first";

Wanda Korzowski, CSPDS, my first preceptor, whose excellence in the field of surgical technology and sterile processing has set the highest standards for others to follow;

Ken Warnock, CST, my colleague, whose dedication and commitment to students and this textbook set standards for all to follow;

Charlene McPeak, PhD, APRN, BC, Dean of Health and Human Services at Macomb Community College, for her commitment and futuristic vision for clinical career ladder educational opportunities for growth and development for students in the fields of central processing distribution technician, surgical technology, and surgical first assisting.

Members of the Macomb Community College Advisory Committee, for their constant support and encouragement to strive to be the best, and for their commitment and dedication to surgical technology students. The members I would like to thank include:

Susan Assaf; Lynne Behrens-Hanna; Rosa Berry; Lori Clifton; Deborah Crilli; Roseanne DiMaria; Constance Fordyce; Connie Franko; Michael Haynes, MD; Wendy Herzog; Anne Marie Kaminski; Wanda Korzowski; Jamie Krupa; Jacqueline McKay; Charlene McPeak; Margaret Mulcrone; Lori Renda-Francis; Donna Sennott; Jane Serra; Jennifer Smith; Erik Stone; Erlie Topacio; Diane Thompson; Barbara Walzak; Ken Warnock; Herman Young; and Nancy Zehnpfennig.

A thank you to all of my family and friends, and a special thank you to the following members of my family…

To my dad, Theodore Van Meter, retired attorney, for his thorough review and assistance on Chapter 3, Law and Ethics;

To my children, Andrew, Matthew, and Michelle, and to my husband, Jim, who have encouraged and supported me for the past two years, patiently allowing me to work on this project.

EN

Preface

Welcome to *Surgical Technology: Principles and Practice, 4th Edition*. With this textbook in hand, you are about to take the first step toward a career filled with many fulfilling opportunities and rewards. As a surgical technologist, you will be able to make a difference in the lives of others and be a part of the ever-changing world of health care. The U.S. Department of Labor's Bureau of Labor Statistics *Occupational Outlook Handbook* (2004) projects that employment for the surgical technologist will increase between 21% and 35% over the next 10 years. This growth can be attributed to the increasing numbers of over-50 Americans who are approaching retirement age and the additional types of surgery that can be performed on an outpatient basis. Rapid advances are occurring in surgery with the development and increased use of fiber optics, laser technology, and robotics, which have created a need for more highly skilled health care professionals.

What does this mean for you? It means that, armed with the solid foundation of theory and procedural knowledge provided in this textbook, you will be prepared to take advantage of the tremendous opportunities that await you in the surgical technology field.

Today's surgical technologists must be thoroughly educated in every aspect of their scope of practice in order to work closely with surgeons, anesthesiologists, registered nurses, and other perioperative personnel in delivering optimal patient care before, during, and after surgery. For over 20 years, this textbook has been a trusted and comprehensive source of the core knowledge and skills you need to achieve a successful career as a surgical technologist. This textbook is the first written by a surgical technologist for surgical technology students. It covers all core content required for instruction in surgical technology programs that are accredited by both the Commission on Accreditation of Allied Health Education Programs (CAAHEP) and the American Board of Health Education Schools (ABHES), so you can be certain that everything you will learn in this textbook reflects best practices in the field. What's more, you can count on this textbook to properly prepare you for surgical technology certification examinations.

The innovative presentation of up-to-date concepts and information in this book will equip you to perform your duties effectively and make the right decisions as you work with other members of the health care team. Clear guidelines help you understand and follow key skills, surgical procedures, common setups, and more to ensure that the operating room environment is safe, that equipment functions properly, and that operative procedures are conducted under conditions that maximize patient safety. Nearly 600 illustrations reflect the latest skills and procedures you need to learn, the instrumentation you will be using, and other vital elements of the job. The humanistic approach woven throughout will help you gain an appreciation for the respect and dignity patients deserve, as well as how to effectively interact with colleagues on the job.

Organizational Structure

Surgical Technology: Principles and Practice, 4th Edition, is written specifically for surgical technology students and organized in a format that teaches the foundational material first, before introducing the surgical procedures. This format better prepares you to learn the core surgical procedures only after you have a solid understanding of the foundational concepts and skills that apply to each of them. The text is divided into two units: *Theory and Techniques in Surgery* and *Surgical Procedures.*

Unit One, Theory and Techniques in Surgery, provides important foundational knowledge surgical technologists need to know in order to function both inside and outside the operating room, including legal and ethical boundaries, professional concepts, the operating room environment, aseptic techniques, and patient preparation and transport. The very latest topics and skills are included, including robotics, endoscopic procedures, computers, and electricity. At the end of each chapter, from chapter 1 to Chapter 20, mini case studies have been added to promote critical thinking and application of concepts learned in the chapters to help you better relate content to real-life situations.

Unit One includes five new chapters. Chapter 2, The Patient, discusses Maslow's hierarchy of needs and its relationship to patient care; how to meet the patient's physiological, psychosocial, and environmental needs; how to practice therapeutic communication; and the importance of culturally appropriate patient care. Chapter 4, Hospital Administration and Organization, discusses how hospitals are administered and the process of accreditation, and it identifies operating room staff members and their duties.

Chapter 6, Communication and Teamwork, discusses how to effectively communicate with other staff members; approaches to solving conflict; active listening skills; and the importance of good teamwork in providing patient care. Chapter 14, Environmental Hazards, identifies proper safety methods to prevent injuries and burns to patients; proper disposal of hazardous waste; and electrosurgical, laser, and chemical safety.

Chapter 18, Endoscopic Surgery and Robotics, describes setup and care of endoscopic instruments and equipment and the components of a robotic surgical system. Chapter 19, Diagnostic Procedures, provides an in-depth overview of the various laboratory tests, examinations, and procedures performed on patients to assist physicians in determining diagnoses and identifying courses of treatment.

Unit Two, Surgical Procedures, presents all the latest core surgical procedures you need to know to be fully prepared to step into the job. Organized by surgical specialty, this portion of the text presents the very latest techniques and equipment and presents procedures in a consistent format that breaks down each procedure into its surgical goal, pathology, technique, and discussion. The technique section is highlighted so that the critical steps involved can be followed. The new Chapter 30, Pediatric Surgery, covers approximately 20 procedures specific to the pediatric patient. Psychological and physiological needs of the pediatric patient are also addressed.

Elizabeth Ness

Acknowledgments

It takes a very dedicated group of individuals to complete a project of this magnitude. I would like to thank Shirley Kuhn for giving me the opportunity to work on this 4th edition. A very special thanks goes to Amy Holmes, a dedicated individual with whom I had the pleasure of working for most of the early production of this textbook. She provided excellent guidance, detailed instructions, and constant encouragement and support throughout this project.

I would also like to thank some particular individuals at Elsevier for their commitment, dedication, and support to the completion of this textbook. First, I would like to thank Dan Smigell, Senior Educational Publisher's Representative, for providing me the wonderful opportunity to be involved as the contributing editor of this 4th edition. I would also like to thank Michael Ledbetter, Publisher, and Laurie Gower, Senior Developmental Editor, who have been instrumental in the final editing and publication of this much awaited textbook.

Elizabeth Ness

Special Features

Learning Objectives and **Terminology,** with glossary-style definitions at the beginning of each chapter, set the stage for student learning.

Learning Objectives

After studying this chapter the reader will be able to:

- Describe the rationale for practicing aseptic technique
- Clearly distinguish among sterile, nonsterile, and aseptic
- Explain surgical conscience
- Explain the concept of barriers
- Practice the rules of aseptic technique
- Explain the relationship between personal hygiene and aseptic technique
- Perform the surgical hand scrub correctly
- Demonstrate aseptic technique by donning gown and gloves
- Don sterile gloves using proper open gloving technique
- Remove gown and gloves using aseptic technique
- Remove contaminated gloves from another person
- Discuss reasons why personnel might not follow the rules of asepsis

Terminology

Airborne contamination—Incident in which microorganisms carried in the air by moisture droplets or dust particles make contact with a sterile surface.

Antiseptics—Chemical agents that are approved for use on the skin and that inhibit growth and reproduction of microorganisms. Antiseptics are used to cleanse and paint the surgical site to reduce the number of microorganisms to an absolute minimum.

Asepsis—The absence of pathogenic microorganisms on an animate surface or on body tissue. Literally, asepsis means "without infection." In surgery, asepsis is a state of minimal or zero pathogens. Asepsis is the goal of many surgical practices.

Aseptic technique—Methods or practices in health care that promote and maintain a state of asepsis. Also called sterile technique.

Chemical barrier—The barrier formed by the action of an antiseptic that not only reduces the number of microorganisms on a surface but also prevents recolonization (regrowth) for a limited period of time.

Closed gloving—A technique of gloving in which the bare hand does not come in contact with the outside of the glove. The sterile glove is protected from the nonsterile hand by the cuff of a surgical gown.

Contamination—Result of physical contact between a sterile surface and a nonsterile surface in surgery. Contamination also can result from airborne dust, moisture droplets, or fluids that act as a vehicle for transporting contaminants from a nonsterile surface to a sterile one.

Handwashing—A specific technique used to remove debris and dead cells from the hands. Handwashing with an antiseptic also reduces the number of microorganisms on the skin.

Latex allergy—Sensitivity to latex, which can cause itching, rhinitis, conjunctivitis, and anaphylactic shock leading to death. Personnel and patients with latex allergy must not come in contact with any articles that contain latex.

Nonsterile personnel—In surgery, team members who remain outside the boundary of the sterile field and do not come into direct contact with sterile equipment, sterile areas, or the surgical wound. The circulator, anesthesia care provider, and x-ray technician are examples of nonsterile team members.

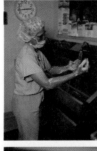
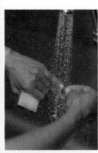
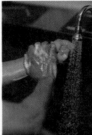
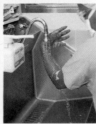

FIGURE 9-9
Surgical hand scrub. (From Perry AG and Potter PA: *Clinical nursing skills and techniques*, ed 5, St Louis, 2004, Mosby.)

Gowning Yourself
Surgical gowns are worn by all sterile personnel. The gown is donned immediately before the start of surgery and may be changed during surgery if it is penetrated by blood or other fluids. Many types of surgical gowns are available, but the most common type wraps around the body and is designed to cover both the front and the back of the wearer. As mentioned earlier, however, *the back is considered nonsterile.*

Most disposable gowns are water resistant. Gowns used in orthopedics, obstetrics, and other specialties in which there

Dynamic, full-color photos provide visual connection and promote student involvement with the material.

---

is very slowly absorbed into the cerebrospinal fluid through the dura mater. It spreads both caudally (toward the feet) and cephalad (toward the head). For a single-shot epidural, the patient's position and the molecular weight of the anesthetic have no effect on its distribution. However, with a continuous epidural, the position of the patient does seem to affect the spread of the local anesthetic. Epidural anesthesia is often used in obstetrical, gynecological, urological, and rectal surgery. It is also used for postoperative pain control.

The patient's skin is prepared as for spinal anesthesia. The epidural needle is advanced through the ligamentum flavum until it enters the epidural space. A thoracic, lumbar, or caudal puncture site is used, depending on the target site of the anesthesia. The anesthetic agent is then injected directly into the epidural space. Lidocaine, chloroprocaine, and bupivacaine are commonly used.

Continuous or intermittent epidural anesthesia is created by the delivery of an anesthetic drug through a small indwelling catheter. This technique also is used for postopera-

Table 12-4 LOCAL ANESTHETICS FOR INJECTION

Generic Name	Trade Name	Local Infiltration or Nerve Block or Epidural Block	Spinal Block (Subarachnoid)	Duration*	Comments
Bupivacaine hydrochloride	Marcaine† Sensorcaine MPF	+	+	Long‡	Produces long-acting epidural anesthesia in labor with no reported effects on fetus. Maximum dose is 200 mg.
Chloroprocaine hydrochloride	Nesacaine	+	0	Short	Little systemic toxicity because of rapid hydrolysis in plasma. No effects reported on fetus after epidural anesthesia in mother. Maximum dose is 800 mg.
Etidocaine hydrochloride	Duranest	+	0	Long	Highly lipid soluble. Onset time for epidural block is 5 min. Profound muscle relaxation is desirable for abdominal surgery but not for labor.
Lidocaine	Xylocaine†	+	+	Intermediate	Widely used local anesthetic. Maximum dose is 300 mg (4.5 mg/kg body weight). Can cause drowsiness, fatigue, and amnesia.
Mepivacaine	Carbocaine†	+	0	Intermediate	Chemically related to lidocaine. Maximum dose is 400 mg (7 mg/kg body weight).
Prilocaine	Citanest†	+	0	Intermediate	Used for dental procedures. Maximum dose is 400 mg.
Procaine hydrochloride	Novocain†	+	+	Short	Noted for its safety because of its rapid hydrolysis in plasma. Maximum dose is 600 mg (10 mg/kg body weight). Duration of epidural block is unreliable.
Propoxycaine and procaine	Ravocaine and Novocain with Neo-Cobefri	+	0	Short to intermediate	Used for dental procedures. Dose is 4 mg propoxycaine and 20 mg procaine.
Ropivacaine	Naropin†	+	0	Long	Used for epidural, field block, and major nerve block anesthesia. Dose is 20-40 mg.
Tetracaine	Pontocaine†	0	+	Long	Most widely used drug for spinal anesthesia. Onset is 5 min. Dose for spinal anesthesia is 2-15 mg. Available in hyperbaric, isobaric, and hypobaric solutions.

From Clark JF and Queener SF: *Pharmacologic basis of nursing practice*, ed 6, St Louis, 1999, Mosby.
+, Suitable use; 0, not suitable use.
*Duration without epinephrine: short, 1 hr; intermediate, 2 hr; long, 3 hr (approximations).
†Available in Canada and the United States.
‡Duration of bupivacaine in nerve block is 6-13 hr.

Information is presented in an **at-a-glance** format through the use of **lists, illustrations, and tables.**

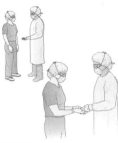

REMOVING THE GOWN

When removing sterile attire, one removes the gown first, according to the following guidelines (Figure 9-17):

1. Grasp the gown at the shoulders, releasing or breaking the ties or snaps, and pull the sleeves downward. This will roll the gown inside out as it slides over your gloved hands.
2. Roll the gown so the contaminated outside surface faces inward.
3. Dispose of the gown in a biohazard bag.

REMOVING GLOVES

The gloves should be removed second according to the following guidelines (Figure 9-18):

1. Grasp one glove at the outer wrist, using the opposite gloved hand.
2. Pull the glove off. It will turn inside out as you remove it.
3. Place your bare fingers *inside* the cuff of the opposite hand and roll this glove off your hand.
4. Dispose of both gloves in a biohazard receptacle *without touching the contaminated outside of the gloves.*

FIGURE 9-16
Removing a contaminated glove during surgery.

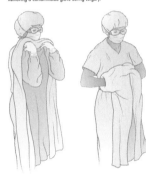

FIGURE 9-17
Removing a contaminated gown after surgery.

Step-by-step instructions with full-color illustrations make it easy to learn skills and procedures.

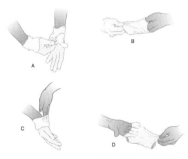

FIGURE 9-18
Removing contaminated gloves aseptically after surgery. **A,** Grasp the edge of the glove. **B,** Unroll the glove over the hand. Discard the glove (not shown). **C,** With the bare hand, grasp the opposite glove cuff on its inside surface. **D,** Remove the glove by inverting it over the hand. Discard the glove (not shown).

CASE STUDIES

Case 1
After you have performed the hand scrub, you enter the surgery suite and proceed to the area where your gown and gloves are located. As you are removing the towel, you notice that some water from your hand has dripped onto your sterile gown. What will you do?

Case 2
During surgery you notice that the surgeon has a hole in his glove. You notify him of this. He replies, "Don't worry about it." How will you respond?

Case 3
When you arrive in surgery, you notice that someone has placed your wrapped sterile instruments next to the heating vent. There is moisture on the outside of the pack. What should you do?

Case 4
During surgery you are moving a heavy instrument tray from one area of the sterile table to another. As you pick up the tray, the corner of the instrument tray accidentally rips the sterile sheet covering the entire back table. What will you do?

Case 5
The surgeon has just spoken abruptly to you about how you hand him sutures. A minute later you rip your glove on the suture, and the surgeon must wait while you remove your contaminated glove and put on a sterile one. The surgeon is visibly irritated. What would you say to the surgeon, if anything, while changing your glove?

Case 6
When you open your sterile basins while setting up a case, you notice moisture on the inside of a sterile basin. What is the significance of this?

Case 7
While you are scrubbed on a vaginal procedure, the mechanical engineer comes in to fix a plug. As he passes by your sterile setup, his nonsterile scrub top brushes against the in-

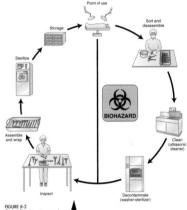

FIGURE 8-2
Cycle of equipment processing.

locks must be opened and hinges extended to their widest adjustment.

The washer-sterilizer operates much the same as the steam sterilizer. The washer-sterilizer sends copious amounts of soapy water over the instruments. Steam under pressure and air are then injected into the water, which activates the water significantly. As the water drains from the chamber, tissue debris and particles are filtered off and steam fills the entire chamber. The temperature is then maintained at 270° F for 3 minutes. Near the completion of the cycle, the steam is released through the exhaust system.

After processing in the washer-sterilizer, all instruments should be placed in the **ultrasonic cleaner** (Figure 8-4). This cleaning further removes particles and debris through a process called **cavitation**. During cavitation, high-frequency sound waves are generated through a water bath in which the instruments are placed along with a neutral to slightly alkaline detergent. Cavitation causes tiny air spaces trapped

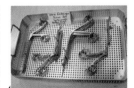

FIGURE 8-3
Instrument tray. (Courtesy of Case Medical, Ridgefield, NJ.)

Almost 600 illustrations and photos have been revised to provide true-to-life, full-color images that reflect the most current techniques and equipment.

Case Studies promote critical thinking and application of concepts. Answers are available in the *Instructor's Curriculum Resource with CD-ROM.*

Contents

SURGICAL
TECHNOLOGY
PRINCIPLES AND PRACTICE

Unit 1

Theory and Techniques in Surgery

Chapter 1

The Surgical Technologist

Learning Objectives

After studying this chapter the reader will be able to:

- Understand the development of the surgical technologist after World War II
- Describe the process of certification for the surgical technologist
- Discuss career opportunities available to the surgical technologist
- List personal attributes for success as a surgical technologist
- Describe the differences among certification, licensure, and registration
- Identify the duties of the surgical technologist
- Describe the difference between delegation and assignment

Terminology

ABHES—Accrediting Bureau of Health Education Schools.

ACS—American College of Surgeons. A professional organization that establishes educational standards for surgeons and surgical residency programs.

AORN—Association of periOperative Registered Nurses. The professional organization for surgical nurses; originally known as Association of Operating Room Nurses.

ARC-ST—Accreditation Review Committee for Surgical Technologists. The professional agency for accreditation of surgical technology programs.

AST—The Association of Surgical Technologists. The professional association for surgical technologists.

Back table—A large stainless steel table that is draped with a sterile sheet before surgery. Equipment and instruments are placed on this table in reserve, available for use during surgery.

CAAHEP—Commission on Accreditation of Allied Health Education Programs. It accredits educational programs in allied health professions.

Case-cart system—Organizational method of preparing equipment and instruments for a specific surgery. Equipment is prepared by the central services or supply department and sent to the operating room for use hours later.

Circulator—The nonsterile surgical team member who assists in gathering additional supplies and equipment needed during the surgical procedure and advocates for the patient.

CST—Certified Surgical Technologist. A surgical technologist who has successfully passed the certification examination distributed by the Liaison Council on Certification for the Surgical Technologist.

CST-CFA—Certified Surgical Technologist–Certified First Assistant. A Certified Surgical Technologist First Assistant who has successfully passed the certification examination distributed by the Liaison Council on Certification for the Surgical Technologist.

Delegation—The transfer of responsibility for an activity from a licensed person to a nonlicensed person; the person initiating the transfer retains accountability for the outcome of that activity.

Dependent tasks—Tasks that are delegated to another person and require direct supervision by the person delegating the task.

Flash sterilize—To sterilize instruments and equipment in a high-pressure autoclave. Used only in an emergency, such as when an instrument is contaminated during surgery and must be sterilized immediately.

Terminology—cont'd

Independent tasks—Tasks that are transferred to another person and do not require direct supervision by the person delegating the task.

LCC-ST—The Liaison Council on Certification for the Surgical Technologist. The professional body responsible for developing and administering the national certification examination.

Open a case—To begin work on a surgical case by opening sterile supplies and equipment using sterile technique. Tables and stainless steel furniture are first draped with sterile sheets, and sterile equipment is opened onto the tables without contamination.

Proprietary school—Private, for-profit school.

Scrub—Member of the sterile team who handles instruments, supplies, and equipment necessary for the surgical procedure. The surgical hand scrub is the process of prescribed, thorough hand cleaning before the donning of sterile gloves and gown.

Sharps—Any objects that can penetrate the skin and have the potential for causing injury and infection, including but not limited to, needles, scalpels, broken glass, broken capillary tubes, and exposed ends of dental wires.

Sterile—Free from living microorganisms.

EVOLUTION OF THE PROFESSION

Since the practice of medicine and surgery began, the profession of surgical technology has evolved into a distinct category of health-care worker with specialized education, certification, and standards of practice. The field of medicine has always had assistants whose jobs varied according to immediate need and the demands of the healer, physician, or surgeon, whether in a war, in an urban setting, or in a rural setting.

History of the Profession

Beginning with the development of effective anesthesia and antisepsis in the late nineteenth century, the role of the nurse in surgery has been easily defined and tracked. In the late 1800s she prepared instruments for surgery, and in the early 1900s she assisted in surgical procedures and in the administration of ether, called "etherizing." Her duties from about the 1920s to the 1940s were those of a **circulator.** She also instructed student nurses in their surgical education. Often the operating room supervisor was the only graduate nurse in surgery, and it was her duty to oversee the student nurses as they completed their rotation in surgery.

The need for assistive personnel in surgery did not arise until World War II. During World War I, army corpsmen worked on the battlefield to offer aid and comfort to the wounded, but they had no role in surgery. World War II dramatically changed that. With the development of antibiotics such as penicillin and sulfa, war surgeons could operate on and save the lives of many more patients than was previously possible. Technological advances also created a need for trained personnel who could assist in applying these advances.

The increase in battlefield survivors created a drastic shortage of nurses. In addition to those nurses needed to staff field hospitals, many more were needed to staff base hospitals, and still more were needed at home to attend to the needs of the wounded who returned from battle. To supply the field hospitals in the Pacific and European theaters, the army began training corpsmen to assist in surgery, a role that previously had been filled only by nurses. By this time, however, corpsmen were expected to administer anesthesia and also act as the first assistant to the surgeon. When nurses were not available, such as on combat ships where women were not allowed, corpsmen worked under the direct supervision of the surgeon. Thus a new profession was born, which the army called operating room technicians (ORTs). From this time on, the military played a significant role in refining the position of the ORT. Each branch of the military (except the Marines) provided specific training and job descriptions for the ORT, who received secondary training after first becoming a medic.

After World War II, the Korean War caused a continued shortage of operating room nurses, and the need for fully trained nurses in the operating room was questioned. At this time the operating room supervisors began to recruit ex-corpsmen to work in civilian surgery. Their primary function was that of a circulator. Registered nurses continued to fill the **scrub** or "instrument nurse" role until about 1965, when the roles were reversed.

Prompted by the need for guidelines and standards in training paramedical surgical personnel, the **Association of Operating Room Nurses (AORN)** published a book titled *Teaching the Operating Room Technician* in 1967. In 1968, the AORN Board of Directors created the Association of Operating Room Technicians (AORT). In its early years the AORT was governed by the joint AORN–AORT advisory board. During this time, the ORT received his or her training only on the job. Formal training for the civilian ORT began in **proprietary schools** across the United States around this time.

Surgical Technologists' Professional Organization

Along with organizational independence came steps toward formalizing the technologist's education. The AORT formed two new committees: **Liaison Council on Certification for the Surgical Technologist (LCC-ST)** and the Joint Review Committee on Education. The first certifying examination for operating room technicians was given in 1970, and those technologists who passed the examination were given a new title: Certified Operating Room Technician (CORT). In

1973, the AORT became independent of the AORN, and soon afterward changed the title of the position to surgical technologist and changed the name of its professional organization to its current title, the **Association of Surgical Technologists (AST)**.

By 1974 it was evident that an accreditation body was needed to ensure quality education of the ORT.

The AST has since worked actively and diligently to promote excellence in the profession of surgical technology. During the 1980s the AST developed a code of ethics and standards of practice, and expanded the professional journal. In the next decade a formal job description was published. The AST continues to be the surgical technologists' professional organization and represents members nationwide. The association promotes professional standards; provides advanced educational and administrative conferences; offers opportunities for continuing education credits, educational materials, and scholarships; and advocates for personal and professional growth. For the student or practicing surgical technologist, it is important to become an active member of AST and become a part in promoting and achieving the highest standards for the profession of surgical technology.

TRAINING, CERTIFICATION, AND EMPLOYMENT

Training and Program Accreditation

Surgical technologists are trained in 2-year colleges and in vocational and proprietary programs. A 2-year accredited program leading to an associate's degree is the preferred path to training and education, but many accredited 9-month and 18-month programs also are available. Currently more than 350 accredited surgical technology programs offer training. Surgical technology programs are accredited through a formal process involving the American Hospital Association (AHA), **American College of Surgeons (ACS)**, and the AST. Curriculums for surgical technology programs are written in accordance with educational guidelines developed by the AST. Surgical technology programs are required to submit to the **Accreditation Review Committee for Surgical Technology (ARC-ST)** written documentation showing that the AST's educational standards have been met. The ARC-ST is the specific professional body that reviews and verifies this documentation. The ARC-ST also schedules on-site visits for programs seeking initial or continuing accreditation.

Surgical technology programs that comply with educational standards in the areas of curriculum, laboratory training facilities, and clinical site training facilities are submitted by the ARC-ST for review by the **Commission on Accreditation of Allied Health Education Programs (CAAHEP)**. The CAAHEP grants formal accreditation to educational programs in allied health professions that meet its criteria. Accredited surgical technology programs seeking continuing accreditation are required to submit an an-

nual report to the ARC-ST for review, to prove continued compliance with the guidelines and standards required for program accreditation.

Effective January 2004, the Liaison Council on Certification for the Surgical Technologist (LCC-ST) voted to grant graduates from surgical technology programs that are awarded accreditation from the **Accrediting Bureau of Health Education Schools (ABHES)** eligibility to sit for the national certification examination. Institutions offering surgical technology programs currently accredited by the ABHES may apply for accreditation through the ABHES for the surgical technology program. The surgical technology program is required to submit written documentation to the ABHES demonstrating compliance with the educational standards and guidelines required by the AST. Surgical technology programs demonstrating compliance with the educational standards earn accreditation from the ABHES.

Certification and Licensure

Certification is acknowledgment by a private agency that a person has achieved a minimum level of knowledge and skill. Certification is voluntary and not regulated by the government, but it is recognized nationally and from state to state. Certification rather than licensure was selected as the preferred method of credentialing for surgical technologists because it allowed employers to evaluate prospective employees by one verifiable national standard.

Graduates from accredited surgical technology programs or previously certified surgical technologists are eligible to sit for the national certification examination. Surgical technologists must apply to the LCC-ST to sit for the national certification examination. The LCC-ST must verify that every candidate seeking to take the examination meets eligibility requirements. A passing grade on the examination demonstrates entry-level competency in the profession, and the surgical technologist earns the title of **certified surgical technologist (CST)**. The LCC-ST examinations for Certified Surgical Technologist (CST) and Certified First Assistant (CFA) are the *only* recognized examinations in the country accredited by the National Commission for Certifying Agencies (NCCA).

Certification is not required in all hospitals or health-care settings to be eligible for all jobs. However, most hospitals prefer to hire certified surgical technologists because a CST has demonstrated commitment to quality patient care and earned a nationally recognized professional credential. Certification is also preferred by risk-management departments, because certification indicates the employee has successfully passed a competency examination. Certification also demonstrates a health-care institution's commitment to quality during an accreditation review. Certification is maintained through continuing education credits granted by the AST. The purpose of continuing education credits (CE) is to ensure that certified individuals keep up-to-date with current information and technology, which helps in providing and improving quality patient care. To continue active certification, 60 CEs must be earned in a 4-year period; the alternative to keeping active certification is to retake the certification examination.

The National Center for Competency Testing (NCCT) has developed certification examinations for surgical technologists and surgical assistants. These examinations were designed for individuals that do not meet the certification eligibility requirements of the LCC-ST. For certification as a surgical technologist, the NCCT requires scrub experience from all applicants with a minimum of 150 validated documented surgical cases. The NCCT requires applicants to have a high school diploma or equivalent and requires any of the following eligibility requirements listed.

1. Be a graduate of an operating room technician, surgical technician, or surgical technologist program of a school or college that is recognized by the United States Department of Education (USDOE).
2. Be a graduate of a formal operating room technician or surgical technology training program, with 1 year of validated work experience in the past 2 years, or 2 years of work experience in the last 4 years.
3. Have 7 years of validated scrub experience within the past 10 years.
4. Medical doctor (MD), registered nurse (RN), licensed practical nurse (LPN), or licensed vocational nurse (LVN) with extensive documented scrub experience.

Individuals who successfully pass the examination receive the credential Tech in Surgery–Certified, TS-C (NCCT). The NCCT also requires individuals to maintain CEs for certification. Those individuals who successfully pass the surgical assistant certification examination earn the credential Assistant in Surgery–Certified, AS-C (NCCT). For eligibility requirements, see the NCCA website listed in the chapter references.

Licensed personnel are those health-care workers who have been given the right to practice by a government agency. Applicants must complete formal education and training in an accredited institution and pass a licensing examination. Examples of government agencies that license health-care workers are the state board of physicians and the state board of nursing. These professionals must be licensed to be allowed to work. Licensed professionals must be registered by the state in which they work and can practice only in the state or states in which they are licensed. Licensed personnel, however, may become certified in a specialty or advanced practice.

There is currently no licensure for surgical technologists, but there is advanced certification, the **Certified Surgical Technologist–Surgical First Assistant (CST-CFA).** No state currently requires licensure of surgical technologists. Several states have begun lobbying successfully for registration and actively investigating licensure of CSTs, and this trend is expected to gain momentum in the coming years. Registration differs from certification in that it is regulated by the individual state and allows CSTs to be held accountable under the state's regulatory structure. Registry differs from licensure in that a licensed professional is allowed to delegate specific tasks to unlicensed personnel while retaining accountability for those tasks.

Specialty Practice and Employment Opportunities

Surgical technologists have many employment choices. In addition to the hospital operating room, they may work in private specialty practices such as ophthalmology, neurosurgery, and orthopedics. Ambulatory surgery centers also employ surgical technologists, as do veterinarians for assistance in surgery. A growing number of surgical technologists work as sales representatives or technical specialists, teaching operating room staffers how to use new equipment, such as orthopedic devices and implants. Surgical technologists also manage central or **sterile** supply departments of a hospital and can receive advanced training in hospital administration. In the field of education, qualified, experienced surgical technologists are needed to train and teach surgical technology in a variety of settings, including 2-year and proprietary programs. A surgical technologist also can be certified by the LCC-ST as a certified surgical technologist–surgical first assistant (CST-CFA).

DESIRABLE ATTRIBUTES FOR SUCCESS

The successful surgical technologist possesses certain personal characteristics and aptitudes that contribute greatly to both good patient care and job satisfaction. Although most skills can be learned, certain characteristics, such as honesty, empathy, and caring, cannot be taught. Novices to the profession likely have many valuable untapped skills and attributes that develop with time and experience.

Success in the profession must be defined by successful patient care and a sense that one has contributed to that care. The surgical technologist can achieve this goal in any setting, whether it is a fast-paced, complex, high-profile institution or a small community-based setting. Everyone has unique talents to bring to the workplace. Some surgical technologists prefer a quiet workplace in which highly cooperative interpersonal relations are emphasized. Others prefer a highly technical, high-pressure environment in which many overtime hours are required and a wide variety of procedures are performed. Perhaps the greatest skill surgical technologists acquire is an appreciation for their own professional niche in which they can deliver the best possible patient care, feel challenged but not overwhelmed, achieve a high degree of satisfaction, and attain professional growth.

Care and Empathy

A person usually has the qualities of care and empathy before he or she enters the health-care field. However, once the professional begins working in the health-care field, he or she can enhance these qualities through personal growth or lose them through job stress. Care and empathy require active communication between caregiver and patient. Providing care in the health domain requires a devotion to humans, in all their states and predicaments. It is nonjudgmental and requires the caregiver to look beyond the external circumstances of the patient and take part in a privileged dialogue between health and illness. Empathy is a response to the emotional or physical experience of another human. It is the dual ability to *comprehend* the other's feelings—grief, joy, sorrow, pain—and to *convey* that comprehension through words, actions, or body language. Trust is an essential component of care and empathy. Without trust, the patient cannot allow the caregiver to participate fully in the healing process.

Having the desire to contribute to the patient's well-being is the most important attribute of any health-care worker. It is important, however, to separate empathy from *pity.* Pity is a singular emotional reaction to another person's condition. Pity evokes strong feelings that may prevent therapeutic communication with the patient. Empathy involves communication between the caregiver and the patient that results in a healing response, whereas pity centers on the emotions of the caregiver only.

Respect for Others

Respect for others is a quality that is universally recognized and admired in all environments. When people are respected, they feel accepted *as they are.* Respect is a form of empathy because it requires protection of another's vulnerability. Showing a lack of respect implies that that a person has little worth as a human being. Giving simple expressions of thanks, acknowledging everyone's contribution to the work environment, and avoiding gossip are just a few ways that health-care workers can demonstrate respect for each other. Respect for the patient is required of all health-care workers. When coworkers do not show respect for each other in front of the patient, the patient may question or mistrust care received from those people.

Emotional Self-Control

The operating room environment can be stressful at times. The stress arises from many sources. Because of its nature, surgery itself can be stressful. Emergency surgeries are not common in most hospitals, but emergencies can arise during routine surgery. Stress in the operating room is common in those situations. The emotional maturity and self-control of operating room personnel contribute greatly to a professional and safe work environment. The surgical technologist who knows his or her own emotional limits and can control outbursts reduces the risk of error and can recover quickly from adverse events. Strong emotional reactions must be expressed at the right time and channeled in a healthy way.

Honesty and Ethical Behavior

In surgery, honesty about one's actions, mistakes, and abilities is called surgical conscience. A strict surgical conscience is one of the most important elements for becoming successful as a surgical professional. When a person makes an error in surgery, he or she *admits the error at the time it is made.* This is vital when there is a break in aseptic technique or a medication has been wrongly administered. *Not admitting an error is a serious breach of ethics and risks injury to the patient and coworkers.* It is difficult to admit an error, particularly in front of others, but doing so and accepting responsibility are signs of professional and emotional maturity. It is a requirement for work in any health-care profession. If you are not honest when you make a mistake, you become a danger to the patient. Always pretend the patient on the operating room table is you or somebody you love, and treat each and every patient in the manner in which you would want to be treated.

Manual Dexterity

The surgical technologist is required to work quickly and deftly with different-sized instruments and equipment, from very small to very large. Small, delicate sutures and fine microsurgical instruments require special handling to prevent damage and maintain functional integrity. This requires skill and keen observation. Excellent hand-eye coordination is required to master the skills needed to prepare for surgery and assist during surgery. Speed is not always the most important skill, and in fact, trying to work *too* fast can result in a breakdown in organization, dropping of instruments, and injury. Actions should not be abrupt or wasted. This avoids the need to repeat a task, which is time consuming and frustrating for everyone.

Organizational Skills

Organization is the ability to prioritize tasks and equipment in a logical and efficient manner. For example, the surgical technologist is required to prepare, assemble, and physically arrange instruments and equipment in order of need. This requires overall knowledge of the surgical objective and all the processes and actions needed to complete the surgery. Any one procedure may require hundreds of items to be organized. Instruments, sutures, sponges, needles, electrosurgical devices, solutions, and medications all must be immediately available. Materials must be organized in a logical and methodical way so that they are readily at hand when needed. This skill is developed with practice and time.

Concentration

Surgery requires *constant focused attention* on the operative site. While there may be periods of relaxed activity, the surgical technologist is in motion during most of the procedure, either preparing equipment for delivery or passing instruments in the correct spatial position. At the same time, he or she must be anticipating the next step of the procedure. This requires moderate to intense levels of concentration during most of the procedure. Lapses in focus can increase risks to the patient and other team members. Many operative accidents, such as needle sticks, accidental cutting or burning, and loss of items in the surgical wound, are not the result of a lack of knowledge or skill, but of a lack of attention. The following short-term and long-term problems represent the most common causes of lost concentration:

▶ Stress
▶ Hunger (hypoglycemia)
▶ Lack of sleep
▶ Illness
▶ Substance abuse
▶ Exhaustion
▶ Lack of interest or burnout

Problem-Solving Skills

The work of the surgical technologist is complex. Problems arise in every workday. Some solutions are technical; other solutions require a combination of "people skills" and environmental adjustments. The person with good problem-solving skills demonstrates the following behaviors:

▶ Prioritizes activities when there are many to consider.
▶ Calmly demonstrates genuine willingness to seek solutions to any and all problems.
▶ Uses time wisely and anticipates problems. Asks, "Can this problem be solved within the time required?"
▶ Assesses own abilities. Asks, "Do I have what I need to solve this problem myself? If not, who can best assist?"
▶ Demonstrates flexibility. Asks, "If the problem cannot be solved within the time required, what alternatives do I have?"
▶ Selects the best alternative to achieve positive results.
▶ Analyzes the result and accepts feedback from others as part of the learning experience.

Sense of Humor

The ability to put events in perspective and enjoy the lighter side of work and life is a great asset. Humor, *when expressed appropriately,* can create ease and relaxation. Not all humor is appropriate. Humor that is sarcastic, mean-spirited, prejudicial, or crude creates tension, disdain, and contempt among team members. The patient should never be the object of inappropriate humor.

SCOPE OF PRACTICE AND STATE JURISDICTION

In all work settings, the surgical technologist performs duties within task boundaries called the scope of practice. The scope of practice is determined by several different regulating agencies to protect the public and ensure a high level of quality medical care. Regulating bodies or instruments that directly or indirectly specify the scope and type of activities in which the surgical technologist may engage include the following:

▶ Written hospital policy (based on the standards and regulations of accrediting and governmental agencies)
▶ State nursing practice acts
▶ State medical boards

▶ State business and professional codes
▶ Department of Health and Human Services
▶ Joint Commission on Accreditation of Healthcare Organizations

Individual institutions determine the activities of their surgical technologists. At the writing of this text, there is not yet any state licensure of surgical technologists. Therefore the duties of the surgical technologist are determined by the employer and specified in the job description. The job description is based on professional requirements and is created according to the standards and regulations of the state. To protect the patient from harm, certain practices are prohibited to those who are not licensed to perform them.

Surgical technologists are often confronted with situations in which they are asked to perform an activity that they are prohibited from performing according to state jurisdiction. It is the responsibility of all members of the surgical team to know their state's practice acts. Many states specify certain tasks that the surgical technologist cannot perform even if a surgeon, a nurse, or another licensed person delegates the task. For example, the surgical technologist can never administer medications of any kind. In other words, **delegation** does not imply permission. Because there are few states that explicitly define the role of the surgical technologist, the surgical technologist's scope of practice is defined by professional organizations and, by default, by the portion of state codes that applies to unlicensed assistive personnel. With cost cutting and efficiency major concerns in hospitals, the role of the surgical technologist is constantly changing. Responsibility and accountability are increasing.

In most states, the unlicensed surgical technologist may not engage in the practice of medicine. For example, the following is a portion of the definition of the practice of medicine as established by the state of Washington:

A person is practicing medicine if he does one or more of the following:
1. *Offers or undertakes to diagnose, cure, advise, or prescribe for any human disease, ailment, injury, infirmity, deformity, pain or other condition, physical or mental, real or imaginary, by any means or instrumentality;*
2. *Administers or prescribes drugs or medicinal preparations to be used by any other person;*
3. *Severs or penetrates the tissue of human beings.*

As with the prohibition against the practice of medicine, in most states the unlicensed surgical technologist may not practice nursing. Prohibited activities include but are not restricted to the following:

▶ Activities that require nursing assessment and judgment during their implementation
▶ Physical, psychological, and social assessments that require nursing judgment, referral, or intervention
▶ Design of a plan of nursing care and evaluation of that plan
▶ Administration of medications by any route

As a general rule, patient or family health teaching is also a nursing duty that cannot be delegated. This includes giving advice about postoperative care.

TASKS AND RESPONSIBILITIES OF THE SURGICAL TECHNOLOGIST

Delegation of Tasks and Responsibilities

Delegation is the transfer of responsibility for an activity from one person to another. In the health care setting, delegation refers to the assignment of tasks that are normally the responsibility of a licensed person. A licensed person may delegate specific tasks to an unlicensed person provided the unlicensed person has the necessary training and knowledge and is legally permitted to carry out the delegated task. The legal accountability for the outcome of the task lies with the person who delegated the task. For example, if the surgeon delegates the task of retraction to the surgical technologist during surgery, it is the surgeon who is accountable for any tissue damage that may occur. A person can only delegate a task to someone who can legally perform the task, has received the proper training, and is competent to perform the task. A task that is *assigned* may not require any special training, while a task that is *delegated* may require special training on the part of the person to whom the task is delegated.

Surgery is a collaborative effort. Each member of the team has specific duties and tasks that complement the other members and achieve common goals. **Independent tasks** are those that the surgical technologist performs without supervision. Activities such as preparing surgical equipment and maintaining the sterile field are independent tasks. The completion of some tasks, however, might require one person to supervise another. **Dependent tasks** are those that require *direct supervision* by a licensed health-care worker—a surgeon, nurse, anesthesiologist, or, in some states, physician assistant. Dependent tasks are those that are delegated.

In the surgical setting, the surgeon is responsible for his or her own actions and those of others to whom he or she delegates tasks (such as a surgical resident who is asked to suture the wound). The surgeon's actions are governed by state medical codes and hospital policy. The RN also has specific duties, some of which are delegable and others are not. For example, the performance of tasks such as assessment and administration of drugs (in most states) requires a license. An RN or surgeon cannot delegate these tasks to someone who does not have a license. The surgical technologist is autonomous in most duties but is supervised in others. Supervision is required only when the task is delegated or the surgical technologist is a student. Otherwise, he or she works autonomously (without direct supervision). The term *direct supervision* is loosely defined in many states.

To learn the tasks and behaviors expected of the surgical technologist, one must view this role in a larger context. This context includes the duties and responsibilities of all members of the surgical team and perioperative personnel (those who contribute to but do not participate directly in the sur-

gical procedure). Table 1-1 is a reference tool that describes the activities of the surgical technologist and others involved in the surgical patient's care.

The tasks of the surgical technologist are described as "sterile" or "nonsterile." Sterile personnel are scrubbed and have donned surgical gown and gloves. Nonsterile personnel do not wear sterile attire. The *circulator* is a nonsterile team member. The circulator may be either a surgical technologist or an RN. The *scrub person* is a member of the sterile team. The surgical technologist performs certain tasks before scrubbing and becoming a member of the sterile team. So that the reader may understand the duties and responsibilities of the surgical technologist in the preoperative, intraoperative, and postoperative roles, this chapter will refer to the surgical technologist before scrubbing and in the circulator role as the *nonsterile surgical technologist;* during the intraoperative role the surgical technologist will be referred to as the *sterile surgical technologist.* The tasks described in the chapter will be discussed in further detail in later chapters.

Duties of the Nonsterile Surgical Technologist—Preoperative

PREPARING SUPPLIES AND INSTRUMENTS

In most hospitals, surgical instruments are wrapped and sterilized in instrument sets. These are groups of instruments that are commonly used in particular procedures. For example, a laparotomy set includes instruments needed for procedures of the abdomen. Other instruments are added as needed. The most common method of equipment preparation is the **case-cart system.** In this system, the sterile supply department collects most of the equipment needed for a procedure and places it on a moveable stainless steel cart. The cart is then delivered to the operating room. Carts are received case by case or stored near the operating room suites in a clean area.

To prepare the supplies and instruments, the nonsterile surgical technologist:

1. Assembles, wraps, and sterilizes instrument sets as necessary
2. Checks the case cart to make sure it is complete
3. Gathers instruments or other supplies as needed
4. Stations the cart in the appropriate area where the risk of contamination is minimized

PREPARING THE OPERATING ROOM SUITE

Each operating room suite is equipped with standard equipment and furniture, an operating table, and anesthesia equipment. Before a case is opened, all equipment must be arranged as necessary for the case, with space being used efficiently (see Chapter 5, Operating Room Environment, for further discussion).

To prepare the operating room suite, the nonsterile surgical technologist:

1. Receives information about the type of case and the side (if applicable) on which the operation will be performed,

Table 1-1   TASKS AND DUTIES OF THE SURGICAL TECHNOLOGIST AND OTHER TEAM MEMBERS

Scrubbed Technologist	Circulator	Surgeon
Before Surgery		
Receives case cart for surgery or selects individual items needed from instrument and supply rooms.	Positions the OR table and prepares foam pads and accessories according to the surgery.	Greets patient in holding area.
Assembles all items needed for surgery according to surgeon's case information.	Assembles needed equipment.	Orients patient and family.
	Connects suction canisters to ceiling or wall mounts.	Answers patient's questions.
Orients furniture in the room in accordance with surgery.	Tests suction and in-line gas.	Ensures that permits are signed and witnessed.
Opens sterile equipment and instruments using aseptic technique.	Keeps the OR doors closed.	Has patient mark operative side and site.
Protects the sterile equipment from contamination.	Obtains radiographs or other diagnostic reports needed during surgery.	If patient is to be placed in prone position, assists in transfer after anesthesia induction. Patient undergoes induction in supine position and is then turned to prone.
Performs surgical hand scrub. After scrub, surgical technologist is a "sterile" team member.	Opens sterile supplies.	
	*Selects medications and drugs for use during surgery.	Along with surgical assistants, performs surgical hand scrub or may scrub after positioning patient following induction.
	*Reviews operative checklist.	
	*Witnesses signing of operative or anesthesia permit.	
	*Checks all permits.	
	Notes operative side and surgeon's mark or signature on operative side.	
	Assesses patient's psychosocial condition.	
	*Measures vital signs and performs assessment.	
	Answers patient's questions about surgery and postoperative care.	
	Transfers patient to OR.	
	Transfers patient to OR bed using safe technique.	
	Applies safety strap over patient.	
	Provides warm blankets for patient.	
Before First Incision Is Made		
Gowns and gloves self using aseptic technique.	Secures scrubbed surgical technologist's gown.	May perform skin preparation.
Drapes Mayo stand.	Secures surgeons' gowns.	With assistants, enters OR suite from scrub area. Along with assistants, is gowned and gloved by surgical technologist.
Places sterile instrument trays in position on back table.	Performs the instrument, sponge, and needle count with the scrubbed surgical technologist.	
Separates sharps (e.g., scalpel blades, needles) from other equipment to avoid injury during setup.	*Distributes medications to scrubbed surgical technologist.	With assistants and surgical technologist, drapes patient.
Sorts drapes and surgical gowns in order of use.	Prepares nonsterile equipment.	
According to the specific surgery, prepares instruments, sutures, devices, solutions, and medications.	*Assists anesthesiologist during anesthesia induction and intubation.	
	*Assists in the correct positioning of the patient for surgery.	
Protects the surgical setup from contamination.	*Carefully applies grounding pads to the patient for use of electrocautery.	
Performs the initial instrument, sponge, and needle count.	*May perform skin preparation.	

ACP, anesthesia care provider; *OR,* operating room; *PACU,* postanesthesia care unit; *RN,* registered nurse.
Tasks in red indicate those that only an RN may perform.
*These tasks may be delegated.

Continued

Table 1-1	TASKS AND DUTIES OF THE SURGICAL TECHNOLOGIST AND OTHER TEAM MEMBERS—cont'd	
Scrubbed Technologist	Circulator	Surgeon

Before First Incision Is Made—cont'd

Scrubbed Technologist	Circulator	Surgeon
Receives medications from circulator using proper technique.	*Completes hook up of suction, power, electrocautery, and light cords to be used.	
When setup is complete, waits *within the sterile field.*	Advocates for patient safety during the procedure.	
Hands each surgeon/assistant sterile towel to dry hands.		
Gowns and gloves each sterile team member.		
Hands individual draping materials to surgeon and assistants. Participates in draping, maintaining sterility.		
Moves Mayo stand into position.		
Secures suction tubing and power and light cords to top drape. Hands or drops ends off OR table for attachment to power sources.		
Hands light handle covers to surgeon.		

From Incision to End of Surgery

Scrubbed Technologist	Circulator	Surgeon
Places two sponges on incision site.	*Records time of incision on patient record.	Marks incision area or begins skin incision.
Passes marking pen or scalpel to surgeon. Gives retractors to assistant after skin incision.	*Distributes sterile solutions and medications to scrubbed person.	Performs surgery according to plan and intraoperative events.
Participates in all instrument, sponge, and needle counts with circulator.	Provides additional equipment as needed by the surgical technologist and surgeons.	Directs the surgical team during emergency.
Passes sterile equipment to surgeons and assistants using correct orientation and technique.	Operates nonsterile equipment.	If count is incorrect and missing item is not found, takes responsibility for further action (e.g., radiography, reopening of wound)
Listens for direction and anticipates each step of the surgery.	Adjusts lighting.	
Maintains a sterile field, notifying others when aseptic technique is broken.	Flash sterilizes instruments as needed.	Removes gown and gloves, signs patient care documents, and gives any instructions to RN and ACP.
Deposits soiled sponges in designated receptacle.	Answers surgeon's pages and relays messages.	Assists in transferring patient to stretcher.
Maintains a safe surgical field by exercising all precautions when electrosurgical devices, lasers, and sharps are in use.	Anticipates flow of surgery and equipment needs of surgeon and surgical technologist.	
Requests additional equipment as needed.	*Monitors urinary output.	
Secures intraoperative tissue and fluid specimens provided by surgeon.	Responds to medical emergencies.	
Obtains grafts and implants as required by the surgery.	Directs instrument, sponge, and needle counts at appropriate times.	
Prepares dressings and begins to separate soiled from clean instruments.	*Labels specimens obtained from the scrubbed person for the pathology department.	
Participates in final instrument, sponge, and needle count.	Wearing gloves, separates sponges and places them in counting area or isolates them in groups of 5 or 10.	
Notifies surgeon if count is incorrect.	Maintains safe environment. Keeps doors closed; maintains quiet.	
	Replaces equipment that is unsafe or malfunctions.	

ACP, anesthesia care provider; *OR,* operating room; *PACU,* postanesthesia care unit; *RN,* registered nurse.
Tasks in red indicate those that only an RN may perform.
*These tasks may be delegated.

Table 1-1	TASKS AND DUTIES OF THE SURGICAL TECHNOLOGIST AND OTHER TEAM MEMBERS—cont'd	
Scrubbed Technologist	Circulator	Surgeon

From Incision to End of Surgery—cont'd

Scrubbed Technologist	Circulator	Surgeon
If count is incorrect, searches for missing item.	Assesses the patient's physical status and assists ACP as needed.	
Applies sterile dressings as directed by surgeon.	Near completion of surgery, calls for next patient.	
Maintains sterility until patient leaves the room.	Checks on equipment for next procedure.	
Keeps basic instruments on Mayo stand in case of emergency. Prepares instruments on back table for decontamination.	Participates in count.	
	Notifies surgeon if count is incorrect.	
	At completion of surgery, assists in removing drapes and disconnecting hoses and tubing. Suction remains connected until patient leaves the room.	
	Applies tape to dressings and connects nonsterile ends of drainage devices.	
	Removes dispersive electrode pad and assesses site.	
	*Completes intraoperative record.	
	Transfers patient to stretcher.	
	Calls for orderlies to prepare for room turnover.	
	*Accompanies patient and ACP to postoperative recovery unit and gives report to PACU nurse.	

After the Patient Leaves the Room

Scrubbed Technologist	Circulator	Surgeon
Separates single-use from reusable items. All soiled disposables are placed in biohazard bags. Linens are also placed in biohazard bags.	Checks on equipment for next case.	Notifies family of patient's condition.
Aspirates all solutions in closed suction containers.	May begin to open the next case after the OR suite is cleaned.	Dictates operative report.
Removes containers from room.	Receives next patient in holding area.	
Places sharps in secure closed sharps container.		
Places all contaminated materials in biohazard bags.		
Removes soiled gown and gloves and places them in biohazard waste bag.		
Removes mask by handling only strings. Removes face shield without touching bare skin.		
Puts on nonsterile gloves to transport covered equipment to decontamination area.		
Follows hospital policy for equipment decontamination. Is responsible for correct destination of instruments and supplies.		
Assists with proper cleaning of OR suite.		

and obtains additional necessary equipment, such as a microscope or video equipment

2. Makes sure the appropriate type of operating table is in the room
3. Arranges the furniture (**back table,** mayo stand, kick bucket, and prep tables) as required
4. Ensures suction and electrocautery units are operational and positioned correctly
5. May check nonsterile equipment and replace items such as light cables or bulbs as needed
6. Consults with the anesthesiologist about the position needed for anesthesia equipment

OPENING A CASE

To **open a case** means to open sterile supplies and begin to create the sterile field. This is performed before the patient is brought into the room. Tables are draped, and sterile supplies are opened onto the sterile surface, via aseptic technique. Linens used for draping, gowns, gloves, and other paper supplies are usually packed as one bundle, which is opened directly onto the back table. Other small supplies are then added. Large instrument trays are placed on smaller tables, and the wrappers are opened via sterile technique. Wrapped basins are placed in a ring stand, and the outer wrapper is removed aseptically. A minimum number of sutures are opened to avoid waste. Before and during the case, the surgeon's preferences about a particular surgery are consulted as needed. The preference book or preference card may be written and contained in a binder, or the information may be computerized and generated with the surgical schedule.

To open a case, the nonsterile surgical technologist:

1. Completes the task independently or with another person
2. Discusses the needs of the procedure with the circulator and looks at the surgeon's preference notes as required
3. Practices aseptic technique, and if contamination occurs, removes the contaminated object from the field and re-drapes the area
4. Creates a sterile field on which to open supplies
5. Opens sterile wrapped supplies using aseptic technique
6. Uses proper body mechanics while opening heavy instrument and equipment trays
7. Takes care to put fragile items on top of heavier supplies
8. Works carefully to avoid dropping and contaminating equipment and supplies while distributing them to the field
9. Opens scrub person's gown and gloves on a separate table

TRANSPORTING AND TRANSFERRING THE PATIENT

An aide, orderly, or surgical technologist usually transports the patient to the preoperative holding area. During this time, the preoperative holding room RN and the circulator check the patient's identity, the operative and anesthesia permits, and the operative checklist (see Table 1-1). *The surgeon must obtain the operative permit* because it is his or her re-

sponsibility to explain the risks of the procedure and ensure that the patient understands the risks before signing. A permit for anesthesia and blood product transfusion is also required. The checklist includes procedures ordered by the surgeon and other important information such as surgical site verification (SSV) and whether the patient wears dentures, has any loose teeth, or has a sensory deficit. The circulator is accountable for ensuring that the preoperative checklist is complete. At this time the anesthesiologist and surgeon may also see the patient.

To assist in this task, the nonsterile surgical technologist:

1. Transports the patient to the holding area from the floor unit using safe transport methods
2. May accompany the circulator while he or she visits the patient and verifies that the checklist is complete
3. Transports the patient to the operating room suite
4. Offers therapeutic communication and emotional support, and ensures the patient's environmental comfort
5. Notifies the circulator, surgeon, or anesthesiologist of any special requests the patient may have
6. Directs the family or other support persons to the waiting area
7. Refers any questions about the length of the procedure or the outcome to the surgeon

TRANSFERRING THE PATIENT TO THE OPERATING ROOM TABLE

The patient is transferred to the operating room table slowly with assistance from enough personnel to avoid injury to the patient or personnel. Once on the operating room table, the patient is secured, mid-thigh, with a wide safety strap.

To assist in this task, the nonsterile surgical technologist:

1. Helps move the patient to the operating room table
2. Secures the safety strap on top of the patient's blanket, allowing three fingers' breadth between the strap and the patient
3. Ensures the environmental comfort, dignity, and safety of the patient by using warm blankets and minimizing exposure

PERFORMING URINARY CATHETERIZATION

Before surgery many patients require insertion of an indwelling urinary catheter. The purpose is to keep the bladder empty and to monitor urinary output, which is a physiological indicator of metabolism and urinary system function. The surgeon, circulator, or surgical technologist performs this task if allowed in his or her current job description. It is a delegated task, and accountability rests with the delegator. Risks involved include infection and tissue injury.

If this task is delegated to the nonsterile surgical technologist, he or she:

1. Gathers supplies needed for catheterization
2. Positions the patient as needed

3. Tests the balloon for inflation and deflation
4. Practices aseptic technique
5. Catheterizes the patient with attention to risk factors
6. Connects the indwelling catheter to a collection bag
7. Notifies the circulator of the characteristics and amount of urine collected at the time of catheterization

POSITIONING THE PATIENT

Positioning the patient is a critical task. It requires advanced knowledge of physiology and anatomy. Specific risks include permanent paralysis of a limb, persistent paresthesia, permanent nerve damage, and persistent pain and suffering. Positioning is a collaborative team task. The anesthesia care provider or surgeon directs and guides other team members during positioning. The anesthesia care provider must give permission before a patient's position is changed while on the operating table.

To contribute to this task, the nonsterile surgical technologist:

1. Gathers needed positioning equipment appropriate for the procedure and the individual patient
2. Positions the surgical patient with other team members
3. Protects the patient from nerve, skin, vascular, and skeletal injury

PERFORMING SURGICAL SKIN PREPARATION

After the patient has been anesthetized and positioned, the surgical site is cleaned with an antiseptic solution to minimize the risk of postoperative wound infection. Skin preparation always adheres to the principles of aseptic technique. Just before the skin preparation is performed, electrosurgical grounding pads are placed on the patient. The circulator usually but not always performs this task. The circulator evaluates the patient's skin before applying the grounding pads or performing the skin prep.

To prep the patient, the nonsterile surgical technologist:

1. Uses a specific skin-preparation technique
2. Uses antiseptic solutions as ordered by the surgeon with prior notification of any patient allergies
3. Prevents pooling of preparation solutions under the patient

DRAPING THE PATIENT

After skin preparation, the patient and surgical site are draped with sterile sheets to create the sterile surgical field. Sterile drapes cover the patient during the surgical procedure to maintain a sterile field. Draping is a systematic process involving surgical coverings for limbs, special fenestrated sheets for the incision and surrounding area, and body drapes to cover any area that is part of the surgical field. Draping is primarily the role of the scrub, surgeon, and assistants. Nonsterile team members assist, however, by handling the drapes only within 1 inch of the edge. They may help position the drapes and observe that all areas of the sterile field are covered.

Duties of the Nonsterile Surgical Technologist (Circulator)—Intraoperative

At the beginning of surgery, the nonsterile surgical technologist:

1. Notes the time when surgery begins (when the first incision is made)
2. Places the kick bucket or other sponge receptacle in close proximity to the sterile field
3. Opens additional equipment as needed during surgery
4. Connects electrosurgical devices, nitrogen, air, and suction hoses to sterile connections
5. Separates discarded sponges and organizes them for an orderly count
6. Answers the surgeon's pages
7. Receives specimens from the sterile field and labels them according to hospital policy
8. Maintains the environment of the room by properly disposing of linens and waste
9. Troubleshoots problems with surgical devices such as suction, video equipment, and lighting sources
10. Assists in the positioning of x-ray equipment or C-arm fluoroscope
11. Maintains the sterile field and notifies team members when a break has occurred
12. Participates in the sponge and needle count *according to hospital policy* (in most hospitals an RN is required to participate in the sponge and needle count)
13. **Flash sterilizes** equipment that has been dropped
14. Communicates messages to others outside the surgical suite
15. Wears nonsterile gloves at all times when handling linens, sponges, or any item that may contain blood or body fluids
16. Immediately cleans the floor of any spills of blood and body substance using the agency-approved disinfectant
17. Anticipates the needs of the current and next surgery and may leave the room to organize equipment *if there is another circulator present*
18. Attends to the needs of the surgeon, such as helping to move the microscope into place, connecting light sources, or adjusting power settings on equipment *as directed by the surgeon*
19. Operates nonsterile video equipment, endoscopic accessories, insufflation devices, and other technological equipment

At the close of surgery, the nonsterile surgical technologist:

1. Removes connections from electrosurgical unit and air hoses (suction must remain operative while the patient is in the room)
2. Assists in applying dressings and connecting wound drainage devices
3. Assists in returning the patient to a neutral position

4. May remove and evaluate the site of the dispersive electrode grounding pad
5. Removes radiographs or other diagnostic films from the view box and places them in the correct envelope, *ensuring that the patient's name matches that on the envelope*
6. Ensures that the patient's bed is ready (if he or she will be transferred to the intensive care unit)
7. Brings the patient's stretcher into the room
8. Notifies environmental services that the room will soon be ready to turn over (clean and prepare for the next case)
9. Stands by the patient during emergence from anesthesia
10. Assists in transferring the patient from the operating table to the stretcher
11. May accompany the anesthesia care provider during patient transport to the postanesthesia care unit as needed
12. Collects all equipment and disposes of waste appropriately
13. Participates in room disinfection and cleanup

Duties of the Sterile Surgical Technologist— Preoperative

SURGICAL HAND SCRUBBING, GOWNING, AND GLOVING

The sterile surgical technologist begins the assigned case by first performing the surgical hand scrub. The hand scrub is performed using antiseptic detergent or other approved agent. The scrub is performed before and after each case or when personnel directly contact (without gloves) body fluids or tissue. After performing the presurgical hand scrub, the surgical technologist enters the surgical suite and proceeds to gown and glove. This is done according to prescribed aseptic technique.

ORGANIZING STERILE SUPPLIES

After gowning and gloving, the surgical technologist will begin to sort and organize sterile supplies that were previously opened. All supplies are organized and prepared without causing contamination. If contamination occurs, the contaminated item is removed and sterility is reestablished.

To organize supplies, the sterile surgical technologist:

1. Drapes the Mayo stand
2. Arranges supplies according to category and order of use in the procedure
3. Places all **sharps** on a magnetic board or sharps holder
4. Prepares sutures for immediate use and retains unopened packages until they are needed
5. Works smoothly and moves items as few times as possible
6. Keeps a mental note of where everything is on the sterile tables

7. Receives medications and solutions from the circulator
8. Immediately labels all medications with name and strength
9. Arranges drapes in reverse order of use
10. Arranges instruments on the Mayo stand in an orderly fashion
11. Requests additional items as needed
12. Participates in the initial sponge, needle, and instrument count

GOWNING AND GLOVING OTHER STERILE TEAM MEMBERS

The surgical technologist hands sterile towels to the surgeon and the assistant(s) after they have completed the surgical hand scrub. He or she then gowns, gloves, and turns them using aseptic technique.

DRAPING THE PATIENT

To participate in draping, the sterile surgical technologist:

1. Prepares the drapes in a neat stack before the procedure so that those needed first are on the top and those applied last are on the bottom
2. Works with the surgeon and assistant to unfold the drapes over the patient
3. Takes care not to become contaminated
4. Anticipates the need for drapes that may not be readily available during the procedure
5. Drapes the microscope or other large nonstationary equipment, assisted by the circulator
6. Uses aseptic technique throughout draping and follows approved guidelines for draping

Duties of the Sterile Surgical Technologist— Intraoperative

The intraoperative period begins when the first incision is made. At the beginning of the procedure, there is much activity. Care must be taken to avoid unnecessary rushing, which can lead to errors or injury.

At the beginning of surgery, the sterile surgical technologist:

1. Adjusts the lights using sterile light handles
2. Adjusts the Mayo stand and back table so that equipment is within reach
3. Remains at the field and anticipates the needs of the surgeon

Because each procedure is different, the tasks of the sterile technician as the surgery progresses do not always occur in the same order. During surgery (and in no particular order), the surgical technologist:

1. Anticipates the need for specific instruments, equipment, and supplies depending on the procedure, and

correctly orients instruments while passing them to the surgeon

2. Receives medications from the circulator in the approved manner and transfers these to the surgeon for administration
3. Keeps the electrosurgical tip stored safely and free of tissue debris
4. Maintains attention to the surgical field
5. Opens and prepares sutures as needed
6. Prepares specialty items such as orthopedic implants or grafts
7. Receives and protects tissue specimens and tissue grafts
8. May cut sutures at the operative site under the supervision of the surgeon
9. Maintains the sterility of the field and alerts the team when contamination has occurred
10. Maintains safety on the surgical field by monitoring the location of all sharps, keeping track of sponges that are on the field and in the surgical wound, placing the electrosurgical pencil in a protective holder, and following all safety precautions when lasers are in use
11. Participates in the sponge, needle, and instrument counts at appropriate times and in the approved manner
12. Requests sterile items from the circulator as needed
13. Deflects outbursts from other team members by reintroducing a calm atmosphere and refrains from argument, verbal conflict, divisive comments, or other unprofessional behavior at the field
14. Responds to intraoperative emergencies according to his or her scope of knowledge and hospital policy

Duties of the Sterile Surgical Technologist— Postoperative

After surgery is completed, the anesthesiologist and circulator transport the patient to the postanesthetic recovery unit while equipment is removed from the room using standard precautions. The surgical technologist collects equipment and places linens and disposable items in designated bags. Sealed suction canisters are removed and placed in the soiled equipment disposal area. After removing soiled items from the room, the surgical technologist may assist in disinfection and cleanup of the surgical suite.

The Surgical Technologist as Preceptor

Surgical technologists are often asked to act as preceptors (personal tutors) while scrubbed. Surgical technology students, new employees, and nursing students who are learning to scrub require a more experienced person to teach them the practical and hands-on aspects of surgical technology. Some people enjoy this role and are natural teachers. Others are uncomfortable with the responsibility or are disappointed that they can no longer handle cases alone. Serving as preceptor requires patience and a willingness to share knowledge and experience (Box 1-1).

When you become a preceptor, it is important to remember your roots; you were once standing in the same spot as the person you are training. Place yourself in his or her shoes, and remember how you felt when you were learning. Remember the attributes your preceptors possessed that improved and accelerated your learning experience when you were a student. Consider it an honor to guide and teach another to become a surgical technologist, as you are helping to shape the future of your profession.

Box 1-1   Guidelines for Serving as a Preceptor

1. If you are a student now, notice the problems you encounter. Think of the preceptors from whom you have learned the most and consider why you learned from them.
2. Develop a plan with the person for whom you are serving as preceptor. Discuss with the learner what each of you will do and how it will be done. For example, as the preceptor you might start the case and then allow the learner to step in and complete it. You might also have the student perform certain tasks while you do others.
3. *Never* try to perform the same task at the same time as your student. For example, if the learner is passing instruments, allow him or her time to think and act. Silently point to the correct instrument but do not reach for it. This would result in hand collisions on the Mayo stand and frustration for everyone.
4. If the learner is struggling, try to help by coaching quietly in the background. If this is insufficient, ask the learner whether you should take over for a while. This allows the student to gain composure.
5. *Never* make a learner feel inadequate or foolish. This will only intensify his or her lack of confidence. Encouragement is much more productive than criticism. If you cannot contain negativity, ask to be excused from preceptor duties.
6. Always introduce the learner to the surgical team before beginning the procedure. This allows the learner to feel like part of the team and encourages confidence.
7. Respect the learner as a person. Remember that the learning phase is only one aspect of this person's life. You have a privileged job in helping the student achieve his or her goals. You are also in a position to hurt the student's confidence. This is especially true of adult learners, who may not be accustomed to steep learning curves.
8. If the surgeon becomes irritated or anxious because of the learner's lack of experience, support the learner. If the situation becomes critical, ask the learner to wait until the critical situation has passed. Then invite him or her back into the case after assessing whether the surgeon is tolerant or not.
9. Show respect for your profession by sharing it with others!

CASE STUDIES

Case 1
As a certified surgical technologist you are scrubbed on a general surgery case. The surgeon asks you to clamp a blood vessel and hold it while he applies a suture at the base. What will you do?

Case 2
After the circulator has removed the dispersive electrosurgical pad, you see a large burn in the area of the pad. The circulator has not mentioned it. What will you do?

Case 3
After taking a job as a surgical technologist, you find that you are asked to perform tasks beyond the scope defined by your state's practice acts. You feel confident to perform these tasks and feel that doing so gives you more experience. What will you do?

Case 4
While you are serving as a preceptor to a student surgical technologist, the surgeon begins to criticize her for her incompetence. You have allowed her to perform tasks that you both agreed she might do. How will you respond to the surgeon's outburst?

Case 5
As a certified surgical technologist, you have been assigned to serve as preceptor to nursing students in their scrub experience. You dislike this task because you find it boring. This conflict is affecting your attitude about work. How will you resolve this?

Case 6
As a surgical technology student, you notice your preceptor is rolling his eyes at you and quietly making rude comments about you. What should you do? From whom will you seek help?

REFERENCES

Accreditation Review Committee on Education in Surgical Technology (ARC-ST) website.

Accrediting Bureau of Health Education Schools (ABHES) website.

Association of Surgical Technologists (AST) website: *Standards of Practice.*

Association of Surgical Technologists (AST) website: *Position statements and reports.*

Bureau of Labor Statistics, United States Department of Labor website: *Occupational outlook handbook, 2002-03 edition, Surgical Technologists.*

The Liaison Council on Certification for the Surgical Technologist (LCC-ST) website.

Litsky W et al: Frances Ginsberg: Educator and advocate of surgical technologists, *J Assoc Surg Technologists,* July/August, 36-41, 1983.

The National Center for Competency Testing (NCCT) website.

Phippen ML et al: Assistive personnel in the perioperative setting: changing the paradigm, *Semin Perip Nurs* 1:2, 1992.

Chapter 2

The Patient

Learning Objectives

After studying this chapter the reader will be able to:

- Describe patient-centered care
- Discuss Maslow's hierarchy of needs and its relationship to patient care
- Define patient-centered care
- Demonstrate how the surgical technologist can meet specific patient physiological needs
- Describe patient environmental needs and how to meet them
- List the needs of specific patient groups
- Describe the psychosocial needs of the patient
- Practice therapeutic communication
- Describe the differences of special needs patients
- Discuss the importance of culturally appropriate patient care

Terminology

Aggression—A forceful physical, verbal, or symbolic action. It may be appropriate (self-protective, indicating healthy self-assertiveness) or it may be inappropriate.

Comorbid disease—A disease or condition that exists simultaneously with another unrelated disease in the same patient.

Critical thinking—The process of analyzing information about the patient, comparing it with similar previous experience, and responding to the unique needs of the current patient. For example, your pediatric patient is 8 years old and is having surgery. You know that the developmental needs at this age include a need for information about the environment. In this particular case, however, the patient has a severe hearing deficit. You must plan some way other than speech to communicate information to the patient to help him cope with his fears about the operating room environment.

Direct care—Care that is usually "hands on." Direct care is often therapeutic or diagnostic.

Indirect care—Patient care that requires skills and knowledge about the patient, the disease, and the procedure, and an appropriate response to the individual patient's needs. Indirect care does not include patient assessment, intervention, or evaluation.

Leads and cues—A therapeutic communication skill that urges the patient to continue speaking or communicating needs. An example of a lead is "I see, tell me more." An example of a cue is nodding one's head as the patient speaks.

Maslow's hierarchy—A model of human achievement and self-actualization developed by psychologist Abraham Maslow. This model is widely accepted in Western medicine and describes human needs on a hierarchical basis starting with the most basic needs first.

Patient—A person who is ill or injured or who is undergoing any type of medical treatment.

Patient-centered care—Therapeutic care, communication, and intervention provided according to the unique needs of the patient. Every patient is treated as an individual, and a care plan is developed to meet specific needs identified in the assessment.

Reflection—Communication with the patient that helps him or her connect current emotions with events in the environment.

Regression—An abnormal return to a former or earlier state, particularly infantile patterns of thought or behavior. This can result from feelings of helplessness and dependency in a patient with a serious physical illness.

Therapeutic communication—A purposeful method of communication in which the caregiver responds to explicit or implicit needs of the patient.

Therapeutic response—Communicative response to the patient. The goal is to encourage the patient to express his or her needs and to show caring and empathy.

PATIENT-CENTERED CARE

The **patient** is the primary reason for the surgical technologist's existence in health care. While performing your assigned duties as a surgical technologist, you must remember to treat and care for the patient in the manner in which you would want to be treated. Each surgical technologist is responsible for ensuring that every patient is given the best care.

In **patient-centered care,** the surgical team bases assessment, planning, and intervention on the unique needs of the individual patient (Figure 2-1). For the surgical technologist to participate fully in patient care while remaining within the scope of practice, he or she should understand the patient's general physical status, developmental stage, and immediate psychosocial needs. The *unique* needs of the individual patient are revealed through information from others, astute observation, and good communication.

Critical Thinking

Critical thinking is a process. It is the application of knowledge and experience gained in the past to solve a current problem. In patient-centered care, this means the health-care provider must analyze and compare past experience and knowledge with the current patient's physical and emotional needs. Past experience and skills provide the tools to solve new problems, even when the problem has never been encountered before.

The steps of critical thinking are illustrated by this practical example:

▶ **Obtain information about the current patient.** For example, a person with a gunshot wound to the chest is scheduled for emergency surgery. Begin to determine the specific equipment needed and plan the sequence of actions based on your skills, experience, and knowledge.
▶ **Consider previous experience in dealing with the same injury.** If you have no experience with the current situation, consider previous situations that were *similar,* such as severe hemorrhage and chest surgery. Consider the possible requirements for procedures involving this specific injury, such as thoracic instruments, extra suction, and extra sponges. The circulator and surgeon also are using critical thinking, even if they have never encountered this type of trauma before. They think about the drugs that may be needed, the best approach to the wound, the priorities, and the sequence in which action should occur.
▶ **Consider any specific needs** *for this unique patient.* For example, perhaps the patient is under the influence of drugs or alcohol and is combative. Will additional help be needed? How might this affect preparations for surgery?
▶ **Perform tasks and seek further information in accordance with your evaluation of the situation.** How should you respond to this *particular* patient? Do you have the supplies that you need? If not, what will you do about it?

Do you have questions about the specific needs of the patient? Whom will you ask?

When a health-care worker is motivated to improve patient care and increase knowledge, critical thinking becomes more acute with time. Because every patient is a unique individual, nothing in surgery is absolute. Critical thinking skills develop a sense of connection among patient needs, priorities, and effective solutions to problems.

Direct and Indirect Care

The concept of patient care is complex. Many separate components contribute to the holistic (multidimensional) care of the person. In general, there are two types of patient care: **direct** and **indirect.** Both are critical to the healing, protection, or palliative care of the patient, and *both require the same level* of professional commitment to patient safety and well-being. Direct care is *hands-on.* Touch is usually involved in direct care. It requires knowledge of the body, including physiology, pathology, risks, and outcomes. The surgeon and nurse routinely provide direct care. The surgical technologist provides both indirect and direct care. Direct care, however, is defined according to state professional practice acts and the rules of delegation (see Chapter 3, Law and Ethics).

Indirect care requires special skills that are preventive and collaborative. For example, if the patient begins to hemorrhage, the surgical technologist rapidly assesses the surgical emergency and gives the surgeon the equipment and instruments needed to stop the hemorrhage. This is indirect care. If the surgical technologist does not know the surgery, the anatomy involved, and the correct instruments to use, the surgeon may lose critical time during the intervention to stop the hemorrhage. In this case, the surgical technologist provides a critical link in the delivery of direct care.

Indirect care includes activities that usually do not involve hands-on care of the patient but are nonetheless important and require a high level of technical, interpretive, and communicative skills. Table 2-1 lists some examples of direct and indirect patient care. For purposes of this chapter we are referring to direct hands-on patient care. However, indirect care also may be provided by personnel from many other ancillary departments, such as central sterile processing, laboratory, pharmacy, x-ray, and medical records.

MASLOW'S HIERARCHY

In the 1970s psychologist Abraham Maslow developed a theory about human needs. His model, named **Maslow's Hierarchy,** is depicted as a triangular hierarchy, with the most important needs at the base levels (Figure 2-2). If a human being's most basic requirements for life are not met, the needs at the next level of existence cannot be fulfilled. Maslow's model for meeting human needs also is a model for patient care in this text. The surgical technologist is involved most often with the first two levels of needs: physiological needs and the need for safety and security. However,

Text continues on p. 23

**SURGERY PATIENT ASSESSMENT
AND PLAN OF CARE FLOWSHEET**

MERCY
St. Joseph's OF MACOMB

Addressograph

DATE: _____ TIME: _____ HT: _____ WT: _____ AGE _____

PRIMARY PHYSICIAN	PHONE #
CARDIOLOGIST	PHONE #
OTHER:	PHONE #

	Yes	No		Yes	No
ADVANCED DIRECTIVE / BROUGHT WITH PT.			USE TOBACCO? _____ YEARS		
ADVANCED DIRECTIVE ON CHART			_____ PACKS A DAY _____ QUIT SMOKING		
ASHD			DRINK ALCOHOL AMT.?		
CARDIAC SURGERY			USE STREET DRUGS		
HEART DISEASE / CHF/ MI			PSYCHIATRIC PROBLEMS		
CHEST PAIN			LMP DATE:		
IRREGULAR HEARTBEAT / PACEMAKER			CULTURAL/RELIGIOUS CONCERNS		
MITRAL VALVE PROLAPSE / HEART MURMUR			DISCHARGE CONCERNS		
HIGH BLOOD PRESSURE			BLOOD THINNER IN PAST MONTH		
LUNG DISEASE / TB			CORTISONE/STEROIDS WITHIN PAST YEAR		
SLEEP APNEA			A BAD REACTION TO ANESTHESIA		
ASTHMA, WHEEZING			MALIGNANT HYPERTHERMIA		
BRONCHITIS/EMPHYSEMA/PNEUMONIA			RELATIVES with MALIGNANT HYPERTHERMIA		
RECENT COUGH OR COLD			ANYTHING TO EAT OR DRINK TODAY - TIME _____		

ASSISTIVE DEVICES ☐ NONE

	Yes	No
SOB AT REST		
SOB WITH EXERTION		
KIDNEY DISEASE / DIALYSIS / STONES		
INDWELLING CATHETER		

☐N/A   ☐PROSTHETICS   ☐CRUTCHES
☐W/C   ☐WALKER   ☐CANE
DO YOU REQUIRE ASSISTANCE WITH ADL? ☐ YES ☐NO

ORIENTATION ☐TIME/PLACE/PERSON ☐SEE REMARKS

COMMUNICATION ☐ HEARING AID ☐RT ☐LT ☐REMOVED

	Yes	No
LIVER DISEASE/JAUNDICE/HEPATITIS A-B-C		
HIATAL HERNIA / HEARTBURN / REFLUX		
DIABETES / HYPOGLYCEMIA		
THYROID DISEASE		
SEIZURES / SYNCOPE		

☐ENGLISH ☐HARD OF HEARING ☐DEAF
☐BLIND ☐ABLE TO UNDERSTAND
☐LEARNING IMPAIRMENT ☐SEE REMARKS

PEDIATRIC: PATIENT UNDER 12 YEAR/ ☐ N/A

	Yes	No
STROKE / TIA / PARKINSONS		
CHRONIC BACK PROBLEMS		
HAVE ANY PHYSICAL RESTRICTIONS		
NEUROMUSCULAR PROBLEMS / DISEASES		
BLEEDING OR BLOOD DISORDER / ANEMIA		
A BLOOD TRANSFUSION IN THE LAST 3 MOS.?		
SICKLE CELL DISEASE		
POSITIVE HIV / AIDS		
SIGNIFICANT WT. LOSS		
SKIN INTEGRITY INTACT		
ADEQUATE GENERAL HYGIENE		
ARTHRITIS		
CANCER		
OTHER: _____		

Pediatric rows:

	Yes	No
HAVE ANY PHYSICAL RESTRICTIONS		
SLEEP APNEA?		
ABNORMALITIES AT BIRTH?		
GESTATIONAL AGE? PREMATURE/TERM		
HEAD CIRCUMFERENCE (For Patients Under 2 yrs)		
BIRTH WEIGHT_____ # _____ OZ		
HEART DISEASE		
MITRAL VALVE PROLAPSE / HEART MURMUR		
IRREGULAR HEARTBEAT		
LUNG DISEASE		
ASTHMA, WHEEZING		
BRONCHITIS/EMPHYSEMA/PNEUMONIA		
RECENT COUGH OR COLD		
HIATAL HERNIA / HEARTBURN / REFLUX		

SURGERIES ☐ NONE

	Yes	No
LIVER DISEASE/JAUNDICE/HEPATITIS A-B-C		
KIDNEY DISEASE		
DIABETES/HYPOGLYCEMIA		
THYROID DISEASE		
SEIZURES FEBRILE ☐		
BLEEDING OR BLOOD DISORDER / ANEMIA		
A BLOOD TRANSFUSION IN THE LAST 3 MOS.?		
SICKLE CELL DISEASE		
POSITIVE HIV		
SIGNIFICANT WT. LOSS		
NEUROMUSCULAR PROBLEMS / DISEASES		
OTHER ILLNESS:		

OTHER	YES	NO	N/A
ADEQUATE GENERAL HYGIENE			
EVIDENCE OF ABUSE / NEGLECT			

IMMUNIZATIONS

ARE YOUR CHILD'S IMMUNIZATIONS CURRENT? _____
☐YES ☐NO ☐UNSURE
IF NOT CURRENT, WHY?

ADULT/CHILD
☐ LAST IMMUNIZATION _____
        DATE _____
VERIFIED BY: ☐PARENT RECORD ☐HISTORY ☐MCIR
HAS YOUR CHILD BEEN EXPOSED TO ANY COMMUNICABLE
DISEASES IN THE PAST 3 WEEKS (E.G. CHICKEN POX, MEASLES,
MUMPS) ☐YES ☐NO DATE OF EXPOSURE _____

ALLERGIES / REACTION	☐ NKDA	REACTION
LATEX _____		
☐ _____		
☐ _____		
☐ _____		
☐ _____		
☐ _____		

MEDICATIONS	☐ NONE		TAKEN TODAY
DRUG/DOSE/SCHEDULE			☐
			☐
			☐
			☐
			☐
			☐
			☐
			☐
			☐
			☐
			☐
			☐
			☐
			☐
			☐
			☐
			☐
			☐
			☐
			☐
			☐
			☐
			☐

PREOP MEDICATION	DOSE	ROUTE	TIME	BY WHOM

Sol _____ cc   IV Cath _____ gauge

—RN:

SITE: _____ RIB TO OR _____ CC

FIGURE 2-1
Perioperative nurse assessment plan. (Courtesy of St. Joseph's Mercy of Macomb, Clinton Township, Mich.)   *Continued*

PAIN ☐YES ☐NO ☐NA

DO YOU HAVE PAIN NOW?_____

SITE_____DESCRIBE_____

	2	4	6	8	10

NO PAIN   MODERATE PAIN   WORST POSSIBLE PAIN

0   2   4   6   8   10

PRE-SURGICAL PROCESS EXPLAINED ☐YES
PRE-OP TEACHING INITIATED ☐YES
POST OP TEACHING INITIATED ☐YES
PAIN MANAGEMENT BROCHURE GIVEN ☐YES

Addressograph

NUTRITION   DENTURES ☐YES ☐NO ☐REMOVED

1. Patient has chewing, swallowing, or mouth problems that make it hard to eat? ☐YES ☐NO
2. Patient has had nausea, vomiting or diarrhea for the last 5 days? ☐YES ☐NO
3. Patient has unintentionally lost or gained 10 lbs or more in the last 6 months? ☐YES ☐NO
4. Patient is unable to afford adequate food or unable to shop, cook, or feed self? ☐YES ☐NO

NUTRITION RISK IDENTIFIED? ☐YES ☐NO
REFERRED TO OP DIETITIAN? ☐YES ☐NO ☐ENTERED INTO COMPUTER
DIET INFORMATION SHEET PROVIDED TO PATIENT? ☐YES ☐NO
* 2 OR MORE YES QUESTIONS INDICATES A NUTRITION RISK EXISTS.

DISCHARGE INFORMATION
☐OTHER_____
☐HOME ☐RESPONSIBLE ADULT
☐LOBBY NAME:_____
PSS RN SIGNATURE
ADMITTING NURSE SIGNATURE & TITLE

PRE-OP NOTES

TIME	

PRE-OP NURSING DIAGNOSIS   POTENTIAL FOR.................

☒ 1. ANXIETY: R/T SURGICAL OUTCOME
NURSING INTERVENTION: Encourage verbalization of fears: Allow family to stay with pt. as long as possible.
PATIENT OUTCOME: Patient will have decreased level of anxiety.

☒ 2. KNOWLEDGE DEFICIT:
NURSING INTERVENTION: Explain procedure and plan of care, complete all pre-op teaching.
PATIENT OUTCOME: Verbalize understanding.

☒ 3. INJURY:
NURSING INTERVENTION: SR x2, Brakes on, monitor and report abnormal labs, x-rays, EKG, or assessment data.
PATIENT OUTCOME: No injury

Addressograph

POST-OP PROCEDURE ASSESSMENT
POST-OP ADMITTING NURSE

ANESTHESIA:
☐ General ☐ Reversal
☐ Spinal ☐ Block_____
☐ Epidural ☐ Local w/ sedation
☐ Local
☐ Conscious sedation

AIRWAY SUPPORT:
☐None ☐Nasal
☐Endotracheal ☐Mandibular
☐Oral ☐Other

CONDITION ON ARRIVAL:
☐alert ☐unresponsive
☐somnolent ☐combative
☐crying ☐orientated
☐confused ☐apprehensive
☐calm ☐uncooperative
☐other_____ ☐drowsy

SAFETY: ☐Ambulatory
☐Rails up ☐Bed
☐Rail pads ☐Bed/ICU
☐Cart ☐Wheelchair
☐ASC Chair
SKIN:
☐Warm ☐Dry
☐Cool ☐Moist

INVASIVE MONITOR
☐Arterial Line
☐Calibrate
Site_____
☐A-Line Flush
☐Discontinued
Pressure Applied
_____mins.
☐Pulse present

O₂ THERAPY
RA - Rm Air
NC - Nasal Cannula
M - Mask
AM - Aerosol Mask
V - Vent
TP - T-Piece
DC - Discontinued
ABB - Aerosol
Blow Bag

ADMISSION VITAL SIGNS

TIME										
BP										
HEART RATE										
RESP / SaO₂										
O₂ THERAPY Mode O₂										
TEMP OTHER										

FIGURE 2-1—cont'd

POST ANESTHETIC ASSESSMENT		TIME	ADM				DC
Activity	Able to move four extremities voluntarily on command	2					
	Able to move two extremities voluntarily on command	1					
	Able to move no extremities voluntarily on command	0					
Respiration	Able to breathe deeply and cough freely	2					
	Dyspnea or limited breathing	1					
	Apneic	0					
Circulation	BP ± 20% Systolic of Preanesthetic level	2					
	BP ± 30–50% Systolic of Preanesthetic level	1					
	BP ± 50% Systolic of Preanesthetic level	0					
Consciousness	Fully Awake	2					
	Arousable on calling	1					
	Not responding	0					
O_2 Saturation	Able to maintain O_2 saturation > 92% on room air	2					
	Needs O_2 inhalation to maintain O_2 saturation > 90%	1					
	O_2 saturation < 90 % even with O_2 supplement	0					
Dressing	Dry	2					
	Wet but stationary	1					
	Wet but growing	0					
Pain	None to mild	2					
	Mild pain handled by oral meds	1					
	Pain requiring parenteral meds	0					
Ambulation	Able to stand up and walk straight	2					
	Vertigo when erect	1					
	Dizziness when supine	0					
Postoperative Emetic Symptoms	None to mild nausea	2					
	Transient vomiting or retching	1					
	Persistent - moderate – severe nausea & vomiting	0					
Urine Output	Has voided	2					
	Unable to void but comfortable	1					
	Unable to void and uncomfortable	0					

Total Score = 20   Score 8–10 indicates readiness for transfer
OPS/Procedure: 16–20 indicates readiness for discharge   **Total**

DISCHARGE SIGNATURE & TITLE

I.V. INTAKE | INFUSED | RIB
TIME | O.R. I.V. FLUIDS TOTAL
| BLOOD PRODUCTS TOTAL

IV LINES: SITE: ___ PATENT ☐YES ☐NO
IV DISCONTINUED @ ___ WITH ___ INFUSED
CATHETER ☐YES ☐NO   STRAIGHT CATHED ☐YES
VOIDED ☐YES ☐NO ☐N/A

TIME	POST OP MEDICATION	ROUTE	SITE	PAIN SCORE	RN SIGNATURE

INJECTION SITE CODE
1. Right Hip 3. Right Thigh 5. Right Arm
2. Left Hip 4. Left Thigh 6. Left Arm
7. Right Abdomen 8. Left Abdomen

MANAGEMENT STRATEGY (MEDICATION / DOSE / OTHER THERAPIES) AND RESULTS OF INTERVENTION
- Heat/Cold - Massage/Healing
- OT/PT - Relaxation Techniques
- Music - Pastoral Care
- Distraction - PT & Family Services

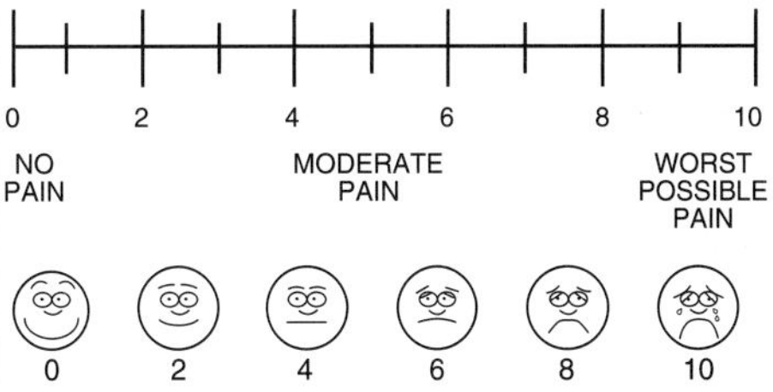

0 2 4 6 8 10
NO PAIN   MODERATE PAIN   WORST POSSIBLE PAIN

0 2 4 6 8 10

REASSESS PATIENT AFTER EACH INTERVENTION AND DOCUMENT.

ICE ☐UE R L ☐LE R L ☐____
Elevation ☐UE R L ☐LE R L
Splint / Cast ☐UE R L
Immobilizer/Sling ☐UL R L

Sensation - Adm.: Site ____
☐normal ☐tingling ☐SNN
☐numb ☐absent
Circulation - Adm.: Site ____
☐pink ☐cyanotic ☐SNN
☐cool ☐warm ☐blanche
Discharge:☐No chg. ☐SNN

POST-OP NOTES   Addressograph

TIME	
	Pulses ☐Absent ☐Doppler ☐Weak ☐Normal ☐Bounding
	Movement ☐Present ☐Absent ☐SNN - document/report ____

POST-OP EKG STRIP

816223(4/02)

FIGURE 2-1—cont'd   *Continued*

Addressograph

POST PROCEDURE NURSING DIAGNOSIS POTENTIAL FOR:

☒ 1. <u>ALTERED HEMODYNAMICS, NEUROVASCULAR, RESPIRATORY STATUS:</u> R/T anesthesia, surgical intervention, hypovolemia, nausea/vomiting.
NURSING INTERVENTIONS: VS as indicated; cardiac monitoring; O_2 therapy and airway management; IV therapy as indicated; watch for S/S of bleeding; position patient as indicated; Rx prn for N/V, hypotension, hypertension; elevation of of affected extremities.
PATIENT OUTCOME: VS WNL; no respiratory complications; minimal N/V; operative site has minimal to no drainage; no circulatory impairment by cast or dressing; maintain effective breathing.

☒ 2. <u>INJURY:</u> R/T anesthesia, surgical intervention.
NURSING INTERVENTIONS: monitor LOC; orient patient prn; bedrest until alert; NPO until gag reflex returns; Rx as needed for pain; hypotension, universal precautions.
PATIENT OUTCOME: VS WNL; able to ambulate as per pre-op or with aids; LOC as per pre-op; be free of injury and in a safe environment.

☒ 3. <u>ALTERED THERMOREGULATION:</u> R/T surgical intervention; OR environment, and/or anesthetics, irrigations, age, fluid replacement.
NURSING INTERVENTIONS: monitor temperature; warming blankets; limit exposures, Rx prn for shivering; assess peripheral circulation if indicated.
POTENTIAL OUTCOME: no shivering; temperature WNL; skin W/D

☒ 4. <u>SKIN INTEGRITY AND POTENTIAL FOR INFECTION:</u> R/T surgical site.
NURSING INTERVENTIONS: assess surgical site for bleeding, swelling, redness; proper positionings; change dressing prn; teach pt to splint incision if indicated; circulatory status of site.
POTENTIAL OUTCOME: operative site dry or minimal drainage; circulation not impaired by cast or dressing; maintains pre-op skin integrity.

☒ 5. <u>COMFORT:</u> R/T surgical procedure.
NURSING INTERVENTIONS: assess for pain; Rx prn; positioning; evaluate effectiveness of interventions; assess circulatory status.
PATIENT OUTCOME: pt verbalizes or demonstrates increased comfort; pain reasonably controlled.

☒ 6. <u>KNOWLEDGE DEFICIT:</u> R/T post-op care.
NURSING INTERVENTIONS: review post-op instructions with patient and/or companion; give copy of instructions/scrips; allow patient to verbalize questions and concerns.
POTENTIAL OUTCOME: pt/companion will verbalize and/or demonstrate understanding of post-op care, instructions, equipment, etc.

☒ 7. <u>ANXIETY:</u> R/T post-op diagnosis, procedure; separation from family; unfamiliar surroundings, changes in lifestyle and/or body image.
NURSING INTERVENTIONS: orient prn: give reassurance, emotional support: encourage pt. to express fears and ask questions; provide privacy.
POTENTIAL OUTCOME: verbalizes orientation to environment; pt expresses feelings and concerns; verbalizes anxiety and understanding of events.

POST ENDOSCOPY NURSING DIAGNOSIS POTENTIAL FOR:

☒ 1. <u>ALTERATION IN COMFORT:</u> pain R/T procedure
NURSING INTERVENTIONS: assess location & nature of pain; observe for S/S of perforation; assess color & amount of any rectal drainage; position for comfort & passing flatus; allow patient to verbalize.
PATIENT OUTCOME: verbalize relief of pain; observe relaxed facial expressions and body positioning; passing flatus.

2. <u>INJURY:</u> R/T sedation.
NURSING INTERVENTIONS: maintain IV fluids; bedrest until alert; medication prn N/V; NPO until gag reflex returns; monitor VS; provide support and comfort.
PATIENT OUTCOME: vs WNL; no aspiration; minimal N/V.

3. KNOWLEDGE DEFICIT:
<u>NURSING INTERVENTI</u>ONS: give printed post procedure instruction and review with pt/family/significant other; give copies; reinforce dr's instructions.
PATIENT OUTCOME: verbalize understanding of post procedure instructions.

RN SIGNATURE _____

DATE _____

____ Operative site is dry/minimal drainage, + circulation is not impaired by casts or drainage.

____ Personal items returned to patient.

____ Mental status oriented x 3

____ Vital sign stable + BP is within 20% of pre-op pressure.

____ Patient has voided if spinal or epidural anesthesia per Dr. orders. (If not: patient given appropriate instructions.)

____ Physician spoke with family / significant other.

____ Patient steady when upright and able to ambulate or equivalent to pre-op status. Demonstrates use of assistive advice

DISCHARGE CRITERIA

____ Pain is reasonably controlled by p.o. medication.

____ PT/Family educated: save/effective use of medications.

____ Discharge instructions reviewed by patient and family members Understanding of instructions verbalized.

____ Discharged in stable condition to the care of family/significant other/ care giver. @ _____ .

☐ W/C   ☐ Ambulatory   ☐ Stretcher

CODE: + = Discharge criteria met.   0 = Discharge criteria not met.
See post-op nurses notes for explanation.
Discharge RN Signature _____

POST PROCEDURE TELEPHONE CALL	Phone #_____ DOS: _____ Procedure: _____		DATE:	TIME:

VERBAL REPORT ON CONDITION PER ☐PATIENT ☐FAMILY MEMBER ☐MESSAGE LEFT ON ANSWERING MACHINE ☐NO ANSWER	ANY BLEEDING: ☐YES ☐NO

FEVER: ☐YES ☐ NO	INCISION INTACT: ☐YES ☐NO ☐N/A	NAUSEA/VOMITING: ☐YES ☐NO	DRESSING REMOVED: ☐YES ☐NO ☐N/A

FOLLOW-UP MEDICAL APPT. MADE: ☐YES ☐NO ☐N/A	DID YOU UNDERSTAND POST-OP INSTRUCTIONS.: ☐YES ☐NO	ABILITY TO REST: ☐YES ☐NO

0–10 CURRENT PAIN SCORE SCORE:	RELIEF FROM PAIN MED: ☐YES ☐NO ☐N/A	REFERRED TO SURGEON: ☐YES ☐ NO

CAN THE HOSPITAL NURSE LEAVE A MESSAGE ON YOUR ANSWERING MACHINE / WITH SIGNIFICANT OTHER / FAMILY MEMBER? ☐YES ☐NO

	RN SIGNATURE _____

FIGURE 2-1—cont'd

Table 2-1   DIRECT AND INDIRECT PATIENT CARE

Activity	Direct	Indirect
Preparing equipment and devices to be used during surgery		X
Performing urinary catheterization	X	
Taking vital signs	X	
Sterilizing surgical supplies		X
Providing the correct instruments at the correct time during surgery		X
Providing therapeutic communication to the patient	X	
Performing the preparation of skin at the surgical site	X	
Demonstrating a high level of organizational skill and quick thinking		X
Assembling and testing complex surgical equipment		X
Monitoring the safe operation of instruments during surgery		X
Transferring the patient to and from the operating table	X	
Anticipating each step of a procedure and the instruments needed for each step		X
Evaluating the integrity of a stainless steel implant		X

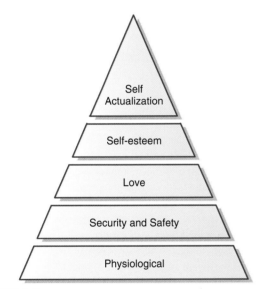

FIGURE 2-2
Maslow's hierarchy of human needs.

because of the individuality of each patient, every case is different. The patient's emotional, psychosocial, and spiritual needs also are addressed at all levels of care.

PHYSIOLOGICAL NEEDS

Physiological needs are the minimum requirements for life. These include nutrition, air, rest, elimination, shelter from the extremes of heat and cold, and the ability to exercise or move one's body. Although as caregivers we may not be consciously thinking of each need, we instinctively know about these needs from our own experience. There are many levels of care that meet these needs. Some care actions are easily performed, such as providing warmth; others are more complex, such as balancing electrolyte and glucose levels to

maintain survival. Each level is performed by skilled and competent caregivers who respond according to their level of training. The simple tasks, such as providing a warm blanket, are often pushed aside in favor of more complicated ones. The *importance* of the simple task does not change, however. Table 2-2 describes critical physiological needs and some of the ways these are met.

To contribute to the patient's physical care, the surgical technologist must know certain information about the patient. Although the surgical technologist does not assess the patient's condition, information is critical to perform required tasks. A complete description of the surgical technologist's duties is given in Chapter 1, The Surgical Technologist.

Weight and Height

Information on the patient's weight and height is critical to safe transport and positioning (see Chapter 10, Transporting, Transferring, and Positioning) and for the proper selection of surgical equipment and instruments *before the start of surgery*. For example, many patients are smaller or larger than expected for their age.

Age

The age of the patient is important information in planning for surgery. For example, age influences the patient's physical condition, mobility, and emotional needs, and affects physiological response during surgery. However, chronological age does not always define a patient's needs. Developmental age is typically a more accurate measurement (Table 2-3).

Condition

The patient's condition may be described as critical, serious, guarded, or stable. If the procedure is an emergency, speed of preparation is critical, sometimes causing protocols to be al-

Table 2-2 BASIC PHYSIOLOGICAL NEEDS OF THE PATIENT

Need	Examples of How Needs Are Met in the Perioperative Environment
Nutrition, water	Administration of intravenous replacement fluids and nutritive or electrolyte fluids
Shelter	Control of temperature through cloth blankets, air heating, or cooling blankets
Air and oxygen	Maintenance of an open airway
	Provision of the proper mix of oxygen with anesthetic or room air
	Attention to signs of oxygen deficit
Rest and sleep	Protection from environmental stress such as noise, light, or cold
Elimination	Catheterization or opportunity to void as needed
	Medical attention to conditions that prevent elimination
Movement	Freedom from restraint and assistance with movement when patient is unable to move on his or her own
Freedom from pain	Observation of the patient for signs of pain
	Administration of pain medication
	Exercise of care when moving the patient

Table 2-3 DEVELOPMENTAL GROWTH THROUGH THE LIFE SPAN

Stage of Life	Milestones of Development
Infancy (birth to 1 year)	▶ Head large in proportion to body; movement uncoordinated; vision unclear; good hearing, smell, and taste senses; teeth begin to erupt at 6 months; physical growth is rapid; decline in amount of "baby fat"; lumbar curvature develops
	▶ Learns to walk, communicate (talk), and understand some words; eats solid foods; forms relationships; sleeps and eats regularly
Toddler (1 to 2 years)	▶ Muscles and nervous system become more coordinated, especially hands; physical growth continues less rapidly
	▶ Learns to communicate with words; becomes less dependent and tolerates separation from person giving primary care; controls bowels and bladder; able to move by crawling, climbing, and running; plays in parallel (not together)
Early childhood (3 to 5 years)	▶ Grows taller; gains little weight; increases coordination; begins to draw and write
	▶ Ability to communicate increases; learns gender difference and modesty; learns right from wrong; plays with others; develops sense of family; provides some care of self
Middle childhood (6 to 8 years)	▶ Grows in height and weight slowly; primary teeth are lost; hand coordination increases, allowing cursive writing; permanent teeth erupt
	▶ Develops skills to play games; gets along with others of same age; learns basic skills of language and math; develops self-image of gender and self-esteem
Late childhood (9 to 12 years)	▶ Muscles increase in strength, coordination, and balance; develops physical skills; grows in height (girls taller than boys); permanent teeth appear; secondary sexual characteristics appear
	▶ Becomes independent; develops peer relationships; develops interest in sexual information
Adolescence (13 to 18 years)	▶ Rapid physical growth; changes of puberty begin; growth uneven (clumsiness); "wisdom" teeth appear
	▶ Rapid psychosocial development; relationships with peers and dating experiences develop
Young adulthood (19 to 45 years)	▶ Little physical growth; bone growth plates close
	▶ Chooses occupation; develops family unit with marriage, children, or others
Middle adulthood (46 to 65 years)	▶ Gradual slowing of metabolism; changes of aging occur
	▶ Lives on own or with adjusted family as children leave and parents age or die; develops leisure activities
Late adulthood (66 years and older)	▶ Declines in physical strength, endurance, and overall health condition
	▶ Adjusts to retirement, reduced income, and death of spouse; accepts own death

From Gerdin J: *Health careers today,* ed 3, St Louis, 2003, Mosby.

tered to meet the immediate problems, such as massive hemorrhage or need for emergency cesarean section.

Musculoskeletal Impairment

The patient with musculoskeletal impairment requires particular care in moving and positioning to avoid pain or further impairment.

Language

The patient who does not speak English cannot participate in his or her own care without an interpreter or translator. To provide *equal care for all,* this service must be available.

Impairment of the Senses

The patient with impairment of sight, hearing, touch, or other sensations deserves the same level of communication as a nonimpaired patient. The impaired surgical patient must have access to the same personnel and technical resources that are available to the impaired *nonsurgical* patient. See Chapter 6, Communication and Teamwork, for specific guidelines.

Pain

Pain is demonstrated by physiological changes and by body language. Respect for the patient's pain during preoperative preparations is essential to patient-centered care. If what you are doing causes pain, ask the patient for more information so that you do not increase the pain. Report the patient's pain to the registered nurse (RN) or anesthesia care provider.

Environmental Stress

Environmental stressors create tension in the patient; they are a source of noxious stimulation and also can affect the body's physiological response to anesthesia. Environmental stressors such as loud talking and frequent opening and closing of doors not only are a source of patient stress but also create a risk of contamination by airborne pathogens (see Chapter 7, The Process of Infection). Room noise should be kept to a minimum whether the patient is awake or asleep. Personal conversations should never be held with the patient in the room. Table 2-4 lists some of the environmental safety and security conditions that can appear in the perioperative environment and the appropriate protective responses. (Specific safety concerns are explained fully throughout the text.)

SPECIFIC PATIENT GROUPS

Certain patient groups require particular interventions and preparation for surgery. These considerations are both physical and psychosocial. Apart from their individual needs, patients who are similar in age or psychosocial group, or who share common pathology, also share common needs.

High-Risk Patient

The high-risk patient is one who requires surgery but has one or more **comorbid diseases** that endanger the outcome of the surgery. The following are patients who are considered at moderate or high risk when undergoing surgery.

Table 2-4   SAFETY, SECURITY, AND ENVIRONMENTAL CONCERNS IN THE PERIOPERATIVE ENVIRONMENT

Concern	Solution or Action
Hazards from electrical equipment	Seek knowledge and adhere to all safety precautions regarding equipment. *Ask questions when in doubt.*
Hazards related to patient transfer and positioning	Proceed according to demonstrated competence.
Risks associated with disease transmission	Adhere to strict aseptic technique and standard precautions. Maintain environment that is free of potential contaminants.
Hazards of body exposure	Keep the patient covered at all times to ensure privacy, warmth, and respect for personal dignity.
Patient feelings of objectification or humiliation	Communicate with the patient and other team members with respect. Use discretion in speech and mannerisms. Routine use of unprofessional or suggestive language and behavior can become normal to staff members. To the patient, it can be horrifying.
Sense of disorder and lack of privacy because staff come in and out of room frequently	Ensure that the patient is covered and request that others avoid unnecessary traffic through the room.
Excessive noise in operating room	Demonstrate the need for quiet to others in the room by modeling quiet work and refraining from loud talking and sudden noises. Keep doors closed.
Noxious, unfamiliar odors detectable to the patient	Communicate with the patient about any odors, such as those from bone cement or other sources. Explain the therapeutic use of an odorous substance in simple terms. Keep doors closed.
Risk of environmental damage to tissues	Know the progression of the surgical procedure and the order in which instruments are needed. This contributes to shorter operative time and reduced environmental exposure of tissues.

MALNOURISHED PATIENT

The malnourished patient lacks the necessary nutritional reserves to support the process of healing. Trauma to the body—whether intentional, such as surgery, or unintentional—requires high metabolic activity during the healing process. Protein and carbohydrates are in particularly high demand by the body to rebuild tissue and meet the physiological demands of organ systems. The patient who enters surgery undernourished (without enough food intake to support health) or malnourished (lacking the right kinds of foods to support body functions) is at high risk. Cancer, alcoholism, metabolic disease, and advanced age are a few conditions that often result in malnutrition or undernutrition.

DIABETIC PATIENT

Diabetes mellitus is an endocrine disease causing disruption in the metabolism of carbohydrates, fats, and proteins. When diabetes is not controlled, the patient experiences severe damage of vascular and neurological tissues. The risks associated with surgery in the diabetic patient are complex. They arise from the healing properties of the vascular system and the efficient use of glucose for tissue metabolism. Because many diabetic patients have compromised vascular systems, their risk of surgical-site infection is higher than in other groups. They are also subject to prolongation of wound healing, hypertension, and peripheral edema.

PATIENT WITH RESPIRATORY DISEASE

The patient with respiratory disease is at high risk for postoperative pneumonia or failure to regain voluntary respiratory function. Examples are chronic smokers and those with chronic pulmonary diseases such as asthma and emphysema.

ALCOHOLIC OR DRUG-ADDICTED PATIENT

Alcoholic and drug-addicted patients are often nutritionally depleted or anemic and may have multiple organ failure or disease in the liver, kidney, and pancreas. This affects the body's ability to metabolize anesthetic agents, defend against postoperative infection, replace lost blood cells, and metabolize carbohydrates.

IMMUNOSUPPRESSED PATIENT

The patient whose immune system is compromised or suppressed is threatened with postoperative infection and delayed healing. A healthy immune system is needed for the body to respond to the trauma of surgery and defend it against pathogens that may have invaded it during surgery. Patients who are being treated with immunosuppressants or antineoplastic agents for cancer are immunosuppressed. Those undergoing organ transplant receive immunosuppressants to depress the body's immune reaction to the new organ. Patients with the human immunodeficiency virus (HIV) or who have acquired immunodeficiency syndrome (AIDS) or other conditions that affect the immune response are also at increased risk for nosocomial (hospital-acquired) infections.

TRAUMA PATIENT

The patient who is rushed into surgery because of physical trauma is at high risk for many reasons. When severe trauma is present, there may be no time to obtain a previous medical history or the patient may be physically unable to provide it. Preexisting conditions may not be known, especially if the patient is unconscious. The patient may have eaten recently. This increases the risk of vomiting, aspiration, and subsequent pneumonia. There may be no witnesses to the trauma. Witnesses can supply important information about the nature of the trauma, which aids diagnosis. Injuries may be undetected, especially if the patient cannot answer questions. The trauma patient may arrive in surgery in a precarious physiological state with extensive blood loss, severe shock, and fluid electrolyte imbalance. Intoxication from alcohol or drugs can alter the physiological response to surgery and complicate the process and method of anesthesia.

PATIENT WITH HIV INFECTION OR AIDS

The patient with HIV or AIDS has multiple barriers to safe postoperative recovery. Because the patient does not have a healthy immune system, the potential for postoperative infection is high. The patient with AIDS has multiple comorbid diseases, which deplete the body's reserves for healing. Skin integrity is often compromised by open sores and lesions. Bacterial or viral infection may already be present. During surgery, infectious microorganisms can gain access to the sterile surfaces of the body and create serious systemic disease. One of the most common disorders associated with AIDS is infection with *Pneumocystis carinii,* a pathogenic microorganism that causes lung disease. Drug-resistant tuberculosis is also common in this population.

With the advent of highly active antiretroviral therapies (HAART), HIV is becoming recognized as a manageable illness. However, many of the medications currently used to treat HIV may have negative effects on a person's metabolism that may impair wound healing. Certain anti-HIV medications also may affect lipid levels in the blood, leading to an increased risk of heart disease and peripheral vascular disease.

The social stigma attached to AIDS is an added source of severe emotional and social trauma. In addition to showing concern and compassion for the patient, we can demonstrate care to others in the operating room who are fearful or unsure of the patient. Fear can be related to a lack of knowledge about the disease or to the social stigma attached to the disease.

Pediatric Patient

The pediatric patient presents particular challenges in both communications and physiological response to surgery. Pediatric patient groups are defined according to approximate chronological age ranges. The age group reflects the developmental stage:

Infant	Birth to 18 months
Toddler	19 months to 3 years
Preschooler	4 to 6 years
School-aged child	7 to 12 years
Adolescent	13 to 16 years

SPECIAL PHYSIOLOGICAL CONSIDERATIONS

The pediatric patient usually undergoes surgery for treatment of congenital malformation. In general, these malformations include anomalies of the gastrointestinal system, craniofacial structures, or vertebral column and spinal cord; renal anomalies; tracheoesophageal malformations; and limb malformations. Injury from accidents is also common in the pediatric population.

The pediatric patient presents special challenges in surgery, including the size of anatomical structures, the relative fragility of the body, and the ratio of surface area to volume. Even a small amount of blood or fluid loss is severe in the pediatric patient. The large surface area compared to mass predisposes the patient to chilling or overheating during surgery. This can result in excess fluid loss or hypoglycemia, especially in the infant.

DEVELOPMENTAL STAGES AND HOSPITALIZATION

Children of different developmental stages have predictable fears, responses, and reactions to hospitalization and the process of surgery. Knowledge of these stages helps the surgical technologist understand the behaviors exhibited by children in the operating room.

Infants need to be physically close to their caretakers. They should be held as much as possible until the procedure begins. Stress is high in infant patients. They have been separated from the familiar feel, smell, and sight of their primary caregiver, and feedings have been stopped before surgery. Because of this they are difficult to comfort and may cry continually.

Toddlers suffer frustration and loss of autonomy as well as extreme anxiety when separated from their primary caretaker. The operating room environment can be terrifying to a toddler, who expresses this by crying and screaming or through **aggression** and **regression**. Toddlers are especially difficult to restrain. They require patience and understanding from their caregivers. Stronger restraint (or more restrainers) usually causes more terror and increased resistance. Taking time to instill calm is the humane way to provide medical intervention. When this is unsuccessful, rapid sedation may be required.

Preschoolers also suffer extreme fear in the operating room environment. It is common for this group to view the hospital and surgical experience as a type of punishment or as *deliberate* abandonment. Prone to fantasy, they may imagine extreme mutilation as a result of surgery. Because they are unable to understand what the inside of the body actu-

ally looks like, they interpret descriptions of surgery literally. They are concrete thinkers and understand words like "cut," "bleed," and "stick," in extreme, literal, and often exaggerated forms. Their primary fear is body mutilation. This is often manifested by regression or aggression.

School-aged children are more compliant and cooperative with health-care personnel, but many tend to withdraw from their caregivers. They fear mutilation but are curious about their bodies and often insist on "helping" with their own care. They are very sensitive about body exposure, which can be extremely stressful. For school-aged children, receiving information is a way of coping with their fears. They welcome explanations and descriptions of how things work and how devices and equipment in the environment relate to their own bodies.

Adolescents are very sensitive about body image and changes in the body. They resent any intrusion of privacy and bodily exposure. They also fear loss of control. At times stoic and curious, they are grateful for concrete information about the surgical environment and the procedure itself. Among their many concerns, potential loss of presence with their peers and fear of being "left out" because of illness or deformity are very important.

Geriatric Patient

The healthy geriatric patient usually has minimal physiological changes. However, he or she is at risk for skin, joint, muscle, and bone injury, especially during transfer and positioning. During the aging process, the body loses adipose tissue, which pads the skeleton and protects it from injury. Connective tissue in joints and skin is lost, which produces increased injury as a result of a loss of skin elasticity. The geriatric patient's skin is often dry and extremely fragile. Appropriate care must be taken to avoid injury to these tissues.

Loss of body heat resulting from a lack of body fat is a special consideration for the geriatric patient. Do not assume that the patient is comfortable because he or she does not say otherwise. Table 2-5 describes physiological changes related to aging.

PSYCHOSOCIAL NEEDS

An early treatise on patient care written by Paul E. Johnson describes the seriously ill hospital patient with clarity and compassion:

> The hospital patient suffers from mental anguish more acute than his physical pain. His emotional condition is one of anxiety and insecurity as he dangles in a chasm of distress between a past he would gladly return to and a future he is reluctant to face. He has lost the values he once had of health, freedom, and power to do and be sufficient to the strenuous joys of active achievement. He can look back but with vain regret. Looking ahead he sees only poignant uncertainty. Am I to live or die? If I live, will I be disabled and have to live in restricted patterns of uncertain health, with faltering steps and hesitant, watchful caution? Can I ever be free again? . . . Am I on borrowed time

Table 2-5	PHYSICAL CHANGES THAT OCCUR WITH AGE
Body System	**Changes**
Respiratory	Chest diameter decreases from front to back (anterior to posterior).
	Blood oxygen level decreases.
	Lungs become more rigid and less elastic.
	Recoil of alveoli diminishes.
Gastrointestinal	Peristalsis diminishes.
	Liver loses storage capacity.
	Motility of stomach muscles decreases.
	Gag reflex diminishes.
Cardiovascular	Capillary walls thicken.
	Systolic blood pressure increases.
	Cardiac output decreases.
Musculoskeletal	Muscle strength decreases.
	Range of motion decreases.
	Cartilage decreases.
	Bone mass decreases.
Sensory perception	Progressive hearing loss occurs.
	Sense of smell diminishes.
	Pain threshold increases.
	Night vision decreases.
	Sensitivity to glare increases.
	Sense of body position in space (proprioception) can decrease.
Genitourinary	Bladder capacity diminishes.
	Stress incontinence in women occurs.
	Kidney filtration rate decreases.
	Reproductive changes in women occur:
	▶ Vaginal secretions decrease.
	▶ Estrogen levels decrease.
	▶ Reproductive organs atrophy.
	▶ Breast tissue decreases.
	Reproductive changes in men occur:
	▶ Testosterone production decreases.
	▶ Testicular size decreases.
	▶ Sperm count decreases.
Skin	Skin loses turgor (elasticity).
	Sebaceous glands become less active.
	Skin becomes thin and delicate.
	Pigment changes occur.
Endocrine	Cortisol production decreases.
	Blood glucose level increases.
	Pancreas releases insulin at a slower rate.

from now on, costing more than I can earn, depriving my family of their necessities, turning over my work to stronger men, trying to look more cheerful than I feel, with a brave pose of gaiety that covers a hollow gulf of threatening insecurity?

From Paul E. Johnson, *Psychology of Pastoral Care,* New York, Abingdon Press, 1953.

As caregivers we cannot presume to meet all the psychosocial needs of the patient, especially in the brief time that we interact with them. Human needs, both inner and demonstrated, are complex. We can, however, be aware of those needs and be aware of *our own feelings* and attitudes about complex psychosocial aspects of care. Knowledge of our own attitudes helps to clarify and prepare our response to the patient. As professionals, we must never allow our own beliefs to interfere with care or cause judgment of another. The role of the caregiver is to support and heal.

Physical Security

Security is a feeling of well-being and protection. Although many patients are confident about the outcome of surgery and even feel relieved to be resolving a medical problem, most have some level of anxiety or fear. This is a normal reaction to pending trauma to the body. Patients develop trust in those who are caring for them when team members demonstrate care by their *actions and communication.* The patient feels greater security when team members explain, honestly and professionally, *what is occurring and why.* For example, the patient safety strap is secured as soon as the patient is transferred to the operating table. Rather than say jokingly, "I'm putting this strap on so you don't get away" or "This strap is to keep you from falling off the table" (the latter introduces a new source of anxiety because it may never have occurred to the patient that he or she might fall off the table), a more reassuring statement might be, "The operating bed is very narrow. I'm putting this strap over your legs to remind you to stay centered on the bed." This statement explains that a safety issue exists and is being addressed.

Spiritual Needs

Spirituality is not necessarily the same as *religion,* although they are often expressed as one entity. Spirituality, however, can be practiced apart from religion. It is a sense or understanding of something more profound than humanity, not perceived by the physical senses. It is an awareness or belief in an energy or power greater than humankind. This power may be referred to as "creator," "spirit," "God," or the patient may have no name for it. When based in religion, spiritual life is integrated into rituals (practices that have special meaning) and ceremonies that are common to those who practice a particular faith. The caretaker may be purposefully invited to play a role in the patient's spiritual life, as when the patient asks for prayer, or may unknowingly be present in times of great spiritual conflict or distress.

The silent patient may be praying or communing with his or her spiritual entity(ies). For many patients, surgery is a deeply troubling event. The patient may question whether he or she will live or die during the procedure. The patient may have fears and unresolved social and emotional conflicts of which no one else knows. Always remember that appearances do not tell the whole story of a patient. We can affect the patient positively or negatively. It is a choice that we make daily in our encounters with those who come to surgery. Our most powerful spiritual support can be silent acknowledgment of and respect for the human life. If the patient requests prayer or other spiritual expression before surgery, team members should support the patient's request.

THERAPEUTIC COMMUNICATION

Today's health-care system often requires that as many surgeries as possible be completed in each 24-hour period. The surgical patient lives in the center of a storm of activity, in a very busy environment that is frightening and authoritative. He or she has no control over what is happening and is handed from one person to the next with scant introductions or knowledge about the roles of people in the environment. The model for health care emphasizes treatment of the patient as a whole individual. However, health-care providers often seem to have little time for providing psychosocial and spiritual support and comfort. The best guide-

line for patient communication is to mentally place yourself in the patient's position. How would you want to be treated? How would you respond to the environment if you were ill or injured? If you were a child, how would you interpret the sights, sounds, and smells of the operating room? Would these experiences deeply affect you? No one can create or teach empathy and caring. One can only train a caregiver to recognize needs and carry out the process of care. From that point on, the caregiver's humanity and connection with the patient govern his or her response to the patient's emotional concerns.

The types of communication in which surgical technologists are likely to engage focus on the surgical environment, physical (comfort) needs, and perhaps the way the patient is feeling. The surgical technologist can greatly affect the patient's well-being by displaying focused, purposeful, and caring communication. Appropriate **therapeutic communication** requires a nonjudgmental and supportive presence (Box 2-1). *Presence* means that the caregiver's attention is focused *on the patient.*

The following are characteristics of therapeutic communication:

▶ **It is goal directed.** It has a specific purpose. The purpose is to comfort the patient, gain information about the pa-

---

Box 2-1   Guidelines for Therapeutic Communication

Listen to the patient attentively. Show your interest by making eye contact (unless culturally inappropriate—for example, in traditional Islamic culture, women do not make direct eye contact with men) and by leaning your upper body slightly toward the patient. Show that you care. Do not allow yourself to be distracted while communicating with the patient. If your attention is split, you will convey a lack of concern. Remember that your thoughts are revealed by your body language, actions, and expressions.

When communicating with the patient, watch for nonverbal cues such as withdrawal, facial expressions, sighing, or crying. A relaxed face shows little strain. A downturned mouth, pursed lips, and stiff jaw may denote anger or resentment. Fear is expressed with wide eyes and downturned outer eyelids.

Explain what you are doing in plain, simple language. Look for cues that the patient understands. Do not assume that because the message was given, it was also received and comprehended.

Do not ask closed-ended questions as a method of communication unless you have a reason to ask specific questions. Closed-ended questions are designed to be answered with very few words and make it appear the caregiver is simply completing a survey. Open-ended questions allow the patient to elaborate on a point, which may produce greater insight into the patient's concerns or current situation. Continual questioning can make a person feel uncomfortable. Therapeutic communication allows the patient to express needs and concerns. Examples of open-ended questions are, "How are you feeling?" and "Do you

have any concerns about your procedure?" Examples of closed-ended questions are, "How long have you been sick?" and "Do you live alone?"

Do not talk about yourself. It is inappropriate for team members to share personal information with the patient or with coworkers in the presence of the patient. Joking and offensive language can have serious effects on the patient's sense of security. Although it is not meant to offend the patient, it is not only disconcerting but also unprofessional. Would you want to hear the details of someone's date while waiting to have abdominal surgery for cancer?

Refer questions when you do not know the answers. Be honest about what you do not know. Patients are often unaware of the professional roles of their caretakers. If you are asked a medical question or one that requires assessment or other nursing skills, refer the question to licensed personnel. Ask the patient if he or she has discussed the issue with the physician. It is better to delay an answer than to mislead or give information that is outside the scope of one's practice.

Do not use innuendoes or stereotyped greetings such as "Hi beautiful" or "How's my best patient?" Patients know when they are not being treated as individuals. Sexual innuendoes spoken among staff workers are quickly perceived by patients awaiting surgery. Patients are not insensitive to their social environment. In another setting, the patient might be unaffected by this type of communication. In the medical setting, it is unprofessional and can be upsetting.

tient's needs, and respond in a way that meets or acknowledges those needs.

▶ **It is unique to each patient.** Every patient is a unique person with individual hopes, fears, and concerns. Therapeutic relationships honor this uniqueness with specific verbal and physical responses, not stock answers and comments that are automatically used for every patient. Therapeutic communication is learned behavior.

▶ **It requires active engagement.** It is not haphazard or casual.

▶ **It requires excellent observation and listening skills.** These are reinforced through experience and guidance. Listening is both an art and a skill. It requires patience, focus, and presence. One can learn important information by observing the patient. One can meet needs by recognizing signs of discomfort, fear, anxiety, or other intense emotion.

Therapeutic Response

Therapeutic responses include cue giving, clarification, restatement, paraphrasing, reflection, and touch. When these responses are used, communication becomes centered on the patient's needs.

Leads and cues are actions and words that encourage the patient to communicate. The goal is to prevent the patient from becoming self-conscious or afraid to express feelings and sensations. Leads and cues include nodding in affirmation and making comments such as "Really?" and "I see."

Example

PATIENT: "*I should have had this surgery a long time ago, but I just couldn't face it.*"
RESPONSE: "*Really?*" (A short verbal cue indicates that the listener cares and invites the patient to continue to share her feelings.)
PATIENT: "*I was so afraid.*"
RESPONSE: "*It must have been very difficult for you.*" (Acknowledges the patient's fear.)

Restatement is not simply parroting the patient but rather restating the patient's comment in a way that takes in the underlying meaning.

Example

PATIENT: "*This is the fifth back surgery in 8 years for me. I just hope this surgeon knows what he is doing.*"
RESPONSE: "*You've been through a lot of surgery—you're hopeful that this surgeon has the knowledge needed to help you?*"

In this case the patient expresses doubts about the expertise of the surgeon. The caregiver acknowledges the patient's anxiety.

Paraphrasing is different from restatement in that the caregiver looks past the patient's stated words and addresses the underlying message. In paraphrasing, the caregiver demonstrates empathy about the *unstated* need for comfort and security.

Example

PATIENT: (Nervously) "*Everyone here is so busy.*"
RESPONSE: "*I know there is a lot of activity. It must seem really fast, but everyone is taking care of his or her patients. Is there anything I can do to help you feel more comfortable while we're waiting for the anesthesiologist?*" (Appropriately addresses the unstated meaning, which is, "I wonder if they will take good care of me—there is so much going on.")

Reflection allows the patient to connect his or her emotions with information provided in the immediate environment or from a different event or situation.

Example

PATIENT: "*It's always so cold in these places. After all the money these hospitals make, the least they could do is turn up the heat.*"
RESPONSE: "*It sounds like you feel frustrated about being here. It is a difficult time. The temperature is low for safety reasons. I'll get you a warm blanket.*"

A skilled caregiver understands that the patient is not only cold but also angry about the helplessness of his or her situation. The patient is unable to meet his or her own environmental needs. The caregiver acknowledges the patient's frustration and responds appropriately.

Nontherapeutic responses are casual and do not assist the patient in coping with anxiety or conflict.

Example

PATIENT: "*Are all those instruments for my surgery?*"
NONTHERAPEUTIC RESPONSE: "*Yeah, we have to have everything ready in case we need it. You never know what the doctor might want.*"
PATIENT: "*Oh.*"
(Thinking): "*It must mean they think there will be complications. Maybe the surgery will be much more extensive than I thought. What if I have cancer and they didn't tell me?*"
CORRECT RESPONSE: "*Our instruments come in preassembled sets. We use only what we need from each set.*" (This response conveys order, knowledge, and professionalism. It answers the question directly and addresses underlying fear.)
PATIENT: "*I'm relieved to hear that!*"

Therapeutic Communication with the Geriatric Patient

When communicating with the patient who has partial hearing loss related to age, speak clearly and slowly, facing the patient while talking. *Speak in a normal voice.* Unless the patient has significant hearing loss, do not yell while talking. Ask the patient if he or she understands and always address the patient by name.

If the patient is visually impaired, introduce yourself to the patient first. Explain clearly what is happening around the patient to reduce fear and anxiety. Orient the patient to the surroundings.

Respect the patient at all times. In American culture, the elderly often do not have the care of extended family and familiar people that is found in other cultures in which the family remains physically close and intact. This may result in feelings of worthlessness and alienation. Loss of health is a particular threat to this population because it often implies loss of independence, which American culture values highly. Loss of independence may mean loss of home and familiar surroundings. The prospect of moving to a care facility is grim to many elderly people who have lived a previously fulfilling life.

When communicating with the elderly patient:

▶ **Do not use clichés.** Do not reach for the first available, easiest response. For example, if the patient says that she is a burden to others in her illness, *do not* respond with, "Oh, I'm sure you're no bother." Instead, support the patient in her feelings. For example, say, "It must be very difficult for you to have surgery right now."

▶ **Do not refer to the patient as "sweetie," "honey," or "cutie."** These titles are offensive to many patients. They convey a lack of respect for the patient as an adult person with a lifetime of accomplishments and knowledge. Always address the patient by his or her proper name. Respect is contagious. Demonstrate to others in the healthcare environment that you acknowledge the fullness of the patient's life.

▶ **Do not assume that a geriatric patient is mentally impaired.** The normal aging process does not preclude dementia. Senile dementia is a disease state. Some geriatric patients are slightly confused or disoriented in the hospital. Help to orient them; do not assume they have organic brain disease. If there *is* evidence or knowledge of organic brain disease, it may be necessary to repeat questions and responses. It is not necessary to speak *louder* in such a case—it is only necessary to repeat the statement.

▶ **Respect the geriatric patient's privacy as you would that of any patient.** Unnecessary exposure is *a violation of the patient's right to dignity.*

Touch

Touch is an important part of therapeutic communication, but it must be used with caution and respect. Some patients do not want to be touched but may not explicitly express that. There are many reasons why a patient may not want to be touched, including cultural beliefs or previous experience with trauma or violation of the body. The caregiver may ask permission to touch a neutral area of the body such as the hand and watch for cues from the patient. If the patient is comforted by touch, he or she will show relaxation and relief by his or her body language and facial expression. When touch is rejected, the patient may pull back or show signs of distrust or fear. Every patient has the right to reject or refuse touch. In this case, the caregiver must seek other methods of offering reassurance and comfort. When touch is acceptable, it can convey deep and tender feelings of empathy and care.

CULTURALLY APPROPRIATE PATIENT CARE

Patients of a wide variety of cultures are common in American hospitals. In many cultures, the concepts of health, sickness, therapy, and behavior are very different from those in the Western model of heath care. These variations often cause confusion and mistrust on the part of patients and caregivers. The most effective way to approach a patient whose cultural beliefs are different from one's own is with knowledge of that culture. What may seem strange or "wrong" to one person is often cherished by a person of a different culture. Health-care professionals have an ethical responsibility to honor and respect those beliefs, just as they would want their own beliefs to be honored in a different culture.

Language barriers often make health care more difficult and frustrating at times for both the patient and the caregiver. However, translators are available. People commonly tend to speak to someone of a different language *louder* than normal, as if difficulty in hearing were the communication problem. This can be degrading to a patient whose hearing is perfectly intact. The use of pictures or gestures is sometimes effective when an interpreter is unavailable. See Table 6-2 in Chapter 6, Communication and Teamwork, for examples of cultural characteristics that affect communication.

CASE STUDIES

Case 1

You are transporting a patient with AIDS to the operating room on a stretcher. The patient is silent. She is cooperative and her facial expression shows anxiety. What will you say to this patient while transporting her to the operating room? What psychosocial needs do you think this patient has? How can you meet these needs?

Case 2

You are preparing equipment for a cardiac procedure. The patient has been brought into surgery and is lying on the operating table. He says to you, "How long do you think this will take?" How will you respond? What possible concerns does this patient have? Is he expressing these concerns to you through his question?

CASE STUDIES—cont'd

Case 3

You are assisting the circulator with a 3-year-old patient about to have a tonsillectomy. The patient is screaming and kicking. He is crying and says he wants his mommy. The circulator calls for more help to restrain the child. When you attempt to soothe him, he kicks you. What will you do? What is this patient experiencing? What needs can you meet for this patient?

Case 4

The patient is a 20-year-old brought to the operating room for an emergency cesarean section. She is crying. She says to you, "I hope I don't lose the baby. When will my doctor be here?" What is your response?

Case 5

The patient is a 40-year-old woman from Southeast Asia. She does not speak English. You overhear a coworker mimicking her attempts to speak to staff. The patient overhears this too and begins to cry silently. How will you respond to her? Will you respond to your coworker?

Chapter 3

Law and Ethics

Learning Objectives

After studying this chapter the reader will be able to:

- Describe sources of the law
- Describe common hospital policies
- List common areas of negligence in the operating room
- Define criminal liability
- Describe and give examples of an incident report
- Describe informed consent
- Describe the advance directive and the living will
- Discuss why documentation is important
- Define the relationship between ethics and the law
- Describe several ethical conflicts

Terminology

Abandonment—The failure to stay with a patient who is under one's care.

Advance directive—A document in which one gives instructions about his or her medical care in the event that he or she cannot speak for himself or herself because of serious illness or incapacity. Examples of this are a living will and a medical power of attorney.

Complaint—The legal document that begins a civil lawsuit and designates who is suing whom and why.

Court (or bench) trial—Trial in which a judge determines factual evidence and makes the final judgment.

Damages—Money awarded in a civil lawsuit to compensate the injured party.

Defamation—A derogatory statement concerning another person's skill, character, or reputation.

Delegate—To assign one's duties to another person. In medicine, the person who delegates the duty retains accountability for the action of the person to whom it is delegated.

Deposition—Testimony of a witness, under oath, and transcribed by a court reporter during the pretrial phase of a civil lawsuit.

Ethics—Standards that govern a specific group of people.

Ethical dilemma—A situation in which ethical choices involve conflicting values.

Hospital policy—A set of rules or regulations that hospital employees are required to follow. They are created to protect patients and employees from harm and to ensure the smooth operation of the hospital.

Informed consent form—A legal document stating the patient's surgical procedure and the risks, consequences, and benefits of that procedure, that must be signed by the patient or the patient's representative before surgery can proceed. Also known as a *patient operative consent form*.

Insurance—A contract in which the insurance company agrees to defend the policy holder if he or she is sued for acts covered by the policy and to pay any damages up to the policy limit.

Jury trial—Trial in which a case is presented to a selected jury and the facts and final judgment are determined by the jury.

Laws—Standards that apply to all people within a given society.

Liable—Legally responsible and accountable.

Libel—Defamation in writing.

Terminology—cont'd

Living will—Legal document stating the patient's wishes to refuse or limit care if the patient becomes incompetent. Living wills are utilized mainly for cases of terminal illness.

Malpractice—Negligence committed by a professional. Malpractice also may be committed if a person deliberately acts outside of his or her scope of practice or while impaired.

Medical power of attorney—Legal document signed by a person giving another person the power to make health-care decisions for the first person if he or she becomes incompetent, unconscious, or unable to make decisions for himself or herself.

Medical practice acts—State laws that define the practice of medicine.

Negligence—"Omission to do something that a reasonable person, guided by those *ordinary* considerations which ordinarily regulate human affairs would *do,* or doing something which a reasonable and prudent person would *not* do."*

Nurse practice acts—State laws that define the practice of nursing.

Perjury—Crime of intentionally lying or falsifying information given during court testimony after being sworn to tell the truth.

Professional license—Governmental permission to perform specified actions.

Retained object—An item that is inadvertently left inside the patient during surgery.

Sentinel event—"A sentinel event is an unexpected occurrence involving death or serious physical or psychological injury, or risk thereof. Serious injury specifically includes loss of limb or function. The phrase 'or risk thereof' includes any process variation for which a recurrence would carry a significant chance of serious adverse outcome. Such events are called 'sentinel' because they signal the need for immediate investigation and response."**

Sexual harassment—Sexual coercion, sexual innuendoes, or unwanted sexual comments or touch.

Slander—Spoken defamation.

Subpoena—A court order requiring its recipient to appear and testify at a trial or deposition. Medical records also can be the subject of subpoenas.

Summons—A court-issued document that is received by a person being sued, notifying the person that he or she is a defendant in the lawsuit.

Tort—A wrong, independent of contract law violations, perpetrated by one person against another person or person's property. Any act of negligence or fraud compensable by money damages. Torts may be intentional or negligent in nature.

SOURCES OF THE LAW AND PRACTICE

Law Versus Morals and Ethics

To understand the law as it applies to health care, one must have a basic knowledge of how **laws** are created and how laws differ from morals and **ethics,** which also affect how a health-care professional acts in specific situations. Laws generally are designed to proscribe conduct that is considered harmful to others. The surgical technologist should understand the basic differences among morals, ethics, and laws in order to provide appropriate care of the surgical patient.

Morals may be described as personal standards. These are standards that persons adopt to govern their personal conduct. Morals are generally instilled in a person from a very young age by parents, religious or spiritual leaders, and other role models. Moral conduct encompasses actions such as lying or cheating. Ethics, on the other hand, may be described as group standards. Specific groups of people create and adopt rules that regulate the conduct of their own members. For example, the Association of Surgical Technologists (AST) has adopted broad guidelines that state how surgical technologists conduct themselves when working in the health-care setting. Nurses, physicians, and many other groups have adopted statements of ethical behavior that guide members of the respective groups. One of the best-known ethical statements is: "First, do no harm." Finally, laws can be described as societal standards. Laws govern the conduct of every member of a society. Laws arise from several sources (as described later in this chapter); however, they are designed to apply to every person in society. A simple example of this is a speed limit. The law states that the posted speed on a stretch of road is the maximum speed one can travel on that road. If an individual exceeds the posted speed, he or she may face criminal sanctions, including fines or jail time. A person who violates ethical standards may face sanctions from the group, including dismissal from the group, but no fines or jail time may be imposed. In certain cases, a conflict may arise among an individual's moral standards, the ethical standards of the group to which the indi-

---

*Creighton H: *Law every nurse should know,* ed 5, Philadelphia, 1986, WB Saunders.

**Association of periOperative Registered Nurses, *AORN position statement on correct site surgery,* Denver, CO.

vidual belongs, and the societal standards or laws that govern their conduct. This chapter will provide guidance for some common dilemmas.

Law Versus Recommended Practice

In the United States, there are four sources of law that regulate society. The first source is known as *constitutional law.* The U.S. Constitution is the supreme source of law in the nation, and no other law may violate provisions of the Constitution. Similarly, each state has a constitution that is considered the supreme law for the state. The second source of law gives rise to *statutory law.* Statutes are laws that are passed by legislative bodies. Generally, bills passed by the U.S. Congress and approved by the president are known as laws, while bills passed by state legislatures and signed into law by the governor of the state are called statutes. Local communities may pass laws, which usually are called ordinances. Another source of law is the agencies and departments of the government that create regulations. This is known as *administrative law.* Examples of administrative laws are the rules established by the Environmental Protection Agency (EPA) for the handling of waste and by the Drug Enforcement Agency (DEA) regarding the prescription of drugs. Other sources of administrative law that affect health-care workers include the Department of Health and Human Services (DHHS), the Occupational Safety and Health Administration (OSHA), and the Department of Energy, which oversees the Nuclear Regulatory Commission (NRC), which regulates the operation of radioactive equipment. The fourth source of law is known as *judicial* or *common law.* In situations of conflict between two parties, the courts may become involved to resolve the dispute. The rulings issued by courts have the effect of law and are binding within the jurisdiction of the particular court.

Each state also has established professional practice acts that govern the actions of those in a given profession. When a state board of practice establishes standards for practice, the board can take disciplinary action against a member who violates the standard. For example, if a professional nurse or physician practices under the influence of drugs or alcohol, the state board may revoke or suspend the person's **professional license,** declare the offense to other professionals, or require rehabilitation. Because it is also *illegal* to practice under the influence of drugs or alcohol, the person also may face criminal prosecution.

Government agencies and established laws are created to protect patients. Professional organizations establish and publish codes of ethics. These codes outline the behaviors expected of any member of the health profession. A health professional is thus expected to act in a certain way and within the ethical standards of the profession and the laws of the state. Health professionals have an unspoken contract to maintain a particular kind of relationship with their patients. The American Hospital Association has developed guidelines to help patients understand their rights and re-

sponsibilities in the hospital setting (see Box 3-1, "The Patient Care Partnership: Understanding Expectations, Rights, and Responsibilities").

Whether a legal action or a disciplinary action is taken against a health professional depends on whether that person has broken a law or violated a recommended standard of practice. Both may occur at the same time. If the health-care worker is licensed (given permission to practice by the government), each state sets precise legal limitations. If the person is unlicensed, such as a certified surgical technologist (CST) or surgical technologist, his or her actions are judged according to the laws of civil or criminal law, like those of any other person in society. Currently, there are no state professional practice acts for the CST because the surgical technologist is not licensed by the government. However, a number of states have begun to take steps to oversee the practice of surgical technologists. Such measures include the establishment of a registry for surgical technologists. A registry allows a state regulatory board to investigate complaints of wrongdoing against the surgical technologist and impose penalties for such wrongdoing. A number of allied health professionals, including x-ray technologists and respiratory therapists, are regulated in this way.

Legal boundaries for unregulated personnel are defined by what is *not* permitted rather than by what *is* permitted. A surgical technologist is *not* a doctor and therefore cannot practice medicine as defined by the law. A surgical technologist is *not* a licensed nurse and therefore cannot practice nursing. Because of their unlicensed status, the surgical technologist works under the direct supervision of a licensed person. However, the surgical technologist remains directly responsible and may be held **liable** for any act of **negligence** or criminal wrongdoing.

FEDERAL REGULATIONS

A number of federal regulations apply to health-care personnel. Those issued by the DHHS prescribe standards for hospitals receiving funds under Medicare. OSHA issues and enforces standards for the protection of employees and patients against risks in the environment. These include hazards such as those caused by noxious chemicals and electrical devices, and risks associated with blood-borne diseases. The EPA regulates the use of chemicals for disinfection and sterilization.

STATE LAW: MEDICAL AND NURSE PRACTICE ACTS

Under the U.S. Constitution, each state has the power to regulate businesses and professions, including the practice of medicine and professional nursing. The laws differ from state to state and are called **medical practice acts** and **nurse practice acts.** These laws require that a person obtain a license before practicing medicine or nursing. As stated previously, a license is official permission given by a governmental agency to perform specific duties such as surgery or to possess or administer pharmaceutical products. For example, physicians may di-

Box 3-1 The Patient Care Partnership: Understanding Expectations, Rights, and Responsibilities

When you need hospital care, your doctor and the nurses and other professionals at our hospital are committed to working with you and your family to meet your health-care needs. Our dedicated doctors and staff serve the community in all its ethnic, religious, and economic diversity. Our goal is for you and your family to have the same care and attention we would want for our families and ourselves.

The following sections explain how you can expect to be treated during your hospital stay. They also cover what we will need from you to care for you better. If you have questions at any time, please ask them. Unasked or unanswered questions can add to the stress of being in the hospital. Your comfort and confidence in your care are very important to us.

What to Expect During Your Hospital Stay

▶ **High-quality hospital care.** Our first priority is to give you the care you need, when you need it, with skill, compassion, and respect. Tell your caregivers if you have concerns about your care or if you have pain. You have the right to know the identity of doctors, nurses, and others involved in your care, and you have the right to know when they are students, residents, or other trainees.

▶ **A clean and safe environment.** Our hospital works hard to keep you safe. We use special policies and procedures to avoid mistakes in your care and keep you free from abuse or neglect. If anything unexpected and significant happens during your hospital stay, you will be told what happened, and any resulting changes in your care will be discussed with you.

▶ **Involvement in your care.** You and your doctor often make decisions about your care before you go to the hospital. Other times, especially in emergencies, those decisions are made during your hospital stay. When decision-making takes place, it should include:

> ▶ *Discussing your medical condition and information about medically appropriate treatment choices.* To make informed decisions with your doctor, you need to understand:

>> ▶ The benefits and risks of each treatment.

>> ▶ Whether your treatment is experimental or part of a research study.

>> ▶ What you can reasonably expect from your treatment and any long-term effects it might have on your quality of life.

>> ▶ What you and your family will need to do after you leave the hospital.

>> ▶ The financial consequences of using uncovered services or out-of-network providers.

>> ▶ Please tell your caregivers if you need more information about treatment choices.

> ▶ *Discussing your treatment plan.* When you enter the hospital, you sign a general consent to treatment. In some cases, such as surgery or experimental treatment, you may be asked to confirm in writing that you understand what is planned and agree to it. This process protects your right to consent to or refuse a treatment. Your doctor will explain the medical consequences of refusing recommended treatment. It also protects your right to decide whether you want to participate in a research study.

> ▶ *Getting information from you.* Your caregivers need complete and correct information about your health and coverage so that they can make good decisions about your care. That includes:

>> ▶ Past illnesses, surgeries, or hospital stays.

>> ▶ Past allergic reactions.

>> ▶ Any medicines or dietary supplements (such as vitamins and herbs) that you are taking.

>> ▶ Any network or admission requirements under your health plan.

> ▶ *Understanding your health-care goals and values.* You may have health-care goals and values or spiritual beliefs that are important to your well-being. They will be taken into account as much as possible throughout your hospital stay. Make sure your doctor, your family, and your care team know your wishes.

> ▶ *Understanding who should make decisions when you cannot.* If you have signed a health care power of attorney stating who should speak for you if you become unable to make health-care decisions for yourself, or a "living will" or "advance directive" that states your wishes about end-of-life care, give copies to your doctor, your family, and your care team. If you or your family need help making difficult decisions, counselors, chaplains, and others are available to help.

▶ **Protection of your privacy.** We respect the confidentiality of your relationship with your doctor and other caregivers, and the sensitive information about your health and health care that are part of that relationship. State and federal laws and hospital operating policies protect the privacy of your medical information. You will receive a Notice of Privacy Practices that describes the ways that we use, disclose, and safeguard patient information and that explains how you can obtain a copy of information from our records about your care.

▶ **Preparing you and your family for your departure from the hospital.** Your doctor works with hospital staff and professionals in your community. You and your family also play an important role in your care. The success of your treatment often depends on your efforts to follow medication, diet, and therapy plans. Your family may need to help care for you at home.

You can expect us to help you identify sources of follow-up care and to let you know if our hospital has a financial interest in any referrals. As long as you agree that we can share information about your care with them, we will coordinate our activities with your caregivers outside the hospital. You can also expect to receive information and, where possible, training about the self-care you will need when you go home.

Box 3-1 The Patient Care Partnership: Understanding Expectations, Rights, and Responsibilities—cont'd

▶ **Help with your bill and filing insurance claims.** Our staff will file claims for you with health-care insurers or other programs such as Medicare and Medicaid. They also will help your doctor with needed documentation. Hospital bills and insurance coverage often are confusing. If you have questions about your bill, contact our business office. If you need help understanding your insurance coverage or health plan, start with your insurance company or health benefits manager. If you do not have health coverage, we will try to help you and your family find financial help or make other arrangements. We need your help with collecting needed information and other requirements to obtain coverage or assistance.

While you are here, you will receive more detailed notices about some of the rights you have as a hospital patient and how to exercise them. We are always interested in improving. If you have questions, comments, or concerns, please contact _____.

---

agnose and treat disease, cut and suture tissue, prescribe drugs, and pronounce death. Nurses may administer medications that are prescribed by a physician. Because of the variation among states, each person must become familiar with the laws of the state in which he or she works.

Health-Care Policy and Procedure

Accredited hospitals and other health-care facilities are required to orient employees and make available to employees printed documents that detail the policies and procedures required by that facility. Each new employee (or student) must become familiar with and understand the procedures that dictate job performance and responsibilities. Policies are constantly updated, and one must keep aware of any changes. Forgetting to read about policy changes does not protect an employee from legal action in case of negligence. Because of the many different areas of liability and practice, each facility categorizes job descriptions according to task and responsibility. In addition, various individual departmental manuals are available to employees.

The **hospital policy** manual or orientation manual describes general administrative and logistical issues of the hospital. It includes an organizational chart that clarifies the chain of command and information on other topics such as the rules pertaining to employee identification, privileges, and salary procedures.

The operating room procedure manual describes safe practices and policies such as aseptic technique, disinfection and sterilization methods, procedure for room turnover, equipment storage, and other topics specific to procedures used in the operating room (other than surgical procedures themselves).

An infection-control manual lists methods and policies for preventing nosocomial infection (caused by hospitalization) and iatrogenic infection (caused by a procedure) in the operating room and hospital. It includes methods of surveillance for infection, surveillance requirements, isolation procedures, and techniques for taking cultures and maintaining a disease-free environment.

The disaster plan includes information that all employees must know in case of a natural or human-caused disaster in the hospital or community. It describes the duties of each person by department, and describes where to go and what to do. Hospitals periodically enact a mock disaster to test the system.

Other manuals also are available. These include the surgeons' preference manual or cards, which details each surgeon's choice of equipment, positioning, and materials for a given surgery. Other manuals contain materials safety data sheets, which describe appropriate measures and precautions for environmental use of hazardous chemicals.

Legal Doctrines

A variety of legal doctrines have been developed to ensure accountability and responsibility for the safety of the patient. Doctrines also have been developed to protect hospitals from being sued. Hospitals historically have been nonprofit organizations that seldom were sued because they were covered by the doctrine of charitable immunity. Charitable immunity protected hospitals from being sued by injured patients to prevent the depletion of money needed to treat many other patients. The hospitals also protected themselves through the borrowed servant doctrine. In the past, the "captain of the ship" doctrine implied that the surgeon was the captain of the ship and picked the crew (borrowed servants) and directed all activities and orders. The operating room staff employed by the hospital was the borrowed servant and worked directly under the surgeon, ultimately holding the surgeon accountable for all activities in the operating room. This would allow the surgeon to be sued and the hospital not to be held accountable for the mistake of the employee. This doctrine no longer holds true, however, as hospitals are now held accountable for the actions of their employees.

Some examples of legal doctrines are:

▶ Doctrine of *respondeat superior liability:* Dictates that the employer can be sued if an employee commits negligence during his or her scope of employment, even though the employer may have done nothing wrong.
▶ Doctrine of *forseeability:* Dictates the extent to which an event or action could have been anticipated and prevented by reasonable and prudent action.

▶ Doctrine of *res ipsa loquitor* ("the thing speaks for itself"): Indicates that in some cases the injury is evident and outside of the control of the patient. An example of this would be someone leaving surgical instruments or sponges in the patient.

▶ Doctrine of *detrimental reliance:* Specifies that a surgeon may in certain cases rely on the professionalism of the scrub and circulator and therefore may deflect responsibility for an injury.

TORTS (CIVIL LIABILITY)

A **tort** is a civil wrong—an act committed against a person or a person's property. Whereas a criminal act can result in fine or imprisonment, a civil wrong can result in a lawsuit in which money is awarded to the injured party. There are two types of torts—intentional and unintentional. An intentional tort is a wrong that is purposefully and knowingly committed against a person. An unintentional tort is one that is committed inadvertently, without intent to harm.

Negligence (Unintentional Tort)

Negligence is an unintentional tort. Negligent torts are the most common example of tort liability in the health-care setting. Negligence is defined as "the commission of an act that a prudent person would not have done or the omission of a duty that a prudent person would have fulfilled, resulting in injury or harm to another person." (*Mosby's Pocket Dictionary of Medical, Nursing, and Allied Health,* ed 4, St. Louis, 2002, Mosby.) Four elements of negligence must be proven:

1. There is a duty to the patient that is initiated the moment that the patient receives treatment or care from a hospital or physician.
2. The duty is breached when there is a failure to meet the standard of care.
3. The breach causes injury to the patient.
4. The breach of duty results in damage to the patient. This is known as *causation* or *proximate cause.*

A party who proves that negligence was committed may be awarded compensation, also called **damages.** The three types of damage are direct damage (current and future medical expenses and loss of wages), indirect damage (pain, suffering, and emotional distress), and punitive damage (intentional conduct or gross negligence; awarded infrequently in medical **malpractice**).

In certain cases a person may not be able to prove each of the four elements. In this situation, the courts rely on the doctrine of *res ipsa loquitur.* This doctrine recognizes that an injury occurred that was beyond the control of the patient. Examples of this are when foreign bodies are inadvertently retained in the patient or when an incorrect medication is administered.

There are many situations in the surgical setting in which negligence can injure patients or coworkers. These injuries can result in lawsuits against the individual as well as the hospital. The hospital, like any employer, is liable for the negligent acts of its employees. The activities that carry the highest risk of harm are discussed in this chapter.

The best way to reduce or avoid risk of harm to others is to:

▶ Be aware of what you don't know. Ask questions. Seek help when you are unsure about the process of a task or its consequences.

▶ Be conscious of what you are doing. Not consciously thinking is one of the major causes of tragic accidents in the operating room.

▶ Come to work mentally and physically prepared for extreme situations. These occur unexpectedly and frequently in the operating room.

▶ Always let your practice be guided by the traditional principles that improve the profession and ensure quality patient care:

　▶ Primum Non Nocere: First, do no harm
　▶ Aeger Primo: The patient first

Areas of common negligence are discussed below.

RETAINED OBJECTS

A **retained object,** such as an instrument or sponge, is one that is unintentionally left in the patient as a result of surgery. A retained object is a foreign substance, and the body reacts as it would to any foreign body. The result is inflammation, tissue destruction, or infection. A retained instrument can migrate through tissue, injuring solid or hollow organs and causing infectious peritonitis or hemorrhage. Delayed healing and unresolved pain are potential consequences of any retained object.

Accountability lies with the entire operating team. The scrub and the circulator are responsible for the surgical counts; however, the physician is the one who actually places items inside the patient, so he or she also may be legally responsible for an item being left in the patient. The surgeon relies on the scrub and circulator to relay critical count information to him or her, so it is very important to make an accurate count of items.

Courts have made decisions holding the scrub, circulator, and surgeon equally liable. Courts also have held that the surgeon relied on the information given to him or her by the staff. This is called the doctrine of *detrimental reliance.* Surgical item counts must be completed according to hospital policy, and extra precautions may be taken according to individual circumstances.

The procedure for counts is described in Chapter 15, Surgical Technique and Wound Management. To reinforce understanding of this critical task, study the following:

▶ Surgical counts are performed during any surgery in which an item can be lost in the patient.
▶ A count is performed by *two people.* The law does not specify the qualifications of those who perform the

count (licensed or unlicensed) or the manner in which it is performed. However, the Association of periOperating Room Nurses (AORN) recommends that a registered nurse and a surgical technologist participate. One person must be in the scrub role. This is a standard that most institutions follow. Refer to Chapter 15, Surgical Technique and Wound Management, for a complete discussion.

▶ Counts are performed at the beginning of surgery, at the closure of a hollow organ, at the closure of a body cavity such as the thoracic cavity or peritoneum, and at the closure of skin. If at any other time there is suspicion of a retained item, a count should be performed.

▶ A count is performed whenever there is a change in personnel performing the scrub and circulating roles, such as during a change of shift.

▶ The standard of practice is for the circulating registered nurse to identify the scrub and circulator on the patient's operative record.

BURNS

Burns occur in the operating room as a result of misuse or negligent operation of electrosurgical equipment, heating blankets, hot solutions, hot instruments, lasers, or chemicals. Every person who works with these devices and agents is responsible for learning about the risks and adhering to safe practices. The following are examples of burn injuries caused by negligence:

▶ During laser surgery of the upper respiratory tract the wrong type of endotracheal tube is used. The endotracheal tube bursts into flames, causing third-degree burns in the patient's trachea.

▶ The patient is improperly grounded and suffers serious electrical burns.

▶ A warm airflow pad that covers the patient's body is improperly connected. The patient suffers massive burns that are not discovered until the end of surgery when the drapes are removed.

▶ An improperly placed dispersive electrosurgical pad allows current to flow to electrocardiograph leads, which results in serious burns under the leads.

▶ Alcohol used during patient preparation pools within the drapes. When the electrosurgical equipment unit is activated, the drapes ignite and the patient catches on fire.

▶ A stainless steel retractor is removed from the autoclave and immediately placed in the patient. The abdominal contents are burned by the hot instrument.

▶ Preparatory solutions are allowed to pool under the patient. After the procedure, the drapes are removed to reveal the patient's blistered skin.

▶ Irrigation solutions are kept in warmers with excessively high temperatures. The cavity in which the irrigation solution is used receives tissue damage from the intense heat of the solution.

FALLS

Falls can result in serious injury to the patient. The following are examples of circumstances that may result in falls:

▶ The side rails are not kept up on a stretcher or a safety strap is not secured on the operating room table.

▶ Children who are left unattended may crawl out of cribs or beds and experience serious falls.

▶ A patient emerging from general anesthesia may struggle and thrash. If left unattended or improperly restrained, the patient can fall off the operating table.

▶ An insufficient number of staff members are present for the safe transfer to and from the operating table.

▶ A sedated or disoriented patient may climb over the side rails or become entangled between the rails.

▶ Unsafe transfer techniques to and from a wheelchair can result in a fall.

IMPROPER POSITIONING

The patient can be seriously and permanently injured as a result of improper positioning. Only those who are specifically trained and competent to position the patient should assist in this task. Overextension of limbs, pressure on bony prominences, loss of circulation as a result of improper padding, and restricted ventilation are some results of improper positioning. An unconscious patient or one who is sedated cannot speak for himself or herself. Fractures, sprains, bruising, and damage to soft connective tissue can occur when such a patient is moved. The surgeon, anesthesiologist, nurse anesthetist, surgical assistant, and circulator should work collaboratively while positioning the patient to ensure safety.

PATIENT IDENTITY AND OPERATIVE SITE

There is no excuse for mistaken identity or operation on the wrong side. Surgeries on a wrong level, wrong site, wrong side, and wrong patient are considered **sentinel events.** To prevent such negligence, the registered nurse checks and rechecks the patient identification card, bracelet, chart, and preoperative record. In addition, the patient is asked to describe what he or she understands the surgery will entail and on which side it is to be done. If there is any discrepancy between records and the patient's report, no action should be taken until absolute surgical site verification (SSV) is ensured. At no time should staff members rely on the surgical boarding schedule for accuracy in this matter.

Individual hospital policy specifies who is to perform marking of the surgical site. Some hospitals now require that the surgeon sign his or her name *on the patient's skin* at the operative site when an operative side applies (e.g., for limbs, eyes, ears) to prevent surgery on the incorrect side; other hospitals require the patient to mark the operative site. In addition, the entire surgical team may take a "time out" immediately before the start of the procedure or incision for a final verification of the surgical procedure and location of the proper surgical incision site.

SPECIMEN HANDLING

Specimens removed from the patient require careful and attentive handling. If the specimen is removed to confirm or rule out malignancy, loss or lack of proper labeling can have disastrous consequences for the patient, including a misdiagnosis or a delay in appropriate treatment. All specimens must be identified by the hospital pathology department. Some are forensic evidence that will be used to prove innocence or guilt in a criminal case. It is one of the responsibilities of the surgical technologist to properly handle specimens and deliver them off the surgical field. The surgical team must identify, label, and ensure delivery of the specimen to the pathology department or other area specified by hospital policy. This procedure is described in Chapter 15, Surgical Technique and Wound Management.

MEDICATIONS

The surgical technologist is not licensed to administer any drug. However, he or she does accept drugs from the circulator. These must then be properly labeled and passed to the surgeon. If a medication is improperly labeled (or not labeled at all), the risk of injury to the patient increases. Accepting and passing the wrong medication to the surgeon can injure the patient and constitutes serious negligence. The scrub should always state the medication name and strength when passing drugs or solutions to the surgeon.

ABANDONMENT

A patient must never be left unattended. Cardiopulmonary arrest or other life-threatening conditions may occur unexpectedly. The licensed person who has responsibility for the care of a patient should never pass that responsibility to another person unless he or she is trained to respond to an emergency. Leaving a patient alone in a hallway or in the operating room suite constitutes **abandonment.** A case for abandonment also can be made if a staff member leaves the operating room at the change of shift *once the patient is on the operating table,* and there is no relief available. Surgical personnel often work many hours of overtime and are committed health-care workers; nevertheless, they are ethically and legally obligated to remain on the job until relieved by another staff member.

FAILURE TO COMMUNICATE

The failure of a medical staff member to communicate a patient's complaint to the appropriate person (either because of forgetfulness or because the patient's communication is ignored) is considered negligence. Failure to communicate can result in serious injury. For example, the patient has had his leg casted and complains of extreme pain in his foot. The communication is not reported. Later the patient requires amputation of the foot as a result of loss of blood supply to the area. The surgical technologist is not trained in assess-

ment or medical evaluation. He or she must report the patient's complaints to licensed personnel who are qualified to make further assessment and take action.

LOSS OF PATIENT PROPERTY

Patients sometimes arrive in surgery with dentures, jewelry, hearing aids, or glasses. Loss of these items can be very traumatic to the patient. Any personal property must be properly labeled with the patient's name and hospital number and sent either to the hospital security department or to another depository according to hospital policy.

Intentional Tort
INVASION OF PRIVACY

The patient has a right to both physical and social privacy. One of the most common offenses against the patient is invasion of privacy. Discussions about patients in public areas of the hospital are common. These are a violation of ethical and legal codes. Vivid descriptions of the patient's surgery or disease, including the names of the attending physicians, are commonly heard in cafeterias, hallways, and elevators. Family or friends overhearing these discussions can be devastated by their content. Any conversation about a patient must take place only within the therapeutic environment and never in public.

The patient's operative record and all other medical records are permanent legal documents. They may not be altered or changed. A **subpoena** can be served for their use in a court of law, and they are considered evidence in the event of negligence or criminal action. The patient has a right to information contained in his or her record, but the public does not. Records must be protected from public viewing at all times.

The Health Insurance Portability and Accountability Act of 1996 (HIPAA), created by the Department of Health and Human Services (HHS), outlines the federal standards for protection of patients' privacy by protecting patients' medical records and other health information. HHS developed the Standards for Privacy of Identifiable Health Information "Privacy Rule" to implement the requirement of the HIPAA. Individually identifiable health information includes any information that relates to the individual's past, present, or future physical or mental health or condition; any provision of health care to the individual, or the past, present, or future payment for the provision of health care to the individual. The goal of the Privacy Rule is to ensure that the individual's health information is properly protected while the individual seeks health care, and at the same time protect the individual's privacy while he or she is seeking and receiving health care. This will promote high-quality health care and protect the patient's health and well being. Individual identifiers commonly used in health care that also need protection are name, address, birth date, and Social Security number. The Privacy Rule applies to any transmission of information through any medium, whether electronic, paper, or oral.

The HIPAA developed regulations for health-care providers, health plans, and health-care clearinghouses that conduct certain financial and administrative transactions (e.g., billing, enrollment, and eligibility verification) by electronic transfer of patient information, to protect the security and confidentiality of patient information. Health-care insurers, pharmacies, doctors, and other health-care providers were required to follow the federal standards beginning in April 2003.

DEFAMATION

Defamation is a derogatory statement made by one person about another. If the statement is made verbally, it is **slander.** If the statement is written, it is **libel.** Medical personnel sometimes witness practices or acts that they consider to be incompetent or dangerous to the patient. It is negligent *not to report incompetence* (or impairment such as intoxication) to the appropriate person. However, it is defamatory to discuss the suspected incompetence in public. The appropriate response to any unusual or dangerous occurrence in the operating room is to inform that person's supervisor verbally and in an incident report. Although claims of defamation are usually made by a health-care worker against a colleague or against the institution, a patient or the patient's family also can claim defamation by health-care workers.

There are two defenses for a claim of defamation. The first is truth. In this defense, although a certain communication may be damaging to an individual's reputation, the statement is factual. A second defense is privilege. Health-care workers are required to communicate certain information to ensure safe and effective care. If the communication is conducted in a private setting and is related to the care of the patient, then the conversation is privileged.

CIVIL ASSAULT

Civil assault is the threat or attempt to strike or harm another, whether or not the threat is carried out, provided the intended victim is aware of the danger. An example of civil assault in the surgical setting would be to threaten to hold down the patient on the operating room table. This is a punishable civil crime, and the victim may sue for mental distress as well as damages resulting from the assault.

CIVIL BATTERY

Civil battery is the actual unlawful touching or striking of someone, even if the injury is slight. Touching or striking a patient in any inappropriate way is battery. The injured party may file suit for damages as a result of the battery.

FALSE IMPRISONMENT

False imprisonment is the act of depriving a person of freedom of movement by holding him or her in a confined space or by physical restraint. A patient not in danger to himself or herself or to others who is wrongfully restrained may therefore be a victim of false imprisonment.

CRIMINAL LIABILITY

Civil liability is not the only risk in the operating room environment. Criminal liability also can occur.

Actions Exceeding Scope of Practice

A person who fraudulently poses as a nurse or physician and proceeds to perform duties associated with that profession commits a criminal offense. However, if an unlicensed person is **delegated** a task that is defined as practicing medicine or nursing, does he or she still commit a crime? The fact that a licensed person grants permission to perform a task to an unlicensed person does *not confer legal status.* This means that if the act is in violation of the law, it does not matter who delegates the task; it remains a violation. Some states may allow the delegation of certain duties to unlicensed personnel, and others specifically forbid it. Hospital policy is usually very clear on this matter. When in doubt, the surgical technologist should seek the advice of the operating room supervisor or the hospital's legal staff. If a lawsuit should arise, the surgical technologist who asked for legal advice is in a more defensible position than one who proceeded blindly.

Any discussion concerning the surgical technologist's scope of practice ultimately becomes an ethical one. Because the surgical technologist often is eager to increase his or her expertise, and because surgeons may offer the surgical technologist the opportunity to perform tasks that exceed the scope of practice, engaging in such activities may seem permissible and harmless. The fact that the task seems harmless, however, does not negate the legal boundary or the safety factors that define it. The professional chooses an ethical path that coincides with both patient safety and legality.

Theft

Theft is the willful taking of another's property with the intention of keeping it. In the operating room, as in any workplace, theft of supplies or equipment is a crime punishable by law.

NEED FOR LEGAL REPRESENTATION

The average surgical technologist or nurse may never need a lawyer. Each person should, however, be able to recognize when one is necessary and be able to select a competent one.

A lawyer is needed if malpractice is suspected and legal papers arrive. If a CST or RN receives any legal document, it should be shown to his or her lawyer or the hospital's lawyer immediately. Almost any lawyer will be able to explain the significance of the document, which usually will be a subpoena or a **summons.**

Subpoena

A subpoena is an order to appear as a witness to an incident (Figure 3-1). If a surgical technologist or nurse is required to testify about an incident at the hospital, he or she should

982(a)(15.1)

ATTORNEY OR PARTY WITHOUT ATTORNEY *(Name, state bar number, and address)*:	*FOR COURT USE ONLY*
TELEPHONE NO.: FAX NO.:	
ATTORNEY FOR *(Name)*:	

NAME OF COURT:
STREET ADDRESS:
MAILING ADDRESS:
CITY AND ZIP CODE:
BRANCH NAME:

PLAINTIFF/PETITIONER:

DEFENDANT/RESPONDENT:

**CIVIL SUBPOENA (DUCES TECUM) for Personal Appearance
and Production of Documents and Things at Trial or Hearing
AND DECLARATION**

THE PEOPLE OF THE STATE OF CALIFORNIA, TO *(name, address, and telephone number of witness, if known)*:

1. **YOU ARE ORDERED TO APPEAR AS A WITNESS in this action at the date, time, and place shown in the box below
   UNLESS your appearance is excused as indicated in box 3b below or you make an agreement with the person named in
   item 4 below.**

   a. Date: Time: ☐ Dept.:   ☐ Div.:   ☐ Room:

   b. Address:

2. **IF YOU HAVE BEEN SERVED WITH THIS SUBPOENA AS A CUSTODIAN OF CONSUMER OR EMPLOYEE RECORDS
   UNDER CODE OF CIVIL PROCEDURE SECTION 1985.3 OR 1985.6 AND A MOTION TO QUASH OR AN OBJECTION HAS
   BEEN SERVED ON YOU, A COURT ORDER OR AGREEMENT OF THE PARTIES, WITNESSES, *AND* CONSUMER OR
   EMPLOYEE AFFECTED MUST BE OBTAINED BEFORE YOU ARE REQUIRED TO PRODUCE CONSUMER OR EMPLOYEE
   RECORDS.**

3. YOU ARE *(item a or b must be checked)*:
   a. ☐ Ordered to appear in person and to produce the records described in the declaration on page two or the attached
      declaration of the affidavit. The personal attendance of the custodian or other qualified witness and the production of the
      original records are required by this subpoena. The procedure authorized by Evidence Code sections 1560(b), 1561, and
      1562 will not be deemed sufficient compliance with subpoena.
   b. ☐ Not required to appear in person if you produce (i) the records described in the declaration on page two or the attached
      declaration or affidavit and (ii) a completed declaration of custodian of records in compliance with Evidence Code sections
      1560, 1561, 1562, and 1271. (1) Place a copy of the records in an envelope (or other wrapper). Enclose the original
      declaration of the custodian with the records. Seal the envelope. (2) Attach a copy of this subpoena to the envelope or
      write on the envelope the case name and number; your name; and the date, time and place from item 1 in the box above.
      (3) Place this first envelope in an outer envelope, seal it, and mail it to the clerk of the court at the address in item 1. (4)
      Mail a copy of your declaration to the attorney or party listed at the top of this form.

4. **IF YOU HAVE ANY QUESTIONS ABOUT THE TIME OR DATE YOU ARE TO APPEAR, OR IF YOU WANT TO BE CERTAIN
   THAT YOUR PRESENCE IS REQUIRED, CONTACT THE FOLLOWING PERSON BEFORE THE DATE ON WHICH YOU ARE
   TO APPEAR:**

   a. Name of subpoenaing party or attorney: b. Telephone number:

5. **Witness fees:** You are entitled to witness fees and mileage actually traveled both ways, as provided by law, if you request them
   at the time of service. You may request them before your scheduled appearance from the person named in item 4.

> **DISOBEDIENCE OF THIS SUBPOENA MAY BE PUNISHED AS CONTEMPT BY THIS COURT. YOU WILL ALSO BE LIABLE
> FOR THE SUM OF FIVE HUNDRED DOLLARS AND ALL DAMAGES RESULTING FROM YOUR FAILURE TO OBEY.**

Date issued:

▶

....

(TYPE OR PRINT NAME)   (SIGNATURE OF PERSON ISSUING SUBPOENA)

_____

(TITLE)

(Declaration in support of subpoena on reverse)   **Page one of three**

Form Adopted for Mandatory Use
Judicial Council of California
982(a)(15.1) [Rev. January 1, 2000]

**CIVIL SUBPOENA (DUCES TECUM) FOR PERSONAL APPEARANCE
AND PRODUCTION OF DOCUMENTS AND THINGS
AT TRIAL OR HEARING AND DECLARATION**

American LegalNet, Inc.
www.USCourtForms.com

Code of Civil Procedure,
§ 1985 et seq.

FIGURE 3-1
Example of a subpoena. (Courtesy of American LegalNet, Inc., Encino, Calif.)

check with the hospital administration before doing so. In some cases the hospital (or its **insurance** carrier) may provide a lawyer to be present during the testimony.

Two types of testimony might have to be given. The most common is called a **deposition.** This is the testimony taken in a lawyer's office or in some other informal location and is given under oath and transcribed by a court reporter. All lawyers involved in the case are allowed to question the witness. The witness may have a lawyer present and will certainly have one if he or she is also directly involved in the lawsuit. The deposition can be read to the jury during the trial if the witness is not available, or it can be read while the witness is testifying during the trial to show that the testimony has changed or to refresh the witness's memory.

The second form of testimony is that given in court during a trial. If required to testify at a trial, a surgical technologist or nurse should inform the hospital administration and consider consulting an attorney, depending on the seriousness of the case and the degree of involvement in the suit. When testifying, it is imperative to tell the truth because you are under oath. To lie under oath is called **perjury,** which is a punishable crime.

Anyone who receives a subpoena should remember that it is a court order requiring his or her presence; to disobey the subpoena can result in criminal penalties.

Summons

A summons differs from a subpoena in that a summons makes its recipient a party to the lawsuit (Figure 3-2). If a person receives a summons, he or she is being sued. Attached to the summons is usually the **complaint** or petition that the lawyer for the injured person has filed with the court to initiate the suit. The person who was injured and is suing is called the plaintiff. The person being sued is the defendant.

All summonses require action by the recipient within a limited time (usually 20 to 30 days). One should take the papers to a lawyer or an insurance company immediately. Failure to do so could cause the defendant to lose the case without ever having the chance to defend himself or herself.

Judgment

A claim for tortuous injury may be pursued in either a **court trial** or a **jury trial.** The trial will determine whether the defendant is liable for the injury to the plaintiff and, if so, the extent of direct damages, indirect damages, and punitive damages. The judgment is the amount of money awarded to the plaintiff based on damages incurred.

DOCUMENTATION

Operative Report

The circulator identifies the personnel who have participated in the sponge, instrument, and needle counts. Implantation of any medical devices in the patient or other infor-

mation about technical material is also documented. Any documents that pertain to the patient's medical or nursing care must be completed by the physician and nurse, respectively.

Informed Consent Form

A patient operative consent form, or **informed consent form** (often called the *surgical permit*), is a legal document that describes the risks, possible complications, benefits, and nature of a medical procedure, including surgery. The consent document also includes the consequences of *not having the surgery.* To ensure that the patient understands the procedure and willingly agrees to it, the patient or the patient's representative must sign the informed consent form. Because of the legal implications of this document, it is the physician's responsibility to verbally explain its contents and to obtain the patient's signature. *Without this signed document, surgery cannot proceed.* The anesthesia provider also must obtain an informed consent document to substantiate that the patient has been informed about the nature and possible risks of anesthesia. A specific consent is needed to administer blood or blood cell products. Other consent forms are used for patients participating in experimental treatments or procedures and for patients undergoing elective sterilization. The consent forms must be signed by a witness and must include the name of the surgeon or anesthesia provider, the details of the procedure, and the date. The forms should be signed before the administration of any medications that might affect the patient's level of consciousness or understanding.

If the patient has questions after signing the document and you suspect that he or she in fact does *not* understand the procedure or its outcome, you must notify the surgeon. For example, the surgical permit may specify the removal of tissue for biopsy *and wide excision* if the tissue is found to be malignant. If the patient states that he or she is only having a small mole removed, you might suspect that the patient does not understand that the surgery could be more extensive, and this should be reported.

WHO CAN SIGN THE CONSENT FORM

There are specific cases in which the patient may *not* sign the surgical consent form. These cases are those in which the patient is a minor or is mentally incompetent. There are also special cases in which certain factors determine who can sign the surgical consent (Box 3-2).

WHO CAN WITNESS THE CONSENT SIGNING

The witness to the consent signing can be a legal guardian, spouse, agency representative, or other authorized person who can attest to the *identity* of the patient, verify that the consent was signed *without any coercion,* and confirm that the patient was *not mentally impaired* at the time of the signing. The attending surgeon *may not* witness the consent because of conflict of interest.

SUMMONS
(CITACION JUDICIAL)

NOTICE TO DEFENDANT:
(Aviso a Acusado)

FOR COURT USE ONLY
(SOLO PARA USO DE LA CORTE)

YOU ARE BEING SUED BY PLAINTIFF:
(A Ud. le está demandano)

You have *30 CALENDAR DAYS* after this summons is served on you to file a typewritten response at this court and have a copy served on your plaintiff. A letter or phone call will not protect you; your typewritten response must be in proper legal form if you want the court to hear your case. There may be a court form that you can use for your response. You can find these forms and more information at the California Courts Online Self-Help Center (www.courtinfo.ca.gov/selfhelp), your county law library, or the courthouse nearest you. If you cannot pay the filing fee, ask the court clerk for a fee waiver form. If you do not file your response on time, you may lose the case by default, and your wages, money and property may be taken without further warning from the court.

There are other legal requirements. You may want to call an attorney right away. If you do not know an attorney, you may call an attorney referral service. If you cannot afford an attorney, you may be eligible for free legal services from a nonprofit legal services program. You can locate these nonprofit groups at the California Legal Service Web site (www.lawhelpcalifornia.org), the California Courts Online Self-Help Center (www.courtinfo.ca.gov/selfhelp), or by contacting your local court or county bar association.

Tiene 30 DIAS DE CALENDARIO después de quele entreguen esta citación y papeles legales para presentar una repuesta por escrito en esta corte y hacer que se entregue copia al demandante. Una carta o una llamada telefónica no lo protegen. Su repuesta por escrito tiene que estar en formato legal correcto si desea que procesen su caso en la corte. Es posible que haya un formulario que usted pueda usar para su repuesta. Puede encontrar estos formularios de la corte y más información en el Centro de Ayuda de lasCortes de California (www. courtinfo.ca.gov/selfhelp/espanol), en la biblioteca de leyes de su condado o en la corte que le quede más cerca. Si no presenta su repuesta a tiempo, puede perder el caso por incumplimiento y la corte le podrá quitar su sueldo, dinero y bienes sin más advertencia.

Hay otros requisitos legales. Es recomendable que llame a un abogado immediamente. Si no conoce a un abogado, puede llamar a un servicio de remisión a abogados. Si no puede pagar a un abogado, es posible que cumpla con los requistos para obtener servicos legales gratuitos de un programa de servicios legales si fines de lucro. Puede encontrar estos grupos sin fines de lucro en el sitio web de California Legal Services (www.lawhelpcalifornia.org), en el Centro de Ayuda de las Cortes de California (www.courtinfo.ca.gov/selfhelp/espanol) o poniéndose en contacto con la corte o el colegio de abogados locales.

The name and address of the court is:
(El nombre y dirección de la corte es)

CASE NUMBER:
(Número del Caso)

The name, address, and telephone number of plaintiff's attorney, or plaintiff without an attorney, is:
(El nombre, la dirección y el número de teléfono del abogado del demandante, o del demandante que no tiene abogado, es):

Date: Clerk, by _____, Deputy
(Fecha)   *(Secretario)*   *(Adjunto)*

(For proof of service of this summons, use Proof of Service of Summons *(Form POS-010).)*
(para prueba de entrega de esta citación use el formulario Proof of Service of Summons *(POS-010)).*

[SEAL]

NOTICE TO THE PERSON SERVED: You are served
1. ☐ as an individual defendant.
2. ☐ as the person sued under the fictitious name of *(specify)*:
3. ☐ on behalf of *(specify)*:

under: ☐ CCP 416.10 (corporation)   ☐ CCP 416.60 (minor)
       ☐ CCP 416.20 (defunct corporation) ☐ CCP 416.70 (conservatee)
       ☐ CCP 416.40 (association or partnership) ☐ CCP 416.90 (individual)
       ☐ other (specify) :
4. ☐ by personal delivery on *(date)*:

Page 1 of 1

Form Adopted for Mandatory Use
Judicial Council of California
SUM-100 [Rev. January 1, 2004]   **SUMMONS**   American LegalNet, Inc.
www.USCourtForms.com   Code of Civil Procedure, §§ 412.20, 465

FIGURE 3-2
Example of a summons. (Courtesy of American LegelNet, Inc., Encino, Calif.)

Box 3-2   Special Cases in Obtaining Informed Consent

1. If the patient is a minor, the parent or legal guardian may sign.

2. If the patient is illiterate, he or she makes an "X," which is followed by the witness's signature and the words "patient's mark."

3. If the patient is mentally incompetent or incapacitated, a responsible guardian, agency representative, or court may sign.

4. In the case of an emancipated minor,* a responsible relative or spouse may sign.

5. In an emergency, consent for immediate lifesaving treatment is *not* necessary. A verbal consent by telephone is permitted but only if *two registered nurses* obtain the verbal permit. The written consent must then be obtained later.

*Be sure to research the state's definition of an emancipated minor for the state in which you practice.

Incident Report

An incident report is a document submitted to the operating room supervisor or other designated individual whenever an event occurs that is unusual or dangerous, or requires further action. In general, an incident report is required whenever an event occurs that *has resulted* or *might result* in death, injury, or harm. Incident reports should be filled out for patients or employees. An employee may become injured during employment and will need to fill out an incident report and follow hospital protocol regarding the particular injury. It is critical that employees complete incident reports so that there is documentation of the incident on record, which helps to protect the employee. An incident report is designed to be a quality-assurance or quality-improvement tool rather than a document that affixes blame. If an incident report is filled out about the patient, the report should never be included as part of the patient's chart.

Incident reports are made in writing with a form. When you are answering questions about the incident, *state only the facts.* Do not give your opinion about the incident. Examples of proper statements are, "Dr. X smelled strongly of alcohol. His speech was slurred" or, "The needle count was found to be incorrect at the close of surgery. A radiograph was ordered, which did not reveal the needle, and the needle was not found outside the patient." Record the date, time, persons present during the event, and other information required on the form. Submit the form *as soon as possible* after the event. If you are uncertain whether an incident report is needed, submit the report. In some circumstances, employees may wish to protect others who were involved. Always use good ethical judgment, keep the safety of the patient in mind, and submit the incident report.

After an incident report is submitted to the risk management or legal department, an informal investigation usually is conducted or the hospital's insurance company is notified. Further action is then taken if needed. The purpose of an incident report is to reduce or prevent further risk. The following occurrences would require an incident report:

▶ Death of a patient
▶ Retention of an object after surgery
▶ Suspected intoxication of personnel
▶ Accidents during surgery such as burns, electrical shock, falls, or unintentional trauma
▶ Suspected malpractice
▶ Extreme inappropriate behavior by medical or other staff
▶ Violation of the patient's rights by another

Advance Directive

An **advance directive** is a document in which you give instructions about your medical care to be followed in the event that you cannot speak for yourself because of serious illness or incapacity. If the patient is incompetent or a minor, a guardian or family member may sign the advance directive. There are different forms of advance directive. For example, an individual may refuse mechanical ventilation but accept medication. If the patient is considered to be in a persistent vegetative state, the guardian may request withdrawal from mechanical support systems. The advance directive must be reactivated with each separate hospital admission in most institutions. The following sections explain the different types of advance directives.

DO NOT RESUSCITATE

A DNR (do not resuscitate) order specifies that cardiopulmonary resuscitation must not be initiated in the event of cardiac or pulmonary arrest. When the patient has DNR status, this is clearly stated on the front of the patient's chart. Because of effects of anesthetic agents on the cardiovascular and respiratory systems, some hospitals suspend a DNR order for the duration of the surgical procedure. The order must be rewritten when the patient is in the post-anesthesia care unit (PACU).

ORGAN DONATION

Patients have the right to refuse the removal of organs for transplantation after their death. A number of different religions do not allow organ transfer (see Chapter 2, The Patient). If this is the case, a written advance directive should be included in the patient's chart.

REFUSAL OF BLOOD OR TISSUE PRODUCTS

Patients may refuse blood or tissue products because of their faith or personal beliefs. For example, Jehovah's Witnesses do not allow blood transfusions or use of other tissue products. Simply stating that one belongs to a certain faith does not automatically restrict medical intervention. If the patient is unable to communicate his or her wishes, lifesaving measures may be initiated. An advance directive is needed if the normal process of patient care, including transfusion, is to be interrupted.

LIVING WILL

A **living will** is a legal document that specifically states the type of medical intervention or treatment the patient wants. Possible interventions included are artificial feeding, transfusions, specific diagnostic tests, pulmonary maintenance on a ventilator, and the use of medications. Living wills can be created with help from the state bar association, state nursing association, state medical association, or hospital. A living will is not the same as a *last will and testament,* which is a legal document used for the distribution of a person's property after death.

MEDICAL POWER OF ATTORNEY

The patient may assign a specific person to act as his or her proxy regarding medical treatment. After the **medical power of attorney** is prepared and signed, the proxy can thereafter speak on behalf of the patient regarding his or her medical treatment. The medical power of attorney does not confer legal authority in any area except medical treatment.

ETHICS

Ethics is the moral or "correct" conduct of people based on their profession, culture, or group association. One's ethical behavior usually demonstrates his or her relationship to other people, ideas, beliefs, or living things. Most cultures and societies define ethics by law and custom. People understand what is acceptable in that society and what is considered unethical. Through training, examination, and demonstration of abilities, the surgical technologist gains the knowledge to provide quality ethical care to patients. The surgical technologist is committed to serving the patient in a way that ensures a high level of protection.

Specific Ethical Behaviors

Ethical behavior is based on a few very powerful directives that have wide implication:

▶ Respect human individuality and uniqueness
▶ Do no harm
▶ Act with beneficence
▶ Act with justice
▶ Respect all confidences entrusted to you
▶ Act with faithfulness to the patient and others
▶ Act with honesty
▶ Respect the free will of the patient

These behaviors might be applied to any situation in life. In the care of patients, they have special meaning.

RESPECT HUMAN UNIQUENESS

Each person is different from all others. Each person has needs that are specific to his or her personality, medical condition, psychological state, emotions, social life, and culture.

Respect for these qualities is demonstrated when we treat the patient as a person with a name, a history, and a lifetime of experiences that are probably very different from our own. We must act without judgment or condemnation.

DO NO HARM

One must maintain constant awareness of the potential for injury to the patient, others, and oneself. Almost every task in the surgical environment requires some form of protection from harm. Aseptic technique, sponge counts, and education about equipment are examples of protection.

ACT WITH BENEFICENCE

It is important to act in the true spirit of doing good deeds. Beneficence implies empathy and commitment to healing. It requires that we move beyond aspects of the patient's condition that offend our senses or make us emotionally uncomfortable and instead focus on the use of our professional and personal skills. Active care of a patient who has a purulent infection, shows self-neglect, or has a disease associated with a social stigma, such as acquired immunodeficiency syndrome, is an act of beneficence.

ACT WITH JUSTICE

All patients have the right to equal treatment regardless of age, physical attributes, mental state, ethnicity, or socioeconomic status. Advocating for justice may mean speaking out in the workplace when equal rights are violated.

RESPECT ALL CONFIDENCES ENTRUSTED TO YOU

Confidential information about the patient should not be shared with others outside the operating room. Confidence among coworkers is also an expected ethical behavior. Gossip is an insidious but common breach of confidentiality. It extracts enormous cost in emotional hurt and can affect the professional and personal lives of people in profound ways that we may never realize.

ACT WITH FAITHFULNESS

It is your responsibility to remain faithful to the patient as his or her advocate. At all times, you must respect the patient's personal and physical privacy, and honor the patient's trust in you. It is important to remain true to your profession, protect the patient's rights, and be faithful to your own beliefs.

ACT WITH HONESTY

If you make an error, it is crucial that you admit it. When you are unsure about a procedure, be sure to ask for help and accept that help without resentment or anger. Falsifying information or records is dishonest, as is embellishing or diminishing your actions or those of others.

RESPECT THE FREE WILL OF THE PATIENT

All patients have the right to refuse care and to participate in their care. They have the right to receive information about their condition from their doctors and nurses and to ask for advocacy. Patients lose almost all physical freedom when they enter the hospital. Although not restrained except in certain circumstances, they lose mobility, the freedom to work and care for other family members, and the ability to participate in a normal life. Health-care workers are expected to respect and respond to patients' freedom to make choices and express needs and concerns.

COMBINED ETHICAL AND LEGAL CONCERNS

Impairment

An impaired team member is a major threat to the safety of the patient and others in the environment. It is illegal to care for others while under the influence of drugs or alcohol. Health-care workers have both a legal and an ethical responsibility to report suspected impairment of a coworker or, if needed, to seek treatment for themselves. Self-destructive behavior such as drug or alcohol dependence reveals not a weakness but an illness. In reporting these behaviors, team members protect not only everyone in the environment but also the abuser. Treatment programs are available to those who need help. The goal is to return the health worker to a productive and satisfying role in the workplace and to enable him or her to resume a stable personal and social life.

Sexual Harassment

Sexual harassment is unwanted sexual coercion, lewd comments, innuendoes, or touching perpetrated by one person on another. Sexual harassment is identified when a person repeatedly says or acts in a sexually aggressive manner that causes discomfort, embarrassment, humiliation, or shame. It is illegal and unethical. In the last 20 years, sexual harassment has become increasingly condemned in the workplace. Incidents that used to be accepted as the norm in team relationships are no longer tolerated by institutions or health-care workers themselves. No one in any profession is obliged to tolerate implied or actual physical or verbal sexual aggression. Because sexual harassment is defined differently by different individuals, it is best to *document* and *report* every instance of harassment as it occurs. The person who is harassed should retain an exact duplicate of the report. If the perpetrator is a superior, the report should be made above his or her administrative level or up the chain of command. Remember that accepting sexual harassment is not an indicator of one's "toughness." Harassment is a violation of one's person and dignity, and is punishable by law.

Refusal to Perform an Assigned Task

The surgical technologist has the right to abstain from participation in certain types of cases (such as abortion or organ transplant cases) that violate his or her ethical, moral, or religious values. The operating room supervisor must know of this, however, when the surgical technologist is hired. It is not ethical to suddenly refuse to perform a task on moral grounds unless the case is one that could never have been anticipated by the staff member. When offered a position, the surgical technologist should submit, in writing, a list of those cases in which he or she feels compelled to refuse to participate.

Occasionally a team member refuses to work with another person based on that person's history of inappropriate behavior. The surgical technologist should report the behavior before the next time he or she may be working with this person. To suddenly refuse to participate in a case, or worse, to walk out in the middle of the case, could be interpreted as abandonment of the patient. If the reason for refusal is a personality clash, steps must be taken to resolve the problem before being assigned to the case (see Chapter 6, Communication and Teamwork).

Any person may refuse to perform a task that is beyond the scope of his or her professional ability, skill, or training. In the case of repeated requests to perform such tasks, the individual should submit a formal report to the operating room supervisor or next person in the chain of command. If the task is in the person's job description, however, it is his or her duty and obligation to learn to perform the task.

ETHICAL DILEMMAS

An **ethical dilemma** is a situation in which a person must choose an action that entails a conflict of ethics. The following are examples of some common ethical dilemmas.

▶ Loyalty. A loyalty dilemma requires that a person be loyal to one person while being disloyal to another. For example, you have been called into the operating room director's office about an incident involving a coworker. During the conversation, the director mentions that they have been trying to get rid of this coworker for quite some time. This coworker is your friend.

▶ Confidentiality. You have been asked to scrub in room 12 by special request. You arrive in the lounge and an OR employee reading the surgery schedule sees a coworker's name on the surgery schedule and loudly announces "Mary K. is having breast surgery today in room 12." Your coworker sees you are assigned to scrub in room 12 and asks you, "What do you think is the matter with her?"

▶ Values. You have refused to participate in abortion procedures. You are called in for an emergency. When you arrive at the hospital, you learn that you will serve as scrub on a case of an incomplete self-induced abortion. There is no one else available to serve as scrub. The patient is hemorrhaging.

▶ Bioethical issues. A patient with advanced metastatic disease has a cardiac arrest during surgery. There is no advance directive. The team begins cardiopulmonary resuscitation. You are asked to help.

One method of resolving ethical conflict is to examine your own beliefs thoroughly and come to a resolution about how you will act in certain circumstances. Not every ethical dilemma is predictable, but surgical technologists are confronted frequently with certain issues such as abortion, organ transplantation, and the right to die. These issues de-

Box 3-3 Code of Ethics of the Association of Surgical Technologists

1. To maintain the highest standards of professional conduct and patient care.

2. To hold in confidence, with respect to the patient's beliefs, all personal matters.

3. To respect and protect the patient's legal and moral rights to quality patient care.

4. To not knowingly cause injury or any injustice to those entrusted to our care.

5. To work with fellow technologists and other professional health groups to promote harmony and unity for better patient care.

6. To follow principles of asepsis.

7. To maintain a high degree of efficiency through continuing education.

8. To maintain and practice surgical technology willingly, with pride and dignity.

9. To report any unethical conduct or practice to the proper authority.

10. To adhere to the Code of Ethics at all times with all members of the health-care team.

Printed with permission and copyright of the Association of Surgical Technologists.

serve thoughtful consideration. Speaking with other health-care professionals or those who have helped mentor you can help you in defining personal values and integrating them into professional ethics.

PROFESSIONAL CODES OF ETHICS AND STANDARDS OF PRACTICE

Professional organizations such as the Association of Surgical Technologists (AST), the American Nurses Association, the American Hospital Association, and the American Medical Association have created codes of ethics that reflect expectations of those professionals as they make decisions involving ethical issues. By acting in accordance with these ethics, professional health-care workers demonstrate their advocacy for human rights, patient protection, and the laws of society. In all situations, the health-care worker is the patient's advocate; the health-care worker is doing what the patient would do, if he or she were able. The AST code of ethics was established in 1985 (Box 3-3).

A standard of practice is a description of standards to which members of a particular profession are expected to adhere. It serves as a model for performance and level of care that reflects the ethical and professional values of the organization and its members. The standards of practice for surgical technologists, written by the AST, appear in Box 3-4.

Box 3-4 Standards of Practice of the Association of Surgical Technologists

Standard I
Teamwork is essential for perioperative patient care and is contingent on interpersonal skills. Communication is critical to the positive attainment of expected outcomes of care. All team members should work together for the common good of the patient. For the benefit of the patient and the delivery of quality care, interpersonal skills are demonstrated in all interactions with the health-care team, the patient and family, superiors, and peers. Personal integrity and surgical conscience are integrated into every aspect of professional behavior.

Standard II
Preoperative planning and preparation for surgical intervention are individualized to meet the needs of each patient and his or her surgeon. The surgical technologist collaborates with the professional registered nurse in the collection of data for use in the preparation of equipment and supplies needed for the surgical procedure. The implementation of patient care identified in the plan of care is performed under the supervision of a professional registered nurse.

Standard III
The preparation of the perioperative environment and all supplies and equipment will ensure environmental safety for patients and personnel. The application of the plan of care includes wearing appropriate attire, anticipating the needs of the patient and perioperative team, maintaining a safe work area, observing aseptic technique, and following all policies and procedures of the institution.

Standard IV
Application of basic and current knowledge is necessary for a proficient performance of assigned functions. The surgical technologist should maintain a current knowledge base of procedures, equipment and supplies, emergency protocol for various situations, and changes in scientific technology pertinent to his or her performance description objectives. It is the responsibility of the surgical technologist to augment his or her knowledge base by studying recent literature, attending in-service and continuing education programs, and pursuing new learning experiences.

Standard V
Each patient's right to privacy, dignity, safety, and comfort is respected and protected. Each member of the operating room team has a moral and ethical duty to uphold strict observance of the patient's rights. The surgical technologist, like all members of the health-care team, is expected to perform as a patient advocate in all situations. This is an accountability issue and should be part of each aspect of patient care.

Standard VI
Every patient is entitled to the same application of aseptic technique within the physical facilities. Implementation of the individualized plan of care for every patient includes the application of aseptic or sterile technique at all times by all members of the health-care team. All patients are given the same dedication in their care.

Printed with permission and copyright of the Association of Surgical Technologists.

CASE STUDIES

Case 1

You are scrubbed on a case involving an exploratory laparotomy. The surgeon has revealed a large tumor involving the pancreas, liver, and mesentery. He calls in another assistant to help with retraction. The case becomes complex very quickly. The surgeon asks you to cauterize ("buzz") bleeders as he clamps them. What will you do?

Case 2

Your patient is a 50-year-old about to undergo breast biopsy with possible mastectomy. Your role is to act as assistant circulator to the registered nurse. He asks you to go to the holding area to see whether the patient has arrived. When you arrive at the holding area, the surgeon is there with the patient. As the surgeon looks over the chart he notices that the patient has not signed the operative permit. He asks you to witness the patient's signing. What will you do?

Case 3

While scrubbed on a case involving repair of carpal tunnel syndrome, you complete the instrument, sponge, and needle count. You are missing a needle. You announce to the surgeon that the count is incorrect. He replies, "Oh, don't worry. The needle can't be in the wound, it's too small. I would be able to see it. Let's close." What will you do?

Case 4

While in the locker room you notice that one of your coworkers is emptying the pockets of her scrub suit. There are two vials of injectable medications. You cannot see what they are. She puts them in her purse and leaves. What do you do?

Case 5

You have been called into the office of the hospital's attorney to answer questions about a case on which you served as scrubbed technologist 2 months earlier. The case involves the retained needle in the patient undergoing carpal tunnel surgery in Case 3, and she is suing the hospital and staff. Based on how you answered question 3, what are your thoughts as you wait to see him?

Case 6

You have been asked to help position an 80-year-old male for hip surgery. He is under general anesthesia and is intubated. After the surgery the anesthesiologist discovers that his right ulna is fractured. The surgeon says, "We'd better fix this ulna now." Think about the events in this procedure. Who is responsible for the fracture? Can the surgeon repair the ulna without a permit? What (if anything) is the appropriate action for you as a surgical technologist at this point? What will you do if you believe that you may have caused the fracture?

Case 7

You are scrubbed on a cholecystectomy case. You have been given sterile saline, Hypaque (contrast media used during radiography to observe strictures inside the ducts of the gallbladder), and thrombin (a coagulant). You have put these in separate medicine containers on your back table. The surgeon asks you to prepare a syringe of 50% Hypaque and 50% saline. Instead you hand him thrombin. Just as he begins to inject the bile duct, you realize that you made an error. What do you do? Who will be responsible for any injury to the patient? How could you have avoided this mistake?

REFERENCES

Association of periOperative Registered Nurses (AORN) website: *AORN position statement on correct site surgery,* Denver, Colo, 2003.

Balcezak TJ et al: *Issues in risk management,* New Haven, Conn, 1998, Yale-New Haven Hospital, Yale School of Medicine and Center for Advanced Instructional Media website.

Bernzweig EP: *The nurse's liability for malpractice,* ed 6, St. Louis, 1996, Mosby.

Brent NJ: *Nurses and the law,* ed 2, Philadelphia, 2001, Saunders.

Christoffel T: *Health and the law: a handbook for health professionals,* New York, 1982, Free Press.

Creighton H: *Law every nurse should know,* ed 5, Philadelphia, 1986, WB Saunders.

Health care decisions: advance directives, Phoenix, Ariz, www.hcdecisions.org/.

Miller-Kovach RD and Hutton RC: *Problems in health care law,* ed 8, Boston, 2000, Jones & Bartlett Publishers.

Personnel Policy Service website: *Sample policy: productive work environment (sexual harassment).*

Regan JJ and Regan WM: *Medical malpractice and respondeat superior, Southern Medical Journal* 95:5, May, 2002.

US Department of Health and Human Services (HHS) website: *Protecting the privacy of patients' health information,* Washington, DC, 2003.

US Department of Health and Human Services (HHS), Office for Civil Rights website: *HIPAA, Medical privacy—national standards to protect the privacy of personal health information,* Washington, DC, 2003.

Chapter 4

Hospital Administration and Organization

Learning Objectives

After studying this chapter the reader will be able to:

- Describe different kinds of health-care facilities
- Discuss how hospitals are administered
- Define hospital policy
- Describe the process of accreditation
- List common hospital ancillary services and describe their functions
- Describe an organizational chart and explain its significance in an organization
- Identify operating room staff members and their duties

Terminology

Accreditation—The process whereby a hospital is evaluated by the Joint Commission for the Accreditation of Healthcare Organizations, which examines the hospital's practices, records, procedures, and outcomes to ensure that minimum standards for patient and employee safety are met.

Chain of command—A hierarchy of personnel positions that establishes both vertical and horizontal relationships between positions.

JCAHO—Joint Commission for the Accreditation of Healthcare Organizations. The accrediting organization for hospitals and other health-care settings in the United States.

Mission statement—A written declaration that defines the central goal of the health-care institution and reflects the organization's ethical and moral beliefs in broad terms.

Nonprofit hospital—A hospital that provides services to the community and that allocates nontaxable profits to the maintenance or improvement of the facility.

Organizational chart—A graphic depiction of an organization's chain of command that shows the lines of vertical (higher and lower) and horizontal (equal) administrative authority.

OSHA—Occupational Safety and Health Administration. Section of the U.S. Department of Labor that establishes rules and standards to protect the safety of employees in the workplace.

Proprietary hospital—A hospital that is owned by shareholders, who receive and pay taxes on the profits made by the institution. Also called a *for-profit* hospital.

Risk management—The process of tracking, evaluating, and studying accidents and incidents to protect patients and employees. Risk management produces change in policy or enforcement of policy if the risk reaches an unacceptable level.

Satellite facilities—Community health-care offices that are administered by a single institution but are located in communities in surrounding urban or rural areas. These facilities offer primary and preventive health-care services in general medicine and other specialties.

HEALTH-CARE FACILITIES

Most large hospitals provide primary health care, inpatient and outpatient services, diagnosis, and outpatient rehabilitation services. Primary or secondary (preventive) medical care is provided in a fixed location such as the community hospital. The community hospital, whether privately or publicly owned, brings together people with different professional skills to provide coordinated services. Larger hospitals or medical centers also operate **satellite facilities** in rural or urban areas away from the central facility. Satellite facilities may deliver various types of care or treatments to patients. Satellite facilities may include, but are not limited to, ambulatory surgery centers, clinics, urgent-care centers, laboratory and radiology centers, physician offices, extended-care centers, and rehabilitation facilities.

Extended-care and rehabilitation facilities offer patients an alternative to hospital-based care. Extended-care facilities offer medical services to patients who require care for longer than 25 days. Rehabilitation clinics are residential or outpatient facilities and offer professional services to the patient recovering from health problems such as stroke, head and spinal cord trauma, and heart disease.

Nonprofit Hospitals

Hospitals are classified by their method of financing, their size, and the populations they serve. A **nonprofit hospital** or not-for-profit hospital is one that is owned by a private group of individuals, usually a corporation. Any financial gains accrued by the hospital are reinvested in the facility for improvements or maintenance. The hospital's revenue is not taxed. A nonprofit hospital also can be owned by the government at the federal, state, county, or city level, and services are managed and delivered by public employees. An example of a governmental hospital would be Veteran Affairs (VA) hospitals. This type of facility is supported by taxes. State university hospitals are public institutions and also belong in this category. The primary goal of public hospitals is to contribute to the overall health of the public and to deliver care to everyone who needs care, regardless of their ability to pay. Many nonprofit hospitals now provide satellite services within the community. These may be acute-care facilities or diagnostic and primary-care clinics. Satellite clinics allow people to seek medical help in their own communities for primary screening and treatment of illness. If acute care is required, they are then referred to the central hospital.

For-Profit (Proprietary) Institutions

A for-profit or **proprietary hospital** is usually owned by a group of private individuals. Profits are taxable and are returned to the shareholders. Most privately owned hospitals serve an insured population, and they seek a reputation of outstanding quality care in all areas of service. For-profit hospitals make up 10% of the hospitals in the United States.

Surgical Facilities

Surgery can be performed in several settings: hospitals, special ambulatory surgical centers, and physicians' offices. Ambulatory surgical centers undertake minor surgery that does not require postoperative hospital recovery. Ambulatory-surgery or outpatient-surgery departments within hospitals also are increasingly popular. In addition, some types of surgery are being performed more frequently in physicians' offices.

Surgery that requires general anesthesia or complex local anesthesia is performed in a hospital facility, where perioperative services are coordinated with the services of other departments and the patient recovers in the hospital. This setting provides continuity of care and ensures that immediate professional care is available in the event of an emergency. The hospital operating room is equipped to handle emergencies and offers a wide range of equipment and instruments for all types of surgical procedures.

HOSPITAL ADMINISTRATION

Mission Statement

The **mission statement** of a hospital or other health-care facility reflects the overall goal and ethics of that institution. It is not a policy or a regulation but a kind of public announcement that communicates the moral or ethical basis on which the hospital was created and its beliefs about how care should be delivered.

Policies created by hospital administrators should reflect the mission statement and consider the capability of the hospital to carry out such policies. If these three are not congruent, then the hospital's commitment to the community cannot reflect the true spirit of the mission statement (Box 4-1).

Organization of Personnel
CHAIN OF COMMAND

The **chain of command** is the hierarchy of administrative positions. These are usually depicted on an **organizational chart**. Vertical alignment of positions indicates the administrative authority that one position has over another. For example, the head nurse has authority over the nurses on her unit. Horizontal alignment indicates equal authority. The

---

Box 4-1 Example of a Mission Statement

St. Joseph's Mercy of Macomb Mission Statement

We serve together at St. Joseph's Mercy of Macomb in Trinity Health, in the spirit of the Gospel, to heal body, mind, and spirit, to improve the health of our communities, and to steward the resources entrusted to us.

Courtesy of St. Joseph's Mercy of Macomb, Clinton Township, Mich.

fact that some positions are lower vertically than other positions does not necessarily mean that all the lower positions are under the authority of a given higher-level person. For example, the chief medical engineer does not have administrative authority over the surgical technologist even though his or her vertical position is higher.

ORGANIZATIONAL CHART

An organizational chart is a graphic explanation of the chain of command. *A clear chain of command is critical to the smooth operation of any group.* It ensures that the correct person is addressed about issues and personnel under his or her control. Failing to adhere to the chain of command by taking your concerns to a person above the appropriate level can be detrimental to group cohesion and smooth operations. All personnel should become familiar with the organizational chart of their institution and department. A sample organizational chart is shown in Figure 4-1.

HOSPITAL MANAGEMENT

Hospital management and operational staff are usually organized into three separate bodies.

The *board of directors* is responsible for hiring the chief executive officer. It determines the hospital's administrative and development policies and mission, and reviews the delivery of safe and ethical patient care.

The *medical staff* delivers services to patients according to the privileges granted them by license and state codes. The medical staff participates in peer review and quality improvement programs to ensure patient safety and coordinates staff activities with the hospital administration to implement medical protocols and policies.

The *administration* designs and implements personnel procedures and policies, and financial systems. The administration also interfaces with the public and handles overall institutional issues such as communication and quality assurance.

HOSPITAL POLICY

There is a fine line between the "perfect" environment and the environment that is acceptable and results in the lowest possible risk to patients and employees. Hospital policies are formed with this goal in mind. Some are dictated by law, others by practice evaluation and outcome. Policies are created by professionals who have studied the outcomes of different methods of practice and have balanced the risk with the resources available and the ability to enforce compliance among personnel. The purpose of any policy is to create a standard that protects the patient, hospital personnel, and public from harm.

Some policies are written to define the administrative rules of the institution so that all personnel understand their

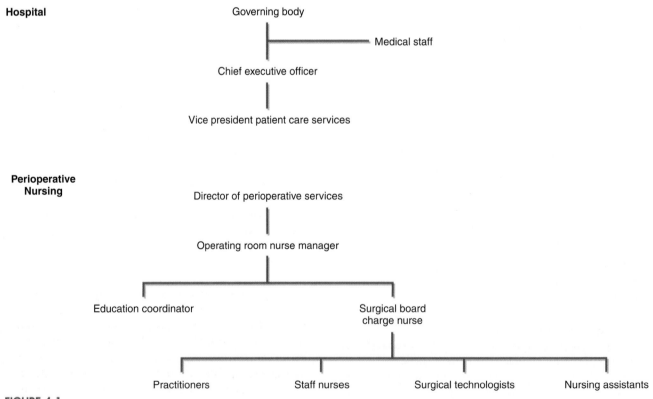

FIGURE 4-1
Sample operating room organizational chart. Administrative lines of authority, responsibility, and accountability are defined to establish working relationships between departments and personnel. (Modified from Phillips N: *Berry & Kohn's operating room technique,* ed 10, St Louis, 2004, Mosby.)

obligations to the institution. The **Joint Commission on Accreditation of Healthcare Organizations (JCAHO)** requires that all hospital policies be available to personnel in written form. These documents are called policy manuals. A hospital may have several policy manuals, each pertinent to a specific aspect of operations, activities, the hospital environment, or administrative issues.

All new employees are required to read and follow the policies applicable to their job descriptions and duties. Failure to comply with hospital policy may result in disciplinary action or termination of employment. Organizations that contribute to the knowledge and research used to create hospital policy are listed in Box 4-2.

HOSPITAL ACCREDITATION

Accreditation is the process in which a team of surveyors visits a health-care facility to inspect practices, policies, and outcomes of patient care. The facility is evaluated based on national guidelines and standards set by health-care professionals. The institution is awarded accreditation when these standards are met. Accreditation is a voluntary process, but government agencies and insurers use accreditation to determine whether an institution qualifies for patient care reimbursement.

Hospitals in the United States are accredited by JCAHO, a private nonprofit organization that evaluates and accredits health-care organizations of all types. It is the dominant accrediting and standard-setting organization in the United States. To become accredited by JCAHO, a hospital must meet or exceed the high standards set by this commission. JCAHO bases its own standards on those of professional and governmental agencies. JCAHO is governed by a Board of Commissioners, which is made up of members of the American College of Physicians, American Society of Internal Medicine, American College of Surgeons, American Dental Association, American Hospital Association, and American Medical Association, as well as nurses, ethicists, and other professionals. JCAHO standards apply to every area of the hospital and focus on patient safety, protection, and quality care. Surveyors evaluate the hospital's *performance,* not its intentions.

HOSPITAL ANCILLARY SERVICES AND DEPARTMENTS

Individual hospital departments offer services to patients and employees. These services are classified by function or by accountability (e.g., administrative, medical, nursing). In this text, we use the term *operating room* to mean the entire surgical department, which includes the individual rooms in which surgery is performed, administrative offices, scrub sink areas, locker rooms, anesthesia department, and other service areas directly involved in the day-to-day performance of surgery. In addition, the term *surgical suite* is used in this text to mean the individual room in which surgery is performed. Every hospital has multiple departments and services. Box 4-3 lists the hospital departments found in most institutions.

Many of the departments listed in Box 4-3 coordinate directly with operating room personnel. The surgical technologist should become familiar with the services these departments offer. When working with personnel from other departments, you should be understand that these departments may provide support to several other departments of the hospital, and not just to the operating room staff. Operating room staff employees sometimes become frustrated when they believe that outside personnel are unresponsive or do not understand the urgency of *their* particular request for supplies or services. In many instances, departments face multiple demands that may exceed their limits of available personnel and time. Patience, respect, and professionalism build good interdepartmental relationships and help reduce stress and interdepartmental conflict.

The following departments directly associate with the operating room.

Pathology

The pathology department receives all tissue samples and other specimens from surgery. A pathologist, who is a medical doctor, examines each specimen to determine the type of tissue, to identify disease within the tissue, and to create a permanent legal record. If the specimen is an object, such as a weapon fragment or bullet, it is preserved as legal evidence. If the surgeon requires an immediate tissue evaluation, as in the case of a suspected tumor, the pathologist is available to perform a frozen section analysis. The specimen is frozen with liquid nitrogen, and thin sections are removed for examination under the microscope.

Box 4-2   Agencies and Organizations Whose Research and Data Are Used to Develop Hospital Policy

AAMI—Association for the Advancement of Medical Instrumentation

AORN—Association of periOperative Registered Nurses

APIC—Association for Professionals in Infection Control and Epidemiology

CDC—Centers for Disease Control and Prevention*

EPA—Environmental Protection Agency*

FDA—Food and Drug Administration*

JCAHO—Joint Commission on Accreditation of Healthcare Organizations

NIOSH—National Institute for Occupational Safety and Health*

OSHA—Occupational Safety and Health Administration*

*Governmental agency.

Box 4-3   Hospital Departments

Patient Medical Services

Diagnostic services
▶ Radiology
▶ Clinical laboratory/pathology
▶ Other diagnostic services (e.g., computed tomography, magnetic resonance imaging)

Patient care units
▶ Cardiovascular
▶ Labor and delivery
▶ Medical surgical
▶ Neonatal
▶ Neurological
▶ Orthopedic
▶ Pediatric
▶ Trauma
▶ Psychiatric
▶ Renal dialysis

Intensive and critical care units (ICUs)
▶ Cardiac telemetry
▶ Cardiac (CICU)
▶ Medical (MICU)
▶ Neonatal (NICU)
▶ Neurological
▶ Operating room
▶ Postanesthesia care (PACU)
▶ Trauma (TICU)
▶ Pediatric (PICU)

Anesthesia and pain management
Blood bank
Outpatient or ambulatory surgery
Emergency department (ED or ER)
Rehabilitation
Physical therapy
Outpatient medical clinics
Nuclear medicine
Food and nutrition services
▶ Dietitian
▶ Outpatient nutrition services

Psychosocial and Outreach Services

Patient education
Community health services

Home health services
Hospice
Adult day services
Hospital chaplaincy
Occupational therapy

Employee and Administrative Services

Human resources
Employee education
Employee health services and insurance
Accounting
Patient accounts
Reimbursement
Managed care
Auditor
Payroll

Environmental Services

Infection control
Maintenance
Bioengineering (clinical engineering)
Housekeeping

Materials Management

Central supply
Distribution

Communications

Switchboard
Paging system
Telecommunications
Mobile radio communications
Electronic communications

Safety

Risk management
Security

Records and Clerical Services

Medical records
Admissions

This examination immediately produces the information needed to determine the need for additional radical surgery. When a surgeon is excising a known malignancy, the pathologist also examines excised tissue to check tumor margins and ensure that all of the malignancy has been removed.

Radiology

Radiology is an important diagnostic tool used in many medical services. X-rays generate an image of body tissues in negative contrast according to density. The radiograph can reveal fractures, organ shape, and the inner contours of hollow organs and structures. Areas of greater density can result from infection, tumor, or fibrous tissue. During many surgeries, a portable x-ray machine is brought into the operating suite and radiographs are taken of the operative site. These radiographs provide views of implants such as orthopedic appliances or other types of connective tissue repair. During surgery of the biliary, circulatory, or other systems that require reconstruction of hollow structures, opaque dye is injected through a fine catheter into the structure to allow visualization of stones or strictures (narrowing of vessels). Surgical technologists and registered nurses (RNs) are sometimes required to assist and scrub in the radiology department during diagnostic procedures.

Infection Control

Infection control personnel are specialists in the prevention and control of nosocomial infections (hospital-acquired infections). The hospital environment is a potential source of many types of infection. Whenever people are in close physical proximity, especially people who are already ill or are debilitated by surgery, nutritional problems, stress, and trauma, the potential for infection is high. The infection control department develops policy based on the standards and recommendations of JCAHO, the Centers for Disease Control and Prevention (CDC), the Association for Professionals in Infection Control and Epidemiology (APIC), the **Occupational Safety and Health Administration (OSHA)**, and the National Institute for Occupational Safety and Health (NIOSH).

The objectives of infection control are to reduce the incidence of nosocomial infections and prevent the transmission of infectious disease in hospitals. Policies affect nearly every department of the hospital. Important goals in infection control include educating staff and patients, tracking policy compliance, and investigating the sources of infection. Infection control professionals also must keep current with the information in their field, as new disease strains and types appear in the population.

A policy manual that describes methods of infection control is available in every operating room. These policies are written by the infection control committee and the operating room supervisor, and follow standards set by organizations such as the Association of periOperative Registered Nurses (AORN), the CDC, APIC, OSHA, and JCAHO.

Sterile Processing

The sterile processing department, sometimes called the sterile supply department, receives soiled materials and instruments from all departments of the hospital. Equipment is decontaminated, wrapped, and sterilized for reuse. The operating room depends heavily on the sterile processing department for instruments and equipment for every surgical procedure. Most hospitals use a case-cart system in which all equipment needed for a particular surgery is placed on a mobile cart and sent to the operating room. Hospitals that have the operating room and sterile processing on separate floors may have a special elevator that connects the operat-

ing room directly to the sterile processing department. Soiled equipment is sent back to the sterile processing department in a separate elevator. Sterile processing personnel are under heavy pressure from all departments to send equipment quickly. Because the operating room and the sterile processing department are separated and one is almost wholly dependent on the other, good communication between the two departments is extremely important.

Central Supply

Disposable items, linens, and equipment are distributed to hospital departments by the central supply department. Items are usually tracked by computer, and distribution is carefully managed to control hospital costs. In some hospitals this department may be responsible for receiving soiled equipment used in surgery. Wrapping and sterilization then are performed in separate areas of the department. Items may be purchased from this department or from a separate purchasing department.

Linen Supply

Linens used in the operating room may be processed by a commercial laundry facility or within the hospital itself. Scrub suits, sheets, blankets, and pillows are provided by the linen supply department after they have been disinfected, washed, and packaged. Clean linens are delivered to the units that use them, usually once daily.

Bioengineering

Because surgery has become increasingly complex and sophisticated, advanced training is required to safely operate and maintain complex equipment. These maintenance services often are provided by technicians in the bioengineering department. This department may be located within the operating room or in a separate department. Technicians are called to the operating room suite in the event of equipment failure during surgery. The operating room staff is required to *remove any equipment that malfunctions* and submit it to the bioengineering department or other designated department.

Nuclear Medicine and Interventional Radiology

Nuclear medical procedures use radioactive materials or radiopharmaceuticals to diagnose and treat disease. The radioactive materials are substances attracted to different organs, bones, or tissues. Nuclear medical procedures produce information about the structure and function of all organs in the body. Nuclear medical studies are used in imaging and diagnosing abnormalities and to diagnose disease process. Examples of nuclear medical procedures are diagnosis and treatment of hyperthyroidism (Graves' disease); bone scans for bone pain and orthopedic injuries; and lung, liver, and gallbladder scans to diagnose clots, blockages, and abnormal function.

Interventional radiology uses x-ray, magnetic resonance imaging (MRI), computed tomography (CT), ultrasound, and other imaging techniques to guide instruments into vessels and organs. Surgical technologists may be required to assist in interventional radiology because sterile technique is required. Examples of interventional radiology procedures are angiography, angioplasty, insertion of a gastrostomy tube, needle biopsy, and stereotactic procedures.

Nuclear medicine and interventional radiological procedures that use radioactive materials or imaging techniques follow hospital, professional, and federal guidelines and policies to ensure the safety of patients and staff.

Pharmacy

The pharmacy distributes medications to patient-care units within the hospital. Medications and anesthetic agents used in the operating room are received from the pharmacy either by regular delivery or by special requisition. Controlled substances are kept in locked storage on all units. Other medications are stored in the sterile or central corridors. Anesthetic agents are usually stored in the anesthesia department or workroom, located within the surgical department.

Laboratory

The laboratory produces essential patient information. Tests performed in the laboratory include chemical, biological, hematological, immunological, microscopic, and bacteriological examinations. Clinical laboratory personnel examine and analyze body fluids, tissues, and cells. Specimens are examined for microorganisms and analyzed for chemical content. The lab types and cross-matches blood specimens for the blood bank. The data and results obtained in the lab are returned to the physician to aid in evaluation and treatment.

Blood Bank

The blood bank provides blood products used for transfusion in the surgical, postanesthesia care, and medical units of the hospital. Because of the fragility of blood and blood products, and because of the strict protocols regulating blood-product transfusion, professionals working in the blood bank must be familiar with the handling, storage, and transport of these products and the strict identification methods that must be used. Whenever blood is transported in the hospital, it must be kept cold. Blood may be transfused only after two licensed personnel have together verified the identification number of the patient and confirmed the corresponding information on the blood unit bag, including contents, type, and other important information required in cross-matching. This identification process is performed at least twice before the blood is administered.

Risk Management

Because of the many environmental risks and the possibility for errors and omissions by personnel, surveillance is required to track the number and exact nature of adverse events in a given time period. The cause of each event is studied, and policies are enacted to prevent future incidents of the same type. For example, if the incidence of chemical burns among staff were increasing, the **risk management** team would investigate the circumstances, time of day, personnel involved (e.g., housekeeping, nursing), and other important aspects to identify the cause. The team then would develop a plan to reduce the number of incidents. The team might change existing policy regulating the use of chemicals or give personnel intensive training. After the plan is implemented, an evaluation is performed to determine whether the measures taken actually did reduce the number of chemical burns. Incident reports (discussed in Chapter 3, Law and Ethics) are very important to risk management because they contain the information needed to analyze incidents and develop a plan of intervention.

Switchboard and Paging Service

The hospital switchboard is the central communication point for the hospital. Calls are received from both inside and outside the hospital. The emergency department communicates with ambulance personnel through a separate radio system. Because of the volume of calls coming in and out of the switchboard, every department should post a directory of numbers near central telephones so that calls can be made directly without going through the switchboard first.

Paging systems are usually set up by individuals. Hospital personnel can be reached through a private paging service or the hospital's own paging service. In a hospital paging system, the caller simply dials the desired party's number followed by a specific in-hospital number. Before beginning surgery, the physician often leaves his or her pager in a convenient location in the surgical suite. When a call comes in, the circulator returns the call and either puts the caller on the room's speaker system or passes the caller's message to the surgeon.

Medical Records

The medical records department is responsible for receiving, maintaining, and transferring all patient records. Because patient records are considered legal documents, strict protocols determine when signatures are required, who may make entries, what must be included, and where the patient's documents should be stored. Loss of a patient's chart is a serious matter. Information in the chart includes the following:

- ▶ Notes on the patient's physical examination, assessment, and history
- ▶ Information on prior hospitalizations
- ▶ Laboratory and diagnostic test results
- ▶ Psychosocial information
- ▶ Advance directive
- ▶ List of allergies
- ▶ Operative reports
- ▶ Nurses' notes
- ▶ Medication orders and records
- ▶ Anesthesia progress sheet
- ▶ Operative permits

Sometimes a patient is transferred from another hospital to receive surgery. Records from the outside hospital may or may not be available at the time of surgery or other medical intervention. The patient's hospital record should stay with the patient during transport within the hospital. When transporting a patient, always hand the chart directly to the person taking responsibility for the patient.

The operative report is filled out by the circulating nurse and signed by members of the operating team. This report becomes the permanent legal record of safety measures taken, the care plan, and any incidents that occurred during surgery. It includes information on the preoperative diagnosis; the operative site; sponge, instrument, and sharps counts; medications; start and completion times; and electrosurgical grounding pad sites. It also records the sites of any injuries that occur during surgery, skin assessments before and after surgery, types of sutures used on closure, and information about prostheses, such as serial and lot numbers, type, and material. The recording of detailed information about the procedure itself is the responsibility of the surgeon, and this documentation is called the *surgical report*. The surgeon usually dictates this report by telephone directly onto a transcription tape as soon as possible after the surgery. The typed transcription is then placed in the patient's chart.

Maintenance

The maintenance department is responsible for environmental systems in the hospital. These include the hospital's power source (regular and emergency), ventilation, in-line gases, suction, electricity, water, light, heat, cooling, and humidity control. Standards for environmental control and safety are established by governmental and private agencies. Failure to comply with these standards increases the risk of infection and accidents in the hospital. Never ignore or try to repair a system that malfunctions. Maintenance personnel should be available at all times to respond to environmental emergencies. Complying with standards for temperature and humidity is particularly important in the operating room.

Housekeeping (Environmental Services)

Housekeeping personnel perform essential cleaning and decontamination services for all departments of the hospital. Control of microorganisms on all surfaces prevents the transmission of disease. Housekeeping personnel must be familiar with the safe use of chemicals and disinfectants to prevent injury to themselves and others. Handling of biohazardous waste in the hospital requires strict attention to protocol to prevent cross contamination to other areas or to people. In the operating room, surgical aides may transport patients as well as ensure a clean environment. They are often responsible for ensuring rapid changeover in the operating room suite from the end of one case to the start of another. They are conscious of their own safety as well as that of their patients and co-workers.

OPERATING ROOM PERSONNEL

The responsibilities and functions of every member of the surgical department are clearly defined in writing in the hospital's *operating room policy* or *procedure manual*. These policies and manuals are written to clarify job descriptions and to establish the accountability of each employee. They comply with state and federal laws and ensure that the hospital meets the minimum standards set by the JCAHO. Policies must be strictly followed because they define the scope of practice necessary to the safe and efficient operation of the department. The number and type of personnel who compose the operating room staff depend on the size of the hospital and of the surgical caseload. The organization, titles, ranking, and educational requirements of staff positions vary from hospital to hospital.

The role of the surgical technologist as a member of the operating room team is discussed in Chapter 1, The Surgical Technologist, as well as throughout the text.

Surgeon

The surgeon is the patient's primary physician in the operating room and is responsible for guiding the surgical team during the procedure. The surgeon operates under the prescribed policies of the hospital in which he or she works and is licensed under the medical practice acts in his or her state. The surgeon is either a Medical Doctor (MD) or a Doctor of Osteopathic Medicine (DO).

The surgeon has completed an undergraduate degree, 4 years of medical school, and a minimum of 5 years of surgical residency.

Anesthesia Care Provider

The anesthesiologist is either an MD or a DO and is a specialist in perioperative medicine. The anesthesiologist is responsible for the meticulous assessment, monitoring, and adjustment of the patient's physiological status during surgery. The anesthesiologist is trained to render immediate care in the event of physiological crisis.

The Certified Registered Nurse Anesthetist (CRNA) is a highly trained registered nurse who renders the same care as the anesthesiologist and may work under the supervision of an anesthesiologist in the operating room. The CRNA also may work as an independent contractor at physician offices.

Operating Room Director

The operating room director is responsible for overseeing all clinical and professional activities in the department. The operating room director generally supervises preoperative, intraoperative, and postoperative departments. He or she helps to set policies concerning major clinical and professional practices in the operating room. The operating room director also is responsible for implementing and enforcing these policies. This position is typically held by an RN who holds a master's degree in nursing or business administration and has at least 3 years of operating room and postanesthesia care unit (PACU) experience.

Depending on the hospital, the operating room director usually reports to a hospital vice president responsible for the perioperative area. The operating room director may represent the department at supervisory meetings, where he or she will help coordinate activities in other departments with those of the operating room.

Nurse Manager

The nurse manager may assist the operating room director with his or her duties. If the director is absent from the department, the nurse manager may assume the role of the director if necessary. The nurse manager is responsible for day-to-day activities of the operating room, which may include altering the surgical schedule in the event of cancellations or emergencies. The nurse manager may or may not participate in operating room activities. The nurse manager is usually a registered nurse (RN) with a baccalaureate degree in science (BSN).

Operating Room Educator

The operating room educator is usually an RN with extensive operating room experience. He or she is generally responsible for developing and implementing educational programs, seminars, and in-services (informational training on new products or techniques) within the department. The operating room educator is also responsible for orientation and assignment of new employees in the operating room. In addition, many operating room educators work directly with surgical technology programs to assist with clinical assignments for the student surgical technologists assigned to their particular clinical site.

Registered Nurse

The RN, or staff nurse, holds a current license in nursing and also may have advanced certification in a clinical specialty. He or she may be a credentialed certified nurse operating room (CNOR) after successfully passing a national certification examination. The staff nurse may act as a circulating nurse or "circulator," may act as the scrub person, or may take additional training and become a registered nurse first assistant (RNFA). The staff nurse always performs his or her duties in accordance with the individual institution's written job description and within the laws regulating practice of licensed personnel for the state in which he or she is employed. The staff nurse reports to the operating room nurse manager.

Physician Assistant

A physician assistant (PA) is a licensed professional who practices medicine with physician supervision. A PA is also required to pass a national certification examination and earn the title of a physician assistant-certified (PA-C). A PA in the operating room has received additional training in surgery.

Certified Surgical Technologist-Certified First Assistant

The certified surgical technologist-certified first assistant (CST-CFA) is a certified surgical technologist who has completed a formal educational program for first assisting, or a certified surgical technologist who had previously been trained to first assist. The candidate must meet the eligibility requirements set forth by the Association of Surgical Technologists (AST) and successfully pass the certification examination distributed by the Liaison Council for Certification for Surgical Technologists (LCC-ST). Upon passing the examination, the individual earns the title of Certified Surgical Technologist-Certified First Assistant. The CST-CFA directly assists the surgeon with the operation. The CST-CFA is specially trained to handle tissue, produce exposure using instruments and suture, and provide hemostasis.

Licensed Practical Nurse and Licensed Vocational Nurse

The licensed practical nurse (LPN) or licensed vocational nurse (LVN) must complete a 1-year program in a vocational or technical school. After completing a state-approved practical nursing program, an LPN or LVN becomes licensed by successfully passing a licensing examination. In the operating room, the LPN or LVN functions in the role of "scrub."

Unit Secretary

The surgical unit secretary receives scheduling requests from the surgeons or their representatives. He or she also must answer the telephone and relay messages within and out of the surgical department. In the event of emergency, he or she must assist the manager in rescheduling any cases that have been canceled (or "bumped") and notify all personnel involved in these cases. The unit secretary is under considerable strain to maintain an orderly schedule and satisfy the scheduling needs of many different surgeons. Consequently, the job requires a composed and efficient personality. He or she must be knowledgeable about medical and surgical terminology, have excellent communication skills, and be able to cheerfully but firmly cope with the many demands made during the workday.

Surgical Orderly or Aide

The function of the surgical orderly or aide depends on the size of the hospital and the availability of other types of paraprofessional personnel. The orderly participates in many types of patient-care services, including the transportation of the patient to and from the surgical department, the preoperative preparation of the wound site, and the transfer of patients on and off the operating table. He or she also may participate in the safe clean-up of the surgical suite after procedures and the restocking of supplies. He or she assists in the preparation of supplies and instruments for decontamination and sterilization. The job of the orderly is demanding because many members of the surgery department make many requests for his or her attention. He or she must be knowledgeable in patient care and Universal Precautions, have a caring attitude toward his or her patients, and be able to shift between job assignments very quickly.

CASE STUDIES

Case 1
You have just had a dispute with your head nurse and were unable to resolve the problem. He asks you to meet with him later in the day and gives you a specific time. Soon after, you pass by the office of the nursing executive. You decide to go in and talk to her about your dispute. Was this the correct thing to do? What do you think will be the result of this conversation with the nurse executive? How will it affect your working relationship with your head nurse in the operating room?

Case 2
You are the lead surgical technologist in your specialty team in the operating room. You have been asked to sit in on a meeting about the rising infection rate in your service. How will you prepare for this meeting? What will you talk about? How can you best represent the interest of the patients? What attitude on your part would be most helpful when you enter the meeting? What attitude would be counterproductive or detrimental? Do you consider the invitation to this meeting to be a reprimand or an opportunity for problem solving?

Case 3
You have been asked to transfer a patient from the postanesthesia recovery unit to her hospital unit. She is awake and oriented. When you arrive on the unit the nurse asks you for the patient's chart. You suddenly realize that you don't have it. What will you do? Whose responsibility is it to protect the patient's chart? What routine will you establish for yourself in the future regarding charts?

Case 4
You are circulating during surgery, and the surgeon's pager sounds. The surgeon asks you to answer the page. You dial the number and learn it is the nurse from the intensive care unit, who tells you that the surgeon's patient from earlier in the day is having severe pain, and she would like an order for stronger medication. The surgeon tells you the drug and dosage to give the patient. What will you do?

Case 5
You are called into an emergency involving a worker who has fallen from a three-story roof. Internal hemorrhage is suspected. When you arrive, your teammate, a circulator, helps you open the case. You both realize that an essential set of vascular clamps is not included in the instrument set. You quickly call central supply. What will you say to them? How will you convey your urgency?

Case 6
You are preparing to scrub on a general surgery case when you discover that one of the electrical outlets sparks when you try to connect a plug. What will you do? Do you call someone immediately? If so, whom do you call?

Case 7
You learn that a JCAHO team will be coming to spend 4 days at the hospital the next week. They will spend a few hours in the operating room, during which time they will question staff members and inspect records and equipment. Does this visit affect you? How will you respond to the news that JCAHO is coming?

REFERENCES
Cutler DM, ed: *The changing hospital industry: comparing not-for-profit and for-profit institutions (National Bureau of Economic Research conference report)*, Chicago, May, 2000, University of Chicago Press.
Groah L: *Operating room nursing: perioperative practice*, ed 2, Norwalk, Conn, 1990, Appleton & Lange.

Chapter 5

Operating Room Environment

Learning Objectives

After studying this chapter the reader will be able to:

- Describe the purposes of the operating room design
- Describe traffic flow patterns in the operating room
- Describe specific design features of the surgical suite
- Differentiate restricted, semirestricted, and nonrestricted areas of the operating room
- Discuss environmental controls in the surgical suite and why they are important

Terminology

Air exchange—The exchange of fresh air for air that has been recirculated in a closed area.

Case-cart system—Organizational method of preparing equipment and instruments for a specific surgery. Equipment is prepared by the central services or supply department and sent to the operating room.

Central core—The restricted area of the operating room in which sterile supplies and flash sterilizers are located.

Contaminated—The condition in which instruments, supplies, or items have been exposed to a nonsterile item, particle, or surface through physical or airborne contact.

Decontamination area—A room or small department in which soiled instruments and equipment are cleaned of gross soil and decontaminated to remove microorganisms.

Efficiency—The economic use of time and energy to prevent unnecessary expenditure of work, materials, and time.

High-efficiency particulate air (HEPA) filters—Filters installed in the operating room ventilation system that remove 99.97% of particles equal to or larger than 0.3 micrometers (μm).

Laminar airflow (LAF) system—A ventilation system that moves a contained volume of air in layers at a continuous velocity, with 800 to 900 air exchanges per hour.

Restricted area—Area of the operating room in which only personnel wearing surgical attire, including masks, shoe coverings, and head coverings, are allowed. Doors are kept closed and air pressure is greater than that in areas outside the restricted area.

Semirestricted area—Designated area in which only personnel wearing scrub suits and hair caps that enclose all facial hair are allowed.

Sterile—Completely free of all microorganisms.

Traffic flow—The movement of people and equipment into, out of, and within the operating room.

Transitional area—Area in which surgical personnel or visitors prepare to enter the semirestricted and restricted areas. This area includes the locker and changing rooms.

Unrestricted area—Area that people dressed in street clothes may enter.

OPERATING ROOM DESIGN PRINCIPLES

The operating room environment includes the work areas, floor plan, and environmental systems such as heat, lighting, and ventilation. It also includes the design of each operating room suite—its storage areas, furniture, and means of entry. There are many different designs that meet the needs of the surgical patient and personnel.

The most important reason for learning about the operating room environment is to increase awareness about patient and employee safety. Operating room design is based on three main principles:

1. Infection control
2. Safety
3. Efficient use of personnel, time, and space

Knowledge about the logic and rationale guiding environmental design allows the surgical technologist to transfer skills from one setting to another.

Infection Control

The design and layout of the operating room create two methods for infection control:

1. Clean and **contaminated** areas should be kept physically separated when possible. An example of physical separation in design is the placing of the central processing **decontamination area** away from the surgical suites. The surgical department itself is separated from hospital corridors and units by doors that remain closed at all times.
2. When complete physical separation is impossible, then contaminated objects are contained. *Containment means confinement.* For example, the air in the surgical suite cannot be completely separated from the air outside the suite, so it is contained by keeping the doors closed and maintaining higher air pressure inside the suite than outside. Scrub attire contains the hair and skin and prevents it from contaminating the clean and **sterile** environments in the operating room. Nonporous materials are used for floors, so that dirt, water, and body fluids remain on the surface, from which they can be removed.

Safety

Both patients and staff face many hazards in the operating room. Some of these are obvious, but others are not. Engineering and mechanical systems in the operating room are maintained by professionals. Maintenance plans and standards guide their operation, so that accidents are prevented and the equipment and environment needed to perform surgery are technically supported. Environmental systems discussed in this chapter include lighting, heating, electrical circuits, ventilation, and in-line gases. Hazards arising from medical devices such as the electrosurgical unit or laser are discussed in later chapters.

Efficiency

Efficiency describes the use of physical effort and materials. It is the economic use of time and energy to prevent unnecessary expenditure of work, materials, and time. *The physical, mental, and emotional efforts of people must never be taken for granted or devalued, regardless of the nature of their work.* Efficient design honors the value of work because it reflects the limits and needs of the human body. Work in the operating room is strenuous. It requires standing for long periods, constant movement, and long periods of concentration, often without breaks. Intelligent design can reduce physical stress by reducing travel or creating work surfaces and systems that minimize strain on the skeletal system.

Efficiency also describes the use of time. The flow of people (traffic pattern) and the way equipment and supplies are moved from one place to another directly affect time efficiency. Saving time is economically efficient, ensures smooth operations, and reduces stress. In an emergency, time is sometimes the most important factor in achieving a good outcome.

Efficient use of space affects the use of time and the health of personnel. Equipment that is stacked too high for safe retrieval or large equipment that is jammed into a storeroom creates the perfect setting for employee injuries. The proper storage of sterile supplies and efficient use of space protects the sterility of the items and allows staff to find what they need quickly and retrieve it safely.

ARCHITECTURAL DESIGN

Floor Plans

Many different types of floor plans meet the goals of environmental safety, efficiency, and separation of clean from hazardous or contaminated areas of the department. Two common floor plans are shown in Figures 5-1 and 5-2. In Figure 5-1, the surgical suites are separated from the workroom by a corridor. The surgical suites are arranged around a "race track." The **transitional areas** are located at one end so that traffic into the department can be controlled at one location. In Figure 5-2, the **central core** contains clean and sterile equipment and supplies. The workrooms where contaminated instruments and equipment are processed are located outside the central core in another area. The primary design goal of the floor plan is to create a clear separation between soiled and clean equipment.

Traffic Flow

Traffic flow is the movement of people and equipment into, out of, and within the operating room. The flow of traffic *into* the operating room from the outside is controlled by the location of the outside doors and by their position relative to the unit office. The use of space and rooms is designed to prevent unauthorized entry of people or equipment that have not been prepared for the surgical environment. The flow of personnel moves from unrestricted to restricted. As equipment is prepared, transported, stored, and used, it

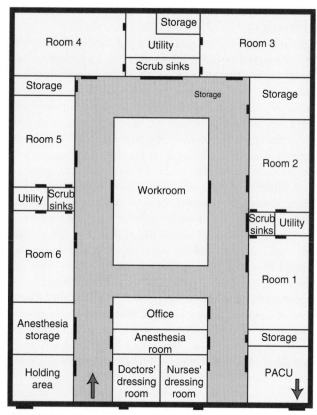

FIGURE 5-1
"Race track" operating room floor plan.

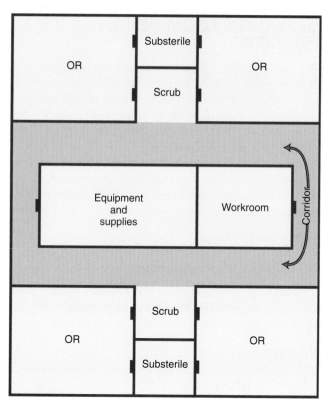

FIGURE 5-2
Operating room floor plan with a central corridor. (Modified from Phillips N: *Berry & Kohn's operating room technique,* ed 10, St Louis, 2004, Mosby.)

must follow the same pattern. The goal, as always, is to prevent contaminated items from coming into contact with clean and sterile goods.

The patient moves from the **unrestricted area** to the **restricted area**. Patients are not required to wear masks unless they harbor a communicable respiratory disease such as tuberculosis. In all cases, they must enter the operating room wearing a clean gown. Stretcher linens must be clean, and the patient's hair must be covered with a surgical cap.

Traffic into and out of the operating suite must be kept to a minimum. Air pressure within the operating room suite is higher than air pressure in surrounding corridors. This design helps to keep out contaminants from outside the room. For this reason, doors to the suite should be kept closed at all times, and traffic flow into and out of the room should be minimized after the room is opened for a surgical procedure. Whenever the door to the operating room suite is opened, air from the outside may enter the room, which disrupts the positive air pressure and carries particulate matter that may contaminate the surgical field.

Design Features
FLOORS AND WALLS
Floors are made of nonporous material that is durable and easy to clean. In most operating rooms, seamless vinyl is used. Tile, asphalt, and terrazzo are also used. Hard surfaces, however, cause extreme fatigue and foot and back problems

among personnel. Because floors are cleaned with a wet vacuum and harsh chemicals, the surface must be durable and must resist corrosion.

When explosive and flammable anesthetic gases were commonly used in the operating room, conductive flooring and shoes were required. Since the use of these agents is now prohibited, conductivity is less important in the surgical suite itself. However, conductive floors may be installed in areas where flammable solutions and chemicals are stored.

Walls are made of nonporous material for easy cleaning and resistance to microbial colonization. A matte finish prevents glare. The walls should be continuous with the floor so that dirt cannot accumulate in crevices.

CEILINGS
Ceilings are made of nonporous, fire-resistant material with a matte finish. Ceilings should be sealed with a filler to prevent flaking or fallout of paint or undersurface material. Any signs of moisture in ceilings (or walls) must be immediately investigated. Cracks and chips in ceilings or walls can serve as a niche for bacterial colonization.

AREAS OF THE OPERATING ROOM
Unrestricted Area
Personnel dressed in street clothes and portable equipment that has not been disinfected are confined to the unrestricted

area. This is a monitored area where people entering the department are stopped and directed to change into surgical attire or remain in the unrestricted area.

Transitional Area
The transitional area is where surgical personnel or visitors prepare to enter the semirestricted and restricted areas. Preparation includes obtaining authorization to enter and changing from street clothes into approved surgical attire.

The transitional area includes a locker room for those who need to change clothes. The locker room contains restrooms, showers, and storage areas for personal belongings. Clean scrub attire must be located in an area protected from contamination by fluids or soil near the locker rooms. Head caps should be available in the same location as scrub attire, because one must put on the head cap before the scrub suit to prevent hair and dander from falling onto the scrub top. Food must not be stored in lockers because it can attract insects. The locker room should be cleaned as thoroughly as any other area of the operating room. Clutter collects dust and creates areas for microbial colonization.

If the locker room leads directly into the lounge area, it should be completely separated from the nonrestricted area. The areas must be clearly delineated so that personnel dressed in street clothes do not frequent the lounge, offices, or other areas used by those who work in restricted zones. The lounge area often presents a problem for infection control because personnel in street clothes may have easy access and traffic control is limited or absent. It is very important that food and drink be limited to the lounge area and never taken into the operating room or restricted areas.

Semirestricted Area
Only personnel wearing surgical attire (scrub suit and hair cap that encloses facial hair) are allowed in the **semirestricted area.** The corridors between various rooms in the department, the instrument and supply processing area, storage areas, and utility rooms are all semirestricted.

PATIENT HOLDING AREA
Surgical inpatients are transported from the medical units to the holding area on a stretcher (also called a gurney). Surgical outpatients are escorted to the holding area after changing clothes in the patient locker room or patient-designated changing area. The holding area is a check-in point where the surgeon, anesthesiologist, and circulator can talk with the patient, confirm that all laboratory and preoperative documentation is in order, and verify all information on the preoperative checklist. If the surgery is an emergency procedure, the patient may be brought directly from the emergency department to the operating room suite.

SURGICAL OFFICES
The front office, which is situated near the main entry doors, is usually a central communication area for the department. General incoming calls are received and referred from this office. Cases may be scheduled here, although this task usu-

ally is handled by a dedicated scheduler in large operating rooms. Because of its location, the main office is a monitoring point for personnel entering the department. Other offices include those of the operating room supervisor, head nurse, educational director, anesthesia director, and chief or specialty technologists. If these offices are located *outside* the operating room, they are designated as unrestricted. The distinction should be made clear to both staff and visitors, however, so that they have no confusion.

CORRIDORS
The corridors usually lead directly into the operating suites, offices, storerooms, scrub areas, and substerile rooms. They also lead to the instrument workrooms and decontamination areas, which must be situated in distinctly separate areas to avoid mixing of contaminated and sterile supplies. Corridors are often collecting areas for equipment such as microscopes, electrosurgical units, and fluoroscopy machines. Hallway clutter is often a consequence when an operating room is expanding its technical capabilities and acquiring additional equipment but is using the same amount of square footage. Clutter presents a hazard and an annoyance to personnel when the rapid and safe movement of patients or equipment is required.

SCRUB SINK AREAS
Scrub sinks are located directly outside the surgical suites so that personnel can proceed directly to surgery immediately after the scrub. Some operating room designs include closed areas for the scrub sinks, and these are restricted (masks are required). These areas contain masks, face shields, protective eyewear, brushes, and surgical soap. The area around the scrub sink should be kept clean and the floors frequently mopped to prevent slips and falls.

EQUIPMENT AND SUPPLY ROOMS
The equipment rooms are used to store large equipment such as the operating microscope, image intensifier, and laser units. When stored in rooms, equipment must be arranged in a way that prevents damage during movement in and out. Delicate optics, controls, and accessories are easily broken. Thousands of dollars of the operating room's yearly budget are spent on equipment repair as a result of careless handling. Damage usually occurs when a person is rushing through a task, but it frequently occurs when pieces of equipment are stored tightly in a small space.

UTILITY WORKROOM AND CENTRAL PROCESSING DECONTAMINATION AREA
Soiled instruments and equipment are decontaminated and washed in either the utility workroom or the central processing decontamination area. Some operating rooms use a combination of systems, holding back certain specialty instruments for decontamination and sterilization in the utility workroom and sending the remainder to central processing. The workroom must be located in an area convenient to the staff but well contained and away from all restricted

areas. Many variations of workroom design are used. Whether the central processing decontamination area is located in the department or outside, connected by a dumbwaiter (elevator shaft) or by a corridor, the important factor is its separation from restricted areas and prevention of cross-contamination of sterile and clean goods.

When a **case-cart system** is used, soiled equipment is loaded onto a stainless steel cart and sent directly to the utility workroom and central processing decontamination area via a dumbwaiter or is delivered by hand (Figure 5-3). The case-cart system is used in most modern hospitals. In this system, sterile supplies such as wrapped instrument sets, linens, disposable suction tubing, canisters, electrosurgical accessories, special disposable items for a given specialty, gloves, and sometimes sutures are loaded onto a closed or open stainless steel cart. The supplies are loaded in the central supply department. The case carts usually are prepared the night before the day's cases and are sent to the operating room. As new cases are added to the schedule, new case carts are assembled. After a case, soiled instruments and equipment are loaded back onto the cart and sent back to the utility workroom and/or the central processing decontamination area. The cart and instruments are decontaminated, and instruments are transferred to be assembled into trays, wrapped, and resterilized. Refer to Chapter 14, Environmental Hazards, for a complete discussion on the safe handling of contaminated materials.

In certain hospitals, the central processing department is on a different floor from the operating room. Case carts are transported to, and returned from, the operating room via an elevator system similar to a dumbwaiter. Care must be taken to ensure that contaminated items are returned to the processing area only via the dirty elevator. Clean case carts are sent to the operating room only on the clean elevator.

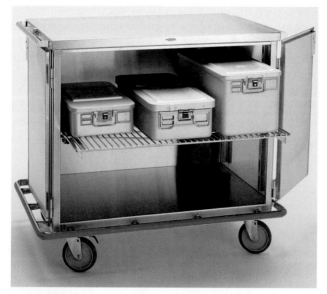

FIGURE 5-3
Case cart. (Courtesy of Pedigo Products, Vancouver, Wash.)

CLEAN PROCESSING ROOM

Any instruments that are not sent out of the department for decontamination and sterilization are brought to a clean processing room for assembly. Items that are particularly delicate or that are used infrequently may be processed in this area. If an item must be reused in a later case and there is not enough time to send it to the central processing department, it also may be cleaned and prepared for flash sterilization in the clean processing room. Generally only rapid flash sterilizers are used in the operating room. These are reserved for unwrapped equipment only. Wrapped instrument sets must be sent to central processing for sterilization.

ANESTHESIA WORKROOM

The anesthesia workroom contains clean respiratory equipment, anesthetic agents, and adjunctive drugs. Tubes, hoses, valves, and other equipment are stored in the workroom and organized neatly to avoid errors and to enable the anesthesia provider and technicians to find items quickly in the event of emergency. This semirestricted area also may contain its own separate office.

POSTANESTHESIA CARE UNIT

Patients are taken directly from the operating room to the postanesthesia care unit (PACU) after surgery. The unit is adjacent to the operating room. Critical care nurses assist the patient in recovering from general or local anesthesia. They assess, monitor, document, and notify the surgeons in the event of an emergency. The patient emerging from anesthesia faces many physiological risks. These include airway obstruction, cardiac arrest, hemorrhage, neurological dysfunction, hypothermia, pain, and malignant hyperthermia. The topic of anesthesia for the surgical technologist is explored in detail in Chapter 12, Anesthesia.

Restricted Area

The restricted area is the cleanest area of the operating room and includes the surgical suites, procedure rooms, and sterile corridor where flash sterilizers and sterile supplies are located. These areas are strictly monitored, and the doors are kept closed. Only personnel in scrub attire, including full cap and mask, may enter.

OPERATING ROOM (SURGICAL) SUITE

Many pieces of equipment and furniture are standard in most surgical suites. A gas anesthesia machine is kept in each surgical suite. Other accessory equipment such as physiological monitors, an anesthesia supply cart, intravenous fluids, and sitting stools are also maintained in each room. Other standard items include suction machines and the electrosurgical unit.

Any furniture in the operating room suite must be made of stainless steel, which is nonporous and easy to decontaminate. Any furniture that is part of the sterile field is covered with sterile drapes before use.

The *operating table* on which the patient is positioned for surgery is adjustable for height, degree of tilt in all directions, orientation in the room, articular breaks, and length (Figure 5-4). This allows manipulation of the patient into any position while maintaining proper body alignment. The surface is covered with a firm pad that may be removed for cleaning. The operating table is discussed in further detail in Chapter10, Transporting, Transferring, and Positioning.

Many accessories to the operating table are available to meet the needs of various types of surgery. *Removable armboards* allow extension of the patient's arms and hands for intravenous lines. The *surgical armboard* is wider and creates a broader surface for surgery on the hand or arm. *Stirrups,* used in gynecological and some general surgical procedures, connect to the mid-break of the table, which is flexed downward or removed altogether. *Leg holders* may be attached to the sides of the table for access to the knee. A special table-top *cassette attachment* that accepts x-ray cassettes is attached to the table surface during operative procedures that require radiographs.

The *back table* is a large table on which all instruments and supplies except those in immediate use are placed during surgery (Figure 5-5). In some cases more than one back table may be required to keep instruments and supplies organized. Back tables come in different sizes. Before surgery a sterile linen pack is opened onto the back table, and sterile supplies are deposited onto the back table. After gowning and gloving, the scrubbed surgical technologist or nurse places the supplies into an orderly arrangement.

The *Mayo stand* is a tray supported by two legs that is placed immediately adjacent to the operative site (Figure 5-6). The scrubbed surgical technologist or nurse places instruments that will be used frequently during a procedure on this stand where they are immediately accessible. The stand is adjustable in height and also may be placed directly over but never in contact with the patient.

The *kick bucket* is used by surgical team members for disposal of soiled sponges during surgery (Figure 5-7). The bucket frame has wheels so it can be moved easily about the suite.

A *single ring stand* is used to hold a large basin for sterile water or saline (Figure 5-8). The sterile basin arrives wrapped. It is placed in the stand, and the drapes are opened out to cover the stand and the basin. A *double ring stand* holds two large sterile basins for larger cases; generally one basin holds sterile water and the other holds normal saline (Figure 5-9).

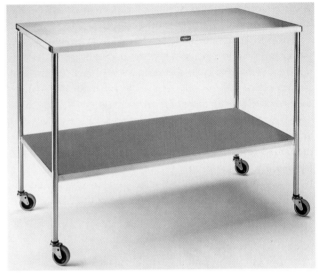

FIGURE 5-5
Back table. (Courtesy of Pedigo Products, Vancouver, Wash.)

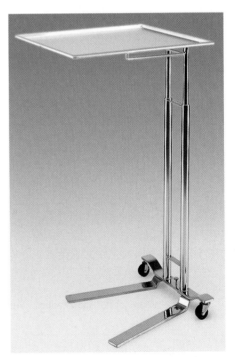

FIGURE 5-6
Mayo stand. (Courtesy of Pedigo Products, Vancouver, Wash.)

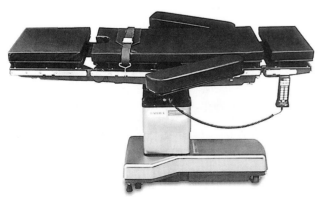

FIGURE 5-4
Operating table. (Courtesy of STERIS Corp, Mentor, Ohio.)

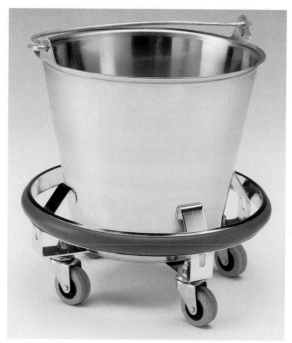

FIGURE 5-7
Kick bucket. (Courtesy of Pedigo Products, Vancouver, Wash.)

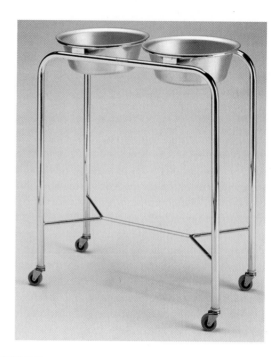

FIGURE 5-9
Double ring stand. (Courtesy of Pedigo Products, Vancouver, Wash.)

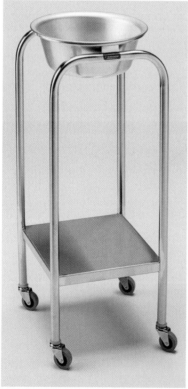

FIGURE 5-8
Single ring stand. (Courtesy of Pedigo Products, Vancouver, Wash.)

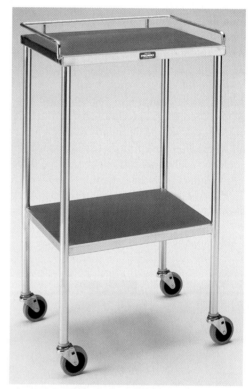

FIGURE 5-10
Preparation table. (Courtesy of Pedigo Products, Vancouver, Wash.)

The *preparation table or prep table* is a small, waist-high table on which skin preparation trays, preoperative injectable medications, and other necessary preoperative supplies are placed (Figure 5-10). The surgeon or circulator works from this table when preparing the patient's skin be- fore surgery. The draped prep table is separated from the sterile back table and Mayo stand used during surgery. After skin preparation is complete, the prep table is moved away from the patient, the patient is draped, and the sterile surgical field is created.

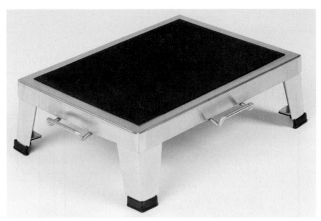

FIGURE 5-11
Step stool. (Courtesy of Pedigo Products, Vancouver, Wash.)

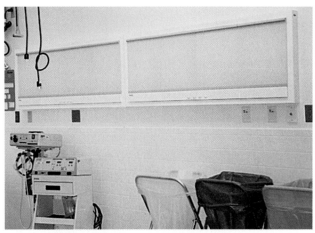

FIGURE 5-13
X-ray viewing box. (*AORN Journal*, 76:1042 December 2002. Copyright © AORN, Inc, 2170 S Parker Road, Suite 300, Denver, CO 80231.)

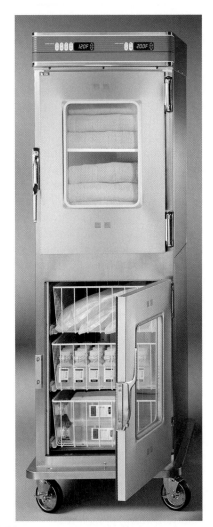

FIGURE 5-12
Blanket warmer. (Courtesy of Pedigo Products, Vancouver, Wash.)

on a "*lift*" or *step stool* to ensure that he or she has access to the field of visualization (Figure 5-11).

Because the temperature is cool in the operating room, warming units called *blanket warmers* are used in the room to store blankets used to keep the patients warm during surgery (Figure 5-12). In smaller operating suites, the warmer may be immediately adjacent to the operating room or in a connected substerile room. Warmers also may be used to keep irrigating solutions warm before they are introduced into the surgical field. Prep solutions should not be stored in warmers because the heat from the warmer tends to reduce the efficacy of the antibacterial solution.

Clocks are mounted on the walls so that the time of day and duration of the procedure may be noted.

The *radiograph* or *x-ray viewing boxes* are located on the wall and are recessed to prevent dust buildup (Figure 5-13).

Computers generally are used for patient charting and documentation. Modern operating room suites have fixed computer stands to allow personnel to directly enter documentation into the patient's medical record. Hospitals that have no computers maintain an area away from the sterile field that is designated for the circulator's task of recording the operative documentation while observing the surgical procedure. This area may be a separate table and chair or a fold-down desk and stool.

Operating rooms also are equipped with *communication systems,* such as overhead paging, telephones, and speakerphones for calls required during the surgical procedure. The communication system is the primary link between the surgical team and personnel outside the surgery suite. A panic button or "code button" also is installed in each room and is used to call for help in case of emergency. This button can be activated by the foot or knee, which allows scrubbed personnel to remain sterile while alerting outside personnel of the emergency.

Supply cabinets located in each room are used to store items such as suture material, dressings, sponges, and other supplies commonly needed during surgery (Figure 5-14).

The operating room table is designed to be raised and lowered, depending on the height of the surgeon, so that the surgeon may operate comfortably and have easy access to areas on which he or she is operating. These adjustments may, however, require the scrubbed surgical technologist to stand

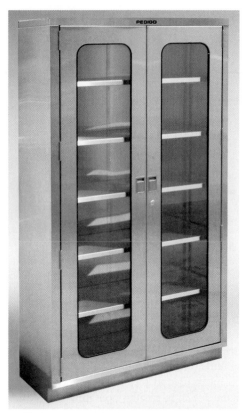

FIGURE 5-14
Supply cabinet. (Courtesy of Pedigo Products, Vancouver, Wash.)

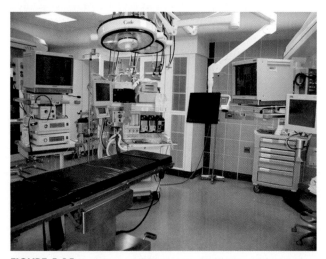

FIGURE 5-15
Modern operating room suite. (Courtesy of Allegheny General Hospital, Pittsburgh, Pa.)

Figure 5-15 shows a typical modern operating room suite.

ENVIRONMENTAL CONTROLS

Airflow

Allowing airflow *from unrestricted to restricted areas* can increase the risk of infection. To reduce this risk, air pressure in the surgical suite is maintained at a level that is 10% higher

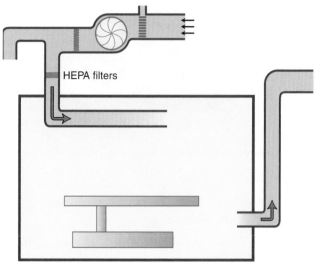

FIGURE 5-16
Ceiling-to-floor air vent. (From Gruendemann BJ and Mangum SS: *Infection prevention in surgical settings,* Philadelphia, 2001, WB Saunders.)

than the air pressure in adjacent semirestricted areas. Surgical suite doors must remain closed to maintain this positive pressure differential. Positive pressure forces air from the operating room into the hallways, thus preventing the potentially contaminated hallway air from entering the operating room.

Air exchange in the surgical suite takes place when filtered fresh air enters through ceiling vents and is combined with existing air in the room (recirculated air). The combined air is vented out through floor ducts (Figure 5-16). All air, whether recirculated or fresh, is filtered before entering the room. The AIA Academy on Architecture for Health (AAH) in collaboration with the U.S. Department of Health and Human Services (DHHS) recommends a minimum of 15 filtered air exchanges per hour, with a minimum of 20%, or 3, of the exchanges being fresh air exchanges. The maximum number of air exchanges allowed is 20 filtered air exchanges per hour with 4 exchanges of fresh air. No more than 20 exchanges per hour should be allowed because the turbulence created by more movement than this would cause dust and bacteria to be swept around the room.

High-efficiency particulate air (HEPA) filters are installed in the operating room ventilation system and remove particles equal to or larger than 0.3μ (micrometers) at an efficiency rate of 99.97%. HEPA filters must be changed regularly to maintain their efficiency. Bacteria and molds can easily colonize in heating and cooling vents and in dirty filters, creating a major source of infection, especially in burn units.

A **laminar airflow (LAF) system** moves a contained volume of air in layers at a continuous velocity. HEPA-filtered exchanges range from 400 to 600 exchanges per hour. The function of LAF is to move large volumes of air containing particulate matter and microorganisms out of the operating room suite. An LAF is very expensive to implement and maintain. Infection-control professionals currently debate the rate of surgical site infections (SSIs) when LAF systems are used compared with the rate when strict aseptic and surgical techniques are meticulously practiced.

Humidity

Air humidity is controlled to reduce the risk of infection and minimize static electricity and consequent ignition of flammable solutions or objects in the operating room. Recommendations by the Joint Commission for the Accreditation of Healthcare Organizations (JCAHO) and the AAH specify a relative humidity of 50% to 55%, and recommend keeping humidity below 60%, which is conducive to bacterial growth. Higher humidity also increases the risk of electrical conductivity, which could lead to electrical shock to staff members or burns to the patient.

Temperature

Temperature control is an important component of patient care and safety. The operating room is maintained at 20° to 23° C (68° to 73° F). This temperature range is less hospitable to the growth of microorganisms and maintains the temperature within the comfort range of patients and personnel. In extreme cases in which the patient's core temperature must be raised, such as for burn or pediatric patients, a warmer environment must be created to prevent hypothermia.

Electricity

Electrical outlets in the operating room must be grounded. Ceiling-mounted columns produce a wide margin of safety and prevent the accidental disconnection and possible damage to cords that extend directly from overhead outlets. All overhead outlets must have a locking device to prevent disconnection. Both 110-volt and 220-volt electricity is available in the modern operating room. The use of electrical devices in the operating room requires constant attention to maintenance and proper use, and immediate termination of use in the event of malfunction. In the event of a power failure, an emergency backup system is activated. Refer to Chapter 14, Environmental Hazards, and Chapter 15, Surgical Technique, for a detailed discussion on risk management and procedures affecting electrical equipment.

In-Line Gas and Suction

Modern operating rooms now have in-line sources of oxygen, nitrous oxide, and compressed air. All outlets should be fitted with a locking device and hung from the ceiling fixtures or mounted directly into the wall (Figure 5-17). Suction and gas lines pass through pressure sensors that produce a read-out on a gauge. Main control valves are located in panels outside the room, usually in the corridor nearby. In the event of malfunction or emergency, in-line gas and suction should be turned off at the main panel (see Chapter 14, Environmental Hazards, for more details). Connectors should never be altered to fit on a certain gas or suction outlet. If a gas line connector does not seem to attach to an in-line gauge, one should obtain assistance to ensure that the correct hose is connected to the correct supply.

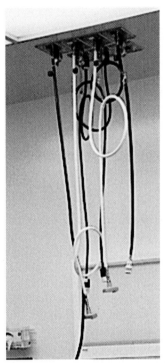

FIGURE 5-17
In-line gas and suction outlets. (*AORN Journal*, 76:1042 December 2002. Copyright © AORN, Inc, 2170 S Parker Road, Suite 300, Denver, CO 80231.)

Compressed air is used as a power source for drills and other medical devices requiring high-speed operation without the danger of electrical cords on the sterile field. Before a compressed-air instrument is disconnected from the hose, any remaining air in the hose should be bled (released from the hose by activating the device). To bleed compressed gases from a line or hose, one must turn off the gas valve at its source and activate the device (hand piece) away from the patient and other staff members. After the compressed gas is released, the scrub person may disconnect the sterile hand piece and the circulator may disconnect the hose from the source. The general rule for turning off valves is to turn the valve clockwise until the valve is closed (to the "right tightens" and to the "left loosens").

Suction is used by both the anesthesia provider and the surgeon. On the surgical field, suction is required to clear blood and fluids quickly and to ensure a clear view of tissues. The anesthesia provider uses suction to clear the patient's airway. Suction should never be turned off until the patient leaves the room.

Lighting

Many different light sources are used in the operating room. Each has a particular purpose and is designed to meet the requirements of that purpose.

Lighting in the operating room is produced by main overhead fluorescent lights (room lighting) and by the surgical spotlights. Surgical spotlights are the lights designed for use during the operation to create illumination specific to the surgical field. The overhead room lights create general lighting and are fluorescent or incandescent lamps. The surgical lights usually are halogen lamps (Figure 5-18). Halogen has a higher color temperature (a measure of the hue that a light emits) than incandescent light. This means that the halogen bulb emits light with a pale bluish cast that is very intense but less fatiguing to the eyes than other types of light of equal intensity. In addition, more of the energy emitted by halogen lighting is given off as light rather than as heat, making it safe to use near delicate tissues.

Most surgical lights create a central focal point surrounded by a wider, less intense area of illumination. The light intensity is controlled via a rheostat. The surgical lights usually are suspended from the ceiling. Sterile light handles are fitted at the center of each light at the beginning of surgery. These handles may be made of reusable aluminum or a disposable material. The sterile light handle allows the sterile team members to adjust the direction of the light into the surgical wound. Some light handles also are designed to allow the surgeon to adjust the focus of the light beam.

Two or three separate surgical lights suspended from the ceiling are usually sufficient to illuminate the surgical field. Surgical lights must be arranged in a logical formation to produce the best lighting. Inadequate light on the field is among the most frustrating environmental problems for the team. When the surgeon is working in deep body cavities, one of the lights must be brought closer to the patient and aimed on a more horizontal plane. If the light seems dim or inadequate for viewing the site, another portable light source must be introduced. One should offer the surgeon an immediate alternative rather than allow surgery to continue under frustrating and dangerous conditions. After surgery, the problem should be analyzed and the appropriate person called in to solve it.

Many surgeons wear headlights to create an additional intense focal point of light (Figure 5-19). The headlight is placed and adjusted comfortably on the surgeon's head before the surgeon begins the surgical scrub. A fiberoptic cable connects the headlight to the fiberoptic power source. The headlight and cord are not sterile. After the patient is draped and surgery is about to begin, the circulator must attach the cord to the power source. Because the cord is often short, it is necessary to bring the power source close to the sterile field. Fiberoptic light is extremely intense. Within the cable are thousands of tiny glass tubes that conduct light and focus it at the tip. The glass tubes are coated so that no light escapes the tubes and is refracted to the tip. The lighted tip of the cable may feel cool to the touch but must never be placed on a flammable surface because it can ignite the surface. The headlight should be turned down and off before the cable is disconnected from the power source. Fiberoptic light also is used during endoscopic procedures. Refer to Chapter 18, Endoscopic Surgery, for a complete discussion of fiberoptics.

COMMUNICATION

Paging and Telephones

Reliable communication with the operating room is essential to a smooth-running environment. Failure to relay messages or inability to find personnel in a large operating room can be frustrating and time-consuming. The operating room is equipped with a voice paging system and a telephone that connects to each surgical suite. These devices can be used to find personnel in the department. Individual pagers also can be used to locate people quickly, as long as personnel are able to *respond* quickly. Cellular telephones are sometimes carried by the nurse supervisors and others who receive many calls during the workday.

Most surgeons leave their pagers with the circulator at the start of a procedure. The circulator then can respond to incoming calls and relay messages to the surgeon without in-

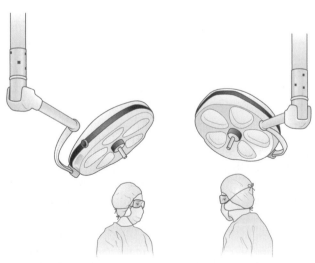

FIGURE 5-18
Surgical spotlights.

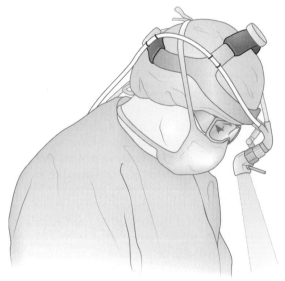

FIGURE 5-19
Headlight.

terrupting the surgery. Speakerphones also are used so the surgeon can speak directly to the caller without breaking scrub (removing gown and gloves).

Closed-Circuit Television

Closed-circuit television is used in many teaching hospitals. Simultaneous transmission allows the procedure to be viewed from a remote location, such as a classroom or conference room. Electronic and computer connections between the camera and the reception screen allow radiographs to be examined and endoscopic procedures to be viewed exactly as the endoscopic camera sees them. As a teaching and documentation tool, closed-circuit viewing is invaluable. It avoids the need for learners to be present in the operating room and documents the procedure on videotape for future reference.

Computers

Today's health-care institutions use computers for a variety of purposes, from managing patient records to controlling inventory. Computers enable operating staff members to find specific patient information rapidly and reduce the incidence of medical errors. Examples of the use of computers in the surgical setting are described below.

DOCUMENTATION

Computer programs allow a great deal of information to be entered directly into the patient's medical record. Operative notes, nursing notes, patient history and physical, laboratory tests, and any other relevant information may be entered into a computer system, giving appropriate personnel access to a patient's up-to-date status. This tool permits rapid decision-making by the nursing staff and physicians as they quickly respond to the patient's condition.

INVENTORY CONTROL

A variety of computer-based technologies allow for accurate management of surgical supplies and equipment. Some programs track surgical instruments through the use of bar-code scanning, which allows the central services department to track specific instrument sets and identify their location at any given time. These programs identify instrument sets that have been used a certain number of times and automatically advise central services personnel to take a routine action, such as holding an instrument set for sharpening of scissors or replacing certain reusable items.

These systems track instruments or instrument sets through each area of the health-care setting. For example, the bar-code on an instrument pan is scanned when the pan is received in the decontamination area. After decontamination, the pan is scanned before it is processed and packaged. The pan is scanned when it is placed into a sterilizer and again when it is placed on the shelf in the case-cart area. When the case cart is being built, the pan is scanned before being placed on the cart. The cart then may be scanned before being sent to a specific operating room. In another ex-

ample, should a specific operating room need an item in a one-of-a-kind instrument set, central services staff members could quickly find the item and deliver it to the room that needs it.

To improve the management of disposable items, special cabinets and carts have been designed that allow a staff person to press a button next to or below an item when removing the item, and the computer records that the item has been removed. A computer printout in a central inventory office will tell the supply or stock personnel to replace that item. These systems may be configured to allow direct billing for these items, listing the items on an itemized receipt and reducing the need for additional staff members to determine what was used in the care of a particular patient.

These systems have the potential for saving thousands of dollars in lost inventory or in wasted time searching for instruments or supplies.

PATIENT TRACKING

The patient who is brought to surgery often has family members or friends present in the waiting areas. Family and friends may anticipate that their loved one is having a $1^1/_2$-hour hernia repair and begin to worry when they do not see the surgeon in 2 hours. In many cases, the boarding time refers to the time the patient is actually in the operating room undergoing surgery. Boarding time does not allow for the time the patient is in the preoperative holding area or in the PACU.

Computer screens set up in waiting areas can allow family or friends of the patient to see the patient's location at any given time. Patient identity is protected by the assignment of an identification number that family members can identify on the screen. Information is updated whenever a patient is transferred from one area to another. This allows family members to learn right away if the start of the procedure has been delayed or when the patient is transferred to the PACU.

SECURITY AND CONFIDENTIALITY

Protection of sensitive information is of utmost importance in the health-care setting. Safeguards have been created to prevent unauthorized access to patient-specific information. Violation of a patient's confidentiality can result in serious sanctions, including the termination of employment. Security measures include the use of passwords or terminal access keys. Computer passwords and keys must never be shared. When selecting a computer password, one should not use personal numbers, such as the user's birth date or telephone number, or names, such as the name of the user or his or her family members. Computer users must log off any computer before leaving the terminal to prevent another person from viewing information by using another's password.

Health-care institutions protect patient information by conducting an electronic audit. Electronic audits identify the information that has been accessed and the person who accessed it. Information that has been accessed is linked to the password of the person who was logged onto the computer at the time the information was accessed. Regardless of who actually accessed the information, the person who was logged on will be held responsible for any breach of patient confidentiality. If a user forgets a password or if a computer access key has been lost or stolen, the authorized user must contact the system administrator or administrative supervisor as soon as possible.

ALTERNATIVE SURGICAL SITES

Not all surgery takes place in the operating room. Special procedure rooms are used to perform cystoscopic and invasive diagnostic procedures. These procedures are sometimes performed in other departments of the hospital, such as the radiology or nuclear medicine department, or even at the patient's bedside. Wherever surgery is performed, the principles of asepsis must be followed. Regardless of the situation, it is always possible to separate sterile from nonsterile and to create a field that the surgical technologist can protect and maintain.

Performing surgery in other departments is sometimes challenging because the work area is often cramped and the usual routines must be changed to maintain a safe environment. This requires flexibility and patience on the part of the surgical technologist. Always make the needs of the patient the top priority, maintain aseptic technique, and deliver assistance as needed. The principles do not change even though the location and circumstances may be unfamiliar or different from usual.

CASE STUDIES

Case 1
You are asked to assist the circulator in surgery on a 5-month-old infant. The anesthetist requests that you increase the room temperature to 80°F before the patient is brought into the room. After surgery begins, the surgeon tells you to lower the temperature because he is too warm. How will you respond to his request?

Case 2
As you are opening a case, you notice that a small piece of paint has flaked off the ceiling and landed on your sterile setup. What will you do?

Case 3
You are scrubbed on a procedure involving the patient's diaphragm, which is accessed through an abdominal incision.

The surgeon complains that the light is terrible. What can you do to assist the surgeon? What can the circulator do to assist?

Case 4
During your case, the suction pressure is very low. You have tried to fix it but are unsuccessful. You are about to leave for the day, and the next team will be using that room. What will you do about the suction?

Case 5
You are called to the Labor and Delivery department to assist on an emergency c-section. The staff insists on leaving the operating room doors open during the procedure. What will you do?

REFERENCES

Bureau of Labor Statistics, United States Department of Labor website: *Occupational outlook handbook, 2002-03 edition,* Clinical Laboratory Technologists and Technicians.

Donley KM: Brushing the surface of disinfectants, *Infection Control Today* website, 11/2001.

National Institute for Occupational Safety and Health, Centers for Disease Control, US Department of Health and Human Services website: *Hazardous waste disposal. Guidelines for protecting the safety and health of health care workers,* Washington, DC, September, 1988.

US Air Force PROACT website: *Fact sheet: management of medical/infectious waste,* October, 1998.

US Environmental Protection Agency website: *Medical Waste.*

Use of cover gowns, shoe covers falls to new low, *Operating Room Manager Journal,* 16:8, September, 2000.

Chapter 6

Communication and Teamwork

Learning Objectives

After studying this chapter the reader will be able to:

- Describe the meaning of content and tone in communication
- Demonstrate body language and describe its meaning
- Discuss the significance of touch in communication
- Role-play situations to demonstrate assertive behavior
- Describe the dimensions of assertive behavior
- Use active listening skills
- Discuss types of problem behavior and how to cope with them
- Define sexual harassment and discuss how to confront it
- Describe the qualities of good teamwork
- Describe how poor teamwork results in poor patient care
- Discuss how to approach problem behavior in the workplace
- Describe three approaches to conflict solving and give examples

Terminology

Aggressive—Behavior that is demanding, loud, sarcastic, or threatening.

Assertiveness—A quality in people with self-esteem; assertive behavior seeks to protect one's own rights while respecting those of others.

Consensus—Agreement among members of a group.

Content—Substance or actual information contained in a message.

Feedback—Physical response to a message; a component of effective communication.

Gossip—The telling and retelling of events about another's personal life, professional life, or physical condition.

Groupthink—In sociology and group behavior theory, the conformity of a group to one way of thinking and behaving. Groupthink creates two factions, those who agree (in-group) and those who disagree (out-group). This generates resentment and conflict in the workplace.

Norms—Behaviors that are accepted as part of the environment and culture of a group. Norms are usually established by custom and popular acceptance rather than by law, although the two may not be mutually exclusive.

Receiver—The person who receives the message communicated by a sender.

Sender—The person who communicates a message to another.

Tone—The expression of emotion or opinion contained in the delivery of a message. It is not explicit but is implied by intonation, emphasis on certain words, or measured delivery of words. Tone also is established by nonverbal communication.

Values—Beliefs, customs, behaviors, and norms that a person defends and upholds.

Win-lose—In conflict resolution, a situation in which one party is satisfied but the other finds the solution unsatisfactory.

Win-win—In conflict resolution, a situation in which both parties in a conflict gain by the solution.

WHY STUDY COMMUNICATION?

Communication is a two-way process whereby one person (the **sender**) expresses ideas and feelings and another (the **receiver**) receives them, processes them, and gives **feedback.** In patient care, effective communication is important in understanding the patient's needs, feelings, and experiences. Clear communication among coworkers is equally important because it produces cohesion and efficiency in the workplace. It gives personnel the information needed to establish priorities and act on them. It also helps to solidify roles so that all individuals know what is expected of them. Clear communication clarifies relationships and helps to establish professional and social boundaries. It increases teamwork and reinforces team goals. Good communication greatly increases the safety of the environment for the patient. Poor communication results in poor patient care, errors, conflict, and stress.

Good communication is not accidental. It requires skill and practice. *Everyone wants to be understood and to have his or her ideas and feelings respected.* Even under the best circumstances, however, communication can be difficult. Many health-care workers are surprised to find that the greatest challenge in their work is not the work itself but the interactions and social climate of the workplace. This chapter is intended to increase the reader's understanding of communication skills and the way communication affects interpersonal relationships and team building.

Among the most important reasons to improve communication skills is to maintain respect, trust, and empathy among coworkers and management. The operating room environment is often rushed, tense, and even brusque. In this atmosphere, people sometimes feel a loss of control over their work. Long hours, insufficient breaks, low pay, and verbal abuse result in a loss of morale and may lead to burnout. This downward spiral can be avoided. When individuals are allowed to express their needs in the workplace and others are willing to listen and respond, conflicts and destabilizing events can be avoided or addressed.

DIMENSIONS OF COMMUNICATION

People express their ideas, needs, and feelings through verbal language, posture, facial expressions, and gestures. Silence and stillness are another form of communication. The purposes of communication include:

▶ Giving information
▶ Sharing feelings
▶ Making requests
▶ Promoting action
▶ Evoking a specific response

Elements of Communication

In all forms of expression, effective communication between people results in understanding and acknowledgment of the information. Communication has three basic components.

The first is the *sender.* The sender is a person who wishes to convey an idea, concept, or feeling to others. Second is the *message.* The message is the concept, thought, idea, or feeling that is being expressed. The third element of communication is the *receiver.* The receiver is the person or group who hears or sees the message.

For communication to be considered *effective,* one additional item is required. This is known as *feedback.* Feedback is a response by the receiver that acknowledges the message that was sent. An example of this is a commercial on television. A company wants to sell a product or service. The company is the *sender.* The company creates a visual and audio display that appears during the intermission of your favorite television program. This is called the *message.* You, sitting in the comfort of your living room, are the *receiver.* The sender obtains *feedback* when you go out and inquire about the product or service. Feedback tells the company whether its advertisement (the message) was effective.

The **content** is the actual information conveyed in a communication. For example, "Please keep the doors closed." This content is simple information. Information can be perceived as negative ("You must work the next two weekends"), positive ("Everyone is getting raises next month"), or neutral ("Shut the door"). The message has an effect based on the content itself.

Delivering the Message

The method used to deliver a message is almost as important as the content of the message. When one refers to communication delivery, he or she is referring to the way the message is expressed, including verbal and nonverbal methods. Appropriate modes of communication delivery must be used to ensure that the message produces its desired effect. For example, you would not send your child a memo requesting that he or she clean his or her room. Likewise, if you wish to communicate a policy change to your employees, one-on-one meetings may not be appropriate.

VERBAL COMMUNICATION

Verbal communication means communication that is spoken or written. Examples of spoken communication include telephone calls and face-to-face discussions. Written communication includes policies and procedures, memos, letters, newspapers, and magazines.

In health care, the ability to convey information is critical to patient care, group morale, and team cohesion. The words that we select in day-to-day communication can have a powerful effect on the listener's reaction. When we speak thoughtlessly, without consideration of how the message is interpreted, we can cause conflict and harm. When we speak *as we would like to be spoken to,* we are more likely to produce an environment conducive to problem solving and collaboration.

Some situations in the operating room require the communication of brief, accurate information with little or no dialogue. Even in these cases, it is important to use language and **tone** that are respectful and polite. Box 6-1 lists important considerations in communicating verbally.

NONVERBAL COMMUNICATION

Nonverbal communication includes a number of factors that affect the way a message is received. Nonverbal communication includes tone of voice or inflection, body posture, gestures, and eye contact. Nonverbal communication can convey a meaning that differs significantly from what was originally intended by the sender when he or she created the message. Even if the sender does not wish to express his or her true feelings about the message, they will probably be conveyed by tone and body language. Most people understand the body language of their own culture. Table 6-1 describes some common examples of body language used by U.S. citizens.

Body language can betray our true feelings. One of the qualities of good communication is genuineness. Watch your own body language. Does it express what you feel? How do you think others read your body language? For example, you might ask the orderly to be available to clean your surgical suite in 15 minutes. Placing your hands on your hips translates into authority and **aggressive** behavior. Saying, "This case is finishing up, can you come in 15 minutes?" may sound like an acceptable way to express your need for help, but does your body language communicate the appropriate tone?

Another example is the manner in which we receive job assignments for the day. Not everyone can be assigned the cases he or she wants. When assignments are made, most supervisors attempt to match the skills of the personnel with the tasks required. Many other elements also must be considered, such as shift changes, low staffing, and break periods. When you receive an assignment, do you respect the need to consider these factors? What does your body language convey? If you were the supervisor, how would you react to the person who rolls his eyes, shakes his head, sighs, or turns abruptly away when given an assignment?

Touch

Touch can be both an expression of comfort and a way of controlling people. Touch, except in social gestures such as handshaking, is almost never neutral. It is a powerful means of communication that can soothe and comfort. It also demonstrates dominance. People who want to show their power over others sometimes use touch in a condescending manner. For example, consider the team leader who lays his hand on a subordinate's shoulder and says, "I *know* you won't mind working overtime tonight since you had *last* weekend off." This person is saying, "You *will work* overtime tonight whether you mind it or not!" Touch also is sometimes used in sexual harassment to overpower another person.

Touch is a very delicate issue for many people. Consider the following behaviors that may be seen in the workplace:

▶ Engaging in horseplay or jostling
▶ Making intimate gestures in view of others (jokingly or not)
▶ Surprising someone from behind by touching or grabbing them

---

Box 6-1 Guidelines for Verbal Communication

▶ Focus on the receiver.
▶ Use concrete words. Avoid descriptions that are vague and require the listener to "fill in the blanks" or guess your meaning.
▶ Do not assume how the receiver will respond. Allow him or her freedom to express personal views and opinion.
▶ Do not judge the receiver or others in your dialogue. This engenders mistrust.
▶ Avoid using strong emotional words. These trigger emotional reaction in others.
▶ When speaking with someone, make eye contact with that person and be alert to cues that he or she is *not* listening or wants to terminate the conversation. These include looking away or from side to side, fidgeting, and backing up.
▶ *On the telephone* do not carry on a background conversation while speaking to the person on the phone. It disrupts the phone conversation and prolongs it unnecessarily. If someone interrupts *you* while you are on the phone, ask him or her to wait until you are finished.

Table 6-1 BODY LANGUAGE USED BY AMERICANS

Element of Body Language	What It Demonstrates
Hands on hips	Authority or anger
Arms folded across chest	Resentment or guarding
Eye contact	Attention and respect for the speaker, confidence
Eye rolling	Discontent, disagreement, or impatience
Lack of eye contact	Lack of social comfort (note that people of different cultural backgrounds may not hold eye contact with the speaker because of their culture or faith)
Eyes cast downward	Contemplation, embarrassment, or contrition
Backing up	Social distance that is too close or desire to leave
Rigid posture	Restrained emotions or tension
Upright posture	Confidence or sense of well-being
Hand brushed over forehead or eyes	Exasperation, despair, or fatigue
One eyebrow raised	Doubt or mistrust
Both eyebrows raised	Surprise
Mouth covered by hand	Shock or sudden grief

To some people, these behaviors seem innocent and acceptable, while others find them repugnant and offensive. Very often, the person who finds the behaviors acceptable cannot understand why others will not "loosen up" and participate. People who lack respect for others' feelings, **values,** and experiences demonstrate this in many ways, and touch is one of them. Many people simply do not want to be touched. No one has the *absolute right* to touch another person. It is a privilege earned by trust and limited by the boundaries of culture and social custom.

Silence and Stillness

Silence and stillness communicate powerful messages. Silence can mean contemplation, shock, inability to speak, disagreement, or simply concentration. Many people misinterpret silence and stillness as "dead space" that must be filled. They are uncomfortable with silence. However, allowing others to think carefully before speaking shows respect and self-confidence. Sometimes a person who is uncomfortable with silence feels the need to provide a running dialogue (or monologue) to avoid silence. In the operating room, silence is encouraged because speaking can promote airborne disease transmission. Even here, however, team members may keep up a constant dialogue. In this case, speech can be a distraction from the flow of surgery, which is a risk to the patient.

Some people are naturally quiet and still, even in a busy environment. Individuals with this trait sometimes cause others discomfort because they behave differently from the norm. All persons have a right to express their individual personalities unless they harm or disrespect the rights of others.

TONE

Tone is the environment of the message. It reflects the sender's emotions, such as respect for the receiver, opinion about the message, or attitude toward the receiver. Most people are familiar with the effect that tone has on the message. Examples include the following:

1. "*Please!* . . . Keep—the—doors—*closed!*"
2. "Would you *mind* keeping those doors *closed?!*"
3. "Please keep the doors closed—*thanks!*"

In the first example the sender emphasizes words by volume and by measured delivery. This conveys impatience and frustration. In the second example, the sender uses a bit of sarcasm to emphasize annoyance. In the third example, the sender simply expresses a need to keep the doors closed and shows appreciation for compliance.

The following sentence can be stated in many different ways to convey additional information about the message:

"I'm scrubbing with you again today, Dr. X . . ." (neutral information)

The sender's *tone* might convey any of the following *additional* meanings:

". . . and I'd rather have a root canal job." (dread)

". . . and I'm really glad, because things go so smoothly in your rooms." (relief)

". . . and if you start yelling today, I'm going to report it." (hostility)

Listening (Receiving Skills)

People find it easy to talk with those who have good listening skills. People with these skills are often placed in management positions because of their ability to communicate ideas in a concise, accurate, and nonjudgmental way. People often seek them out for advice because they know they will be heard fairly and with respect.

Listening requires active participation. Passive listening frequently leads to inaccurate interpretation or an inability to respond to the information. Parts of the message may be lost because the listener is distracted or impatient to speak. Most people begin to formulate a response before they have heard everything the sender has said. Their thoughts are fo-

---

Box 6-2   Positive Listening Skills

▶ Focus on the sender. Avoid listening to background noise or other conversations.

▶ Avoid listening for what you *want* to hear. You may misinterpret the message.

▶ Do not judge the sender. If you are preoccupied with personal details about the sender, you cannot interpret the message accurately.

▶ Watch for nonverbal cues such as facial expressions and body language. These help clarify the sender's attitude about the message and help you understand important aspects of the information.

▶ Ask for clarification!

▶ Rephrase the sender's content so that both of you know that the message is understood. For example, "You mean that . . ."

▶ If the sender begins to get sidetracked from the topic, redirect the conversation. Do this by asking questions about the original issue or asking the sender to return to the topic.

▶ If you find that your attention has drifted, ask the sender to repeat what was just said.

▶ Don't *assume background information* unless you know it. If the message seems unreasonable, there may be circumstances of which you are unaware. Be open to the possibility that there is a much bigger picture than the one you know about.

▶ If you find the sender's language or comments in bad taste or offensive, say so without judgment. For example, "I feel uncomfortable when you talk about Dr. X that way," or "I wish you wouldn't use that kind of language, it's offensive to me." When asking another to change his or her tone or language, be sure to state your own feelings about it. For example, "When you get angry with me in front of everyone, I feel very uncomfortable. Can we talk in your office instead?"

cused on what they want to say, and they fail to receive the message.

Refer to Box 6-2 for elements of positive listening skills.

Cultural Differences

Culture reflects the values, social practices, and communication methods of a group of people. Important considerations in cross-cultural communication include but are not limited to:

- Acceptable social distance between people
- Gender value
- Preference for collective versus independent action
- Methods of coping with conflict and uncertainty
- Ways of expressing emotion
- Body language

Communication with people of different cultures requires sensitivity and an open mind. Most people have heard some people make comments about newcomers to the United States such as "They should act like we do," or "They should learn the way we do things," or, worse, "If they don't like the way we do things, they should go back where they came from." These statements show a lack of sensitivity and knowledge about how cultural **norms** are formed and maintained. Social and interpersonal norms are imbued in people from the time they are born. Cultural beliefs are based on tradition and value systems that cannot be switched off and on. All people esteem their cultural values and deserve to have them respected by others. Refer to Table 6-2 for examples of cultural characteristics that affect communication.

QUALITIES OF GOOD COMMUNICATION

Assertiveness

Assertiveness is the ability to express one's own needs and rights while *respecting the needs and rights of others*. It is *not* aggression or confrontation. Aggression is the exertion of power over others by intimidation, loudness, or bullying—qualities that ignore others' feelings or take advantage of another's vulnerabilities. The aggressive person puts his or her own needs and wants above those of everyone else. By contrast, the assertive person communicates self-worth without showing arrogance or "pulling rank." The assertive person does not submit to the aggression of others but serves as a self-advocate by stating his or her needs clearly, without hesitation or self-effacement.

You can convey assertiveness through nonverbal or verbal language. To show assertiveness using body language:

- Maintain good posture.
- Use eye contact when speaking and listening. In maintaining relaxed eye contact, shift your gaze on the other person from one eye to the other. A fixed stare can convey emotional intensity.

- Stand still and do not fidget or shift your weight. This conveys ambivalence.
- Place your arms at your sides. This communicates acceptance and genuineness.
- Curb annoying actions such as knuckle cracking and foot tapping, which can create distraction.

To express assertiveness through verbal language:

- Do not interrupt people. Patience shows respect.
- State your question, request, information, or comment without hesitation. Try to avoid an apologetic tone unless it fits the situation.
- State your message without blame or criticism.
- State your own needs or feelings in a straightforward manner.
- Accept the consequences of your message. Remain calm and deliberate in your speech. Remain open to the responses.
- Remain engaged and attentive during conversation.
- If you are emotionally upset, *take time to calm down* before speaking (unless the patient or a coworker is in direct harm). Strong emotions cloud the ability to think and speak coherently.
- Never assume that, because the work environment is intense, your own intensity has no effect on others—it does.

Consider the following examples:

Example 1

A. "I came to ask you for the weekend off. My brother's coming in from overseas. I really want to spend time with him before he leaves again."

B. "Uh, oh, I was thinking about this weekend. I, well I've been on call for the last two weekends. I mean, I know you are short staffed, but I was wondering if I could have this weekend off. I don't know, maybe it'll throw your schedule off. I just thought I'd ask."

Example 2

A. "I want to report that Dr. X threw another bloody sponge across the room today. It hit the wall and barely missed the circulator. Please speak to him."

B. "I was in a room with Dr. X. You know how he is. But, well, I think maybe someone might need to talk to him. Maybe he shouldn't throw sponges. I mean, he did it again today. I know he's chief of surgery, but, well, isn't it bad practice? I mean, couldn't someone get hepatitis or something?"

C. "This operating room is so awful. I mean, to let someone like that get away with throwing bloody sponges all over the room. No wonder people get hepatitis. Why don't you do something? You make these policies but no one ever does anything about them!"

These examples demonstrate several ways to make a request. In statement B of both examples, the sender is not confident about the request. He or she has needs but is reluctant

Table 6-2 CROSS-CULTURAL DIFFERENCES AMONG MAJOR ETHNIC GROUPS

Cultural Element	European/American	Asian	Pan-American Indian	Arabic or Islamic*	African
Communication	Verbal orientation; use of eye contact more common in men than in women; women tend to facilitate communication with questions; men tend to be more direct and declarative.	Use of silence and nonverbal cueing; no eye contact; communication based on contextual cues, gender, and social position; formal communication used with those outside intimate circle.	Increasing use of tribal languages, also Spanish and English; use of silence, nonverbal cues; limited eye contact; respectful silence; reserved manner and "small talk" common until rapport is established; tact and diplomacy valued.	Personal; verbal orientation with same gender; close eye contact (staring); communication is easier with peers, more reserved when there is a difference in social status.	Oral; verbal orientation; use of verbal rhythms, feedback from listener; truth is expected; facial and hand gesturing and intonations create emphasis and emotive expression.
Space	Consider close proximity and touch a sign of intimacy; use of touch more common between women; displays of affection between men and women and kissing are present in media and in public.	Close personal space tolerated for long periods without social engagement; use of touch and space has subtle and distinct communication aspects and varies based on intimacy; touch occurs between those of same sex and between parent and child but not with those of opposite sex.	Group orientation prevails with touch among intimates; spaces carry social and religious/symbolic significance—each space may have appropriate uses or carry behavioral expectations.	Personal space is close; touch is between parent and child and those of same sex, with limited touch between members of opposite sex; hand holding or arm linking is between members of same sex only.	Personal space is close in company of familiars; individuals may be guarded and reserved until rapport is established; touch may signify familiarity.
Time orientation	Monochronic—see time in a linear, segmented way; task orientation, concern with punctuality; future orientation; consider concerns about the past old-fashioned.	Polychronic—see time as flowing with several simultaneous tasks; future orientation in work and technology; achieve harmony and present orientation in social situations.	Strong orientation to present; relationships and present interactions must be handled well; consideration of the patient's orientation with regard to ancestry and tradition.	Strong orientation to present; no social regard for appointments and interactions; social expectation is that people will be tended to when someone is available; trustworthiness expected.	Polychronic; orientation depends on adoption of dominant world view; continuity is seen from past to future; may tend toward orientation to present.
Social organization	Nuclear families; Judeo-Christian religion is hierarchical; relationships and groups organized around similarities.	Hierarchical, with obligations and duties to those above and below; filial piety important, with loyalty and duty to male household head, superior; hierarchy based on gender and age; devotion to tradition varies by generation.	Family oriented; nuclear families with extended kinship ties; hierarchy based on age and gender; family pride and honor regulate behavior.	Organized by group affiliation, especially affiliation to political/religious groups, also by lineage and tribe; born into established social status; affiliations are generally for life; hierarchical by age, sex, lineage, and social status.	Social pattern greatly affected by history of discrimination; family oriented, with family extended to nonkin dependents and community members; community emphasized.

Modified from Varcarolis EM: *Foundations of psychiatric mental health nursing,* ed 3, Philadelphia, 1998, WB Saunders.
HIV, Human immunodeficiency virus; *STDs,* sexually transmitted diseases; *TB,* tuberculosis.

Table 6-2	CROSS-CULTURAL DIFFERENCES AMONG MAJOR ETHNIC GROUPS—cont'd				
Cultural Element	European/American	Asian	Pan-American Indian	Arabic or Islamic*	African
Relation to environment	Value science and technology; action oriented; tend to attempt to manipulate environment to adapt to human needs.	Adjust to physical and social world; believe that order is predetermined and accept what is valued; individuals are expected to recognize consequences of actions and adjust behavior accordingly.	Being oriented; focus on harmony with forces outside the person, including community, nature, and spirits or deities; show concern for balance and moderation in relations with nature and others.	Give limited emphasis to personal control; control and authority are obtained from those with established power and wealth; expectation is that those with power and control will care for their dependents; rely on benevolence of others.	Focused on interrelationship between person and external world; relationships, nutrition, religious observances, and respect for those who came before affect health and well-being; history of social injustice may affect view of ability to alter social environment.
Biological aspects	Dominant focus in medicine is heart and lungs; fast-paced lifestyle promotes stress-related diseases such as hypertension, migraines, ulcers, cancers.	Dominant focus is chest and abdomen; "belly" is seat of soul or mind; mental distress is given somatic expression in form of dizziness, shoulder pain, stomach distress; subject to diseases of industrialization; tropical diseases vary by region.	Forced migration and reservation residence altered healthy traditional habits; currently plagued by diseases of poverty—alcohol abuse, STDs, TB, depression, and suicide; may be genetically predisposed to diabetes and alcohol addiction.	Orientation is to abdomen and chest area; may express feelings nonverbally through abdominal pain or joint and muscle pain.	Discrimination and unemployment have led to diseases of poverty—substance abuse, STDs, TB, malnutrition; urbanization of poverty has created increased susceptibility to urban problems—violence, asthma, hypertension; cultural lack of comprehension of meanings of bloodborne diseases, HIV infection, and organ donation.

to express them directly. In statement A of both examples, the messages are polite, clear, and to the point. They state a need, show respect for the receiver, and are delivered without hesitation. The receiver *knows* exactly what the request is and can make a decision. Statement C in example 2 communicates disrespect for the receiver and anger at the situation, without actually stating what the problem is or who is involved. This type of approach is aggressive, not assertive.

Respect

Respect for others communicates the recognition of value—*both our own and that of other people.* It shows that although we may not agree with another's opinion or beliefs, we value that person's right to express and act on them, as long as the person does not cause harm to others.

People immediately sense when another person respects them. The person's actions and speech clearly show it. The respectful person:

▶ Does not judge others
▶ Does not **gossip**
▶ Does not reveal personal or confidential information about others
▶ Speaks directly and listens attentively to others
▶ Responds with empathy to others
▶ Does not interrupt

▶ Acknowledges the value of different opinions and ideas
▶ Does not use others to gain personal advantage
▶ Does not *disparage* another person to appear smarter, more skilled, or better
▶ Does not demand another's attention

Respectful people are well liked because others feel accepted in their presence. This quality is developed from one's past experiences and one's own self-esteem. Sometimes people do not realize that their behavior shows a lack of respect. They do not see the cues or have never been told that their communication is offensive or hurtful. Others feel entitled to treat people in a disrespectful manner because they were treated this way at some time in their lives. This type of person is often self-centered and may be socially isolated. Such a person seeks out others who find their behavior acceptable and validate it.

Clarity

Clarity means that the important aspects of the message are delivered without ambiguity or unnecessary information. Consider the following examples:

Example 1. "You know, I just went to sterilize Dr. X's curettes—you know, the ones he always wants on his total knee surgeries . . . and when I closed the door I hit "Start" and a little steam kept coming out from around the door and the buzzer never went off, and I tried to turn it off and I couldn't. These old sterilizers . . . I think the seal is broken; maybe someone should look at it. Can you call someone? I need those curettes and I don't have time."

Example 2. "Sterilizer number 3 is leaking steam around the door, it won't open, and Dr. X's curettes are inside. Would you mind calling engineering? I need to scrub."

When reporting a problem such as that in the previous examples, give the right person the necessary information, as in example 2. In that example, the receiver knows exactly what and where the problem is. He or she also understands the level of urgency and can act on this information without further questioning.

Feedback

Feedback is the response to the sender's message. Effective communication includes clear feedback. Poor communication results when a message is delivered but the receiver does not acknowledge that additional information is needed. In this case, feedback is missing. This may happen when the receiver is distracted, in a hurry, or reluctant to seek clarification.

Look for cues that the receiver understands the message. When the message is understood, the receiver should seek additional information or indicate the appropriate action. Just as the sender has a responsibility to clarify the message, the receiver must give direct, specific feedback. In health care, feedback is critically important when one is discussing or reporting safety issues. In the previous examples, a request is made to solve a problem with a flash sterilizer. The person who asks for help must not assume that the other person will follow through. He or she must determine whether the coworker really will be able to call engineering. Asking a follow-up question is one way to receive feedback.

PROBLEM BEHAVIORS

Coping with problem behaviors in the workplace is always a challenge. Because of the unique environment of the operating room, problem behaviors can lead to open conflict. Following are some characteristics of operating room work that contribute to problem behaviors:

▶ **The work is stressful.** As a critical care unit, the operating room requires personnel to work at a high level of mental, physical, and emotional strength. Because of the demanding schedules, strong lines of authority, and wide diversity of behavior and personality types, excellent communication skills are required.

▶ **Close teamwork is necessary** even when team members have little knowledge of each other's work styles and personalities. This is especially true in a teaching hospital where surgical residents and medical, nursing, and surgical technology students rotate through the department regularly. Even when communication is good among team members, working under intense conditions with new people can be challenging.

▶ **The chain of command is defined.** Some people are not accustomed to this type of structure. Their responses are varied. While some people are content to work within an established chain of command, others resent it, especially if they lack respect for those in authority.

▶ **People and departments compete for time, space, materials, and personnel.** All operating rooms, whether in a large metropolitan area or in a small community, must meet the needs of the patients with fixed staff, equipment, and time. When the patient load requires more resources than are immediately available, there is potential for conflict over available staff, equipment, and rooms. Conflict arises when the needs of one person overpower those of the others without sound rationale.

▶ **The model for team relationships is in transition.** The social model for team interaction traditionally has been authoritarian, hierarchical, and intended to put people "in their places." Many of these social traditions are no longer tolerated by administrators and professional associations. Whenever there is a major change in a social structure—for example, turnover in staff and management—and a major change in what is acceptable and what is not, there is a period of testing and adjustment, which is stressful.

Problem behaviors cause mistrust and frustration in others, and interpersonal conflict. Everyone has a unique combination of personality traits that promote or inhibit the achievement of life goals and sense of well-being. The person with problem behavior, however, uses extreme defensive or aggressive tactics to achieve a level of social comfort. Supervisors cannot resolve every conflict that arises. Each person on the unit must make an effort to communicate effectively and assertively. On the other hand, if everyone avoids responsibility for resolving a problem, the problem will be referred to a higher administrative level than might be appropriate or effective. However, administrative intervention *is* appropriate in extreme cases.

When working with people with problem behaviors, one must remember to *focus on the behavior, not the person.* Difficult people relate poorly to each other, their environment, and themselves because they have not learned how to meet their needs in socially acceptable ways. They have not learned to cope. This does not dismiss the frustration and even humiliation that others experience in their presence. However, it is neither productive nor helpful to attack the *person* in order to cope with the behavior. This usually exacerbates the defensive behavior and alienates the person even more.

Verbal Abuse

Verbal abuse is communication that is rude, demeaning, and thoughtless. It includes ridicule, blaming, or deliberate personal attack. It may be accompanied by physical behaviors such as throwing things. Several studies have shown that verbal abuse is a frequent occurrence in the operating room. In one study, verbal abuse accounted for 94% of all disruptive behavior in the OR; in more than half of those cases, surgeons were the perpetrators. This study also showed that 44% of operating room managers stated that, at some point, they considered a patient to be at risk because of disruptive behavior such as verbal abuse (Pat Patterson, Disruptive Abuse, *OR Manager,* 12:12, Dec, 1996).

Verbal abuse doubtlessly has a negative effect on patient care because it causes staff to become tense, upset, and distracted. Morale also is affected. In another study, 81% of the participants reported a decrease in morale and even physical illness as a result of verbal abuse (Helen Cox, Verbal abuse nationwide, part II: impact and modification, *Nursing Management,* 22:3, March, 1991). Verbal abuse also reduces productivity and increases errors and staff turnover.

CAUSES OF VERBAL ABUSE

Verbal abuse by surgeons increases when they are allowed to show favoritism toward particular staff members. Others who are obligated to work with these surgeons on emergency calls or under other circumstances are often the targets of severe verbal abuse because they lack the "inside knowledge" of the select group. This type of treatment leads to conflict and resentment among staff members and increases the scope of the problem. People in the select group who feel secure in their positions sometimes use their power to belittle and criticize others, especially students or new employees. This behavior damages self-esteem and inhibits the newcomer's ability to fit into the group.

Verbal abuse is sometimes built into the operating room culture. When the administration does not address and act on the problem in a serious manner, the administration implies that it approves of the situation. Victims who cannot seek sympathy from or action by those who can affect policy are left with little recourse. They may leave the job or suffer the abuse silently as their stress level increases. Administrative support is very important to changing operating room culture.

Rude, vulgar, and offensive behavior is *not* a natural reaction to stress. It is a choice made by those who perpetrate it. The job stress carried by surgeons and other operating room personnel is no greater than that of people in many other professions, such as firefighters, rescue workers, and police officers. Yet in these groups one finds *increased* cohesion and support rather than abuse among coworkers. A culture of verbal abuse and passive aggression does not flow naturally from the environment; it comes from individuals who use their authority to hurt others.

Remember, as a student it is important to inform your instructor if you are the recipient of verbal abuse, and allow them to help in resolving the situation.

COPING WITH VERBAL ABUSE

Assertive behavior is one of the most effective ways to counteract verbal abuse. The following guidelines describe specific coping behaviors:

▶ **Remain calm.** To deescalate rising tension and disarm the abuser, you must prepare yourself to address him or her. This is often very difficult, especially when the outburst is extremely demeaning and loud, and contains foul language. Tell yourself the following:
  ▶ "I have the right to confront this person."
  ▶ "I have the right *not* to take this abuse."
  ▶ "There is no acceptable excuse for this behavior."

▶ **Make an assertive statement.** Do not engage in sarcasm or personal attack; this usually escalates the situation. Instead, state *what you feel and what you want:*
  ▶ "Dr. X, please don't speak to me like that. It is rude and demoralizing."
  ▶ "Dr. X, it is not necessary to scream at me. When you do that, I can't work."
  ▶ "Dr. X, if I make an error, tell me what the error is. It's not necessary to yell and curse at me."

  After you have made your statement, proceed with your work. If the abuser continues, it is sometimes helpful just to ignore him or her. The abuser will soon realize that you are not listening. The important fact is that *you have stated your rights and are in control of yourself.* If the situation continues, restate your position calmly.

▶ **Do not become aggressive.** When you act aggressively in the face of aggression, it escalates the conflict and may cause a major crisis. This creates a risk to the patient and is not acceptable. The patient must *never* bear the consequences of anyone's behavioral problems. If you cannot stop the behavior, wait until after surgery, then confront the abuser.

▶ **Stand up for your coworkers.** If you are in a room where your coworker is being abused, defend him or her. Your silence is approval of the abuser's behavior.

▶ **If the abuse gets completely out of hand, call for the supervisor.** Do not allow abuse or other disruptive behavior to continue. Do not be afraid to request the presence of others who are in an administratively stronger position to stop the abuser.

After an abusive situation has occurred, it is natural to want to tell the first person you see what has happened. However, pick the correct time and place. The operating room corridor is not the appropriate place to vent your feelings. Patients can overhear talk and become frightened and insecure. File a complaint with the operating room supervisor. You can do this face to face or in a written report, stating when the abuse occurred, what was said, and who was in the room. If you choose to meet with your supervisor, *make an appointment.* Do not burst into the supervisor's office demanding that he or she "do something about Dr. X." If you need to vent your anger, avoid lashing out at others. This only spreads the effects of the abuse and multiplies the abuser's ability to demoralize people. If possible, take a break and write down your feelings. Vent your stress in physical activity or other appropriate ways.

When you work with the abuser again, continue to reinforce your position—that he or she is the abuser and that you have the right to tell him or her to stop. Continue to file appropriate written reports of the abusive behavior.

Complaining
LEGITIMATE VERSUS CHRONIC COMPLAINING
Legitimate complaints about conditions in the workplace are important and should be addressed. Legitimate complaints often lead to creative solutions that produce a safer and more efficient operating room. However, when people complain without the intention of seeking solutions, they erode morale and sometimes cause conflict. Chronic complaining can be contagious. When it becomes part of the workplace culture, it spreads discontent and feelings of helplessness or despair. Habitual complaining usually is not about occasional incidents. Habitual complainers are usually unhappy about many aspects of their lives. They do not look for solutions; they simply want everyone to know how they feel and seek out others to hear and validate their many complaints. It *is* helpful for people to share their feelings about incidents. By sharing their thoughts and emotions, they find support and empathy. Chronic complainers, however, have little regard for or knowledge about the unhappiness that they spread in the work environment.

COPING WITH PEOPLE WHO COMPLAIN
Here are some guidelines for dealing with chronic complainers:

▶ **Do not become a complainer yourself.** Often we are tempted to jump in and agree with a complainer. This only perpetuates the problem. Offer a solution or suggest how the person might solve the problem. If the complainer rejects the solution immediately or gives more examples of how bad things are, you know that he or she is not interested in seeking solutions but simply wants to state and restate the negative aspects of work or of his or her personal life.

▶ **Just listen.** Sometimes silence has a powerful effect on the complainer. Listen without emotion and then simply leave. This is not a satisfying response to the complainer, and he or she may stop.

▶ **Confront the complainer.** Complainers often dominate locker room conversation or complain in front of patients. If you are in the presence of a patient, simply say, "Not now . . ." or "This isn't the time . . ." Speak to the complainer *in private* and tell him or her how you feel about the complaining and the effect it has on the team. Ask the person to curb the behavior. *It is not necessary to speak harshly or unkindly to this person.* The individual does not complain out of maliciousness. The complainer is unhappy and does not know how to cope with this unhappiness.

▶ **If possible, remove yourself from the situation.** If other solutions do not work, simply do not stay with the complainer. Understand that listening to the complainer regularly is frustrating and tiring. Do not allow this person to increase your stress.

Gossip and Rumors
Gossip is the telling and retelling of events about another's personal life, professional life, or physical condition. It is insidious behavior that hurts people, erodes teamwork, and damages group ethics. Gossip is *not* the same as the normal sharing of news or events that occur in people's lives. It is communication about another person or event that is confidential or personal. The goal of gossip is to shock or evoke intrigue. As gossip spreads, the story may change slightly and facts may become blurred, so that the only importance of the story is its ability to entertain, at the expense of someone else.

A rumor is information whose validity is in question. The damaging effect of a rumor is that, after the story begins to circulate, people assume that it is true and they react as if the rumor were fact. If the rumor is unpleasant news, conflicts arise and people may become resentful, angry, or even fearful. Ironically, people who spread rumors often fail to validate the rumor. As with gossip, the value of the rumor lies in its effect on others during the telling and retelling, not in whether it is based on reality.

COPING WITH GOSSIP AND RUMORS
Adapt the following rules in coping with gossip and rumors:

▶ **Don't participate.**
▶ **Call attention to the behavior.** One very effective way to do this is to make a remark such as, "We shouldn't be talking about Dr. X. That's his personal business." (Note that

it is important not to accuse the other person; that is, do not say, "*You* shouldn't . . .") You might also say, "It's not fair to talk about someone when he can't defend himself." The point is to reinforce to the gossiper that the behavior is damaging and that you are not going to participate.

If you find yourself participating in rumors or gossip, ask yourself whether *you* would want others to discuss the details of *your* personal life or other private news in public.

Groupthink

Groupthink is collective behavior and thinking. It is based on peer pressure and occurs when members of a group are polarized in their opinions, ways of doing things, and means of expression. It produces two categories of people: those who are "in" and those who are "out." Whether the values of the group are positive or negative, people avoid becoming isolated and strive to become part of the "in" group. They change their own values to fit those of the "in" group. In this way group culture is created and maintained.

Groupthink establishes unwritten, unspoken rules. Those who do not follow the rules may be criticized or ostracized by their peers. Standards of practice are deeply affected by groupthink. When the group sets high standards, groupthink is a positive force, but when aseptic technique and other practices slide, the people in the "out" group may be the only ones trying to uphold the high standard.

Groupthink is usually a negative force because it does not allow freedom of speech or action without the implied threat of isolation. As a surgical technologist one should be an independent and critical thinker, uphold high standards, and act in a professional manner in every situation.

Criticism

Criticism is a helpful tool in correcting work habits or raising awareness about harmful or unsafe situations. When offered appropriately, criticism is specific, nonjudgmental, and focused on the task, not on the person. When criticism is used to exercise power over others or boost one's self-confidence, however, it can be very destructive. People who criticize are usually insecure in their own lives. They use criticism as a way to soothe the anxiety they experience as a result of self-dissatisfaction. Nevertheless, this does not give them the right to demoralize or demean others. Some critics are expert at finding vulnerabilities in their coworkers and using these to demonstrate their superiority. Staff members must not tolerate their behavior.

COPING WITH CRITICISM

Habitually critical people often are defensive and may become resentful when confronted with their behavior. However, it is important to point out when their criticism is causing conflict. When confronting the critical person, you should:

▶ State that you find the person's behavior distressing rather than helpful.

▶ Tell the person that if he or she wishes to discuss your work you will do so in private. This formalizes the critical process and removes its ability to cause embarrassment in front of others.

▶ Ask the person to be *specific* about the problem. Respond with a request for clarification or simply state without emotion or further discussion your reason for behaving as you did.

Example

COMMENT: "*The way you stacked these things I can't find anything. You're so sloppy.*"
RESPONSE: "*Tell me how you would like them arranged.*"
COMMENT: "*I don't know, that's not my job.*"
RESPONSE: "*I can't improve the situation unless you can identify the problem.*"

Example

COMMENT: "*Why can't you ever loosen up in surgery? You're so serious.*"
RESPONSE: "*What bothers you about it?*"
COMMENT: "*You never laugh at any of my jokes.*"
RESPONSE: "*I don't find them amusing and I prefer not to talk during surgery.*"

Sexual Harassment

In spite of increased awareness and the enactment of laws and policies regarding sexual harassment, it continues to be a problem in the workplace, including the operating room. Sexual harassment is an extreme misuse of power in which a person engages in the following types of behavior:

▶ Expects sexual favors in exchange for personal or professional gain.
▶ Participates in any kind of sexual coercion.
▶ Directs sexually explicit comments toward another.
▶ Makes unwanted sexual or casual physical contact with another person.
▶ Directs vulgar or sexual innuendoes at another.

The legal implications of and responses to sexual harassment are discussed in Chapter 3, Law and Ethics. Behavioral responses to aid in coping with this behavior are discussed in this chapter.

COPING WITH SEXUAL HARASSMENT

Sexual harassment is illegal. However, because the victims are humiliated and embarrassed and often feel powerless to do anything, incidents go unreported and perpetrators continue the behavior. The perpetrator often considers sexual harassment to be innocent behavior, and any one event may be open to interpretation (unless the sexual content is blatant), so the victim may feel that she or he has no grounds on which to make an incident report. *Any incident that evokes a sense of sexual invasion, humiliation, shame, or guilt should be reported.* Documentation of an incident is the best way to elicit disciplinary action by those in a position to take it.

Box 6-3　Defenses Against Sexual Harassment

▶ If the institution does not have policies covering reporting and discipline, request that the process of developing such policies be initiated.

▶ Do not engage in sexual jokes or conversation yourself. Walk away from the scene or simply change the subject. If you are scrubbed and cannot leave, confront the person either at that time or later. If you are afraid to make the report, ask another person who was present to do it. Explain why.

▶ Inform your coworkers that you recognize a given behavior as sexual harassment. If they agree, ask them to participate in a confrontation. If you are not the subject of the harassment but are present, help others by confronting the perpetrator as your coworker's advocate, especially if the victim is so humiliated that he or she cannot respond.

▶ Report all incidents of sexual harassment even if you are not the victim.

▶ Stand up for your rights. If you feel victimized, others probably feel they are too. Seek others out for support in taking appropriate action.

▶ If your supervisor does not respond to repeated reports, write a letter or speak to the person at the administrative level directly above the supervisor.

Although it is sometimes difficult, the victim should confront the perpetrator *when sexual harassment occurs* and afterward submit a written report. Examples are as follows:

▶ "Don't touch me again. *I don't like it and I won't tolerate it.*"
▶ "Don't use those kinds of sexual references around me. Your comments are inappropriate."
▶ "My personal life is not open for discussion."

See Box 6-3 for specific proactive defenses that personnel can use, in addition to confrontation, to prevent and stand up against sexual harassment.

TEAMWORK

Types of Teams

A *team* is a group of people who come together to reach a common goal or set of goals. The surgical team is only one type of team that plans and implements patient care in the operating room. In some large hospitals certain personnel work within a surgical specialty such as cardiology or orthopedics. In this type of structure, surgical technologists work with their peers to design instrument sets, order equipment, and update the surgeons' procedural changes. There may or may not be a team leader.

The surgical technologist also may participate in other types of interdepartmental teams or groups to improve care or produce information for surveillance and monitoring. Within a team, different personalities, work styles, values,

and cultures are brought together. The team must identify and prioritize the steps of the process in order to reach the desired goal of a positive patient treatment outcome.

The surgical team includes the surgeons, anesthesia caregiver, assistants, surgical technologist, and registered nurse. They all work together on a single procedure. Communication is usually focused, task oriented, and at times intense.

A *group* does not have a common goal, but the people in the group share common professions, task requirements, or other characteristics. Group work and teamwork are very similar. Interpersonal relationships and the ability to resolve differences are equally important whether in a team or a group. When people work on the same shift in the operating room, they form a group. There is an understanding among everyone that people will help each other with certain tasks and try to resolve work-related obstacles.

Qualities of Good Teamwork

Good teamwork is the result of healthy relationships within the team. This does not mean that conflicts do not arise. Conflict in groups is normal because people have different ideas, problem-solving skills, values, and beliefs. The qualities of a good team reflect how conflict is managed. Individuals should retain valued traits such as genuineness, self-assertion, and empathy while at the same time being willing to discuss, yield, and accept change.

DISCUSSION OF CONFLICTS

Conflict cannot be managed unless people communicate about their problems. Discussion means that the group must admit that a problem exists. Identifying the problem requires sharing of experiences and interpretation of events *without judgment*. Members of successful groups do not accuse others of wrongdoing. They simply state the facts and relate the effect. Although people's perceptions of events, situations, or problems may be different, it is important to focus on the problem, *not the people*. Attacks on others in the group lead to defensive behavior, which is counterproductive to creating solutions.

YIELDING

Yielding in teamwork does not mean giving up one's values or beliefs. It means accepting the fact that there are other valid points of view and conceding when one has made incorrect assumptions or conclusions. People who are able to yield are open-minded and retain a sense of fairness during team interaction. A team member who tries to gain control of all decisions and conversations is unable to yield to other people's right to express their views. Such individuals cannot imagine any way but *their* way and make little or no attempt to broaden their thinking.

ACCEPTANCE OF CHANGE

The ability to accept change is crucial to good teamwork. Many people experience change as a positive event, but others face it with dread. One of the purposes of a team is to adjust to a changing environment such as unfolding events during a surgical procedure, a change in instrumentation, or new responsibilities. When groups or teams are confronted with change, they must adjust their ways of working to accommodate the change. Team members must identify new tasks or procedures and implement them with as little disruption as possible. This requires personal flexibility, one of the positive character traits identified in the successful surgical technologist.

POLITENESS

Politeness concerns the manner in which people speak to and behave toward each other. The attributes of acceptable behavior include respect, gratitude, and acceptance. The operating room culture does not always promote these attributes. This does not mean that they are unimportant. On the contrary, teams that *do* honor and practice these qualities have a pleasant work atmosphere, are efficient, and show a high level of professionalism. They experience fewer conflicts, and team members exhibit high self-esteem. Unfortunately, group thinking and aggressive behavior often overcome civility in the operating room. The most powerful way to instill civility in a group is to model it.

Polite behavior is not complicated or difficult. Saying "Thank you" or "Please" makes people feel appreciated and respected. Offering to help another person even when you are not asked and responding to requests for help without resentment creates an atmosphere of cohesion and empathy among coworkers. Speaking with others in an even and calm manner without sarcasm promotes evenness and reduces stress.

COLLABORATION

Collaboration is people working together for a common purpose. In the operating room, personnel contribute their skills, time, and energy to the care of the surgical patient. Collaboration requires that everyone solve problems and obstacles as a group. Cooperation and the ability to accept one another's individual personalities contribute to successful collaboration. Successful patient outcomes result when each team member understands the relationship among his or her own responsibilities and the tasks of the other members. Each person sees that his or her own contribution is one of many and that problems or strengths in one area affect the entire collaborative effort.

Team Problems

CONFLICT BETWEEN TEAM MEMBERS

Personality clashes, attempts to gain control of the group, and power plays are some causes of team conflict. When stress occurs between two or more people on a team, all team members feel the tension. Other members feel frustrated because they cannot solve the problem. Team cohesion disintegrates, and members worry about productivity, safety, and accountability. Resolving the conflict may require mediation if the individuals involved cannot resolve their differences.

Particularly in health care, the overall goal (patient care) must not suffer because of individuals' inability to get along or resolve differences.

CONFLICT BETWEEN TEAM GOALS AND PERSONAL GOALS

On the surface, a team's goals might seem obvious. Although each person is aware of the final outcome (i.e., the surgery is completed), the manner in which each person contributes to the final outcome is affected by personal goals. For example, if a student is scrubbed with a surgical technologist, the role of the surgical technologist is to be a teacher (preceptor). The overall goal remains the same—completion of the surgery in a safe and efficient manner. The goals of the student, however, are to learn about the procedure and practice skills so that he or she can work independently. The surgical technologist may not want to give up control of the case. The surgical technologist may be concerned that the surgeon will blame him or her if the surgery is slowed or errors are made. Perhaps the surgical technologist wants to show the student how much he or she knows rather than allow the student to participate actively. In such a case, the student becomes frustrated because there is a conflict of goals. In this type of conflict, the needs of each person must be discussed. The most favorable outcome is for each person to recognize the overall priority of needs and to be willing to yield to these priorities.

CONFLICTING PRIORITIES

Setting team priorities requires **consensus,** agreement on what the goals are and how they will be reached. Everyone may know the goal, but people may disagree on how to reach it. For example, during surgery the surgeon's goal is to work quickly without pauses in the flow of the procedure. The surgical technologist's goal is to remain ahead of the surgeon, anticipating what will happen next and what instruments and supplies will be needed, while at the same time providing what is needed in the present. To do this, the surgical technologist must use every moment to prepare as well as work in the present.

Consider a scenario in which the surgeon places used instruments out of the surgical technologist's reach. Suction devices, hemostats, and needle holders soon pile up at the opposite end of the work area from the surgical technologist. The surgeon has created a situation in which the surgical technologist cannot do his or her work. The surgical technologist reminds the surgeon of the need to return instruments. This causes interruption. The surgeon is frustrated because he or she must periodically retrieve the instruments, and the surgical technologist must expend time requesting the instruments and sorting them. Cooperation is lacking. The solution, of course, is for the surgeon to place the used instruments within the surgical technologist's reach immediately after using them, but this is not the surgeon's main priority. In this case it would be helpful for the surgical technologist to point out that the procedure would go more quickly and more smoothly if the used instruments were placed within reach. The surgeon may be unaware of this need or may not have thought about the effect of his or her work habits on achievement of the overall goal.

ROLE CONFUSION

Role confusion occurs when individuals are uncertain of what is expected of them. The following comments are common expressions of role confusion:

▶ "That's not *my* job."
▶ "I thought *you* were supposed to do that."
▶ "What am *I* supposed to do about that?"
▶ "No one told me that was part of *my* job description."

Most role confusion is a result of poor communication. Another common problem occurs when one person assigns a task to another who does not have the knowledge or time to complete the task. In cases of delegation, it is the responsibility of the person who delegates the job to evaluate the outcome and assist if help is needed. When a task is transferred from one person to another with the same qualifications, however, the person completing the task must have both the *freedom to work independently* and *the authority to carry out the task*. Never assign a task to someone else just to get rid of it yourself. Learn whether that person is qualified, is capable of doing the job, *and* has the time to do it. Always request a specific job description when beginning employment. When working on a team, ask for clarification of what is expected of each person. Do not give up responsibility for a task after you have accepted it. If you cannot complete it, you must pass the task to someone else who agrees and is qualified to complete it.

Conflict Resolution

The goal of conflict resolution is to attempt to find a solution that is acceptable to all parties. This is called a **win-win** solution. The other type of resolution is a **win-lose** solution, in which one party is satisfied but the other is not. This is not a satisfactory resolution because resentment and frustration will continue.

In a win-win resolution, both parties are satisfied with the result. The goal of conflict resolution is to find a win-win solution. This requires behaviors such as a nonbiased approach, flexibility, willingness to yield, and ability to focus on the problem, not the people.

The following are some steps for resolving conflicts:

▶ **When discussing the problem, try not to consider your personal opinion or bias about the situation.** Consider the *problem* and the objective (e.g., to provide smoother turnaround between cases).
▶ **Remain open-minded about solutions.** Do not get stuck on a single fact or solution.
▶ **Gather information about the problem before discussing it.** Then assess the information and how it relates to the problem.
▶ **View the problem as a group problem, not as your problem.** Even interpersonal conflict is a group problem because it affects everyone.
▶ **Brainstorm for solutions.** Offer suggestions without deep analysis. Brainstorming allows people to suggest creative or different solutions without fear of judgment.
▶ **Address any interpersonal conflicts in the group before other problems are solved.** Tension in the group competes for energy needed for other types of problem solving.
▶ **Formulate a plan for improvement** that includes necessary behaviors and rationale for changes.
▶ **Try to reach a win-win conclusion.** If such a conclusion is not reached, go back over the plan and evaluate whether concessions can be made to achieve a more satisfactory resolution.
▶ **Seek mediation** if the conflict cannot be resolved.

CASE STUDIES

Case 1

You have repeatedly been the victim of verbal abuse by one member of the surgical team. You avoid working with this person, as does almost everyone else. When you are assigned to work with her, you are tense and upset even before the case begins. How will you prepare yourself to work with this difficult person?

Case 2

In the situation described in the previous example, you have made repeated complaints to the operating room supervisor, who tells you that she can't really do anything about it. What steps will you take next?

Case 3

You are among six surgical technologists on an orthopedics team in a large hospital. The team leader is aggressive and rude to you. You feel that his technical expertise is lacking and that he was made team leader because of his relationships with the sales representatives. How will you handle your working relationship with this person? How can you reduce your own stress?

Case 4

You are a new employee in a large hospital operating room. You have been assigned a preceptor with whom you have difficulty working. You are not learning much because she

CASE STUDIES—cont'd

won't let you do anything except observe. When you tell her you would like to do more, she declares, "You're not ready to do anything—just watch." After several weeks the situation has not changed. What will you do?

Case 5

You are a student scrubbing in with your preceptor. When draping begins you reach for the drapes and he pushes you out of the way, saying, "Dr. X likes me to do this." What will you do?

REFERENCES

Cox H: Verbal abuse nationwide, part I: oppressed group behavior, *Nursing Management*, 22:2, Feb, 1991.

Cox H: Verbal abuse nationwide, part II: impact and modifications, *Nursing Management*, 22:3, March, 1991.

Maun C: Conflict management: what really works, *Surgical Services Management*, 6:6, June, 2000.

Patterson P: Verbal abuse most common problem, OR managers say, *OR Manager*, 12:12, Dec, 1996.

Thorsness R and Sayers B: Systems approach to resolving conduct issues among staff members, *AORN Journal*, 61:1, Jan, 1995.

Chapter 7

Microbiology
and the Process
of Infection

Terminology

Acquired immunity—Disease immunity established through cellular memory. Specific protein antigens cause the immune system to create protein antibodies. Antibodies initiate a cascade of host-protective mechanisms that destroy disease organisms when encountered at a later time.

Aerosol droplet—A droplet of moisture that is small enough to remain suspended in air and can carry microorganisms within it.

Antibiotic resistant—The ability of a microorganism to resist destruction by antimicrobial therapy. Antibiotic-resistant strains of microorganisms arise through genetic mutations induced by the use of antibiotics in animal feed, improper use of antimicrobial drugs, overprescription of antibiotics, and environmental factors.

Antibodies—Complex glycoproteins produced by the immune system, formed in response to antigens. An antibody makes contact with an antigen to destroy or control it.

Terminology—cont'd

Antigens—Macromolecules, such as proteins, glycoproteins, lipoproteins, and polysaccharides, on the surface of cells that identify them as part of the organism ("self") or foreign ("nonself"). Antigens can trigger a response by the immune system, which seeks out and destroys the marked cell. Surface antigens in bacteria include the flagellar (H), somatic (O), and capsular (K or Vi) antigens.

Bacteria (pl); Bacterium (sing)—Unicellular microorganisms with a rigid cell wall, classified with respect to motility, reaction to staining with particular dyes, and their pathogenicity for other living organisms including man. Bacteria are classified as belonging to one of the three domains: Bacteria, Archaea, and Eukarya. They are one of the two domains that are classified as prokaryotes (cells that lack nuclear membrane). All of the prokaryotes of medical importance are in the domain bacteria. They are categorized according to different staining techniques (Gram's stain or the acid fast stain) and fall into three categories: gram-positive bacteria, gram-negative bacteria, and acid-fast bacteria.

Colonization—The process of a group of bacteria living together.

Convalescence—The stage of disease in which damaged cells are repaired and the patient recovers from the effects of the illness or operation.

Cross-contamination—The transmission of microorganisms from one source to another.

Dehiscence—The separation of the layers of the surgical wound; it may be partial and superficial only, or complete, with disruption of all layers.

Direct transmission—The transfer of microbes from their source to a new host by direct physical contact, for example, exhalation by one individual of a water droplet containing respiratory virus and its inhalation by another.

Droplet nuclei—Dried remnants of previously moist secretions containing microorganisms. Droplet nuclei are an important source of disease transmission.

Endospore (spore)—The dormant stage of some bacteria that allows them to survive without reproducing in extreme environmental conditions, including heat, cold, and exposure to many disinfectants. When conditions are favorable for reproduction, the spore again becomes active and produces bacterial colonies.

Endotoxin—Bacterial toxin, associated with the outer membrane of certain gram-negative bacteria. Endotoxins are not secreted but are released when the cells are disrupted or broken down.

Evisceration—The protrusion of an internal organ through a wound or surgical incision.

Exotoxin—A toxic substance produced by microorganisms and excreted outside of the bacterial cell. Exotoxins differ in the particular tissues of the host that they may affect. Examples of these would be Pseudomonas and tetanus.

Fomite—An intermediate, inanimate source in the process of disease transmission. Any object such as a contaminated surgical instrument or medical device can become a fomite in disease transmission.

Gram stain—A method of differential staining of bacteria that separates them into one of two groups, gram-positive or gram-negative. Each group has common characteristics that identify its members and aid in diagnosis and treatment.

Host—The organism that harbors or nourishes another organism (parasite).

Indirect transmission—Transmission of microorganisms by an intermediate nonliving source, such as a nonsterile instrument or surgical implant (see *fomite*).

Infection—State or condition in which the body or body tissues are invaded by pathogenic microorganisms that multiply and produce injurious effects.

Inflammation—The body's nonspecific reaction to injury or infection that causes redness, heat, swelling, and pain.

Innate immunity—A nonspecific body response to foreign proteins, substances, tissues, viruses, or microorganisms. It includes the process of inflammation and vascular and cellular responses.

Nonpathogenic—Refers to an organism that does not cause disease in a healthy individual. About 95% to 97% of all bacteria are nonpathogenic.

Nosocomial infection—An infection that is acquired as a result of being in a hospital or other health-care facility.

Obligate aerobe—A microorganism that requires oxygen to live and grow.

Obligate anaerobe—An organism that must live in the absence of oxygen to survive.

Parasite—An organism that lives within, upon, or at the expense of another organism, known as the host, without contributing to the survival of the host.*

Pathogens—Disease-causing microorganisms.

Phagocyte—Any cell capable of ingesting particulate matter and microorganisms.

Portal of entry—In microbial transmission, the sites where microorganisms enter the body (e.g., an anatomic passage such as the nose or mouth, or the skin).

Prion—A protein-like microbe that is highly resistant to common sterilization methods. A common example of a prion-based illness is Creutzfeldt-Jakob disease.

Prodromal—Referring to the period between the first symptoms and the acute phase of a disease in the process of infection. Many diseases have prodromal symptoms specific to that disease, whereas in others the symptoms are more generalized.

Prokaryote—Cellular organism lacking a true nucleus or nuclear membrane. The microorganisms included in this classification are bacteria and blue-green algae.

*Venes D and Thomas CL, eds: *Taber's cyclopedic medical dictionary,* ed 19, Philadelphia, 2001, FA Davis.

Terminology—cont'd

Reservoir—In epidemiology, a possible source of disease transmission. A reservoir can be a person or an inanimate surface. For example, soil is a reservoir for tetanus bacteria. A health worker who sheds *Staphylococcus aureus* also is a reservoir of transmission.

Resident microorganisms—Also called normal flora, these are microorganisms that normally live in certain tissues of the body.

Retrovirus—A group of viruses whose genetic information is coded in RNA rather than in DNA. Human immunodeficiency virus is a retrovirus.

Standard Precautions—Guidelines recommended by the Centers for Disease Control and Prevention (CDC) to reduce risk of transmission of blood-borne and other pathogens.

Transient microorganisms—Organisms that do not normally live in the host tissue. Transient microorganisms are crowded out by resident flora, washed off, or find their new environment unsuitable for colonization. Infection can occur when the transient microorganism overwhelms the body's defenses.

Transmission—The transfer of microorganisms from one source to another.

Vector—A living intermediate carrier of microorganisms from one host to another. An example is the transmission of the bubonic plague. The vector is a flea, and the bacterium is transmitted to the human by a bite from an infected flea. Fleas may cause a similar disease in rodents.

Virulence—The degree to which a microorganism is capable of causing disease.

Virus—A genetic element containing either DNA or RNA that replicates in cells but is characterized by having an extracellular state. It is parasitic in that it is entirely dependent on nutrients inside cells for its metabolic and reproductive needs. They differ from other microbes in that they cannot reproduce their genetic material, but must produce within a living host.

INTRODUCTION TO MICROBIOLOGY AND THE PROCESS OF INFECTION

It is important to know not only how **infection** is transmitted, but how it is contracted and who is likely to succumb to an infection. The process of infection has been studied for centuries (Box 7-1). This chapter discusses important concepts related to disease **transmission** in the health-care setting. It is not intended to cover the broad field of microbiology. Rather, it focuses on the causes, consequences, results, and prevention of infectious diseases.

Microorganisms are minute organisms capable of reproduction that cannot be seen by the naked eye. Although there are many disease-producing organisms (called **pathogens**), those most commonly studied in the health-care environment are **bacteria, viruses,** and fungi. Bacteria, which are responsible for many diseases, grow in groups of multiple organisms. Their proliferation is often referred to as **colonization**.

An infection is the proliferation and growth of any microorganism or virus in any area of the body. Not all infections cause disease. An infection is harmful only if it causes an illness. Such an infection is an invasion in which the particular microorganisms attack or injure different areas of the body. Infectious diseases range from mild to lethal. The term **virulence** is used to describe the disease-evoking capability of a microorganism. A virulent microorganism is one that has a high potential to cause disease.

Disease is a state of altered health. There are many different sources of disease, such as genetic mutation, the environment, and stress. The disease can be *localized* (confined to one area of the body) or *systemic* (spread throughout the body by the bloodstream and lymphatic system). Infectious diseases are categorized by the period of time they are present in the body. A *chronic* disease is a long-term disease. If inflicted with a *persistent* disease, the body's immune system is unable to completely eliminate the microorganism, although the disease may not be active at all times. An *acute* infection

Box 7-1   Important Events in the History of Microbiology

1677: Anton van Leeuwenhoek develops the light microscope and observes "little animals" under magnification.

1796: Edward Jenner develops the first smallpox vaccination.

1850: Ignaz Semmelweis discovers the association between handwashing and a decrease in puerperal infection.

1861: Louis Pasteur disproves the theory of spontaneous generation and develops the germ theory of infection.

1867: Joseph Lister first practices surgery using antiseptic practices.

1876: Robert Koch offers the first proof of the germ theory using *Bacillus anthracis*.

1882: Robert Koch develops the **Koch postulates.** Paul Ehrlich develops the acid-fast stain.

1884: Christian Gram develops the Gram stain.

1885: Louis Pasteur develops the first rabies vaccine.

1892: Dimitri Iosifovich Ivanovski discovers the virus.

1900: Walter Reed proves that mosquitoes carry yellow fever.

1910: Paul Ehrlich discovers a cure for syphilis.

1928: Alexander Fleming discovers penicillin.

1995: The first microbe genome sequence (for *Haemophilus influenzae*) is published.

is an infection with a sudden onset and may be brief or prolonged.

MICROBE-HOST RELATIONSHIPS

Biological advances in the last decade have led to a new understanding of how microorganisms interact with the human body to cause disease. The traditional model described organisms as beneficial, neutral, or harmful. We now understand that the microbe-host relationship changes according to specific conditions. These include the following:

1. The number of microbes in the body (called the dose).
2. The physiologic environment in the body, such as the pH, temperature, amount of moisture, pressure, or presence of chemicals or immune proteins.
3. The location of entry into the body (called the **portal of entry**).
4. The strength of the body's immune system, which determines the body's ability to recognize and destroy harmful organisms.
5. The disease-producing potential of the bacteria, known as its virulence. Virulence depends on the following:
   ▶ The number of pathogenic microorganisms that have penetrated the body.
   ▶ The pathogen's ability to adhere to the target tissue and secrete enzymes that destroy the target cells.
   ▶ The pathogen's ability to evade the body's defense system by chemical or physical means, or by mutation.

The process by which organisms of two different species live together is called symbiosis. If neither organism is harmed, the association is called commensalism; if the association is of benefit to both, it is mutualism; and if one is harmed and the other benefited, it is parasitism.

Parasitism

A **parasite** is an organism that lives on or within another organism (the **host**) and causes it harm. The human immunodeficiency virus (HIV), which causes acquired immunodeficiency syndrome (AIDS), is an obligate intracellular parasite that invades the human cell and "instructs" the T-helper leukocyte cell's (white blood cell's) DNA to changes its transcription. HIV expends nearly all of its energy on reproduction because the host meets its metabolic requirements, with tragic consequences. Some parasites, like viruses, depend completely on the host for survival, whereas others have a less dependent or more flexible relationship with the host.

Only about 3% to 5% of all microorganisms are defined as pathogenic (causing disease under most circumstances). However, **nonpathogenic** microbes (those that do not usually cause disease) that live in and on the body can *become* pathogenic when the dose, the portal of entry, or the environment changes. When this occurs, the microorganism is described as opportunistic. A compromised host is a person whose body is weakened metabolically or physically, such as

by preexisting disease. Compromised patients are particularly at risk for infection.

Commensalism

In commensalism, one organism uses another to meet its physiologic needs but causes its host no harm. For example, the human intestinal tract contains many different types of bacteria that are essential for the body's metabolism, such as *Escherichia coli (E. coli).* The bacteria survive in physiologic balance as long as they remain in the intestine. If *E. coli* enters the sterile tissues of the body, however, such as when the bowel is perforated by trauma or disease, the result can be deadly. When it is in the bloodstream, *E. coli* bacteria destroy vital organs and can cause death very quickly. This is an example of how a change in the environment of a **bacterium** changes its relationship with the host from commensal to parasitic.

Mutualism

In mutualism, both organisms benefit from the relationship. For example, vaginal lactobacilli create an acidic environment, which discourages the growth of bacteria that prefer a higher pH. Both the human and the lactobacilli benefit. If the environment changes, however, such as under hormonal influence when the pH of the vaginal tissue increases, the lactobacilli reproduce in large numbers, causing disease.

TYPES OF MICROORGANISMS

The binomial classification system differentiates microorganisms (microscopic entities that reproduce independently of a host) into two groups—**prokaryotes** and eukaryotes. Prokaryotes are all bacteria and archaea (prokaryotes that live in extreme conditions). Eukaryotes include the protozoa, fungi, arthropods, and helminths. Eukaryotic and prokaryotic cells are illustrated in Figure 7-1. Bacteria and viruses cause most infectious diseases that affect humans. This chapter focuses mostly on these agents and on other microorganisms significant in the health-care setting.

Bacteria

Bacteria are single-celled organisms that have no nucleus or specific metabolic organelles. Each bacterium is surrounded by a single wall, bilayer, or unit membrane made up of phospholipids. Some bacteria also produce an extracellular capsule that resists destruction of the bacteria by the host. Capsules are virulence factors because they may protect successful phagocytosis. The interior cytoplasm contains the genetic material and substances needed for cell reproduction and metabolism. Bacteria synthesize both DNA and RNA. The genetic material is contained in a single chromosome that is coiled inside the cell (Figure 7-2). Extrachromosomal circular DNA material called plasmids also is located within the cytoplasm. Plasmids replicate inside the bacterial cell but are not necessary for reproduction of the bacterial cell itself. Bacteria require a host to meet their nutritional and environmental needs.

Prokaryote

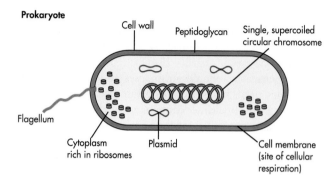

Eukaryote

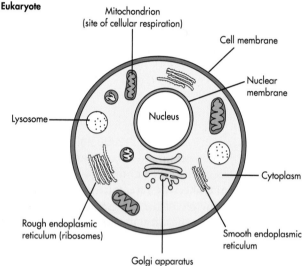

FIGURE 7-1
Prokaryote and eukaryote cells. (From Murray PR et al: *Medical microbiology,* ed 4, St Louis, 2002, Mosby.)

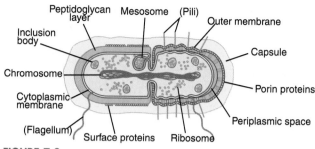

FIGURE 7-2
Diagrammatic structure of a generalized bacterium. (Modified from Murray PR et al: *Medical microbiology,* ed 4, St Louis, 2002, Mosby.)

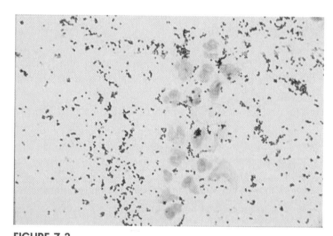

FIGURE 7-3
Gram stain of pus from patient with a wound infected with *Staphylococcus aureus.* (From Hart T, Shears P: *Color atlas of medical microbiology,* London, 2000, Mosby.)

Bacteria are partially identified by their structure. The study of form and structure is called morphology. There are three separate forms or shapes of bacteria:

▶ spherical (cocci)
▶ rod-shaped (bacilli)
▶ spiral or curved (spiral forms)

In addition, each type of bacteria may group together in a particular way, such as in small clusters or long chains.

Upon **Gram staining,** certain bacteria retain the stain (gram-positive bacteria) while others do not (gram-negative bacteria). The Gram staining procedure requires two dyes: crystal violet as the primary stain and safranin as the counter stain. Under the microscope, gram-positive bacteria appear dark purple, and gram-negative bacteria are pink (Figure 7-3). The nature of the bacterial cell membrane determines the bacterium's Gram stain classification and its response to specific antibiotics. Antibiotics are described as effective against gram-negative organisms, gram-positive organisms, or both types of bacteria. Gram staining reveals the shape of individual bacteria and aids in identification.

Bacilli are rod shaped and occur singly or in pairs, chains, or filaments. Examples of pathogenic bacilli and the diseases

they cause are *Mycobacterium tuberculosis* (tuberculosis), *Clostridium perfringens* (gas gangrene), and *E. coli* (tissue and organ necrosis).

Spirochetes are curved or spiral shaped. Pathogens in this group include *Treponema pallidum* (syphilis) and *Vibrio cholerae* (cholera).

Cocci are spherical bacteria that occur singly (micrococci), in chains (streptococci), in pairs (diplococci), or in clusters (staphylococci). Examples of pathogenic cocci are *Streptococcus pneumoniae* (pneumonia) and *Neisseria gonorrhoeae* (gonorrhea).

Tail-like appendages called flagella allow bacilli and spirochetes to move freely in their environment. The cocci are incapable of independent movement.

Flagella are responsible for bacterial motility and can help certain bacteria cause disease. In gastric ulcers, *Helicobacter pylori* uses its powerful flagella to penetrate the viscous mucous coating of the stomach lining.

Pili are shorter than flagella and function in twitching and gliding motility, in transferring DNA between cells, and in attaching bacterial cells to the surface lining of epithelial cells. Some *E. coli* have adhesives that attach to receptors on the surface of the epithelial cells lining the small intestine, causing a severe watery diarrhea. These pili are called fimbriae.

A bacterium reproduces through a process known as binary fission in which the cell simply splits apart. Before undergoing this process, however, the bacterium must duplicate its genetic material. Genetic material can be transferred from one bacterium to another and from bacteria to virus to bacteria. All of these evolutionary adaptations improve the bacteria's ability to survive. The bacterial **endospore** (commonly called a spore) is a vegetative or dormant phase in the reproductive cycle of some bacteria. In this stage, the bacteria form a thick, multilayered protein wall around their genetic material. This wall resists extreme environmental conditions such as boiling, drying, chemical destruction, and high pressure. When environmental conditions are favorable, the spore becomes active and begins normal colonization. Examples of bacteria that form endospores are *Clostridium tetani* (tetanus) and *Bacillus anthracis* (anthrax). Any method used to sterilize an object must be capable of destroying spores. This is the highest standard for all sterilization processes.

Bacteria are capable of surviving in hospitable environments. Important environmental parameters for reproduction include temperature, oxygen level, pH, moisture, and atmospheric pressure. Bacteria are ubiquitous in the natural world, living under a wide variety of conditions. Those that reproduce in humans generally require more moderate conditions. Some bacteria can produce a spore form that resists extreme conditions like temperature ranges of −20 to 90 degrees Celsius. Archaea that closely resemble bacteria in size and shape have not been reported to cause disease in man or animals. Archaea live under extreme conditions such as high-salt, low-pH, and high-temperature environments. Archaea bacteria can be found in frozen environments, thermal hot springs, high-salt areas of an ocean, and decaying organic matter.

Oxygen requirements for bacteria vary widely. An **obligate aerobe** is a microorganism that needs oxygen to live and grow. An **obligate anaerobe** does not require oxygen for reproduction. Some anaerobes can live in the presence of varying concentrations of environmental oxygen, while others are very sensitive to any amount. The latter are called strict anaerobes. The significance of anaerobes in infection is their ability to proliferate in deep traumatic or surgical wounds. Facultative anaerobes can reproduce with or without environmental oxygen.

The normal pH in the body increases its resistance to invading microorganisms, while a change in pH can destroy defensive resident flora and allow pathogens to proliferate. However, bacteria have evolved to withstand both ends of the pH spectrum. For example, the normal pH of blood is between 7.35 and 7.45. Another example is the pH of *Helicobacter pylori*, which can invade the gastric mucosa and reproduce at a pH of 2.

Bacteria that are significant in infectious disease prefer a moist environment. One method of destroying bacteria is desiccation (drying). Desiccation is used for preservation of bacteria as well as for destruction. Resistance to drying makes bacteria such as myobacteria a public health problem, because it can spread through dried sputum.

Bacteria are not usually subjected to extremes of barometric pressure. However, pressure is a critical parameter in ensuring their destruction in the hospital setting. The spore form of bacteria can withstand very high pressure and temperature. All critical medical devices must undergo a sterilization process that kills spores. This includes steam under high pressure (see Chapter 8).

Pathogenic Microorganisms

The following section describes some major groups of pathogenic microorganisms and the diseases they cause. The pathogens discussed represent the most common forms and those seen most often in the hospital setting. Table 7-1 lists specific organisms and their associated diseases.

PYOGENIC BACTERIAL INFECTIONS

Bacteria that cause infection are termed pyogenic. Included in this group are streptococcal, staphylococcal, meningococcal, pneumococcal, and gonocococcal organisms, and the coliform (intestinal) bacilli. These organisms typically cause suppuration and tissue destruction and may lead to systemic involvement, resulting in death.

STAPHYLOCOCCAL INFECTIONS

Staphylococcal bacteria are bacteria commonly carried in the skin.

Staphylococcus aureus

Staphylococcus aureus (S. aureus) is the most widespread cause of surgical site infections. It is a gram-positive resident bacterium of the skin transmitted to the surgical wound by direct or indirect contact with a health worker, contaminated object, or another patient. *S. aureus* can easily invade the circulatory system from the skin or upper respiratory tract and spread throughout the body. From 30% to 70% of people are skin carriers and 30% to 50% are nasal carriers of *S. aureus*. The organism causes endocarditis when it colonizes heart valves and osteomyelitis when it invades bone. When confined to the surgical wound itself, it produces copious amounts of pus, which spreads and erodes tissues. *S. aureus* is also responsible for causing boils, carbuncles, and abscesses.

Methicillin-resistant *S. aureus* is a separate strain of *S. aureus* that is **antibiotic resistant** to penicillin (the drug usually used to fight a *Staphylococcus* infection). Emergence of a new semi–antibiotic resistant strain, vancomycin-intermediate-resistant *S. aureus,* may eventually result in evolution of complete vancomycin antibiotic resistance as well. Superinfections with these organisms are increasingly common in the hospital environment. Identifying the cause of antibiotic-resistant strains is a major goal of health-care providers.

Table 7-1A GRAM-POSITIVE COCCI

Organism	Major Infection	Less Common Infection	Vaccine Preventable	Incubation Period	Period of Inactivity
Staphylococci					
S. epidermidis	Bacteremia in immuno-compromised	Most often associated with indwelling devices	No		
S. saprophyticus	Urinary tract infections		No		
S. aureus	Boils, impetigo, wound infections, osteomyelitis, septicemia	Pneumonia, endocarditis, toxic shock syndrome, food poisoning	No		
Micrococcus	Occasional contaminant of clinical specimens.				
Streptococci					
a) Beta hemolytic					
S. pyogenes (group A)	Tonsillitis, impetigo, cellulitis, scarlet fever (rheumatic fever, glomerulonephritis)	Puerperal sepsis, erysipelas, septicemia	No	1-3 days	
S. agalactiae (group B)	Neonatal sepsis	Puerperal sepsis, osteomyelitis	No		
S. zooepidemicus (group C)	Bacteremia		No		
b) Alpha hemolytic					
S. pneumoniae	Pneumonia, otitis media	Meningitis, septicemia	Yes (some serotypes)		
S. viridans	Dental caries	Subacute bacterial endocarditis	No		
c) Group D streptococci					
S. faecalis (enterococci) (Enterococcus faecalis)	Urinary tract infections, wound infections, intraabdominal abscess	Bacteremia, endocarditis	No		
S. bovis	Endocarditis, bacteremia		No		
Other streptococci					
S. milleri	Intraabdominal sepsis, wound infections, brain abscess		No		

Sources and Transmission of Bacteria

Organism	Reservoir			Transmission				Comments
	Man	Animal	Environ	Fecal/oral	Droplet	Direct	Nosocomial	
Staphylococcus epidermidis	+					+	+	
S. saprophyticus	+					+		
S. aureus	+	+	±	+	+	+	+	Methicillin-resistant strains are important hospital problem
Micrococci	+		+			+	±	
Streptococcus pyogenes	+				+	+	+	

Table 7-1A   GRAM-POSITIVE COCCI—cont'd

Sources and Transmission of Bacteria

Organism	Reservoir			Transmission				Comments
	Man	Animal	Environ	Fecal/oral	Droplet	Direct	Nosocomial	
S. agalactiae	+				+	+		
S. zooepidemicus	+	+		+	±			Outbreaks have resulted from unpasteurized milk
S. pneumoniae	+				+			Penicillin-resistant strains increasing
S. viridans	+				+/	+		
E. fecalis	+					+	+	Occasional vancomycin-resistant strains
S. bovis	+	+				+		
S. milleri	+					+	+	

From Hart T, Shears P: *Color atlas of medical microbiology,* London, 2000, Mosby.

Table 7-1B   GRAM-NEGATIVE COCCI AND COCCOBACILLI

Infections

Organism	Major Infection	Less Common Infection	Vaccine Preventable	Incubation Period	Period of Inactivity
Neisseria					
N. meningitidis (13 serogroups)	Meningitis, septicemia	Arthritis	Yes (serogroups A/C)	2-10 days	Until 24 hours after Rifampicin (rifampin) prophylaxis
N. gonorrhoeae	Gonorrhea, pelvic inflammatory disease	Arthritis, conjunctivitis	No	2-7 days	Months if untreated
Moraxella					
M. catarrhalis	Pneumonia	Conjunctivitis, otitis media	No		
M. lacunata	Conjunctivitis		No		
Francisella					
F. tularensis	Tularemia		Yes	2-10 days	Not directly transmitted

Sources and Transmission of Bacteria

Organism	Reservoir			Transmission					Comments
	Man	Animal	Environ	Insect	Fecal/oral	Droplet	Direct	Nosocomial	
Neisseria meningitidis	+					+			Epidemics of serogroup A occur in Africa
N. gonorrhoeae	+						+		Penicillin-resistant strains increasing
Moraxella catarrhalis	+					+			
M. lacunata	+						+		
Francisella tularensis		+	+	+	+	+	+		Category III pathogen

From Hart T, Shears P: *Color atlas of medical microbiology,* London, 2000, Mosby.

Continued

Table 7-1C AEROBIC GRAM-POSITIVE BACILLI

Organism	Major Infection	Less Common Infection	Vaccine Preventable	Incubation Period	Period of Inactivity
		Infections			
a) Spore forming					
Bacillus					
B. anthracis	Anthrax		(Yes)	2-5 days	
B. cereus	Food poisoning	Wound infections, endocarditis	No		
b) Non-spore forming					
Listeria					
L. monocytogenes	Neonatal sepsis, meningitis	Septicemia in immuno-compromised	No	No	3 days to 3 weeks
Corynebacterium					
C. diphtheriae	Diphtheria	Skin infections	Yes	2-5 days	Up to 4 weeks
C. urealyticum	Cystitis				
C. jeikeium	Infection associated with prosthetic devices and intravenous or CSF catheters		No		
Erysipelothrix					
E. rhusiopathiae	Erysipeloid	Bacteremia, endocarditis	No		
Lactobacillus spp.		Rarely associated with endocarditis, abscesses	No		

From Hart T, Shears P: *Color atlas of medical microbiology,* London, 2000, Mosby.

Staphylococcus albus

Staphylococcus albus is a harmless resident bacterium often found on the hands. However, in a person in a debilitated or weakened condition, *S. albus* may become opportunistic and pathogenic.

Staphylococcus epidermis

Staphylococcus epidermidis is an opportunistic pathogen that is commonly spread by means of medical devices such as catheters, prosthetic valves, and artificial joints. Although it is a normal resident of the skin, it can cause serious disease when it penetrates the body and enters sterile tissue. It is often multidrug resistant.

STREPTOCOCCAL INFECTIONS

The streptococci cause several clinically significant infections. The lesions of a streptococcal infection appear as watery, blood-stained abscesses. The streptococci are responsible for diseases such as rheumatic fever, impetigo, bacterial endocarditis, tonsillitis leading to otitis media, and severe postoperative wound infection. Transmission is by direct contact with a contaminated source, by droplet, and by dust particles.

Streptococcus pyogenes

Many nosocomial streptococcal infections are caused by *Streptococcus pyogenes* (Group A Beta Hemolytic streptococ-

cus). These potentially lethal pathogens cause surgical site infection and can spread via the lymphatic system to other sites in the body, causing anaerobic cellulitis (infection of the subcutaneous tissue) and tissue necrosis. Toxic enzymes produced by the bacteria facilitate the spread of infection. Burn patients also are particularly susceptible to streptococcal infection. *Streptococcus pyogenes* is normally found in the upper respiratory tract and skin. Surgical site infection is most commonly caused by **direct transmission.**

Streptococci are responsible for other serious diseases such as scarlet fever, rheumatic heart disease, and upper respiratory tract infection. *S. pyogenes* is referred to as a flesh-eating bacterium because it produces an enzyme called hyaluronidase or "spreading factor" that breaks down hyaluronic acid, the substance that holds human cells together.

COLIFORM BACTERIAL INFECTIONS

The coliform bacteria normally reside in the intestines of healthy persons, where they cause no harm. If, however, they are released from the bowel, as during rupture or injury of the intestine, severe peritonitis or other localized, suppurative infections may result.

Escherichia coli

Escherichia coli (E. coli) is a gram-negative resident flora of the gastrointestinal tract. It is the third most frequent cause of surgical site infections. Contamination generally occurs by **indirect transmission** via a contaminated object such as a urinary endoscope or catheter. Direct transmission occurs when the gastrointestinal tract is entered purposefully or accidentally during surgery and bowel contents spill into the sterile peritoneal cavity. Because of the close proximity of the urinary meatus to the lower gastrointestinal tract, especially in females, *E. coli* is the most frequent cause of urinary tract infection. In the bloodstream *E. coli* can seed to other organs and cause severe tissue destruction.

Pseudomonas aeruginosa

Pseudomonas aeruginosa (*P. aeruginosa*) is an aerobic gram-negative organism found in the normal gastrointestinal tract and in sewage, dirt, and water. It has emerged as an increasingly important pathogen affecting patients. It can infect nearly all body systems. Burn patients are particularly susceptible to *Pseudomonas* infection. It can cause septicemia (systemic vascular infection), osteomyelitis (bone infection), urinary tract infection, and endocarditis (infection of the membrane lining the heart). Patients are infected by direct or indirect contact with the bacteria in their environment. The bacteria are resistant to antibacterial agents and are controlled only with several powerful drugs, most of which are toxic in doses large enough to eradicate the disease from the body. Some strains of *P. aeruginosa* are drug resistant.

Klebsiella

Klebsiella are opportunistic gram-negative organisms that usually cause disease only in a compromised host. They are a frequent cause of nosocomial urinary, pulmonary, and wound infections.

The medically significant *Klebsiella* are:

- *K. oxytoca:* Urinary tract infections, bacteremia in babies
- *K. ozaenae:* Chronic diseases of the respiratory tract
- *K. pneumoniae:* Infections of the respiratory tract and urinary tract infections
- *K. rhinoscleromatis:* Found exclusively in patients with rhinoscleroma and their contacts
- *K. planticola:* Septicemia
- *K. serratia:* Infections of the endocardium, blood, wounds, and urinary and respiratory tracts in immunosuppressed patients

The spread of *Klebsiella serratia* and *Klebsiella pneumoniae* is controlled by following strict aseptic technique and proper handwashing.

ANAEROBIC BACTERIAL INFECTIONS

Anaerobic bacteria are those that can live in an oxygen-free environment. Most anaerobic bacteria are spore forming and may normally reside in the intestine of the healthy person. These bacteria often are found in soil, a significant factor for the patient who has suffered injury in the presence of dirt.

Clostridium perfringens

Gas gangrene, initiated by the bacillus *Clostridium perfringens*, is the result of a complex process aided by the presence of other clostridial organisms. This relatively rare disease must not be confused with the type of gangrene caused by vascular insufficiency, which results in the necrosis of an organ or limb. (For example, we often refer to a "gangrenous" foot or leg seen in cases of severe atherosclerosis, where major blood vessels are so occluded with plaque that they are unable to transport blood to the lower limbs.)

In true gas gangrene, the injured tissues of the wound are destroyed by the toxins of the *C. perfringens* bacillus. The *C. novyi* bacilli, another type, invade the necrotic tissue and release toxic gases within the tissue, and absorption of these gases leads to death. The disease is transmitted directly from a contaminated substance to an open or penetrating wound.

Clostridium tetani

Tetanus (commonly called "lockjaw") is primarily a disease of the nervous system caused by the bacillus *Clostridium tetani*. The toxins released by this bacillus travel along the peripheral nerve pathways, eventually reaching the central nervous system. Painful muscle spasms, convulsions, and eventual involvement of the respiratory system lead to death from asphyxia. The bacillus is commonly found in soil and in the normal intestinal tract. Transmission is through direct contact of the bacillus with an open or penetrating wound.

Clostridium difficile

Clostridium difficile is a gram-positive anaerobic rod. It is spore forming and causes antibiotic-associated diarrhea. It is easily spread among patients who are compromised, and the infection can be rapidly fatal. Strict attention to **standard precautions** (see Chapter 14) is needed to control its spread in the health-care setting.

MYCOBACTERIAL INFECTIONS

The bacillus *Mycobacterium tuberculosis* is the cause of the disease tuberculosis. There are two strains of the bacteria, the human strain and the bovine (i.e., deer and cow) strain. The human strain causes dense nodules or tubercles to form in localized areas of the body, including the liver, spleen, and bone marrow. Lung involvement occurs in all cases, and the lung is the organ most affected by the disease.

Mycobacterium tuberculosis

Tuberculosis is a serious concern in public health and health-care facilities. Multidrug-resistant strains of *Mycobacterium tuberculosis* are increasingly common throughout the world. Tuberculosis kills about 3 million people and infects about 9 million every year worldwide. The organism primarily causes a respiratory disease, but it also can infect other areas of the body, including vital organs. Infection is spread by inhalation of the bacteria in **aerosol droplet** or dust containing dried mycobacteria. It can be introduced into the body via medical equipment such as respiratory diagnostic equipment or anesthesia equipment.

After the bacteria have entered the respiratory system, they are engulfed by macrophages. The bacteria are detectable in the body by intradermal injection of purified protein derivative of the tuberculosis bacteria. The injection site becomes erythematous (reddened) and puffy within 72

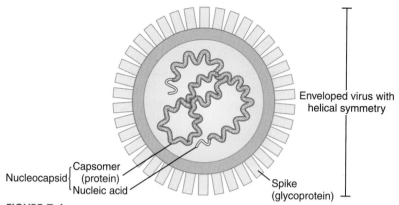

FIGURE 7-4
Nucleocapsid. (Redrawn from Bergquist L and Pogosian B: *Microbiology: principles and health science applications*, Philadelphia, 2000, Saunders.)

hours. Those mycobacteria that are not destroyed by phagocytosis become encased in granular tubercles that remain in the lungs. These heal but become calcified and fibrotic. If the infected person becomes immunocompromised or weakened through disease (such as AIDS), the bacteria again become active and cause serious disease. The treatment for tuberculosis requires prolonged therapy with multiple drugs for a minimum of 6 months to 1 year. However, there is currently no cure for tuberculosis caused by some multidrug-resistant strains.

Viruses

Viruses are nonliving infectious agents ranging in size from 10 to 300 nm. They are the smallest obligate intracellular pathogen (pathogen found within the cell of another organism). A complete virus particle is called a virion (enveloped virus) and consists of a double or single strand of either DNA or RNA, but never both. This genetic material is surrounded by a protein coat (capsid) made up of protein molecules. The total structure is called a nucleocapsid (Figure 7-4). Depending on the type of virus, the nucleocapsid can take on many different complex geometric shapes.

Although viruses contain genetic material, they cannot replicate without a host cell. To replicate, they inject their DNA or RNA into the host cell and break apart the cell's genetic material. The virus then uses the host cell's physiologic mechanisms to replicate its own genetic material, synthesize new capsids, and assemble new virions. When the host cell ruptures, the newly formed virions are released (Figure 7-5). The host cell also may slowly release the virus particles over time. This is known as a persistent infection. Not all viruses destroy the host cell. Some remain inside the host cell in latent form. In this state the virus is not infective but it continues to replicate. Then, under certain conditions favorable to the virus, it begins to replicate more actively and produces disease symptoms, perhaps years later. Examples of viruses that follow this cycle are herpes simplex virus and poliovirus. Viruses also may be oncogenic, meaning they can cause tumors.

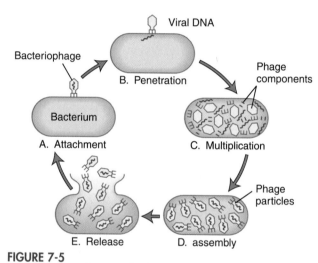

FIGURE 7-5
Stages in the infection of a host's cell and replication of a virus. (Redrawn from Bergquist L and Pogosian B: *Microbiology: principles and health science applications*, Philadelphia, 2000, Saunders.)

Blood-Borne Pathogens

Blood-borne pathogens are a direct threat to hospitalized patients and all health-care personnel. Because of the high risk of transmission through contact with blood and body fluids, the CDC has developed strict protocols for handling patients, medical waste, body fluids, and soiled equipment in the hospital environment. These protocols are called Standard Precautions. All employees are required to follow Standard Precautions. These precautions can be found in Chapter 14. Exposure to blood-borne pathogens in the workplace requires immediate attention. The CDC produces guidelines for management of exposure based on the type of exposure and the nature of the pathogen. These guidelines also are found in Chapter 14.

In the health-care setting, HIV, a **retrovirus,** and other viral blood-borne pathogens such as hepatitis virus are health risks to patients and health-care workers.

Box 7-2 Global and National HIV Statistics and Estimates

Worldwide Statistics

▶ There are 40 million people living with HIV/AIDS.

▶ AIDS is the leading cause of death in Africa and the fourth leading cause of death worldwide.

▶ In 2001, there were 3 million AIDS deaths and 5 million HIV infections worldwide.

Kaiser Global Projections

▶ 45 million HIV infections by the year 2010 (two-thirds could be prevented).

▶ Cumulative death toll could reach 100 million by 2020.

▶ Falling life expectancy, reversing steady gains over the last century. By 2010, life expectancy could drop below 30 years in some countries.

▶ More than 25 million children under the age of 15 likely will lose one or both parents to AIDS by 2010.

▶ The number of young people ages 15-24 living with HIV/AIDS could rise from a current estimate of 12.4 million to 21.5 million in 2010.

United States Estimates

▶ Almost 1 million Americans living with HIV/AIDS.

▶ 40,000 new infections in 2001, holding constant for more than a decade.

▶ Close to half a million AIDS-related deaths in the U.S. to date.

▶ Leading cause of death for African Americans, ages 25 to 44; fourth leading cause of death for Latins in this age group.

▶ Half of the new infections in the United States are among teens and young adults.

▶ As many as one third of people infected with HIV do not know it.

Data from the Catholic Relief Services, www.catholicrelief.org.

HUMAN IMMUNODEFICIENCY VIRUS (HIV)

Human immunodeficiency virus (HIV) is a retrovirus that attacks and destroys the immune system T-helper leukocytes. It is the cause of acquired immunodeficiency syndrome (AIDS). See Box 7-2 for global and national HIV statistics and estimates.

HIV infection has been associated with certain social and economic groups, and historically the victims have received little sympathy. The global effect of AIDS has changed practices and procedures in health care dramatically. The care of individuals who are stricken with HIV requires our utmost ethical and humanitarian consideration. To give less is to deny our commitment to alleviate the suffering of all people, regardless of the nature or cause of that suffering.

HIV is transmitted via blood-to-blood contact, sexual contact, and contact with certain body fluids. The following fluids are known to transmit HIV:

▶ Blood
▶ Semen
▶ Vaginal secretions
▶ Breast milk
▶ Cerebrospinal fluid
▶ Synovial fluid
▶ Amniotic fluid
▶ Any body fluid containing blood

HIV is transmitted when the body fluids of an infected person are deposited onto the mucous membranes or into the vascular system of another person. Sexual contact and use of contaminated needles are primary modes of transmission in the general public. The risk of transmission during sexual contact increases when partners also are infected with another sexually transmitted disease. Transmission through the transfusion of whole blood, plasma, platelets, or blood cells presents a small risk (1% in adults, 5% in children). HIV can be transmitted to the fetus in utero and to the infant who receives breast milk from an infected mother. A neonate also may be infected during the process of labor and delivery.

Casual contact with an infected person does not transmit the virus. Although HIV has been found in saliva, tears, and sweat, the number of pathogens found in these body fluids has been very small. Contact with these fluids has *not* been shown to result in the transmission of HIV.

Occupational risk to health-care workers is highest in needle-stick and other sharps injuries. There is little risk of transmission from an infected health-care worker to a patient, unless an infected health-care worker has a needle stick during a procedure.

HIV genetic information is carried in RNA rather than DNA. When the virus is transmitted, it attacks a specific type of lymphocyte called CD4 lymphocytes (CD4 cells) or T helper lymphocytes (T cells). This lymphocyte is necessary for the immune system to recognize foreign **antigens** and to activate other lymphocytes (B lymphocytes), which produce **antibodies.** As HIV disease progresses, increasing numbers of CD4 or T cells are killed, which releases more virus into the bloodstream (recall that viruses need a host cell to survive). Gradually the number of CD4 or T cells declines until the infected person is no longer protected from microorganisms or cancer cells.

A person with HIV infection may be asymptomatic (not exhibiting symptoms) yet still transmit the disease to others. This is because early in the disease process the body's immune system is able to attack the virus. As long as the person is not tested, he or she may continue to transmit the disease to others without realizing that he or she is infected. Weeks after the initial infection, mild illness occurs, followed by increasingly serious disease manifestations. Years may pass before symptoms of AIDS begin to appear. The conversion

Box 7-3 Opportunistic Infections and Tumors in AIDS

Viruses

▶ Disseminated cytomegalovirus (lungs, retina, brain)
▶ Herpes simplex virus (lungs, gastrointestinal tract, CNS, skin)
▶ JC papovavirus (brain: progressive multifocal leukoencephalopathy)
▶ Epstein-Barr virus (EBV) (tongue or buccal mucosa: hairy leukoplakia)

Bacteria*

▶ Mycobacteria (e.g., *Mycoplasma avium, Mycobacterium tuberculosis:* disseminated, extrapulmonary)
▶ *Salmonella* (recurrent, disseminated; septicemia)

Protozoa

▶ *Toxoplasma gondii* (disseminated, including CNS)
▶ *Cryptosporidium* (gastrointestinal tract: chronic diarrhea)
▶ *Isospora* (gastrointestinal tract: diarrhea, persisting longer than 1 month)

Fungi

▶ *Pneumocystis carinii* (lungs: pneumonia)
▶ *Candida albicans* (esophagus, lung)
▶ *Cryptococcus neoformans* (CNS)
▶ *Histoplasma capsulatum* (disseminated, extrapulmonary)
▶ *Coccidioides* (disseminated, extrapulmonary)

Tumors

▶ Kaposi sarcoma[†]
▶ B-cell lymphoma (e.g., brain; some are EBV induced)

Other

▶ Wasting disease (cause unknown)
▶ HIV encephalopathy (AIDS dementia complex)

Data from Mims C et al: *Medical microbiology,* ed 2, London, 1998, Mosby.
AIDS, acquired immunodeficiency syndrome; *CNS,* central nervous system; *HIV,* human immunodeficiency virus.
*Also pyogenic bacteria (e.g., *Haemophilus, Streptococcus, Pneumococcus*) causing septicemia, pneumonia, meningitis, osteomyelitis, arthritis, abscesses, etc.; multiple or recurrent infections, especially in children.
[†]Associated with human herpesvirus 8, an independently transmitted agent; 300 times more common in AIDS than in other immunodeficiency conditions.

from HIV infection to AIDS-related complex to AIDS is poorly understood. HIV infection is confirmed by the presence of specific antibodies.

AIDS is not a separate disease organism but a syndrome that results from infection with the HIV virus. The AIDS patient lacks normal immune response, and certain diseases are common in this population. A true diagnosis of AIDS is made when the presence of one or more of these diseases is confirmed (Box 7-3). There is currently no cure for AIDS. For extensive information about AIDS and its treatment, contact the Centers for Disease Control and Prevention (CDC).

VIRAL HEPATITIS

Hepatitis is a disease of the liver that is caused by one of three significant viruses. Hepatitis A, B, and C are significant in the hospital setting.

Hepatitis A Virus

Hepatitis A virus is transmitted by ingestion and by close contact with an infected person. Fecal and oral routes are the common modes of transmission. This virus cannot be cultured, but hepatitis can be diagnosed through a serologic test that shows the presence of antibodies to hepatitis A virus. This disease is rarely fatal, and one infection causes permanent immunity to the disease.

Hepatitis B Virus (HBV)

Infection with the hepatitis B virus (HBV) causes chronic hepatitis, cirrhosis, and massive liver necrosis. Each year about 200,000 to 300,000 new cases of hepatitis B and 1 million to 1.25 million new HBV carriers appear in the United States. Hepatitis B is responsible for 4000 to 5000 deaths per year. Like HIV, HBV is transmitted through blood and body fluids and represents a threat to both patients and health-care personnel. It can be spread by oral or sexual contact and is found in most body secretions. Infected mothers also pass it to infants in 70% to 90% of births. Infected infants have a 90% chance of becoming chronic carriers.

The incubation period of HBV is 10 to 12 weeks, during which time the virus can be detected through serologic testing. The disease has three phases: preicterus, icterus, and **convalescence.** General weakness, arthralgia, myalgia, and severe anorexia characterize the preicteric phase. Icterus is a yellowing of the skin also called jaundice. It is caused by the destruction of red blood cells and the release of the pigment bilirubin. The liver usually breaks down bilirubin, which is then excreted from the body. When the liver is diseased, it can no longer perform this function. Fever and upper-abdominal pain also may be present. Many patients develop jaundice as the serum bilirubin level rises. The convalescent stage is characterized by a resolution of symptoms and a return to well-being. Some patients, however, develop cirrhosis and liver cancer as a complication of the disease. Treatment is symptomatic. An effective and safe vaccine is available, and *all health-care workers* and those coming in contact with blood products or body fluids should be vaccinated.

Hepatitis C Virus (HCV)

The hepatitis C form of viral hepatitis (HCV) is transmitted by blood transfusions and blood products. The virus also is found in saliva, urine, and semen. Health-care workers, those who receive blood transfusions, intravenous drug abusers, organ transplant recipients, and hemodialysis patients are at high risk for the disease. Symptoms are similar to but milder than those of hepatitis B. About 50% of patients develop chronic hepatitis and cirrhosis and may require liver transplant. The highest rates of infection are found in transfusion recipients and intravenous drug abusers. HCV is a causal agent of liver cancer. There is currently no vaccine against or cure for HCV infection.

Prion Agents

Creutzfeldt-Jakob disease (CJD) is a rare transmissible disease that is progressive and always fatal. The disease attacks the central nervous system, and symptoms include progressive dementia, spasm of muscles or muscle groups, motor disturbances, and distinctive electroencephalogram (EEG) changes. The disease is very slow to develop, with an incubation period of up to 20 years. CJD initially was thought to be a slow virus, but current research has found that the transmissible agent responsible for CJD is actually a **prion** (short for proteinaceous infectious particle). The prion protein replicates by converting the normal host protein into prion protein, which creates more prion protein molecules. The prion protein is "infectious" as it catalyzes the conversion of normal protein to prion protein by changing the properties of the protein. Only if the cell is synthesizing normal protein is the prion protein able to replicate.

There is no vaccine for CJD and no cure. Although the disease is not contagious, it is transmissible. The mechanism of transmission currently is unknown. CJD represents a threat in the health-care setting because it is known to be transmissible via contaminated electrodes during neurosurgical stereotactic surgery, via corneal grafts, and via direct contact with neurosurgical instruments that have been used on CJD patients. Therefore current infection-control standards require the use of disposable instruments for these types of surgical procedures or specialized decontamination procedures.

Fungi

Fungi are found worldwide on living organic substances, in water, and in soil. They are classified into two groups, molds and yeasts. Yeasts are unicellular, and molds are multicellular and may reproduce sexually or asexually. Like the bacterial endospore, fungal spores are resistant to extreme environmental conditions including heat, cold, drying, and attempted destruction with acids or other chemicals. In the health-care setting, fungi can survive in the heating and cooling ducts of the ventilation system, releasing spores into the environment from which patients and workers can become infected.

Fungal (mycotic) diseases occur as superficial or deep mycoses. Superficial mycoses are transmitted by direct contact with the source and cause mild disease symptoms. Deep mycosis, however, can be fatal. Patients who are immunosuppressed or who are weakened by metabolic disorders, infectious diseases, or trauma are at high risk for serious mycotic disease.

ASPERGILLUS FUMIGATUS

Aspergillus fumigatus causes opportunistic infections in immunosuppressed patients (those whose immune systems are unable to perform their normal functions because of disease or immunosuppressive drugs). This fungus invades the body through the lungs and blood vessels and can cause thrombosis (blockage in the bloodstream) and partial blockage of the airways. In the compromised patient, invasive *Aspergillus* infection is usually fatal.

CANDIDA ALBICANS

Candida albicans is a common opportunistic infection in patients who are compromised by disease. When localized in the oral cavity or vagina, this infection usually can be treated successfully with antifungal drugs. Systemic infection, however, can spread to any location in the body, including the heart, kidney, and other vital organs. Candidiasis is a common disease in AIDS patients and is difficult to treat.

PNEUMOCYSTIS CARINII

Pneumocystis carinii (*P. carinii*) pneumonia is a common respiratory disease among AIDS patients. *P. carinii* infection is widespread in the general population but usually results in only mild symptoms. However, *P. carinii* causes serious disease in immunosuppressed patients, including those receiving immunosuppressive drugs for organ transplant. The infection is difficult to diagnose because the symptoms are nonspecific and the fungus cannot be isolated from the patient's sputum through normal methods.

Protozoa

Protozoa are a group of non-photosynthetic single-celled eukaryotic organisms that lack cell walls. They consist of a single cell or of an aggregation of nondifferentiated cells, loosely held together and not forming tissues.

Protozoa are found free-living in a variety of freshwater and marine habitats. A large number are parasitic in animals, including humans. Some are found growing in soil or in animal habitats, such as on the surface of trees.

Protozoa are usually single-celled, free-living microorganisms. They inhabit soil and water, and can infect other organisms, causing mild to lethal disease. Most have complex life cycles with intermediate hosts that facilitate their transmission and reproduction. They can infect any tissue or organ of the body. Infection usually enters through an insect bite or by ingestion of the protozoa themselves.

Protozoal diseases are generally associated with public health hazards such as dirty water, improper sanitation, and inattention to food safety. Populations in remote or underserved communities are particularly vulnerable. However, a number of significant protozoal diseases also can be found in developed areas. These are not detected until an outbreak of the disease occurs. Protozoal diseases appear most often in tropical climates, but some organisms, like *Giardia*, survive and proliferate in cooler, moist environments. Protozoal disease is not usually found in the hospital environment and is not a cause of concern in the surgical setting.

Arthropods

Arthropods include insects such as biting flies, fleas, ticks, lice, and mosquitoes. These insects transmit disease through their bites. Many ingest human blood as a source of nutrition, spreading bacterial, viral, and rickettsial pathogens to the bite victim. Diseases such as yellow fever, Lyme disease, typhus, and malaria are spread via arthropods. Rickettsiae are very small bacteria that are carried by arthropods. All the rickettsial diseases except Q fever (caused by *Coxiella burnetii*) are transmitted to humans by arthropods. Another example of a rickettsial disease is Rocky Mountain spotted fever.

Helminths

Helminths are multicellular (flat or round) parasitic worms. Those that are significant in the human population are the tapeworms, flukes, and roundworms. Worms can enter the body via penetration through the skin, through the bite of an intermediate insect host, or via fecal-oral contamination.

PROCESS OF INFECTION

Infectious disease is the abnormal *presence* of pathogenic microorganisms in the body. Although the body may become infected, it also has the capacity to defend itself. The process of infection can be thought of as attack and counterattack by the pathogen and the body. The infectious process depends on many conditions. These include the physiologic and immunologic integrity of the host, the dose of invading organisms, and the microorganism's ability to resist or debilitate the body's defenses.

One can study the process of infection by examining distinct events. A typical disease process occurs in these phases:

1. *Transmission:* entry of the pathogen into the body from an external source or movement from one location to another in the same person
2. *Incubation:* the period between entry of the organism and the first signs of infection
3. *Prodromal phase:* the first appearance of symptoms
4. *Acute phase:* the phase of greatest physiologic impact of the pathogen
5. *Convalescence:* period of tissue repair, death or dormancy of the pathogen, and reduction of symptoms
6. *Resolution:* absence of infection, completion of tissue healing

From the pathogen's point of view, the disease process is successful if the microorganism continues to reproduce. This is achieved through chronic disease in the host or transmission to a new host.

Disease Transmission

Now that we are familiar with the environments favored by bacteria, we can study how bacteria or other microorganisms are transferred from one source to another. Disease is transmitted in many ways, and these should be studied by all operating room personnel so that they can take steps to prevent the spread of infection.

For bacteria to be transmitted from one surface to another, they must be carried by an intermediate source. When a living organism carries pathogenic microorganisms from one source to another, it is called a **vector.** Plants and food items are not allowed in the operating room because they can attract and harbor vectors. An inanimate (nonliving) carrier source that is capable of harboring and transmitting disease is called a **fomite.**

A nonsterile surgical instrument can become a fomite by transmitting microorganisms into sterile tissue during surgery. Instruments can harbor pathogenic bacteria encased in dried blood and body tissue that was not removed during the cleaning process. A contaminated surgical implant such as an artificial joint or heart valve can become a fomite. Examples of other common fomites in the hospital are bed linens, wound dressings, and contaminated surgical instruments. Fomites in the everyday environment include objects such as money, eating utensils, toys, and clothing.

Disease transmission requires a source of potential pathogens, the **reservoir** (source), and a host (Figure 7-6). Pathogens can enter the body through one system, such as the surgical incision site, and migrate to other parts of the body. The entry site is called the portal of entry. Most pathogenic microorganisms are environmentally suited to a specific body system. The portal of entry and the exit site are usually but not always the same. For example, organisms causing respiratory infections enter the body via the nose and mouth by direct contact (usually from the hands) or by inhalation of droplets from an infected person's nose and mouth. Unless the pathogens are destroyed in the host or reservoir, there is a potential for transmission.

The following are examples of how an infection can be directly transmitted:

▶ *Respiratory transmission* can occur via aerosol droplet when microorganisms are transmitted from the respiratory tract of one person to that of another person after water droplets are forcefully expelled during talking, coughing, or sneezing. The most effective distance for transmission by droplet from one person to another is 3 feet or less. Airborne transmission also occurs via dust and **droplet nuclei** (dried remnants of previously moist secretions containing microorganisms). Droplet nuclei can be infective for long periods and can remain suspended in the air because of their small size (usually 1 to 5 μm). Bacteria can be attached to droplets of moisture that remain suspended in the air or to droplets that settle on a surface. This is called an aerosol effect. For this reason talking is kept to a minimum while surgery is being performed.
▶ *Gastrointestinal transmission* occurs by ingestion (eating or drinking food or water contaminated with infectious microorganisms). The body usually can combat these invasions through normal defense mechanisms.
▶ *Urogenital infection* almost always results from an outside source. The female urogenital tract is especially vulnerable to infection because of its anatomic configuration.

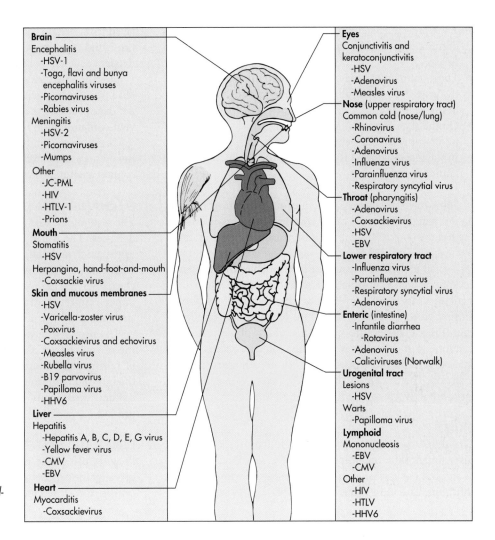

Brain
Encephalitis
-HSV-1
-Toga, flavi and bunya
encephalitis viruses
-Picornaviruses
-Rabies virus
Meningitis
-HSV-2
-Picornaviruses
-Mumps
Other
-JC-PML
-HIV
-HTLV-1
-Prions
Mouth
Stomatitis
-HSV
Herpangina, hand-foot-and-mouth
-Coxsackie virus
Skin and mucous membranes
-HSV
-Varicella-zoster virus
-Poxvirus
-Coxsackievirus and echovirus
-Measles virus
-Rubella virus
-B19 parvovirus
-Papilloma virus
-HHV6
Liver
Hepatitis
-Hepatitis A, B, C, D, E, G virus
-Yellow fever virus
-CMV
-EBV
Heart
Myocarditis
-Coxsackievirus

Eyes
Conjunctivitis and
keratoconjunctivitis
-HSV
-Adenovirus
-Measles virus
Nose (upper respiratory tract)
Common cold (nose/lung)
-Rhinovirus
-Coronavirus
-Adenovirus
-Influenza virus
-Parainfluenza virus
-Respiratory syncytial virus
Throat (pharyngitis)
-Adenovirus
-Coxsackievirus
-HSV
-EBV
Lower respiratory tract
-Influenza virus
-Parainfluenza virus
-Respiratory syncytial virus
-Adenovirus
Enteric (intestine)
-Infantile diarrhea
-Rotavirus
-Adenovirus
-Caliciviruses (Norwalk)
Urogenital tract
Lesions
-HSV
Warts
-Papilloma virus
Lymphoid
Mononucleosis
-EBV
-CMV
Other
-HIV
-HTLV
-HHV6

FIGURE 7-6
Portals of entry for disease in the body. (From Murray PR et al: *Medical microbiology*, ed 4, St Louis, 2002, Mosby.)

▶ *Skin penetration* can result in local, regional, or systemic infection. Postoperative infection can result when bacteria on the skin are introduced into the surgical wound.

▶ *Sexually transmitted diseases* (STDs) are spread when the mucous membrane of an infected person comes into contact with the mucous membrane of an uninfected person. Transmission of STDs is limited to intimate physical contact, generally during sexual intercourse. There are also nonsexual means of transmission:

▶ Herpes simplex type I (HSV): transmitted by kissing or exchange of saliva

▶ Mother to infant: vertical transmission occurs, from one generation to another prenatally or perinatally. Transmission of syphilis, gonorrhea, hepatitis B, and HIV can occur.

BODY DEFENSES

Innate Immunity

Innate immunity is nonspecific. The protective mechanisms are invoked against any pathogen or foreign substance. Innate immunity is present from birth but can be affected by

health status, age, and genetics. Mechanisms of innate immunity include the following:

▶ The physical and chemical protection provided by skin, mucous membranes, and resident microflora

▶ Responses by the vascular and lymphatic systems: **inflammation** and phagocytosis

NORMAL (RESIDENT) FLORA

Shortly after birth, an infant's body begins to acquire a wide variety of bacterial colonies that live in symbiosis with the host within certain tissues of the body. These are called normal or resident flora. Resident flora or **resident microorganisms** are found in areas of the body that communicate with or are exposed to the outside environment. These include the skin, scalp, mouth, throat, nose, gastrointestinal tract, and urogenital tract. All other tissues in the body are normally sterile.

Throughout a person's life the number and type of microorganisms in the resident population grow and recede according to environmental exposure. The following are important functions of resident flora:

▶ They prevent the colonization of invading organisms by dominating the "ecologic niche" provided by the host tissue.

▶ They maintain the pH of the skin and mucosa to prevent the growth of harmful microorganisms (e.g., lactobacilli in the vagina).

▶ On the skin they produce fatty acids, which are a barrier to other bacterial species.

▶ In the intestinal tract they facilitate the production of vitamins B and K.

Some microorganisms come in contact with the body but do not remain. These are called **transient microorganisms.** In the healthy body, transient microorganisms are overwhelmed by the body's normal flora, are washed off with soap and water, or fail to survive because of inhospitable environmental conditions such as unsuitable temperature or pH. Some transient microorganisms can withstand the body's defense mechanisms, either because of their own pathogenicity (ability to cause disease) or because of the vulnerability of the host. They continue to form colonies and cause infection. Thus not all microorganisms cause disease and not all pathogens cause an infection. There are more than 3000 different varieties of bacteria, but only 1% to 3% of these are pathogenic.

SKIN
The skin is perhaps the body's greatest protective mechanism. Intact skin, including the mucous membranes, serves as an excellent barrier against the transmission and spread of infection. The indigenous flora of the skin, fatty acids derived from perspiration, excretions of sebaceous glands, and the rapid growth of keratin prevent bacterial entry into deeper tissues (Figure 7-7).

Specific skin tissues are specialized in their ability to defend the body against infection. For example, skin appendages such as the eyelashes and nasal and ear hair prevent contamination by dust and droplets.

The lacrimal glands produce tears and continuously irrigate the eyes, washing away debris and microorganisms. Tears also contain a natural bacteriostatic agent and lubricating fluid.

MECHANICAL AND CHEMICAL DEFENSES
The respiratory tract employs extensive barrier and chemical defenses. The mucous membranes, cilia, secretions of the upper tract, and coughing and sneezing trap dust, droplets, and other particles and then sweep them out of the nose, trachea, pharynx, larynx, and bronchi. The resident flora of the upper respiratory tract also prevent colonization by transient flora.

The primary defenses in the *gastrointestinal tract* include the normal bacterial flora throughout the system, the flow of saliva in the mouth, peristalsis, acid pH in the stomach, the bile and lymphoid tissue in the small intestine, and mucus and shedding of epithelium in the large intestine (Figure 7-8).

LYMPHATIC SYSTEM
Phagocytosis is the response of the lymphatic system triggered by the process of inflammation (Figure 7-9). In phagocytosis, specialized leukocytes rush to the site of the foreign

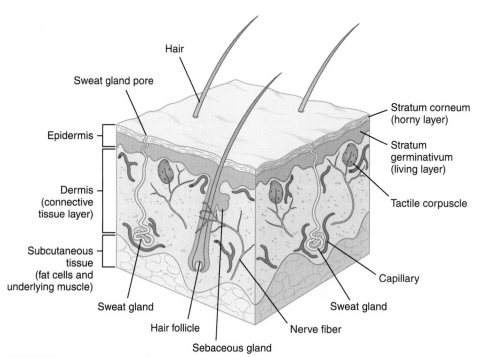

FIGURE 7-7
Skin. (Redrawn from Bergquist L and Pogosian B: *Microbiology: principles and health science applications,* Philadelphia, 2000, Saunders.)

pathogen, bind to the wall of the microorganism, and surround and engulf it. Once the microorganism is inside the leukocyte, the leukocyte's lysosomes fuse with the microorganism and digest it. Nonviable remnants of the microorganism are then released out of the leukocyte. Two types of **phagocyte** are involved in this process. Neutrophils are carried to the site of infection within 90 minutes. Within about 5 to 48 hours, macrophages arrive and continue to engulf and digest large amounts of bacteria. The neutrophil has a shorter life span than the macrophage but is quicker to respond.

As part of the nonspecific immune process, regional lymph nodes collect cellular debris and act as centers for more intensive phagocytic activity. Pus at the site of an infection is composed of dead cells, lymphocytes, and living and dead pathogens. The cellular immune system is closely connected with the second type of defense, the adaptive immune system.

Adaptive Immune System

Acquired immunity or adaptive immune response is specific to a given pathogen or foreign substance. In this process the body forms distinct cell components that are programmed to attack a particular pathogen or substance. Acquired immunity can be active or passive.

Active immunity develops when the body is stimulated to *form its own* antibodies against specific disease antigens. In this process, T and B lymphocytes are activated to bring about the production of antibodies (proteins that remain in the immune system memory). When the body is reexposed to the disease pathogen, the antibodies are reactivated, quickly bind to the invading microorganisms, and rapidly destroy them. Immunity can last for years or a lifetime.

One can develop active immunity in two ways: by being infected by the disease agent or by receiving vaccine containing a small amount of disease antigen. The antigen is modified to prevent the recipient from becoming diseased but is effective in stimulating the formation of antibodies. In some types of immunization, several injections are required to create sufficient antibody levels, while in others one dose is effective.

Passive immunity develops when the body receives the specific disease antibodies from an outside source, which eliminates the need for the body to synthesize them. The fol-

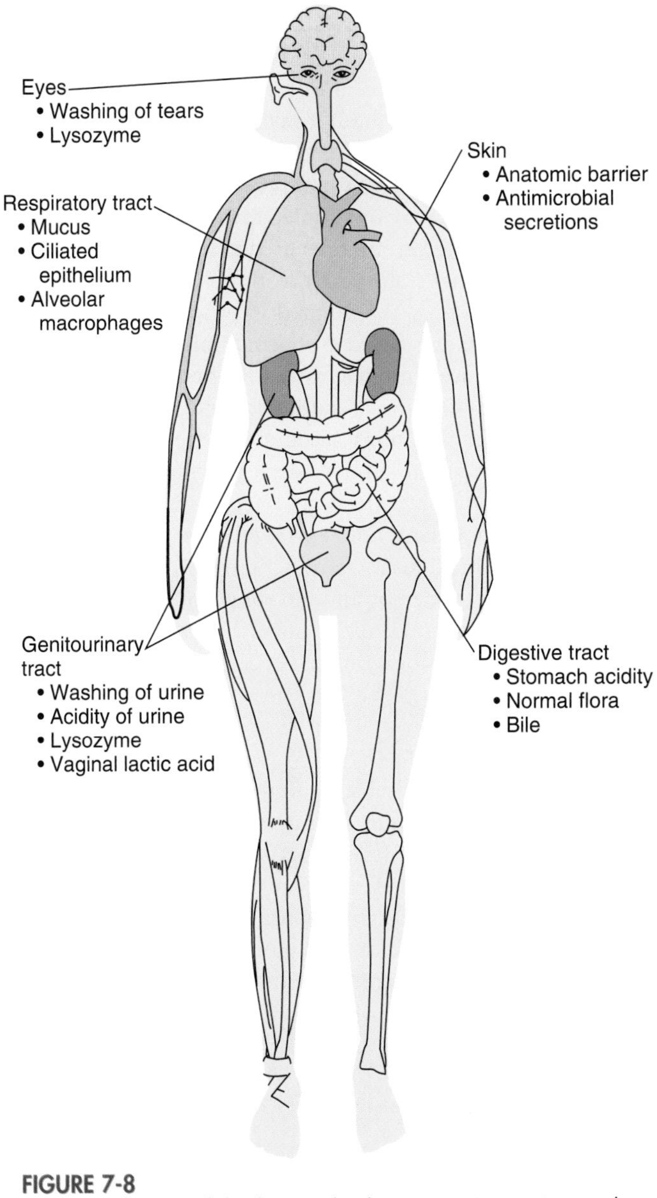

Eyes
• Washing of tears
• Lysozyme

Respiratory tract
• Mucus
• Ciliated epithelium
• Alveolar macrophages

Skin
• Anatomic barrier
• Antimicrobial secretions

Genitourinary tract
• Washing of urine
• Acidity of urine
• Lysozyme
• Vaginal lactic acid

Digestive tract
• Stomach acidity
• Normal flora
• Bile

FIGURE 7-8
Barrier defenses of the human body. (From Murray PR et al: *Medical microbiology*, ed 4, St Louis, 2002, Mosby.)

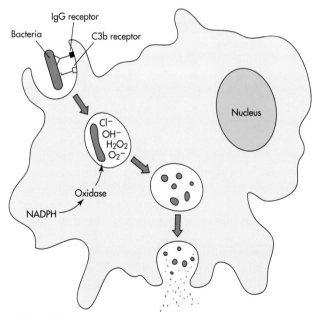

FIGURE 7-9
Phagocytosis. (From Murray PR et al: *Medical microbiology*, ed 4, St Louis, 2002, Mosby.)

lowing are three examples of the development of passive immunity:

▶ The fetus receives antibodies in utero from the mother's immune system.
▶ The infant receives antibodies from the mother's breast milk.
▶ A person receives antiserum that contains antibodies for a specific disease, or α-globulin that contains non–disease-specific antibodies.

MICROBIAL ACTION

Evasion of the Immune System

Microorganisms have developed means of evading the body's immune system. For example, viruses, most notably HIV, can use defensive T lymphocytes as their host cells, allowing the virus to hide within the cells meant to detect them. They also cause the T lymphocytes to synthesize more viral DNA instead of the DNA needed to carry out the host's defensive mechanisms. HIV also has the ability to mutate rapidly, which allows it to avoid damage by virucidal drugs.

Another method of immune system evasion is used by tuberculosis mycobacteria. These bacteria encase themselves in a protective granuloma or tubercle that is physically resistant to immune system attack.

Antibiotic Resistance

Certain strains of pathogens have evolved that are either partially or completely resistant to the most powerful antimicrobial agents available. Certain gram-negative rods are of grave concern because they are easily transmitted, colonize rapidly, and can be lethal. The cause of antibiotic resistance is natural selection. In the presence of antimicrobial agents, some pathogens are destroyed, but the more resistant microbes survive and are transmitted to other hosts. The resistance is passed to succeeding generations of microbes through simple replication or via plasmid exchange, which carries the genes of the resistant strain to other microbes.

Natural selection of resistant strains has been exacerbated by overprescription and underprescription of antibiotics and their improper use by patients. Feeding of antibiotics to meat animals also contributes to the problem. The most threatening resistant microorganisms in the United States currently are vancomycin-resistant enterococci, methicillin-resistant *S. aureus* (MRSA), vancomycin-intermediate-resistant *S. aureus,* and multidrug-resistant *M. tuberculosis.* These microorganisms often are found in the hospital environment, especially in patients who are critically or chronically ill.

Microbial Toxins

Endotoxins (*endo* means "inside") are lipopolysaccharides (LPS) of the gram-negative bacteria contained within the cell wall of the microorganism. When the cell ruptures, endotoxins are released into the bloodstream and spread to dif-ferent organ systems. Endotoxin toxicity stimulates release of many cytokines. The toxic effects include fever, increased or decreased number of white blood cells, diarrhea, shock, extreme weakness, or death.

Exotoxins are proteins, usually enzymes produced by gram-positive bacteria and gram-negative bacteria. The activity of some toxins breaks down tissue surrounding the toxin. This allows the pathogen to spread and colonize freely. Exotoxins enter specific body cells and disrupt the cell's chemical and physical structure. For example, *Clostridium botulinum* produces a highly concentrated toxin that damages the nerve-muscle mechanism and causes paralysis in the host. One gram of botulinum toxin is enough to kill 10 million people. Table 7-2 lists important disease organisms that produce exotoxins and the effects of these toxins.

NOSOCOMIAL INFECTION

A **nosocomial infection** is an infection acquired while the patient is in a hospital. About 2 million patients per year in the United States acquire infections, including surgical site infections, as a result of hospitalization. Seventy percent of the bacteria that cause these infections are resistant to at least one of the drugs commonly used to treat that infection. About 14,000 patients die yearly from hospital-acquired infections. When a hospital-acquired infection is spread from person to person, it is called **cross-contamination.** If the infection is introduced into one part of the body from another, it is termed self-infection or autoinfection.

Urinary tract infections account for the most nosocomial infections, followed by surgical wound infections, lower respiratory tract infections, bacteremia (bacterial invasion of the circulatory system), and other types that do not fit into the previous categories. Many of these infections can be resistant to therapy and can spread to multiple organ systems of the body. Even the normally harmless resident microorganisms can overwhelm the body's immune system and lead to death.

Inflammatory Response

Injury, infection, chemical and thermal burns, extreme cold, and tissue necrosis result in inflammation—either acute (short term) or chronic (long term). This discussion focuses on inflammation caused by tissue trauma and infection. These inflammations are usually acute except in the case of chronic infection, which can last months or years.

The four classic signs of inflammation are:

1. Heat
2. Redness
3. Swelling
4. Pain

In the period immediately after trauma, blood vessels temporarily constrict at the site of injury. Constriction of capillaries helps reduce bleeding and restricts the movement of any microbial toxins present. This is rapidly followed by localized

Table 7-2   EXOTOXINS OF IMPORTANCE IN DISEASE

Organism	Exotoxin	Tissue Damaged	Action	Disease
Bacteria				
Clostridium tetani	Tetanospasmin	Neurons	Spastic paralysis	Tetanus
Clostridium perfringens	α-Toxin	Erythrocytes, platelets, leukocytes, endothelium	Cell lysis	Gas gangrene
Clostridium botulinum	Neurotoxin	Nerve-muscle junction	Flaccid paralysis	Botulism
Corynebacterium diphtheriae	Diphtheria toxin	Throat, heart, peripheral nerve	Inhibits protein synthesis	Diphtheria
Shigella dysenteriae	Enterotoxin	Intestinal mucosa	—	Dysentery
Escherichia coli	Enterotoxin	Intestinal epithelium	Fluid loss from intestinal cells	Gastroenteritis
Vibrio cholerae	Enterotoxin	Intestinal epithelium	Fluid loss from intestinal cells	Cholera
Staphylococcus aureus	α-Toxin	Red and white cells (via cytokines)	Hemolysis	Abscesses
	Hemolysin	Red and white cells (via cytokines)	Hemolysis	Abscesses
	Leukocidin	Leukocytes	Destroys leukocytes	Abscesses
	Enterotoxin	Intestinal cells	Induces vomiting, diarrhea	Food poisoning
	TSST1	—	Release of cytotoxins	Toxic shock syndrome
	Epidermolytic	Epidermis	—	Scalded skin syndrome
Streptococcus pyogenes	Streptolysin O and S	Red and white cells	Hemolysis	Hemolysis, pyogenic lesion
	Erythrogenic	Skin capillaries	Skin rash	Scarlet fever
Bacillus anthracis	Cytotoxin	Lung	Pulmonary edema	Anthrax
Bordetella pertussis	Pertussis toxin	Trachea	Kills epithelium	Whooping cough
Legionella pneumophila	Numerous	Neutrophils	Cell lysis	Legionnaire's disease
Listeria monocytogenes	Hemolysin	Leukocytes, monocytes	Cell lysis	Listeriosis
Pseudomonas aeruginosa	Exotoxin A	Cell lysis	Cell lysis	Various infections
Fungi				
Aspergillus fumigatus	Aflatoxin	Liver	Carcinogenic	Liver damage/cancer
Protozoa				
Entamoeba histolytica	Enterotoxin	Colonic epithelium	Cell lysis	Amebic dysentery

From Mims C et al: *Medical microbiology,* ed 2, London, 1998, Mosby.

arterial and venous dilation. As a result the injured area becomes red and warm. Local capillaries become more permeable, and this allows plasma to escape into the surrounding tissue. The plasma dilutes any toxins in these tissues and also increases the viscosity of the local blood supply, which encourages clotting. As a consequence, however, the injured person experiences swelling, pain, and impaired function.

Surgical Site Infection

Surgical site infection is the second most frequent type of hospital-acquired infection in hospitals in the United States. About 60% to 70% of surgical site infections are confined to the incision, while the remaining spread to distant or adjacent sites. Bacteria are the most common cause of surgical site infections. Physiologic complications of surgical site infections include the following:

▶ Tissue destruction or necrosis
▶ Wound **dehiscence** (splitting apart of deep and superficial wound edges)
▶ **Evisceration** (protrusion of visceral contents outside the body through a surgical incision)
▶ Incisional hernia (protrusion of tissue through a weakened area of the abdominal wall at the site of a previous incision)
▶ Septic thrombophlebitis
▶ Single or multiple organ failure
▶ Recurring pain

▶ Increased metabolic requirements that result in malnutrition and bacteremia (circulatory involvement)
▶ Disfigurement
▶ Loss of function

Surgical site infection occurs when a pathogenic or non-pathogenic microorganism gains entry to sterile tissues and colonizes there. Some wound infections are minor, involving only the skin, while others occur in deep tissue or body cavities. The infection may remain localized or spread throughout the body, especially if the causative microorganism is resistant to antimicrobial therapy. The general preoperative condition of the patient may directly affect the extent and severity of the infection. Factors include the integrity of the immune system, the dose and type of microorganism in the wound, and the portal of entry. Certain surgical patients are particularly at high risk for infection (Box 7-4).

Surgical wounds are classified according to risk of contamination and infection *at the time of the surgery* (Box 7-5).

CHARACTERISTICS OF SURGICAL SITE INFECTION

When a surgical site infection begins to develop, the patient's temperature becomes elevated soon after surgery. The patient may experience pain at the incisional site or deep within the wound. Exudate (accumulation of pus, drainage, dead cells, and serum) may appear around the incision. The wound site becomes extremely tender, and the patient's white blood cell count increases. If the infection is localized, antimicrobial therapy may be initiated and the infection eradicated. Deep infections, however, lead to localized or widespread areas of tissue necrosis, accumulation of pus,

---

Box 7-4 Physiologic Risks for Surgical Site Infection

Age: The immune system of an elderly patient is less responsive than that of a younger patient. Tissues heal more slowly, and innate body defenses are less effective. Elderly patients are often undernourished.

Undernourishment or malnourishment: Essential proteins required for tissue healing and body defenses against infection are often missing in the diet of these patients. Low body fat predisposes the patient to lowered body temperature, which increases physiologic stress.

Diabetes mellitus: The diabetic patient is at extremely high risk of infection because of problems with the circulatory system, which must be properly functioning to have a healthy immune system. Poor peripheral and visceral circulation prevents the flow of nutrients and oxygen to traumatized tissue, which increases the overgrowth of both resident and disease-producing microorganisms.

Substance or alcohol abuse: These patients are often malnourished. Liver damage related to substance abuse and alcohol abuse leads to poor conversion of glycogen to glucose, which is necessary for cellular metabolism. Immune function is often depressed.

Immune suppression: Patients with acquired immunodeficiency syndrome (AIDS) or other immune diseases, those undergoing cancer therapy, and those who have been prescribed high doses of corticosteroids have impaired immune function.

Long preoperative stay in hospital: A prolonged preoperative stay allows the body to incubate and colonize bacteria and other microorganisms commonly found in the hospital environment, especially antibiotic-resistant forms

Surgical wound classification: Certain classes of wounds are associated with a higher risk of infection in the postoperative patient. Wound classifications are determined in the operating room by the variables listed in Box 7-5.

Long operative procedure: Long procedures put the patient at higher risk for exposure to airborne pathogens and direct contact with contaminated medical devices and instruments.

Box 7-5 Classification of Surgical Wounds

Clean wound (1% to 5% risk of postoperative infection)

Examples: total hip replacement, vitrectomy, nerve resection
▶ Uninfected
▶ Clean
▶ No inflammation
▶ Closed primarily (all tissue layers sutured closed)
▶ Respiratory, gastrointestinal, genital, and uninfected urinary tracts not entered
▶ May contain closed drainage system

Clean-contaminated wound (3% to 7% risk of postoperative infection)

Examples: cystoscopy, gastric bypass, removal of oral lesion
▶ Respiratory, gastrointestinal, genital, or urinary tract is entered without unusual contamination
▶ No evidence of infection or major break in aseptic technique
▶ Includes operations of the biliary tract, appendix, vagina, and oropharynx

Contaminated wound (10% to 17% risk of postoperative infection)

Examples: removal of perforated appendix, removal of metal fragments related to an explosion
▶ Open, fresh, accidental wound
▶ Surgical procedure in which a major break in aseptic technique has occurred
▶ Gross spillage from the gastrointestinal tract
▶ Acute, nonpurulent inflammation

Dirty or infected wound (>27% risk of postoperative infection)

Example: incision and drainage of an abscess
▶ Old traumatic wounds with devitalized tissue
▶ Existing clinical infection
▶ Perforated viscera

and breakdown of the sutured tissue layers. Infection usually results in the breakdown of the surgical repair that was the focus of the surgery. As suture materials degrade in the presence of bacteria, the wound may dehisce (split open). An abdominal wound can split open and the contents eviscerate (spill outside the wound). A large accumulation of pus leads to the spread of infection into adjacent tissues. An uncontrolled infection in a body cavity results in inflammation of the lining of that cavity, such as peritonitis in the abdomen. This can rapidly become fatal as vital organs are infected and become unable to function.

TREATMENT OF SURGICAL SITE INFECTION
If the surgical wound is caused by trauma, becomes grossly contaminated during surgery, or is infected post-operatively, treatment with antimicrobial agents is usually initiated immediately. The agent used depends on the type of infecting organism. In addition, the wound may be incised again, and pus and necrotic (dead), devitalized tissue removed. This procedure is called an incision and drainage (I & D). The wound may be continuously irrigated during convalescence to prevent the buildup of pus that prevents wound healing. When infection is present, the wound cannot be sutured, because infected tissues cannot withstand the tension of sutures and bacterial toxins rapidly break most suture material. Rather, the wound is packed with gauze dressings and allowed to heal from the bottom to the exterior. This is called healing by granulation. Wound management is covered in detail in Chapter 15.

CASE STUDIES

Case 1
The patient is a 23-year-old man who has suffered multiple injuries in an automobile accident. He has penetrating wounds from the gas pedal and multiple abrasions caused by the air bag and seat belt. A portion of the gearshift is lodged in his right subcostal area. How would you classify this procedure?
What would the surgical wound classification be labeled for this procedure?

Case 2
The patient is an 85-year-old man who has suffered a ruptured diverticulum. He is in toxic shock and requires immediate surgery to close the defect in the bowel. How do you classify this surgery?

Case 3
What are the possible consequences of contamination of a heart valve placed in the patient?

Case 4
You are scrubbed on a known hepatitis B or C case. The circulator, while emptying the urine from the catheter bag, accidentally spills it all over your lower legs and shoes. You have a large cut on your lower leg. What should you do?

Case 5
How would you design a system to handle contaminated waste in the hospital? How important is such a system? What would you classify as contaminated wastes?

Case 6
You are in the restroom and observe a fellow employee leaving the restroom without washing his or her hands. What should you do?

Case 7
You are scrubbed on a known HIV case. The surgeon punctures his or her finger with a contaminated needle, so you offer to have the circulator begin to fill out an incident report. The surgeon says not to worry about it. What should you do?

Case 8
You are going to transport a patient to the operating room for surgery. You notice on the chart that the patient has methicillin-resistant *Staphylococcus aureus* (MRSA). Are there any precautions you need to take? How will you handle the transport of the patient?

REFERENCES
Bach T: The bloodborne pathogens standard and disinfection, *Infection Control Today*, Sept, 2000.
Centers for Disease Control and Prevention, National Center for Infectious Diseases website: *Questions and answers regarding Creutzfeldt-Jakob disease infection-control practices.*
Fogg DM: Clinical issues, *AORN Journal*, 72:4, October, 2000.
Garner JS: Guideline for isolation precautions in hospitals, *Infection Control and Hospital Epidemiology*, 17, 1996, and *American Journal of Infection Control*, 24, 1996.
Goodner B: *The OSHA handbook: interpretive guidelines for the bloodborne pathogen standard*, El Paso, 1993, Skidmore-Roth Publishing.

National Institute for Occupational Safety and Health (NIOSH): *NIOSH alert: preventing needlestick injuries in health care settings,* Cincinnati, Nov, 1999, National Institute for Occupational Safety and Health.

Nester et al: *Microbiology, a human perspective,* ed 4, 2003, McGraw Hill.

Occupational Safety and Health Administration: *OSHA regulations, occupational and safety health standards, bloodborne pathogens,* standard number 1910.1030.

Rutala WA: *APIC guidelines for infection control practice,* Washington, DC, 1996, Association for Professionals in Infection Control and Epidemiology.

Rutala WA and Weber DJ: Creutzfeldt-Jakob disease: risks and prevention of nosocomial acquisition, *Infection Control Today,* August, 2001.

Rutala WA and Weber DJ: New disinfection and sterilization methods, *Emerging Infectious Diseases,* 7:2, Mar-Apr, 2001.

Chapter 8

Disinfection, Decontamination, and Sterilization Standards and Practices

Learning Objectives

After studying this chapter the reader will be able to:

- Distinguish between disinfection and sterilization
- Understand the classification of patient-care equipment
- Recognize the hazards associated with the use of chemical disinfectants
- Be familiar with different disinfectant agents
- Understand what sanitation is and how it is accomplished
- Understand the process of instrument decontamination
- Understand the postoperative duties of the surgical technologist
- Understand Standard Precautions as they apply to decontamination
- Understand what personal protective equipment is
- Define and understand sterility
- Distinguish between the process of sterilization and other processes that render objects clean or disinfected
- Describe the different methods of sterilization used in the operating room
- Properly load the steam sterilizer
- Understand and practice safety precautions when using any type of sterilizer
- Determine which sterilization process is approved for which equipment
- Understand the principles of gas sterilization
- Describe the environmental concerns associated with the use of the gas sterilizer
- Prepare equipment for sterilization

Terminology

Antisepsis—A process that destroys most pathogenic organisms on animate surfaces.

Bactericidal—Able to kill bacteria.

Bacteriostatic—Capable of inhibiting the growth of bacteria but not killing them.

Bioburden—Contamination of an item from debris or microorganisms.

Biological indicators—A mechanism for measuring sterility assurance that determines the presence of pathogenic bacteria on objects subjected to a sterilization process.

Cavitation—A process in which air pockets are imploded (burst inward), releasing particles of soil or tissue debris.

Chemical indicators—Methods used to verify that an item has been exposed to a particular sterilization process. Chemical indicators ensure that specific parameters of a sterilization process have been met.

Chemical sterilization—A process that uses chemical agents rather than steam to achieve sterilization.

Cleaning—A process that removes organic or inorganic soil or debris.

Cobalt 60 radiation—A method of sterilizing prepackaged equipment; ionizing radiation.

Critical items—In medicine, those items that must be sterilized before use on a patient; items that penetrate body tissues or the vascular system.

Decontamination—A process of disinfection.

Disinfection—A process that destroys most but not all pathogenic microorganisms on inanimate objects.

Ethylene oxide—Highly flammable, toxic gas that is capable of sterilizing an object.

Event-related sterility—The interference of environmental conditions or events with the integrity of a package; sterilized items are otherwise assumed sterile between uses.

Fungicidal—Able to kill fungi.

Germicidal—Able to kill germs.

Gravity displacement sterilizer—Type of sterilizer that removes air by gravity.

High-level disinfection—Disinfection process that destroys many forms of microorganisms, not including bacterial spores.

High vacuum sterilizer—Type of steam sterilizer that removes air in the chamber by vacuum. Also known as a pre-vacuum sterilizer.

Inanimate—Nonliving.

Lumen—The inside portion of a hollow tube.

Noncritical item—Items that are not required to be sterile as they do not penetrate intact tissues (e.g., bedpans, blood pressure cuffs).

Peracetic acid—Chemical capable of rendering objects sterile.

Plasma sterilization—Sterilization process that uses the form of matter known as plasma (e.g., hydrogen peroxide plasma) to achieve sterilization of an item.

Sanitation—A process that cleans an object.

Semicritical items—Items that are required to be free of most pathogenic organisms including *Mycobacterium tuberculosis,* as these items contact mucous membranes (e.g., respiratory equipment, endoscopes).

Shelf life—The amount of time a wrapped item will remain sterile after it has been subjected to a sterilization process.

Sporicidal—Able to kill spores.

Sterilization—A process by which all types of microorganisms, including spores, are destroyed.

Ultrasonic cleaner—Equipment that cleans instruments through cavitation.

Virucidal—Able to kill viruses.

Washer-sterilizer—Equipment that washes and sterilizes instruments after an operative procedure.

DISINFECTION

Disinfection is a process by which *most but not all* pathogenic microorganisms on **inanimate** (nonliving) surfaces are destroyed. This process is clearly distinguished from **sterilization**, which is the destruction of *all* microorganisms on an object. In the operating room, sterilization is used to destroy all microorganisms on all objects that enter the body, such as instruments, catheters, and needles. Quite different from disinfection and sterilization is **antisepsis**, which is a process that destroys most pathogenic microorganisms on animate (living) surfaces.

The distinction between these terms is critical. Disinfection is used in the operating room and elsewhere in the hospital to render objects nearly free but not completely free of microorganisms. Patient-care objects such as respiratory therapy equipment and patient furniture are examples of objects that are disinfected. Antiseptics, used only on living tissue, are used on the skin of the surgical site and for the surgical hand and arm scrub of sterile team members. These do not sterilize the skin but do kill many pathogenic microorganisms.

Several other terms are important to the understanding of disinfection. The suffix -*cidal* means to destroy or kill. Thus, if a product is **bactericidal,** it destroys bacterial cells. A sporicide destroys bacterial spores, the vegetative form of the bacteria that is very difficult to kill by any means. Generally, if a product is **sporicidal,** it is highly effective against all types of microbes and is said to achieve a *high level of disinfection.* A virucide is a product that is effective in killing viruses, and a germicide (**germicidal**) is any agent that kills microorganisms. A tuberculocidal agent is one that kills tubercle bacilli. The suffix -*static* refers to a process of controlling or inhibiting growth. Thus, a **bacteriostatic** disinfectant is one that inhibits the growth of bacteria on a surface but does not necessarily destroy the bacteria. After the disinfectant is removed, the bacteria freely proliferate. A hospital-grade disinfectant is one that has proven effectiveness against *Salmonella, Staphylococcus aureus,* and *Pseudomonas aeruginosa.* These are all significant microorganisms in the hospital setting.

Classification of Patient-Care Equipment

The following is a system of classification for items that are commonly disinfected or sterilized in the hospital. Although many of these items are not encountered in the operating room setting, it is important to understand the distinctions made and why they fall into various groupings. These distinctions were developed in the past 2 decades and remain in use today. The categories are based on *the degree of risk of infection* associated with each item. Items in categories II and III are disinfected according to their classification. That is, they are disinfected with a specific process and substance to achieve the needed level of disinfection. **High-level disinfection** is a process that destroys all forms of microorganisms except bacterial spores. *Intermediate-level disinfection* is a process that inactivates *Mycobacterium tuberculosis,* vegetative bacteria, most viruses, and most fungi, but may not destroy bacterial spores. *Low-level disinfection* is a process that destroys some virus and fungi and most bacteria. However, this process is not reliable in killing tubercle bacilli or bacterial spores.

CATEGORY I: CRITICAL ITEMS

Critical items are those that must be sterile. These objects enter sterile tissue or the vascular system. In most cases, sterilization requires special equipment and critical monitoring. Examples of critical items include:

▶ Surgical instruments and supplies
▶ Vascular and urinary catheters
▶ Implants
▶ Needles

CATEGORY II: SEMICRITICAL ITEMS

Semicritical items are those that come in contact with mucous membranes or skin that is not intact. The items in this category must be completely free of microorganisms except for bacterial spores. This is because mucous membranes are resistant to bacterial spores but have little or no defense against bacteria such as tubercle bacilli and viruses. Semicritical items are disinfected away from patient-care areas, and require some special equipment for disinfection. This group of items includes:

▶ Respiratory therapy and anesthesia equipment
▶ Endoscopes

CATEGORY III: NONCRITICAL ITEMS

Noncritical items are those that come in contact with skin but not mucous membranes. Skin is effective in protecting the inner tissues of the body against bacteria and viral inva-

sion; thus this category includes items that are commonly found in patient-care areas:

▶ Blood pressure cuffs
▶ Bed linens
▶ Bedside tables
▶ Crutches
▶ Some food utensils
▶ Bed frames
▶ Floors
▶ Walls

Selection and Use of Disinfectants

In the operating room and elsewhere in the hospital, the most common disinfection process uses a liquid disinfectant. Disinfectants commonly used in patient care fall into chemical types. These are discussed below and in Table 8-1. The *selection* of a disinfectant is based on the result required. Some disinfectants are effective in destroying a limited number of microorganisms; others are very effective in killing all organisms, including bacterial spores. Some are extremely corrosive, while others are relatively harmless to common materials found in the hospital.

Factors that affect a disinfectant's activity (or "-cidal" ability) include the concentration of the solution, the number of microorganisms present on the object being disinfected, water hardness and pH, temperature of the solution, and presence or absence of organic matter. Most disinfectants have a dilution factor that is critical to their efficacy. Therefore it is very important to follow mixing instructions *exactly*. Some disinfectants can be extremely harmful to materials such as plastics, rubber, and tile. Mixing errors can be costly in terms of both destruction of equipment and simple economic use of the product. Nearly all disinfectants are considerably weakened in the presence of organic material such as blood, sputum, or tissue residue. Therefore items to be disinfected must undergo **cleaning** (removal of organic debris and soil) and thorough drying before the disinfection process. Cleaning is performed with detergent, water, and mechanical action and should never be confused with disinfection or sterilization.

Precautions and Hazards

Many disinfectants are *unsafe for use on human tissue including skin.* This means that employees must be extremely cautious when handling certain liquid disinfectants. Warnings and instructions for use must be strictly followed. *Do not be misled by the mild odor of some disinfectants.* Many chemicals are preferred for commercial or medical use because they do not give off noxious fumes. *This is not an indication of any lack of toxicity to skin or the respiratory system.* Because of the toxicity of some disinfectants, the following precautions always should be exercised:

1. All disinfectants should be stored in well-ventilated rooms and their containers kept *covered.*

Table 8-1   SUMMARY OF DISINFECTION AND STERILIZATION PROCESSES

Definition	Items and Devices	Processes Used*	Products Used
Critical items			
Enter vascular systems or sterile tissues, or have blood flowing through them	Surgical instruments Implants Needles Catheters (vascular and urinary) Laparoscopes and arthroscopes (if sterilization is not feasible, should receive at least high-level disinfection) Endoscopy accessories (e.g., biopsy forceps, cytology brushes) Some dental instruments (e.g., scalers, burrs, forceps, scalpels)	*Sterilization* Heat (steam, dry) Chemical gas, vapor, plasma Radiation Peracetic acid with hydrogen peroxide *NOTE:* Longer exposure times required for sterilization than for disinfection.	*Liquid chemicals, sporicidal sterilants* Aldehydes (e.g., glutaraldehyde) Hydrogen peroxide Peracetic acid
Semicritical items			
Contact mucous membranes or nonintact skin	Gastrointestinal endoscopes Laryngoscopes Bronchoscopes Endotracheal tubes Respiratory therapy and anesthesia equipment Dialyzers Diaphragm-fitting rings Cryosurgical probes Some dental instruments (e.g., amalgam, condensers, air/water syringes) Hydrotherapy tanks (if used for patients with intact skin) Tonometers (5-min immersion recommended) Thermometers (alcohols preferred)	*High-level disinfection* ≥20-min minimum required; 12 min for orthophthalaldehyde (Cidex OPA) *NOTE:* sterilization may be preferred.	*Wet pasteurization agents or liquid chemicals* Aldehydes (e.g., glutaraldehyde) Cidex OPA Hydrogen peroxide Peracetic acid Peracetic acid with hydrogen peroxide Chlorines (sodium hypochlorite, 1000 ppm, 1:50 dilution)
		Intermediate-level disinfection ≤10-min immersion *NOTE:* with label claim for tuberculocidal activity	Alcohols (70%-90%) Iodophors Phenolics Chlorines
Noncritical items			
Contact intact skin (not mucous membranes)	Stethoscopes Blood pressure and tourniquet cuffs Electrocardiogram leads Bedpans Linens	*Intermediate-level disinfection* *NOTE:* required if contamination is heavy or there is significant blood contamination	Alcohols (70%-90%) Iodophors Phenolics Chlorines
	Environmental surfaces (e.g., tabletops, bedside stands, furniture, floors)	*Low-level disinfection* *NOTE:* adequate for most noncritical items and surfaces	Alcohols (70%-90%) Iodophors Phenolics Chlorines (sodium hypochlorite, 100 ppm, 1:500 dilution) Quaternary ammonium compounds ("quats")

From Gruendemann BJ, Mangum SS: *Infection prevention in surgical settings*, Philadelphia, 2001, WB Saunders.
ppm, Parts per million.
*Using products approved by the Environmental Protection Agency and the Food and Drug Administration and following manufacturers' instructions.

2. The following personal protective equipment (PPE) must be worn when employees handle a chemical disinfectant (Figure 8-1):
   ▶ Protective eyewear
   ▶ Gloves
   ▶ Masks
   ▶ Full protective body wear such as a jumpsuit, apron, or cover gown
3. Data concerning the safe use of chemical disinfectants are kept by every hospital.
4. The dilution ratio of a liquid chemical should never be changed unless an appropriate supervisor so orders.
5. Always use a measuring device designated for mixing liquid disinfectants with water. Do not rely on haphazard technique or guesswork when preparing solutions.
6. Two disinfectants never should be mixed together. This could create toxic fumes or unstable and dangerous compounds.
7. Dispose of liquid chemicals as directed by hospital and label instructions. Some chemicals are unsafe for disposal through standard sewage systems.
8. An unlabeled bottle or container never should be used and should be discarded. Be aware of what chemical is being used and its specific purpose.

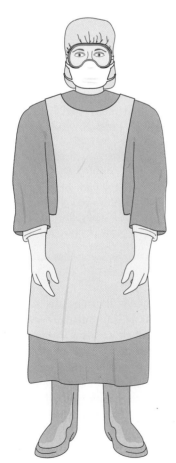

FIGURE 8-1
Personal protective attire. (Redrawn from Reichert M, Young J, eds: *Sterilization technology for the health care facility*, ed 2, Gaithersburg, 1997, Aspen Publishers.)

Disinfectant Chemicals

The following are disinfectants that are commonly used in the hospital environment. These are regulated and registered by the Environmental Protection Agency (EPA). See Table 8-2 for properties of disinfectants listed below.

ALCOHOL

Alcohol is a commonly used disinfectant that is composed of two components: ethyl alcohol and isopropyl alcohol. Both are water soluble (mix easily in water). Alcohol is not sporicidal but is bactericidal, tuberculocidal, and **virucidal.** It is effective against cytomegalovirus and human immunodeficiency virus. Alcohol's optimum disinfection ability occurs at a 60% to 70% dilution. Alcohol must never be used on surgical instruments because it is not sporicidal and is very corrosive to stainless steel. In the hospital, alcohol is most often used to disinfect patient thermometers and medication vial stoppers. It is damaging to shellac mounting on lensed instruments and must never be used repeatedly on rubber or plastic tubing because it causes swelling and hardening of these substances.

Alcohol also is often used as a topical antiseptic to cleanse patient injection sites. It greatly reduces the number of bacteria on skin when used as a hand rinse in the absence of water and antiseptic soap. However, toxicity has been reported when it is used on children as a sponging liquid to reduce fever. Alcohol is extremely drying to skin and irritating to mucous membranes.

Because it is *highly flammable and volatile,* alcohol must never be used in the presence of electrocautery or lasers. Alcohol must be stored in a *cool, well-ventilated area.* Skin prep solutions that contain alcohol must be allowed to dry completely before they are applied to surgical draping material, and care must be taken to prevent pooling of these prep solutions under the patient to prevent fires.

SODIUM HYPOCHLORITE

Sodium hypochlorite (household bleach) is a broad-spectrum disinfectant that is limited in use because of corrosiveness to metal. However, it is commonly used to clean floors and countertops. The Centers for Disease Control and Prevention (CDC) has recommended this product for use in spot cleaning of blood spills because it is very fast acting. However, it is deactivated in the presence of organic material, so the area must be cleaned first before application of hypochlorite. When hypochlorite solution comes in contact with formaldehyde, bis-chloromethyl ether, a carcinogen, is produced. When hypochlorite is mixed with an acidic solution, toxic chlorine gas is produced.

FORMALDEHYDE

The common form of formaldehyde is formalin, a 37% solution of formaldehyde in water. It is bactericidal, tuberculocidal, **fungicidal,** virucidal, and sporicidal. Its primary use in the hospital is in the preservation of tissue specimens, although it has been used to disinfect renal dialysis equip-

Table 8-2   PROPERTIES OF DISINFECTANTS

Chemical	Level of Disinfection	Kills Spores	Kills HIV	Kills *M. Tuberculosis*	Kills HBV	Uses	Risk
Isopropyl alcohol 70%-90%	Intermediate (some semicritical and noncritical items)	No	Yes	Yes	Yes	Limited. No longer used as general disinfectant.	Flammable. Can damage lensed instruments.
Phenolic detergent compounds	Low	No	Yes	Yes	No	Environmental cleaning only.	Highly toxic.
Glutaraldehyde 2%	High (critical items)	Yes	Yes	Yes	Yes	Endoscopes, respiratory equipment, anesthesia equipment, immersible items. Long shelf life. Disinfectant active for long periods when used properly.	Vapor causes eye, skin, nasal irritation. Improperly rinsed endoscopes can cause tissue damage.
Stabilized hydrogen peroxide 6%	High (critical items)	Yes	Yes	Yes	Yes	Must contact all surfaces when used as a sterilant.	Can cause tissue irritation.
Formalin (37% formaldehyde)	High	Yes	Yes	Yes	Yes	Currently used for specimen preservation.	Highly noxious fumes. Carcinogenic.
Iodophor (free iodine in a detergent-disinfectant solution)	Intermediate to low depending on concentration	No	Yes	Yes	Yes	As a disinfectant limited to use in cleaning hydrotherapy tanks and thermometers, environmental cleaning.	May cause reaction in sensitive individuals.
Quaternary ammonium detergent	Low (noncritical items)	No	Yes	No	No	Limited effectiveness. Used for low-level environmental disinfection.	May cause reaction in sensitive individuals.
Sodium hypochlorite 5%, 500 ppm	Low (noncritical items)	No	Yes	No	Yes	1:100 ppm for spot disinfection and blood spills. Environmental cleaning.	Fumes can cause irritation to skin and mucous membranes.

ment. Formaldehyde emits extremely irritating fumes and is toxic to tissue. Formaldehyde in a combination with isopropyl alcohol (8% formaldehyde and 70% isopropyl alcohol) may be used as a chemical sterilant. Sterilization is achieved in 3 hours. However, because of its toxicity and noxious odor, this method of sterilization is rarely used. When used, formaldehyde is employed to produce high-level disinfection. Items must be thoroughly rinsed after submersion in formaldehyde before patient contact.

GLUTARALDEHYDE

Glutaraldehyde is a widely used high-level disinfectant that is sporicidal, bactericidal, and virucidal. It is completely safe to use on instruments, such as endoscopes, which is how it is mainly used in hospitals. It can be used safely on respiratory therapy and anesthesia equipment. This agent is a chemical relative of formaldehyde and is active in a lower concentration (2% glutaraldehyde vs. 8% formaldehyde). It is less destructive to instruments when used for high-level disinfection. Like formaldehyde, this agent requires prolonged exposure to achieve sterilization and therefore is rarely used for this purpose. As with formaldehyde, items submerged in a glutaraldehyde solution must be thoroughly rinsed after disinfection and before use on a patient.

To render glutaraldehyde effective as a sterilant, the item must soak in the solution for 10 hours. It is tuberculocidal, however, in 20 minutes. Instruments must be thoroughly dried before being placed in the solution. This disinfectant is weakened considerably by unintentional dilution, which occurs if instruments are wet when placed in an immersion bath of glutaraldehyde, and by the presence of organic matter. When glutaraldehyde solutions are mixed and kept for repetitive use, the solution must be completely renewed after 14 days because it is ineffective after that time. In addition, during its time in use, the solution must be tested with test strips often to ensure that proper concentration is maintained at 2% glutaraldehyde. If the test strips do not indicate that the solution is effective, it must be changed immediately before use.

Occupational hazards of glutaraldehyde are most commonly found when the solution is kept in open immersion baths in a poorly ventilated work area. The safe levels of formaldehyde or glutaraldehyde in the air are under 0.2 ppm. Any amount over that level causes irritation to the eyes and nasal passages. Glutaraldehyde is toxic to tissue; items that have been disinfected or sterilized in glutaraldehyde must be completely rinsed with sterile distilled water before use on the patient. After employees rinse the items, they also must change their sterile gloves before using items on the patient during a procedure.

ORTHO-PHTHALDEHYDE

Ortho-phthaldehyde 0.55% (Cidex OPA) is a non–glutaraldehyde-based high-level disinfectant that can be used for medical devices that can be immersed in the solution. Instruments or equipment are thoroughly cleaned, dried, and placed in the solution for 12 minutes (moisture retained on items not thoroughly dried will dilute the solution, which could render the solution ineffective). The items must be thoroughly rinsed with water three times after submersion, with fresh water each time. Items not properly rinsed will stain the skin of the handler or the patient. Ortho-phthaldehyde has a **shelf life** of 14 days; however, the manufacturer's recommendation is for daily testing to ensure that the concentration of the disinfectant is at the required level.

PHENOLICS

Phenol (carbolic acid) is available in detergent form for use in routine hospital cleaning. It is not sporicidal but is tuberculocidal, fungicidal, virucidal, and bactericidal. Because not many data are available on the specific effects of phenol on microorganisms, its use is restricted to disinfection of non-critical items. It is extremely important to follow the manufacturer's label instructions for dilution and mixing because phenolic mixtures have been indicated in a number of studies involving toxicity to certain patients. Phenol has a very noxious odor and causes skin lesions and respiratory irritation. Phenol is extremely corrosive to the skin, and appropriate protective attire must be worn. Skin that contacts phenol must be immediately rinsed with copious amounts of isopropyl alcohol to neutralize the agent and prevent serious skin injury.

QUATERNARY AMMONIUM COMPOUNDS

The quaternary ammonium compounds (commonly called "quats") are sensitive to environmental conditions such as hardness of water, soap, and some types of soil, which may render them ineffective. Benzalkonium chloride and dimethyl benzyl ammonium chloride have been widely used as disinfectants. Although the quats have traditionally been used on the skin, the CDC advised that this practice be discontinued because of the incidence of infection associated with their use as an antiseptic.

Quats developed more recently, such as twin-chain or dialkyl quats, are much more effective in hard water than those traditionally used in the hospital. They are reported to be fungicidal, bactericidal, and pseudomonacidal, but not effective in sporicidal or tuberculocidal disinfection. In addition, the disinfectant qualities are greatly reduced when they are used in conjunction with items such as gauze or sponges; the sponge or gauze absorbs the active ingredient in the quat and thus renders the disinfection process ineffective.

DECONTAMINATION

To render the operating room environment, which includes all cleanable surfaces, as disease free as possible, certain regimens are followed on a scheduled basis. The routines are the general responsibility of everyone in the department. In certain settings, the responsibility belongs to specific personnel assigned by the nurse manager or by the job description given to them by the hospital. At present, the emergence of human immunodeficiency virus (HIV) and other blood-borne pathogens has produced an element of urgency and extreme focus on the practices of **sanitation** and **decontamination**. The duties and tasks associated with sanitation and decontamination must never be taken lightly. The devastating results of carelessness in this area testify to its importance, as discussed in Chapter 7.

Disinfection or sanitation is the process by which *any* surfaces, materials, and equipment are cleaned with specific substances (disinfectants) that render them safe for their intended use. The term decontamination implies that a surface or object is assumed to harbor pathogenic microorganisms and is cleaned and disinfected in a manner that renders it safe for its intended use. Therefore any item that is soiled with organic matter such as blood, tissue, or any body fluids is considered *contaminated*. The process that renders the surface or item safe is decontamination. The disinfection or sanitation process may achieve the same result as decontamination. One must assume that all items are contaminated, and clean all items properly. Cleaning refers to the process by which any type of soil, including organic material, is removed. This is accomplished with detergent, water, and mechanical action. *Cleaning precedes all disinfection processes. The purpose of sanitation and disinfection is to prevent cross-contamination between patients and between patients and personnel.*

Decontamination of the Surgical Suite
BEFORE THE WORKDAY

All furniture, surgical lights, and fixed equipment used in the operating suites must be damp dusted with a clean, lint-free cloth and a hospital-grade chemical disinfectant. Environmental dust falls to flat surfaces, carrying disease-causing microorganisms with it. Therefore all horizontal surfaces must be wiped.

DURING SURGERY

The principles of Standard Precautions apply to all surgical procedures, and all cases are considered contaminated and treated accordingly. During surgery it is the duty of the circulator and his or her assistants to ensure that the environment in the surgical suite is kept as disease free as possible. They do this by *confining and containing* all potential contaminants. The following activities describe how this is accomplished. These activities are called Standard Precautions and must be performed to prevent cross-contamination with blood-borne pathogens:

1. Any blood spills or contamination of other organic material should be *promptly* removed with a hospital-grade disinfectant. The use of household bleach for this purpose is discouraged because of its potential to damage certain equipment and instruments.

2. All articles used and discarded in the course of surgery must be placed in leak-proof containers. This prevents spilling of contaminated liquid onto other surfaces.

3. Any contaminated or suspect item must be handled in a manner that protects personnel from contamination. Nonscrubbed personnel must wear personal protective equipment (PPE). This includes gloves, cover gown, face shield or mask, and protective eyewear. It is permissible to use an instrument (called no-touch method) to transfer contaminated articles to a waste or other receptacle.

4. Tissue specimens, blood, and all other body fluids must be placed in a leak-proof container for transport out of the department. The outside of any specimen container that is passed off the surgical field to the circulator must be cleaned with a hospital-grade disinfectant.

5. Because paper products are difficult or impossible to decontaminate, all attempts should be made to keep patient charts, laboratory slips, x-ray reports or radiographs, and other paper documentation free from contamination.

6. Contaminated sponges must be collected in a kick bucket in which a plastic bag or liner has been previously placed. Sponges must not be lined up on the floor for counting. Sponges should be counted and immediately placed in plastic bags representing increment numbers such as 5 or 10 sponges.

7. Instruments that fall off the surgical field must be retrieved by the circulator (with gloves protecting the hands) and placed in a basin or pan containing a non-corrosive hospital-grade disinfectant. In this way organic debris on the instrument is prevented from drying and becoming air-borne. If the instrument is needed to continue surgery it may be cleaned in the decontamination room and flash sterilized. The circulator must wear gloves and take precautions while cleaning the instrument.

During surgery, the scrubbed surgical technologist should periodically wipe blood and tissue from instruments. Those that are difficult to clean, such as orthopedic rasps, drill bits, and suction tips, should be kept moist at all times to prevent blood, tissue, and body fluids from drying on the surface. Small bore cannulas and suction-tip **lumens** should be flushed frequently to prevent interior buildup of debris. If a suction tip becomes completely occluded, use a metal stylet to remove the debris before flushing. When blood and tissue are allowed to dry on an instrument, they stick to the surface and may pass intact through subsequent phases of processing, including vigorous mechanical washing. Any organic debris or residue that remains is a potential source of pathogenic microorganisms, even if the item has been through the sterilization or disinfection process. A basin of sterile water should be available during surgery to aid in keeping instruments clean. Never soak instruments in saline as it causes the metal to corrode.

At the close of surgery after the final count, the scrub prepares equipment and instruments for transport out of the surgical suite. Instruments are separated by weight and structure. Delicate instruments and those with sharp tips must never be mixed with heavy instruments or equipment. This dulls cutting edges and can bend or break the tips. Any instrument exposed to the sterile field must be processed, whether it appears soiled or not.

AFTER SURGERY

After a surgical procedure, duties are shared between the scrub person, who handles equipment and instruments directly related to the performance of the surgery, and the personnel responsible for case cleanup. These can be housekeeping personnel, scrub persons, circulators, or surgical aides. Regardless of the type of personnel participating in the cleanup, all must be attired in PPE.

All linen used during the case, soiled or not, should be removed from the surgical field with as little activity as possible. This prevents contaminants from spreading via lint or other air-borne particles.

One disconnects disposable suction containers from their units and disposes of them in accordance with hospital policy. There may be regulations affecting these containers to prevent them from contaminating sanitary sewer systems; these regulations are based on specific state laws.

All disposable sharp instruments (e.g., knife blades, sutures, trocars) are placed in a designated sharps container in a manner that will not injure personnel handling the container next. If other personnel are responsible for cleaning up the back table, the scrub person should verbally communicate the presence of sharps on the table and visually identify them to the other personnel. The disposal of sharps containers is dictated by hospital policy. As a general rule, sharps disposal containers should be replaced when they are three-quarters full to prevent injury to personnel.

The scrub person then removes his or her gown and gloves, places them in the appropriate receptacles, and puts on clean protective gloves.

When all supplies, instruments, and linens have been contained, linen and trash bags then are sealed and transferred to the appropriate disposal area.

Soiled instruments and equipment then are transported from the surgical suite in a closed contained cart or open draped cart away from the restricted area. The purpose of the closed cart or an open cart draped with plastic is to reduce contamination of other areas during transport. Always confine and contain contaminated equipment during transport. Equipment is transported to a central processing area in the operating room or sent to the central processing area in a separate department. If both clean and contaminated dumbwaiters are available, place the soiled equipment in the contaminated dumbwaiter.

CASE-CART SYSTEM

The case-cart system is a method of transporting all surgical and hospital equipment from the central processing area to the outside departments, and from the outside departments back to the central processing department for reprocessing. The cart system may require specific architectural planning to ensure a means of transporting contaminated equipment *separately* from sterile-wrapped or decontaminated equipment. If elevators are used (commonly called dumbwaiters), two separate elevators, one for clean and one for contaminated equipment, are used to transport goods to and from the operating room. The central processing department may be on a separate floor or adjacent to the operating room.

The case-cart system uses one of several types of stainless steel carts for transportation of goods. Case carts that contain doors are more efficient in preventing contamination of goods than open, unprotected carts. After a surgical procedure, all contaminated equipment is loaded onto the cart, which is transported directly to central processing, where trained personnel decontaminate, assemble, wrap, sterilize, store, and distribute the equipment. All equipment to be used for a particular surgical procedure is noted on written preference cards or on computer-generated preference sheets. This method provides the information needed to help ensure that assembly of the case carts is uniform. This method requires communication between personnel in the operating room and the central processing department. In addition to standard case carts, emergency carts are maintained. The goals and advantages of a case-cart system are as follows:

1. The risk of cross-contamination and disease is reduced through separate handling and transport of sterile versus contaminated goods.
2. Quality control measures are more efficiently followed when designated personnel and work areas are centralized.
3. Packaging standards are consistent when processing is centralized.

4. The need for duplicate surgical equipment throughout the hospital is eliminated, thus reducing expense.
5. Duplication of processing equipment by different departments in the hospital is eliminated.
6. When operating room personnel are relieved of decontamination and reprocessing duties, more of their working time can be spent on patient care.

DECONTAMINATION OF FURNITURE AND FIXED EQUIPMENT

After all equipment, instruments, and supplies have been contained after surgery, the room itself and its furniture and fixed equipment can be cleaned and disinfected. One disconnects disposable suction containers from wall units and disposes of them in accordance with hospital policy. As previously mentioned, there may be regulations affecting these containers to prevent them from contaminating sanitary sewer systems; these regulations are based on specific state laws.

All equipment and furniture used during a surgical procedure are thoroughly cleaned with a hospital-grade disinfectant. During the cleaning process, mechanical friction is instrumental in the destruction of microorganisms.

The floors should be mopped between cases as specified by hospital policy. The following procedure may be used:

1. Fill bucket with disinfectant/detergent.
2. Use decontaminated mop heads or disposable mop heads (used once only) in the operating room suite.
3. Change solutions and mop heads for each suite, and clean the buckets before new solution is mixed.

The pads of the operating table are removed to expose the undersurface of the table. All surfaces of the table and pads are cleaned with particular attention to hinges, pivotal points, and castors. The table must be moved so one can clean under the supporting post and castors.

Doors and walls are spot cleaned with disinfectant. Additional attention should be paid to supply cabinet doors in the area around the latches or handles.

Linen bags are sealed and removed to the appropriate disposal area.

The surgical spotlights should be cleaned only after they have been allowed to cool, to prevent them from cracking. Some light manufacturers recommend a specific type of cleaner to prevent buildup of detergent or disinfectant film over the light's surface. Surgical spotlights are very expensive, so it is important to follow the manufacturers' guidelines and recommendations for cleaning them.

Decontamination of Other Areas in the Operating Room
DAILY CLEANUP

Areas around the surgical suite are cleaned according to need during the day. Scrub sink areas need particular attention during the day, particularly because water, a vehicle for bacterial contamination, is frequently splashed on the floors and walls. Scrub areas are frequented by surgeons who may or may not have removed protective shoe covers between cases. In the course of a busy schedule, blood and debris often are tracked from one surgical suite to another through pooled water at the scrub sinks.

The halls and doorways of the operating room experience heavy traffic and also need particular attention. Studies have shown that sticky mats placed outside the doorways of the operating room actually transfer bacteria from the mat to the shoes of those entering the department rather than the reverse; thus their use is discouraged.

Other areas that may be cleaned daily according to operating room policy include:

- Locker rooms
- Dictation and conference rooms
- Lounges
- Special equipment storage areas
- Soap dispensers: Because soap dispensers have been found to contain significant numbers of microorganisms, these must be completely disassembled and disinfected before refilling. Disposable, one-time-use soap dispensers are growing in popularity.
- Outpatient areas: Including treatment and holding areas, including all furniture and equipment. The outpatient areas often become "orphaned" because of their location away from the operating room in some hospitals, but their decontamination and sanitation must not be neglected.
- The floors of the operating room suite: These are cleaned at the end of each day with a wet vacuum system. This can be either a centralized system or a portable wet vacuum system.

At the end of each day, each operating suite should undergo terminal disinfection. In this process, all items within the suite, including walls, ceilings, floors, and equipment, are cleaned with a particular focus on wheels, castors, and other crevices. Before beginning this process, one should remove all porous items from the room to prevent splashing with cleaning solutions. One begins the process by wiping ceilings and floors with a sponge-mop and disinfectant solution.

Next, all equipment, including table legs and castors or wheels, is wiped down with disinfectant solution. The OR table should be raised to its highest level, and all pads and attachments removed. All surfaces of the OR table are cleaned with disinfectant solution as are pads and attachments. These items should be allowed to air-dry before reassembly. Ancillary equipment, including the electrosurgical unit, suction units, anesthesia gas machines, supply carts, stools, desks, and kick buckets, also is cleaned.

Finally, equipment is moved to one side of the room and the floor is saturated with disinfectant, scrubbed, and wet-vacuumed. Equipment is then shifted to the other side of the room, and the remaining floor is cleaned and wet-vacuumed. After the floor is dry, equipment is repositioned for the next day's surgical procedures.

WEEKLY CLEANUP

According to operating room and hospital policy, the following surfaces and areas are cleaned and disinfected each week:

1. Ventilation and air conditioning/heating duct grills must be vacuumed to prevent the release of bacteria-laden dust into the surgical environment.
2. Inside shelves of supply cabinets must be cleaned.
3. In some hospitals, utility and supply carts are steam cleaned.
4. Utility rooms, including those used to store housekeeping supplies, sewer hoppers, and linens, must be cleaned.

Decontamination of Surgical Instruments

To avoid risk of contamination by pathogens (especially blood-borne organisms), personnel working in cleaning and decontamination areas must don personal protective attire. This includes head cap, face shield, impermeable gown or apron, gloves, and shoe covers or boots.

When instruments are received in the processing area, they are fully sorted (Figure 8-2). Sharp instruments are placed in cleaning trays or basins so that the tips face down and are easily visible. Any equipment that is needed right away is separated for immediate reprocessing. Any instrument with detachable parts is disassembled. This exposes all areas to be properly cleaned. When the instruments are disassembled, small parts should be kept together to avoid loss.

Surgical instruments represent a significant threat of cross-contamination between the patient and surgical personnel. Therefore they merit special discussion. It is extremely important to clean the surgical instruments properly. After the instruments are received for decontamination, they must be thoroughly inspected and cleaned.

The most common method of decontaminating stainless steel surgical instruments uses the **washer-sterilizer**. The washer-sterilizer not only cleans but also sterilizes instruments. However, before being processed through the washer-sterilizer, some hard-to-clean areas of the instruments must be scrubbed to remove bits of tissue and debris. Of special concern are the serrations of hemostatic and other tissue clamps, rasps, blades that contain bits of bone and tissue, and items with lumens, all of which must be thoroughly cleaned. One washes instruments by placing them in a basin with a mild detergent that is neutral or slightly alkaline. Extreme care must be taken to prevent splashing and spraying of contaminated material; when a brush is used to clean the instruments it must be kept below the level of the water.

Personal protective attire must be worn during the washing procedure. After cleansing, instruments may be placed in the washer-sterilizer in mesh trays (Figure 8-3). All box

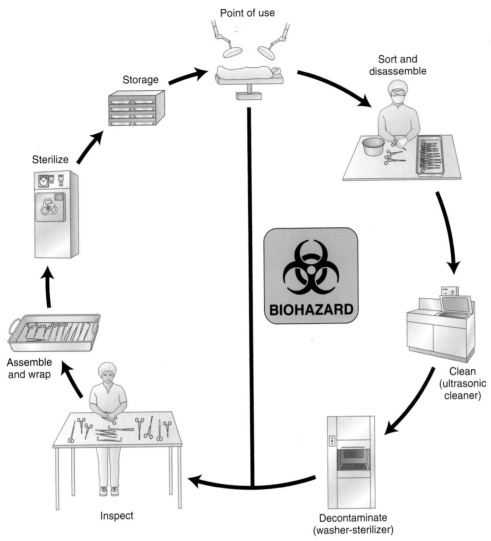

FIGURE 8-2
Cycle of equipment processing.

locks must be opened and hinges extended to their widest adjustment.

The washer-sterilizer operates much the same as the steam sterilizer. The washer-sterilizer sends copious amounts of soapy water over the instruments. Steam under pressure and air are then injected into the water, which activates the water significantly. As the water drains from the chamber, tissue debris and particles are filtered off and steam fills the entire chamber. The temperature is then maintained at 270° F for 3 minutes. Near the completion of the cycle, the steam is released through the exhaust system.

After processing in the washer-sterilizer, all instruments should be placed in the **ultrasonic cleaner** (Figure 8-4). This cleaning further removes particles and debris through a process called **cavitation**. During cavitation, high-frequency sound waves are generated through a water bath in which the instruments are placed along with a neutral to slightly alkaline detergent. Cavitation causes tiny air spaces trapped

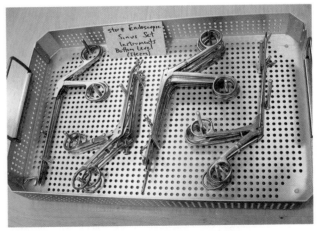

FIGURE 8-3
Instrument tray. (Courtesy of Case Medical, Ridgefield, NJ.)

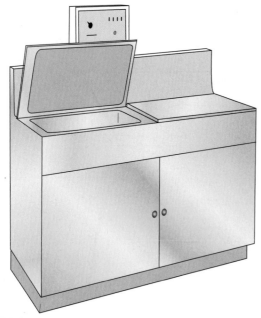

FIGURE 8-4
Ultrasonic cleaner. (Redrawn from Reichert M, Young J, eds: *Sterilization technology for the health care facility,* ed 2, Gaithersburg, 1997, Aspen Publishers.)

within debris to explode inwardly (implode), and this causes their release from the surface of the instrument.

After cavitation, instruments are rinsed thoroughly and dried. Because cavitation is *not* a disinfecting or sterilizing process, all instruments subjected to cavitation must first be processed by the washer-sterilizer. In addition, if the washer-sterilizer has not been used to process instruments before their ultrasonic cleaning, the immersion bath of the ultrasound cleaner must be rinsed and cleaned between cycles of instruments, because it may contain tissue debris that can culture potentially harmful microorganisms.

STERILIZATION

Sterility is defined as the absence of any living microorganism, including bacteria, viruses, and spores. An object is either sterile or not sterile. Because the inner tissues of the body are sterile, any instruments or items that come in contact with these tissues also must be sterile. The purpose of disinfection and sterilization is to reduce the probability of disease transmission to the lowest possible level. Contamination of body tissues with nonsterile items can lead to serious infection. It is therefore critical that all personnel working in surgery or those working with surgical supplies and equipment understand the process of sterilization. One point is of critical importance: *disinfection does not render an item sterile.* The several methods used to sterilize equipment are discussed in this chapter.

All methods of sterilization require three elements to be effective: concentration, time, and temperature. Concentration refers to the amount or percentage of sterilization

agent used during the process. Time is the minimum amount of time a sterilizing agent must remain in contact with all surfaces of the item being sterilized to achieve sterility. Each agent used during sterilization has an effective temperature range that is specific to the particular agent. When selecting a method of sterilization, one must consider the item to be sterilized. Some items may be damaged by excessive heat and therefore may not be processed through high-temperature sterilization methods. Certain sterilizing agents are damaging to particular instruments and must not be used to process those items. Safety and cost-effectiveness of sterilization processes also are of concern to health-care managers.

Steam Sterilization

The boiling point of water is 212° F (100° C). When water exceeds this temperature, it converts to steam. Steam alone is inadequate for sterilization, but when steam is pressurized, its temperature rises. Steam under pressure (moist heat sterilization) is the most common method of sterilization for instruments and supplies used in the operating room and elsewhere in the hospital. Steam sterilization is the most cost-effective and safest, and is least damaging to most items.

For pressurized steam to be effective, a specific amount of moisture must be present within the sterilizer chamber. It is this moist, pressurized heat that causes the destruction of microbes by coagulation and denaturation of the protein within the cells. The relationship among temperature, pressure, and exposure time is instrumental in the destruction of microbes. When steam is contained in a closed compartment and the pressure is increased, the temperature will increase provided the volume of the compartment remains the same. If items are exposed to steam long enough at a specified temperature and pressure, the items will be rendered sterile. The unit used to create this atmosphere of high-temperature pressurized steam is called an *autoclave.*

TEMPERATURE AND STEAM STERILIZATION

Steam sterilization is typically performed at 250° F (121° C) or 270° F (132° C), depending on the items being sterilized. Water is converted to steam at 212° F (100° C). This temperature is inadequate to achieve destruction of bacterial spores. However, when steam is placed under pressure, its temperature is raised to an acceptable level that will destroy spores. During the process of raising the temperature within the sterilizer (autoclave) chamber, heat is transferred to the objects being sterilized. This process of heat transfer increases the time required to achieve sterilization.

The term heat (or heating) describes the transfer of energy from one substance (steam) to another (item to be sterilized). Temperature refers to the amount of energy present in an object and is described according to a designated scale (Fahrenheit or Centigrade). During steam sterilization, sufficient energy (heat) must be transferred from the steam to the item being sterilized to ensure destruction of all microbes.

PRESSURE AND STEAM STERILIZATION

Pressure is used to raise the temperature of steam to a level sufficient to destroy all microbial life. Pressure is typically expressed as atmospheric (barometric) pressure. Standard atmospheric (barometric) pressure is expressed as 14.7 pounds per square inch (psi). Atmospheric pressure is measured with a barometer, a gauge that uses the element mercury (Hg) and identifies the height of a column of mercury raised by air pressure at a given time. This measurement is expressed in inches or millimeters. Standard atmospheric (barometric) pressure at sea level is 29.92 inches of mercury (29.92 in/Hg) or 760 millimeters of mercury (760 mm/Hg) in height.

A steam sterilizer is simply an enclosed vessel that is designed to allow steam to become pressurized. The pressure within the sterilizer chamber is measured by a pressure gauge. A pressure gauge measures the difference between chamber pressure and the external atmospheric pressure. The standard pressure gauge measures pressure in pounds per square inch and vacuum in millimeters of mercury. This is expressed as pounds per square inch gauge (psig) and indicates absolute pressure minus standard atmospheric pressure. During installation, the gauge is set to record zero at normal atmospheric pressure.

The pressure (psig) required to achieve a temperature of 250° F (121° C) is 15 pounds (per square inch gauge) within the chamber. The pressure within the chamber must reach 27 psig to increase the temperature to 270° F (132° C). Remember, at sea level, normal atmospheric pressure is 14.7 psi. Keep in mind that at higher elevations atmospheric pressure decreases. This is important to remember when considering the pressure required to increase the temperature of steam to an acceptable level to destroy microbial life. A general rule is that the pressure required within the sterilizer chamber must be increased 0.5 psi for every elevation in altitude of 1,000 feet above sea level to maintain appropriate sterilization temperatures.

TIME AND STEAM STERILIZATION

In steam sterilization the minimum time required for sterilization depends on the temperature used and whether the cycle being used is a gravity displacement sterilizer or a high-vacuum sterilizer, along with manufacturer's recommended guidelines (Table 8-4).

CONCENTRATION AND STEAM STERILIZATION

Effective steam sterilization requires a specific concentration, or quality, of steam. This factor depends on the amount of moisture present in the steam. If too little moisture is present, items become superheated and can eventually be damaged. Too much moisture will leave items wet and prone to strike-through contamination after removal from the chamber. The quality of steam used for sterilization should exceed 97%. This means that no more than 3% liquid water is present in the sterilizer; 100% quality means that no water is present in liquid form. Steam quality of less than 97% can result in wet packs, which can lead to strike-through contamination.

Water is converted to steam at 212° F (100° C). Steam at this temperature is ineffective for sterilization. As the steam at this temperature contacts instruments and other items in the load, the items to be sterilized draw heat from the steam, thus lowering the temperature of the steam initially. When this happens, the steam is converted back to its liquid state. This is known as condensation. Steam of this quality is called saturated steam. That is to say, the moisture content of the steam is high. Heat transfer and condensation allow items to reach the sterilization temperature more quickly than is noted with dry-heat sterilization.

CONTAMINANTS AND STEAM STERILIZATION

Although water that is used during steam sterilization is filtered, contaminants are still present. These usually consist of minerals that are too small to be trapped by filters. These minerals become deposited on the surfaces of sterilized items and on the internal surfaces of the sterilizers. Water that contains excessive mineral content is frequently called "hard water." The presence of orange, white, brown, or black spots on items removed from the steam sterilizer may indicate the presence of excess minerals in the water supply. Trained personnel should check water quality to correct this problem. As these minerals become deposited in the box locks of surgical instruments, they can impair the function of these instruments. Mineral deposits also lead to dulling of scissors and the breakdown of fabrics.

TYPES OF STEAM STERILIZERS

Gravity Displacement Sterilizer

The **gravity** (or "downward") **displacement sterilizer** uses the principle that air is heavier than steam (Figure 8-5). Within the sterilizer there is an inner chamber where goods are loaded and an outer jacket-type chamber that injects steam forcefully into the inner chamber. Any air in the inner chamber blocks the passage of pressurized steam to the surface of the goods and thus prevents sterilization. All the air must be removed from the inner chamber because all surfaces of the items must be exposed to the pressurized steam to ensure sterilization. Therefore the sterilizer is constructed in such a way that air is pushed downward by gravity (hence the name "gravity displacement sterilizer").

The air exits the chamber through a temperature-sensitive valve. As the amount of steam builds up in the chamber, the temperature increases, and when the sterilization temperature is reached, the valve closes. Careful loading of items in this type of sterilizer is critical because if the load is too dense or improperly positioned, air may get trapped in pockets. Items in these air pockets will not be sterilized because the steam cannot displace the air, which acts as an insulator.

Prevacuum Sterilizer

The prevacuum sterilizer does not rely on gravity to remove air from the inner chamber. Instead, the air is pulled out of the chamber using a special vacuum apparatus built into the sterilizer. This evacuates all air within the chamber. Steam is

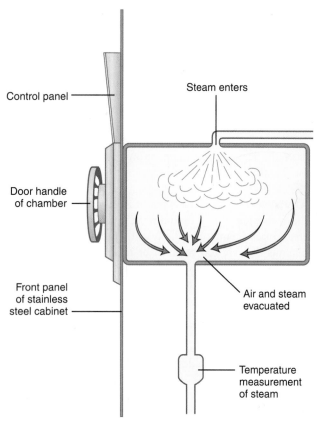

FIGURE 8-5
Steam sterilizer. (Redrawn from Phillips N: *Berry & Kohn's operating room technique,* ed 10, St Louis, 2004, Mosby.)

then injected into the chamber to replace the air. This type of sterilizer offers greater steam penetration in a shorter time than the gravity displacement sterilizer. When the designated time, pressure, and temperature have been reached and maintained, the steam is removed through a filter and the chamber is reduced to normal (atmospheric) temperature and then cooled to a level at which personnel may safely handle the sterilized goods. There is an alternative process in which the air is removed by a process of steam flushes and pressure pulses at *above atmospheric level.* This process is not affected by air leaks that may occur through the valves and around the door seal and thus produces a more reliable method of sterilization.

Flash Sterilizer

The flash sterilizer has traditionally been used in the operating room and in other areas of the hospital to quickly sterilize items that are unwrapped. It had been common practice to flash sterilize any instrument that had become contaminated during surgery. If the instrument was still required to complete the surgery, it was flash sterilized and returned to use. However, this type of sterilizer should now be used only when no other alternative is available. The efficacy of the flash sterilization is constantly scrutinized. When unwrapped goods are sterilized in the flash sterilizer, the risk of contamination of the processed items is great because of the process of transferring the sterile items. When any item is

flash sterilized, its manufacturer's recommendations for time and temperature must be followed. Implants should never be flash sterilized. See Table 8-3 for flash sterilization parameters and Box 8-1 for recommended practices for flash sterilization.

Ideally, items to be flash sterilized should be in a specially designed covered tray. Items that are flash sterilized must not be wrapped. Linen and paper prevent adequate contact time for steam sterilization in a flash sterilizer. Institutions that do not use covered flash-sterilization trays will have special transfer handles that are sterilized and allow for the aseptic transfer of trays from the flash sterilizer to the OR.

Items that have been sterilized in a flash sterilizer are removed with sterile handles individually packaged and used by a team member who is not in sterile gown and gloves. The sides of the mesh tray in which the items were sterilized are grasped with the sterile transfer handles, and the tray is offered to a scrub assistant for transfer to the surgical field. When the instrument tray is removed from the sterilizer and carried to the surgical team, the surgical technologist's arms and hands must be positioned away from the tray to prevent fallout contamination. The scrub should remove the sterile item from the tray with care to prevent contamination of her or his gown or gloves. The tray should not be left on the sterile field, and *under no circumstances should the scrub leave the sterile field or room to retrieve the item from the sterilizer.*

When removing a sterile tray from a flash sterilizer, remember that the walls of the inner chamber are very hot. If the sterilizer has just completed its cycle, be extremely cautious when removing trays or items.

LOADING AND OPERATION

Because steam sterilization depends on direct steam contact with all surfaces of the items, the sterilizer must be loaded so that the steam will penetrate through each pack (Figure 8-6, *A* and *B*). Instrument pans with mesh or wire bottoms are sterilized flat on the sterilizer shelf. Linen packs, because of their density, require special attention. Linen packs are best sterilized by placing packs on their sides. Packs and instrument trays should be placed so they touch loosely, and small items should be placed crosswise over each other. Heavy packs should be placed at the periphery of the load, where steam enters the chamber. Basins, jars, cups, or other containers should be placed on their sides with the lids slightly ajar so the air can flow out of them and steam can enter. Any item that has a smooth surface on which water can collect and drip during the cooling phase of the sterilization cycle should be placed at the bottom of the load.

Most modern steam sterilizers are controlled via push buttons that are clearly labeled. The operator sets the temperature and time and then initiates the cycle. The sterilizer passes through its phases automatically. Some sterilizers are equipped with a graph adjacent to the time and temperature panel that registers the maximum temperature and pressure reached during the cycle. This graph must be monitored to ensure that the items in the sterilizer have been adequately

Table 8-3   TIME-TEMPERATURE PARAMETERS FOR FLASH STEAM STERILIZATION

Type of Sterilizer	Load Configuration	Temperature in °C (°F)	Time in Minutes
Gravity displacement	Metal or nonporous items only (no lumens)	132-135 (270-275)	3
	Metal items with lumens and porous items (e.g., rubber, plastic) sterilized together	132-135 (270-275)	10
Prevacuum	Metal or nonporous items only (no lumens)	132-135 (270-275)	3
	Metal items with lumens and porous items sterilized together	132-135 (270-275)	4 or manufacturer's instructions
Pulsing gravity	All loads	Manufacturer's instructions	Manufacturer's instructions
Abbreviated prevacuum	All loads	Manufacturer's instructions	Manufacturer's instructions

From Rothrock JC, ed: *Alexander's care of the patient in surgery,* ed 12, St Louis, 2003, Mosby.

Box 8-1   Recommended Practices for Flash Sterilization

▶ Implants should never be flash sterilized before use. If an implant must be sterilized in an emergency, a rapid-readout BI must be used.

▶ The manufacturer's specifications for exposure time and temperature must be followed.

▶ If a covered sterilization container is used to flash sterilize instruments, parameter values specified by the manufacturers of both the container and the sterilizer must be compared and the specifications followed as directed.

▶ Never flash sterilize any power equipment or cords without first verifying the manufacturer's recommendations. Many pneumatic or battery-operated power instruments cannot be safely sterilized by steam under pressure.

▶ Flash sterilizers must be located in an area where unwrapped sterile items can be transported directly from the sterilizer to the sterile field.

▶ Never wrap items for flash sterilization unless permitted by the manufacturer's specifications. If wrappers are permitted, always follow prescribed exposure time and temperature.

▶ Sterilization monitors must be used with every load.

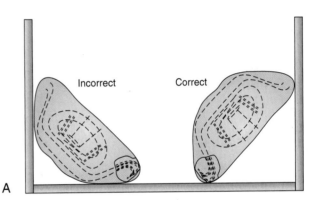
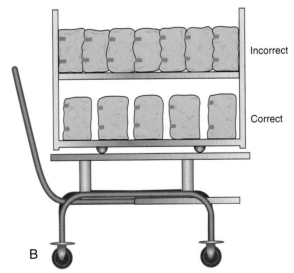

FIGURE 8-6
A, Placement of basin sets in chamber. **B,** Drying packs on carts. (Courtesy of STERIS Corp, Mentor, Ohio.)

exposed to the prescribed amount of heat, pressure, and time. The total time necessary to expose goods to pressurized steam and sterilize them depends on the density of the goods and on the temperature within the sterilizer. The minimum temperature-time standards are listed in Table 8-4.

These exposure times and temperatures do not reflect the entire time needed to include all phases of the sterilization process. These minimum standards apply only to the amount of time necessary for the pressurized steam to contact all surfaces of the load. Total exposure time includes the warm-up phase, holding phase (sometimes called the "kill time"), a factor of safety time, and an exhaust phase. Some sterilizers also

include a drying phase. Because these times may vary from load to load, depending on the items to be sterilized, the operator should always check the specifications of the item's manufacturer, not the sterilizer's manufacturer, for recommended sterilization times and temperatures. Many items, es-

Table 8-4   MINIMUM EXPOSURE TIME STANDARDS FOR STEAM STERILIZATION AFTER EFFECTIVE STEAM PENETRATION AND HEAT TRANSFER

	Gravity Displacement		Prevacuum
Materials	250° F (121° C)	270° F (132° C)	270° F (132° C)
Basin sets—wrapped	20 min	Not applicable	4 min
Basins, glassware, and utensils—unwrapped	15 min	Not recommended	3 min
Instruments, with or without other items—wrapped as set in double-thickness wrappers	30 min	Not applicable	4 min
Instruments—unwrapped but with other items, including towel in bottom of tray or cover over them	20 min	10 min	4 min
Instruments—completely unwrapped	15 min	3 min	3 min
Drape packs—12 × 12 × 20 inches (30 × 30 × 50 cm) maximum size, 12 pounds (5.5 kg) maximum weight	30 min*	Not applicable	4 min
Fabrics, single items—wrapped	30 min*	Not applicable	4 min
Rubber and thermoplastics, including small items and gloves but excluding tubing—wrapped	20 min*	Not applicable	4 min
Tubing—wrapped	30 min	Not applicable	4 min
Tubing—unwrapped	20 min	Not applicable	4 min
Sponges and dressings—wrapped	30 min	Not applicable	4 min
Solutions—flasked	(Slow exhaust)	Not applicable	Automatic selector determines correct temperature and exposure period for solutions
75-ml flask	20 min		
250-ml flask	25 min		
500-ml flask	30 min		
1000-ml flask	35 min		
1500-ml flask	45 min		
2000-ml flask	45 min		

From Phillips N: *Berry & Kohn's operating room technique*, ed 10, St Louis, 2004, Mosby.
*Fabrics and rubber deteriorate more quickly with repeated sterilization for prolonged periods in gravity displacement sterilizer.

pecially heavy instruments and power-driven orthopedic tools, require longer periods of sterilization and cooling.

PRECAUTIONS AND HAZARDS

In spite of safety features that are built into the steam sterilizer, *accidents occasionally happen.* The operator should be particularly careful when opening or closing the door. It is held in the lock position by a pressure-sensitive valve that prevents the door from being opened when the chamber is under pressure. Because the door has a tremendous amount of pressure inside exerted on it by the steam, the valve is designed to withstand very high temperatures and force from within. If the valve malfunctions for any reason, the operator may be able to open the door while the chamber is partially pressurized with steam. If this happens, he or she will be exposed to a rapid burst of hot steam when the door is opened. *Always check the pressure gauge on the control panel*

before opening the door! If the pressure has not dropped to atmospheric (0) level at the completion of the sterilization cycle, wait for it to do so. If the pressure remains elevated, do not attempt to open the door. Do not attempt to resolve the malfunction. The malfunction should be reported so that trained personnel can be called for assistance.

Occasionally the operator may fail to close the door all the way. This is usually caused by the misalignment of the spoke-like locks that are mounted on the front of the door. When this happens, a constant flow of steam escapes from around the edges of the door. This is often associated with a loud "whistle" from the escaping steam. The escape of steam may be so great that the operator cannot approach the sterilizer control panel to turn the unit off. Most models have a steam shutoff valve located close to the floor, below the sterilizer. The valve can be turned to the "off" position only if it is approachable without risk of injury. Steam should then be

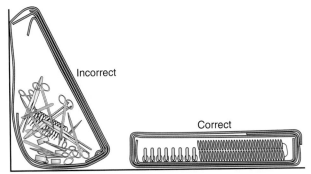

FIGURE 8-7
Placement of instrument trays in chamber. (Courtesy of STERIS Corp, Mentor, Ohio.)

allowed to dissipate from the sterilizer until it is safe to open the door completely. Do not attempt to reach the valve unless the area around it is completely cool and free of steam.

PREPARATION AND INSPECTION OF ITEMS

Steam sterilization should be used only for items that can withstand high temperatures and pressures. Some items are impenetrable by steam, and these should be sterilized through another method. If unsure about which method to use on a particular piece of equipment, the operator should always check the manufacturer's specifications. Below is a list of items commonly sterilized by steam under pressure. This discussion assumes that the item has already been thoroughly cleaned and is ready for sterilization.

Stainless steel instruments must be open (unlocked) and strung together by means of an instrument stringer designed to hold the instruments in an open position during the sterilization process (Figure 8-7). When assembling instrument trays, make sure that any sharp or pointed items are turned down to avoid injury or glove puncture when the pack is opened and sorted at the sterile instrument table.

Most operating rooms keep computerized file cards that list the various types of instruments to be included in particular trays. Make sure that all instruments listed on the card are included in the tray. If an item is missing, locate the item before processing the instrument tray. Do not simply leave it out of the tray. Instrument trays should have a mesh bottom so that steam can circulate up through the tray and adequately cover all surfaces of the instruments. Be sure that no instrument tips are caught in the perforations where they could become damaged. Towels may be placed on the bottom of the pans to prevent damage to the instrument tips during the sterilization process. Remember, towels or linen must not be used during flash sterilization. Always place heavy instruments on the bottom of the tray and pack or nest the instruments so that they cannot shift and damage each other during processing.

All instruments must be examined to ensure that all tissue debris, fats or grease, and soil have been removed. At the same time, instruments must be checked for proper function and for mechanical and structural soundness. Different guidelines must be followed for different instruments.

Instruments should be checked periodically for proper function. When inspecting instruments, first examine all areas of the instrument. The shanks of instruments such as hemostats, needle holders, and scissors should be straight. The instrument should be opened and shut several times. If the instrument is stiff while opening and closing, it should be lubricated with an instrument milk solution. While examining the instrument, consider the following: Do the ratchets mesh properly? Does the instrument stay shut after it is closed? With time, hemostats and needle holders may spring open unexpectedly. This is dangerous. To determine whether the instrument is "sprung" (will not stay closed), close the jaws and lock the ratchets in place. Rap the edge of the finger rings gently on a firm surface. An instrument that is sprung will pop open when bumped. This occurs if the shanks are bent or the ratchets are out of alignment.

Cutting instruments such as scissors, curettes, osteotomes, rongeurs, and shears should be examined for pitting along the cutting edge. Sharp instruments should be inspected to ensure that the blade surfaces meet smoothly and properly. Forceps must be tested for spring. When the tips are compressed and then released, they should immediately return to the open position. The tips of forceps should close freely, and the tips should meet precisely in alignment.

Microsurgical instruments are very expensive to purchase and very expensive to repair or replace. Microsurgical instruments should never be mixed with heavier instruments. The tips of micro instruments always should be inspected under magnification to ensure that the sharp points are smooth, sharp, and in proper alignment. Any instrument that is found to be malfunctioning should not be packaged and sterilized. It should be sent for repair.

Linen must be freshly laundered when it is used as a wrapping material or is the item being wrapped. The minute amount of water trapped between the individual fibers of linen vaporizes and pushes the air out of the fabric when steam sterilized. Fabric that is not freshly laundered contains no moisture, and thus air trapped within the fibers prevents adequate steam penetration. The largest acceptable linen pack size is 12 × 12 × 20 inches and should have a maximum weight of 12 pounds.

Basins should be stacked together with a towel or absorbent cloth between each separate basin (Figure 8-8, *A* through *C*). This allows steam to penetrate the cloth and wick to all surfaces of the container. Bowls or cups should be prepared in the same manner.

Items with a lumen should have a small amount of sterile de-ionized (distilled) water flushed through them immediately before sterilization. This water vaporizes during sterilization and forces air out of the lumen. Any air that is left in the lumen may prevent sterilization of its inner surface.

Powered surgical instruments (e.g., drills, saws) should be sterilized only according to the manufacturer's specifications. The equipment always should be disassembled before sterilization. Hoses can be coiled loosely during packaging, and all delicate switches and parts should be protected during preparation. Before sterilization, power instruments

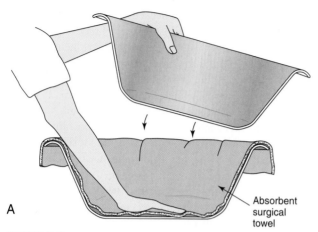

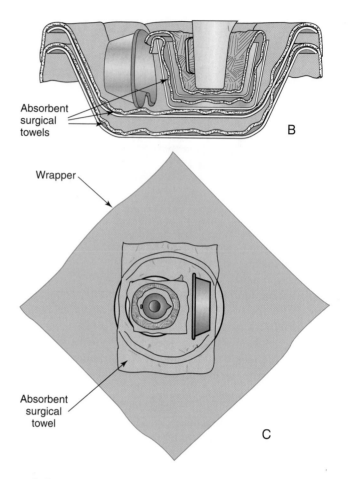

FIGURE 8-8
A and **B,** Stacking basins together with towels between them. **C,** Preparing basins for wrapping. (Courtesy of STERIS Corp, Mentor, Ohio.)

should be lubricated according to the manufacturer's specifications. Some instruments require that the motor be operated during lubrication to distribute the lubricant through the internal mechanism. Always consult the manufacturer's specifications before choosing a lubricant. Do not operate the instrument unless you have been specifically taught how. Excessive pressure (expressed in pounds per square inch [psi]) can irreversibly damage the instrument. Finally, before processing, ensure that all switches and control devices are in the *safety* position.

Stainless steel, linens, and other substances and devices that can withstand high temperature, high pressure, and moisture are steam sterilized. Rubber and latex products cannot be steam sterilized because steam is unable to penetrate the material.

Items that should not be sterilized by steam include items made of rubber (steam does not penetrate rubber), wood items (such as tongue depressors), or any item that would obviously be severely damaged by high temperature and pressure, such as lensed instruments, those with delicate parts, or those that contain materials that could melt. Synthetic materials, such as Silastic, Teflon, polyethylene, polypropylene, and other complex polymers, must be sterilized according to the manufacturer's instructions. When in doubt about whether an item can tolerate steam under pressure, *wait, seek assistance, and follow instructions.*

To assist in the removal of moisture and to prevent "wet packs," the sterilizer operator may use a dry cycle as part of the steam sterilization process. Regardless of whether a dry cycle is employed, items that have been steam sterilized should be allowed to remain in the sterilizer chamber for 15 to 30 minutes after the cycle to prevent formation of condensate.

Ethylene Oxide Sterilization

Ethylene oxide (EO) is a highly flammable liquid that, when blended with inert gas, produces effective sterilization by destroying the DNA and protein structure of microorganisms.

Ethylene oxide is used to sterilize items that cannot withstand high temperatures, high pressure, or moisture. In the past, ethylene oxide was blended with chlorofluorocarbons (CFCs) or Freon for stabilization. Since the passage of the Clean Air Act, however, CFC-12 and Freon are no longer options. Alternative ethylene oxide mixtures and sterilization methods have been developed. Ethylene oxide is now used in 100% pure form, blended with carbon dioxide gas, or mixed with hydrochlorofluorocarbons.

At this time, no sterilization method matches ethylene oxide's penetrability. Ethylene oxide's primary advantage is its ability to penetrate wrappers and other materials and to disinfect objects that cannot tolerate the heat, moisture, and pressure of steam sterilization.

Ethylene oxide is toxic and poses serious risks to patients and personnel. Prolonged occupational exposure to ethylene oxide gas is known to cause leukemia and may result in neurological dysfunction, respiratory damage, or spontaneous abortion. Ethylene oxide may be teratogenic (capable of causing birth defects). It is a stable compound with a long half-life. Its advantage as a penetrating sterilant also poses hazards. It is difficult to remove, and the level of ethylene oxide residue is not the same in different materials. In addition, it reacts with many different substances, causing their disintegration or creating other toxic compounds such as ethylene glycol and ethylene chlorohydrins. These chemicals also are difficult to remove from the environment.

Table 8-5	MINIMUM AERATION TIMES AFTER ETHYLENE OXIDE STERILIZATION AT DIFFERENT TEMPERATURES			
		Ambient Room Air	Mechanical Aerator	
Materials		65°-72° F (18°-22° C)	122° F (50° C)	140° F (60° C)
Metal and glass				
Unwrapped		May be used immediately		
Wrapped		2 hr	2 hr	2 hr
Rubber for external use—not sealed in plastic		24 hr	8 hr	5 hr
Polyethylene and polypropylene for external use— not sealed in plastic		48 hr	12 hr	8 hr
Plastics except polyvinyl chloride items—not sealed in plastic		96 hr (4 days)	12 hr	8 hr
Polyvinyl chloride		168 hr (7 days)	12 hr	8 hr
Plastic and rubber items—those sealed in plastic and/or those that will come in contact with body tissues		168 hr (7 days)	12 hr	8 hr
Internal pacemaker		504 hr (21 days)	32 hr	24 hr

From Phillips N: *Berry & Kohn's operating room technique*, ed 10, St Louis, 2004, Mosby.

Ethylene oxide kills microorganisms and their spores by interfering with the metabolic and reproductive processes of the cell. The process is intensified with both heat and moisture. The ethylene oxide (EO) sterilizer operates at a low temperature. The temperature of the gas directly affects the penetration of items in the chamber. Operating temperatures range from 85° F to 100° F for a "cold cycle," and 130° F to 145° F for a "warm cycle." Dried spores are resistant to sterilization by ethylene oxide. For this reason, moisture is added to the sterilization cycle. The preferred humidity (moisture content) for EO sterilization is 25% to 80%. The length of exposure depends on the type and density of material to be sterilized, temperature, humidity, and concentration of the gas. Exact time is specified by the sterilizer's manufacturer.

Unlike steam sterilization, items sterilized with ethylene oxide require *aeration* to dissipate any residual gas remaining on the items. *The manufacturer's recommendations for aeration are critical to the safety of the patient and to hospital personnel handling equipment that has been gas sterilized.* Aeration takes place in a special aeration chamber or may be accomplished with room air provided that safety precautions are followed. In many newer models, aeration takes place within the sterilizer chamber through the addition of an aerator that evacuates the gas from the chamber and flushes the chamber with room air. The aeration time for an object depends on its porosity and size (Table 8-5).

Observing the following precautions reduces occupational and patient risk:

▶ After the sterilization process is finished, keep the sterilizer door opened slightly for about 15 minutes.
▶ Be sure goods transported from the sterilizer to the aerator remain on a transport cart.
▶ Always wear protective gloves when handling un-aerated items.

▶ Always pull the transport cart rather than pushing it. Pushing the cart places personnel in back of the air flowing from the un-aerated items.
▶ Follow the manufacturer's specifications for aeration exactly.

PRECAUTIONS AND HAZARDS

The environmental and safety hazards associated with ethylene oxide are many and grave. Any employee who is involved with this sterilization process should follow all recommended guidelines to prevent injury to himself or herself, patients, and others in the hospital environment. Ethylene oxide is suspected of being carcinogenic and mutagenic. It is also teratogenic and can have other serious physical effects. Ethylene oxide can cause the following:

▶ Burns to skin and mucous membranes
▶ Nausea, vomiting, headache, weakness
▶ Irritation of the respiratory system
▶ Destruction of blood cells (when undissipated gas contacts the circulatory system)

To prevent injury from ethylene oxide exposure, the Occupational Safety and Health Administration (OSHA) requires air sampling in areas that are likely to contain high concentrations of ethylene oxide. The level of ethylene oxide must not exceed 0.5 ppm in any area. Sampling is documented in accordance with federal, state, and local regulations. Personal dosimeter badges measure ethylene oxide exposure. Air samples should be taken regularly in the sterilization area. Water combines with ethylene oxide to form ethylene glycol. Other safety precautions include the installation of an exhaust system that vents the gas to the outside of the building through an exhaust vent located above the chamber door. Six to ten exchanges of fresh air per hour are delivered to the sterilization area.

Never retrieve an instrument from the aerator before completion of the approved aeration period. Likewise, do not ask anyone else to do this, even if the surgeon requests it.

PREPARATION AND INSPECTION OF ITEMS

All items to be gas sterilized must be *clean* and *dry.* Any moisture left on equipment will bond with ethylene oxide gas and produce a toxic residue. This residue can cause burns or toxic reaction to those who contact it. Any organic material or soil that is exposed to ethylene oxide also may produce toxic residues; therefore all items processed for EO gas must be completely clean. Items are loaded in the sterilizer loosely, so that the gas is free to circulate over every surface. Every attempt should be made to load items that have similar aeration requirements. Some items must not be gas sterilized. These include acrylics and some pharmaceutical items. Because ethylene oxide does not penetrate glass, solutions contained within a glass vial or bottle will not be rendered sterile by this method.

Any instruments that have fittings or parts should be disassembled before ethylene oxide sterilization. This facilitates their exposure to the gas.

A general rule when preparing any equipment for gas sterilization is that loose is better than restricted. For example, rubber sheeting, such as that used in the manufacture of Esmarch bandages, always should be loosely folded rather than tightly rolled. Any two surfaces that are held tightly together will not be exposed to the gas and thus will not be rendered sterile.

Wrapping techniques for ethylene oxide sterilization are the same as those for high-pressure steam sterilization. However, some wrapping materials are not suitable for ethylene oxide processing. These include wrappers of natural fiber combined with nylon and rayon, polyester, and polyvinyl chloride. Double-wrapped peel-apart pouches are not suitable for some ethylene oxide sterilizers. The manufacturer's recommendations always should be followed.

The ethylene oxide sterilizer is loaded in such a way that gas can penetrate all surfaces of the packages. Packages must not touch the bottom or top of the chamber and must be placed loosely on their sides.

Sterilization by Ionizing Radiation

Most equipment available prepackaged from the manufacturer has been sterilized by ionizing radiation (**cobalt 60**). This process is restricted to commercial use because of the expense. Items such as sutures, sponges, and disposable drapes are just a few of the many types of presterilized products available. Also included are anhydrous materials such as powders and petroleum goods. These products traditionally have been sterilized by dry heat in the hospital setting. However, there is a trend to move away from dry-heat sterilization because of its inconvenience and because these substances are now available as single-use items, packaged in one-dose containers to prevent cross-contamination. Items intended for single use, whether they are supplies for use in the surgical field or substances meant for single use, must

never be resterilized by conventional methods (steam sterilization, ethylene oxide, or chemical sterilization) without the manufacturer's express recommendation to do so. The item might change in composition or deteriorate and could become a hazard to the patient or personnel.

Wrapping Products for Sterilization

All items to be sterilized by pressurized steam, ethylene oxide, or plasma methods must be wrapped *in a prescribed manner.* The procedure for wrapping goods is not based on convenience or personal preference. It is based on the principle *of enhancing the ease of sterilization and of preserving the sterility of the item.* In achieving these two goals, certain standard methods must be used. These methods have been subjected to challenge and proven to be effective.

Several different materials are available for wrapping items and equipment to be sterilized. All materials have been chosen because they meet certain specifications. Some materials are better for certain processes than others, and these always should be used with the intended process in mind. The wrapper should protect the item from dust, vermin, and penetration. It should resist tearing or delamination (separation of layers). It should be easy to handle to facilitate wrapping and delivery.

Fabric wrappers are made from high-quality cotton muslin (commonly referred to as "linen"). Muslin has sufficient density to protect goods from contamination and yet is porous enough to allow the penetration of steam or gas. The thread count (number of threads per square inch) must be at least 140 to be effective. Two double-thickness muslin wrappers or the equivalent (one double-thickness wrapper of 280-count muslin) are used to wrap items.

Paper and nonwoven fabrics (such as those used in the manufacture of disposable drapes) also are used. These wrappers should be durable and flexible and are intended for *one time use only.* After being used once during sterilization, they may lose their ability to prevent contamination. Always check with the manufacturer's specifications to determine whether wrapping material can be used more than once. Nonwoven fabrics must be used in accordance with their thickness. Lightweight fabrics require the same treatment as muslin (i.e., four thicknesses for complete protection). Heavier fabrics may be used according to the manufacturer's specifications. These are valuable for wrapping heavy instruments and flat-surfaced items such as basins and trays or heavy linen. When wrapping goods in linen or nonwoven fabric, the most common method is the envelope technique (Figure 8-9).

Combination plastic and paper wrappers commonly called *sterilization pouches* or *peel pouches* are available in various compositions and styles (Figure 8-10). Sterilization pouches are used for steam or gas sterilization of lightweight instruments or small items. Pouches are made of a number of different synthetic materials that meet the standards for the sterilization process. Double pouching or packaging is commonly employed for all but very light instruments. Some institutions use combination wrappers that are manufactured on a large roll that resembles a sleeve. The paper

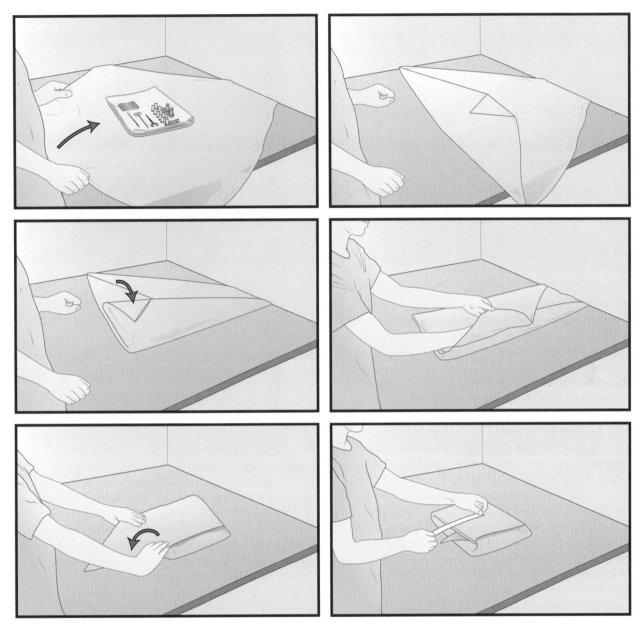

FIGURE 8-9
Envelope style wrapping.

and plastic are laminated back to back along their edges. A designated length is cut from the roll, the item is placed within the sleeve, and the ends are heat sealed or taped.

When this type of wrapper is used, it is critical that as much air as possible be evacuated before sealing. Failure to do this can cause the package to split open during sterilization. When a mechanical heat-sealing device is used, the seal should be checked very carefully to ensure that there are no air pockets along the seal. Other institutions use self-sealing pouches, which have a self-adhesive strip at the bottom of the wrapper that seals the pouch. After placing items in the pouch, push the excess air out and seal the open end. The process for wrapping items for sterilization is the same, regardless of the type of pouch your institution uses. All pouches must contain an internal disinfection monitor.

Manufactured containers also are used to hold equipment for sterilization. These must not be used for flash sterilization but are convenient and safe for both gas and conventional steam sterilization. These containers incorporate disposable filters within the construction of the container, and these must be in place after sterilization to maintain the sterility of the enclosed items.

Regardless of the type of packaging or wrapping system used, each package must be marked with both the current date and the date of expiration. The name of the item must be *clearly* marked, and a lot control number must be included. The lot control number is used to identify items that have been included in a sterilization load that may have yielded a positive biologic or mechanical control test. All packages must identify the type of sterilization—gas or steam—that is appropriate.

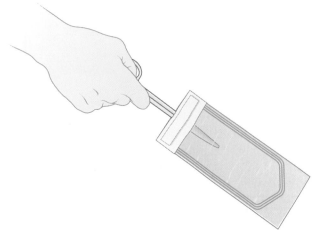

FIGURE 8-10
Sterilization pouches.

Sterilization and Control Monitors

Several methods are used to determine whether the sterilization process used on any given day or on any piece of equipment has been effective. Because contamination of items used in surgery and in other areas of the hospital is a critical problem, monitoring of the sterilization process is exacting and vital. Subjecting items to the process of sterilization does not ensure that the items are sterile. Simply placing an item in a sterilizer and initiating the process does not ensure sterility of the item. Objective testing or monitoring is needed to verify both the mechanical process and outcome.

Failure to achieve sterility may be caused by mechanical failure of the system used, improper use of the equipment, failure to wrap or load the items properly, or misunderstanding of the concepts involved. The best method for preventing human error is education and proper attitude. An attitude that always puts the patient first produces efficient and positive results. One can minimize mechanical failures through a complete understanding of the sterilization process and of the equipment used.

An external indicator used to monitor the sterilizer is the combined temperature-time graphs that are installed within the control panel of the sterilizer. The temperature-time graphs produce a permanent written record of duration of exposure to sterilization and the temperature exposure for each load that has been processed. Newer sterilizers may be equipped with a computer printout that records the parameters of each phase of the sterilization process.

Control monitors offer a way to check on the efficiency and efficacy of a sterilization. A *chemical monitor* is an object that is treated with material that changes its characteristics when sterilized. This may be in the form of special ink that is impregnated into paper strips or tape and placed on the outside of the package (Figure 8-11), or it may be a substance that is incorporated into a pellet contained in a glass vial. Chemical monitors are available for both steam and ethylene oxide sterilization.

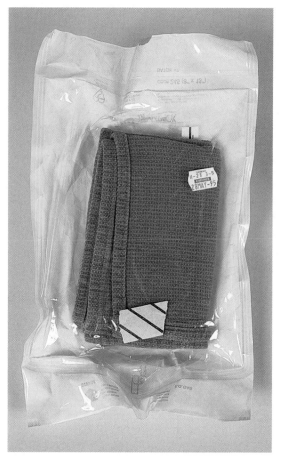

FIGURE 8-11
Chemical monitors. (From Elkin MK, Perry AG, Potter PA: *Nursing interventions and clinical skills,* ed 3, St Louis, 2004, Mosby.)

The important fact to remember about all **chemical indicators** is that *they do not indicate sterility, only that certain conditions for sterility have been met.* In other words, the chemical responds to conditions such as extreme heat, pressure, or humidity but does not take into consideration the duration of exposure, which is critical to the sterilization process. A chemical monitor should be placed within and on the outside of all packages to be sterilized, even if it is only one item.

To test and monitor the efficiency of the **high vacuum sterilizer,** a test called the *Daily Air-Removal Test (DART)* is performed each day. Commercially available *Bowie-Dick tests* also are available. High vacuum sterilizers are monitored to detect air in the chamber during the exposure phase. In these tests, a special package of properly wrapped towels is taped with heat-sensitive chemical monitor tape and stacked to a height of 10 or 11 inches. The package is then placed *by itself* in the sterilization chamber and run for the appropriate time. An unsatisfactory DART indicates a failure in the vacuum pump system or a defect in the gasket of the sterilizer door. Unsatisfactory results must be reported to biomedical engineering so they can inspect the vacuum system and door seals.

Internal monitors or indicators are chemically treated strips that are placed inside wrapped instrument trays, linen packs, and pouches. These items verify that the inside of a given package reached the parameter values necessary for sterilization and determine the penetration of the sterilization medium. The scrubbed technologist must check each internal indicator of all packs opened on the sterile field to ensure that each and every pack has an internal indicator that has reached the required parameters for exposure to sterilization. To be of any value, the indicators must be read by the scrub.

Each package must contain a monitor on both the inside and the outside of the package. Some chemical monitors are available in the form of tape that is placed outside of the package.

To verify that the sterilization method has effectively destroyed all microorganisms, including spores, a third type of biological monitor is required. This is the **biological indicator** (BI). A biological indicator has been impregnated with microorganisms and is used to verify that all of the conditions for sterilization have been met. The number of microorganisms and their resistance to sterilization far exceed the number and resistance of the microorganisms (**bioburden**) expected to be on the items to be sterilized (American Hospital Association).

For steam sterilization, spores of the bacteria *Bacillus stearothermophilus* are used. The gas sterilization and **peracetic acid** processes use bacterial spores of *Bacillus subtilis*. **Plasma sterilization** generally uses the bacterial spores of *Bacillus subtilis var. niger* for monitoring purposes.

Biological indicator kits include the test spore itself contained in a vial, paper strip, or disk, and a control BI that is not sterilized at the time of monitoring. The monitor is placed in the most challenging location for sterilization. For steam sterilizers this is usually at the lowest point of the chamber near the drain. In EO monitoring the biological test pack is positioned in the center of the load. Manufacturer directions address placement in other types of sterilizers. The monitor is recovered after sterilization, and both the BI and the control spore are cultured for results.

During culturing, the bacterial spores are allowed to grow in a sterile culture medium for at least 24 hours. Growth of bacteria in the test monitor culture indicates that the sterilization process was ineffective. If no bacteria grow, it is presumed that sterility of all items within the load was achieved. Biological controls should be administered at least once weekly. They always should be used whenever an artificial implant or prosthesis is sterilized and the item withheld from use until the results are known to be negative. If any biological indicator test result is positive, all items included in that load must be retrieved and resterilized. If the items have already been used in surgery, the physician must be notified.

Rapid biological monitoring detects an enzyme that binds to spores. The monitoring system is used for both high-pressure steam and EO sterilization. Results can be obtained in 1 to 4 hours, depending on the sterilization process. The monitoring system is self-contained, and the results are easily read.

Storage and Handling of Sterile Supplies
SHELF LIFE
Shelf life is defined as the amount of time a wrapped sterile package remains sterile when in storage. The shelf life of an item or pack depends on many conditions. Whether a package remains sterile depends completely on the conditions under which it is stored and on the handling of that package.

After an item is processed and sterilized, consideration must be given to how the item can be kept sterile. Time-related sterility measures (based on the amount of time since sterilization) are no longer commonly used. **Event-related sterility** or terminal sterilization is the accepted standard. Event-related sterility or terminal sterilization is based on the principle that sterilized items are assumed sterile between uses, unless environmental conditions or events interfere with the integrity of the package.

Sterile items should be stored in areas that are separate from those used to store clean nonsterile items. The area must be dust and lint free. Closed cabinets are preferred to open storage areas. Sterile items should be stored in critical areas or in the sterile core when possible. They should be placed in a draft-free area away from vents and windows. Sterile items must never be stored near sinks or other areas where they can be exposed to water. Strike-through contamination can occur in areas of high humidity as well as through direct splashing. Packages should be placed loosely on shelves to avoid crushing, tearing, or damaging items and wrappers. Heavy items must never be stacked on top of lighter ones. Stacking heavy instrument trays poses a risk that wrappers will be torn as the top tray is removed. Seldom-used items can be wrapped in protective dust covers.

Events that cause contamination occur often during handling. Obviously, the more an item is handled, the greater the risk of contamination. The more a package is handled, the greater the chance of weakening, tearing, or creating pinholes in the wrappers. These defects may not be obvious and may not be seen by the person opening the package. Paper pouch wrappers can develop small holes in stress areas. Pouch wrappers stored in bins are particularly likely to become contaminated because staff frequently rummage through the bins looking for items. One must closely inspect the integrity of all packages. *Items commercially prepared and sterilized by manufacturers* may be considered sterile indefinitely. An expiration date printed on the package shows the maximum time the manufacturer can guarantee product stability and sterility on the basis of test data approved by the Federal Drug Administration (FDA).

STORAGE
Ideally, sterile supplies should be stored in an area that prevents their exposure to the adverse conditions listed earlier. They should be stored in areas of restricted traffic, away from ventilation ducts, sprinklers, and heat-producing light. If items are stored in open bins, the bins or drawers should be shallow to prevent excess handling of the items. Closed

cabinets are ideal for storage. Mesh or basket containers are preferable over those with a solid surface where dust and bacteria can collect. The area should be cleaned frequently and protected from exposure to dampness. The temperature and humidity should be controllable. Items should never be stored around scrub sinks, in hallways, or near nonrestricted areas. Packs should be handled as little possible. They should be inspected for wrapper integrity before they are opened for use. Any suspicious pack should be rewrapped before being resterilized. *Always check the expiration date of an item before offering it for use.*

In most hospitals, the Central Sterile Processing Distribution (SPD) Department is responsible for the decontamination, disinfection, sterilization, storage, distribution, and inventory control of all sterile supplies, equipment, and case carts. Some hospitals, however, may have a sterile storage area for specialty instrumentation that will be readily available for use in emergency situations.

Cold Chemical Sterilization

A number of liquid chemical agents available today can sterilize an item immersed in it. A liquid sterilizing agent is one that kills all microorganisms, including bacterial spores. The safe use of liquid sterilants requires adherence to the manufacturer's directions. However, most of these chemicals are so corrosive and damaging to the equipment being sterilized that they cannot be used for this purpose. The products that can be safely used for sterilization are a 2% solution of *glutaraldehyde* (discussed earlier in the chapter), *peracetic acid,* and *hydrogen peroxide.*

Glutaraldehyde is noncorrosive when used as directed and offers a safe means of sterilization of delicate lensed instruments such as cystoscopes and bronchoscopes. Most equipment that is safe for immersion in water is safe for immersion in 2% glutaraldehyde. Because of the amount of time required to achieve sterilization, glutaraldehyde is used primarily for high-level disinfection of endoscopes. Some items such as fiberoptic endoscopes have a control head that cannot be immersed in liquid. The insertion tube (the part that enters the body), however, is the critical part and can be sterilized with a liquid chemical. Other instruments such as the cystoscope can be completely immersed in solution because the delicate optical portions can be separated. The preparation of an item for cold **chemical sterilization** requires that it be clean and dry. Any organic matter such as blood or sputum may prevent the liquid from penetrating crevices or joints of the instrument. If the item is wet, the moisture will dilute the sterilizing solution and render it ineffective.

Peracetic acid (Steris) is used to sterilize immersible flexible and rigid endoscopes, some types of cameras, and microinstruments. Peracetic acid 35% and surface-active buffering agents are contained in a premixed canister, which is placed in the sterilizer unit. The unit produces continuous chemical irrigation of exposed surfaces in the chamber for 30 to 45 minutes at low temperatures of 122° to 133° F (50°

to 55° C). Instruments processed in the system must be used immediately after the sterilization process. Sterility cannot be assured if the items are stored.

Before processing, all surfaces of the instrument must be thoroughly cleaned. All tissue and organic debris must be removed from channels, gaskets, and stopcocks, and detachable parts must be disassembled.

After precleaning, the instrument must be tested for leaks. It is then positioned in the sterilization tray to ensure that all surfaces of the instrument come in contact with the sterilizing agent. In sterilizing an endoscopic lumen, the endoscope is secured to the system fluid path with connectors. *Failure to secure these connectors correctly results in sterilization failure and may break the valves or lumens of the instrument.* The sterilant is delivered to the unit along with filtered tap water. After exposure, there are four rinse cycles. The covered tray containing the instrument is then removed from the unit and delivered to the sterile field.

Safety precautions required to prevent peracetic acid injury include the use of protective eyewear, gloves, and skin protection. Although peracetic acid is nontoxic and noncorrosive at the dilution (0.2%) at which it is generally used, in its concentrated form (35%), it can cause *severe burns and permanent blindness.* Repeated exposure to peracetic acid may cause tissue irritation to sensitive individuals. In case of skin contact, the skin should be immediately flushed with copious amounts of running water.

Hydrogen Peroxide

Low-temperature hydrogen peroxide units use ionized air in a low-moisture environment to achieve sterilization. The sterilization process includes two phases. Dry, precleaned items are wrapped in nonwoven polypropylene or Tyvek® pouches and placed in the chamber. Air is removed from the chamber to create a vacuum, which is replaced by air plasma (ionized air), which removes any remaining moisture in the chamber. The sterilant is contained in a cartridge that automatically releases hydrogen peroxide, which vaporizes in the chamber. The ionized air is then exposed to radio-frequency energy in the chamber. This breaks down the hydrogen peroxide into free radicals, which combine with pathogens or parts thereof and destroy them. Any free radicals that remain uncombined after the exposure period are converted into water and oxygen. At the end of the cycle, filtered air enters the chamber and items can be removed. Total cycle time is 55 minutes. No aeration is required.

The Sterrad J hydrogen peroxide sterilization system can be used on many new video camera systems, rigid and flexible endoscopes, and endoscopic accessories. Because of the limitations of this system, one must check the manufacturer's specific statements about sterilization of a particular product using a hydrogen peroxide system. This system cannot be used for cellulose material, linens, or liquids, and the gas cannot penetrate lumens or channels more than 12 inches (31 cm) in length or less than $1/4$ inch (6 mm) in diameter.

CURRENT ISSUES IN STERILIZATION AND DISINFECTION

Reprocessing of Single-Use Items

The current emphasis on cost cutting in the health-care system has led many hospitals to propose the reprocessing (resterilization) of disposable items (single-use devices or SUDs). Increased use of SUDs has reduced the risk of disease transmission but created a disposal problem.

Patient and employee safety remains the central issue. Other points of current discussion include the patient's right to be informed when reprocessed SUDs are used, the number of reuses that should be allowed, the reprocessing method, and the tradeoff between cost savings and the risks of reprocessing. Despite ongoing discussion, one standard is clear: No item should be reprocessed if its integrity and safety cannot be assured.

There is currently little conclusive evidence to discourage or endorse reprocessing of SUDs. The FDA has issued standards and regulations for reprocessing. Third-party outsourcing of reprocessing is available, and these processors must meet FDA standards and requirements for reprocessing outcome. Hospitals that currently reprocess SUDs within the institution must produce extensive data to support the safety of reprocessing, including but not limited to proof of sterilization, proof that the item has not been structurally or mechanically damaged in any way, information on quality control of the process, detailed records of processing parameters, and documentation of any incidents involving reprocessed items. The FDA continues to examine all issues concerned with reprocessing.

Prevention of Transmission of Creutzfeldt-Jakob Disease

Creutzfeldt-Jakob disease (CJD) is a fatal neurodegenerative disease. It is believed to be caused by a prion, a cellular glycoprotein. CJD is classified as a human transmissible spongiform encephalopathy. The disease has been transmitted from one patient to another through contaminated medical equipment. The CJD prion agent has a high rate of infectivity for brain, spinal cord, and eye tissue. Tissues or fluids with lower infectivity rates are cerebrospinal fluid, kidneys, liver, lungs, lymph nodes, spleen, and placenta. The CJD prion cannot be destroyed by routine methods of sterilization and disinfection.

To prevent the transmission of CJD, a stringent protocol must be followed. Sodium hypochlorite and heat in a gravity displacement steam sterilizer are effective against prions. Sodium hypochlorite is very corrosive, however. Disposable instruments currently are often used for *high-risk procedures* to ensure that the patient is not exposed to the disease agent. Disposable waste is securely contained and incinerated at high temperature. The World Health Organization and the CDC issue guidelines for the handling of equipment and prion-contaminated waste. These are updated as more research is completed. Contact the World Health Organization and the CDC for more information.

CASE STUDIES

Case 1

While scrubbed you open a basin set and find a small amount of water pooled in the bottom of the basin. What are the possible causes of this? What will you do?

Case 2

During the setup for a case, you notice one of the indicator strips in a pan of instruments on your back table has not changed color. What should you do?

Case 3

You are employed in a small community hospital. In your first week you are scrubbed on a laparotomy case. The circulator opens a single-use electrosurgery pencil that has been resterilized with EO in the hospital's central processing department. What will you do?

Case 4

You are the afternoon shift relief scrub on a plastic surgery case. About an hour into the case on which you have relieved, you happen to notice the chemical sterilization monitor at the bottom of the instrument tray, which is on the sterile back table. The monitor has not changed color. The surgeon is using instruments from this tray. What do you do?

Case 5

You are about to scrub on an orthopedic case in which a stainless steel implant will be inserted into the patient's hip. The surgeon wants to see the implant before surgery. He opens the package and examines it with bare hands. He then instructs you to flash sterilize the implant. What will you do? Who is responsible? What are the risks associated with flash sterilization of implants?

Case 6

You have been assigned to work in the gastrointestinal laboratory for the day. You will use gastrointestinal endoscopes. When you arrive in the laboratory, you notice that the endoscope to be used first is soaking in disinfectant solution that has expired (has been held beyond the date approved for disinfection). The doctor tells you that he will use the endoscope anyway. What is your response?

CASE STUDIES—cont'd

Case 7

While scrubbed on a total-hip-replacement procedure, you are setting up the case. You notice that one of the rasps in the orthopedic instrument set is full of dried blood and tissue. You bring this to the attention of the circulator, who says, "Oh, that's okay, it's sterile tissue. Just wash it off in the basin." What is your response?

Case 8

While opening sterile goods for a case, you find a basin set that has been wrapped in one wrapper. You are able to open the basin set using sterile technique. Is it sterile?

Case 9

You are assisting in a sigmoidoscopy using the flexible endoscope. The surgeon wishes to take a biopsy of the sigmoid colon mucosa. After removing the biopsy tissue, he returns the instrument to you. He then asks you for the same instrument again to remove another piece of tissue in a different location in the sigmoid colon. Is the biopsy instrument still sterile? What is the significance of this?

REFERENCES

Alvarado CJ and Reichelderfer M: APIC guideline for infection prevention and control in flexible endoscopy, *American Journal of Infection Control,* 28:2, April, 2000.

Bach T: The bloodborne pathogens standard and disinfection, *Infection Control Today,* Sept, 2000.

Conviser S: The future of ethylene oxide sterilization, *Infection Control Today,* June, 2000.

Descoteaux JG et al: Residual organic debris on processed surgical instruments, *AORN Journal,* 62:1, July, 1995.

Dunn D: Reprocessing single-use devices—regulatory roles, *AORN Journal,* 76:1, July, 2002.

Fogg DM: Clinical issues, *AORN Journal,* 72:4, October, 2000.

Fogg DM: Clinical issues, *AORN Journal,* 71:5, May, 2000.

Furman, PJ: New regulations clear the way for third-party reprocessors, *Infection Control Today,* October, 2001.

Garner JS: Guideline for isolation precautions in hospitals, *Infection Control and Hospital Epidemiology,* 17, 1996, and *American Journal of Infection Control,* 24, 1996.

Gruendemann BJ: Taking cover: single-use vs. reusable gowns and drapes, *Infection Control Today,* March, 2002.

Kern B: Preventive instrument maintenance, *Infection Control Today,* Sept, 2000.

Lind N: Using indicators, *Infection Control Today,* June, 2000.

Occupational Safety and Health Administration: *OSHA regulations, Occupational and Safety Health Standards, Bloodborne Pathogens,* standard number 1910.1030.

Reichert M and Young J, eds: *Sterilization technology for the health care facility,* ed 2, Gaithersburg, 1997, Aspen Publishers.

Rutala WA: *APIC guidelines for infection control practice,* Washington, DC, 1996, Association for Professionals in Infection Control and Epidemiology.

Rutala WA and Weber DJ: Creutzfeldt-Jakob disease: risks and prevention of nosocomial acquisition, *Infection Control Today,* August, 2001.

Spry C: Low-temperature sterilization, *Infection Control Today,* May, 2001.

Chapter 9

Aseptic Technique

Learning Objectives

After studying this chapter the reader will be able to:

- Describe the rationale for practicing aseptic technique
- Clearly distinguish among sterile, nonsterile, and aseptic
- Explain surgical conscience
- Explain the concept of barriers
- Practice the rules of aseptic technique
- Explain the relationship between personal hygiene and aseptic technique
- Perform the surgical hand scrub correctly
- Demonstrate aseptic technique by donning gown and gloves
- Don sterile gloves using proper open gloving technique
- Remove gown and gloves using aseptic technique
- Remove contaminated gloves from another person
- Discuss reasons why personnel might not follow the rules of asepsis

Terminology

Airborne contamination—Incident in which microorganisms carried in the air by moisture droplets or dust particles make contact with a sterile surface.

Antiseptics—Chemical agents that are approved for use on the skin and that inhibit growth and reproduction of microorganisms. Antiseptics are used to cleanse and paint the surgical site to reduce the number of microorganisms to an absolute minimum.

Asepsis—The absence of pathogenic microorganisms on an animate surface or on body tissue. Literally, asepsis means "without infection." In surgery, asepsis is a state of minimal or zero pathogens. Asepsis is the goal of many surgical practices.

Aseptic technique—Methods or practices in health care that promote and maintain a state of asepsis. Also called sterile technique.

Chemical barrier—The barrier formed by the action of an antiseptic that not only reduces the number of microorganisms on a surface but also prevents recolonization (regrowth) for a limited period of time.

Closed gloving—A technique of gloving in which the bare hand does not come in contact with the outside of the glove. The sterile glove is protected from the nonsterile hand by the cuff of a surgical gown.

Contamination—Result of physical contact between a sterile surface and a nonsterile surface in surgery. Contamination also can result from airborne dust, moisture droplets, or fluids that act as a vehicle for transporting contaminants from a nonsterile surface to a sterile one.

Handwashing—A specific technique used to remove debris and dead cells from the hands. Handwashing with an antiseptic also reduces the number of microorganisms on the skin.

Latex allergy—Sensitivity to latex, which can cause itching, rhinitis, conjunctivitis, and anaphylactic shock leading to death. Personnel and patients with latex allergy must not come in contact with any articles that contain latex.

Nonsterile personnel—In surgery, team members who remain outside the boundary of the sterile field and do not come into direct contact with sterile equipment, sterile areas, or the surgical wound. The circulator, anesthesia care provider, and x-ray technician are examples of nonsterile team members.

Terminology

Open gloving—A gloving technique in which the bare skin does not touch any part of the outside of the glove. Open gloving is generally used when a health worker does not wear a sterile gown.

Pathogenic—Having the potential to cause disease.

Physical barrier—In surgery, a barrier that separates a sterile surface from a nonsterile surface. Examples are sterile surgical gloves, gowns, and drapes. A physical barrier, such as a clean surgical cap, also can prevent a bacteria-laden surface, such as the hair, from shedding microorganisms.

Resident flora—Microorganisms that are normally present in specific tissues of people. Resident flora is necessary to the regular function of these tissues or structures. Also called normal flora.

Scrub—Member of the sterile team who handles instruments, supplies, and equipment necessary for the surgical procedure. The surgical hand scrub is the process of prescribed, thorough hand cleaning before the donning of sterile gloves and gown.

Scrubbed personnel—In surgery, members of the surgical team who work within the sterile field. Also called sterile personnel.

Sharps—Any objects that can penetrate the skin and have the potential for causing injury and infection, including but not limited to, needles, scalpels, broken glass, broken capillary tubes, and exposed ends of dental wires.

Spatial relations—One's physical relation to sterile and nonsterile areas or surfaces. Concepts considered in spatial relationships include the varying heights of sterile team members, distance between a nonsterile team member and a sterile surface, and movement within a sterile area.

Sterile field—An area that includes the draped patient, all sterile tables, and sterile equipment in the immediate area of the patient. The patient is considered the center of the sterile field.

Sterile item—Any item that has been subjected to a process that renders it free of all microbial life, including spores.

Sterility—A guarantee of the absence of all microbial life, including spores. Sterility is assured when an item is properly packaged and subjected to a sterilization process. Items are considered sterile unless they have been exposed to air or another event that renders the item unsterile. An item that is properly opened onto a surgical field is then considered *surgically clean* because it is then exposed to the air or to patient tissues. Sterility is considered absolute.

Strike-through contamination—An event in which water, fluids, or blood act as a vehicle to carry microorganisms from a nonsterile to a sterile surface. It occurs, for example, when the outside wrapper of a sterile instrument becomes wet and the water conveys bacteria to the inside of the wrapper and contaminates the instrument, or on the surgical gown, when the gown becomes saturated with blood or other fluids.

Surgical conscience—In surgery, the ethical motivation to practice strict aseptic technique to protect the patient from infection. The team members place the highest emphasis on safe delivery of care for the patient.

Surgical hand scrub—A specific technique for washing the hands before donning surgical gown and gloves before surgery. The scrub is performed with timed or counted strokes using detergent-based antiseptic. The surgical hand scrub is designed to remove dirt, oils, and transient microorganisms, and reduce the number of resident microorganisms.

Surgical site infection (SSI)—Postoperative infection of the surgical wound, most commonly caused by the normal bacteria found on the patient's skin or shed from the skin or hair of surgical team members. The goal of the surgical skin preparation is to prevent postoperative wound infection.

Surgically clean—An item that was considered sterile but is now in use in the surgical field, has become exposed to air or patient tissues, and is no longer considered absolutely sterile. For convenience, items in use within a surgical field are usually called *sterile* instead of *surgically clean.*

Topical antiseptics (antimicrobials)—Agents applied to skin or mucous membrane that temporarily reduce or prevent the growth of microorganisms.

Transient flora—Microorganisms that do not normally reside in the tissue of an individual. Transient microorganisms are acquired through skin contact with an animate or inanimate source colonized by microbes. Transient flora may be removed by routine methods of skin cleaning (see *handwashing* and *surgical hand scrub*).

IMPORTANT CONCEPTS OF ASEPTIC TECHNIQUE

Aseptic technique is:

▶ A method of "doing and thinking" that is used during the entire surgical experience.

▶ A method of performing tasks that reduces the risk of infection in patients and staff.

▶ A method based on the central principle that microorganisms transmit disease from objects, surfaces, air, and dust to patients and personnel.

▶ A method that results in containment, confinement, reduction, or elimination of microorganisms to prevent their contact with the **sterile field.**

The techniques and rationales described in this chapter are the foundation of surgical practice. A sound understanding of aseptic technique is at the center of many skills the surgical technologist uses in professional practice. Developing good aseptic technique takes time and practice, and *everyone* makes inadvertent mistakes. However, minor breaks in aseptic technique usually can be corrected *if they are reported.* Aseptic technique requires constant self-monitoring. All surgical personnel should observe their own practices and ask, "Are my practices consistent with my professional and ethical responsibility? Are my standards consistent with what I would want for myself or my family?"

Activities That Promote Asepsis

Asepsis is a condition in which the body is considered "sterile" and is free of *infectious organisms.* Literally defined, asepsis means *without infection.* Asepsis is a *goal,* whereas aseptic technique involves the *methods used* to achieve that goal. The following are examples of important activities and environmental controls that promote and maintain asepsis:

- The **surgical hand scrub**
- Patient skin preparation
- Air filtering in the surgical suite
- Sterilization of surgical instruments
- Containment of hair and the use of surgical attire
- Use of sterile gowns, gloves, and drapes
- Separation of soiled instruments from clean instruments during processing
- Strict environmental cleaning between surgical cases
- Heating and air venting, control of traffic patterns, and creation of restricted areas to confine microorganisms
- Protection of the surgical wound with sterile dressings
- Draining of the wound to prevent a medium for bacterial growth in the body

Sterility

When an object is sterile, it is completely free of *all* living microorganisms, including bacterial spores. The term *sterile* is absolute. An item either *is* sterile or it *is not* sterile. The process of sterilization is detailed and exact. After an item has been sterilized, its **sterility** is maintained by aseptic technique. Items exposed (opened) to the surgical field are considered **surgically clean** after they have been exposed to the air or to a patient's tissues and must be resterilized before being used on another patient. In the health-care setting, all nonsterile surfaces are considered potentially contaminated with **pathogenic** microorganisms.

Contamination

A contaminated object is an object or body tissue that is not sterile or that has come in contact with a nonsterile object or surface. Recall from Chapter 7 that microorganisms are spread by direct contact, moisture, dust, and droplet nuclei. These are sources of **contamination.**

Gross contamination is the major contamination of the surgical wound or sterile site. This might result when bowel contents spill into the peritoneal cavity or when a wide area of external tissue is damaged, such as might occur in a penetrating or crushing injury. Gross contamination can lead to sepsis (life-threatening infection) because of the number and type of microorganisms that enter the body. Even in cases of gross contamination, aseptic technique is maintained, because wound contamination with one type or strain of microorganism does not eliminate the pathogenic potential of others in the environment.

Surgical Conscience

Aseptic technique is based on **surgical conscience**—*the ethical and professional motivation that regulates one's aseptic technique.* It is the joint responsibility of all members of the surgical team to report and respond to breaks in aseptic technique so that steps can be taken to mitigate the risk of infection. In the case of gross contamination, this may mean starting the patient on intravenous antibiotics. If a glove or drape is contaminated, the appropriate action is to change the glove or re-drape. If fluids are contaminated, they are discarded and new sterile basins and fluids obtained. Admitting and reporting any break in technique demonstrate a high level of professional maturity and surgical conscience.

Aseptic technique is closely associated with one's motivation to protect the patient. The rules of aseptic technique are a model for the highest *standard* of practice.

Concept of Barriers

The principles of aseptic technique are based on the establishment of barriers between a source of contamination and a sterile surface. To better understand and practice aseptic technique, consider the concept of *containment and confinement.* Sterile objects are contained or confined to avoid contact with nonsterile objects and surfaces or other sources of contamination such as air and water droplets.

A **physical barrier** prevents a nonsterile surface from touching a sterile surface. For example, sterile drapes are a barrier between the patient and all **sterile items** and surfaces that contact the top of the drape during surgery. A physical barrier is one that contains (encloses) or separates a *source* of contamination. Hair caps and masks are examples of barriers that contain sources of contamination. Back table covers, Mayo stand covers, and surgical drapes all separate contaminated areas from surgically clean areas.

Distance is another type of barrier. As the distance between a sterile surface and a nonsterile surface increases, the risk of contamination decreases. When learning aseptic technique, visualize an imaginary space around sterile objects and the sterile field. This space is perceived, first consciously and then unconsciously, as "off limits" to nonsterile objects and personnel. Over time, surgical personnel develop a sense of intrusion when nonsterile objects are too close to the field. This concept is called **spatial relations.** Generally, **nonsterile personnel** must remain at least 1 foot (30 cm) from a sterile field.

A **chemical barrier** may be produced by some **antiseptics** used during the surgical scrub and during surgical skin preparation. Some agents produce a residual bacteriostatic effect.

STANDARDS FOR ASEPTIC TECHNIQUE

In all professional health practices, standards define the optimum level of patient care.

The standards for aseptic technique have been set by the following agencies:

▶ Association of periOperative Registered Nurses (AORN)—the professional organization for operating room nurses that sets standards and recommends procedures for operating room practice.
▶ Association for Professionals in Infection Control and Epidemiology (APIC)—performs research and recommends standards and procedures in the area of infection control.
▶ Centers for Disease Control and Prevention (CDC)—official U.S. government agency that researches public health issues and educates the lay public and professionals about disease transmission, origin, and prevention.
▶ Occupational Safety and Health Administration (OSHA)—sets standards for safe environmental conditions for workers in all fields, including health care.
▶ Joint Commission for the Accreditation of Healthcare Organizations (JCAHO)—the official private agency that accredits health-care facilities according to approved standards for outcomes, procedures, and safe environmental conditions within the health-care institution.

Standards for Personal Hygiene and Attire
PERSONAL HYGIENE
Surgical personnel should be free from any contagious illness that might be transmitted to the patient and others in the surgical environment. Bacterial shedding from the nasopharynx and skin is a particular risk. There is evidence that open sores, cuts, or small skin wounds harbor bacteria, which are shed in the course of handling surgical equipment. Research also demonstrates that bacteria in open sores are resistant to elimination through **handwashing.** Surgical personnel should maintain good personal hygiene habits. Handwashing is of particular importance. Keeping hair clean and nails short helps prevent the transmission of *Staphylococcus aureus.*

Fingernails
The subungual area (under the fingernails) hosts a greater number of bacterial colonies than any other area of the hand. This area requires specific cleaning during normal handwashing as well as during the surgical hand scrub. Nail tips must be level with the tip of the finger. Long nails easily puncture gloves and make handling of equipment more difficult. **Scrubbed personnel** sometimes wear gloves that are too large in order to protect long manicured nails. Gloves that are too large for the hand can become caught in equipment and make handling delicate sutures and other supplies difficult and time consuming. With regard to the patient's

comfort, long nails can scratch or dig into the patient's skin during transfer and positioning.

Nail polish itself has not been proven to be a source of bacteria, but if the polish has chips or is flaking, it can be a site of bacterial growth. Nail polish is often worn over artificial or long nails, both of which are unacceptable in the operating room.

Artificial nails harbor pathogenic bacteria (particularly gram-negative bacteria) and fungi such as *Candida* and *Pseudomonas* between the real and synthetic nails, especially when the artificial nail is chipped or cracked. Bacterial counts remain high even after hand scrubbing of artificial nails with antiseptic solution. Personnel with artificial nails tend to avoid thorough scrubbing to avoid damaging the nails, which allows for the proliferation of bacterial and fungal colonies.

JEWELRY
Jewelry of any kind is a potential source of pathogens. Surgical personnel must remove all rings, bracelets, and wristwatches. Microorganisms proliferate freely under rings and bracelets and may resist destruction during handwashing. Necklaces and earrings that are not confined under scrub attire pose a risk of falling onto the surgical field or even into the surgical wound. Exposed necklaces or earrings may become contaminated with blood or other aerosolized particles that may pose a risk to the health-care worker and others who come into contact with these items. The recommended standard is to remove *all* jewelry. For example, the Illinois Department of Public Health dictates standards that allow no jewelry in the operating room.

SCRUB ATTIRE
Scrub Suit
The scrub suit is worn by both sterile and nonsterile surgical personnel. The suit is designed to prevent the release of skin particles and hair into the environment and to protect the wearer from contact with soil and body fluids. Perspiration and normal exudate from sebaceous glands in the skin contain large colonies of bacteria that are released with friction and movement. The scrub suit helps to prevent the release of these substances into the surgical environment. The process used to launder surgical scrub suits in the hospital is vigorous and effective in lowering bacterial counts.

The scrub suit consists of a shirt and pants. It is made of lint-free material and should fit closely to the body. The suit should not be so tight as to produce chafing, however, which increases the release of skin and hair particles laden with bacteria. If the top is not tunic style, it should be tucked into the pants to prevent contact with sterile surfaces (Figure 9-1). The drawstring ties should be tucked into the pants and not allowed to dangle freely because they could accidentally brush the sterile field. A clean scrub suit is donned whenever personnel enter the restricted or semirestricted area of the operating room, and the suit must be changed if it is contaminated by blood or body fluids.

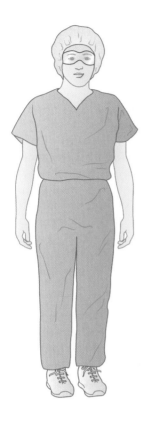

FIGURE 9-1
Scrub attire.

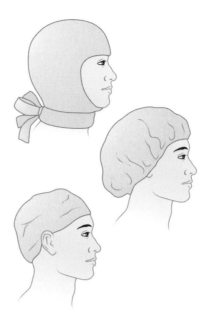

FIGURE 9-2
Head caps.

In some facilities surgical personnel are required to wear a cover gown or laboratory coat over the scrub suit whenever they leave the department to protect the scrub suit from microbial contamination. This is a policy decision of each individual institution.

When removing a scrub suit that has been penetrated by blood or body fluid, surgical personnel must do so in a way that avoids skin contact with the soiled area. Soiled scrub suits must be placed in a marked laundry receptacle so that they do not spread contaminants.

Nonsterile Cover Jacket
In the past, OSHA recommended that all nonsterile personnel wear a long-sleeved cover jacket. The purpose was to prevent shedding from bare arms and to protect skin from the splash of blood and body fluids. However, data collected by the CDC do not suggest that the risk of microorganisms spreading and causing infection in patients or staff increases without a cover jacket. Jackets may, however, be required by the individual facility.

Head Cap
Head caps or hoods are worn to reduce contamination of the surgical field by loose hair and dander from the scalp. Surgical site infections have been traced to *S. aureus* and group A *Streptococcus* from the hair or scalp of surgical personnel. Caps are meant to contain *all hair* and cover the scalp line and sideburns completely (Figure 9-2). Males with facial hair should wear a cap that is specifically designed to cover this hair. One should put on the cap before donning the scrub suit to prevent shedding of hair onto the clean scrub top or dress.

Most hospitals use disposable caps. They are inexpensive and readily available in the operating room. The use of cloth (home-laundered) caps is not recommended, but their use is governed by the policy of the individual institution or state. Cloth caps that are reused day after day are a *source of gross contamination* rather than a barrier against contamination.

Shoe Covers
Shoe covers protect shoes from contamination by blood and body fluids, and should be worn when one can reasonably anticipate that splashes or spills may occur. There is no evidence that their use reduces the risk of surgical site infection, and the primary purpose of shoe covers is to facilitate sanitation. If shoe covers are worn, they should be changed daily; when they become torn, wet, or soiled; and before leaving the surgical suite. If there is a possibility of gross contamination or pooling of blood, body fluids, or other liquids, such as during some orthopedic or obstetrical cases, impervious shoe covers that extend to the knee should be worn.

Mask
Masks are worn to protect the intraoperative environment from contamination by aerosol droplets generated by the mouth, oropharynx, nose, and nasopharynx. Talking, coughing, and sneezing forcefully spread droplets onto the sterile field and surrounding environment. When used properly, masks block droplets and filter air. They also protect the nose and mouth of the wearer from contact with particles of tissue and body fluids, especially during drilling, sawing, cutting, and tissue liquefaction. Masks should be worn at all times by all surgical personnel in restricted areas and in locations where sterile instruments and supplies are stored or processed.

Masks are made of lint-free synthetic material that is woven loosely enough to allow the breath to pass through effectively but tightly enough to filter 99% of particles of 5 μm or larger.

To protect the patient or the wearer, masks must be worn properly:

▶ The mask must cover both the nose and the mouth. Any pliable insert over the nose bridge of the mask should be molded over the nose to fit snugly.

▶ Ties must be secured at the crown of the head and around the neck. Crossing the ties at the back of the head allows the sides of the mask to tent, which causes the breath to bypass the mask and escape from the sides.

▶ Double masking is not recommended. When two masks are worn, the open spaces of the material are doubled so that the wearer must exert more respiratory force during inhalation and exhalation. This causes air to be forced in and out of the sides and defeats the filtering process.

▶ One must remove and dispose of masks immediately upon leaving any restricted or semirestricted area. Even after a short time, bacterial colonization increases to a very high level on the inside surface of the mask. Masks are to be changed between surgical procedures. When masks are worn around the neck between cases, they present a significant source of contamination.

▶ To remove the mask properly, untie the top strings, then the bottom strings, without handling the portion that covers the face. Dispose of the mask in the proper waste receptacle and wash hands thoroughly. Fresh masks are to be worn for each surgical procedure.

▶ Masks should either be left on or left off, and never worn around the neck with the ties dangling.

▶ Specialized masks are worn during laser procedures. These masks are designed to filter out particles that are smaller than those filtered by standard surgical masks; these smaller particles arise when cells are destroyed by laser energy.

Protective Eyewear and Face Shield

All surgical team members must wear impervious protective eyewear or face shields during all procedures and *whenever* there is a risk that blood, body fluids, or particles of tissue can splash on the face. When power equipment is used, bone chips, liquefied tissue, and other debris splatter into the air and onto personnel. Eyewear must cover the eye area from the brow to the top of the surgical mask and must extend over the temples (Figure 9-3). This protects the eyes from the front and sides. Impervious face shields offer increased protection.

A variety of different goggles and face shields are available. One's choice should be based on visual clarity, expense, and comfort. Personnel are less likely to comply with regulations requiring eyewear and face shields when the equipment is uncomfortable or causes glare or visual distortion. Specialized protective goggles may be required with the use of specific types of lasers. In addition to protecting the wearer from laser injury, these goggles also must comply with splash-protection requirements mentioned above.

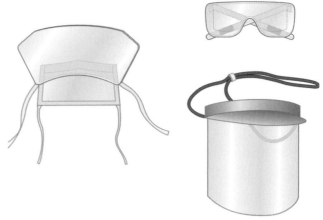

FIGURE 9-3
Protective eye wear.

Standards During Surgery

The following standards and rules apply while in the operating room and are universally accepted by all members of the surgical team:

1. **Sterile surfaces contact only sterile surfaces; nonsterile surfaces contact only nonsterile surfaces.**

   Contamination of a sterile surface occurs when a nonsterile surface touches a sterile surface (such as the circulator's bare hand accidentally touching the surgical technologist while delivering sterile items to sterile personnel).

2. **A sterile item is considered sterile only after it has been processed using methods that are proven effective and that yield measurable results.**

   Before any sterile item is distributed to the sterile field, the integrity of the wrapper and the reading of chemical sterility indicators must be verified. Biological indicators are used to verify the correct functioning of a sterilizing system. Although an item has been through the process of sterilization, it might not be sterile. Many conditions and events can alter the sterility of the item, including puncture holes or tears in the wrapper, moisture, or failure of the sterilizer system.

3. **Certain areas of the body cannot be adequately decontaminated using antiseptics or antibiotics. Aseptic technique helps to prevent the transmission of potentially pathogenic microorganisms (resident flora) from these areas into other areas where these microorganisms may cause infection.**

   The skin, upper respiratory tract, perineal area, and gastrointestinal (GI) tract each harbor microorganisms that are considered helpful to the survival or function of these structures. These microorganisms are called normal or **resident flora**. Extreme care is taken to prevent the introduction of normal (resident) flora from one area of the body into another area of the body.

4. **Sterile drapes, gowns, gloves, and table covers are barriers between a nonsterile surface and a sterile surface.**

Materials used as barriers against contamination are chosen for their density, strength, ability to resist moisture, and ease of use. Materials that do not meet minimum standards for patient safety should not be used.

5. **The edge of any sterile drape, wrapper, or covering is considered nonsterile.**

    When a sterile item is opened, the edge of its wrapper must not touch the item. Maintaining a wide margin between the sterile item and the edge prevents possible contamination of the item as it is being delivered to the field. A one-inch (2.5-cm) margin from the perimeter of a sterile wrapper is considered unsterile. When sterile items are opened and distributed, the nonsterile hand is protected under the wrapper. A specific technique is used to open and distribute sterile goods.

    Sterile liquids in bottles with an edge (lip) that is protected with a sealed sterile cap may be delivered directly from the bottle into a sterile container on the field. Medication vials often are sealed with aluminum caps. When the metal cap is pried open, the edge of the vial is considered contaminated. This is because there is no way to remove the top without dragging the nonsterile cap across the lip of the vial. When you begin to pour sterile solution into a container, do not stop pouring until the container is empty. Pull the container away from the sterile field so that no residual liquid can drip down the nonsterile side of the container into the sterile receptacle below.

6. **If there is any doubt about the sterility of an item, consider it contaminated.**

    Before opening the wrapper of any sterile item, inspect it for signs of contamination. Tears, holes, wear marks, or water spots on any wrapper are signs of questionable sterility. When in doubt, do not use the item.

    If a wrapped item is dropped on the floor, there is a risk of contamination. If an item is dropped on the floor, it should not be used. No questionable item should be distributed to the sterile field. It should be unwrapped and placed aside so that others do not take it to the sterile field. "When in doubt, throw it out."

7. **The draped patient is the center of the sterile field. Other draped items and sterile personnel form the periphery of the field. Nonsterile items are not positioned inside this area.**

    Sterile drapes create a barrier between a nonsterile surface and the working area of the sterile field. For example, the operating microscope, ring basin, and back table are draped. Equipment that is not draped must remain *outside* the sterile field, with at least 12 inches allowed between the sterile and nonsterile surfaces.

8. **Sterile gowns are considered sterile only in front from the axillary line to the waist.**

    Sterile personnel should not drop their forearms or hands below waist level nor raise them above the axillary line. The axilla itself is considered nonsterile even though protected by a gown. This is because of the large population of bacteria in the axillary region.

Sterile personnel must pass other sterile personnel *back to back and front to front.* Even though wraparound gowns are used in most surgical settings, the sterility of the back cannot be guaranteed because the person wearing it cannot observe it.

9. **Sterile tables are considered sterile only at table height.**

    The top of a sterile table is the only surface considered sterile. Suture ends must not hang over the table edge. Table drapes must not be repositioned once they have been placed because this changes the level of the sterile area. After tubing, cords, and hoses are secured to the patient's drape, they must *not* be pulled up to create additional slack. This brings the nonsterile portion of the tubing up to the sterile field. It is the duty of the **scrub** to measure and allow for necessary slack before securing these items in place when they are first brought onto the sterile field.

10. **Sterile personnel remain within the immediate area of the sterile field.**

    Scrubbed personnel must not move away from the sterile field. As personnel move outside the periphery, they increase the risk of contamination. Sterile personnel are sometimes required to move around the periphery of the field to perform their tasks. However, *moving outside the immediate sterile area is a compromise in aseptic technique.* Sterile personnel should not leave the room to retrieve items from another area, even if that area is restricted (such as the sterile core where supplies are flash sterilized). Nonsterile team members are responsible for delivering supplies to the sterile field. This is performed in a prescribed manner to avoid the risk of contamination.

11. **Nonsterile team members never lean over or reach over a sterile surface to distribute sterile goods to the field. They do not pass between two sterile surfaces.**

    When sterile packages are opened, one must hand items to personnel or deposit them on sterile surfaces in such a way that one avoids reaching over previously opened goods. Many commercially prepared surgical items are packaged so that they can be flipped onto the sterile field from a safe distance. If the wrapper does not permit this technique to be used, nonsterile personnel must pass the item directly to scrubbed personnel.

12. **Movement is kept to a minimum during surgery.**

    Team members should move about the operating suite as little as possible. This applies to both scrubbed and nonsterile personnel. Traffic into and out of the surgical suite creates air currents that conduct contaminated particles into the operating room, where they settle on the surgical wound site and sterile surfaces (a process known as **airborne contamination**). Doors to the operating room suite should remain closed when sterile supplies are opened and when surgery is in progress.

    Drapes and linens should be handled as little as possible and with a minimum of movement. This prevents the release of lint and dust particles, which create a vehicle for transmission of airborne bacteria.

13. **Talking is kept to a minimum during surgery.**

    The mouth is a major reservoir for bacteria. Talking forces the breath into the air and immediate environment. Masks worn to prevent the release of bacteria-laden moisture are not 100% effective, and when improperly worn, produce little protection against the dissemination of aerosol droplets containing microorganisms.

14. **Moisture carries bacteria from a nonsterile surface to a sterile surface.**

    When water comes in contact with a sterile drape or gown, it can cause **strike-through contamination**. This occurs when moisture from either side of the drape serves as a vehicle for bacteria to infiltrate the drape from the nonsterile surface. Most disposable drapes are tightly woven to prevent strike-through. With continuous contact, blood and fluids can penetrate gowns and drapes. Woven (reusable) drapes are treated with a chemical that resists moisture but are not completely impervious.

15. **The sterile field is created as close as possible to the time of surgery and is monitored throughout the procedure.**

    When sterile supplies have been opened, the sterile setup is vulnerable to contamination. The longer a sterile setup remains exposed, the greater the risk of contamination. Sterile supplies should be opened as close to the time of surgery as possible. In reality, however, cases often are delayed or even canceled. It is not recommended that supplies be left open before a case for more than 2 hours; after 2 hours the items should be considered contaminated, and the room should be broken down. No data are currently available to suggest that leaving a sterile setup exposed increases the risk of **surgical site infection** (SSI). After a room is opened, it must be constantly monitored to prevent accidental contamination.

As surgical personnel develop experience, they clarify their own practices and compare them with those of the people around them. Even after acquiring excellent technique, people may consciously (or unconsciously) disregard certain practices because of lack of peer or administrative support, lack of professional motivation, or simple apathy. SSIs are the result of poor technique. On a statistical level, the numbers may seem small. On a human level, however, each surgical site infection represents increased suffering for the patient and family, increased costs, extended hospital stay, lost workdays, inability to meet one's personal goals, and caretaking responsibilities for the family.

Standards vary slightly according to the practice setting and the policies of individual institutions. Surgical personnel *can and should* challenge the aseptic technique practices of their team, department, or institution as long as they have evidence to demonstrate that these practices are below the normal safety standard.

The activities that take place before and during surgery have a cumulative effect on the outcome. Each patient entering surgery has a physical and psychosocial background that predisposes him or her to a positive or negative surgical outcome. Each step of surgery, from the opening of surgical supplies until the patient's departure from the recovery room, affects the outcome.

PRACTICE OF ASEPTIC TECHNIQUE

Opening a Case
OPERATING ROOM PREPARATION

Before a surgical case is opened and before the patient arrives in the operating room, preliminary room preparations must be performed. The furniture surfaces and operating room lights should be damp dusted before opening for the first case of the day. The surgeon's preference card and the case-cart supplies must be checked to ensure that all instruments, supplies, and equipment necessary for the surgical procedure are available. One must prepare the operating room by arranging the furniture in the desired locations for the procedure. Patient positioning equipment should be in the room before the patient arrives.

WHEN TO OPEN STERILE ITEMS

Depending on the complexity of the surgery, the amount of equipment to be prepared, and the degree of emergency, the scrub and circulator open the case about 15 to 20 minutes before the start of surgery. In extremely large cases, more time may be needed to allow for opening of supplies and setting up of the case.

After the case is opened, the sterile items should be constantly monitored. The ideal technique is to have someone physically in the room to observe the sterile setup and verify that nothing is contaminated. Covering the setup with a sterile drape is *not* recommended because of the risk of contamination when the cover is removed. Leaving a room vacant and posting a sign on the door advising staff that the room is open is not an acceptable practice.

OPENING LARGE PACKS ONTO A TABLE

Large packs are included in almost all surgical setups. These include linen or nonwoven gowns, towels, sponges, and other items. Preassembled case packs can be custom designed by the institution to include surgical supplies routinely used during specific types of surgery. Some commonly preassembled packs include abdominal, orthopedic, and minor surgery packs. The large case pack is the first to be opened. For each package or item to be opened, be sure to check the integrity of the outside of the package and the external chemical indicators for verification of exposure to the sterilization process. In addition, every item to be opened must be visually checked for package integrity.

Any packages with tears, holes, or water marks are contaminated and should be removed from the room and replaced with new packages. The large pack is opened on the back table, because that is the center of the scrub's work area. After the large pack is unwrapped, instruments, suture packs, and other sterile items are opened onto the draped surface and later organized and set up in logical order.

The following technique is used by nonsterile personnel to open the large pack (Figure 9-4):

1. Center the pack on the table and orient it so the long ends of the outside drape line up with the long end of the table.
2. If the pack is very large and has been square wrapped, grasp the folded edge of the top fold with both hands and pull the edges toward you.
3. Move to the other side of the table and repeat this process on the opposite top fold. Allow 1 inch of margin between the edge of the drape and your nonsterile hand. Remember, *nonsterile team members must never lean over or reach over a sterile surface.*
4. Do not readjust the table drape after it is placed.

OPENING INSTRUMENT TRAYS

The following technique is used by nonsterile personnel to open an instrument tray properly (Figure 9-5):

1. When opening large instrument trays or other heavy equipment, set the tray on a small table and then open in place.
2. Orient the item so that the flap farthest away from the body is grasped first. The flap is opened away from the body and gently pulled down.
3. Open each side flap. Open the flap closest to the body last, pulling it toward you. This prevents the nonsterile arm from reaching across the sterile surface inside the pack.
4. Drape small tables in the same manner. Place the drape on the table. Grasp only the edges of the drape and unfold the top corner or edge of the drape away from you. After the first flap has been pulled back, subsequent flaps must be opened in such a way that the nonsterile arm and hand do not reach across the sterile surface. Move around the table if necessary, always bringing the edge of the drape *toward you.*
5. As sterile items are opened, use more tables if necessary.
6. Do not stack heavy sterile instruments precariously high or in such a way that they might be dropped.
7. Avoid holding a heavy instrument tray in one hand and removing the wrapper with the other. This puts excessive strain on the wrist, and you may drop the tray. Put the tray on a nonsterile table before opening the wrapper.

Delivering Sterile Goods and Solutions during Surgery
PASSING AND RECEIVING ENVELOPE-WRAPPED ITEMS

When items are opened during the setup and the scrub is sterile, the circulator opens these items and delivers them aseptically. One opens envelope-wrapped trays or other small items by grasping the top flap and pulling it back, away from the

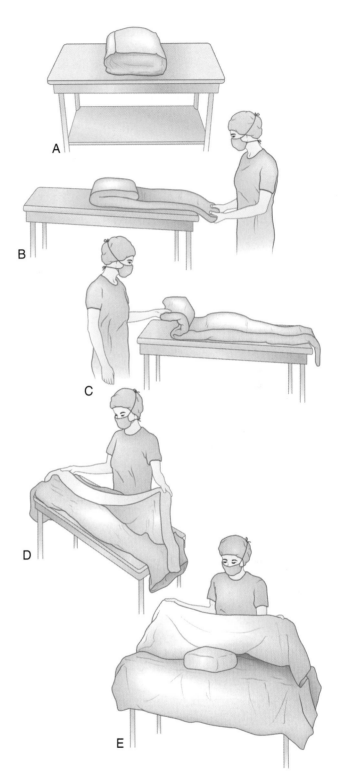

FIGURE 9-4
Opening a table pack. **A,** The large linen pack is placed in the center of the back table. **B** and **C,** Layers are always pulled toward the person opening the pack so that the hand and arm do not extend over the sterile area. **D,** Handle only the edge of the linen. **E,** Follow the same procedure for the final fold.

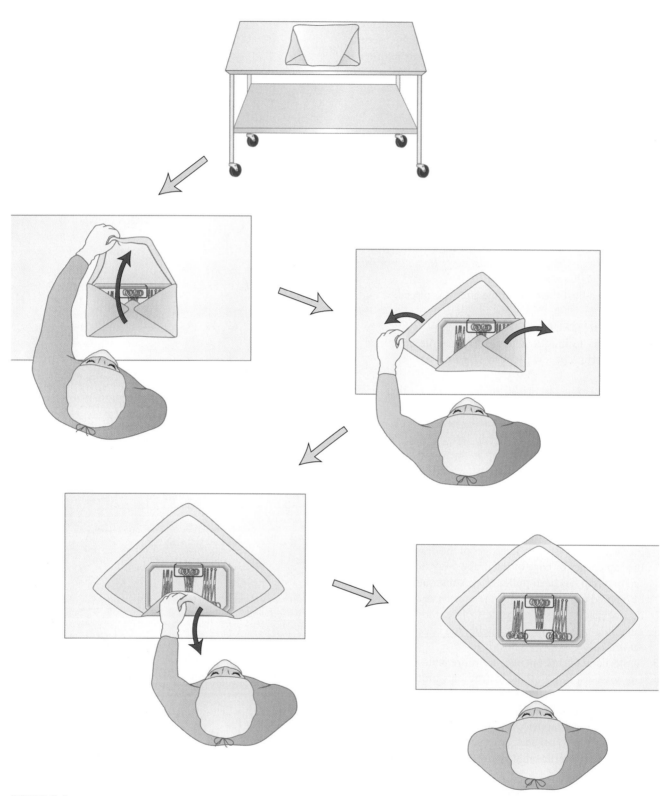

FIGURE 9-5
Opening large instrument trays.

person opening, and under the item. Side flaps are opened next, followed by the near flap. The scrub may take the item directly as shown in Figure 9-6, or the circulator may carefully set the item on a sterile surface *without allowing contamination of the object (e.g., tray, instrument) or the sterile surface.*

OPENING PEEL POUCHES
Items wrapped in sealed pouches are delivered directly to the scrub as shown in Figure 9-7, *A.* Suture packets also may be flipped onto the field (Figure 9-7, *B*). One does this by opening the peel pouch halfway and then quickly popping the

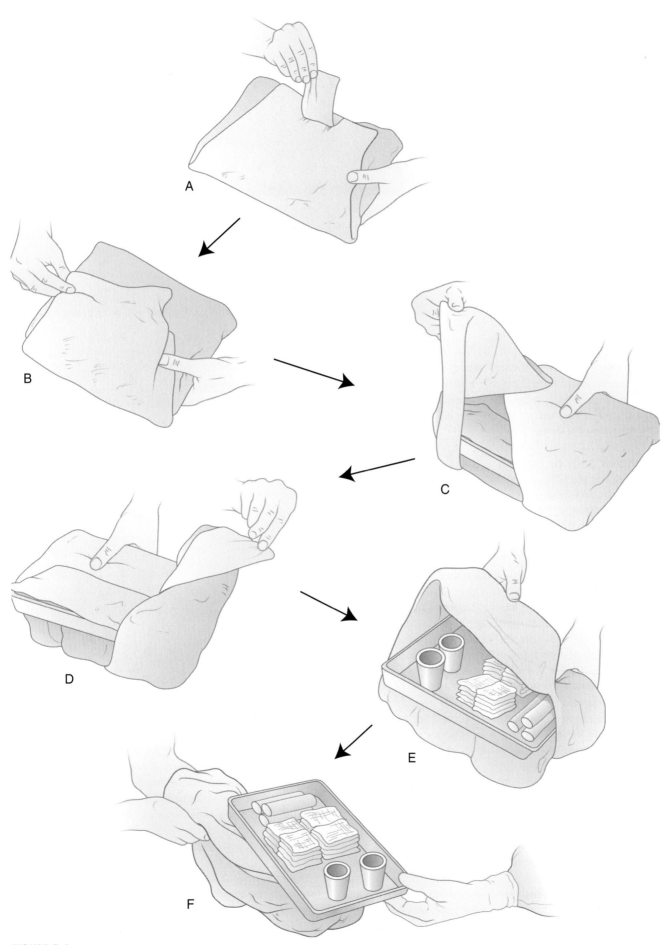

FIGURE 9-6
A through **F,** One opens small packages by grasping the corners of the wrapper and bringing them back over the hand, as shown.

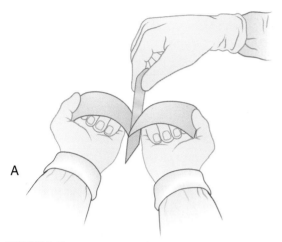
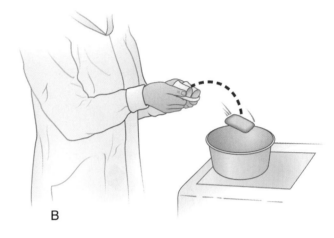

FIGURE 9-7
A, Opening a sterilized pouch. **B,** Flipping items onto a sterile field. (Redrawn from Phillips N: *Berry & Kohn's operating room technique,* ed 10, St Louis, 2004, Mosby.)

wrapper open the rest of the way to propel the contents out of the package and onto the sterile field. One must take extreme care when flipping items onto the field to avoid reaching over the sterile field or flipping the item past the sterile field and onto the floor.

OPENING BASINS
Basin sets are placed on a ring stand and opened in the same manner as large instrument trays. Open the flap farthest away from you first, then the side flaps. *Pull the last flap toward you* to avoid reaching over the sterile basin.

OPENING SMALL ITEMS
Follow these guidelines when opening small items:

▶ Suture packs and small items are opened onto the back table or other location according to institutional policy.
▶ Scalpel blades and other **sharps** should be passed directly to the scrub or unwrapped in an open area where they are easily seen. Blades and other sharps are not to be opened into instrument trays because the sharps can be hidden by other instruments.
▶ Items should never be opened so that sharps are hidden from plain view. If a sharp item is accidentally covered during opening, warn the scrub of its location to avoid injury during the setup.

DISTRIBUTING SOLUTIONS
To distribute solutions, follow these guidelines:

▶ The lip of a solution bottle is considered sterile only if it is covered with a sterile top that extends over the edge of the container.
▶ The recommended method of distributing a solution is to pour the solution directly into a container set close to the edge of the table or held in the hand of the scrub (Figure 9-8).

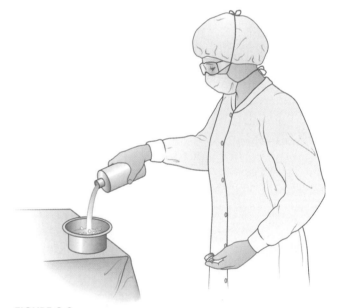

FIGURE 9-8
Pouring solutions. (Redrawn from Phillips N: *Berry & Kohn's operating room technique,* ed 10, St Louis, 2004, Mosby.)

▶ When pouring sterile liquids, empty the entire container and move the down-turned container away from the sterile field. This prevents any liquid from running over the edge of the container and contaminating the field. After the bottle has been opened and its contents poured, the lip of the bottle is no longer considered sterile.

As previously discussed, it is considered poor technique to pry off the metal cap of a medication vial and pour the liquid into a sterile container because the lip of the vial is *not considered sterile.* Refer to Chapter 13 for a complete discussion of the sterile distribution of drugs.

Handwashing

Handwashing is the simplest and most important preventive measure for reducing infection in the workplace. It is performed to remove organic debris and reduce the number of transient microorganisms (**transient flora**) on the skin. All health personnel are at high risk for acquiring and transmitting infectious disease. Attention to handwashing can significantly reduce this risk.

Handwashing is *event related* (performed before and after a specific task or event). Handwashing requires a specific method. Inadequate handwashing increases the risk of infection to patients and personnel.

For handwashing to be effective one must employ adequate friction, adequate time, and an effective washing agent.

Table 9-1 describes the purpose of and methods used for hand cleansing and disinfection in the health-care setting.

AGENTS USED FOR HANDWASHING
Plain Soap
Soap is available in solid bars or liquid form. When used properly, soap is effective in removing soil and debris. It has *little or no antimicrobial activity*. The effectiveness of soap *depends on friction* to remove organic and inorganic matter from skin. Reservoir-type refillable liquid-soap containers can harbor pathogenic microorganisms, and their use is discouraged. Soap holders that are stocked with fresh individual packets are recommended.

Topical Antiseptic Combined with Detergent
Antiseptic detergents (**topical antiseptics**) are used for handwashing and the surgical scrub (Table 9-2). They reduce the number of bacterial colonies, and some produce *barrier protection* that inhibits growth of bacteria over time. This action is produced when the antiseptic binds chemically with the stratum corneum of the skin. Detergents are among the most destructive agents routinely used on skin. Increased amounts of surfactant (an agent that lowers the surface tension of a liquid) cause more rapid and extensive skin damage. Damaged skin is more resistant to antimicrobial action and harbors greater numbers of microbes. Detergent anti-

septics that contain skin emollients are available to prevent the breakdown of skin.

Alcohol-Based Skin Cleaner
Ethyl or isopropyl alcohol combined with skin emollients is now available in the form of foams and creams for use in health-care settings. When employed correctly, these products destroy both gram-positive and gram-negative bacteria at high levels. The effect continues for several hours after gloving. Although pure alcohol is drying and can cause skin irritation and breakdown, commercially prepared alcohol foams and creams used for surgical hand scrubs contain skin conditioners to prevent drying.

WHEN TO HANDWASH
Handwashing should be performed at the following times:

- Before the surgical scrub and at the conclusion of a surgical case.
- Before and after *any contact* with a patient.
- Between contacts with potentially contaminated areas of the same patient.
- *Immediately after contact with blood or body fluids, regardless of whether gloves were worn at the time of contact.*
- Before and after eating.
- After personal hygiene care.
- Before the beginning and at the end of the workday.

HANDWASHING TECHNIQUE
Use the following technique for washing hands:

1. Remove jewelry from hands and fingers.
2. Wet the hands thoroughly under running water and apply sufficient antiseptic agent to cover all surfaces of the hands and wrists.
3. Clean the subungual area with a stiff nail cleaner. Rub the hands together vigorously and include the backs of the hands, interdigital spaces, and wrists. To ensure that the spaces between the fingers are adequately washed, spread the fingers and weave the two hands together, rubbing continuously.

Table 9-1 HAND ANTISEPSIS

Type of Antisepsis	Purpose	Method
Handwash	To remove soil and transient microorganisms	Wash with soap or detergent for at least 10-15 sec.
Hand antisepsis	To remove or destroy transient microorganisms	Wash with antimicrobial soap, detergent, or alcohol-based hand rub for at least 10-15 sec.
Surgical hand scrub	To remove or destroy transient microorganisms and reduce resident flora	Wash with antimicrobial soap or detergent preparation using brush to achieve friction for at least 120 sec, or with alcohol-based preparation for at least 20 sec.

Reprinted from Larson EL: APIC guidelines for handwashing and hand antisepsis in health care settings, *American Journal of Infection Control* 23(4):257, 1995, with permission from the Association for Professionals in Infection Control and Epidemiology.

Table 9-2 SURGICAL HAND SCRUB AGENTS

Agent	Residual Protection	Bactericidal Activity		Toxicity	Comments
		Gram-Negative Organisms	Gram-Positive Organisms		
Povidone iodine (iodophors)	Minimal	Moderate	Moderately good	Possible irritation, allergy, and toxicity. Can be absorbed through skin.	Commonly used. Effective against mycobacteria, fungi, and viruses. Effective in the presence of organic substances. Must be rinsed thoroughly from skin. Caution: do not allow iodophor detergents to splash into eyes.
Chlorhexidine gluconate (alcohol-detergent based)	Good with repeated use	Good	Good	Nonirritating to skin. Highly ototoxic. Causes severe eye damage on contact with cornea.	Not absorbed by skin. Not effective in the presence of organic debris except in detergent base.
Alcohol-based skin cleaners	None	Excellent	Excellent	Damaging to mucous membrane and eyes. Nontoxic on skin. Can be very drying.	Contain skin emollients to prevent drying. If used as a surgical hand cleaner, should be preceded by thorough mechanical cleaning.
Triclosan	Moderate with repeated use	Inhibits growth	Inhibits growth	Nontoxic on skin. Is absorbed through skin.	Not fungicidal. Virucidal activity unknown. Effective against *Mycobacterium tuberculosis*. Least effective of surgical hand scrubs. Use only when personnel cannot use other skin scrub agents.

4. Continue the hand scrub for 10 to 15 seconds, increasing the time after gross contact with known pathogenic surfaces, blood, or body fluids.

5. Rinse all soap from hands and forearms. Avoid shaking fingers and hands in an attempt to dry, as this spreads droplets.

6. Dry hands by blotting with a towel.

Surgical Scrub

The surgical scrub *does not sterilize the skin;* it only renders the skin surgically clean. Living tissue cannot be sterilized, but the use of certain antiseptics along with the standardized scrub technique reduces the number of microbes on the skin and may produce continuous antimicrobial action. This is important because bacteria proliferate quickly in the moist environment between the skin and glove. Scrub brushes impregnated with antimicrobial agent are available individually wrapped. If nondisposable brushes are used, they must be sterile. During the scrub, avoid harsh friction with the brush because it breaks down skin. Repeated skin irritation encourages colonization of both resident and transient bacteria on the hands and arms.

Sterile members of the surgical team perform the surgical scrub immediately before sterile gowning and gloving as well as after direct skin contact with blood or body fluids. Scrubbed personnel scrub before the rest of the sterile team to prepare all sterile supplies and equipment that have been previously opened. Before beginning the surgical scrub, the surgical technologist or scrub nurse opens the sterile gown, towel, and gloves onto a small table on which *no other sterile supplies have been opened.* Never don gown and gloves directly from the back table or Mayo stand, and do not allow anyone else entering the sterile field to do so. The reason is to prevent the contamination of sterile instruments, table covers, and other equipment by water that drips from the hands and arms onto sterile goods.

Government and professional organizations have researched the amount of time required for an effective surgical scrub. In its recommended practice established in 2002, the AORN states that a timed scrub or counted stroke method may be used, and that research in the United States has shown that a 2- to 3-minute scrub is effective. However, the length of time for the surgical scrub is an individual institutional policy. The length of the scrub should be the same for both the initial surgical scrub and all scrubs that follow during the day. The APIC recommends a scrub of at least 2 minutes. Manufacturers of antiseptic agents recommend a specific scrub time for a particular agent. These recommendations should be followed.

Surgical Scrub Technique

When performing the surgical scrub, begin with the hands and proceed to the wrists and arms, *without returning to a previously scrubbed area.* Point the fingers upward and hold the hands above the elbows at all times to prevent water from the unscrubbed area from running down over an area that has been previously cleaned.

Follow these steps to perform a surgical scrub properly (Figure 9-9):

1. Prepare for the surgical scrub by ensuring that the scrub suit top is tucked into the scrub pants or is sufficiently snug so that it remains dry. Remember to adjust the surgical mask and protective face shield or eyewear before starting the scrub.
2. Perform routine washing of hands and arms (as described previously in the section on handwashing) according to institutional policy using antiseptic soap. Rinse hands and arms thoroughly.
3. Unwrap a sterile scrub brush packet and remove the nail cleaner. Hold the brush in one hand while carefully cleaning the subungual area on each finger under running water. Discard the nail cleaner. Moisten the sponge with antiseptic soap, create a lather, and begin with the nails. Keep the surfaces of the fingers, hands, and arms in mind as you begin the scrub. If using the counted method, scrub the nails with 30 strokes. Scrub each side separately on one hand, then the other. Proceed to the three surfaces of one arm (20 strokes on each surface) and then the other without returning to previously scrubbed areas. Extend the scrub to 2 inches above the elbow.
4. Do not allow the scrubbed hand or arm to contact any part of the sink, faucet, or scrub suit. Avoid splashing water on the scrub suit. Donning a sterile gown over a wet

scrub suit is not acceptable because of the danger of strike-through contamination.
5. Keep hands higher than elbows at all times. When the scrub is completed, rinse the hands and arms by passing first the hand and then the arm under running water. Keep the elbows flexed. Do not move the arms back and forth through the water. Try to remove all residual soap because it can harbor debris and also make gloving more difficult. Proceed to the operating room. Enter by pushing the door open with your back, keeping the elbows flexed. Proceed to drying, gowning, and gloving. Be sure to dry hands well, as gloves are difficult to apply when there is moisture, and moist environments are a breeding ground for bacteria.

Alcohol-Based Brushless Scrub

The use of alcohol-based preparations in a brushless scrub is gaining popularity in some institutions both in the United States and in other countries. Because the application of these products does not remove debris, the hands, including the subungual area, must be thoroughly washed before the product is applied. A number of studies have demonstrated that, when appropriate amounts of the product are applied to the hands and arms and friction is used to completely moisten all surfaces, an alcohol-based skin scrub is as effective as a standard surgical scrub. When scrubbing with these products, consult the manufacturer's instructions about recommended use.

DRYING, GOWNING, AND GLOVING

Drying Your Hands

The following is the proper technique for drying (Figure 9-10):

1. After entering the operating room from the scrub sink area, proceed to the gowning and gloving table.
2. Remove the towel by grasping only the edge, and lift it up and away from the sterile gown and gloves. Do not hesitate, because water may drip from the hands onto the sterile gown and gloves, which would contaminate them.
3. Allow the towel to unfold so that the long edge hangs down between your two hands. Bend forward slightly at the waist so the sterile towel does not touch the scrub suit. Use one end of the towel for one hand and arm and the other end for the other hand and arm.
4. Blot the skin, working from hand to wrist to arm *without moving back over a previously dried area.*
5. Keep the towel out in front of you where you can see it to avoid touching the towel to the scrub suit. After drying one hand and arm with one end of the towel, begin drying the other hand by placing the wet hand at the *other end* of the towel while confining it to its own side.
6. Dry the second hand and arm using the same blotting technique. When you are finished, drop the towel into a nearby receptacle. Proceed immediately to gowning.

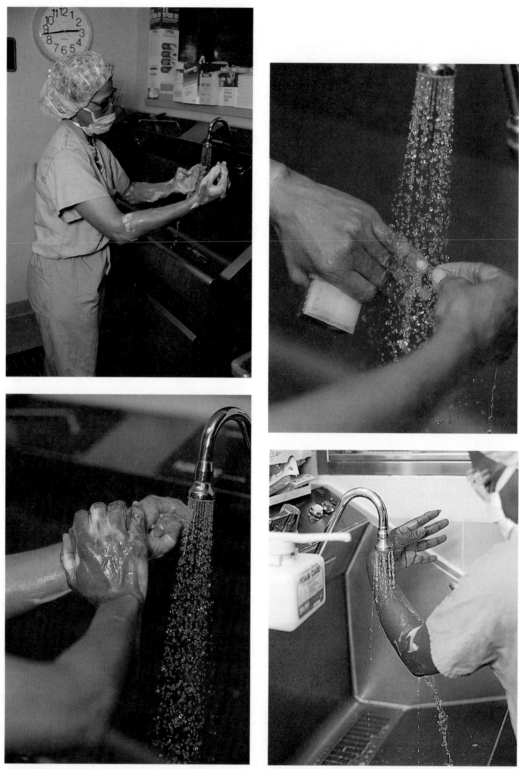

FIGURE 9-9
Surgical hand scrub. (From Perry AG and Potter PA: *Clinical nursing skills and techniques*, ed 5, St Louis, 2004, Mosby.)

Gowning Yourself

Surgical gowns are worn by all sterile personnel. The gown is donned immediately before the start of surgery and may be changed during surgery if it is penetrated by blood or other fluids. Many types of surgical gowns are available, but the most common type wraps around the body and is designed to cover both the front and the back of the wearer. As mentioned earlier, however, *the back is considered nonsterile.*

Most disposable gowns are water resistant. Gowns used in orthopedics, obstetrics, and other specialties in which there are copious amounts of blood or irrigation fluids on and around the sterile field have a waterproof or reinforced shield laminated to the front of the gown.

The surgical technologist or scrub nurse dons a sterile gown immediately after drying the hands. When gowning, consider the gown as having two surfaces: an *inside* surface that will contact the nonsterile scrub suit and bare skin of hands and arms, and an *outside* surface that will be considered sterile only from the waist to the axillary line, and from the hands to the elbows.

Surgical gowns are folded before packaging so that the inside surface faces outward (inside out). This allows scrubbed personnel to grasp the presenting side of the gown with bare hands to put it on, because that surface will be the nonsterile side. Use caution not to grasp the gown at the neckline, because one may contaminate the sterile (outer) section of the gown by handling the gown this way.

Gowning should be performed according to the following guidelines (Figure 9-11):

1. After drying the hands and arms, grasp the gown just below the neckline and lift it up and away from the table, without touching anything else with bare hands. Remember, the *inside* surface of the gown faces outward.
2. Step away from the table and allow the gown to unfold. Do not touch the (outside) surface facing away from you.
3. Being careful not to lower the gown, look for the armholes and place your hands and arms inside the sleeves. Advance your hands, pushing them through horizontally from your shoulders, not above your head, to within about an inch of the knitted cuff edge. At this time the circulator may secure the neck and *inside* ties and assist in securing the back wrap. Glove immediately, using the closed technique.

Gloving Yourself

Many types of surgical gloves are commercially available. The common considerations in choosing gloves are the glove material (**latex allergy** is a major concern), tensile strength, thickness, and economy. Tactile sensation is important, especially in surgical specialties that require the use of fine instruments and in which delicate tissues are encountered. Thicker gloves are more appropriate, however, when there is repeated contact with heavy instruments or there is copious bleeding, such as during orthopedic surgery.

Double gloving has been shown to be effective in reducing glove failure from 51% to 7%. The statistical probability of glove failure increases with increased surgical time and increased handling of tissues and supplies. Glove punctures are associated with the transmission of blood-borne pathogens to health-care workers. Double gloving reduces the risk of contact with blood and body fluids and is encouraged in the following cases:

▶ Orthopedic and vascular procedures
▶ Procedures involving patients known to be carriers of an infectious transmissible virus

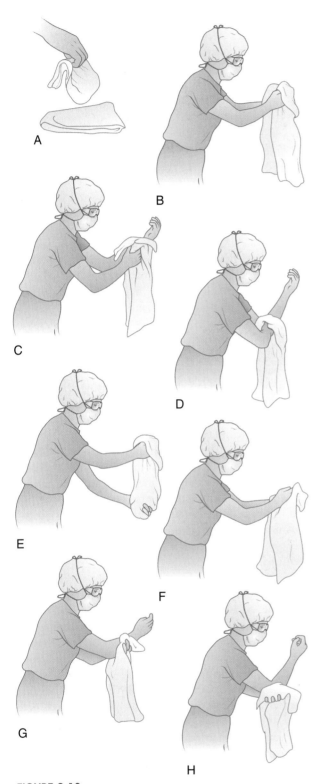

FIGURE 9-10
Drying the hands and arms. **A,** Pick up a sterile towel from the table, being careful not to drip water on the gown beneath it. **B,** Fold the towel lengthwise. **C,** Use one end of the towel only to dry one hand. **D,** Rotate the arm as you proceed to dry it, working from wrist to elbow. Do not allow the towel to contact the scrub suit. **E** and **F,** After the arm is dried, bring the dry hand to the opposite end of the towel and begin drying the other hand. **G,** Dry the arm using the blotting rotating motion. **H,** Proceed to the elbow. The towel may be discarded in the linen hamper or kick bucket.

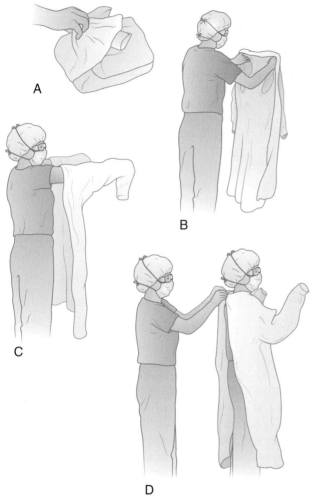

FIGURE 9-11
Gowning self. **A,** Grasp the gown firmly and bring it away from the table. It has been folded so that the outside faces away. **B,** Holding the gown at the shoulders, allow it to unfold gently. Do not shake the gown. **C,** Place hands inside the armholes and guide each arm through the sleeves by raising and spreading the arms. Do not allow hands to slide outside cuff of gown. **D,** The circulator assists by pulling the gown over the shoulders and tying it.

▶ Procedures lasting longer than 2 hours
▶ Procedures in which blood loss is expected to be greater than 100 ml.

To reduce constriction when double gloving, the first or innermost pair of gloves should be one size larger than is normally worn. However, this is a matter of individual preference, and one should try different combinations of glove sizes to see which is the most comfortable.

CLOSED GLOVING

The **closed gloving** technique is used by a person wearing a sterile gown. It is the most effective method to prevent contact between skin and the outside of the sterile glove. When learning the closed gloving technique, think of the glove as having two surfaces or planes—the inside and the outside.

Before the gloves are touched, the entire glove is sterile, inside and outside. As soon as gloving is initiated, however, the inside surface is considered nonsterile.

Gloves are packaged in a paper wrapper. The top of the glove is folded over to form a 2- to 3-inch cuff. The exposed side of the cuff is continuous with the inside of the glove and is considered the nonsterile side.

Packaged gloves are oriented with the *palm of the glove facing upward.* Thus, when handling the gloves, think first about the orientation and position of your hand. Glove with the knitted cuff of your gown pulled over your hand, which is positioned palm up to match the orientation of the glove.

Use the following technique to perform closed gloving (Figure 9-12):

1. Begin closed gloving after donning a sterile gown. Do not allow your fingers to protrude outside the knitted cuff of the gown. You will maneuver sterile gloves onto your hands with your hands hidden from view under the gown's cuffs.
2. Open the glove wrapper, handling only the edge. Open the wrapper carefully so that it stays open and does not snap back when you release the edges.
3. Position your left hand with the palm facing upward, as if you are about to receive an object in your hand. Pick up the left glove with your right hand and place the glove, palm to palm and cuff to cuff, over the left hand.
4. Working inside the gown cuff, pinch the under edge of the glove cuff between your left thumb and fingers. Then, grasp the uppermost edge of the glove cuff. The palm of the glove should still be oriented to your palm. If it is not, you will have difficulty sliding the hand into the glove—a common problem at this point. To correct misalignment of the glove, grasp it at the cuff and realign it correctly, palm to palm.
5. Keep the hidden fingers within an inch of the outside edge of the knitted cuff, and make sure your thumb is beyond the seam of the cuff. This prevents another common obstacle, which occurs when the left hand slips back into the gown sleeve. This makes it very difficult to work the fingers and hand through the knitted cuff and glove, which is now tight around the hand.
6. Pull the glove on. Grasp the left glove cuff and advance your left hand into the glove. After gloving, check both hands for any sign of punctures or tears.
7. Take your time when learning to glove. It is better to be methodical and slow at first. Speed and efficiency will follow with practice if you use the same technique repeatedly.
8. Repeat with the other hand.

OPEN GLOVING

The **open gloving** technique is used during sterile procedures that do not require donning a sterile gown, such as urinary catheterization and patient skin preparation. The hands are not usually scrubbed before open gloving, although they always should be washed. When gloving, consider the two surfaces of the glove—the outside and the in-

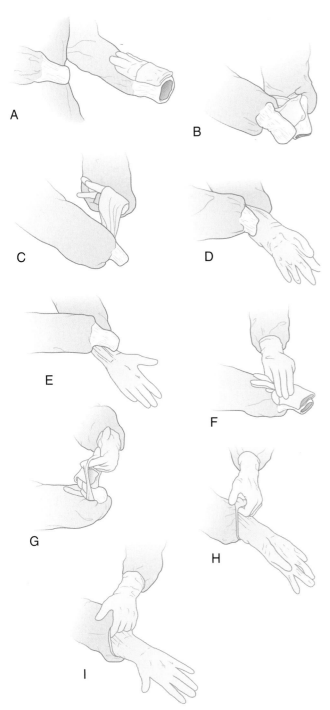

FIGURE 9-12
Gloving self, closed technique. **A,** Lay the glove palm-down over the cuff of the gown. The fingers of the glove face toward you. **B** and **C,** Working through the gown sleeve, grasp the cuff of the glove and bring it over the open cuff of the sleeve. **D** and **E,** Unroll the glove cuff so that it covers the sleeve cuff. **F** through **I,** Proceed with the opposite hand, using the same technique. Never allow the bare hand to contact the gown cuff edge or outside of glove.

side. Remember that each glove has a cuff that exposes the inside surface of the glove. This inner surface is considered the nonsterile surface, even though it is sterile until touched. The *outside surface will remain sterile. The wrapper is considered sterile to within 1 inch of the edges.*

The following is the technique for performing open gloving (Figure 9-13). In this description, the right hand is gloved first.

1. Open the outer nonsterile wrapper and deliver the inner sterile wrapped gloves onto a clean, dry surface.
2. Grasp the edges of the glove wrapper with bare hands and expose the gloves. Before releasing the glove wrapper, ensure that it will stay open. The palms of the gloves should be facing upward, thumbs to the outside.
3. Using your left hand, grasp the upper folded lip of the right glove cuff. Do not to touch the wrapper underneath or the outside of the glove. Pick up the glove and slide your right hand into the glove, keeping your hand palm up, oriented to the palm of the glove. Leave the cuff turned down until you glove the other hand.
4. To glove the left hand, slide the fingers of your sterile, gloved hand *under* the cuff. This positions your gloved hand (sterile) in contact with the outside (sterile) surface of the other glove. Keep the palm up as you slide your bare hand into the glove. You may unroll the cuff carefully, but do not allow the gloved hand to touch any bare skin.

While learning to glove, personnel sometimes experience difficulty in removing the glove from the open sterile wrapper. Very thin or short-cuffed gloves are difficult to don without contaminating the sterile side of the glove or the glove wrapper. Another common problem is caused by sliding the hand into the glove with the palm facing *down*. This places one's thumb in a position opposite to the glove thumb and necessitates repositioning of the hand inside the glove. One can avoid these problems by thinking about each step and working methodically and *slowly.*

Gowning and Gloving Other Team Members

After the surgical technologist has set up sterile supplies and instruments, the other members of the surgical team enter from the scrub sink area. Gowning and gloving of the other team members precedes all other activities and is as much a social tradition as a necessary part of the surgical routine. During gowning and gloving, the surgeon greets the scrub, circulator, and anesthesiologist, and may introduce other members of the team. This time allows formal acknowledgment of the team members and what is to be done before the actual start of surgery. The surgeon also may clarify the need for special instruments or equipment at this time. Interaction among team members during the process of gowning and gloving often sets the tone for the entire surgery.

When the sterile team members enter the operating room, the scrub hands a towel to the surgical team leader (lead surgeon or surgical resident) and then to the other members of the team. Whenever possible, be certain that you have the correct gowns and glove sizes available *before* the team members enter the room.

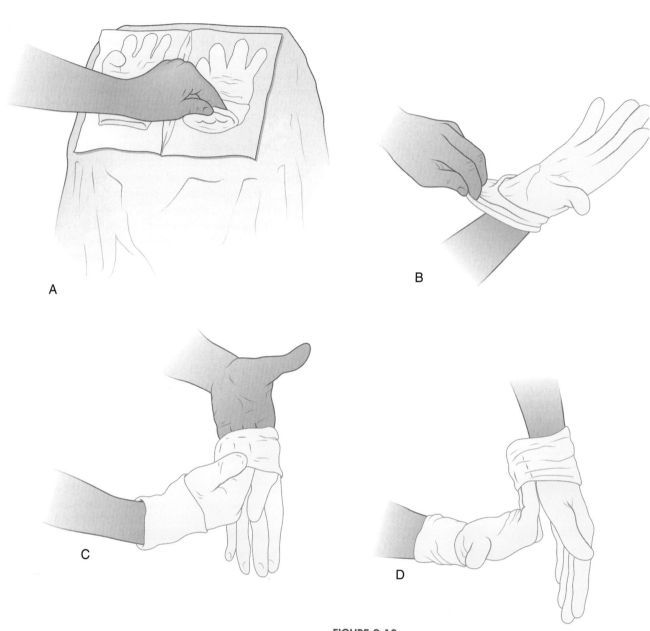

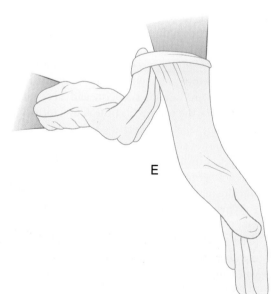

FIGURE 9-13

Gloving self, open technique. **A,** Pick up the glove by its *inside* cuff with one hand. Do not touch the glove wrapper with the bare hand. **B,** Slide the glove onto the opposite hand. Leave the cuff down. **C,** Using the partially gloved hand, slide the fingers into the outer side of the opposite glove cuff. **D,** Slide the hand into the glove and unroll the cuff. **E,** With the *gloved* hand, slide the fingers under the *outside* edge of the opposite cuff and unroll it gently, using the same technique.

GOWNING OTHER TEAM MEMBERS

Use the following technique to gown other team members (Figure 9-14):

1. When the team member reaches out for a towel for drying, pass the sterile towel over the team member's hand so that the long edge of the towel falls between his or her two hands.

2. Grasp the folded gown, step away from any nonsterile surface, and allow the gown to unfold. Cuff your hands under the shoulders of the gown so that the *outside* of

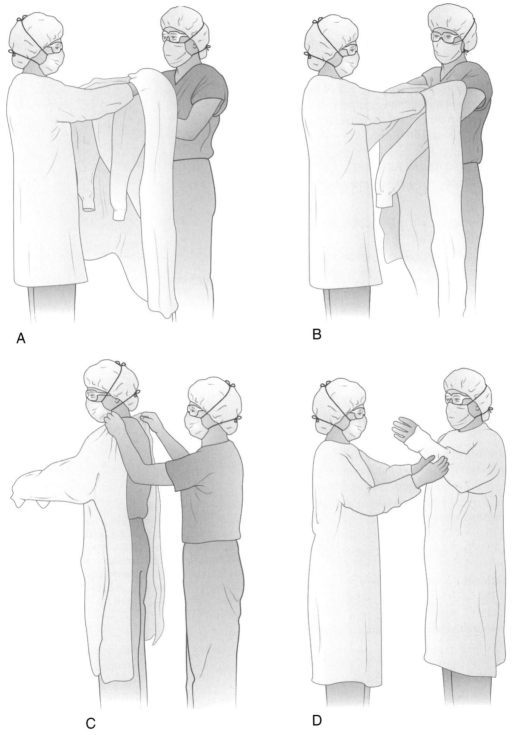

A

B

C

D

FIGURE 9-14
Gowning another. **A,** Grasp the gown so that the outside faces toward you. Holding the gown at the shoulders, cuff your hands under the gown's shoulders. **B,** The surgeon steps forward and places his or her arms in the sleeves. Slide the gown up to the mid upper arms. **C,** The circulator assists in pulling the gown up and tying it. **D,** Gently pull the cuffs back over the surgeon's hands. Be careful that your gloved hands do not touch his or her bare hands.

the gown (the part of the gown that will remain sterile) faces *you*. Position the gown so that the person you are gowning can easily insert his or her hands into the armholes.

3. After the team member has stepped forward and placed his or her arms into the sleeves, pull the gown over the elbows toward the shoulders, and then step back and away and grasp the gloves.
4. Glove the team member (see next section).
5. The circulator secures the neck closure and ties located on the *inside* (nonsterile) surface of the gown.
6. After the team member is gloved, grasp one of the sterile outside ties of the gown while the surgeon turns toward the wrap that encircles the front of the gown. Hand the tie to the wearer to be secured in front.

GLOVING A GOWNED TEAM MEMBER
Use the following technique to glove a gowned team member (Figure 9-15):

1. Open the glove wrapper and place gloves and wrapper near you on the sterile table.
2. Grasp the glove under the cuff and spread the opening with your thumbs held well away from the glove or tucked securely under the cuff.
3. Orient the glove so that the *palm* of the glove *faces the person you are gloving*. Offer the right glove first, then the left.
4. Make sure the sterile team member inserts his or her hand into the glove by pointing all fingers downward. Allow the cuff edge to recoil gently. Repeat the process with the other glove. The surgeon may try to help by placing a finger in the cuff to hold the glove open wider.

When a glove tears or is punctured by a sharp instrument or needle during surgery, small holes or tears may go unnoticed until blood appears underneath the glove. Even if there is no visible sign of a tear, a glove should be changed whenever there is a chance it was punctured.

REMOVING A CONTAMINATED GLOVE DURING SURGERY
The following technique is used to remove a contaminated glove (Figure 9-16):

1. The team member presents the contaminated hand to the circulator *palm upward.*
2. The circulator, wearing nonsterile gloves, grasps the contaminated glove below the wrist and removes it.
3. The cuff of the gown is no longer considered sterile after the glove is removed.
4. The scrub regloves the team member as described previously.
5. If it is the scrub who has a contaminated glove, he or she must have the glove replaced by another sterile team

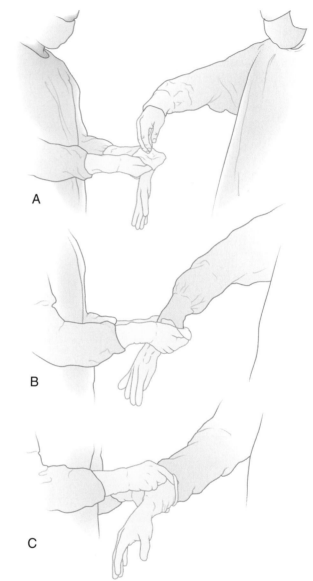

FIGURE 9-15
Gloving another. **A,** Pick up the *right* glove and place the palm away from you. Slide the fingers under the glove cuff and spread them so that a wide opening is created. Keep thumbs under the cuff. **B,** The surgeon thrusts his or her hand into the glove. Do not release the glove yet. **C,** *Gently* release the cuff (do not let the cuff snap sharply) while unrolling it over the wrist. Proceed with the left glove, using the same technique.

member. If the scrub is double gloved, he or she may replace his or her own outer glove.

Removing Gown and Gloves After Surgery
When removing contaminated gown and gloves, follow Standard Precautions. Do not let the contaminated gloved hands or outside of the gown touch bare skin. Gown and gloves are removed in a manner that contains the contaminated portion by folding or rolling the glove and gown inward.

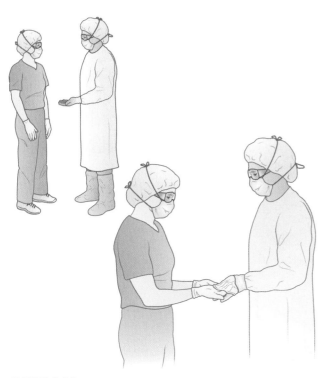

FIGURE 9-16
Removing a contaminated glove during surgery.

REMOVING THE GOWN

When removing sterile attire, one removes the gown first, according to the following guidelines (Figure 9-17):

1. Grasp the gown at the shoulders, releasing or breaking the ties or snaps, and pull the sleeves downward. This will roll the gown inside out as it slides over your gloved hands.
2. Roll the gown so the contaminated outside surface faces inward.
3. Dispose of the gown in a biohazard bag.

REMOVING GLOVES

The gloves should be removed second according to the following guidelines (Figure 9-18):

1. Grasp one glove at the outer wrist, using the opposite gloved hand.
2. Pull the glove off. It will turn inside out as you remove it.
3. Place your bare fingers *inside* the cuff of the opposite hand and roll this glove off your hand.
4. Dispose of both gloves in a biohazard receptacle *without touching the contaminated outside of the gloves.*

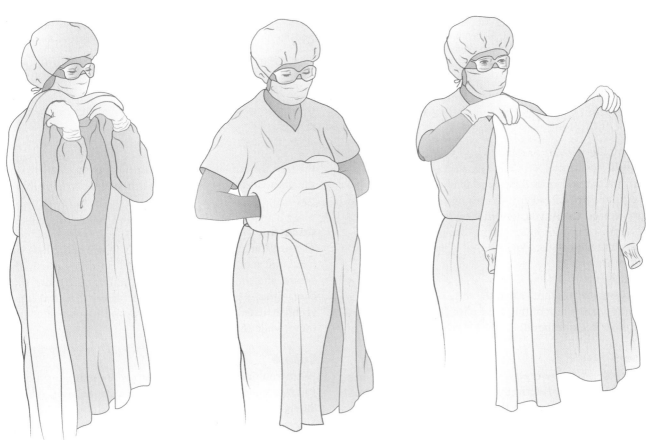

FIGURE 9-17
Removing a contaminated gown after surgery.

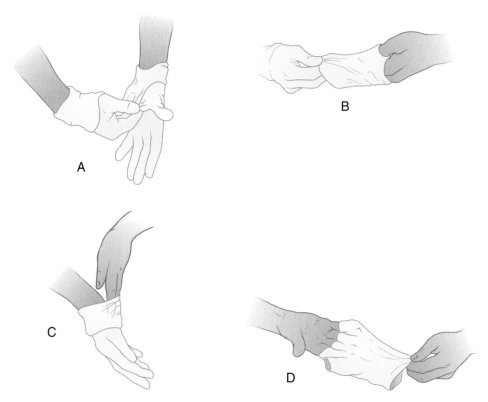

FIGURE 9-18
Removing contaminated gloves aseptically after surgery. **A,** Grasp the edge of the glove. **B,** Unroll the glove over the hand. Discard the glove (not shown). **C,** With the *bare* hand, grasp the opposite glove cuff on its inside surface. **D,** Remove the glove by inverting it over the hand. Discard the glove (not shown).

CASE STUDIES

Case 1

After you have performed the hand scrub, you enter the surgery suite and proceed to the area where your gown and gloves are located. As you are removing the towel, you notice that some water from your hand has dripped onto your sterile gown. What will you do?

Case 2

During surgery you notice that the surgeon has a hole in his glove. You notify him of this. He replies, "Don't worry about it." How will you respond?

Case 3

When you arrive in surgery, you notice that someone has placed your wrapped sterile instruments next to the heating vent. There is moisture on the outside of the pack. What should you do?

Case 4

During surgery you are moving a heavy instrument tray from one area of the sterile table to another. As you pick up the tray, the corner of the instrument tray accidentally rips the sterile sheet covering the entire back table. What will you do?

Case 5

The surgeon has just spoken abruptly to you about how you hand him sutures. A minute later you rip your glove on the suture, and the surgeon must wait while you remove your contaminated glove and put on a sterile one. The surgeon is visibly irritated. What would you say to the surgeon, if anything, while changing your glove?

Case 6

When you open your sterile basins while setting up a case, you notice moisture on the inside of a sterile basin. What is the significance of this?

Case 7

While you are scrubbed on a vaginal procedure, the mechanical engineer comes in to fix a plug. As he passes by your sterile setup, his nonsterile scrub top brushes against the in-

CASE STUDIES—cont'd

strument table. You tell the circulator that the side of the instrument table has been contaminated. He replies, "Oh, don't worry about it, this isn't a clean case anyway." How would you respond?

Case 8
After gowning, you are donning your sterile gloves, and you puncture the glove with a large hole. What should you do?

What is the proper aseptic technique to correct this problem?

Case 9
After gowning the surgeon, you notice a large tear in the sleeve of the surgeon's gown. What should you do? What is the proper aseptic technique to correct this problem?

REFERENCES
Bach T: The bloodborne pathogens standard and disinfection, *Infection Control Today,* Sept, 2000.

Garner JS: Guideline for isolation precautions in hospitals, *Infection Control and Hospital Epidemiology,* 17, 1996, and *American Journal of Infection Control,* 24, 1996.

Goodner B: *The OSHA handbook: interpretive guidelines for the bloodborne pathogen standard,* El Paso, 1993, Skidmore-Roth Publishing.

Leonas KK and Jinkins RS: The relationship of selected fabric characteristics and the barrier effectiveness of surgical gown fabrics, *American Journal of Infection Control,* 25:1, Feb, 1997.

National Institute for Occupational Safety and Health (NIOSH): *Guidelines for protecting the safety and health of health care workers: hazardous waste disposal,* Washington, DC, Sept, 1988, National Institute for Occupational Safety and Health.

Chapter 10

Transporting, Transferring, and Positioning

Learning Objectives

After studying this chapter and laboratory practice the reader will be able to:

- Identify how to incorporate safe body mechanics into patient transport, transfer, and positioning
- Describe the responsibilities of the surgical technologist in patient transport and transfer
- Use the correct procedure to identify a patient
- Demonstrate how to assist a patient from a bed to a wheelchair
- Identify how to ease a patient to the ground in the event of a fall
- Identify the steps to transport a patient by stretcher safely
- Demonstrate the transfer of a patient from a bed to a stretcher
- Identify the proper transport for a pediatric patient
- Demonstrate the transfer of a patient from a stretcher to the operating table
- Describe the use of common operating table accessories
- Demonstrate the transfer of a semiconscious patient from the operating table to a stretcher
- Describe the consequences of nerve and blood vessel compression
- Describe the principles of safe positioning
- Identify methods to prevent shearing injury
- Describe the stages of decubitus ulcers and how to prevent them
- Participate in commonly used methods of patient positioning
- Describe compartment syndrome and how to prevent it
- Describe how to do the following when positioning a patient:
  - Prevent brachial plexus injury
  - Prevent ulnar nerve and cubital tunnel injury
  - Prevent injury to the face, ear, and eye during positioning
  - Prevent injury to the breasts and genitalia in prone position
  - Turn a patient from supine to prone position

Terminology

Abduction—Movement of a joint or body part *away* from the body.

Embolism—Obstruction or occlusion of a blood vessel by a blood clot or trapped air that migrates through the systemic circulation. An embolus may lodge in small vessels of the body, including vessels of the lung, brain, or heart, blocking circulation and causing local ischemia and tissue death.

Fowler position—Sitting position used for cranial, facial, and some reconstructive breast procedures.

Hyperextension—Extension of a joint beyond its normal anatomical range.

Hyperflexion—Flexion of a joint beyond its normal anatomical range.

Ischemia—Loss of blood supply to a body part by either compression or blockage within the blood vessels. Prolonged ischemia causes tissue death resulting from lack of oxygen to the tissue.

Jackknife or Kraske position—A type of prone position in which the patient lies on his or her abdomen with the hips flexed into an inverted-V position.

Lateral position—Position in which the patient is positioned on his or her side on the operating table or bed.

Lithotomy position—Position used for vaginal, perineal, and rectal surgery. The patient's legs are positioned on stirrups that hold them in place.

Log roll—A technique for moving the patient in which one rolls the patient onto his or her side using a bed sheet or draw sheet.

Necrosis—Tissue death.

Neuropathy—Permanent or temporary nerve injury that results in numbness or loss of function of a part of the body.

Prone position—Lying position with the abdomen downward.

Reverse Trendelenburg position—Position in which the prone or supine patient is tilted with the feet down.

Semi-Fowler position—Semi-sitting position used for surgery on the neck and thyroid.

Shear injury—Tissue injury or necrosis that results when two tissue planes are forcefully pulled in opposite directions. Shearing usually occurs when the body is pulled or slides by gravity across a high-friction surface such as a bed sheet. Shearing can lead to a decubitus ulcer.

Supine position—Lying on the back with the face upward.

Table break—Hinged joint between sections of the operating table that can be flexed in any direction.

Thoracic outlet syndrome—A group of disorders attributed to compression of the subclavian vessels and nerves. Such compression can cause permanent injury to the arm and shoulder.

Thromboembolus—A blood clot that breaks loose and enters the systemic circulation, causing obstruction or occlusion of a blood vessel. Also referred to as a thrombus.

Traction injury—Nerve injury caused by stretching or compression of the nerve.

Transfer board—A thin Plexiglas, fiberglass, or roller board that is placed under the patient to move him or her from the operating table to the stretcher or bed.

Trendelenburg position—Position in which the prone or supine patient is tilted with the head down.

BODY MECHANICS

Health-care workers are at high risk for back injury and other types of musculoskeletal injury while caring for, moving, and transferring patients. Workers are injured because these tasks are unpredictable. A weak or sedated patient lacks muscle tone, which results in flaccid limbs and general unwieldiness. The adult human body is asymmetric and heavy, and unlike a large inanimate object, the human body cannot be held close to the health worker's center of gravity when moved.

When a patient is moved, there is always an element of unanticipated mishap. The patient can fall, equipment can become entangled during transfer, or the patient may become agitated. A sudden shift of weight and center of gravity can be required to prevent injury to patients or health-care workers. Hospital rooms are small and crowded, which may necessitate some twisting motions. These motions put the assistant off balance, which increases risk to the back.

Injuries are reduced when health-care providers use proper body mechanics and patient-transfer devices. (See Chapter 14 for a complete discussion of body mechanics.) To prevent injury, follow these guidelines:

▶ Always have sufficient help when moving the patient.
▶ Know your limits, and do not exceed them.
▶ Be prepared for possible weight shifts.
▶ Maintain the spine in a neutral position whenever possible.
▶ Avoid twisting the spine, especially while lifting or bending.
▶ Position yourself as close to the patient as possible. This greatly reduces spinal load.
▶ Keep feet well apart to provide a wide base of support.
▶ When performing horizontal moves, such as transferring the patient from one surface to another, do not bend the knees.
▶ For vertical moves (up or down), do bend the knees.
▶ Avoid awkward positions that reduce your base of support.
▶ Never try to lift or maneuver the patient while reaching forward away from your center of gravity. If necessary, place one knee on the stretcher to bring the patient's weight closer to your center of gravity.

▶ Use abdominal, arm, and leg muscles when lifting the patient. The abdominal muscles can support the trunk much more efficiently than the lower back muscles.

PRINCIPLES OF SAFE PATIENT TRANSPORT AND TRANSFER

Many risks are associated with patient transport and transfer. A weak, disoriented, or pediatric patient may attempt to climb out of the stretcher or crib and fall or become entangled in side rails. Catheters, tubing, and other medical devices can cause severe tissue trauma or injury to the patient if pulled out of the body. The patient can sustain **shear injury** (see the section on positioning injuries later in the chapter) when dragged across a high-friction surface such as bed linens or a draw sheet. Changes in posture can result in severe hypotension or elevated cerebral pressure. Even when transfers are slow and deliberate, accidents can occur.

Transport and transfer injuries occur more often when:

▶ There is insufficient help.
▶ Personnel assisting in the transfer or transport do not have a plan.
▶ Personnel are rushed.
▶ The patient is disoriented or combative.

The following principles apply to all types of patient transport and transfer:

▶ *Know the risks.* To keep the patient safe, one must understand exactly what the risks are and how to prevent injury.
▶ *Protect the patient's personal dignity at all times.* The patient has a right to be protected from exposure and embarrassment. Many patients fear that their personal rights, such as a right to modesty, are forfeited at admission.
▶ *Perform all patient movement deliberately and carefully.* You must have a plan before you begin. Prepare for the unexpected. Think ahead.
▶ *When a patient is transferred, one person should be in charge of the move and guide the others.* Because of the risks involved in patient movement, coordination is absolutely necessary. This requires one person to guide the action of others so that all are working together during each step.
▶ *Know your equipment.* Before moving any patient, know how to operate patient-care equipment. This prevents mechanical injury, falls, and other mishaps.
▶ *Think about what you are doing while you are doing it.* As you move the patient, maintain your focus on the task at hand. Do not allow yourself to become distracted. Think ahead and be prepared for each step of the process.
▶ *Never leave the patient alone.* Leaving the patient unattended on a stretcher or in a wheelchair constitutes abandonment (see Chapter 3) and puts the patient at high risk for injury.
▶ *Protect the patient from environmental stress.* The patient should be adequately covered with blankets. Try to avoid passing through crowded areas while transporting the patient. This is not always possible but is desirable. Use a patient elevator instead of visitor elevators during transportation.
▶ *Identify the patient properly.* Check the name and number on the wrist or ankle band, identification card, and chart.
▶ *Explain the process to the patient before and as the transfer is occurring.* This may relieve the patient's anxiety and make him or her more relaxed during the transfer.

Patient Identification

Patient identity is a critical issue in patient care. It is the responsibility of the health-care assistant to identify the patient using a standard policy. No patient should be transported and no procedure initiated until the protocol for identification has been completed, *even if the patient is known to the health-care assistant.*

All patients are identified in at least three ways. The patient wrist or ankle band is imprinted with the patient's name and hospital number, and the physician's name. Many bands are color coded to indicate allergies or other conditions. The patient identification card is used to stamp all paperwork and matches the patient's identification bracelet. This card must be firmly attached to the chart during transport and must remain with the chart until the patient returns to his or her hospital unit. The patient chart must accompany the patient whenever the patient is transported off of the unit.

The appropriate way to verify the patient's identity is to do the following:

▶ Examine the patient's identification band. Compare both the name and the number with those on the patient chart.
▶ Ask the patient to state his or her full name. Do not call the patient by name before asking the patient to state his or her name.
▶ Ask the patient to tell you what procedure he or she is undergoing and to point to the side on which the surgery will take place.

The following are examples of improper and proper ways of verifying identity:

Example
WRONG: *"Good morning Mr. X, I'm here to take you to surgery."*
CORRECT: *"Good morning, my name is —. I'm here to take you to surgery. Can you tell me your name?"*

Example
WRONG: *"So, Dr. X is planning to fix your arm today."*
CORRECT: *"What surgery will you be having today?"*

If the patient's name, hospital identification number, surgery, and surgical site do not match the chart or operative documents, you must report this to the unit charge nurse. Do not transport the patient if patient information does not match the chart. Call the operating room to let personnel know about the delay and the reason.

If the patient has no identification band, you must report this to the unit charge nurse. Under routine circumstances an identification band must be obtained before the patient leaves the unit.

ASSISTING THE AMBULATORY PATIENT

Transferring a Patient from a Bed to a Wheelchair

Transfer of a patient from bed to wheelchair is performed in distinct steps. First, help the patient to a sitting position, then to a standing position, and finally back to a sitting position in the wheelchair. Explain these steps to the patient *before* beginning the transfer. During the transfer, reinforce and prepare the patient for the next step. This increases the patient's confidence and reduces fear. Remember that weak or elderly patients often are afraid of falling. Seek help when transferring a patient who is at high risk of falling (heavy, unstable, or encumbered with medical devices).

Before beginning the transfer, familiarize yourself with the patient's equipment. Make certain that the wheelchair brakes and steering mechanism are functioning properly. Do not transport a patient in a wheelchair that has no foot supports or other safety attachments. The wheelchair must fit the patient's size and weight.

Check the patient's identification as described previously in the chapter. Free up any tubes or lines and make certain that there is enough slack between the patient and the wheelchair to prevent entanglement or restriction during the transfer. Transfer equipment first, then the patient.

ASSISTING A PATIENT FROM A LYING TO A SITTING POSITION

Whenever you are responsible for transporting the patient, always be aware of the location of the call bell in case you might need assistance or emergent help.

To assist a patient in moving from a lying to a sitting position, follow these steps:

1. Verify the identity of the patient before taking any actions. Bring the wheelchair to the side of the bed so that it is lined up with the bed. *Lock the wheels.* Ensure that the wheels on the bed also are locked, and lower the bed to its lowest position.
2. If the patient is weak on one side, place the wheelchair on the opposite side of the bed. Raise the head of the bed slowly.
3. If the patient reports dizziness or any other changes, seek nursing help before proceeding. Dizziness may be caused by rapid hypotension that results in cardiac arrhythmia or sudden loss of blood to the brain. The patient should be immediately returned to a **supine position.**
4. To assist the patient to a sitting position, support the patient under the shoulders and thighs if necessary.
5. Pull the patient's legs gently over the side of the bed to a sitting position. Allow the patient to remain in the sitting position for a few moments. Do not proceed if the patient exhibits or reports any physical or mental changes.

ASSISTING A PATIENT FROM A SITTING TO A STANDING POSITION

To assist a patient in moving from a sitting to a standing position, follow these steps:

1. Standing directly in front of the patient, place your hands around the patient's torso and under his or her arms to support the shoulder blades.
2. Slightly bend your forward leg while placing your opposite foot in a bracing position (Figure 10-1, *A*).
3. Slowly rock back and raise the patient to a standing position (Figure 10-1, *B*).

ASSISTING A PATIENT FROM A STANDING POSITION TO A WHEELCHAIR AND TRANSPORTING THE PATIENT

To assist a patient in moving from a standing position to a sitting position in a wheelchair and then to transport the patient, follow these steps:

1. One small step at a time, rotate your entire body as the patient does the same until his or her back is lined up with the wheelchair.
2. Slowly lower the patient into the wheelchair. Spread your feet so they are approximately shoulder-distance apart. Use your abdominal muscles to support your back as you lower the patient. Do not allow the patient's weight to pull your torso downward.
3. Bend your knees, use the larger thigh muscles, and *use your abdominal muscles* to support your upper body. Lower the patient when your spine and body are in alignment with the patient and wheelchair (Figure 10-2).
4. Place the patient's feet on the footrests and cover the patient with a blanket or sheet. Secure the safety strap.
5. Proceed to your destination. When entering an elevator or doorway, *pull the patient into the elevator.* Secure doorways in the open position before passing through them. Make certain you have the patient's chart before leaving the area.

Transferring a Patient from a Wheelchair to a Bed or Operating Table

Follow these guidelines when transferring a patient from a wheelchair to a bed or operating table:

1. Place the table or bed at its lowest height.
2. Reverse the steps used to transfer the patient to the wheelchair. Place the wheelchair in line with the bed and lock the wheels.
3. If the patient can put weight on his or her hands, ask the patient to push down. At the same time, lift the patient by placing your arms under his or her arms and securing your hands over the patient's shoulder blades.
4. Place your bracing foot back and rotated slightly outward.
5. As you lift the patient up, rock back on your bracing foot and, step by step, rotate your body with the patient's until he or she is positioned to sit on the edge of the table.

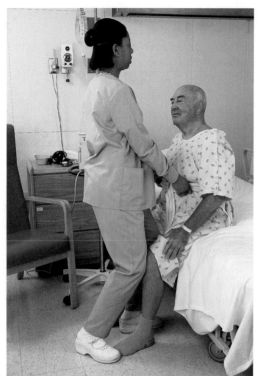 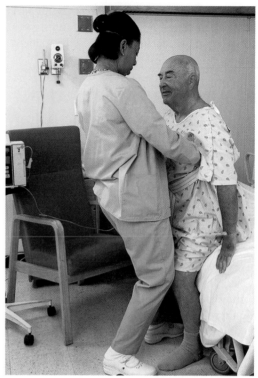

A   B

FIGURE 10-1
Lifting the patient to a standing position. (From Potter PA and Perry AG: *Basic nursing: essentials for practice,* ed 5, St Louis, 2003, Mosby.)

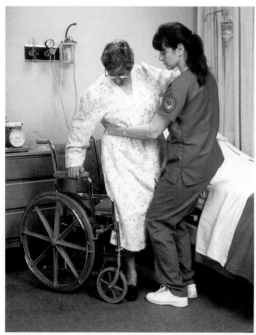

FIGURE 10-2
Lowering the patient into a wheelchair. (From Harkreader H and Hogan MA: *Fundamentals of nursing,* ed 2, St Louis, 2004, Saunders.)

6. Remember to keep your spine and the patient's back in alignment while turning. Ease the patient down to a sitting position on the operating table or bed.
7. One person should support the patient's back and head while another assists in bringing the legs to a horizontal position on the operating table or bed. A third assistant should stand at the opposite side of the operating table or bed to keep the patient from falling.
8. Ease the patient to a lying position. Place a blanket or sheet over the patient and secure the safety strap immediately.

Assisting a Falling Patient

In the ambulatory care setting, patients walk or are transported by wheelchair from the holding area to the surgical area. The surgical technologist may be responsible for assisting. During ambulation there is risk that the patient may fall. He or she may suddenly experience a drop in blood pressure or become light-headed. Always anticipate the possibility of a fall even when the patient is mobile and seems able to walk without assistance.

Patient falls can be dangerous for both the patient and the health-care worker. The weight of the falling person can cause you to lose your own balance, which can result in a twisting injury or fracture. The patient may experience a hip, arm, or knee fracture.

To assist a falling patient, follow these rules:

1. Position yourself slightly behind the patient's shoulder while helping him or her walk. This places you in a position to support the patient in the event that he or she becomes weak or falls. If the patient seems unsteady, use a wheelchair.
2. To assist the falling patient, *do not try to hold up the patient.* Instead, ease the patient to the floor while *protecting his or her head* (Figure 10-3). Spread your feet to create a

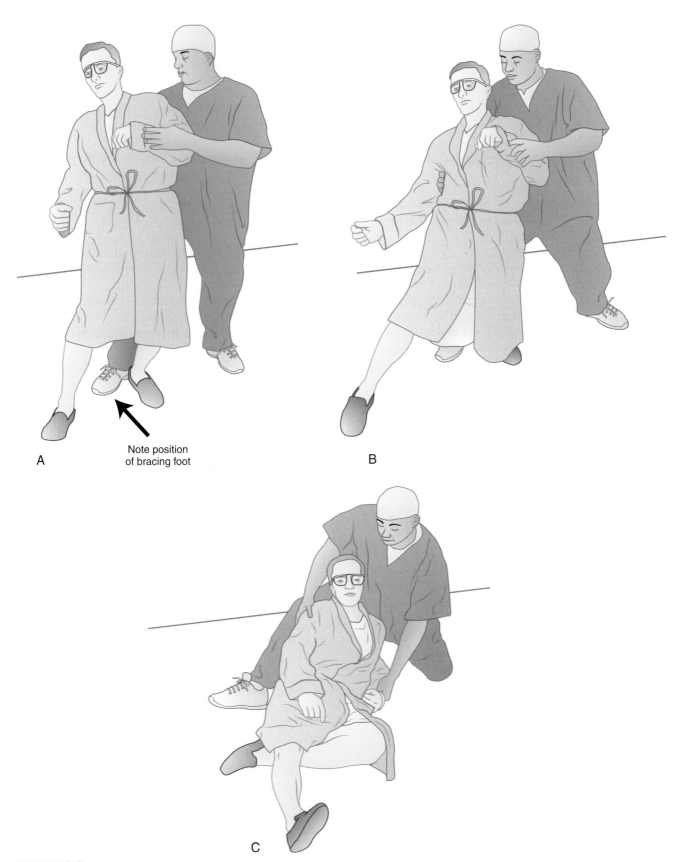

A

Note position
of bracing foot

B

C

FIGURE 10-3
A through **C,** Helping the falling patient. (Redrawn from Sorrentino SA: *Mosby's textbook for nursing assistants,* ed 5, St Louis, 2000, Mosby.)

wide base of support. Bend your knees, and use your thigh muscles for support.

3. Follow the patient's movements with your own body to prevent the patient from dropping.

4. Immediately call out for assistance while remaining with the patient.

5. Do not abandon the patient under any circumstances.

ASSISTING THE INPATIENT

Transferring a Mobile Patient from a Bed to a Stretcher

Inpatients usually are transferred to the operating room by stretcher through the following steps:

1. Before bringing the stretcher into the patient's room, notify the unit clerk that you have arrived to transport the patient to surgery. Collect the chart and any other informational items for the patient.

2. Knock on the patient's door before entering. *Do not simply enter the patient's room with the stretcher and announce that you are taking him or her to surgery.*

3. After introducing yourself, verify the patient's identity.

4. Arrange the furniture so that there is adequate space in which to place the stretcher. Patient rooms often are very small. It is easier to make a path for the stretcher *before* entering with the stretcher. At least two people are required to transfer the patient to the stretcher.

5. Lower the bed rails on the stretcher side.

6. Align the stretcher with the bed and *lock the wheels on both the bed and the stretcher.* Under no circumstances should you move a patient to an unlocked stretcher. Align the bed to the height of the stretcher.

7. *Identify and free up all tubing, drainage bags, or other objects* that can restrain the patient or pull out during the transfer. Drainage bags must remain lower than the patient's body at all times, and intravenous (IV) lines should be higher than the patient's body.

8. Guide the patient slowly across the bed to the stretcher.

9. Proceed from step number 3 in the following section, Moving a Conscious Patient with Limited Mobility.

Moving a Conscious Patient with Limited Mobility

In moving a patient with limited mobility, one manually transfers the patient to the stretcher (Figure 10-4, *A*) using a draw sheet, which is a folded bed sheet or thick torso pad placed under the patient.

This move requires the participation of at least three people. If the patient is unable to support his or her head, one person must guide the head and neck together, making sure that the cervical spine is in neutral position during the move, while two people assist from each side of the patient.

To move a patient with limited mobility, one uses the following procedure:

1. Lower the bed rails on the stretcher side.

2. Align the stretcher with the bed and *lock the wheels.* Under no circumstances should a patient be moved to an unlocked stretcher. Align the bed to the height of the stretcher (Figure 10-4, *B*).

3. Make sure that all tubing and medical devices have been freed.

4. Transfer medical equipment and devices first, and then transfer the patient.

5. Roll the sides of the draw sheet toward the patient and grasp it firmly with both hands (Figure 10-4, *C*).

6. On the count of three, all assistants move the patient horizontally to the stretcher.

7. Cover the patient and raise the side rails.

8. Place a pillow under the patient's head unless directed otherwise. Some patients must be transported flat.

9. Apply the safety strap midway between the knees and hip on top of the blanket or sheet. Allow two fingers' breadth between the strap and the patient. *Do not* place the safety strap over the patient's bare skin.

10. If the patient is cooperative, have the patient place his or her hands over the abdomen, with elbows away from the side rails. The patient's feet must not protrude over the edge of the stretcher.

11. Notify the unit nurse that you are leaving the unit. The patient's chart must stay with the patient at all times.

12. Proceed directly to your destination. If the patient is going to the operating room holding area, wait for the attending nurse to accept the patient before you leave. Do not leave the patient unattended at any time.

Transporting a Patient by Stretcher

Use the following guidelines when transporting a patient by stretcher:

1. When transporting the patient by stretcher, stand at the patient's head and push the stretcher forward. Look ahead as you move. Try to anticipate obstructions, sudden hallway traffic, and corners.

2. When rounding blind corners, be careful of oncoming traffic. Check first before proceeding. Stopping a rolling stretcher is difficult, especially when the patient is heavy and medical devices are attached to the frame. If two people are available for transport, one pushes from the head of the stretcher and the other guides the stretcher from the foot.

3. Make sure to tell the conscious patient to keep hands and arms within the stretcher rails. Patients often try to "help" during transport, which exposes them to the risk of injury.

Anticipation prevents accidents. Stretcher rails do not protect the patient from injury. The patient can easily bruise or even fracture an elbow, fingers, or wrist on walls or doorways. The transporter is responsible for protecting the patient from these injuries. Maintain watch on the patient and remind him or her to keep hands and arms well within the boundaries of the side rails.

Ramps, doors, and elevators present various obstacles when one is transporting a patient on a stretcher. Rules es-

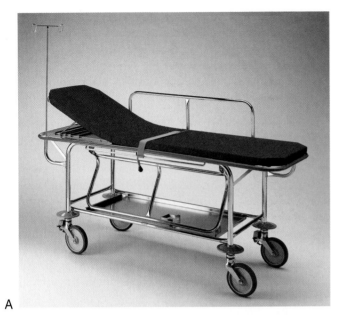

A

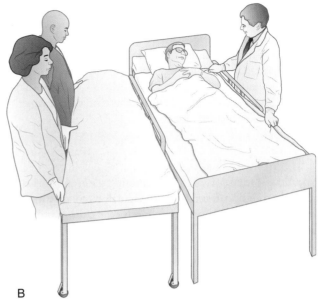

B

C

FIGURE 10-4
A, A standard stretcher. **B,** Aligning the bed with the stretcher. **C,** Moving the patient with a draw sheet. (**A** courtesy of Pedigo Products, Vancouver, WA; **B** and **C** redrawn from Sorrentino SA: *Mosby's textbook for nursing assistants,* ed 5, St Louis, 2000, Mosby.)

tablish the procedure for handling each of these obstacles. If possible, raise the head of the stretcher so the patient can see where he or she is going. Always warn the patient of bumps or other unfamiliar movements that will be encountered, such as entering or exiting an elevator.

RAMPS
When rolling the stretcher down a ramp, do not rely on your strength to hold the stretcher against gravity. *Ask for assistance.* One person should stabilize the foot of the stretcher while the second is at the head. Traveling up the ramp also requires two people: one to push, the other to pull.

DOORS
Remember the following when transporting a patient through doors:

1. When passing through manually operated doors, *open the doors first and secure them open.* Do not push the foot of the stretcher forward against the closed doors, which would allow the doors to slam against the stretcher and drag. This is unacceptable patient care.

2. Stand at the head of the patient and push the patient through the open doors or pull the patient through from the head of the stretcher.

ELEVATORS
When transporting a patient on an elevator:

1. Use the patient elevator. Do not transport the patient in an elevator full of visitors.
2. When the elevator doors open, lock the doors open.
3. Standing at the patient's head, *pull the stretcher headfirst* into the elevator.
4. Do not unlock the doors until you are certain that the foot of the stretcher has cleared the threshold.
5. Locate the emergency alarm and know how to use it.

Dealing with an Emergency During Transport
The patient may suffer sudden hypotension, cardiac arrest, seizure, or another emergency during transport. The effects of moving the patient from bed to stretcher can cause vascular or fluid shifts that may not manifest symptoms immediately.

If an emergency occurs during transport:

▶ Maintain verbal contact with the patient. If he or she reports dizziness or lightheadedness, or if you suspect a problem, call for help immediately.
▶ If you are in the corridor, shout for help.
▶ If you are in an elevator, activate the emergency alarm system, which is clearly marked.

Transferring a Conscious Patient from a Stretcher to an Operating Table

The patient is transported to the operating room shortly before the start of the procedure. The circulator and anesthesia care provider should be present to receive the patient and assist in the transfer to the operating table. At least two and preferably three people should be present during the transfer of a mobile and alert patient. As the stretcher is lined up next to the operating table, one person must stand on the opposite side so that the patient does not move too far and fall. The second person stands alongside the stretcher to brace it against the operating table. If a third person is available, he or she should stand at the head of the table. Make certain that the brakes on the stretcher and the operating table are locked before beginning any transfer.

To transfer a conscious patient from a stretcher to an operating table:

1. Align the head of the stretcher with the head of the operating table. Lock the wheels of the stretcher and the operating room table.
2. Free up any IV line, urinary catheter, or other device. Transfer medical equipment and devices first, and then transfer the patient.
3. Ask the patient to slide slowly onto the operating table while taking the top sheet with him or her.
4. Open the back of the patient's gown.
5. Center the patient on the table and apply the safety strap immediately. Apply the safety strap midway between the knee and hip on top of the blanket or sheet. Allow two fingers' breadth between the strap and the patient. Do not place the safety strap directly over the patient's bare skin. The patient should always be secured on the operating table except during transfer.

Transferring an Immobile or Unconscious Patient from a Stretcher to an Operating Table

Transferring a patient who is unable to control movement to an operating table requires four to six people. Additional personnel are required if the patient is morbidly obese or requires turning from **prone** to supine position, or if there are other restrictions such as spinal injury or special orthopedic considerations. Teamwork is absolutely essential.

Several methods are available for manually transferring an unconscious patient from the stretcher to an operating table. A **transfer board,** which is a roller board or Plexiglas,

usually is used. The patient is transferred to the board, which is then pulled from one bed to the other. The board has a surface that slides easily across the operating table or stretcher. In addition to preventing shear injury, it reduces the vertical exertion required to move the patient.

To use a transfer board:

1. Align the stretcher with the operating table and make sure the wheels are locked on both the stretcher and the operating room table. Never move a patient onto an operating table with wheels that do not lock! The patient may fall to the floor between the stretcher and the table if the wheels are not locked.
2. Before beginning the move, always tell the patient what you are going to do. Begin by freeing up all tubing and monitoring leads to allow slack during the move. To free up tubing and leads, follow the attachment at the patient's body to the source, making sure that nothing is pinched or tangled.
3. Transfer drainage tubes, IV bags, and other attached medical equipment items first and then move the patient.
4. One assistant, usually the anesthesia care provider, guides and directs the move. He or she remains at the patient's head to protect the airway and prevent cervical injury.
5. Another person should assist with the feet while two others assist at each side of the patient.
6. To use a transfer board, one must **log roll** the patient (Figure 10-5, *A*). Two to three people stand at the patient's side and grasp the opposite edge of the bed sheet or draw sheet.
7. The edge of the draw sheet is pulled toward the assistants to log-roll the patient into a position on his or her side with the front of his or her body facing the assistants.
8. The anesthesia care provider protects the patient's neck and airway. The transfer board is placed to the back side of the patient, and those supporting the patient gently ease him or her back into supine position on the board.
9. By grasping the board and pulling it across the stretcher, personnel can easily transfer the patient to the table (Figure 10-5, *B*).
10. Make sure the patient, IV lines, and drainage bags are all secured before unlocking the stretcher wheels for removal of the stretcher from the room.

Whether the patient is conscious or unconscious, the same precautions are used when moving the patient from the operating room table to the stretcher after surgery.

Transporting Children

Children are transported to the operating room by wagon, stretcher, crib, or bassinet. All safety and procedural considerations apply to children as well as to adults. Young children are capable of climbing out of cribs with amazing speed and dexterity. The crib must always be equipped with a Plexiglas cover

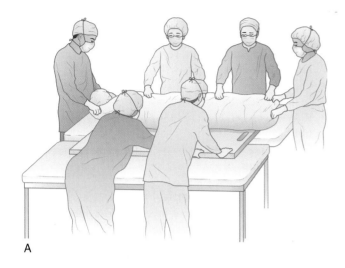

A

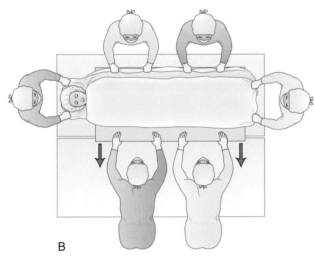

B

FIGURE 10-5
A, Log rolling the patient on the operating table. **B,** Transferring the patient with a transfer board.

during transportation. However, this may not prevent a small toddler from climbing between the top rail of the side bars and the crib cover. *Never leave a child unattended or unobserved.*

Remember the following when transporting a child:

▶ Caregivers may accompany the child to the holding area, and in many hospitals, a parent or other caregiver is permitted to stay in the operating suite during anesthesia induction.

▶ Most young children, especially toddlers and preschoolers, suffer extreme anxiety when separated from their caregivers. Converse with the child during transport and explain what the child sees and hears in simple, nonthreatening terms. Children from ages 5 to 9 years are curious about their environment. Preteens want to take part in their care. Teenagers are likely to show stoicism but appreciate explanations of the environment.

▶ Always allow caregivers to soothe the child during transport. As you converse with the child, remember that children understand the meanings of words in their most literal sense.

▶ Do not treat the child like a small adult. *Provide a calm, supportive presence, showing respect for the child at all times.* Children are quick to understand when they are being falsely reassured.

▶ Refrain from saying, "Oh, don't be afraid; this won't take long." A child who *is* afraid will not be reassured by being told to calm down. A more comforting approach would be to evaluate the child's understanding of what is happening and to clarify his or her perception in simple, concrete terms. Remember that many children view surgery as a punishment, and their fear of mutilation is enormous.

▶ The developmental age of the child is critical to communication. The trip between the safety of the hospital room or holding area and the operating room can either cause great distress or provide a means for the child to integrate the experience of surgery into the hospital stay. A child who arrives in the surgical suite in a state of dread and terror is often more difficult to treat and to anesthetize. Your calming presence during transport can make an enormous difference.

POSITIONING THE SURGICAL PATIENT

Patients are placed in specific surgical positions for many reasons:

▶ To reduce adverse physiological effects and mechanical injury to an irreducible minimum.
▶ To allow optimal access to the operative site.
▶ To permit optimal access for the anesthesia care provider. This includes venous, arterial, and respiratory access, and access to monitoring sites.

Use of a specific surgical position gives the surgeon unobstructed access to the operative site. The needs for physiological stability, protection from injury, and access to the surgical site all affect positioning decisions.

The following elements are important in safe positioning of patients:

▶ *Knowledge of anatomy, physiology, and the individual patient's specific medical condition.* Positioning is not a regimented routine. Each patient is unique and has specific considerations such as age, joint mobility, and disease. Because of the high risk of serious and permanent injury, the surgical team must be guided and directed in the positioning process. The anesthesia care provider, surgeon, and circulator draw this direction from their knowledge of the patient's status.

▶ *Planning.* Planning promotes an organized and efficient effort by everyone involved. All necessary equipment must be assembled ahead of time. Padding, pillows, positioning devices, table accessories, and transfer devices must be on hand before positioning begins. Adequate personnel must be available to complete the task safely.

▶ *Teamwork.* Teamwork is needed to create smooth, step-by-step coordination. Coordinated activities are those that complement each other.

The surgical technologist has specific responsibilities when positioning the patient. He or she must:

▶ Become knowledgeable about normal *range of motion*
▶ Understand common positions and the surgeries for which these positions are used
▶ Know ahead of time the position that will be used for each assigned surgical procedure

▶ Be familiar with adverse events that can occur during positioning
▶ Practice measures for preventing accident or injury during positioning
▶ Question any aspect of the patient's position that appears to have risk potential
▶ Remain alert and focused on patient safety during positioning
▶ Communicate clearly with the entire team as the process is proceeding

General Operating Table

The general operating table is used for most operative procedures (Figure 10-6, *A*). It can be configured into many po-

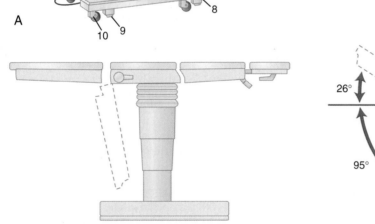

A

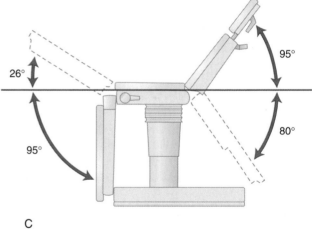

C

FIGURE 10-6
A, Operating table: (1) Removable head section. (2) OR table pad (mattress). (3) Kidney elevator. (4) Perineal cut-out. (5) Radiolucent top and removable head section. (6) Hand control unit. (7) Hydraulic lift cylinder. (8) Table base. (9) Floor locks. (10) Locking swivel casters. (11) Side rail locking system. **B** through **E,** Positions of the operating table. (Modified from Martin JT and Warner MA: *Positioning in anesthesia and surgery,* ed 3, Philadelphia, 1997, Saunders.)

B

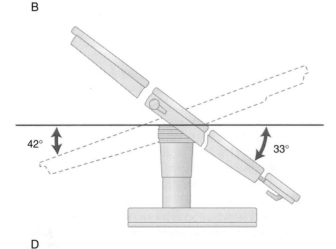

D

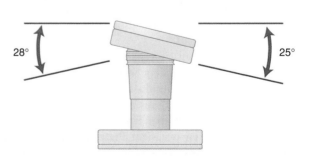

E

sitions and accommodates accessories for different types of surgery (Figure 10-6, *B* through *E*). The frame is stainless steel and attaches to a hydraulic lift. Weight restrictions for operating tables vary. Extremely large or heavy patients require a table that is specifically designed to safely accommodate excess weight and girth.

TABLE FEATURES

Table pads are covered with thick synthetic material and protect the patient from the hard metal surface of the operating room table. Pads are removable for cleaning. The top of the table can be rotated, flexed, or disassembled. The handheld *remote control* unit allows the anesthesia care provider to change the position of the table at any time. The *headboard* and *footboard* can be flexed or removed. The *base* is centered on the frame or may be offset to accommodate X-ray and C-arm fluoroscopy equipment. The *kidney rest* can be elevated to raise the flank and offer wide exposure. A *perineal cutout* allows unrestricted access when the patient is in the **lithotomy position.**

TABLE ATTACHMENTS

The standard *arm board* is used when the patient's arms are outstretched (Figure 10-7, *A*). At least one arm is abducted during surgery to create access to IV and monitoring sites. The arm is secured by means of a padded strap, semirigid brace, or rigid cradle.

The *toboggan* (Figure 10-7, *B*) (also called a *sled*) is a stainless steel or Plexiglas attachment that slides under the patient and holds the arm at his or her side.

Shoulder braces (Figure 10-8) are fixed to the head of the table to prevent the patient from sliding downward when he or she is in a **Trendelenburg position.**

Stirrups are used to elevate and abduct the legs for access to the perineal area. The type of stirrups used depends on the procedure, the surgeon's preference, and the patient's tolerance for the position (see Lithotomy Position). Figure 10-9 illustrates three types of low lithotomy stirrups used for endoscopic, gynecological, genitourinary, and obstetric procedures.

The *headrest* is attached to the operating table and stabilizes the head and neck during craniotomy or when the patient is in **Fowler** or **sitting position.** The horseshoe rest is a padded, U-shaped attachment that supports the forehead in the prone position. Other attachments such as the Gardner and Mayfield headrests penetrate the skull with sterile pins and hold the head in precise position (see Prone Position).

Braces or *padded frames* are used when the patient is in the prone position to create access to the spine and back. Several types of patient braces have been designed to overcome the many risks of prone positioning. Most frames have two raised lateral pieces attached to a base that rests on the operating table. Other styles have lateral crosspieces that extend at right angles to the long axis of the body. All frame styles must be checked carefully to ensure that they *fit the patient* and that areas intended to be protected are not, in fact, experiencing impingement on nerves and blood vessels.

The *footboard* attaches at a right angle to the foot of the operating table. It prevents the patient from sliding downward when the table is tilted into a foot-down (reverse Trendelenburg) position.

Padding is used to distribute the weight of the body, especially where vulnerable areas contact the operating table or table pad. Gel, foam, and deflatable "beanbag" pads are avail-

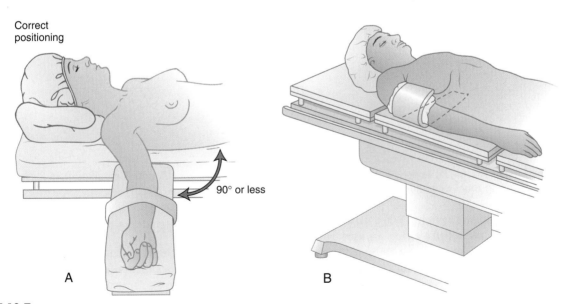

Correct positioning

90° or less

A

B

FIGURE 10-7
A, Armboard. **B,** Toboggan arm holder. (**A** redrawn from Phillips N: *Berry & Kohn's operating room technique,* ed 10, St Louis, 2004, Mosby; **B** redrawn from Martin JT and Warner MA: *Positioning in anesthesia and surgery,* ed 3, Philadelphia, 1997, Saunders.)

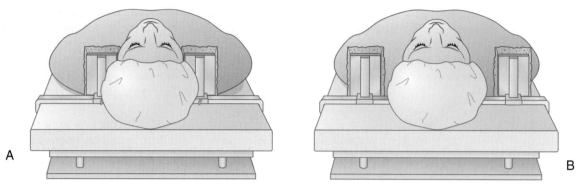

FIGURE 10-8
A and **B,** Shoulder braces. (Redrawn from Martin JT and Warner MA: *Positioning in anesthesia and surgery*, ed 3, Philadelphia, 1997, Saunders.)

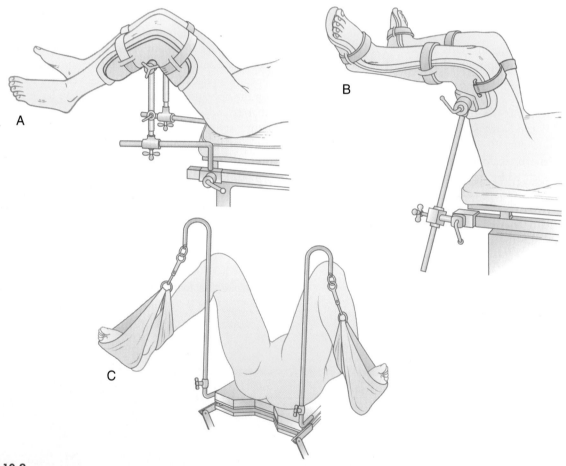

FIGURE 10-9
Stirrups. **A,** Knee-crutch stirrups. **B,** Boat-type stirrups. **C,** Candy cane or sling stirrups. (**A** and **B** modified from Phillips N: *Berry & Kohn's operating room technique*, ed 10, St Louis, 2004, Mosby.)

able to conform to the patient's anatomy. When these are not available, pillows, towels, and rolled blankets are used. However, the rough surfaces of linen pads can cause patient injury. In an older person who has little collagen in the skin, indentations can lead to skin breakdown and sloughing. Improperly placed padding causes skin and deep-tissue injury and creates pressure in areas that are subject to compression injury. Remember that the purpose of padding is *weight distribution, not just cushioning.*

PATIENT INJURIES AND POSITIONING
Principles of Safe Positioning
Research demonstrates that positioning injuries are a result of pressure on neurovascular structures. These injuries are related to the failure of a mechanical accessory, inattention to detail, haste in meeting the demands of a full (or unreasonable) schedule, and lack of adequate help. A shortage of personnel must never be allowed to interfere with patient safety.

Injury awareness is the first step in prevention. When workers participate in patient positioning, it is not just desirable but *necessary* that they have specific knowledge of anatomy, range of motion, risks of pulmonary compromise, and effects of intravascular fluid shifts. Positioning is not a "cookbook" process. Although each position requires the body to assume a certain posture, the positioning team must have specific information about the patient's *individual needs and medical condition.* This information requires medical and nursing assessment skills and is provided by the anesthesia care provider, surgeon, and circulator.

The following guidelines apply to all positioning:

▶ All equipment needed for positioning must be assembled and prepared for use before the patient is brought into the room.

▶ Adequate personnel must be available to assist before positioning begins. *Do not risk the patient's safety because of a crowded surgical schedule.*

▶ Before positioning begins, all team members should be familiar with the position, and each person must understand his or her role in positioning.

▶ The patient should not be moved except on the instruction of the person directing the move. Everyone must be aware of the motion direction, movement process, and resting point of the body. Positioning is a collaborative task. Although everyone involved is responsible for the patient's safety, one person—usually the surgeon, anesthesia care provider, or circulator—guides and directs the others. This ensures that movements are coordinated and reduces injury to both the patient and team members. The anesthesia care provider must give permission before any change in a patient's position.

▶ Do not attempt to move or position a patient without adequate help.

▶ Always check equipment before using it. Tighten the locking devices of all weight-bearing accessories.

▶ Make sure the table is locked securely in position and do not assume that any accessory equipment is in working order.

▶ Move slowly when positioning the patient.

▶ Never move any part of the body against resistance.

▶ Always move the body within its normal structural range. This requires knowledge of joint types and normal anatomical range of motion.

▶ When positioning an unconscious, sedated, or weak patient, make certain that you have complete control of the part you are moving before you start.

▶ Before moving the patient, make sure that all tubing, leads, and other medical devices are untangled. Move devices first, then the patient.

▶ Begin positioning only after the anesthesia care provider reports that it is safe.

Nerve and Blood Vessel Injury

Nerves are injured when they lose their blood supply or are stretched or compressed. During general anesthesia, central nervous system depressants and muscle relaxants are administered, and muscles lose their normal tone. This allows the joints to assume exaggerated positions that the patient normally would not be able to tolerate. **Hyperextension** (greater than normal extension) and **hyperflexion** (greater than normal flexion) can result in nerve injury called **traction** (or stretching) **injury.** Continuous pressure on the nerve or its blood supply can cause tissue **necrosis** (tissue death). A damaged nerve is unable to conduct impulses to the brain, which results in loss of sensation (feeling) or motor function.

Vascular injury and tissue death can develop within 2 hours when there is continual weight over an unpadded area. Compression of vessels restricts blood supply to the tissue, which is called **ischemia.** Loss of oxygen to the tissue causes necrosis. Pressure injuries may not be readily apparent because underlying tissues such as muscle and fascia are more susceptible to damage than skin (Box 10-1). Ischemia is *time and weight related.* To prevent ischemia and necrosis, all bony prominences and dependent areas (areas of the body under gravitational force) must be adequately padded and the weight distributed over a large area. Large blood vessels and nerves of the upper and lower limbs are illustrated in Figure 10-10.

LOCATIONS OF COMMON NERVE AND VESSEL INJURIES

Nerve and vessel injuries often occur at the following locations:

▶ The ulnar nerve where it passes through the condylar groove of the elbow (Figure 10-11). Here the nerve is cov-

---

Box 10-1   Classification of Pressure Damage and Stages of Pressure Ulcers

The National Pressure Ulcer Advisory Panel has developed a ranking system for evaluating the extent of damage caused by pressure. Pressure damage is a risk for the surgical patient as well as for the bedbound, debilitated, and elderly patient.

Stage I—Nonblanchable erythema of intact skin, the heralding lesion of skin ulceration. NOTE: Reactive hyperemia normally can be expected to be present for one-half to three-fourths as long as the time that pressure occluded blood flow to the area.

Stage II—Partial-thickness skin loss involving epidermis and/or dermis. A superficial ulcer evolves and develops clinically as an abrasion, a blister, or a shallow crater.

Stage III—Full-thickness skin loss involving damage to or necrosis of subcutaneous tissue that may extend down to, but not through, underlying fascia. The ulcer presents clinically as a deep crater with or without undermining of adjacent tissue.

Stage IV—Full-thickness skin loss with extensive destruction, tissue necrosis, or damage to muscle, bone, or supporting structures (e.g., the tendon of a joint capsule). NOTE: Undermining and sinus tracts also may be associated with stage IV pressure ulcers.

From Martin JT, Warner MA: *Positioning in anesthesia and surgery,* ed 3, Philadelphia, 1997, WB Saunders.

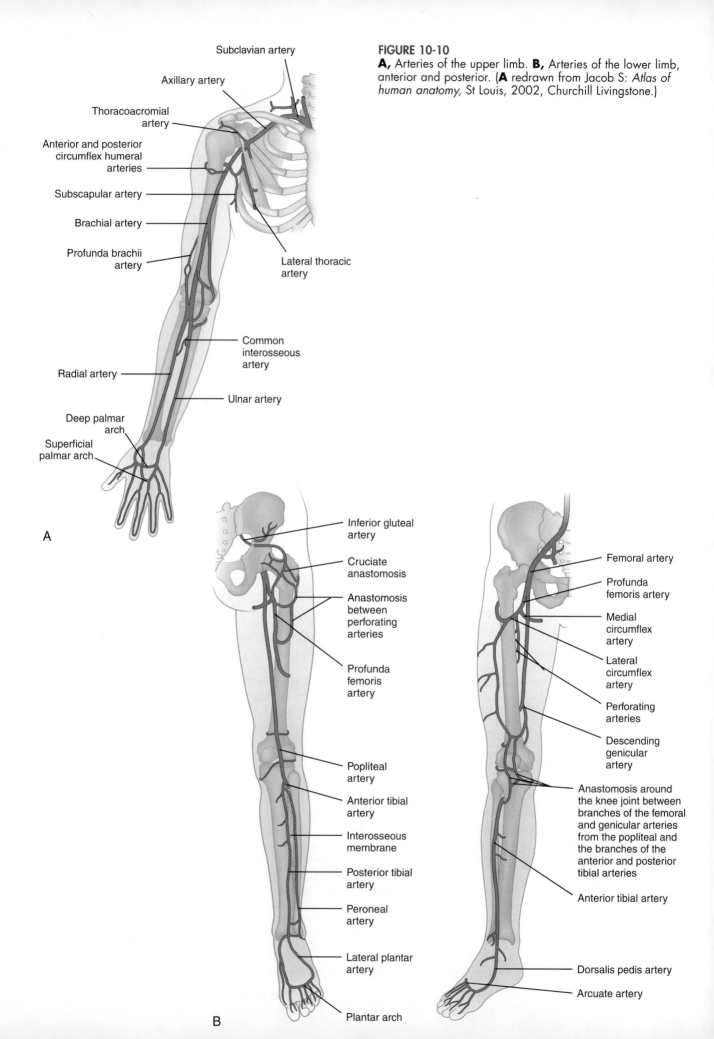

Subclavian artery

Axillary artery

Thoracoacromial artery

Anterior and posterior circumflex humeral arteries

Subscapular artery

Brachial artery

Profunda brachii artery

Lateral thoracic artery

Common interosseous artery

Radial artery

Ulnar artery

Deep palmar arch

Superficial palmar arch

A

FIGURE 10-10
A, Arteries of the upper limb. **B,** Arteries of the lower limb, anterior and posterior. (**A** redrawn from Jacob S: *Atlas of human anatomy,* St Louis, 2002, Churchill Livingstone.)

Inferior gluteal artery

Cruciate anastomosis

Anastomosis between perforating arteries

Profunda femoris artery

Popliteal artery

Anterior tibial artery

Interosseous membrane

Posterior tibial artery

Peroneal artery

Lateral plantar artery

Plantar arch

B

Femoral artery

Profunda femoris artery

Medial circumflex artery

Lateral circumflex artery

Perforating arteries

Descending genicular artery

Anastomosis around the knee joint between branches of the femoral and genicular arteries from the popliteal and the branches of the anterior and posterior tibial arteries

Anterior tibial artery

Dorsalis pedis artery

Arcuate artery

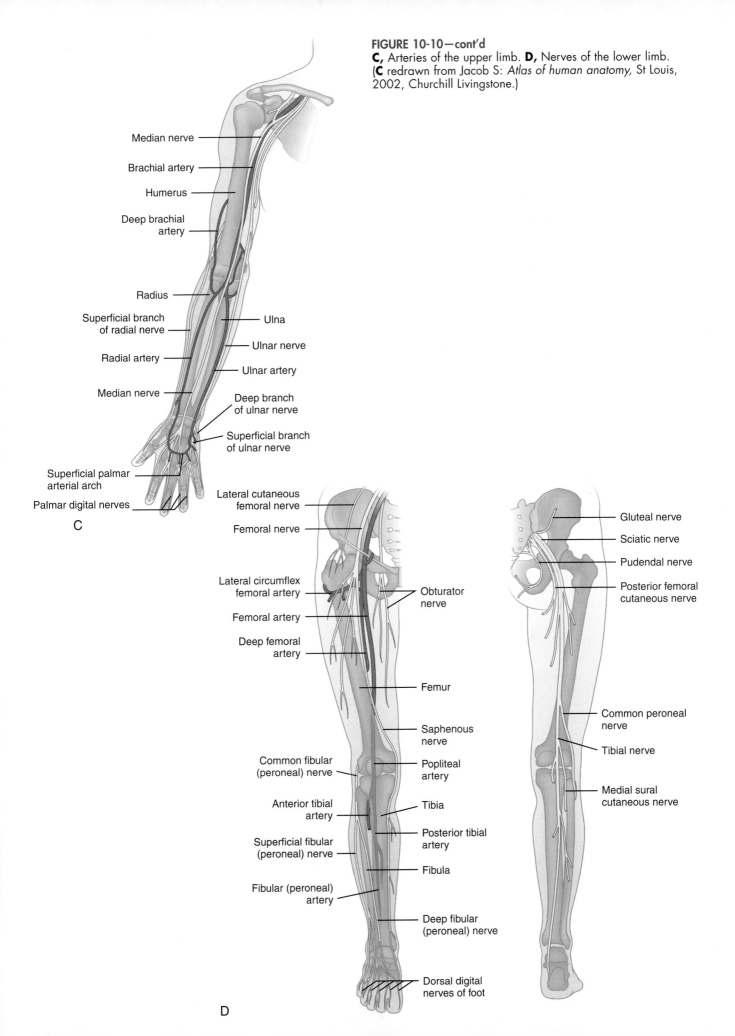

FIGURE 10-10—cont'd
C, Arteries of the upper limb. **D,** Nerves of the lower limb.
(**C** redrawn from Jacob S: *Atlas of human anatomy,* St Louis, 2002, Churchill Livingstone.)

Median nerve

Brachial artery

Humerus

Deep brachial artery

Radius

Superficial branch of radial nerve

Radial artery

Median nerve

Superficial palmar arterial arch

Palmar digital nerves

Ulna

Ulnar nerve

Ulnar artery

Deep branch of ulnar nerve

Superficial branch of ulnar nerve

C

Lateral cutaneous femoral nerve

Femoral nerve

Lateral circumflex femoral artery

Femoral artery

Deep femoral artery

Obturator nerve

Femur

Saphenous nerve

Popliteal artery

Tibia

Posterior tibial artery

Fibula

Deep fibular (peroneal) nerve

Common fibular (peroneal) nerve

Anterior tibial artery

Superficial fibular (peroneal) nerve

Fibular (peroneal) artery

Dorsal digital nerves of foot

Gluteal nerve

Sciatic nerve

Pudendal nerve

Posterior femoral cutaneous nerve

Common peroneal nerve

Tibial nerve

Medial sural cutaneous nerve

D

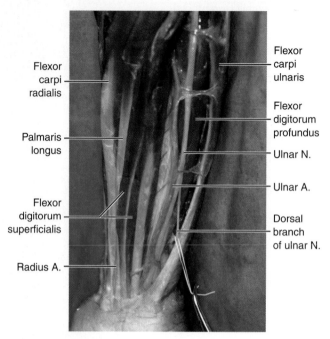

Flexor carpi radialis

Palmaris longus

Flexor digitorum superficialis

Radius A.

Flexor carpi ulnaris

Flexor digitorum profundus

Ulnar N.

Ulnar A.

Dorsal branch of ulnar N.

FIGURE 10-11
Ulnar nerve. (From Kline DG, Hudson AR, and Kim DH: *Atlas of peripheral nerve surgery,* St Louis, 2001, Saunders.)

ered only by skin and subcutaneous fat and is subject to compression (pressure) injury when the elbow is tightly flexed or when there is direct pressure from the edge of the operating table.

▶ The ulnar nerve where it passes through the condylar groove and then at the cubital tunnel. Injury in this area is the second most common cause of postoperative **neuropathy** (temporary or permanent nerve injury).

▶ The common peroneal and tibial nerve and vessels where they pass through the popliteal fossa at the back of the knee.

▶ The brachial plexus, which is a complex anatomical area where the branches of nerve roots from C5 to T1 or T2 merge. The plexus becomes the brachial nerve (Figure 10-12), which then becomes the median nerve and the subscapular, axillary, thoracodorsal, and radial nerves. The brachial plexus is subject to injury because the nerves and blood vessels lie close to bony structures and are subject to direct compression. Injury in this area can be caused by shoulder braces, arm boards, and wrist supports.

▶ Lumbosacral nerve roots at the base of the spine.

PREVENTION OF COMPRESSION INJURY
To prevent compression injury, follow these guidelines:

▶ Padding can distribute weight over a larger surface area, or it can impinge on a vulnerable space. Make sure that in

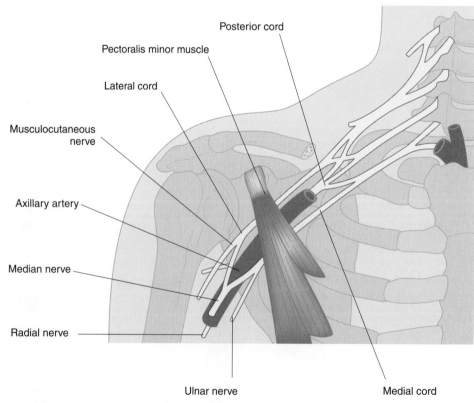

Posterior cord

Pectoralis minor muscle

Lateral cord

Musculocutaneous nerve

Axillary artery

Median nerve

Radial nerve

Ulnar nerve

Medial cord

FIGURE 10-12
Brachial plexus. (From Jacob S: *Atlas of human anatomy,* St Louis, 2002, Churchill Livingstone.)

preventing one type of injury you do not cause another. Rolled blankets must be used with caution because uneven folds in the outer covering may cause skin or compression injury, especially in older or debilitated patients. Axillary rolls must never be placed in the axilla, as this increases pressure on the axillary nerve and vessels. The axillary roll actually is positioned slightly inferior to the axilla when the patient is in the **lateral position.**

▶ All linens and padding must be smooth. Wrinkles can deform the skin and cause skin breakdown.

▶ Extreme joint flexion or extension should be avoided. This can cause tension injury to nerves and injury to the joint itself.

▶ Arm **abduction** must be limited to less than 90 degrees *or less than the angle the patient can tolerate awake.* Avoid using shoulder braces when the patient is in steep Trendelenburg position (head down).

▶ If shoulder braces *must* be used, they should be liberally padded and positioned at the *acromion* rather than at the base of the neck or clavicle. Pressure close to the cervical spine can damage peripheral nerves and muscle. When the braces are placed wide apart, pressure over the shoulders can cause enough compression to force the clavicle into the first rib and damage the subclavicular vessels and brachial nerve plexus (Figure 10-13, *A*).

▶ Wrist restraints are not used when the patient is in Trendelenburg position.

▶ The cervical spine and head are kept in neutral position at all times (Figure 10-13, *B*).

Shear Injury and Pressure Ulcers

Shear injury is associated with pressure injury. It occurs when two parallel tissue planes are forced in opposite directions. The most common cause of shear injury is sliding the

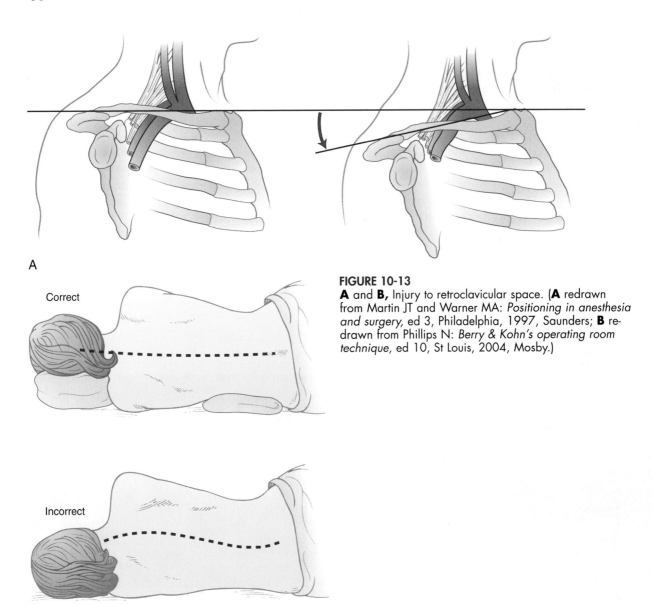

A

Correct

Incorrect

B

FIGURE 10-13
A and **B,** Injury to retroclavicular space. (**A** redrawn from Martin JT and Warner MA: *Positioning in anesthesia and surgery,* ed 3, Philadelphia, 1997, Saunders; **B** redrawn from Phillips N: *Berry & Kohn's operating room technique,* ed 10, St Louis, 2004, Mosby.)

patient across a high-friction surface. Shearing also is associated with particular positions, including the Trendelenburg and **reverse Trendelenburg** positions.

Shearing causes blood clots and tissue death. Tissue damage that begins as a shearing injury can easily progress to a pressure ulcer. Pressure (decubitus) ulcers occur in dependent areas of the body. The skin and underlying tissues slough as a result of compression and loss of blood supply. Any pressure on the ulcer causes continued breakdown until the bone is exposed (Figure 10-14). Exposed tissues become infected and can be very resistant to healing. In extreme cases, skin grafts are required to close the defect. Pressure ulcers are classified by stage and progress rapidly from mild to severe.

Continuous compression or extreme flexion can result in vessel compression and severe swelling below the area of compression. This is called *compartment syndrome.* In this situation blood cannot return to the heart but pools in the extremity. As the surrounding tissues become more and more swollen, there is a risk of complete loss of blood supply to the whole limb and even distant organs. Treatment of compartment syndrome requires an emergency procedure called a fasciotomy to relieve the pressure on deep tissues. In fasciotomy, deep incisions are made in the long axis of the limb to open the tissues and relieve pressure.

Skeletal Injury

Skeletal injury occurs when the joint is manipulated out of a neutral position or is stressed beyond a tolerable load. Sudden dislocation can occur when the limb of a sedated or anesthetized patient is allowed to drop over the table edge. This can happen when positioning is hurried or there are too few workers to maintain safety during positioning. Skeletal

injury also can occur when the patient is not restrained properly. *Do not position the patient unless adequate help is available.*

Safe joint manipulation requires knowledge of the joint capacity, including its type and range of motion, and specific knowledge of the patient's condition. To avoid exceeding normal ranges of motion, one must know what those ranges are. Avoid skeletal injury by referring to the range-of-motion illustrations shown in Figure 10-15. Remember that the unconscious body can be manipulated into positions that would not be tolerable to a conscious patient, and this must be avoided.

Determine whether the patient has any skeletal conditions such as a previous injury, joint implants, or arthritic disease. Remember that *every patient is unique.*

NORMAL RANGE OF MOTION

The joints of the human body allow a specific type of movement or range of motion. For example, the elbow joint is hinged—it can move freely in only one direction. Its movement is described by the angle created by the upper and lower arm. The movement of this joint is called extension or flexion. As the elbow is bent closer to the body, the angle becomes smaller. This is called *flexion.* As the arm straightens, the angle becomes wider or larger. This is termed *extension.* Some joints, such as the ball-and-socket joint in the hip, allow rotation of a body part inward and outward. Such inward and outward rotation is called *internal* and *external rotation.*

In the positioning of the patient, it is critical not to exceed the normal limits of any joint. Some patients are unable to tolerate even normal limits without severe pain or injury. During positioning, you must understand the language of

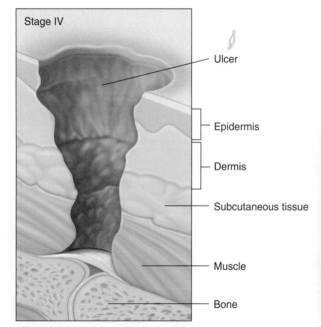

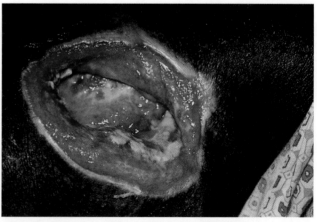

FIGURE 10-14
Pressure ulcers. (From Harkreader H and Hogan MA: *Fundamentals of nursing,* ed 2, St Louis, 2004, Saunders.)

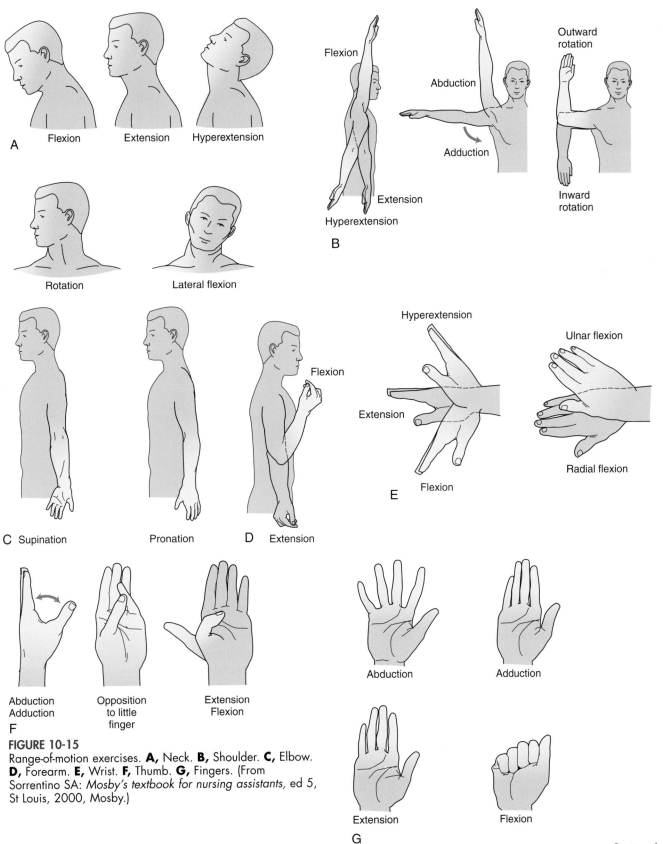

FIGURE 10-15
Range-of-motion exercises. **A,** Neck. **B,** Shoulder. **C,** Elbow.
D, Forearm. **E,** Wrist. **F,** Thumb. **G,** Fingers. (From
Sorrentino SA: *Mosby's textbook for nursing assistants,* ed 5,
St Louis, 2000, Mosby.)

Continued

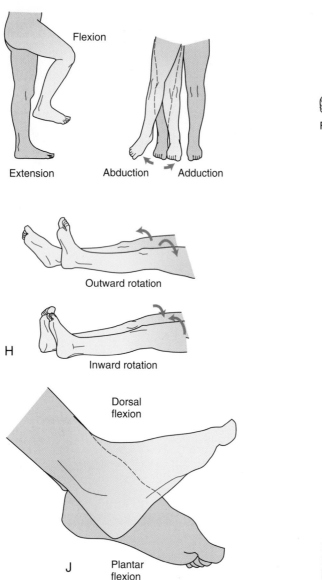

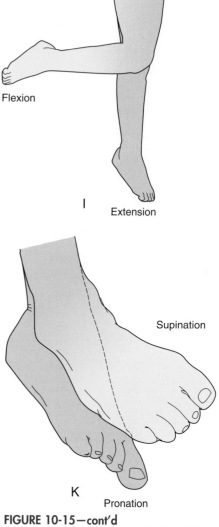

FIGURE 10-15—cont'd
Range-of-motion exercises. **H,** Hip. **I,** Knee. **J,** Ankle. **K,** Foot. (From Sorrentino SA: *Mosby's textbook for nursing assistants,* ed 5, St Louis, 2000, Mosby.)

body movement. If you are asked to "pronate the hand" or "abduct the leg," you must understand what this means to avoid injuring the patient. Most joint movements are described in degrees of movement. For example, in the positioning of the patient's arm on an arm board, it is critical to restrict abduction to less than 90 degrees. This means that the angle between the side of the patient's body and the arm is less than 90 degrees. Figure 10-15 illustrates directions of motion and the proper terms to describe them.

Embolism

A **thromboembolus** (or thrombus) is a blood clot that circulates in the vascular system and lodges in a vessel, causing obstruction or occlusion. Circulating blood normally does not form clots. When blood is allowed to slow or pool, however, as can occur during surgery, clots form in the lower extremities and migrate through the systemic circulation. A circulating thrombus can lodge anywhere in the body. When it blocks blood supply to the lung, brain, or heart, these vital tissues are deprived of oxygen and the tissue dies. Antiembolism stockings or a sequential compression device (SCD) are placed on patients' legs before long procedures or on patients predisposed to clot formation. The SCD wraps around the leg much like a large blood pressure cuff. It sequentially fills with air and then deflates. During the inflation phase the cuffs push venous blood toward the heart, and during deflation the vessels refill. This reduces the risk of blood pooling (stasis) and thrombus formation.

Respiratory Compromise

Positioning can affect the patient's ability to ventilate (fill the lungs with air). Patients in the prone position and steep Trendelenburg position are particularly vulnerable to ventilation problems. Both gravity and the position of the chest wall determine the amount of gas that enters the lungs. The prone position must allow expansion of the abdominal wall. Different types of open braces have been developed to raise the thorax from the operating table (see Prone Position). This increases ventilatory capacity by taking pressure off the abdominal wall.

Falls

Although a patient fall from the operating table to the floor is uncommon, it is a devastating occurrence. Falls can result in major fractures and serious injury to the head and soft tissue. To avoid a patient fall, study and adhere to the following guidelines:

▶ *Never leave a patient unattended—not for any reason or any period of time.*

▶ When transferring the patient between the stretcher and the operating table, *lock both the table and the stretcher firmly in place.*

▶ Make sure at least one person is standing at the receiving side of the operating table or stretcher to prevent the patient from moving too far over the edge.

▶ Do *not* position or move a patient without adequate help. Administrative support may be necessary to establish strict safety standards.

▶ Do not rush while moving an unconscious patient. Likewise, allow a conscious patient to move slowly during any move from one surface to another.

▶ As soon as the patient has moved to the operating table, secure the safety strap halfway between the knees and hips (as described earlier in the chapter).

▶ Position a morbidly obese patient on a specialty table built to carry extreme weight and size. Know the limits of the standard surgical table. A very heavy patient can tilt the tabletop to one side, which may cause the patient to roll off the table and onto the floor.

Physical Conditions That Increase Risk of Injury

Physical examinations by the anesthesia care provider and physician reveal preexisting conditions that affect positioning, including the initial positioning and repositioning that takes place during the procedure (intraoperatively). Workers assisting in positioning may not be aware of these conditions. Therefore those who have assessed the patient medically must guide the team. Box 10-2 describes physical conditions that affect patient positioning.

SURGICAL POSITIONS

Supine Position

The supine position or *dorsal recumbent* position is used for procedures of the abdomen, thorax, and face, and in orthopedic and vascular surgery (Figure 10-16). The patient is positioned with the head and spine in alignment. When an arm board or toboggan is not used, the arm is placed in a natural

---

Box 10-2   Patient Conditions That Influence Positioning

▶ Preexisting nerve compression syndrome
▶ Neuropathy (nerve disorder)
▶ Diabetes mellitus
▶ Osteoarthritis (progressive arthritic disease)
▶ Venous stasis (pooling of blood resulting from inactivity or cardiovascular disease)
▶ Preexisting decubitus ulcer (pressure-sore injury)
▶ Previous traumatic injury
▶ Alcohol abuse
▶ Vitamin deficiencies
▶ Malnutrition
▶ Renal disease
▶ Hypothyroidism
▶ Previous joint fractures
▶ Rheumatoid arthritis
▶ Corticosteroid use
▶ Contractures (scar tissue that restricts joint movement)
▶ Poor skin turgor (lack of skin and tissue firmness)
▶ Peripheral edema (intracellular fluid swelling in legs and arms)
▶ Reduced range of motion
▶ Weakness in extremities

Modified from Martin JT and Warner MA: *Positioning in anesthesia and surgery,* ed 3, Philadelphia, 1997, WB Saunders.

---

position at the patient's side, and the draw sheet is tucked smoothly underneath. The patient's feet must not extend over the edge of the table, and the legs must not be crossed one over the other.

The patient's weight is distributed over the occipital bone, back, sacrum, heels, and posterior legs. Patients with spinal or pelvic malformation or total joint prostheses may require special padding to support irregular curvatures and prevent hyperextension. A foam or gel pad is used to support the head. The safety strap is placed midway between the knees and thighs.

To keep the patient safe in the supine position, be sure to:

▶ Keep the cervical spine and head in neutral alignment.
▶ Distribute weight evenly over the ulnar nerve area—remember that padding may not be sufficient to prevent nerve damage and may even compress the nerve and cause injury.
▶ Protect the brachial plexus. Arm boards must not be abducted more than 90 degrees.
▶ Prevent decubitus ulcer formation at the lumbosacral area in elderly or debilitated patients. Place a soft, pliable surface under this dependent area.
▶ Protect the popliteal fossa from impingement. Do not place pillows directly under the knee joint. Pillows or rolls

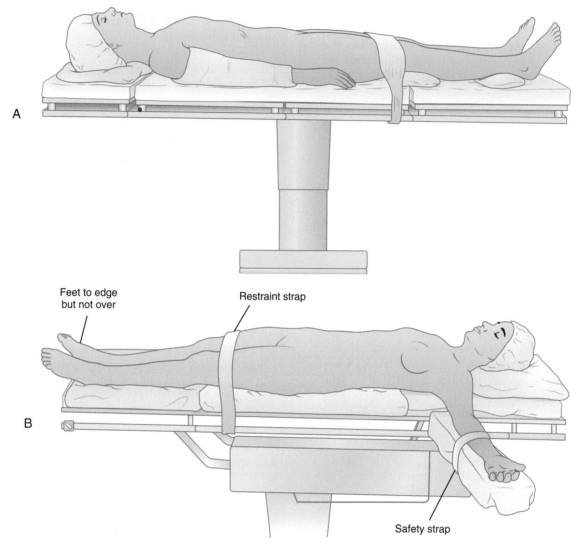

Feet to edge
but not over

Restraint strap

Safety strap

FIGURE 10-16
Supine position. **A,** With arms tucked. **B,** With arms positioned on arm boards; safety strap is applied. (**A** redrawn from Phillips N: *Berry & Kohn's operating room technique,* ed 10, St Louis, 2004, Mosby.)

are placed just proximal to this area. Distribute weight over the area.

▶ Separate the patient's feet so that they do not touch each other. Padding under the heels may be advised.

▶ Avoid the use of knee crutches (leg holders) during extended orthopedic surgery. Compartment syndrome and severe vascular damage can result.

▶ Give the patient an SCD to prevent **embolism.**

▶ Make sure that the patient's legs are not crossed, as this puts pressure on the peroneal nerve and blood vessels of the posterior leg.

Trendelenburg Position

The Trendelenburg position is a variation of the supine position in which the operating table is tilted head down (Figure 10-17). Use of this position permits greater access to the lower abdominal cavity and pelvic structures by allowing gravity to retract organs such as the small intestine, proximal large

bowel, and omentum toward the head. The position is commonly used during lower gastrointestinal surgery and pelvic surgery. It can cause hypertension, respiratory restriction, and increased intracranial pressure. Shoulder braces may be used to prevent the patient from sliding. Shoulder braces are very dangerous, however, and may cause injury to the brachial plexus. If it is necessary to use them, they should be well padded and placed over the acromion process of the scapula, rather than over the soft tissue overlying the brachial plexus.

To keep the patient safe in the Trendelenburg position, be sure to:

▶ Distribute the weight of the elbow and upper arm evenly in the area of the ulnar nerve.

▶ Protect the brachial plexus. Arm boards must not be abducted more than 90 degrees.

▶ Check that shoulder braces do not impinge on the cervical muscles or vascular and nerve bundles.

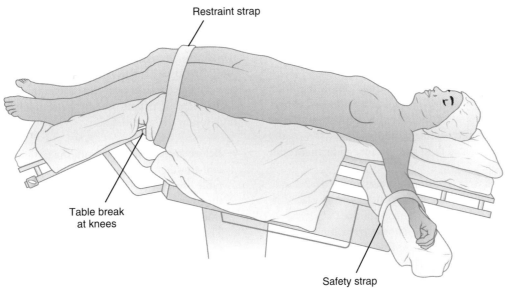

FIGURE 10-17
Trendelenburg position.

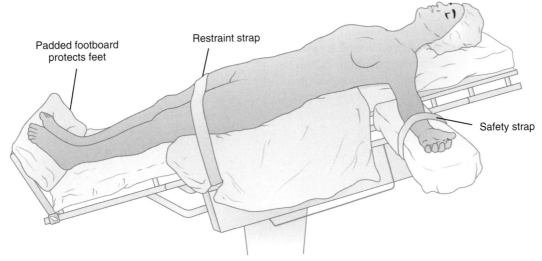

FIGURE 10-18
Reverse Trendelenburg position.

▶ Keep the patient from slipping downward during tilting. This can cause shear injury and lead to decubitus ulcers. Use shoulder braces correctly.

▶ Keep the Mayo stand from coming into contact with the patient's body, if the Mayo stand is positioned over the patient's legs during surgery. If the patient's position is altered in any way, always check the Mayo stand to make sure it is not touching the patient.

▶ Anticipate the onset of severe hypertension or respiratory depression during intraoperative positioning from level supine to Trendelenburg position. Surgery may be halted until the patient's condition is stabilized.

▶ When the patient is returned to the supine position from the Trendelenburg position after surgery, move the patient very slowly, because returning the patient to the supine position too quickly may result in hypotension.

Reverse Trendelenburg Position

The reverse Trendelenburg position, or foot-down position, is used when the surgeon requires unobstructed access to the upper peritoneal cavity and lower esophagus (Figure 10-18). When the operating table is tilted toward the patient's feet, gravity drops the viscera into the lower cavity, which allows a clear view of the diaphragm, cardiac sphincter, and esophagus.

During intraoperative positioning to reverse Trendelenburg position, all instruments lying on the surgical field must be secured by a magnetic pad or pocket holders. Take special care to ensure that endoscopes and all accessories are removed to prevent them from sliding to the floor. All tubing should be well secured at the beginning of surgery. The Mayo stand may be moved to accommodate the shift in patient position.

To keep the patient safe in the reverse Trendelenburg position, be sure to:

▶ Follow all safety precautions applicable to the supine position.
▶ Prevent the patient's body from sliding toward the floor, which can cause shearing injury. Use a footboard if necessary, but employ soft padding or protective foam boots to prevent nerve and vascular compression.
▶ Watch for the onset of fluid and vascular shifts that result in hypotension.
▶ Ensure that the weight of the leg is distributed over a wide area at the popliteal fossa if the patient will be placed in reverse Trendelenburg–lithotomy position. *Do not rely on padding alone to protect the patient from compartment syndrome or nerve or vessel damage!* Use of a low conforming stirrup with moldable gel or foam inserts helps prevent impingement on the back of the knee.

Lithotomy Position

The lithotomy position is a variation of the supine position. The patient's thighs are abducted, and both the knees and hips are flexed. The feet are suspended in stirrups, or the legs rest on low leg braces. Lithotomy position is used for gynecological, obstetrical, and genitourinary procedures.

Standard lithotomy position is used for gynecological procedures (Figure 10-19). During pelvic laparoscopic surgery, incorrect placement in the lithotomy position can cause severe tissue injury; therefore it is critical that protocol be followed. Attention to pressure points is very important. Patients with limited range of motion in the hip, spine, or knee joints are at particular risk. Respect the patient's dignity by placing a cover sheet over the perineum during positioning.

To keep the patient safe in the standard lithotomy position, follow these guidelines:

▶ Before anesthesia induction, the patient receiving a general anesthetic is positioned with the sacrum at the lower **table break**. This places the patient's calves on the edge of the lower section of the table and risks vascular compression, nerve compression, and compartment syndrome. The legs must not remain in this position. The buttocks must not extend beyond the break in the table.
▶ When the patient is unconscious and sufficiently relaxed, the anesthesia care provider announces when it is safe to elevate the legs. The lower portion of the table is flexed downward, or the end section is removed.
▶ *Both legs must be elevated simultaneously by two people.* Raising both legs at the same time keeps the body in alignment and prevents torsion of the lumbar spine, which can cause debilitating postoperative pain. If the patient's arms are tucked at his or her side, care must be exercised to ensure the patient's fingers do not become impinged as the lower table portion is flexed or raised.

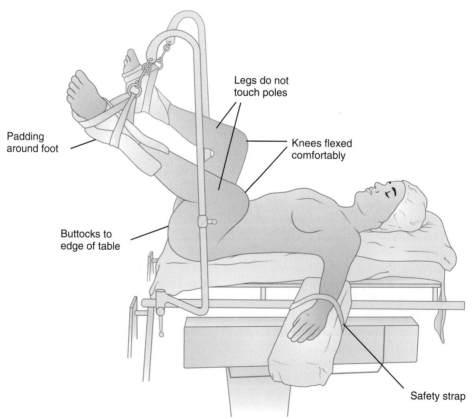

Legs do not touch poles

Padding around foot

Knees flexed comfortably

Buttocks to edge of table

Safety strap

FIGURE 10-19
Lithotomy position.

▶ When placing the legs in stirrups, the knees must be flexed first, keeping them in midline position, and then the thighs *abducted* while keeping the knees flexed. The feet or legs should be secured in stirrups.

▶ Sudden shifts in blood pressure and spinal injury can occur as the legs are positioned in, or removed from, stirrups. To prevent this, the maneuver must be performed very slowly.

▶ Legs should not be allowed to abduct against resistance.

▶ Standard lithotomy stirrups should be attached securely to the table frame. When attaching the stirrups, make certain that the locking device is tight and that no portion of the patient's legs rests against the vertical extensions (Figure 10-20).

▶ The femoral vessels are at risk of compression during lithotomy when the angle of hip flexion is severe. When femoral vessels are compressed, blood supply to the lower legs and abdominal viscera can be reduced significantly.

▶ Protect the peroneal nerve when stirrups are used. Do not place the stirrup sling directly over the Achilles area. Distribute the weight of the leg between both slings on the stirrup.

▶ After the legs are positioned, the hinged lower section of the operating table is flexed downward or removed altogether. When the patient's arms are positioned at the sides, there is a risk of amputating the fingers when the lower table section is restored to level position.

▶ Two people are required to lower the legs after surgery. Release the feet from the stirrups or leg rests, slowly bring the knees together on the midline, and gradually extend the hips and knees. Coordination between both people lowering the legs prevents lumbar torsion.

▶ Slow manipulation is necessary to allow blood to flow back into the limbs gradually. When the legs are lowered too quickly, a sudden shift of blood to the lower extremities and hypotension (severe drop in blood pressure) can occur.

Low lithotomy position is maintained by stirrups or knee crutches that allow the surgeon access to the perineum and pelvic structures. Many endoscopic abdominal surgeries also require low lithotomy position.

A cystoscopy or urology table is used during endoscopic procedures involving the genitourinary tract (Figure 10-21). The patient is positioned in the low lithotomy position. Be-

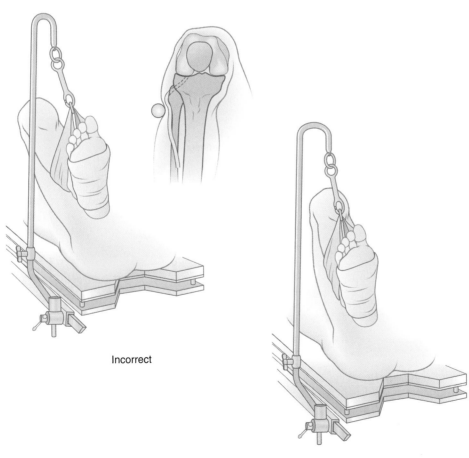

Incorrect

Correct

FIGURE 10-20
Lithotomy injuries. (Redrawn from Martin JT and Warner MA: *Positioning in anesthesia and surgery,* ed 3, Philadelphia, 1997, Saunders.)

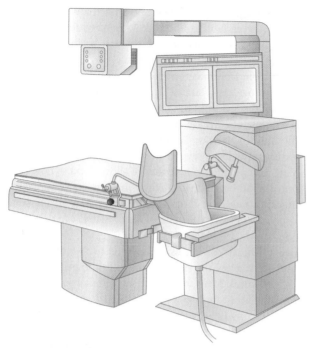

FIGURE 10-21
Cystoscopy table. (Redrawn from Martin JT and Warner MA: *Positioning in anesthesia and surgery,* ed 3, Philadelphia, 1997, Saunders.)

cause copious amounts of fluid are used during urological procedures, the table contains a drain path that exits the end of the table and passes directly into the floor drainage system. The table is also constructed to accommodate video and fluoroscopy imaging processes. Patients are often awake during positioning for urological procedures.

To keep the patient safe in the low lithotomy position, follow these guidelines:

▶ Follow all precautions described for the standard lithotomy position.
▶ Using knee rests in the low lithotomy position can risk compartment syndrome of the lower leg because the popliteal artery and vein lie close to the surface and rest directly on the table attachments. The angle of the knee and distribution of weight in the popliteal fossa must be carefully planned.
▶ The patient's arms must be maintained on arm boards with precautions taken to protect the ulnar nerve and cubital tunnel. If the patient receives only a local anesthetic, the arms can be placed on the patient's abdomen.

Orthopedic Table Position

The orthopedic or fracture table allows the patient to be positioned for hip nailings and other orthopedic procedures. The orthopedic table or fracture table allows circumferential access to the patient's leg while producing horizontal traction during surgery (Figure 10-22). The patient rests with

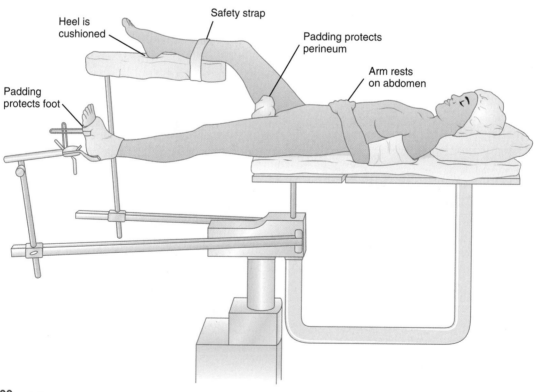

Heel is cushioned

Safety strap

Padding protects perineum

Arm rests on abdomen

Padding protects foot

FIGURE 10-22
Orthopedic table.

the injured leg restrained in a boot-like device. The leg may be rotated, pulled into traction, or released, as the surgery requires. The unaffected leg rests on an elevated leg holder. The open structure of the table allows intraoperative fluoroscopy and radiography. Many different types of attachments are available depending on the complexity and needs of the surgery. Placement of the patient in the orthopedic table position requires at least four people to assist.

Patients requiring orthopedic surgery often are sedated for the positioning procedure. To keep the patient safe in the orthopedic table position, follow these guidelines:

▶ When moving the patient from the stretcher to the orthopedic table, maintain the spine and head in neutral position at all times.
▶ The center post of the orthopedic table must be removed *before* the patient is moved. The post is repositioned, and the patient's genitalia are protected with padding during positioning.
▶ Pressure points on the sacrum, heels, and unaffected lower leg must be adequately padded, and weight must be distributed. The extended leg is held by a boot or a combination of boot and straps.
▶ The perineal area and genital structures must not rest against the center post.
▶ Traction on the affected leg is adjusted by the surgeon who directs the positioning team.

▶ Because of its design, this table is used for patients with fractures of the hip. Moving and transfer of the injured patient must be carried out slowly and carefully to avoid causing further injury.

Sitting (Fowler) Position

The sitting or Fowler position occasionally is used for facial, cranial, or reconstructive breast surgery (Figure 10-23). In the past this position was used for anterior spine procedures. Its use has declined significantly in the last decade because of the many complications and risks associated with it. Use of the position requires experienced personnel who are familiar with the protocol and who practice it frequently enough to prevent accidents. When this position is used, the general operating table is flexed to allow a Fowler or **semi-Fowler position.** The head may be secured by a craniotomy headrest or stabilized with a doughnut-shaped gel or foam pad.

Lateral Position

The lateral position is used for procedures involving the renal system and for cardiothoracic surgery (Figure 10-24). When the lateral position is described, the side named is the side lying on the table. For example, in the left lateral position, the left side lies on the table. The opposite side is the operative or "up" side.

When general anesthesia is used, the patient is anesthetized in supine position and maneuvered into the lateral

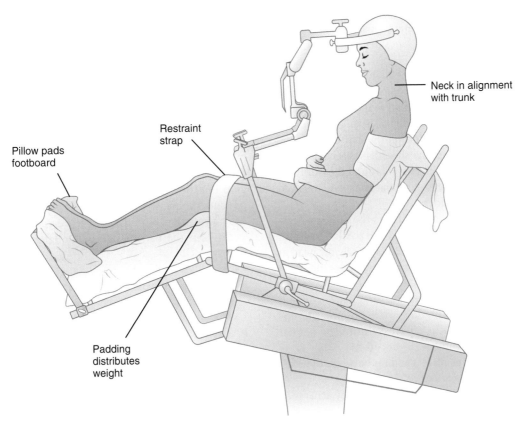

Pillow pads footboard

Restraint strap

Padding distributes weight

Neck in alignment with trunk

FIGURE 10-23
Sitting or Fowler position.

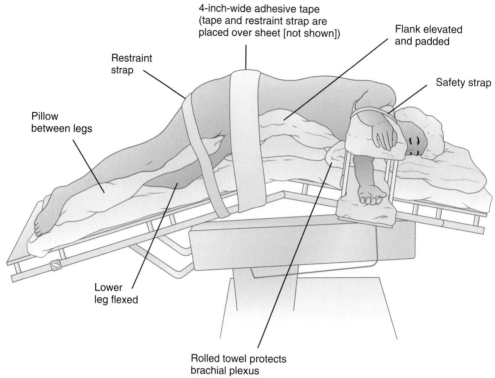

4-inch-wide adhesive tape
(tape and restraint strap are
placed over sheet [not shown])

Flank elevated
and padded

Restraint
strap

Safety strap

Pillow
between legs

Lower
leg flexed

Rolled towel protects
brachial plexus

FIGURE 10-24
Lateral position.

position after intubation. At least three assistants manage the torso, pelvis, and arms.

To turn the patient into the lateral position, follow this technique:

1. Abduct the down-side arm so that it does not become compressed under the trunk. To put the patient in a left lateral position, the assistants stand at the patient's right.
2. The assistant at the hips places his or her *right* hand under the pelvis and the left hand on the iliac crest. At the same time, the assistant at the shoulders reaches around the *back* of the patient's neck (never around the front, because this would compress the patient's airway) and grasps the patient's shoulder.
3. The anesthesia care provider manages the head and cervical spine. If the patient does not have a risk of cervical injury, the anesthesia care provider may rotate the head in advance of the body. The move is directed by the anesthesia care provider.
4. At the count of three, the assistants simultaneously pull the down-side hip and shoulder while pushing the upside hip and shoulder. This effectively turns the patient while maintaining alignment (Figure 10-25).
5. Flex the lower leg and place padding between the legs. The upper leg remains extended.
6. Protect the brachial plexus with padding. The arms may be extended on double arm boards, or the down-side arm, which is the most vulnerable, may be placed in front of the body. An overhead arm sling also may be used.

7. In addition, use flank padding and a head stabilizer.

Use of the flexed lateral position may require stabilization of the hips and/or shoulders with wide tape. The tape is placed *on top of the top sheet, not on the patient's skin.* It is secured to the table frame on both sides and passes over the pelvic rim or the shoulder. The tape is meant to stabilize, not to secure the patient's entire weight. Excess compression by the tape can cause tissue damage. The safety strap is placed midway between the thighs and knees. Flexing the middle table break widens the operative exposure. The kidney elevator, located under the table pad, is used to lift the flank region but must be used with caution. It can cause excessive pressure on the deep blood vessels of the abdomen, and its use may result in vascular injury or hypotension.

To keep the patient safe in the lateral position, follow these guidelines:

▶ During the move from supine to lateral position, the patient's shoulders and pelvis must be moved *in the same plane without any torsion.*
▶ The anesthetized patient must be moved as one unit—head, neck, spine, pelvis, and legs all must be moved together to prevent twisting injury to joints.
▶ The down side of the face should rest on an *open* horseshoe pad to protect the facial nerves, ear, and eye from compression.
▶ When the patient is turned from supine to lateral, the head and neck must be kept in alignment at all times.

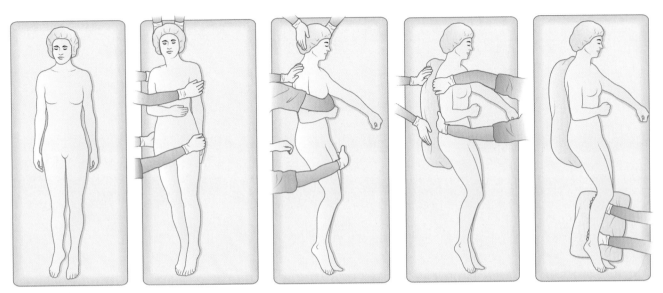

FIGURE 10-25
Turning patient to lateral position.

▶ Padding to protect the brachial plexus is placed under the chest wall, *not in the axillary area!*

▶ The patient's arms should be protected by extending them on double arm boards or positioning them with the up-side arm flexed at an angle of 90 degrees or less and the down-side arm lying close to the torso. The down-side arm can be flexed (no more than 90 degrees). The weight of the upper torso must be distributed evenly with padding.

▶ When the patient is in a flexed lateral position, the angle of flexion and padding must be meticulously checked to avoid pressure damage to vessels and nerves in the flank.

▶ Padding always should be placed between the legs so that it extends the full length of the leg. The up-side ankle must not rest directly on the down-side leg.

Prone Position

A number of different variations of the prone position are used that allow access to the spine, cranium, and perianal region. This position can compromise physiological and structural mechanisms in the body, and its use requires extreme caution. The pressure exerted on the abdomen restricts normal ventilation, and the cervical spine may be forced into a position that would be intolerable to the patient if he or she were conscious. There is risk to nerves, eyes, genitalia, breasts, and spine. In the prone position, the patient's upper body rests on a raised padded frame or elongated pads placed on each side of the patient's thorax.

When placing the patient in prone position, he or she is anesthetized in supine position on the stretcher. After intubation the patient is repositioned on the operating table into the prone position. Four to six people are required to turn the patient. If the patient is turned on the operating table (Figure 10-26, *A*), two people lift and pull the patient close to them and then slowly rotate the body onto the arms of the other two helpers. The spine is maintained in alignment, and the head is controlled by the anesthesia care provider. The female patient's breasts should be placed between the chest rests (Figure 10-26, *B*). Check that the breasts are free from any unnecessary pressure from the chest rests. If the patient is a male, the genitalia must be checked for any unnecessary pressure that could cause injury. The endotracheal tube and eyes must be checked to make certain there is no pressure that can lead to injury.

To turn the patient into the prone position (pronation), follow these steps:

1. Align the stretcher with the operating table.
2. If the patient is to be catheterized, perform catheterization before turning the patient.
3. When the anesthesia care provider is ready, he or she will temporarily disconnect the patient's airway.
4. Two people positioned on the receiving side of the table reach across, while those on the other side slowly lift and rotate the patient's body onto the arms of the receiving personnel. The head is controlled by the anesthesia care provider and the feet by another helper.
5. Reconnect the airway, and make adjustments in the position.
6. Place the arms on arm boards with the elbows flexed.

A laminectomy brace is used to elevate the trunk and allow expansion of the lungs during spinal or back surgery. The patient is turned from the stretcher directly onto the padded brace (Figure 10-27).

Surgery of the posterior spine or cranium often is performed with the patient in prone position and the head in a Mayfield headrest. The head is secured by sterile tongs that attach to the head brace (Figure 10-28).

Jackknife or Kraske position is a modification of prone position (Figure 10-29). The lower table break is flexed downward to achieve a simultaneous head-down and foot-down posture. This position may be used for anorectal sur-

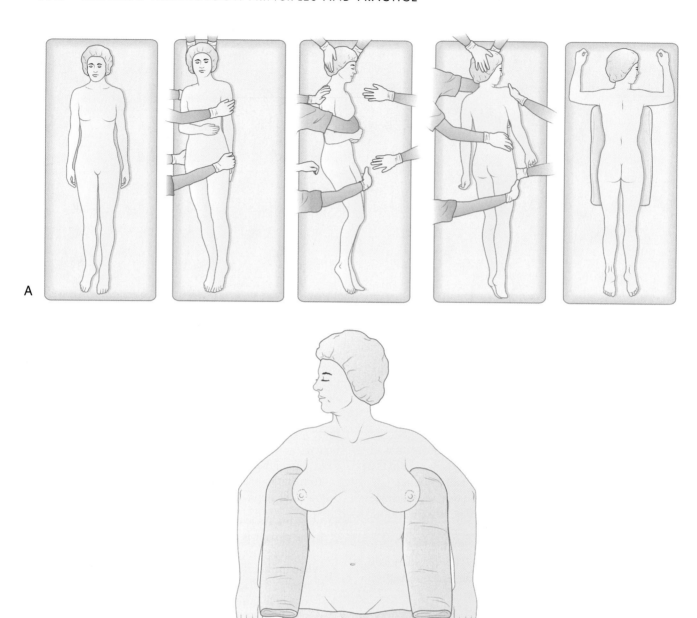

FIGURE 10-26
A, Turning patient to the prone position. **B,** The female patient's breasts should be displaced laterally between the chest rests.

gery. The lower legs may be elevated or may rest on pads to distribute the weight.

The *knee-chest position* is a modification of the jackknife position (Figure 10-30). It is used in ambulatory surgery for rectal procedures that do not require anesthesia.

To keep the patient safe in any prone position, attend to the following guidelines and cautions:

▶ The spine must be kept in a neutral position at all times during positioning.

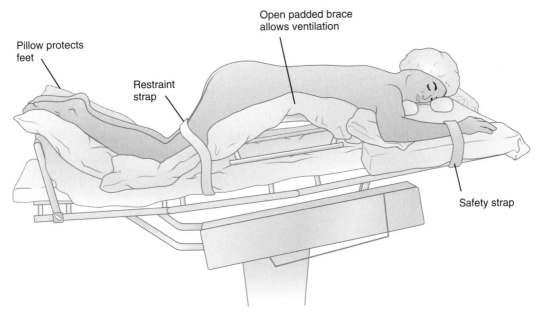

FIGURE 10-27
Laminectomy brace position.

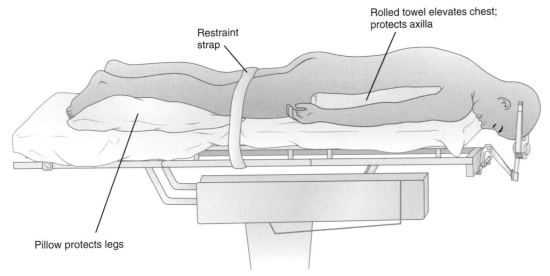

FIGURE 10-28
Craniotomy position using Mayfield headrest.

▶ One must protect the patient's airway by ensuring sufficient elevation from the table to allow deep lung inflation. When a brace is used, the two sides of the brace should not impinge on the abdomen.

▶ Corneal abrasion can result from compression on the globe of the eye and can cause blindness. This can be prevented through the use of a hollow headrest.

▶ A female patient's breasts must be protected. A patient with heavy breasts is likely to be unstable on the operating table because of the lack of firm support in the upper thorax.

▶ *Forcing the breasts laterally during positioning can cause bleeding and tearing at the breast margins.*

▶ Whenever possible the breasts should be directed medially and cephalad (toward the head). When a brace is used, do not force the breasts to the sides of the lateral supports.

▶ Particular care must be given to positioning patients who have had a mastectomy or radiation treatment to the chest wall because the skin and underlying tissues are tender and may be painful.

▶ The male genitalia must be protected from compression. When a brace is used, the genitalia must be clear of any

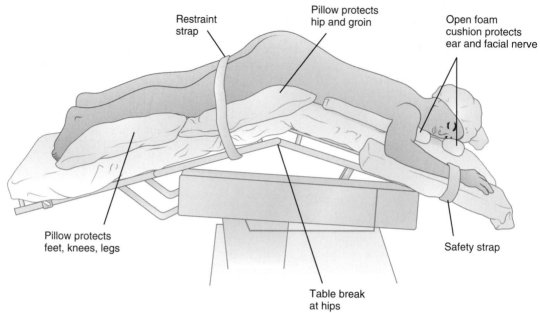

FIGURE 10-29
Jackknife or Kraske position.

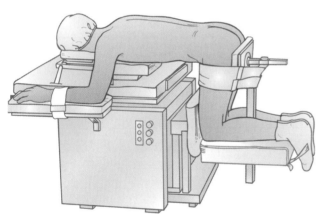

FIGURE 10-30
Knee-chest position. (Redrawn from Phillips N: *Berry & Kohn's operating room technique,* ed 10, St Louis, 2004, Mosby.)

part of the frame. Pads placed across the thighs must not entrap the scrotum and penis.

▶ If the patient has an intestinal stoma, this area must be completely free of contact with the brace or padding.

▶ Pressure on the subclavian artery and brachial plexus when the head is turned to the side with the arms raised can lead to **thoracic outlet syndrome.** The result can be permanent injury causing pain and loss of sensation along the ulnar nerve.

▶ Severe risk of injury to the brachial plexus and cervical spine occurs when the patient's arms are extended above the head. To prevent brachial plexus injury, the upper arms should be placed at an angle of 90 degrees or less to the trunk with the forearms parallel to the trunk.

▶ When the patient's head is rotated to the side, the risk of traction and compression injury to the brachial plexus is increased. Many patients cannot tolerate this degree of cervical rotation. Preoperative evaluation must include an assessment of this area to prevent temporary or permanent injury.

▶ A wide area around the ulnar nerve must be amply padded.

▶ In the knee-chest position, ventilation is a primary concern. Lateral padding of the chest is required in this position, even during short procedures performed under local anesthesia.

CASE STUDIES

Case 1

You are asked to bring a patient from the medical unit to surgery. When you arrive on the unit, the patient is not in his room or in the hallway. What will you do?

Case 2

You are transporting a patient from the medical unit to the operating room. You discover that the patient elevator is out of order. What will you do?

Case 3

While turning the patient into the lateral position, you suddenly realize the patient is falling off the table in your direction. What will you do? What precautions can be taken to avoid falls?

Case 4

You are assigned to act as circulator in a procedure in which the patient is placed in the lithotomy position. The patient emerges quickly from anesthesia, and she begins to struggle. Her legs are still elevated in stirrups. What are the risks to the patient in this situation? What will you do?

Case 5

You are scrubbed on a laparotomy case. A number of medical students have been brought in to observe. One of the medical students is scrubbed and is holding a retractor. You notice the student has placed his elbow on the patient's shoulder and he is resting his weight on the patient. The surgeon has said nothing. What will you do?

Chapter 11

Surgical Preparation and Draping

Learning Objectives

After studying this chapter the reader will be able to:

- List the characteristics of common surgical prep solutions
- Identify necessary precautions to prevent injury associated with skin preparation
- Identify the use of a "no-touch" preparation technique
- Explain the concepts of body hair management prior to surgery
- Identify the proper procedure to perform the surgical skin preparation for all areas of the body
- Identify the proper aseptic technique to catheterize male and female patients
- Identify the proper technique for draping the patient for torso, limb, and lithotomy procedures

Terminology

Antiseptics—Chemical agents that are approved for use on the skin and that inhibit the growth and reproduction of microorganisms. Antiseptics are used to cleanse and paint the surgical site to reduce the number of microorganisms to an absolute minimum.

Barrier drape—Drape intended to separate a contaminated area from the incision site. For example, a barrier drape is placed across the perineum between the vagina and anus during gynecological procedures. The barrier drape is plastic and may have a sticky surface along one edge. This edge is placed at the site where a barrier is needed.

Debridement—The physical removal of devitalized tissue, debris, and foreign objects from a wound. Debridement is performed on trauma injuries, burns, and infected wounds either before surgery or as a part of the surgical procedure.

Desiccation—Tissue drying. Alcohol is a desiccating skin preparation solution. It causes the destruction of tissue protein and therefore is never used around the eyes or on mucous membranes.

Drape—Sterile materials, including towels and sheets, placed around the prepared surgical incision site to create a sterile field.

Fenestrated drapes—Sterile body sheets with a hole or "window" that exposes the surgical incision site. The fenestrated drape is positioned after other drapes and towels have been placed in keeping with the procedure. Fenestrated drapes are differentiated by type, such as laparotomy, thyroid, kidney, eye, ear, and extremity drapes.

Head drape—A turban-style drape created with two surgical towels that covers the patient's head and eyes. Knowing how to prepare and place this drape is a valuable draping skill.

Impervious—Not able to be penetrated.

Incise drapes—Plastic self-adhesive drapes that are positioned over the incision site after the surgical skin preparation. The drape creates a sterile surface over the skin. The incision is made directly through the incise drape and skin.

Prep—The use of antiseptic solutions for cleaning, reducing microbial count, and preventing unnecessary contamination of an area for a sterile invasive (skin incision) or sterile noninvasive (urinary catheterization) procedure.

Residual activity—The microbicidal activity that remains after an antiseptic or disinfectant has dried.

Retention catheter—A urinary catheter with an inflatable balloon that is used to drain the bladder continuously during surgery. Also called an indwelling or Foley catheter, it is placed in the patient before surgical skin preparation.

Terminology—cont'd

Skin preparation sponge—A gauze that does not contain a radioopaque marker and that is used to apply solution during skin cleansing. These sponges are available in many different sizes and types, according to size, configuration, and location of the preparation area.

Sterile field—An area that includes the draped patient, all sterile tables, and sterile equipment in the immediate area of the patient. The patient is considered the center of the sterile field.

Straight catheter—A nonretention catheter used to drain the bladder just before surgery.

Surgical site infection (SSI)—Postoperative infection of the surgical wound, most commonly caused by the normal bacteria found on the patient's skin or shed from the skin or hair of surgical team members. The goal of the surgical skin preparation is to prevent postoperative wound infection.

OBJECTIVES OF SURGICAL SKIN PREPARATION AND DRAPING

Unbroken skin, including mucous membranes, is the body's primary defense against infection. A surgical incision breaks this barrier, creating a portal of entry for microorganisms. Healthy skin contains colonies of microorganisms (normal flora) that compete with and usually overcome foreign or transient bacteria. When normal or transient flora are introduced into the surgical wound, however, they can cause a **surgical site infection (SSI)**.

The most common cause of surgical site infection is the normal bacteria found on the skin of the patient and surgical team members, particularly *Staphylococcus aureus*. Skin is colonized by both superficial bacteria and bacteria that live in deeper skin structures such as sweat and sebaceous glands, hair follicles, and deep pores. Before surgery the skin must be cleansed with **antiseptic** solution to reduce the number of transient and normal microorganisms to an absolute minimum. Because bacteria inhabit both the dermis and epidermis, the skin is prepared both the day before surgery and just before the procedure. The skin **prep** also is designed to remove dirt and oils that also harbor pathogenic microorganisms. After skin preparation, the patient is covered with sterile sheets (**drapes**) that expose only the surgical site and create the center of the **sterile field**. This is the area defined by the draped patient and all sterile surfaces in close proximity.

PREOPERATIVE PATIENT PREPARATION

Bathing

The surgical preparation may begin the day before surgery. The patient may be required to shower at least once the day before and the morning of surgery, using an antiseptic soap. Chlorhexidine gluconate has been proven to be the most effective cleansing preparation for use during showering.

Patient Jewelry

As part of the preparation, the patient *must remove all body jewelry.* Body-piercing jewelry can be lost in body cavities. Mouth and nose jewelry can be dislodged during surgery and block the patient's airway. The patient should sign a written release if he or she chooses not to remove jewelry.

Jewelry such as necklaces, bracelets, watches, and earrings also must be removed before surgery. Many facilities allow patients to continue wearing their wedding rings during the procedure. The facilities that allow this exception have written policies requiring that jewelry left on the patient must be taped.

Patient Clothing

In some outpatient settings, patients are permitted to wear their clothing during surgery, as long as it does not impinge on the sterile field. In the hospital's acute-care operating room, the patient must wear only a clean hospital gown. All other clothing should be removed before the patient arrives in the operating room holding area.

Hair Removal

Hair generally is not removed from the surgical site unless ordered by the surgeon. If hair *is* removed, the following guidelines should be followed:

▶ Hair should be removed as close to the time of surgery as possible. If the skin is to be shaved, this should be done *immediately* before surgery.

▶ Hair is best removed with electric clippers or a chemical depilatory. Shaving the hair results in injury to the skin that may not be visible. Small skin abrasions create a site for bacterial colonization and become a source of potential postsurgical infection. Studies have shown that the incidence of surgical site infection increases when the skin is shaved. If disposable shaver heads are used, these should be considered a biohazard and must be placed in a sharps container after use.

▶ If a depilatory is used, the patient must first be tested for sensitivity to the agent to be applied. This sensitivity test takes a minimum of 12 hours to perform.

▶ Cranial procedures often are performed with minimal hair removal. However, in some cases that require removal of a great deal of hair, the patients may want to have a wig made from their own hair. Hair removed from the patient's head is considered the patient's property and should be returned to the patient after surgery. The surgeon often performs hair removal as part of the skin preparation.

▶ Hair removal requires an order from the physician, and the exact procedure used follows operating room policy.

▶ Eyebrows are never to be shaved as these may fail to regrow or may grow abnormally after surgery.

URINARY CATHETERIZATION

In the health care setting, the dignity and privacy of patients is important. One way to respect the patient's dignity and prevent patient discomfort is to insert the urinary catheter after the patient is transferred to the operating room table and is anesthetized.

During many surgical procedures the urinary bladder must remain empty, or urinary output must be carefully monitored. This is acheived by performing urinary bladder catheterization with a retention catheter. Catheterization is performed by the surgeon, registered nurse, or circulator. Only personnel who have been trained to perform urinary catheterization may carry out this procedure.

Equipment and Supplies

Catheterization is performed immediately before preparation of the surgical skin. If the surgeon chooses continuous urinary drainage throughout the surgery, a **retention** (or indwelling) **catheter** is used. This type of catheter is commonly called a Foley catheter or simply a Foley (Figure 11-1, *A*). A Foley catheter is a flexible tube with a balloon at the tip of the catheter. After the catheter is inserted, this balloon is inflated and prevents the catheter from becoming dislodged from the bladder. The drainage port of the catheter is attached to a length of flexible tubing that connects to a self-contained gravity drainage bag.

If the surgeon requires that the bladder be drained only at the beginning of surgery, a nonretaining or red Robinson

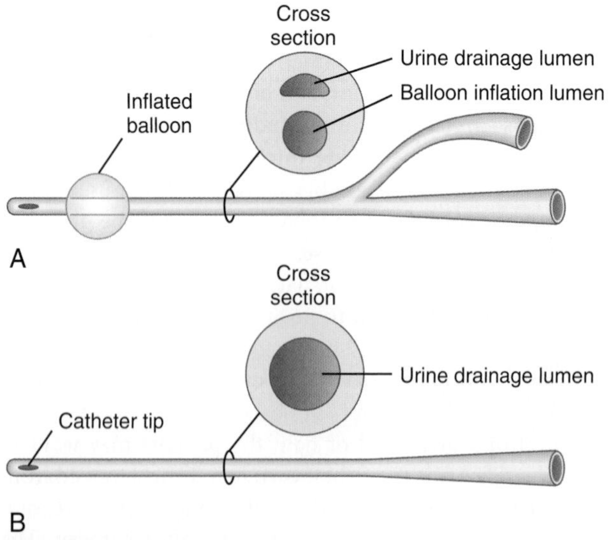

FIGURE 11-1
A, Foley catheter. **B,** Straight catheter. (**A** and **B** redrawn from Harkreader H and Hogan MA: *Fundamentals of nursing,* ed 2, St Louis, 2004, Saunders.)

catheter is used. This is often called a **straight catheter,** and the insertion procedure is called a straight urinary catheterization (Figure 11-1, *B*).

Commercial urinary catheterization kits that contain all of the necessary supplies are available. All catheterization supplies must be sterile. These include a 10-ml syringe prefilled with water to inflate the retention balloon on a Foley catheter, water-based lubricant, small perineal drapes, disposable forceps, cotton or gauze swabs, skin preparation solution, sterile gloves, and the catheter and drainage system. Commercial urinary catheter kits usually contain a 16 French, 2-way, 5 cc balloon catheter.

Patient Risks

Urinary catheterization is a *sterile procedure.* The urinary bladder and proximal urethra are sterile, and contaminants introduced by catheterization increase the risk of urinary tract infection. Because of its close proximity to the rectum (especially in the female patient), the urinary meatus can be easily contaminated with *Escherichia coli,* which may be introduced into the urinary system during catheterization. Urinary tract infection can progress to systemic infection with serious consequences. Urinary tract infection is a major risk and is one of the most common types of nosocomial infections. *In the pregnant patient, urinary tract infection can cause premature birth or fetal death.*

Catheterization can cause trauma to the urethra and bladder. Repeated attempts at catheterization can produce mucosal abrasions that can cause pain and increase the risk of infection. Damage to the urethra and sphincter muscle can result in prolonged urinary retention and inability to urinate. In elderly males, enlargement of the prostate gland also can make urinary catheterization difficult. Consultation with a urologist may be required in a situation in which catheterization is difficult or unsuccessful.

The female patient is placed in a supine position with the hips externally rotated and the knees flexed, commonly called the "frog leg" position. The male patient is catheterized in the supine position. If the patient will be placed in the prone position, catheterization must be performed before the patient is turned. All positioning rules and precautions must be followed (see Chapter 10).

Figures 11-2 and 11-3 illustrate the technique for urinary catheterization of women and men.

SURGICAL SKIN PREPARATION AGENTS

The surgical skin preparation is performed immediately before the start of surgery and after the patient is positioned and anesthetized. The surgical site and a wide area around the site are cleansed and painted with antiseptic solution.

Only agents approved for use on skin surfaces may be used to prepare the patient's skin. While disinfectants also reduce or eliminate microorganisms on surfaces, they are not approved for use on body tissue.

Three antiseptics are commonly used for the surgical skin preparation: alcohol, chlorhexidine gluconate, and iodophors. Two others, triclosan and parachlorometaxylenol (PCMX), are used less frequently.

Alcohol

Alcohol solution contains ethyl or isopropyl alcohol. At 70% concentration, isopropyl alcohol is 95% effective against both gram-negative and gram-positive bacteria, mycobacteria, fungi, and viruses. It is not completely effective against bacte-

rial spores. Isopropyl alcohol is extremely flammable and volatile. In the presence of laser energy, electrosurgical energy, and oxygen, alcohol can ignite drapes and the patient's oxygen delivery system with tragic consequences. All traces of alcohol must be completely dry on the skin before drapes are applied. Alcohol destroys microorganisms through **desiccation** (drying out) of the cell proteins. For this reason, alcohol is never used on mucous membranes or the eyes, or in any open wound. Alcohol preparation solutions are available in liquid or gel form and are combined with other antiseptics.

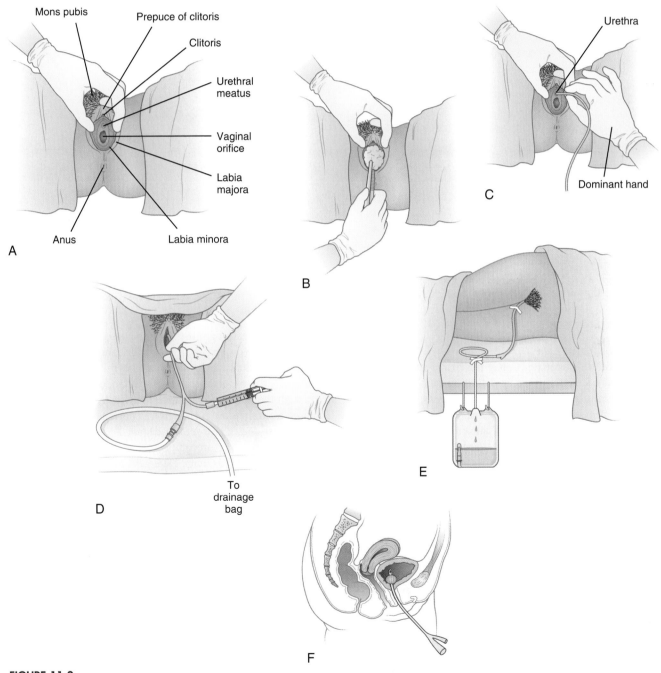

FIGURE 11-2
Urinary catheterization of the female. **A,** Parts of the female genitalia. **B,** Cleansing the genitalia. **C,** Inserting the Foley catheter. **D,** Inflating the balloon. **E,** Drainage bag secured to the leg. **F,** Anatomical position of the Foley catheter.

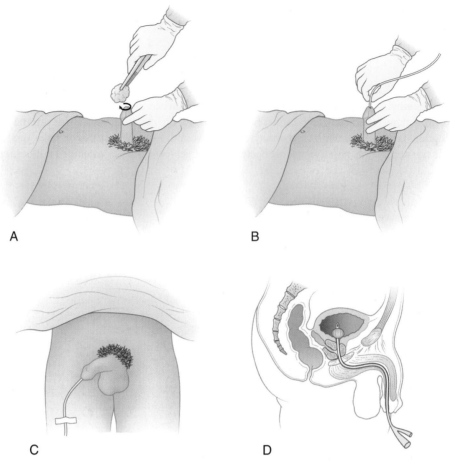

FIGURE 11-3
Urinary catheterization of the male. **A,** Cleansing the penile meatus. **B,** Inserting the Foley catheter. **C,** Foley catheter secured to the leg. **D,** Anatomical position of the Foley catheter.

Chlorhexidine Gluconate

Chlorhexidine gluconate (CHG) is a broad-spectrum antiseptic that has better microbicidal action than povidone iodine. This antiseptic provides **residual activity,** which means that it continues to kill microorganisms after application. It is not absorbed by the skin. A disadvantage of chlorhexidine gluconate use is that it is not effective in the presence of soap and organic debris such as skin oils, blood, and body fluids. If it is used for preoperative bathing, the patient must first bathe and shampoo the hair normally, then rinse off all traces of soap. Chlorhexidine solution is used as a final wash.

CHG has been linked to hearing loss when accidentally introduced into the middle ear. For this reason it should never be used during preparation of the ear. CHG also should be avoided in preparation of the eye and is not recommended for use on large open wounds, such as burns.

Iodophor

Iodine alone is irritating to tissue, but when combined with *povidone* (a synthetic dispersing agent), it becomes *iodophor,* commonly used as a surgical preparation solution. Iodophor is combined with detergent and used for the surgical hand scrub.

It is effective against gram-positive bacteria but weaker against gram-negative organisms, mycobacteria, fungi, and viruses. It has some residual activity and retains its microbicidal action in the presence of organic substances. Iodophor is absorbed through the skin and may cause toxicity. After use, it must be rinsed from the skin. Although it is normally nonirritating to tissue, first-degree and second-degree chemical burns can result when improper preparation technique is used or the patient has iodine sensitivity. Detergent forms are not used on mucous membranes or near the eyes. Iodophor is sometimes commercially formulated with 70% alcohol as a preparation solution. Gel and spray preparations also are available.

Triclosan

Triclosan 1% solution is an antiseptic commonly found in deodorants, antibacterial soaps, and other proprietary goods. Its use in surgery is limited because its full microbicidal effect occurs only with repeated application. It is safe for ophthalmic use and for use on the face.

Parachlorometaxylenol

Parachlorometaxylenol (PCMX) has limited use in surgery at this time. It is nontoxic and can be used in the area of the eyes and ears. It has limited bactericidal, tuberculocidal, virucidal, and fungicidal properties.

PATIENT RISKS RELATED TO SURGICAL SKIN PREPPING

Chemical Burn

Chemical burns result when preparation solutions are allowed to pool under the patient. Pressure and contact with the chemical over time can result in severe blistering and skin loss. To prevent burns, one must frame the preparation area with dry towels to absorb the excess solution at the periphery of the preparation area. One must check the entire site for pooling or dampness before drapes are applied.

Fire

Alcohol and alcohol-based preparation solutions are volatile and flammable. When alcohol solution or volatile fumes come in contact with heat sources, they can easily cause a fire on or inside the patient. In the presence of concentrated oxygen, or in an oxygen-enriched environment such as the operating room, the risk is even greater. Ignition sources include the electrosurgical pencil, the laser, or the intense light of a fiberoptic light cord. Closed cavities such as the throat are particularly at risk because they are small, contained areas. Preventing alcohol-related fires requires vigilance and action on the part of all members of the surgical team. Do not let skin preparation solutions pool around the patient. All skin preparation areas must be completely dry before draping.

Dislocation or Fracture

General anesthesia includes the use of muscle relaxants, and as a result, fracture or dislocation can occur when the arms and legs are manipulated during the surgical prep. During patient preparation, often one assistant must hold the extremity while a second person performs the preparation. It is the responsibility of the person controlling the limb to keep it in anatomical position. If a leg support is used during preparation, remove the leg from the holder after the preparation is completed. Use of a leg holder can result in compression injury and compartment syndrome, because the weight of the leg rests on a small area.

Injuries from Warming of Preparation Solutions

Preparation solutions must *not* be warmed in a microwave unit, an autoclave, or hot water. Heating in this manner is *uncontrolled,* and the exact temperature is unknown. This can increase the risk of thermal burns, especially for patients with delicate or sensitive skin. When iodine is heated in a closed container, it combines with free oxygen and is lost from the solution, which reduces its concentration. When iodine is heated in an open container, water evaporates, which causes an *increase* in concentration and a risk of chemical burn. The manufacturer's recommendations must be followed.

SKIN PREPARATION PROCEDURE

General Guidelines

Before the surgical skin preparation is begun, all supplies must be gathered and placed on a small preparation table (prep table) near the patient. The skin preparation is a sterile procedure. Sterile gloves are worn, and all supplies are sterile. Manufactured sterile preparation trays are available and contain all of the necessary supplies to perform the skin preparation. The preparation tray supplies will vary among institutions, depending on the type of prep tray used at each facility. Before preparation is begun, the preparation table is draped or the sterile outside wrapper is folded down over the table, and a sterile field is created. Prep solutions are poured into a basin, and all other supplies are placed on the table. Do not use radiologically detectable surgical sponges to perform the patient prep because the sponges may be discarded or otherwise become lost. Because radiologically detectable sponges are part of the sponge count, they must not be used except in the course of surgery. After the preparation, used prep sponges are placed in a bag and kept separate from surgical sponges.

SKIN MARKING

Many surgeons outline the incision site with an indelible skin marker. Before the preparation is begun, the operative site should be cross-checked with the patient's chart to confirm that the *surgical site* is correct.

DEFATTING AGENTS

Natural water-resistant secretions can prevent the preparation solution from penetrating to the skin. Pre-preparation solutions are available to remove buildup of these secretions.

MULTIPLE PREPARATION SITES

When more than one procedure is planned during the same surgery, one must prepare each site separately, using a different preparation setup for each site. This scenario occurs during multiple trauma procedures and during procedures that require access through multiple areas of the body. For example, during coronary artery bypass graft surgery, the saphenous vein often is removed and used to replace the coronary vessels. In this case, the leg may be prepared separately from the thorax. In addition, when skin is harvested to produce a graft, the donor site often is located in an area distal to the recipient site.

Technique

Before the preparation, the area to be prepped must be exposed. The proper technique for the skin preparation procedure is as follows:

1. After application of sterile gloves (using open glove technique) and before beginning the preparation, bank the boundary of the preparation site with sterile towels to absorb excess preparation solution. For example, if the

patient is in the supine position, place towels at the juncture of the patient and the operating table along the patient's lower thorax and abdominal region. When squaring the preparation site, make a wide cuff in the towel to protect your sterile gloves. Place each towel using the cuff to protect your hands as you tuck the towel along the border of the preparation site where it contacts the operating table. After a towel has been placed, do not contaminate the upper side or move the towel. The most common sites of chemical burns are along the ribs and sides of the patient, at the coccyx (when the patient is in lithotomy position), and beneath a pneumatic tourniquet.

2. Preparation (cleansing) is performed in a *spiral pattern.* The exact incision site itself is the center of the spiral. The spiral is created in *one direction only*—from the center *outward.* When the pattern is begun, the **preparation sponge** (prep sponge) may not move in reverse and touch an area previously prepped. A new preparation sponge is used to widen the spiral as needed or to repeat the spiral pattern. After a sponge is used, it must be discarded in the sponge bucket.

3. *No-touch* technique is recommended for the skin preparation. This means that the preparation sponges are not held in the hand during the preparation. Instead, sponges are mounted on sponge forceps. When the eyes, ears, and face are cleansed, sponges can be handheld for greater control.

4. Any area that is highly colonized with microorganisms (*contaminated area*), such as a colostomy opening, the anus, skin ulcers, the vagina, or a foreign body, is prepped with fresh sponges after the surrounding area has been cleansed. This type of preparation is performed from the clean area to the dirty, to avoid cross-contamination.

The following sections describe the procedural steps for preparing different areas of the body. NOTE: When performing the skin prep on any conscious patient, always explain to the patient what you are doing and what they should expect to feel.

EYE
Sterile Supplies
▶ Gloves
▶ Lint-free cotton balls
▶ Small basins with warm saline solution and preparation solution
▶ Towels
▶ Bulb syringe

Procedure
1. Explain the procedure to the conscious patient. Instruct the patient to keep his or her hands away from the face during and after the preparation.
2. Turn the patient's head slightly toward the operative side.
3. Don sterile gloves.

4. Start the preparation at the eyelid. Prep in a circular pattern around the eye to within an inch of the hairline, including the nose, cheek, and jaw on the affected side. If the procedure includes both eyes, prep both sides of the face.
5. Do not allow preparation solutions to drain into the patient's ear. Iodophor and chlorhexidine solutions can cause severe damage to the middle ear. Although the tympanic membrane separates the external auditory canal from the middle ear, solutions may enter through a rupture or tear in the membrane. A cotton swab can be used to plug the external canal.
6. Discard each sponge after reaching the periphery of the prep area.
7. Repeat the prep using fresh sponges at least three times.
8. Rinse the prepped area using warm saline and cotton balls. Discard each used cotton ball and obtain a fresh one. Rinse the area at least twice.
9. Use a bulb syringe and small basin to flush the conjunctiva. Using one finger, pull the conjunctival sac slightly downward while flushing with normal saline solution or a solution ordered by the surgeon.
10. Blot any excess fluid from the periphery of the site with a sterile towel. Do not allow the towel to touch the prepared area.

EAR
Sterile Supplies
▶ Gloves
▶ Mild preparation solution such as triclosan or PCMX
▶ Normal saline
▶ Towels
▶ Small plastic drape with adhesive edge
▶ Cotton-tipped applicators

Procedure
1. Don sterile gloves.
2. Place a sterile plastic drape to exclude the eye on the affected side.
3. Do not use alcohol, iodophor, or chlorhexidine preparation solutions around the ear. Follow the surgeon's written order for the correct preparation solution.
4. If it is ordered, place an adhesive towel at the level of the cheek to protect the eye from preparation solution.
5. Cleanse and rinse the folds of the pinna (external ear) with cotton-tipped applicators.
6. Extend the prep area with sponges to the edge of the hairline, face, and jaw. Remember that the hair is a rich source of bacteria. Discard preparation sponges after they touch the hairline. Do not bring a sponge back over the previously prepped face or ear.

FACE
Apply only nonalcohol solutions to the face. Triclosan is a mild antiseptic commonly used in this area.

The hair contains a high concentration of bacteria. If the procedure is elective, the patient is asked to wash his or her hair with an antiseptic solution before surgery. Because of the rapid recolonization of bacteria, the hairline is still considered a contaminated area.

Sterile Supplies
▶ Gloves
▶ Nonalcohol preparation solution such as triclosan
▶ Warm normal saline
▶ Cotton swabs
▶ Cotton-tipped applicators
▶ Towels
▶ Comb and water-soluble hair gel (nonsterile supplies)

Procedure
1. Apply gel to the hair if necessary before combing it back away from the face. Use clips if necessary to hold the hair away from the face and ears.
2. Place a towel on each side of the neck to prevent water from dripping onto the bed sheet.
3. Don sterile gloves.
4. Prepare the face from the neck or chin up to the hairline. The ears may be included in the face preparation.
5. Cotton-tipped applicators are used to cleanse the folds of the pinna. Do not allow prep solution to drain into the ear canal.
6. Prep the face from the incision area outward. Prep the incision site again with fresh sponges. No prep sponge that touches the hairline should be brought back over the skin. Rinse the skin with cotton swabs dipped in warm normal saline solution.

NECK
The neck and throat area is prepared for thyroid surgery, tracheotomy, carotid artery surgery, lymph node biopsy, or radical dissection of the mandible, shoulder plexus, and mediastinum. If radical dissection is anticipated or scheduled, the preparation area extends from the chin to the nipple line or waist and around the side of the body to the operating table on each side (Figure 11-4).

Sterile Supplies
▶ Gloves
▶ Preparation solution
▶ Gauze sponges
▶ Towels

Procedure
1. Turn down the patient's gown to below the preparation area, according to the procedure.
2. Don sterile gloves. The patient's gown is considered contaminated, so do not touch it with gloved hands.
3. Place sterile towels at the periphery of the preparation site. Make a wide cuff in the towel and tuck it between the patient and the bed sheet.
4. Begin the prep at the midline of the throat, applying prep solution in a circular motion to the periphery of the

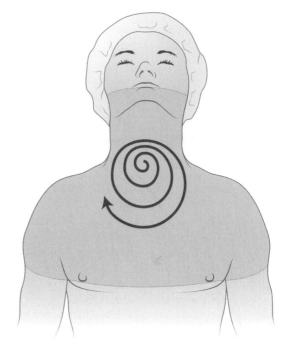

FIGURE 11-4
Neck and throat preparation.

preparation site. Discard each sponge after reaching the periphery.

BREAST AND THORACIC AREA
The breast is prepared for reconstructive surgery or removal of a mass or tumor. The boundaries of the preparation area depend on the extent of the surgery and patient position. In reconstructive surgery, the patient is in semi-Fowler or supine position. The preparation area is chin to umbilicus and around the side of the body to the operating table on each side.

When preparation is for removal of a mass without the possibility of more extensive surgery, the breast is prepped from the clavicle to the midthorax and from the midline around the side of the body to the operating table on the affected side. The prep area is extended into the axilla for lesions in the upper lateral quadrant of the breast.

Surgery that includes both a biopsy of a mass and the possibility of mastectomy requires a much wider preparation area. A radical mastectomy requires a preparation boundary that encompasses the neck, shoulder of the affected side, thorax to the operating table surface, and midpelvic region (Figure 11-5). If the patient is placed in lateral position, the back is also prepped to the level of the sacrum.

Tissue that is suspected to be cancerous must be prepared gently. The area should be painted with as little friction and pressure as possible. This is to prevent tumor cells from migrating into surrounding tissue (called *seeding*).

Skin preparation for surgery of the thoracic cavity uses a bilateral extension of the boundaries for radical breast surgery.

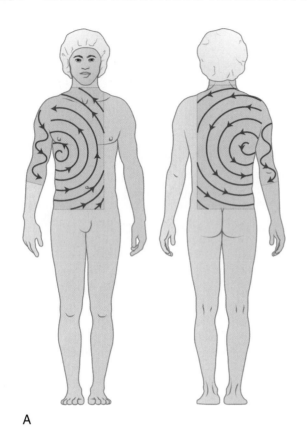

A

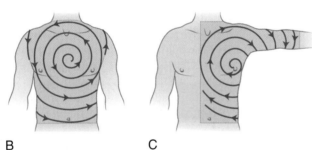

B   C

FIGURE 11-5
Thoracic and breast preparation. **A,** Lateral thoracic prep.
B, Sternal chest prep. **C,** Breast surgery prep. (**A** modified
from Phillips N: *Berry & Kohn's operating room technique,*
ed 10, St Louis, 2004, Mosby.)

Sterile Supplies
▶ Gloves
▶ Towels
▶ Preparation solution
▶ Cotton-tipped applicators

Procedure
1. Remove the patient's gown from the preparation area.
2. Don sterile gloves.
3. Square the preparation boundary with sterile towels.
4. If the umbilicus is included in the prep, clean it with cotton-tipped applicators.
5. Prep the operative area in keeping with the surgery to be performed.
6. If the shoulder is included in the prep, an assistant should abduct the arm so that solution can be applied circum-

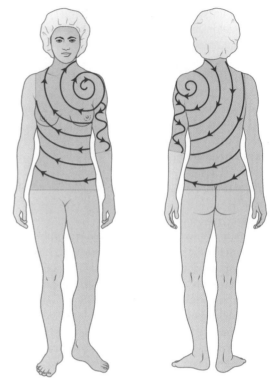

FIGURE 11-6
Shoulder preparation.(Modified from Phillips N: *Berry &
Kohn's operating room technique,* ed 10, St Louis, 2004,
Mosby.)

ferentially. Exercise caution to avoid dropping the arm or allowing it to dislocate.

SHOULDER
The shoulder preparation extends to the chest, neck and shoulder, upper arm, and scapula on the affected side (Figure 11-6). One assistant is required to elevate the patient's arm. The subscapular and midback area also may be elevated on a pad, depending on the surgeon's orders.

Sterile Supplies
▶ Gloves
▶ Preparation solution
▶ Gauze sponges
▶ Towels
▶ **Impervious** sheet

Procedure
1. Remove the patient's gown to the umbilicus.
2. Don sterile gloves.
3. Place sterile prep towels at the periphery of the preparation area.
4. Place an impervious sheet between the operating table and the subscapular area.
5. Have an assistant elevate the arm by holding the patient's hand and wrist.
6. The hand may be excluded from the preparation. Some surgeons wrap the hand in an occlusive drape after the prep.

7. *Do not pull the patient's shoulder laterally to expose the scapular area.* This can cause dislocation of the shoulder or further injury. Seek guidance from the surgeon about the exact nature of the injury or repair to prevent damage.
8. Begin the prep at the site of the incision and extend it to the boundaries in a circular path.

ARM

The full arm is prepared for most procedures of this limb. If the operative area is very small, the preparation may extend only to the joints nearest the operative site.

If Bier block anesthesia is used (discussed in Chapter 12), the entire arm usually is prepped because the block area also must be aseptically clean.

The hand is laden with transient and resident bacteria. It may be prepped but then excluded from the operative site by an occlusive drape. If the operative site is on the upper arm, the preparation might extend to the shoulder and axillary region.

In all cases, the arm must be prepped circumferentially. Two people are required to perform the prep. An assistant must hold the arm and hand away from the operating table while the surgical technologist performs the prep. The arm of an adult is quite heavy. If the arm is fractured or if pulling the arm up risks skeletal or soft-tissue damage, two people may be needed to hold the arm during the prep.

Arm preparation should not be attempted by only one person. This carries the risk of dropping the arm and dislocating the joints or avulsing the arm or hand (tearing away tissue parts).

Sterile Supplies
▶ Gloves (two pairs—one for the assistant)
▶ Preparation solution
▶ Preparation sponges
▶ Impervious sheet

Procedure
1. Don sterile gloves.
2. Elevate the arm carefully, keeping it in anatomical alignment.
3. Place an impervious sheet under the arm, covering the operating table and the patient's torso, to prevent preparation solution from dripping down the arm and soaking bed linen.
4. Using aseptic technique, place sterile towels under the shoulder or anywhere that solutions might pool under the patient.
5. Begin the preparation at the incision site and move outward, coating the arm on all sides as you move outward from the prep site. Discard sponges as they reach the periphery.
6. If the hand is included in the preparation, prep it first. It is the most contaminated area of the prep. The hand is prepped first and isolated with an impervious occlusive drape. Refer to the procedure for hand preparation in the next section.

7. Repeat the prep.
8. When the prepped area is dry, remove the impervious sheet and towels. Do not remove the towels or impervious sheet if the preparation solution is dripping.
9. Continue to elevate the arm during draping.

HAND

The hands require extra attention during preparation to treat the subungual area. The subungual is the area under the nails, which harbors debris and bacteria and must be scrubbed before surgery. If the surgery is elective, the patient should have been instructed to clean under the nails before surgery. However, an elderly, disabled, or trauma patient may arrive in surgery without prior nail cleansing.

The hand with trauma damage such as finger avulsion, crushing injuries, or other types of open wounds is usually prepped by the surgeon to preserve delicate nerves and blood vessels.

The routine hand preparation begins at the fingernails with a thorough cleaning (similar to the surgical hand scrub). After the hand is cleaned, prep solution is applied as usual, beginning at the incision site and moving outward and circumferentially. The upper boundary is a few inches above the elbow unless Bier block anesthesia is used (in which case upper arm preparation is required to the level of the tourniquet).

Sterile Supplies
▶ Gloves (two pairs—one for the assistant)
▶ Preparation solution
▶ Preparation soap
▶ Preparation sponges
▶ Nail cleaner
▶ Scrub brush
▶ Towels
▶ Impervious sheet

Procedure
1. Don sterile gloves.
2. Elevate the hand carefully, keeping it in anatomical alignment.
3. Place an impervious sheet under the arm and hand, covering the operating table and the patient's torso, to prevent prep solution from dripping down the arm and soaking bed linen.
4. Follow the surgeon's written orders regarding preparation solution. If it is ordered, scrub the hand gently, including the nails. Clean the subungual areas with a nail cleaner.
5. Blot the hand dry with sterile towels.
6. Beginning at the incisional area, apply preparation solution in the usual manner, moving outward. Include the interdigital spaces, fingertips, and all four sides of each finger.
7. Extend the prep to the arm, covering all sides.
8. Remove the impervious drape used for the prep, as the drape will be replaced when draping with a new sterile drape during the draping process.

9. Hold the hand until draping begins and the surgeon takes control of it.

ABDOMEN

The abdominal preparation extends from the nipple line to midthigh, and around the side of the body to the operating table on each side. This prep is used for all procedures of the abdominal cavity (Figure 11-7). If a pelvic laparoscopy is planned, a vaginal prep may be included. This is necessary if a uterine manipulator will be inserted into the cervix. Two separate preparation setups are necessary.

Sterile Supplies
▶ Gloves
▶ Towels
▶ Preparation sponges and sponge sticks
▶ Preparation solution
▶ Cotton-tipped applicators

Procedure
1. Remove the patient's gown to the level of the umbilicus.
2. Don sterile gloves.
3. Begin the preparation at the umbilicus. The folds and crevices of this area contain body secretions and bacteria, which must be removed before the abdominal preparation begins so that bacteria are not spread over the surgical site during the preparation.

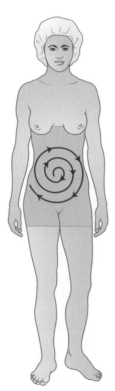

FIGURE 11-7
Abdominal preparation. (Redrawn from Phillips N: *Berry & Kohn's operating room technique,* ed 10, St Louis, 2004, Mosby.)

4. Prepping the umbilicus first seems to violate the rule of cleansing the most contaminated area last. In the case of the abdomen, the umbilicus must be rendered as clean as the rest of the abdomen. Because it is not an entrance to a hollow area or organ but simply a blind pouch, it can maintain a state of antisepsis throughout the surgery as long as it is thoroughly cleansed first.
5. After cleaning the umbilicus, get a new prep sponge and prep the abdomen, beginning at the incision site and move outward using circular strokes of the prep sponge. Discard the prep sponge when it reaches the preparation boundary.
6. Repeat the skin prep at least once more with clean prep sponges.
7. Remove the prep towels and examine the area to make sure that prep solution has not pooled under the patient.

FLANK OR BACK

The flank and back areas are prepped in the same manner as the abdomen, starting at the incision site and moving outward around the side of the body to the operating table on each side. An upper flank incision extends from the shoulder to the iliac crest, back, and midabdominal wall. The frontal prep boundary depends on accessibility in the lateral position. The back preparation extends from the neck to the sacrum with the patient in prone position.

Sterile Supplies
▶ Gloves
▶ Preparation solution
▶ Gauze sponges
▶ Towels
▶ Cotton-tipped applicators

Procedure
1. Remove the patient's gown and cover sheet to the iliac crest.
2. Don sterile gloves.
3. Square the periphery of the preparation site with sterile towels.
4. Begin at the incision area and apply prep solution in a circular pattern, continuing to the periphery. Complete this pattern at least twice, beginning again at the incision site and working outward to the surface of the operating table.
5. Allow prep solutions to dry before applying drapes.

VAGINAL AREA

The vaginal preparation is performed with the patient in the lithotomy position. The patient may be anesthetized or awake for the prep. If she is awake, normal saline and preparation solutions should be at room temperature. After the patient has been placed in lithotomy position, the lower table break is rotated downward. Before beginning the prep, place the sponge bucket at the foot of the table to receive used sponges. *Make sure that the patient's fingers are not in the table break. They can be crushed or amputated when the lower table section is rotated back to flat position.*

An impervious pocket drape may be placed under the buttocks to prevent prep solution from seeping between the coccyx and the table. The coccyx is a common site of chemical burns when the patient is in the lithotomy position. If a single impervious sheet is used, place the tail of the sheet in the sponge bucket to drain excess prep solution.

The vaginal prep is performed in two stages. The pelvis, labia, perineum, anus, and thighs are prepped as one stage, and the vaginal vault is prepped as a separate stage (Figure 11-8).

If the patient is having an abdominoperineal resection, in which a portion of the large intestine including the sigmoid colon and rectum is to be removed, the perineal area must be prepped separately from the abdomen. In this case, the *vaginal vault is not prepped* but all other aspects of the vaginal preparation are the same except that a separate abdominal preparation is added.

Sterile Supplies

▶ Gloves
▶ Preparation solution
▶ Sponge clamps
▶ Gauze sponges
▶ Impervious sheet
▶ Towels

Procedure

1. Fold the lower half of the patient's sheet or blanket onto the abdomen.
2. Don sterile gloves.
3. Start the preparation at the pubis, using *back-and-forth* strokes. This area is prepped to the level of the iliac crest.
4. Apply preparation solution at the labia majora using *downward strokes* only, including the perineum and anus. Discard the sponge after the anus is prepped. Do not return to the area previously prepped.
5. Using clean sponges, prep the inner aspects of the thighs. Start at the labia majora and move laterally, using back-and-forth strokes. Discard the sponge as it reaches the periphery. Remember not to return to previously prepped areas with the same sponge.

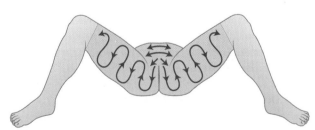

FIGURE 11-8
Vaginal preparation. (Redrawn from Phillips N: *Berry & Kohn's operating room technique,* ed 10, St Louis, 2004, Mosby.)

6. Prepare the vaginal vault last. Use sponges mounted on forceps and ample preparation solution to enter the folds of the vaginal rugae. Prepare the cervix and continue toward the exterior of the vagina, including all parts of the external genitalia. Discard the sponge and repeat.
7. Use a dry mounted sponge to blot excess fluid from the vaginal vault.
8. At this time, perform catheterization if it has been ordered.

PERIANAL AREA

The perianal preparation is performed with the patient in jackknife or knee-chest position. Because the anus is a contaminated area, the surrounding area is prepared first and the anus last. This preparation is used for minor rectal procedures such as hemorrhoidectomy, anal fistula repair, and removal of rectal lesions.

Sterile Supplies

▶ Gloves
▶ Preparation solution
▶ Sponge clamps
▶ Gauze sponges

Procedure

1. Remove the patient's gown and cover sheet to expose the lower trunk. Keep the patient's legs and upper body covered.
2. Don sterile gloves.
3. Begin the preparation outside the anal mucosa and extend the prep area outward about 12 inches in all directions.
4. Prep the anus. Do not penetrate the anus itself. In some institutions anal prep is omitted.

LEG AND FOOT

Leg preparation is similar to that of the arm. The boundaries of the leg preparation are from the ankle to the groin (Figure 11-9). The limb must be elevated by an assistant. Alternatively, the leg may be placed in a special leg holder, which is a vertical table attachment with a U-shaped segment that holds the leg up and off the table. Use a leg holder with extreme caution, because it can cause serious injuries. If the leg holder is not strong enough to support the leg of a heavy patient, it can rotate or slip, causing dislocation, avulsion, and severe soft-tissue injury. One of the most common problems with the leg holder is failure to tighten the attachment securely. This causes the vertical section to slip down, taking the leg with it.

The lower extremity is prepared in the same fashion; however, different areas are prepped for the knee and hip.

For knee surgery, prep the entire leg, but wrap the foot in an occlusive drape before surgery.

Hip surgery requires circumferential prep from the midcalf to the iliac crest, excluding the groin (Figure 11-10).

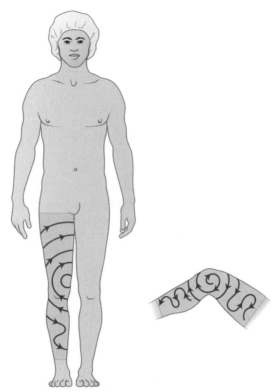

FIGURE 11-9
Leg preparation. (Redrawn from Phillips N: *Berry & Kohn's operating room technique*, ed 10, St Louis, 2004, Mosby.)

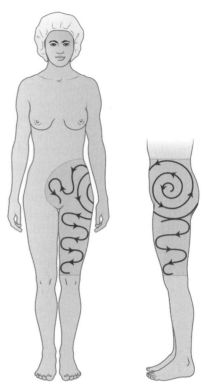

FIGURE 11-10
Hip preparation. (Modified from Phillips N: *Berry & Kohn's operating room technique*, ed 10, St Louis, 2004, Mosby.)

Sterile Supplies
▶ Gloves (two pairs—one for the assistant)
▶ Preparation solution
▶ Preparation soap
▶ Preparation sponges
▶ Nail cleaner (foot)
▶ Scrub brush (foot)
▶ Impervious sheet

Procedure
1. Remove the patient's blanket to the level of the groin, keeping the upper body covered.
2. Don sterile gloves.
3. Place a towel between the groin and the fold of the upper leg to prevent solution from seeping into this area. Severe burns can result if solution collects here.
4. Have an assistant elevate the leg (or use a leg holder).
5. Place an impervious sheet under the leg and over the patient's nonoperative leg. The drape should be tucked under the patient's buttock on the operative side.
6. If the foot is to be included in the prep, scrub it as you would a hand. Remember that because the leg is elevated, the preparation must begin at the highest level and move to the lowest level circumferentially.
7. If the foot is excluded from the preparation, perform wide skin preparation around the operative site.

8. At the conclusion of the preparation, make sure that no preparation solution can drip into the groin area. Keep the leg elevated until draping has started.

PREPARATION IN TRAUMA CASES
Patients who have been injured and who have penetrating and open fractures, or who have metal fragments or other foreign objects protruding from the wound, are usually prepped by the surgeon. The entire site is contaminated, and small pieces of bone and foreign material must be washed from the wound. A pressurized water system may be used to clean the wound. This requires a system for collecting runoff. Specialized drapes with drainage pouches that attach to suction are commercially available. During the cleansing process, the surgeon removes all foreign material and trims away devitalized tissue. This is called **debridement** and requires forceps and small tissue scissors. The surgical technologist should collect any foreign bodies and place them in a cup or basin. After debridement the wound may be surgically prepared and sterile drapes may be applied.

SKIN GRAFT SITE PREPARATION
The collection site for a skin autograft (graft taken from the patient's own body) is prepped with clear solution. This is necessary to maintain a clear view of the vascular bed of the graft. Because iodophor preparations leave a brown stain on

the skin, alternative solutions must be used. Two sites are prepared separately with two skin preparation kits.

PATIENT DRAPING

Draping Materials and Supplies

Drapes are made of woven (cotton or cotton-synthetic blend) or nonwoven (synthetic) material. Sterile drapes must produce a moisture barrier between the patient and the sterile field. Nonwoven drapes are commercially prepared single-use items. They are impervious to moisture and breathable to prevent the patient from becoming hyperthermic. Many different types of nonwoven draping materials are available, designed for specific uses according to type of surgery.

Woven cotton and cotton-blend drapes are reinforced around the fenestration and chemically treated for moisture resistance to help prevent strike-through contamination. They are more pliable and easier to handle than nonwoven drapes but require laundering and repair. Whenever woven drapes are used, extra precautions are needed to prevent penetration with irrigation solutions and blood during surgery.

SURGICAL TOWELS

Towels are used in nearly every draping procedure. They are arranged to frame the incision site. This is called *squaring off* the incision. Towels are made of fabric or synthetic nonwoven material (single use). Single-use towel drapes have an adhesive strip along one border. When handing self-adhesive drapes to the surgeon, hold them with the sticky side facing your body. Woven towels are folded over at the top edge and handed to the surgeon so that the fold will lie against the patient's body. Towels are held in place with nonpenetrating towel clips or an adhesive drape.

PROCEDURE DRAPE

The procedure drape is sized and shaped to fit a specific area of the patient's body. A reinforced window called a *fenestration* is centered over the incision site, and the drape is unfolded so as to maintain the position of the drape. Many different **fenestrated drapes** are available, each designed so that the fenestration is located in the proper position in relation to the rest of the body. Procedure drapes are folded in a way that centers the fenestration within the folds. The fenestration is placed directly onto the incision site, correctly oriented to the patient's head and feet. The drape is then opened out fold by fold. Disposable drapes usually are marked with pictures to indicate proper alignment and placement, and also are marked with arrows to indicate the order in which the drapes should be unfolded.

The *laparotomy drape* covers the patient's body and may include extensions for arm boards. It has a single reinforced fenestration (Figure 11-11, *A*).

The U-shaped drape or *split sheet* is a square drape designed to cover the patient or the surgical table on one end and wrap around the patient's limb at the other (Figure 11-11, *B*). When the drape is opened out, the split divides the drape into two sides or "tails." Single-use split drapes have a self-adherent strip along the edge of the tails.

The *craniotomy drape* may be split and includes a small round fenestration for the skull (Figure 11-11, *C*).

The *lithotomy drape* is a large fenestrated drape that fits over the patient's body, exposing only the perineal area (Figure 11-11, *D*). Some lithotomy drapes contain inserts for the legs. Separate leggings are used in conjunction with a simple fenestrated body drape.

The *eye drape* is a small fenestrated sheet (Figure 11-11, *E*). A similar drape is used for ear surgery. A larger body sheet usually is used with these drapes.

The *tube stockinette* is a rolled stocking made of stretch muslin and usually is lined with impervious plastic. One applies it by placing the rolled stocking over the limb and unrolling it to cover the patient's skin. After application of the stockinette, a U-shaped drape or split sheet is applied.

Plain sheets are nonfenestrated drapes that are used to extend the sterile field or are placed under a limb. These are available in different sizes according to need.

Incise drapes are self-adhering plastic sheets that are placed directly over the incision site. Incise drapes are either clear in appearance or impregnated with iodine for additional antiseptic protection. The incision is made directly through the drape and into skin and deeper tissue. These drapes are available in many different shapes and sizes. One commonly used plastic drape is self-adherent along one folded side of the drape only. This drape is used as a barrier (**barrier drape**). For example, when the patient is in lithotomy position, the adherent towel drape is placed along the superior edge of the anus to separate it from the vagina.

Aluminum-coated drapes are employed when lasers are in use, especially around the head and neck, to help prevent ignition in the presence of oxygen. No drape is fireproof if exposed to laser energy. Wet towels must be placed over an impervious drape for protection from fire.

Draping Techniques

The specific drapes used and the order in which they are applied vary according to the procedure planned, the rules of asepsis, and the surgeon's preference. After the principles and techniques of draping are understood, one can apply any combination of drapes successfully.

The rules of asepsis are followed throughout all draping procedures. When draping, visualize the drape as having two surfaces—one that contacts the patient and one that becomes part of the sterile field. To prevent contamination of sterile surfaces during draping, review the rules of asepsis and apply them to draping technique. Use these guidelines for draping:

▶ Handle drapes with as little movement as possible. Open them by layers. This reduces the risk of contamination and prevents release of airborne particles that can become vehicles for bacteria.

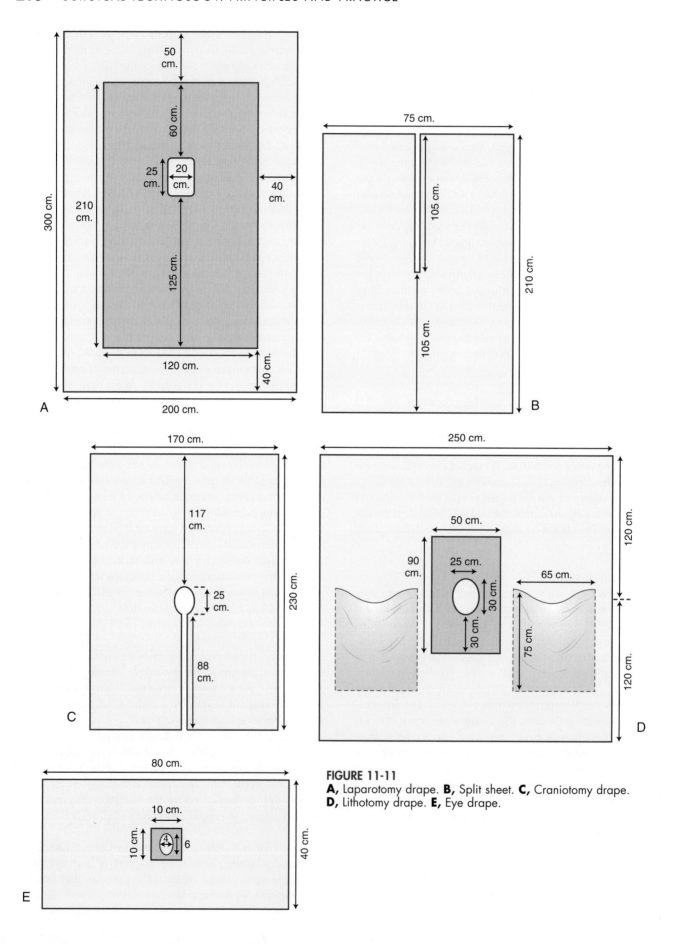

FIGURE 11-11
A, Laparotomy drape. **B,** Split sheet. **C,** Craniotomy drape.
D, Lithotomy drape. **E,** Eye drape.

▶ Always make sure that the preparation site is dry before applying drapes. Prep solutions should be allowed to dry on their own, as duration of contact is important for adequate microbicidal activity. Wet preparation solution can ignite and cause patient fire. Incise drapes or drapes with adhesive strips do not adhere to wet surfaces.

▶ When placing a drape, do not touch the patient's body or any other nonsterile surface. Remain a safe distance from the patient to avoid contamination of your gown.

▶ After a drape has been placed, do not shift or move the drape. To protect the gloved hand during draping with flat sheets, grasp the edge of the sterile sheet and roll your hand inward. This forms a cuff. Position the drape and release the edge of the cuff, keeping your hands on the sterile side of the drape or towel.

▶ Use only nonpenetrating towel clamps for draping. A hole in a drape allows a passageway for bacteria to contaminate the sterile field. When drapes are stapled to the patient's skin, the stapled area should be covered by an impervious drape.

▶ After a drape has been placed, remember that any portion that falls below the edge of the operating table is considered contaminated. If an area of the drape is suspected of being contaminated, the area may be covered with another impervious sterile drape, or, depending on the circumstances, the drape may need to be replaced.

▶ After a drape has been placed, remember that the edges are considered nonsterile.

▶ Remember that strike-through contamination occurs when a drape becomes soaked during surgery and solution penetrates to a nonsterile surface. Whenever possible, use only impervious drapes. If these are not available, an impervious sterile sheet must be placed between the sterile field and the drape.

▶ If necessary, use special, commercially prepared drapes that are fitted with a pocket reservoir and drainage system for use in cases in which runoff from bleeding or excess solutions is anticipated during the surgery. Orthopedic and gynecological procedures are two examples. These drapes must be oriented so that runoff is directed into the collection system.

Before surgery, plan ahead for draping. Verify the surgeon's procedure at the start of draping and stack drapes on the back table in reverse order of application. Have extra sterile towels and sheets available but unopened in case they are needed during draping.

Three common techniques for draping are torso draping, extremity draping, and lithotomy draping. Most areas of the body can be draped with the techniques employed in these three procedures.

TORSO, FLANK, AND BACK DRAPING

The procedure for draping the abdomen can be used to drape many other surgical sites when a fenestrated sheet is to be centered over the surgical site (Figure 11-12). Follow these steps:

1. Unfold towels carefully to avoid spreading particles in the air.
2. Remove strips from the adhesive portion of nonwoven towels.
3. Keep a safe distance from the nonsterile surfaces of the operating table and patient.
4. Place the cuffed towel at the edges of the incision site without touching the patient's skin or contaminating your gown.
5. After the towels are in place, do not move them.
6. Remember that if towel clamps are used, only nonpenetrating types are permitted. Some surgeons use skin staples to secure the towels.
7. Place an adherent incise drape over the towels. Two people are required to perform this step. One person holds one end of the drape while the other pulls the paper backing away.
8. Make sure one person smooths the plastic drape over the contours of the patient's skin. The incise drape also may be placed over the fenestrated drape.
9. To apply the body sheet, place the fenestration over the incision site.
10. Fanfold body or procedure drapes so they can be unfolded easily over the patient.
11. Make a cuff in the drape to protect your sterile glove.
12. Do not drop the drape over the table edge until the patient is covered. After the procedure drape is in place, it may not be moved.
13. When using paper drapes, one should consider the protective removable paper covering the incision site to be contaminated and remove it from the field by touching

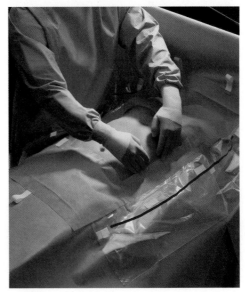

FIGURE 11-12
Torso draping. (© Kimberly-Clark Worldwide, Inc. Used with permission.)

only the outer (top) surface, after the drape has been applied.

EXTREMITY DRAPING

During preparation and draping of an extremity, the limb must be held up and away from the operating table. Two people are needed to perform this procedure. After the skin is prepared, draping begins immediately while the limb is still suspended (Figure 11-13, *A* and *B*). The use of limb holders is discouraged because of the potential for neural and vascular damage. Follow these steps for extremity draping:

1. The circulator holds the limb while the surgeon or assistant applies preparation solution to the lower limb. A sterile impervious sheet is placed under the limb.

2. With the limb still suspended, a sterile team member places an impervious stockinette over the foot or hand, depending on the extremity being draped. It is placed over the foot or hand first to isolate bacteria from the nails.

3. A U-shaped drape is wrapped around the proximal portion of the limb. Nonwoven drapes adhere to the skin.

4. The limb is placed through the fenestrated sheet, and the sheet is draped over the body.

5. When extensive irrigation or blood loss is expected, a sack drape with a drainage system is attached below the limb.

6. After draping is completed, if a pneumatic tourniquet is required for the procedure, the scrub elevates the limb and the surgeon wraps it in a flexible Esmarch bandage from distal to proximal end (Figure 11-3, *C*). This pushes

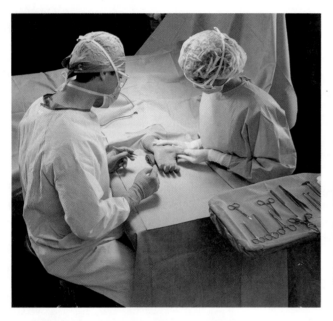

A

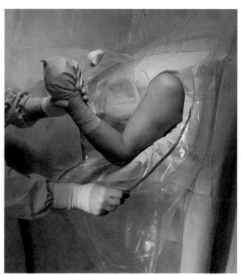

B

FIGURE 11-13
A, Hand draping. **B,** Shoulder draping. **C,** Use of an Esmarch bandage. (**A** and **B** from © Kimberly-Clark Worldwide, Inc. Used with permission.)

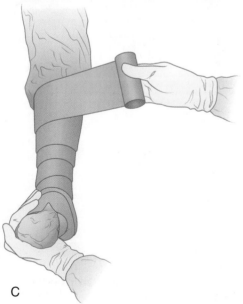

C

blood out of the limb toward the heart. The pneumatic tourniquet is then inflated, and the Esmarch bandage is removed. This produces a bloodless surgical field. Refer to Chapter 15 for discussion of the procedure and risks associated with use of the pneumatic tourniquet.

LITHOTOMY DRAPING

A patient in the lithotomy position often is awake during the surgical procedure. Always respect the patient's modesty. Do not expose the patient unnecessarily.

Lithotomy draping may require isolation of the anal area from the rest of the surgical site (Figure 11-14). Follow these steps for lithotomy draping:

1. An impervious drape is placed under the patient's buttocks to begin draping. Be careful not to contaminate your gown or the sleeves of your gown on the unprepped legs of the patient as you place your cuffed hands under the edge of the drape.
2. The bottom of this drape may be placed in the sponge bucket. Alternatively, a drainage bag drape may be used to collect blood and fluids.
3. A barrier between the anus and the vaginal vault may be created. If a barrier drape is used, a small plastic drape with an adhesive edge is placed across the perineum.
4. Leggings are used to cover the patient's legs in stirrups. Maintain a wide cuff over your hand as you apply the leggings. If the patient is in high lithotomy position, be careful not to contaminate your gown as you bring the leggings over the top of the foot.
5. A fenestrated body sheet is centered over the perineal area and extended over the patient's abdomen and upper body. The top is secured to the anesthesia screen.

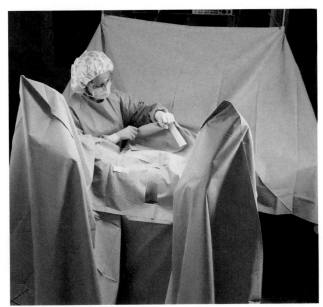

FIGURE 11-14
Lithotomy draping. (© Kimberly-Clark Worldwide, Inc. Used with permission.)

6. Many patients are uneasy and uncomfortable in this position. Offering comfort and reassurance is an important role of the circulator.

HEAD DRAPING

The **head drape** occasionally is used in procedures of the nose and throat. It protects the eyes during surgery and produces a sterile barrier over the head. The surgical technologist creates the head drape with two towels or plain draping sheets. The head is slightly elevated, and both towels are placed under the patient's head as shown in Figure 11-15. One brings the top towel over the face using aseptic technique. Each corner of the towel is brought to the center over the hairline, well back from the eyes, and secured with a nonpenetrating towel clamp. The head drape resembles a turban when completed and secured.

Removing Drapes

At the close of a procedure, all instruments and equipment are removed from the top drape. Make certain that nothing prevents the drapes from being removed smoothly, such as towel clamps, cords, or other objects connected to air hoses,

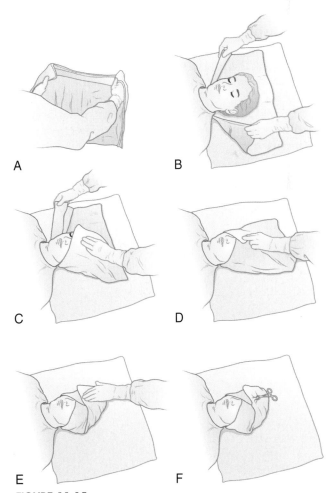

FIGURE 11-15
A to **F,** Application of the head drape. The corners of the towel must be handled carefully to avoid contamination.

electrosurgical equipment, and other devices. The surgeon places sterile dressings over incisions and any drain sites and holds them in place while the drapes are removed. When removing the drapes, pull them slowly away from the patient, starting at the patient's head and proceeding downward. Remove one layer at a time. Be careful not to dislodge any wound drains. Drapes should be contained with as little movement as possible, with the ends wrapped toward the inside to confine blood and body fluids to the inner surface. The drapes then are placed in a biohazard disposal bag. The circulator tapes the dressings in place and connects all wound drainage systems.

CASE STUDIES

Case 1

You are scrubbed on a gynecological procedure with the patient in the lithotomy position. As you observe the circulator preparing the patient, you see that he is using alcohol for the vaginal vault. Will you say anything? How will you handle this situation, knowing that you are part of the team and must protect the patient from injury? What would stop you from saying anything?

Case 2

The patient is brought from the emergency department with multiple traumas. These include a possible ruptured spleen and penetrating fracture of the tibia. The procedures to address these injuries will be performed simultaneously. How do you think this patient should be draped?

Case 3

After bringing the patient to the operating room, you are asked to perform a urinary catheterization. You have never performed one. Do you proceed?

Case 4

You are asked to prepare the patient for a laparotomy with iodophor. You complete the preparation, satisfied that you have taken all precautions to prevent a burn. Draping already has started. You happen to notice that the patient's chart states that the patient is allergic to iodine. What should be done?

Case 5

You have prepared a laparotomy patient with iodophor. When the drapes are removed after surgery, a large blistered area is discovered under the patient's flank. What will you do? What will be the consequences and ramifications of this burn?

Chapter 12

Anesthesia

Learning Objectives

After studying this chapter the reader will be able to:

- Describe the types of anesthesia care providers and their training
- Describe the information that is obtained in the preoperative assessment and explain why this information is necessary
- List the categories of the American Society of Anesthesiologists classification system and give an example of a patient in each category
- Explain why preoperative fasting is important
- List and describe biophysical monitoring devices and procedures
- Describe inhalation anesthesia
- Differentiate among analgesia, sedation, unconsciousness, and amnesia
- Differentiate among levels of consciousness
- Explain why gas scavenging is necessary
- List the physiological requirements for surgery
- Describe the physiology of nerve transmission and the way the body responds to stimuli
- Discuss intravascular fluid balance and the way in which it is achieved during surgery
- Describe the surgical technologist's possible tasks during a cardiopulmonary arrest in surgery
- Describe the circulating surgical technologist's role during an episode of malignant hyperthermia
- Identify the role of the scrub when assisting the surgeon during injection of local anesthesia
- Recognize early signs of central nervous system toxicity
- Describe the risks of anesthetics, including cardiovascular and central nervous system complications

Terminology

Amnesia—Loss of recall of events or sensations. In anesthesia, amnesia is a desirable component produced by specific drugs such as the benzodiazepines. Patient recall of surgery is seen in about 0.2% of all cases performed under general anesthesia.

Analgesia—The absence of pain, produced by specific drugs.

Anesthesia—Literally, "without sensation." In medicine, anesthetic agents block nerve impulses that conduct sensation; these agents also may produce loss of consciousness.

Anesthesia care provider (ACP)—A professional licensed to administer anesthetic agents and medically manage the patient throughout the period of anesthesia.

Anesthesia machines—Machines that are capable of delivering anesthetic gases or volatile liquids. An anesthesia machine delivers titrated amounts of an agent mixed with oxygen. Positive pressure ventilation can be controlled mechanically with a ventilator or manually with a bag and mask. The device monitors the patient's vital physiological signs, such as heart rate, heart rhythm, oxygen saturation, and carbon dioxide level.

Anesthesiologist—A physician who is a specialist in anesthesia and pain management.

Anesthetic—A drug that produces a lack of sensation. A general anesthetic produces a state of unconsciousness, while a regional anesthetic blocks nerve conduction in a specific area of the body without producing loss of consciousness.

Antagonist—A term used to describe a drug that is designed to counteract the effects of another agent.

Terminology—cont'd

Anterograde amnesia—In anesthesia, the patient's inability to recall events that occur while under the effects of certain drugs. After the drug is metabolized in the body, normal recall returns.

Anxiolysis—Reduction in anxiety.

Apnea—Cessation of breathing.

Bier block—Regional anesthesia administered by intravenous injection, used for surgical procedures performed on the arm below the elbow or on the leg below the knee; performed in a bloodless field maintained by a pneumatic tourniquet that also prevents the anesthetic from entering the systemic circulation.

Bronchospasm—An involuntary smooth muscle spasm of the bronchi. Like laryngospasm, it can occur as a complication of anesthesia. Patients with a difficult airway, anatomical malformation, and bronchiole disease are prone to bronchospasm. Certain anesthetic agents cause bronchospasm and laryngospasm.

Certified registered nurse anesthetist (CRNA)—A registered nurse trained and licensed to administer anesthetic agents.

Controlled hypothermia—Deliberate lowering of the patient's core body temperature during general anesthesia in selected cases. This reduces the oxygen requirements of tissues. It can be used in cardiac surgery, procedures that require occlusion or blockage of large blood vessels, and organ transplantation.

Cricoid pressure—Direct manual pressure on the patient's cricoid cartilage, which compresses the trachea, helps to prevent aspiration, and can facilitate intubation.

Delirium—A state of confusion and disorientation. Delirium is a stage of anesthesia induction that produces struggling, coughing, gagging, and possible airway obstruction resulting from bronchospasm or laryngospasm. Delirium, on induction, is seldom observed with the use of modern induction drugs that rapidly bypass this stage.

Drug—Chemical substance that, when taken into the body, changes one or more of the body's functions.

Emergence—A stage in general anesthesia in which delivery of the anesthetic agents is stopped. The patient emerges from a state of unconsciousness into a state of wakefulness. Emergence can be an unstable period that is similar to induction except that physiological and somatic events occur in reverse order.

Endotracheal tube—A hollow airway inserted into the patient's trachea to maintain patency and allow delivery of oxygen and anesthetic gases.

Esmarch bandage—A roller bandage made of rubber or latex. It is wrapped around a limb starting at the distal end and extending to the proximal end. The bandage pushes blood away from the limb. A pneumatic tourniquet located at the proximal end is then inflated to prevent the return flow of blood into the extremity. See *Bier block* above.

Gas scavenging—The capture and safe removal of anesthetic gases that escape from the anesthesia machine and other devices such as a patient face mask. Repeated exposure to anesthetic gases is known to be a risk to surgical personnel. The Occupational Safety and Health Administration and the Joint Commission for the Accreditation of Healthcare Organizations require effective scavenging systems.

General anesthesia—Anesthesia associated with a state of unconsciousness. General anesthesia is not a fixed state of unconsciousness but ranges along a continuum from semiresponsive to profoundly unresponsive.

Homeostasis—A state of balance between the body's environmental and physiological stimuli and its responses. Homeostasis is maintained through the body's intricate feedback systems. For example, when blood volume decreases, the heart rate increases to push available blood more efficiently.

Induced hypotension—The deliberate lowering of the patient's blood pressure during surgery to control hemorrhage, produce a more bloodless operative field, or control intracranial pressure.

Induction—The time from the beginning of administration of an anesthetic agent until the patient reaches the sur-

gical level of loss of consciousness. Sensation is lost, and the patient is unaware of the environment.

Intubation—The process of inserting an endotracheal tube. Insertion requires adequate muscle relaxation to prevent spasms of the larynx and pharynx. Endotracheal intubation is performed after anesthesia induction.

Laryngeal mask airway (LMA)—An airway consisting of a tube and small mask that is fitted internally over the patient's larynx. It has advantages over an endotracheal tube in that it does not require the use of muscle relaxants to facilitate insertion and it can be used in a patient whose anatomy makes endotracheal intubation technically difficult.

Laryngoscope—A lighted instrument consisting of a blade and removable handle or a fiberoptic light. It is used to assist in endotracheal intubation. The lighted end of the laryngoscope allows direct visualization of the airway to facilitate correct positioning of the endotracheal tube. After the endotracheal tube is in place, the laryngoscope is gently withdrawn.

Laryngospasm—Involuntary spasm of the smooth muscles of the larynx. Some drugs cause laryngospasm, and some patients are prone to spasm because of a medical or anatomical condition. Severe laryngospasm can restrict or block the patient's airway. It can occur during intubation, during induction and emergence from deep sedation, or in periods of relatively light anesthesia.

Malignant hyperthermia—A rare condition that occurs in conjunction with general anesthesia. The patient experiences extremely high body temperature, muscle rigidity, seizures, and cardiac arrhythmia. The condition is reversible with specific drugs and management of symptoms but can be fatal if left untreated. Patients with a history of muscular disease are particularly at risk for malignant hyperthermia. Most general anesthetic inhalation agents carry a risk of producing malignant hyperthermia.

Terminology—cont'd

Medication—A naturally occurring substance or a chemical compound (drug) that is used to treat a specific condition.

Neuromuscular blocking agents—Drugs that block conduction of nerves that control striated muscle tissue. Muscle relaxation or paralysis may be needed to allow access to the operative site during general anesthesia.

Patent—Open or unobstructed, in reference to a tubular or hollow structure. It is usually used to describe the patient's airway, a blood vessel, or a duct.

Pneumatic tourniquet—A balloon cuff similar to a blood pressure cuff in design. The pneumatic tourniquet is used to produce a bloodless operative site or to prevent blood flow to an extremity

for injection with local anesthetic in a procedure called a Bier block.

Pulse oximeter—A device that measures the patient's hemoglobin oxygen saturation through the use of spectrometry.

Regional block—Anesthesia and analgesia of a specific area of the body. Regional blocks may be produced by interruption of impulses of one major nerve or a group of nerves. Adjunct drugs usually are administered to sedate and provide anxiolysis.

Sedatives—Agents that induce a state of sedation. The depth of sedation is controlled by the administration of specific agents. Levels of sedation range from slight calming to unconsciousness in which the patient is unrespon-

sive even to repeated deep, painful stimulation.

Synergistic—Term used to describe two drugs that, when combined, produce an effect that is greater than the sum of the effects produced by each drug acting separately.

Ventilation—Movement of gases into and out of the lungs. Positive pressure ventilation is produced by the anesthesia care provider when deep general anesthesia and neuromuscular blocking agents inhibit the patient's normal breathing mechanisms. The reservoir bag on the anesthesia machine allows the anesthesia care provider to manually force oxygen or gases into the patient's lungs. This is called "bagging" the patient.

ANESTHESIA CARE PROVIDER

Training of the ACP

The **anesthesia care provider** (ACP) is a professional trained to administer **anesthetic** agents, perform physiologic monitoring, and respond to anesthetic and surgical emergencies.

An ACP can be trained and certified through several different processes. An **anesthesiologist** is a medical doctor with additional training in the specialty of **anesthesia**. A registered nurse who also holds a Bachelor of Science degree in nursing may enter a nurse anesthetist program after 1 year of acute-care nursing. The **certified registered nurse anesthetist** (CRNA) program requires at least 2 years of specialty training in anesthesia. The final degree conferred may be a master's-level degree, through a school of nursing or allied health, or CRNA credentialing through community-based hospital programs.

A physician's assistant may become an anesthesiologist's assistant (AA). He or she must hold a Bachelor of Science degree and have completed a 2-year training course at an approved medical school offering the AA degree.

Specialty areas within the field of anesthesia care include chronic pain management and clinical anesthesia specialties such as obstetric, cardiac, pediatric, and ambulatory anesthesia.

Role of the ACP

The role of the ACP during surgery is to do the following:

- Manage the patient's pain.
- Maintain **homeostasis.**
- Monitor and document all drugs and agents delivered to the patient.

- Establish, protect, and maintain the patient's airway at all times.
- Communicate with the surgeon about the patient's responses to intraoperative stimuli. This includes communicating information on hemodynamic changes, fluid and electrolyte balance, level of muscle relaxation, and level of consciousness.
- Respond to any surgical or anesthetic emergency.

The primary role of the ACP is to manage the patient's physiologic responses to surgery and to protect the patient from injury. The ACP continually assesses and monitors the patient's physiologic and physical responses to surgery. The only information available to the ACP is measurable or observable responses to the surgical process.

Collaboration and communication between the ACP and the surgeon are essential. The surgeon gives information to the ACP about the patient's physical responses during surgery, such as level of muscle relaxation, hemostasis, and movement. The ACP communicates information to the surgeon about intravascular pressure, oxygen saturation, cardiovascular status, and other physiologic parameters. All work together to maintain an appropriate anesthetic level and homeostasis.

PREOPERATIVE PATIENT CARE

Patient Assessment

When *any* anesthetic administration is planned, the ACP assesses the patient one to several days before surgery. He or she interviews and examines the patient to determine the patient's specific needs and risk factors for anesthesia. The assessment must consider the components described in the following sections. A sample pre-anesthetic evaluation (Fig-

Addressograph

Breath Sounds

A - Absent ☐
C - Clear ☐
D - Decreased ☐
R - Rales ☐
RH - Rhonchi ☐
W - Wheezes ☐
SNN - See Nurses Notes ☐

P.S.S. VITAL SIGNS BP_____ P_____ R_____ T_____ SaO₂_____ (presedative room air)

VITAL SIGNS BP_____ P_____ R_____ T_____ SaO₂_____ (presedative room air)

DATE:_____ TIME:_____

PRE-ANESTHETIC EVALUATION

PRIMARY PHYSICIAN/SURGEON:

PRE-OP DIAGNOSIS:

SCHEDULED OPERATION:

MEDICATIONS:

CIGARETTES: ☐ QUIT SMOKING _____
ETOH:
DRUG ABUSE: _____

REMARKS / FAMILY HEALTH HISTORY:

CARDIOVASCULAR: ☐ ASHD ☐ CHF ☐ H.V.D.
☐ ANGINA ☐ ORTHOPNEA ☐ VALVULAR DISEASE
☐ PREV. M.I. ☐ EDEMA ☐ MVP
☐ ARRHYTHMIA ☐ CYANOSIS ☐ OTHER
☐ THROMBOEMBOLISM ☐ PVD ☐ NEG

RESPIRATORY: ☐ PNEUMONIA ☐ COPD ☐ TRACHEOSTOMY
☐ URI ☐ COUGH ☐ ASTHMA
☐ SOB AT REST ☐ BRONCHITIS ☐ OTHER
☐ SOB W/EXERTION ☐ WHEEZING ☐ NEG

NEUROLOGIC: ☐ SYNCOPE ☐ TIA ☐ LOW BACK PAIN
☐ SEIZURES ☐ COMATOSE ☐ OTHER
☐ CVA ☐ NEUROPATHY ☐ NEG

ENDOCRINE/METABOLIC/RENAL/ HEPATIC: ☐ CIRRHOSIS ☐ DIABETES
☐ ANEMIA ☐ HEPATITIS ☐ HYPOGLYCEMIA
☐ BLEEDING ☐ JAUNDICE ☐ OTHER
☐ SICKLE CELL ☐ CRF ☐ NEG

OTHER: ☐ HIATAL HERNIA ☐ FULL STOMACH ☐ PREGNANCY
☐ H/O MH-FAM ☐ PSYCHIATRIC ☐ NEG

PREVIOUS SURGERIES:
☐ NONE

PREVIOUS ANESTHETIC COMPLICATIONS:
☐ NO KNOWN FAMILY HISTORY OF ANESTHESIA COMPLICATIONS
☐ NONE

REASSESSED IMMEDIATELY PREOP ☐
COMMENTS:

NPO since _____

P.E. AIRWAY MALLAMPATI CLASS 1 2 3 4

ROM: NECK:
TEETH: ☐ DENTURES ☐ CAPS ☐ LOOSE TEETH ☐ CHIPS ☐ RAGGED DENTAL EDGE ☐ PERMANENT BRIDGE
LUNGS:
HEART:
NEURO:

LABS: HGB:_____ ECG ☐ NORMAL
☐ ABNORMAL
HCT:_____ CXR ☐ NORMAL
☐ ABNORMAL
Na+:_____ SMA ☐
K+:_____ CREATININE_____
FBS:_____ PT_____
DOS:_____ PTT_____
PREG TEST: ☐ NEGATIVE
☐ POSITIVE

ASA CLASSIFICATION
1 2 3 4 5 6 E

PROPOSED ANESTHESIA
☐ REGIONAL
☐ IV ☐ EPIDURAL
☐ SPINAL ☐ OTHER
☐ GENERAL
☐ LOCAL W/ SEDATION
☐ LOC/GENERAL
☐ RAPID SEQUENCE INDUCTION

PROPOSED MONITORING
☐ A-LINE
☐ CVP
☐ SWAN

☐ PATIENT CONFUSED, UNABLE TO INTERVIEW
☐ PATIENT RELATIVE INTERVIEWED
☐ RELATIVE UNAVAILABLE
☐ MINOR - MOTHER OR FATHER INTERVIEWED

RISKS/BENEFITS: ☐ DISCUSSED AND UNDERSTOOD
☐ ALL QUESTIONS ANSWERED

SIGNATURE _____

FIGURE 12-1
Sample pre-anesthetic evaluation. (Courtesy of St. Joseph's Mercy of Macomb, Clinton Township, Mich.)

ure 12-1) is used, in addition to the assessment and plan of care flowsheet for the surgery patient (see Figure 2-1).

AMERICAN SOCIETY OF ANESTHESIOLOGISTS STATUS

The American Society of Anesthesiologists (ASA) has developed a risk-assessment system that classifies patients accord-

ing to their individual potential for anesthesia-related problems. This classification system is shown in Box 12-1.

HISTORY OF ADVERSE REACTIONS TO ANESTHETICS

A previous reaction to anesthetics and other medications increases the patient's risk for an adverse or unexpected reac-

Box 12-1 American Society of Anesthesiologists Classification System

ASA 1	The patient is normal and healthy.
ASA 2	The patient has mild systemic disease that does not limit his or her activities (e.g., controlled hypertension or controlled diabetes without systemic sequelae).
ASA 3	The patient has moderate or severe systemic disease that does limit his or her activities (e.g., stable angina or diabetes with systemic sequelae).
ASA 4	The patient has severe systemic disease that is a constant potential threat to life (e.g., severe congestive heart failure, end-stage renal failure).
ASA 5	The patient is morbid and is at substantial risk of death within 24 hours, with or without intervention.
E	Emergency status: In addition to noting his or her underlying ASA status (1-5), one identifies any patient undergoing an emergency procedure by adding the suffix "E." For example, a fundamentally healthy patient undergoing an emergency procedure is classified as 1-E. If the patient is undergoing an elective procedure, the "E" designation is not used.

From Hata T et al.: *Guidelines, education, and testing for procedural sedation and analgesi*a, University of Iowa, 1992-2003. Used with permission of the authors and the University of Iowa's Virtual Hospital, www.vh.org.

tion during surgery and helps the ACP identify the techniques and medications to use and to avoid.

ALLERGIES

One must document the patient's true medication allergies or sensitivities to avoid administering specific medications or classes of drugs that might harm the patient.

CURRENT MEDICATIONS

To avoid interactions between anesthetic agents and drugs prescribed by the patient's physician, a list of the medications the patient is currently taking must be obtained and recorded. Over-the-counter, herbal, and illicit drugs and medications should be included.

CARDIOPULMONARY DISEASE

During anesthesia, many agents are used that can depress cardiopulmonary function or otherwise alter the biochemistry of the cardiopulmonary system. The presence of cardiopulmonary disease increases patient risk.

KIDNEY OR LIVER DISEASE

Many anesthetic and adjunct agents are toxic to the kidneys and liver or are metabolized or excreted by these organs. A patient with preexisting liver or kidney disease may have problems with medication clearance. This results in a longer medication action or increased sensitivity. In patients with certain disease conditions, normal medication dosages may

need to be changed and additional, more invasive intraoperative monitoring may be necessary.

AIRWAY ANOMALIES

A patient with a difficult airway management issues presents a respiratory risk during deep sedation or **general anesthesia**. The patient's airway can become unstable during the period between **induction** (the beginning stages of unconsciousness) and insertion of an artificial airway. It is important to establish this artificial airway quickly so that the patient can be oxygenated in the event of respiratory failure or **bronchospasm**.

MOBILITY

Impaired mobility, skeletal injuries, and other structural problems might lead to patient injury during positioning. The ACP documents any joint replacements, previous skeletal injury, disease, and areas of nerve damage. This information is available in the patient chart, or the ACP may provide specific information during patient positioning.

SUBSTANCE ABUSE

It is important to know whether the patient has used an illicit substance or alcohol habitually or is under the influence of such a substance at the time of surgery. Patients with a history of substance abuse have a high tolerance for **sedatives,** while those who are under the influence of drugs or alcohol may experience a **synergistic** effect (the combined effect of the abused substance and an anesthetic drug is stronger than the sum of their separate effects).

FEARS AND CONCERNS

Patients often fear anesthesia more than the surgery itself. Many worry that they will not wake up or that they will suffer some permanent damage as a result of anesthesia. Another major fear is that the person will be able to feel pain but will be unable to move or talk. The ACP documents the patient's fears and the teaching used to address these concerns. The ACP also explains the anesthetic process as well as the risks involved in different types of anesthesia.

Patient Education

Patient education is an important preoperative tool to help the patient recover from surgery as quickly as possible. Teaching is primarily a nursing intervention. The patient is instructed in deep breathing and coughing, which reopen the lung alveoli and help to clear secretions from the lower respiratory tract. The patient performs these maneuvers as soon as possible after **emergence** from deep sedation or general anesthesia.

Preoperative Fasting

A period of fasting precedes the administration of a general anesthetic or any type of sedative anesthetic. The physician's orders for fasting are "non per os" (NPO) or "nothing by mouth." Fasting is required because under sedation the patient loses normal protective gag and cough reflexes that prevent food and liquids from entering the respiratory tract (aspiration). Aspiration is a serious complication of anesthesia. Because of the low pH (high acidity) of stomach fluid, aspiration of stomach contents can cause lung injury and result in pneumonitis or aspiration pneumonia, which can be fatal. Fasting periods apply to all surgery patients. During emergency surgery, these NPO guidelines are excused because of the greater risk to the patient in delaying surgery. In these situations, the ACP administers a histamine–2 blocking agent, which reduces the production of stomach acid, and a nonparticulate antacid, which increases the pH of the stomach contents.

Preoperative Medications

Preoperative **anxiolysis** is necessary in selected patients. In the past, sedatives and anticholinergic agents (drugs that reduce airway secretions and other secretions) were routinely administered within an hour of surgery. The current trend is to allay the patient's fear and anxiety during the preoperative visit and to prescribe preoperative anxiolytics only as needed.

Patients whose preoperative history is unknown are at risk of vomiting and aspiration. For patients who have esophageal disorders, have not fasted, are obese, are diabetic, are taking narcotic analgesics, or are pregnant, premedication might be required to minimize this risk. Preoperative medications are given so that their peak effect coincides with surgical intervention or are administered immediately before or after the patient arrives in the surgical suite.

Arrival in the Holding Area

When the patient arrives in the surgical holding area, the ACP usually meets with the patient. During this meeting, the ACP performs a brief assessment of the patient's level of consciousness and physical and psychological condition. Any operative permits must have been signed *before the patient receives preoperative medications.*

If the patient has received any drug that alters consciousness or produces sedation, he or she may not give informed consent to a procedure.

Before the patient arrives in the surgical suite, the ACP has already arranged needed equipment and drugs. Intravenous access is established, and monitoring devices are placed on the patient. During this time, the circulator assists the ACP as needed, in accordance with his or her knowledge and skill level and within the state's practice acts. The circulator usually is required to be present during induction.

Arrival in the Surgical Suite

The patient is transported to the surgical suite and transferred to the operating table. The ACP and circulator adjust the patient's position as needed for comfort and safety. The patient is covered with warm blankets to promote comfort and maintain normal core temperature. This is especially critical for pediatric, elderly, or debilitated patients and trauma patients. Throughout the surgical intervention, the ACP monitors the patient's homeostatic functions extensively. Monitoring devices are put in place and some procedures initiated as soon as the patient arrives in the surgical suite.

Biophysical Monitoring

Biophysical monitoring is a critical aspect of general anesthesia. Blood pressure, oxygen and carbon dioxide levels, heart rate and rhythm, and level of muscle relaxation are routinely monitored. Electrical activity in the brain also may be monitored in selected cases. Modern **anesthesia machines** are capable of performing most of these functions, but older models may require external monitors. Routine monitoring consists of many elements, as described in the following sections.

VASCULAR ACCESS AND MONITORING

Vascular access is required for all surgical patients, and establishing this access is one of the first tasks of the ACP. One or more intravascular lines are inserted for intravenous drug administration. Measuring direct arterial blood pressure and assessing arterial blood gases require catheterization into an artery. Additional lines may be placed in large branches of the great vessels of the heart for precise measurement of pressure in the heart chambers.

ELECTROCARDIOGRAPHY

Electrocardiography (ECG) produces a representation of *electrical* activity in the heart. Heart rate and rhythm are measured. ECG is subject to interference by outside electrical sources such as the electrosurgical unit. Accurate monitoring requires that the electrical leads be secure, have good skin contact, and be positioned properly for optimum accuracy. ECG leads are placed on the chest or other area. Lead placement depends on the type of surgery being performed. The ESU dispersive electrode should be placed in such a way as to cause minimal interference with the ECG monitoring process. ECG leads are generally placed on the thorax in a pattern that accurately detects and transmits the electrical impulses of the heart to the monitor.

TRANSESOPHAGEAL MONITORING

A transesophageal ("through the esophagus") stethoscope may be inserted to monitor heart rhythm, intensity, pitch, and frequency during general anesthesia. Respiratory sounds and rate also are monitored through the tubular stethoscope, which is attached to a small earpiece. A temperature probe located on the stethoscope measures the patient's core temperature. The esophageal stethoscope is inserted after the patient is anesthetized.

TEMPERATURE MONITORING

To monitor the patient's core temperature, esophageal, bladder, or rectal monitoring probes may be used. During cardiac surgery, probes can be inserted into the myocardium to monitor the temperature of the heart. With less invasive interventions, skin, external auditory canal, or axillary temperature probes are sufficient for monitoring temperature trends intraoperatively.

PULSE OXIMETRY

The **pulse oximeter** measures the arterial oxygen saturation of blood as well as the pulse rate. It operates by the principles of spectrometry, in which the amount of light that passes through a solution reveals its density. A small light source implanted in an adhesive strip or finger clip is placed in a vascular area such as the fingertip, earlobe, or toe. This produces continuous monitoring of these parameters. Interference by outside light sources or changes in the patient's circulatory volume can reduce accuracy.

BLOOD PRESSURE MONITORING

Blood pressure is measured manually with a mechanical sphygmomanometer and blood pressure cuff, automatically using a computerized blood pressure monitoring system, or is measured directly through an arterial line, or central venous line. Values are displayed on a light-emitting diode (LED) readout, one component of the anesthesia machine, monitor system or a separate electronic monitor.

CAPNOGRAPHY

The capnometer assesses pulmonary function indirectly by measuring the level of carbon dioxide and other anesthetic gases in expired air. The level is transduced into a waveform visible on an LED display.

MONITORING OF NEUROMUSCULAR RESPONSE

Neuromuscular blocking agents are used to produce muscle relaxation during balanced general anesthesia. A peripheral nerve stimulator is used to monitor the level of neuromuscular blocking. The stimulator delivers four electrical impulses at 0.5-second intervals. This is called a *train of four* or TOF test. Muscle twitching in response to the stimuli produces a means of evaluating the degree of neuromuscular blockade.

PHYSIOLOGICAL REQUIREMENTS FOR SURGERY

In order to facilitate performance of the surgical intervention, general anesthesia must produce heavy sedation (superficial or profound loss of consciousness), **analgesia** (loss of pain response), **amnesia** (loss of recall of events that occur during the action of the drug), and muscle relaxation. No single drug produces all these effects. Rather, the ACP uses a variety of agents to achieve the desired physiological balance.

Sedation

Sedation is a state of consciousness that can be described along a continuum from full awareness of one's surroundings to unconsciousness in which the patient has little or no response to external stimuli. Drugs that cause sedation often lead to loss of consciousness. The level of sedation depends on the dose and is affected by environmental factors, including the synergistic effect of other drugs used. Characteristics of different levels of sedation are outlined in Table 12-1.

Analgesia

Analgesia is loss of pain sensation. Specialized nerves in the body normally respond to painful stimuli. To produce a state of analgesia, a drug must interrupt the pain-nerve pathway. Different agents act differently at the cellular level to produce an analgesic response. All general anesthetic agents have the potential to produce analgesia.

Amnesia

Amnesia is loss of recall of events and is a desirable component of anesthesia. Some drugs such as diazepam produce **anterograde amnesia.** This is the loss of memory during the period when the drug is present in the body, particularly during the period of peak action.

Muscle Relaxation

Muscle relaxants act only on skeletal muscles, so the heart is not affected. Because the diaphragm is a skeletal muscle, however, it is paralyzed during profound anesthesia so that controlled **ventilation** is required. Nondepolarizing agents are used most often for muscle relaxation. These block the release of acetylcholine, the neurotransmitter found at the neuromuscular junction that causes muscle contraction. An

Table 12-1 LEVELS OF SEDATION AND THEIR CHARACTERISTICS

Sedation Level	Level of Consciousness	Airway	Verbal Response	Response to Touch
No sedation	Aware of environment and self	Normal or adequate	Normal or adequate	Normal or adequate
Light sedation	Sedated but aware of environment and self	Normal or adequate	Adequate or limited Abnormal	Normal or adequate
Moderate sedation	Sleepy but easily aroused, slight awareness of environment	Airway support may be needed Oxygen may be needed	Limited or none	Adequate or limited Abnormal
Deep sedation	Unaware of environment or self	May be mildly abnormal or absent	None	Only partially responsive to pain
Surgical general anesthesia	Unconscious; does not respond to pain	Limited to absent	None	*No* response to touch or pain

important consideration for the ACP is the adequate dosing of muscle relaxants since some agents last for only short periods of time and are redosed frequently throughout the surgical intervention. Anesthetic agents act synergistically with depolarizing agents. A *peripheral nerve stimulator* is used to test the electrical activity of muscle fibers and determine their reactivity.

BALANCED ANESTHESIA

Modern anesthesia techniques include many different drugs used in combination to achieve the desired results. This is called balanced anesthesia. Depending on the needs of the surgical intervention and the required level of consciousness, the ACP controls the patient's normal physiological functions and metabolism. Rapid physiological changes occur during anesthesia administration and surgical intervention and may result in surgical emergencies. These changes occur during positioning and manipulation of certain tissues, and depend on aspects of the patient's physical condition, such as the presence of cardiovascular disease. Combinations of drugs used in balanced anesthesia minimize the occurence of negative events during surgery.

Inhalation Anesthesia

Inhalation anesthesia is the delivery of gaseous anesthetic agents through the respiratory tract. After the gas has been inhaled, it is absorbed across the alveoli in the lungs, enters the vascular system, and is transported to the brain.

The chemical properties of a liquid determine the temperature and atmospheric pressure at which it simultaneously evaporates (loses volume) and becomes a gas (vapor). Volatile liquids are those that convert easily from liquid to gaseous state. Alcohol is an example of a volatile liquid. All inhalation anesthetic agents except nitrous oxide are volatile liquids that are vaporized (turned to gas) in the anesthesia machine and then delivered to the patient. Explosive gaseous anesthetics such as cyclopropane and ether are still in use in some areas of the world. However, these have been banned for use as anesthetics in the United States.

Action of Anesthetic Gases

Anesthetic gases are delivered from the anesthesia machine directly through the patient's **endotracheal tube, laryngeal mask airway (LMA),** or face mask to the lungs. The actions of all inhalation anesthetics are dose dependent. Increasing the dose of the drug also increases the effects, both intended and adverse. The following are factors that affect the concentration of the gases in the blood and rate of absorption:

▶ The solubility of the agent in blood
▶ The concentration of anesthetic delivered
▶ The rate of pulmonary blood flow (the greater the blood flow, the higher the amount of anesthetic absorbed)
▶ The solubility of the gas in the tissue

The amount of anesthetic that crosses the alveolar membrane varies depending on the type of anesthetic and the pa-

tient's condition. Monitored anesthesia care (MAC) is defined as the concentration of an inhaled anesthetic at 1 Atmosphere of pressure that prevents skeletal muscle movement in response to a noxious stimulus in 50% of patients. It is used as a standard to compare the strength of inhaled anesthetics. MAC values are *increased* by hyperthermia (abnormally high body temperature), alcohol abuse, and long-term use of drugs such as cocaine, amphetamines, and agents used to control Parkinson's disease. MAC values are *decreased* by hypotension (low blood pressure), acute alcohol intoxication, pregnancy, hypothermia (decreased body temperature), opioid drugs, and increased age.

Loss of consciousness is not an isolated event. It occurs on a continuum and is identified by the absence of *specific* responses and reflexes that becomes more profound as the amount of anesthetic agent or sedative delivered increases.

Levels of Consciousness

Levels of consciousness are not distinct or well defined. Modern sedatives reach the target tissues so rapidly that the phases or stages of anesthesia do not have the clinical significance that they used to have.

INDUCTION

Anesthesia induction is the passage from consciousness to loss of consciousness. Induction drugs are carefully selected in accordance with the patient's age, medical history, allergies, and drug sensitivity. Induction may be achieved with intravenous or inhaled drugs. Intravenous drugs are used more often in adults, but inhalational anesthetics are used more often in children. Levels of unconsciousness deepen as increased amounts of induction drugs are administered. The patient retains the ability to hear during early induction even though body movements cease. All noises in the room must be kept to a minimum.

Just before induction, the ACP administers oxygen via a face mask and encourages the patient to breathe deeply. This produces full oxygen saturation of the hemoglobin. The patient's blood is nearly fully oxygenated while he or she is breathing room air. Breathing 100% oxygen raises the saturation very little, but it does increase the PaO_2 significantly, which produces a margin of safety in patients with a difficult airway. In cases in which the patient has a difficult airway or experiences bronchospasm or **laryngospasm,** full oxygen saturation creates a margin of safety until an unobstructed artificial airway can be secured. During this time the circulator stands by to assist as needed. All ambient noise in the room must be reduced to an absolute minimum. Induction and general anesthesia begin when all team members are present and the patient is physiologically prepared and stable.

DELIRIUM

During anesthesia induction, the patient passes through a **delirium** or excitability phase. Signs of this phase may or may not be exhibited because newer drugs act rapidly enough to suppress many of the negative events associated with this phase. The excitability phase may be prolonged, however, when the induction drug is given slowly. Struggling, hypoxia, vomiting, and cardiac arrhythmia are characteristic of this phase and can lead to a medical emergency. Bronchospasm can obstruct the patient's airway if it occurs before an artificial airway is placed. Vomiting can lead to aspiration of the stomach contents, which are highly acidic. This can result in aspiration pneumonia. Struggling may result in patient injury or a fall from the operating table.

Certain drugs and patient conditions are more likely to cause some of these symptoms than are others. These events usually occur before **intubation,** when the patient is at greater risk. However, this is not clinically significant because of the newer, faster-acting medications. Delirium is only a legitimate concern during an inhalation induction, as this is a much slower process.

DEEP SEDATION AND UNCONSCIOUSNESS

After induction, the surgical level of anesthesia must be maintained throughout the operative procedure. Anesthetic gas and oxygen are delivered through the patient's airway or face mask. Muscle relaxants and central nervous system (CNS) depressants also are administered. These medications reduce the amount of anesthetic gas required. The ACP controls the patient's level of consciousness through biophysical monitoring and observation of autonomic and somatic responses.

EMERGENCE

Near the close of surgery, the ACP begins to withdraw anesthetic agents, and the patient emerges from the anesthetic. This period follows a pattern that is the reverse of that during induction. Struggling and delirium may be observed as consciousness returns. Recently developed anesthetic drugs allow rapid emergence, however, and the patient often is fully awake shortly after withdrawal of the drugs. When the patient can breathe independently of the ventilator, the endotracheal tube is removed (extubation). The duration of the emergence phase depends on the agents used, the duration of the anesthetic, the size of the patient, and the presence of surgical and anesthetic complications. In some cases, antagonist agents are used to reverse the effects of narcotics or muscle relaxants.

Balanced Anesthesia Equipment
ANESTHESIA MACHINE

General anesthesia requires the use of an anesthesia machine (Figure 12-2). Newer models have greater capabilities in both safety and precision of delivery of a gas or volatile liquid. The basic mechanism is a circular flow system that includes the patient's inspiratory and expiratory functions. Nitrous oxide and oxygen coming into the system are available from tanks mounted on the machine or from in-line systems (those that provide flow from a continuously available outside source, similar to water from a tap). Volatile liquid anesthetics are converted to gaseous state by a vaporizer.

The patient can be mechanically ventilated or hand ventilated with the reservoir bag. Gases enter the bag and then are delivered to the patient through corrugated gas hoses. The system is described as *semiopen, closed,* or *semiclosed,*

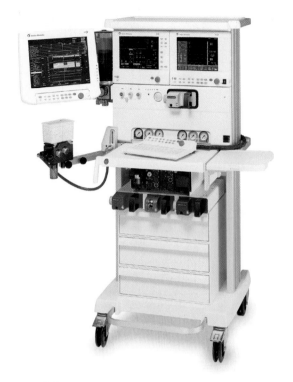

FIGURE 12-2
Anesthesia machine. (Courtesy of Datex-Ohmeda, Madison, WI.)

depending on the level of expired carbon dioxide and gases rebreathed by the patient.

Breathing circuits are classified by type, reservoir, and use of rebreathing (Table 12-2).

In an open system, patients have access to the atmosphere, as almost all of the exhaled gas is vented out of the circuit. This system usually is used in pediatric surgery. A closed system is a system in which the patient rebreathes expired CO_2 and anesthetic. A closed system uses less anesthetic gas and also helps to maintain core body temperature and respiratory humidity. A semiclosed system allows the escape of some exhaled gases. In both the semiclosed and open systems, exhaled gases are taken up through a **gas scavenging** system. To prevent the patient from rebreathing carbon dioxide through the circuit, it is captured and absorbed by a soda lime reservoir. This reservoir is an integral part of the circuit. The circular system is used most often in the United States because it prevents rebreathing of CO_2 while allowing rebreathing of all other gases. The circular system can be adjusted so that the patient is ventilated with air, oxygen, and anesthetic gas (Figure 12-3).

Cleaning, disinfection, and basic trouble shooting are the responsibilities of the anesthesia technician or aide. Maintenance and testing of the anesthesia machine are the responsibilities of the bioengineering department. All equipment that comes in contact with the patient must be decontaminated to prevent cross contamination. Standard precautions are used whenever equipment is handled. The hoses, soda canister, masks, and airways are sources of high bacterial contamination. The intricate valve mechanisms also may harbor large colonies of disease-causing microorganisms.

Table 12-2 CLASSIFICATION OF BREATHING CIRCUITS			
Type	Reservoir	Rebreathing	Example
Open	No	No	Open drop, insufflation, nasal cannula
Semiopen	Yes	No	Nonrebreathing circuit; circle at high fresh gas flow
Semiclosed	Yes	Yes (partial)	Circle at fresh gas flow less than minute ventilation
Closed	Yes	Yes (complete)	Circle at extremely low fresh gas flow, with adjustable pressure-limiting valve closed

From Nagelhout JJ and Zaglaniczny KL: *Nurse anesthesia*, ed 3, St Louis, 2005, Saunders.

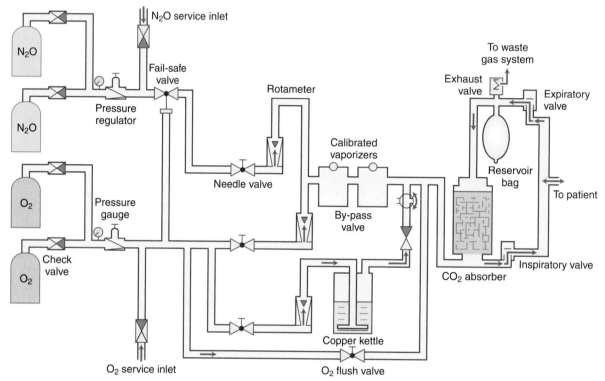

FIGURE 12-3
Anesthesia machine circuit. (Redrawn from Murphy FL and Longnecker DE: *Dripps-Eckenhoff-Vandam introduction to anesthesia*, ed 9, Philadelphia, 1996, Saunders.)

Use of disposable patient air hoses, masks, and airways is preferred whenever possible. Bacterial filters can be used on the anesthesia circuit to prevent contamination of the ventilator and anesthesia machine. All nondisposable items are decontaminated and sterilized.

SCAVENGING SYSTEM FOR WASTE GASES

Escape of anesthetic gas into the surgical suite is an environmental hazard for health workers. Recommendations from the National Institute for Occupational Safety and Health (NIOSH) and the Occupational Safety and Health Administration (OSHA) state that there must not be more than 0.5 parts per million of halogenated agents per hour **maximum value for the OR environment (i.e., escaped gas)** for the anesthesia system itself when used with nitrous oxide. Scavenging equipment can reduce health worker exposure up to

95%. Scavenging systems capture escaped gases and vent them either actively through a vacuum line, or passively to the outside environment.

MEDICAL GAS CYLINDERS

Medical gases to be administered to the patient are obtained through an in-line hose from wall outlets, or from cylinders. Medical gases include oxygen, nitrogen, air, and nitrous oxide. In the United States the color of the tank is correlated with the gas contained inside. There is no international standard, however, and no regulation of color codes. In general, oxygen cylinders are green, nitrous oxide tanks are blue, and nitrogen tanks are gray. However, the safest method to identify the contents of any gas cylinder is to *read the label*. Refer to Chapter 14 for a complete discussion of gas cylinder safety.

INTRAVENOUS SUPPLIES

When starting, maintaining, and using an intravenous (IV) line, the ACP needs gloves, assorted needles and syringes (1, 3, 5, and 10 ml), alcohol wipes, tape, sterile gauze pads, tourniquets, intravenous catheters, and intravenous fluids.

LARYNGOSCOPE

The **laryngoscope** is a rigid instrument used to light the larynx and assist in guiding the endotracheal tube during intubation (Figure 12-4). The laryngoscope consists of a handle and various sizes and styles of blades that are used to depress the tongue.

PERIPHERAL NERVE STIMULATOR

The peripheral nerve stimulator delivers a very low, pulsing electrical current to the skin. It is used to monitor electrical activity in skeletal muscles and determine the level of muscle relaxation (see the earlier section, Biophysical Monitoring).

OXYGEN DELIVERY SYSTEMS

Many systems are available to deliver oxygen to the patient. The nasal cannula is a plastic tube with short flexible prongs that insert into the nares (Figure 12-5, *A*). This

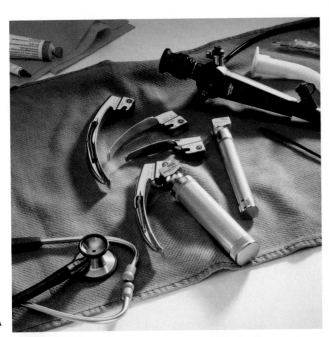

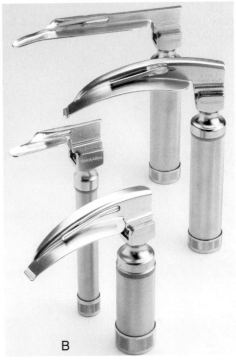

FIGURE 12-4
A and **B,** Types of laryngoscopes. **C,** Use of a laryngoscope during intubation. (Courtesy of Welch Allyn, Skaneateles Falls, NY.)

A

B

C

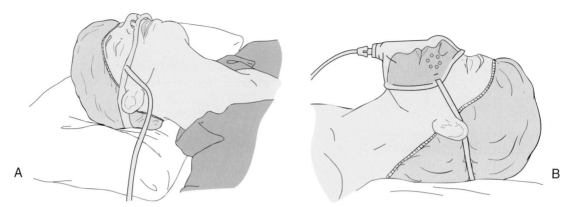

FIGURE 12-5
A, Nasal cannula. **B,** Oxygen face mask. (**A** and **B** modified from Sorrentino SA: *Mosby's textbook for nursing assistants*, ed 5, St Louis, 2000, Mosby.)

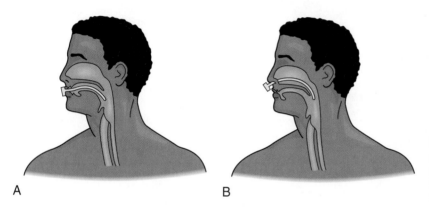

FIGURE 12-6
A, Oropharyngeal airway. **B,** Nasopharyngeal airway. (**A** and **B** modified from Sorrentino SA: *Mosby's textbook for nursing assistants*, ed 5, St Louis, 2000, Mosby.)

system delivers a small amount of oxygen combined with room air. Face masks cover both the nose and mouth and can be fitted tightly to regulate the oxygen intake precisely (Figure 12-5, *B*). Oxygen is delivered in liters per minute.

AIRWAYS
An airway is any device that fits in the nose, mouth, or throat to support and hold open a patient's airway. Oropharyngeal airways and nasopharyngeal airways do not enter the trachea (Figure 12-6, *A* and *B*). These are available in different styles, sizes, and materials. A variety of sizes are selected and prepared before the patient arrives in the operating room. The LMA is inserted orally and covers the larynx (see Figure 12-11). The endotracheal tube is inserted orally or through the nose (see Figure 12-9).

ANESTHESIA FACE MASK
The anesthesia face mask is used to deliver positive pressure ventilation with anesthetic gas and oxygen from the anesthesia machine. It may be used when endotracheal intubation is not possible. An anesthesia face mask generally is not used in place of an invasive airway device except for very brief and light sedation because of the risk of laryngospasm (spasm of the larynx). If laryngospasm should occur while the patient is wearing an anesthesia face mask, there is no way to adequately ventilate the patient.

In pediatric patients, anesthesia induction is sometimes performed with a face mask to avoid the struggling associated with establishment of intravenous access (Figure 12-7).

SELF-INFLATING BREATHING BAG AND VALVE
The breathing bag with valve adapter is attached to the endotracheal tube or proximal LMA to ventilate the patient with oxygen or air.

After induction, an artificial airway is inserted into the patient's airway by mouth or through the nose. These supportive airways prevent tracheal collapse and provide a means of administering anesthetic gas and oxygen, and ventilating the patient. Under extreme circumstances, the patient may be intubated while conscious.

SUCTION DEVICES
Suction must be available to the ACP at all times. As long as the patient is in the operating suite, the suction device must remain operative. In-line suction is available from ceiling posts, cables, or wall outlets. When connecting suction cables, match the two ends of the connector, push, and turn the connector to secure it. This locking mechanism prevents the cables from separating.

Suction is routinely used to remove secretions from the mouth and throat. The Yankauer suction tip is semirigid with a rounded end (Figure 12-8). It is used when secretions

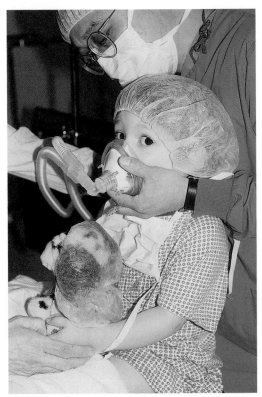

FIGURE 12-7
A child being anesthetized with mask. (From Liebert PS: *Colour atlas of pediatric surgery*, ed 2, Philadelphia, 1996, Saunders.)

are thick or copious. The softer, flexible suction catheter is a tube with perforations at the tip. It can be inserted through the nasopharynx or throat and into the esophagus and stomach.

INTRAOPERATIVE MANAGEMENT OF THE PATIENT

Airway Management

Management of the airway is the first priority in patient care. In both emergencies and routine care, the airway is the vital link supplying oxygen to maintain tissue life. During anesthesia of all types, the patient's airway is managed with a variety of medical devices. Some support the airway and are invasive, such as the endotracheal tube or LMA, while others deliver oxygen passively through a healthy, responsive respiratory system. Devices such as the nasal airway or simple oxygen mask are in the latter category. Positive pressure airway management is achieved with a tight-fitting mask and bag or a forced pressure system such as that connected to the anesthesia machine or a bag-mask system. Not only must oxygen delivery mechanisms be used, but the patient also must have a clean airway to receive air, oxygen, and volatile anesthetics. Secretions must be cleared from the nose and throat. This is performed with a suction tip or catheter.

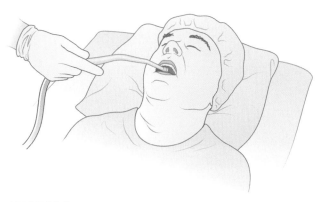

FIGURE 12-8
Yankauer suction. (Redrawn from Sorrentino SA: *Mosby's textbook for nursing assistants*, ed 5, St Louis, 2000, Mosby.)

ENDOTRACHEAL INTUBATION

The endotracheal tube is inserted through the mouth or nose into the patient's trachea. An inflatable balloon near the distal end serves as a barrier between the upper and lower airways and prevents aspiration of fluid into the respiratory tract (Figure 12-9). The balloon does *not* hold the endotracheal tube in place; rather the tube is secured with tape or a face guard. An adapter at the proximal end secures the tube to the gas hose of the anesthesia machine or oxygen delivery system.

The process of inserting the endotracheal tube is called intubation. The patient is intubated only when he or she is in a state of deep CNS depression. Before endotracheal intubation, intramuscular blocking agents are given to relax the jaw muscles. To insert the tube, a rigid or fiberoptic laryngoscope is guided into the oropharynx, and the tube is inserted along its length.

During intubation the ACP may ask the circulator to apply **cricoid pressure.** Pressure over the cricoid cartilage occludes the esophagus and stabilizes the trachea (Figure 12-10). The maneuver is particularly important when there is risk of aspiration of stomach contents.

INSERTION OF THE LARYNGEAL MASK

The LMA is positioned manually without the aid of muscle relaxants. It is placed into the oral cavity and advanced to cover the larynx (Figure 12-11). The inflatable ridge forms a seal. Gases are administered through the tube. When endotracheal intubation is difficult because of the patient's anatomy or medical condition, the LMA provides a less traumatic alternative means of inserting and maintaining a **patent** (open) airway. It is important to note that the seal of the LMA does not produce the same protection against aspiration as the seal of an endotracheal tube; thus LMAs are contraindicated in patients who are at risk for aspiration.

Environmental Control
THERMAL DEVICES

A thermal heating blanket is used to help maintain the patient's core body temperature. A common type of heating

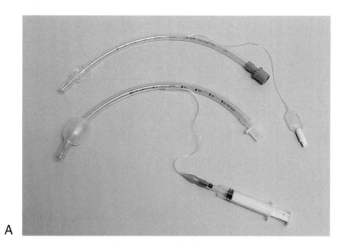

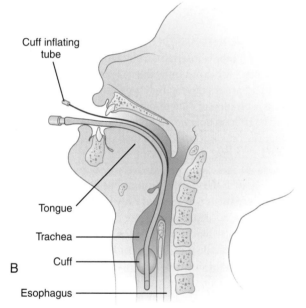

FIGURE 12-9
A, Endotracheal tube. **B,** Endotracheal tube in patient. (**A** from Elkin MK, Perry AG, Potter PA: *Nursing interventions and clinical skills,* ed 3, St Louis, 2004, Mosby. **B** redrawn from Rothrock JC: *Alexander's care of the patient in surgery,* ed 12, St Louis, 2003, Mosby.)

blanket is a baffled air mattress that rests lightly on the patient's body (Figure 12-12). Warmed air is pumped into sections of the blanket via a flexible hose. These blankets are an excellent source of warmth during long procedures.

As with any medical device, improper use or faulty mechanisms create risk. These risks are greatest when the patient is unconscious or semiconscious and unable to respond to pain. Of particular importance are the temperature setting and the air-hose–to–blanket connection. One should check the setting before the unit is activated, and the device should be turned on only after the correct temperature has been verified with the ACP. The design feature that forces hot air into the blanket can result in patient burns. If the connection is loose and the air hose becomes detached during surgery, the hot air will blow over the patient's bare skin, which can lead to second- or third-degree burns. This often goes unnoticed because, after the surgical drapes have been put into place, the connection (or loss of connection) is not in view.

Pediatric patients and those who are thin or debilitated are at particular risk for burns from any heating device. Meticulous attention to any device that creates heat is the collaborative responsibility of everyone on the operating team.

CONTROLLED HYPOTHERMIA
Deliberate lowering of the patient's core body temperature slows the body's metabolism and produces beneficial effects in selected surgical procedures. A lowered metabolism results in lower oxygen requirements in body tissues. This effect is desirable when blood flow must be interrupted or when normal blood flow presents a severe, uncontrollable risk. In cardiac surgery, surgical repair of large vessels, organ transplantation, and neurosurgery, **controlled hypothermia** produces a margin of safety while performing particular surgical procedures.

Hypothermia can be achieved through a number of methods. Blood may be diverted to a cooling system, as during cardiopulmonary bypass. Other methods include intravenous

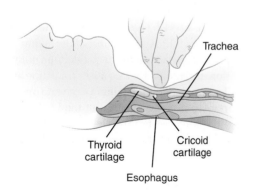

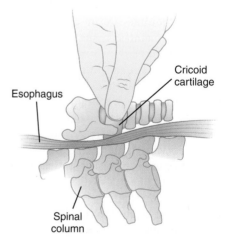

FIGURE 12-10
Cricoid pressure. (Modified from Phillips N: *Berry & Kohn's operating room technique,* ed 10, St Louis, 2004, Mosby.)

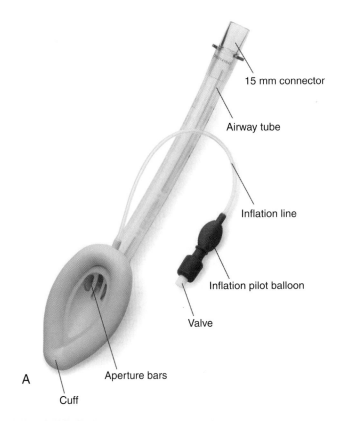

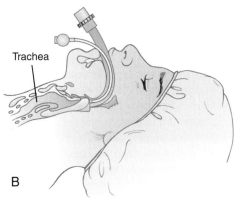

FIGURE 12-11
A, Laryngeal mask (LMA). **B,** LMA in patient. (**A** courtesy of LMA North America. **B** redrawn from Phillips N: *Berry & Kohn's operating room technique,* ed 10, St Louis, 2004, Mosby.)

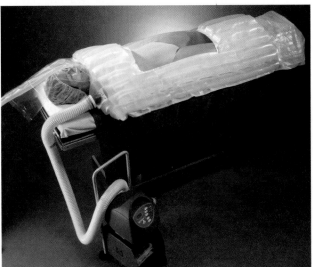

FIGURE 12-12
Thermal heating blanket. (Courtesy of Augustine Medical, Eden Prairie, MN.)

administration of cold solution and irrigation of body cavities with cold fluid. During cardiac surgery, saline ice slush is packed around the heart to produce localized cooling. Target temperatures are no lower than 26° C (78.8° F).

Complications of induced hypothermia include cardiac arrhythmia, which occurs when normal conduction is interrupted. This can lead to heart block and cardiac arrest. Other organs of the body also may suffer damage as a result of inadequate blood supply.

Rewarming is achieved with a heating blanket, heating mattress, warm intravenous fluids, and warm cotton blankets. Shivering, which increases the body's requirements for oxygen, is controlled with muscle relaxants, selected analgesics, and further rewarming. The patient is rewarmed slowly to reduce the risk of circulatory collapse or sudden dilation or constriction of blood vessels.

Maintenance of Intravascular Volume and Electrolyte Balance

The ACP maintains blood pressure and intravascular volume using both drugs and intravenous solutions. Venous access must be available at all times during surgery so that drugs can be administered immediately in case of emergency and intravascular fluid levels can be maintained. Intravenous solutions are classified as hypertonic (greater solute concentration than plasma), hypotonic (lower solute concentration than plasma), and isotonic (equal in solute concentration to plasma). These solutions move fluid in and out of the vascular system depending on solute concentration. Remember that fluid travels across a semipermeable membrane to the area of greater solute concentration.

Solutions that are administered during surgery to maintain physiological balance are intravenous lactated Ringer's solution; normal (isotonic) and hypertonic saline; albumin; and electrolytes. The most common intravenous fluids are lactated Ringer's solution and normal saline, both of which are isotonic.

Blood products are transfused when blood loss is extensive. Whole blood is rarely given unless there is massive hemorrhage. Packed red cells are administered more often because the patient's immediate need is *oxygen-carrying capacity.* Blood products must be matched with the patient's blood type. A precise protocol has evolved to prevent the administration of blood of the wrong type. Patients who schedule their surgery may give their own blood weeks before the surgery. Whether the patient's own blood or banked blood is used, meticulous attention is given to patient identification, blood group, registration number, and date of expiration.

Conditions of blood storage also are critical. Fresh frozen plasma, packed cells, and whole blood must be stored at 1.0° C to 6.0° C (33.8° F to 42.8° F). Blood is warmed within the transfusion mechanism. Blood usually is brought from the blood bank shortly before surgery or, in an emergency, is brought immediately. Blood must be stored in a location known to all personnel and protected from direct heat. Unused blood must be returned immediately to the blood bank.

INDUCED HYPOTENSION

Induced hypotension is the deliberate lowering of the patient's blood pressure to control hemorrhage and reduce the presence of blood at the surgical site. It is used in selected procedures in which blood loss is expected to be high. Examples are spinal surgery, in which a nearly bloodless operative site is important, and orthopedic surgery. However, the ACP adjusts anesthetic agents for individual patient safety; for example, a patient who is normally hypertensive might become ischemic and suffer a stroke during the process of attempted controlled hypotension.

Hypotension is maintained at approximately 70 mm Hg in a patient with normal blood pressure. The systolic pressure is controlled with the use of selected drugs that directly dilate blood vessels and control the sympathetic nerve impulses causing vasodilation. Examples are sodium nitroprusside, nitroglycerin, and nifedipine. The patient with chronic hypertension may arrive at the operating room with a systolic blood pressure of 160 to 180 mm Hg. The ACP adjusts hypotension to the appropriate safe level for each individual patient.

PHYSIOLOGY OF CENTRAL NERVOUS SYSTEM AGENTS

When surgery is performed, drugs are administered to produce a safe environment for the patient, produce deep sedation, control pain, and cause muscle relaxation. The narrow definition of anesthesia is "loss of sensation." In surgery, anesthesia is a much broader and more complex process. It is the *monitoring and rebalancing of the body's responses to surgery.*

Most drugs used to produce or enhance general anesthesia are CNS agents.

Stimulus and Response

The human body is capable of responding to many different types of environmental stimuli. Subjective responses are those reported by the patient. These are called *symptoms.* These subjective experiences differ in quality and intensity among different people depending on their age, past experiences, emo-

tional state, culture, and biochemistry at the time of stimulation. For example, the sensation of pain often is heightened in individuals who have had previous experiences of uncontrolled pain. Feelings of warmth and cold are affected not only by the body's core temperature but also by one's level of consciousness. An inebriated person may have a dangerously low core temperature without feeling cold. This is because alcohol depresses the CNS. By *measuring* the person's core temperature, one can assess whether the person is at risk. Measurements taken during surgery produce *objective* data.

Homeostasis

In a state of well-being, the body responds to stimuli in ways that maintain life. Many complex biochemical, physical, and metabolic processes are required to maintain the balance between stimuli and responses. Examples are shivering when the body's temperature drops and vasoconstriction when blood pressure falls. This maintenance of physiological balance is called homeostasis.

To perform surgery, medical workers must control the body's normal responses to noxious (harmful or painful) stimuli. When these responses are controlled, however, the body's ability to maintain homeostasis also may be reduced.

Under deep general anesthesia or sedation, the patient loses the ability to breathe spontaneously. The ACP must actively ventilate the patient's lungs. Thus the ACP not only administers anesthetic and adjunct agents but also must also maintain the body's homeostasis, or control the reaction to the drugs and surgery itself.

Nerve Transmission

Knowledge of nerve transmission is basic to an understanding of how anesthetics and other CNS drugs work. The following basic description of how stimuli are transmitted provides useful background for the study of anesthesia.

The transmission of nerve impulses (signals) is a complex biochemical process. In simple terms, impulses are chemical and electrical. Chemicals that carry impulses from nerve cell to nerve cell are called neurotransmitters. The biochemical work of the neurotransmitter is to transport the signal from one nerve cell to the next until the signal reaches the target tissue.

Each nerve cell (neuron) is separated from an adjacent nerve cell by a synapse (also called the synaptic cleft). The synapse is the small space in which the neurotransmitter passes from one nerve cell to another. For the neurotransmitter to transport a signal, it must be released from the presynaptic neuron (the neuron before the synapse) and be received by the next neuron in line (the postsynaptic neuron). The neurotransmitter is contained in small vesicles (cell sacs). The receptor for the given neurotransmitter is a specific molecule in the postsynaptic neuron (Figure 12-13).

There are many different types of neurotransmitters, each carrying a different type of impulse. About 30 known neurotransmitters occur in specific tissues of the body.

One type of neurotransmitter can be *blocked* without affecting the others. For example, the neurotransmitter for motor control can be blocked by a muscle-paralyzing agent,

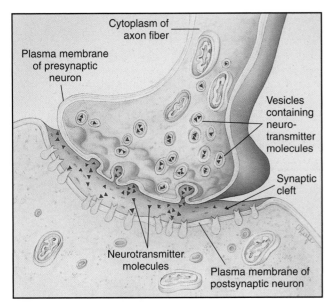

FIGURE 12-13
Synapse. (From Thibodeau GA and Patton KT: *Structure and function of the body,* ed 11, St Louis, 2000, Mosby.)

while the neurotransmitter for pain remains unaffected. This would result in the ability to feel pain but the inability to withdraw from the agent causing it. Likewise, one can achieve sedation or loss of consciousness without reducing the sensation of pain.

One method used to block neurotransmission is to administer a drug that has an affinity for the postsynaptic receptor. A limited number of receptors are available for the neurotransmitter molecule. Thus, when the drug attaches to the receptor site, the neurotransmitter cannot continue on its path because there are no unbound receptors. The neurotransmitter remains in the space between the two neurons (the synapse) and eventually is reabsorbed by the presynaptic cell or broken down by enzymes in the synapse, so that the path of transmission is broken. Drugs that work in this manner are called competitive antagonists.

Certain drugs can increase the availability of postsynaptic receptors and the movement of neurotransmitters. If a drug potentiates release and/or uptake of a particular neurotransmitter, it is called an agonist.

AUTONOMIC NERVOUS SYSTEM
Stimuli in the autonomic nervous system produce specific *involuntary responses in specific body organs and tissues.* The responses occur in smooth muscle tissue, including cardiac smooth muscle and glands. Examples of autonomic responses are changes in heartbeat, release of glandular secretions (such as insulin in the pancreas), and intestinal contractions (peristalsis).

Two types of response can occur within the autonomic nervous system. These responses are classified as sympathetic and parasympathetic. These are often called "fight or flight" responses. Figure 12-14 illustrates sympathetic and parasympathetic responses. The sympathetic and parasympathetic re-

sponses generally produce opposing effects, such as increasing or decreasing heart rate and decreasing or increasing bronchiole dilation. The neurotransmitter for sympathetic nerves is called an *adrenergic.* Agents that block the sympathetic nerves are called *antiadrenergics.* Those that increase the sympathetic response are known as *sympathetic stimulants.*

The neurotransmitter for parasympathetic nerves is *acetylcholine.* Drugs that increase the effects of the parasympathetic nervous system or mimic acetylcholine are called *cholinergic agents.* Drugs that block the action of acetylcholine in the parasympathetic system are called *anticholinergic agents.*

SOMATIC NERVOUS SYSTEM
The somatic nervous system is under direct voluntary control. Neurotransmitters of the somatic nervous system conduct impulses to the striated muscles of the body. This results in voluntary (consciously controlled) coordinated muscle activity that produces movement. When nerve impulses are interrupted, paralysis results. Neuromuscular blocking agents are used during surgery to relax muscles for easier intubation and tissue manipulation. A discussion of neuromuscular blocking agents is found later in this chapter.

CONSCIOUS SEDATION

Conscious sedation is accomplished through administration of a combination of sedatives, hypnotics, and analgesics. The patient can respond and breathe independently but is sedated to tolerate the procedure. The level of sedation forms a continuum from consciousness to unconsciousness. Therefore only qualified personnel are permitted to administer sedating drugs. This restriction protects patients in the event that medical assistance is required during deeper stages of sedation and anesthesia. The ACP must evaluate the patient before the procedure, and the ACP must be present during deep or moderate sedation. Specially trained and certified nurses may administer inducing drugs and manage the patient during minimal and moderate sedation.

Minimal Sedation
Minimal sedation is a state in which the patient can respond to verbal commands. Cognitive function and muscular coordination may be impaired. The patient's ventilatory and cardiovascular systems remain unaffected.

Moderate Sedation
In moderate sedation, the patient's consciousness is depressed. However, he or she can respond to verbal commands when stimulated. Airway support is not needed, and the patient can breathe independently. The cardiovascular system usually is unaffected.

Deep Sedation
During deep sedation the patient cannot be aroused easily. Painful stimulation produces a response. Ventilatory function may be compromised. The patient may require airway

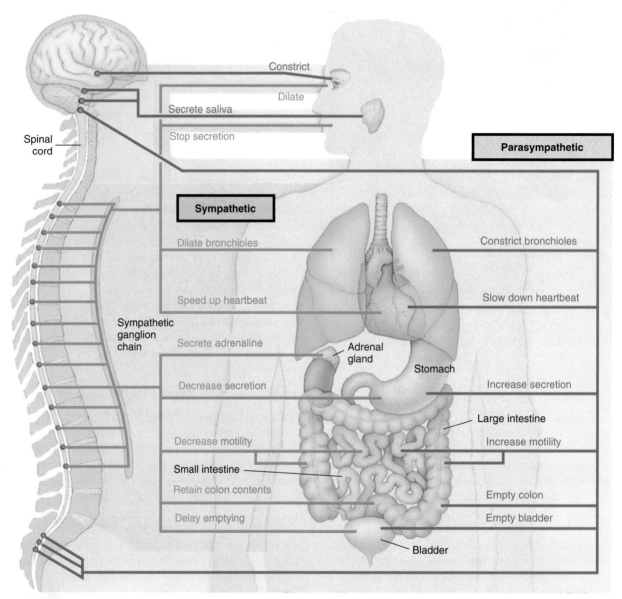

FIGURE 12-14
Sympathetic and parasympathetic systems. (From Thibodeau GA and Patton KT: *Structure and function of the body,* ed 11, St Louis, 2000, Mosby.)

assistance, and spontaneous breathing may be inadequate. Cardiovascular functions remain intact.

Unconscious Sedation

Unconscious sedation is used every day in the operating room and is one step greater in depression of the central nervous system than is deep, conscious sedation. Many people call this a "light general anesthetic."

INHALATION ANESTHETICS

Risks and Selection of Inhalation Anesthetics

All inhalation anesthetics have characteristic effects that are both desirable and undesirable. The adverse effects associated with a specific agent determine the suitability of that agent for a particular patient. Choosing an agent is a complex process requiring the patient to undergo a complete physical examination and history taking. Cardiovascular and respiratory status, presence of metabolic disease, age, nutritional status, drug allergies, lifestyle, and environmental health all are considered. Because of the complex issues involved in the selection of an anesthetic, the suitability of one anesthetic versus another for specific situations cannot easily be summarized.

The life-threatening risks associated with inhalation agents include the following:

▶ **Malignant hyperthermia** (MH) (in susceptible individuals; it is very rare and occurs in less than 150,000 anesthetics); it is associated with all inhalation anesthetics except nitrous oxide (N_2O); it is associated with the use of succinylcholine (Anectine)

▶ Increased respiratory rate and heart rate
▶ Cardiac arrhythmia
▶ Decreased pulmonary resistance and decreased systemic vascular resistance
▶ Hypotension
▶ Depressed response to elevated blood levels of carbon dioxide (carbon dioxide levels determine respiratory rate and inspiratory volume)
▶ Decrease in renal blood flow and urine output
▶ Decrease in hepatic blood flow
▶ Cerebral vasodilation, which leads to increased intracranial pressure

Types of Inhalation Anesthetics

DESFLURANE (SUPRANE)

Advantages

▶ Offers rapid elimination and emergence
▶ Useful for ambulatory surgery
▶ Does not affect cardiac output
▶ Eliminated by the lungs
▶ Undergoes little metabolism in the liver

Disadvantages

▶ Requires heated vaporizer
▶ Causes respiratory irritation, secretions, **apnea**, laryngospasm
▶ Increases heart rate

ENFLURANE (ETHRANE)

Enflurane (Ethrane) is not used often.

Advantages

▶ Smooth emergence
▶ Rapid induction

Disadvantages

▶ Increased intracranial pressure
▶ Increased seizure risk
▶ Cardiovascular depression
▶ Hypotension

HALOTHANE (FLUOTHANE) (not used frequently)

Halothane (Fluothane) is not used often.

Advantages

▶ Rapid induction
▶ No postoperative nausea and vomiting

Disadvantages

▶ Reduced cardiac output
▶ Possible cardiac arrhythmias
▶ High liver toxicity
▶ Poor muscle relaxation

ISOFLURANE (FORANE)

Advantages

▶ Rapid, smooth induction
▶ Good muscle relaxation
▶ 0.25% metabolized

Disadvantage

▶ Hypotension related to peripheral vasodilation

NITROUS OXIDE

Nitrous oxide is a nonflammable gas that supports combustion. It is a weak anesthetic used in combination with other anesthetic gases during general anesthesia to supplement their action. In the United States nitrous oxide is commercially available in blue gas cylinders.

Advantages

▶ Rapid recovery time
▶ No hypotension

Disadvantage

▶ Poor muscle relaxant

SEDATIVES AND ADJUNCT DRUGS

Benzodiazepines (Sedative Hypnotic)

USES AND EFFECTS

Benzodiazepines produce anterograde amnesia (loss of recall of events) for up to 6 hours from the onset of drug action. In combination with other CNS depressants, benzodiazepines can cause significant respiratory and cardiac depression. They have no analgesic (pain reduction) effect and can increase anesthetic recovery time.

Benzodiazepines are used before and during surgery to produce sedation and semiconsciousness, especially when analgesia is not required.

Benzodiazepines are used:

▶ In combination with opioids and muscle relaxants to achieve balanced anesthesia
▶ For preoperative anxiolysis
▶ During endoscopy
▶ During cardioversion
▶ During cardiac catheterization

The effects of benzodiazepines are:

▶ Anxiolysis
▶ Sedation
▶ Amnesia
▶ Anticonvulsant action

These problems can occur when benzodiazepines are used:

▶ Respiratory and cardiac depression
▶ Increased anesthesia recovery time
▶ Synergistic action with CNS depressants

Examples of benzodiazepines are:

▶ Diazepam (Valium)
▶ Midazolam (Versed)
▶ Lorazepam (Ativan)
▶ Alprazolam (Xanax)

REVERSAL OF EFFECTS

Benzodiazepine reversal is necessary in emergency situations of severe respiratory depression and apnea. Flumazenil (Romazicon) binds to the benzodiazepine receptor site and prevents its action on the CNS. Flumazenil is used to reverse sedation, amnesia, and respiratory depression. Adverse effects include anxiety, tremors, nausea, and resedation resulting from the shorter half life of flumazenil versus some of the benzodiazepines.

Miscellaneous Sedative Hypnotics

The agents discussed in the following sections are sedative hypnotics that are not related to the benzodiazepines. They are used for induction and mild or deep sedation. Diphenhydramine (Benadryl) is used for mild sedation only.

PROPOFOL (DIPRIVAN)

Propofol is used in induction and sedation for short operative procedures.
The effects of propofol are:

▶ Sedation to unconsciousness
▶ Quick metabolization, rapid emergence

Three main disadvantages of the use of propofol are:

▶ Pain on injection
▶ Respiratory and cardiac depression
▶ Hypotension

DIPHENHYDRAMINE (BENADRYL)

Diphenhydramine is used in sedation.
The effects of diphenhydramine are:

▶ Blocking of histamines
▶ Synergistic action with CNS depressants
▶ No analgesia
▶ Reduction of mucous membrane secretions

These problems can occur when diphenhydramine is used:

▶ Hypotension
▶ Tachycardia
▶ Urinary retention
▶ Nausea and vomiting

KETAMINE (KETALAR)

Ketamine is a rapidly acting sedative that produces isolation of the sensory parts of the brain, including those mediating sight, hearing, and pain sensation. The result is a dissociative or trancelike state. Ketamine is used in deep sedation. A benefit of ketamine is bronchodilation.

The effects of ketamine are:

▶ Dissociative anesthesia
▶ Sedation
▶ Analgesia
▶ Amnesia

These problems can occur when ketamine is used:

▶ Clonic seizure
▶ Increased secretions
▶ Respiratory depression
▶ Hypertension
▶ Hallucinations or delirium during emergence
▶ Increased intracranial pressure
▶ Nausea, vomiting
▶ Copious secretions

ETOMIDATE (AMIDATE)

Etomidate is an intravenous-induction anesthetic. Unconsciousness occurs about 1 minute after administration. The drug has no analgesic effect but may be combined with narcotics and used intravenously to produce anesthesia.

Neuroleptanesthetic Agents

Neuroleptanesthesia refers to the anesthetic state induced by a combination of droperidol (Inapsine), an opioid such as fentanyl, and nitrous oxide gas. This combination of drugs produces unconsciousness. Its primary use is in older patients and those who are poor anesthetic risks. Side effects include hypotension, bradycardia, and respiratory depression. Neuroleptanesthetic agents are not used often.

Intravenous Barbiturates

Intravenous administration of barbiturates causes rapid induction and unconsciousness (within 30 seconds). Recovery also is rapid. However, these drugs may cause bronchospasm and profound respiratory depression at high doses. Bronchospasm is caused by the release of histamine that occurs with barbiturates. Intravenous barbiturates are poor analgesics and actually may increase pain sensitivity at low dosage (e.g., thiopental).
Intravenous barbiturates are used for:

▶ Induction
▶ Deep sedation for general anesthesia

Intravenous barbiturates produce the following effects:

▶ Sedation and unconsciousness
▶ Amnesia
▶ No analgesia

These problems can occur when intravenous barbiturates are used:

▶ Respiratory depression, synergistic action with CNS depressants
▶ Bronchospasm
▶ Cardiac arrhythmia, tachycardia

▶ Hypotension and peripheral vasodilation
▶ CNS excitement (during "excitement" phase of induction)

The following are examples of intravenous barbiturates:

▶ Thiopental (Pentothal)
▶ Pentobarbital (Nembutal)
▶ Methohexital (Brevital)
▶ Thiamylal sodium (Surital)

Narcotic Analgesics
USES AND EFFECTS
Narcotics are classified according to source. Opium is the source of many different alkaloids (opium derivatives), including morphine. Opium derivatives are sometimes called *opiates.* Three subcategories of alkaloid make up the narcotic analgesics. These are purified alkaloids of morphine, semisynthetic morphine (codeine), and synthetic narcotics. The CNS has many receptors for narcotic analgesics. These agents mimic the brain's naturally occurring endorphins, which are similar in structure to morphine. All narcotics produce analgesia by altering the patient's *perception* of pain and also produce unconsciousness.

When the analgesic effects of narcotics are rated, morphine is used as a reference. For example, fentanyl is 100 times more effective as an analgesic than morphine.

Narcotic analgesics are used in surgery for:

▶ Pain control
▶ Sedation

The effects of narcotic analgesics:

▶ Analgesia
▶ Sedation
▶ Euphoria

These problems can occur when narcotic analgesics are used:

▶ CNS depression
▶ Hypotension, shock
▶ Respiratory depression
▶ Drug interactions with alcohol, amphetamines, antihistamines
▶ Profound sedation, coma
▶ Nausea and vomiting

The following are examples of narcotic analgesics:

▶ Morphine sulfate
▶ Meperidine (Demerol)
▶ Hydromorphone (Dilaudid)
▶ Sufentanil (Sufenta)
▶ Alfentanil (Alfenta)
▶ Fentanyl (Sublimaze)

REVERSAL OF EFFECTS
Agents to reverse the effects of narcotic analgesics displace opiates from their receptor sites in the CNS and arrest their action. However, if additional opioids are administered, they can displace the inhibitory drug. Repeated doses of the reversal drugs may be necessary to restore full respiratory function. The most commonly used opiate reversal agent is naloxone (Narcan). Adverse effects include sudden analgesic reversal causing tachycardia and hypertension (signs of pain), pulmonary edema, withdrawal symptoms in opiate-dependent individuals, and cardiac arrhythmia.

Anticholinergic Agents
Anticholinergic agents inhibit parasympathetic nerve transmission and the effects of acetylcholine. Most are derived from alkaloids of belladonna (a naturally occurring anticholinergic). Anticholinergics have many different effects that correlate with interruption of parasympathetic impulses.

In the past, potent anticholinergics such as scopolamine and atropine were given routinely to all surgical patients. Now, however, these agents are used more selectively and can be administered intravenously for rapid results. In surgery, anticholinergics are usually used to control airway secretions and to regulate heart rate in selected patients. In ophthalmic surgery they are used to produce mydriasis (dilation of the pupil) and cycloplegia (paralysis of the ciliary muscles).

Anticholinergics are used in surgery for:

▶ Prevention of aspiration
▶ Regulation of heart rate
▶ Relaxation of smooth muscles in selected ophthalmic procedures
▶ Drying of secretions

The effects of anticholinergics are:

▶ Reduction of gastrointestinal secretions
▶ Reduction of bronchial and nasopharyngeal secretions
▶ Emergency treatment of cardiac conduction block and sinus bradycardia
▶ Prevention of bronchospasm

These problems can occur when anticholinergics are used:

▶ Hypertension
▶ Tachycardia
▶ Increased intraocular pressure
▶ Increased gastric acid production, vomiting
▶ Many harmful drug interactions

The following are examples of anticholinergic agents:

▶ Atropine sulfate (Isopto Atropine)
▶ Scopolamine (Hyoscine)
▶ Glycopyrrolate (Robinul)

Drugs to Reduce the Effects of Aspiration
To minimize the effects of gastric secretions on the lungs in the event of aspiration, preoperative administration of drugs that suppress gastric acid production, reduce nausea, or raise the pH of the gastric contents may be prescribed.

Sodium citrate with citric acid (Bicitra) increases the pH of gastric secretions. Histamine antagonists (blocking agents) are administered to suppress the release of gastric acids. Examples are cimetidine (Tagamet), ranitidine (Zantac), and omeprazole (Prilosec).

Skeletal Muscle Relaxants

Skeletal muscle–relaxing agents are used in balanced general anesthesia to permit easier endotracheal intubation and tissue manipulation (such as during orthopedic or abdominal surgery). Two categories of muscle relaxants are used: *depolarizing agents* and competitive or *nondepolarizing agents.* Depolarizing agents initially depolarize the postsynaptic membrane, causing the muscles to respond and put them in a refractory state so that further stimulation does not create a response. Nondepolarizing agents occupy the receptor sites for acetylcholine and are the agents primarily used in surgery. The depth of neuromuscular blocking is monitored with a peripheral nerve stimulator (see the earlier section, Biophysical Monitoring).

Skeletal muscle relaxants are used in surgery as an adjunct to general anesthesia to permit tissue manipulation, especially during intubation. Muscle relaxants are classified as depolarizing or nondepolarizing, depending on how the neuroceptor of the skeletal muscle responds.

The effects of skeletal muscle relaxants are:

▶ Relaxation and paralysis of skeletal muscles
▶ No analgesia or sedation

These problems can occur when the skeletal muscle relaxant succinylcholine (Anectine) is used (however, they are not a concern for the more commonly used nondepolarizers):

▶ Respiratory depression and apnea (cessation of voluntary breathing) at high and even low doses
▶ Tachycardia, bradycardia, cardiac arrest
▶ Adverse effects in patients with conditions such as glaucoma, eye injury, anemia, burns, and multiple trauma
▶ Malignant hyperthermia
▶ Bronchospasm, only in those relaxants that cause the release of histamine (i.e., atracurium and mivacurium)
▶ Synergistic effects with some inhalation anesthetics

The following are examples of skeletal muscle–relaxing agents:

▶ Turbocurarine (prototype of the naturally occurring substance curare)
▶ Atracurium besylate (Tracrium)
▶ Cisatracurium besylate (Nimbex)
▶ Rocuronium (Zemuron)
▶ Doxacurium chloride (Nuromax)
▶ Pancuronium bromide (Pavulon)
▶ Metocurine iodide (Metubine)
▶ Succinylcholine chloride (Anectine, Quelicin)
▶ Succinylcholine is the only depolarizing muscle relaxant used in surgery. The rest of these are nondepolarizing agents.

COMPLICATIONS OF GENERAL ANESTHESIA

Cardiopulmonary Arrest

All health-care workers should maintain current certification in cardiopulmonary resuscitation and be able to respond in case of a cardiopulmonary arrest. All hospitals are required to have a specific, well-written protocol for dealing with this complication. Cardiopulmonary arrest can occur during any surgical procedure. The risk increases during sedation or general anesthesia. When arrest occurs, the surgical team responds immediately. If the patient is intubated, oxygen is delivered through the airway. If no airway is in place, the patient may be immediately intubated, cardiac compressions are initiated, and resuscitative drugs are immediately administered. Although the primary responsibility of the scrubbed surgical technologist is to maintain the sterile field, both the circulator and scrubbed technologist should be prepared to assist in closed or open cardiopulmonary resuscitation if necessary.

Other responsibilities of the surgical technologist may include assisting in an immediate thoracotomy for cardiac massage. If this should occur, a basic thoracotomy tray, suction device, extra sponges, and sutures are quickly distributed. The ACP usually directs the resuscitation efforts, and additional help is called as needed to distribute supplies or assist in resuscitation.

Malignant Hyperthermia

Malignant hyperthermia is a *rare* condition that is not clearly understood. The patterns, symptoms, and onset vary among patients. Possible early signs are contracture of the masseter muscle, cardiac arrhythmia and tachycardia, increased carbon dioxide expiration, muscle rigidity, and flushed skin. Late signs include hypoxemia (low oxygen saturation), hypotension, complex cardiac arrhythmias, and hyperthermia.

To stop the reaction, volatile anesthetics are withdrawn and 100% oxygen is administered. Anesthesia is deepened with opioids, benzodiazepines, barbiturates, or propofol. Dantrolene is the antidote and must be given in very high doses. This drug comes as a powder and requires lots of help from ancillary personnel to mix and prepare for administration to the patient. Antiarrhythmic drugs are administered as needed, and sodium bicarbonate is given as indicated by the results of blood gas analysis. Cooling is achieved through delivery of ice water via nasogastric tube as well as the use of ice packs. Surgery is halted as soon as possible, and the patient is transferred to the intensive care unit.

The scrubbed technologist remains sterile to assist in protecting the surgical incision. The circulator assists in obtaining and preparing ice or iced slush solution and other supplies as directed by the ACP.

All inhalation anesthetics with the exception of nitrous oxide are associated with malignant hyperthermia events. The preoperative anesthesia history should identify any family history of problems during anesthesia.

Massive Hemorrhage

In the event of massive uncontrolled hemorrhage, specific surgical equipment is needed immediately. The scrubbed technologist must be prepared for this event, think clearly and methodically, and remain absolutely attentive to the needs of the surgeon and changing conditions.

Extra suction tubing and tips are passed onto the field. An autotransfuser or cell saver system may be set up by the circulator. The surgical technologist must be familiar with this device (refer to Chapter 15). Wide retractors may be necessary, and the means to arrest bleeding may be vascular clamps and suture ligatures. Sponges are required to pack the surgical wound. In extreme emergency, these sponges may not be counted according to normal policy, but the surgical technologist must keep track of how many have been placed in the surgical wound. Blood products and intravenous fluids may be infused via pressure devices to maintain intravascular volume.

It is critical that the scrubbed technologist verify and accurately count the amount of irrigation that is used by the surgeon, and communicate that information to the ACP, so that the ACP can more accurately predict blood loss.

The most important priority during hemorrhage is *visibility and control of the bleeding vessel.* This requires retraction, clamps, and sutures. If the hemorrhage occurs in a large vessel such as the aorta or one of its branches, arterial clamps are distributed to the field immediately. The surgical technologist should place vascular clamps on the Mayo stand as soon as they are available. Appropriate sutures should be loaded and ready for immediate use.

REGIONAL ANESTHESIA

Regional anesthesia is a reversible loss of sensation in a specific area of the body produced by drug delivery. Motor, sensory, and autonomic responses also may be suppressed.

All regional anesthetics are absorbed into the body, metabolized, and excreted. The rate of metabolism of a local anesthetic in relation to the absorption rate is important in terms of patient safety. If absorption is more rapid than metabolism, the risk of toxic reaction increases. Some anesthetics are metabolized by the liver, and others are degraded by enzymes.

The degree of absorption is directly related to the vascularity of the area. One can alter absorption by adding epinephrine to the drug. Epinephrine constricts the blood vessels in the local area and controls bleeding. As part of the anesthetic drug formula, epinephrine prevents dissipation but also creates risks because levels of epinephrine are elevated in the bloodstream as the anesthetic compound dissipates.

Drug Dosage

The effective dosage of an anesthetic must be calculated according to the individual patient's ability to absorb and metabolize the drug. The "normal" or safe dosage depends on many factors. Therapeutic ranges for all local anesthetics are readily available. However, these are considered with knowledge of the patient's physical condition, especially the presence of cardiac disease, concurrent use of prescribed or illicit drugs, age, weight, and vascular status. Dosage is adjusted based on concurrent patient assessment during the procedure.

The rate of metabolism and response to the drug determine whether dangerous levels are being reached. *External monitoring serves as an objective method of detecting signs of toxicity.* This is especially critical in patients who require a wide area of anesthesia, nerve block, or field block. A much larger amount of anesthetic agent is needed in these cases, and consequently the risk of adverse reactions or an emergency situation is much greater.

Anesthetic dosage is calculated *by weight.* For example, the maximum dose of lidocaine (Xylocaine) is 5 mg/kg. A 1% solution of lidocaine contains 10 mg of anesthetic per ml of fluid. Therefore, a 75-kg (165-lb) person should receive no more than 375 mg (37.5 ml) of 1% lidocaine. The addition of epinephrine to lidocaine will increase the amount of solution that can be administered safely because the vasconstricting properties of the epinephrine slow the rate of absorption of the anesthetic. For example, the maximum dose of lidocaine 1% solution with epinephrine is 7 mg/kg. Therefore, a 75-kg (165-lb) patient should receive no more than 525 mg (52.5 ml) of solution.

The surgical technologist has an intermediary role in the delivery of drugs in surgery. He or she receives the drug from licensed personnel and passes it to another person licensed to administer the drug. In playing this intermediary role, the surgical technologist must exercise the same care taken by all personnel in handling drugs.

Because the surgical technologist does not perform nursing or medical *assessment,* his or her critical role is to *know at all times how much drug has been delivered to the field and in what concentration.*

The surgical technologist should plan ahead and consult with the ACP or surgeon to establish a safe level of drugs for the patient. He or she must then inform the ACP, surgeon, and circulator when that level is being approached.

Drug Toxicity and Allergic Response

Toxic reactions to local anesthetics arise most often during **regional block** and epidural anesthesia. This is because of the large amount of drug administered and the proximity to the vascular system. Local anesthesia of the intercostal region is associated with the highest blood level of anesthetic, followed by local anesthesia of the caudal epidural space and the brachial plexus. Toxic reactions from local anesthetics occur in two forms: CNS toxicity and cardiovascular toxicity.

CNS REACTIONS

CNS toxicity occurs in three phases. The *excitation phase* produces light-headedness, restlessness, confusion, perioral tingling (tingling around the mouth), metallic taste, tinnitus (ringing in the ears), and a sense of impending doom. The patient may become talkative. This phase is followed by the *convulsive phase.* In this phase grand mal seizures can occur. The *depressive phase* is characterized by CNS depression, drowsiness, and unconsciousness. Respiratory depression, apnea, and death follow.

CARDIOVASCULAR REACTIONS

The first phase of cardiovascular toxicity is excitation. The patient develops tachycardia, hypertension, and convulsions. This is followed by the depressive phase, which is characterized by reduced blood pressure, reduced cardiac output and stroke volume, bradycardia, and complete heart block (loss of electrical conduction) and arrest. Vasodilation caused by local anesthetics results in severe hypotension, which may or may not be reversible through cardiac drugs.

ALLERGIC REACTIONS

True allergic reactions, which are different from reactions caused by toxicity, range from local skin irritation and itching to severe anaphylaxis, which produces life-threatening changes in the cardiovascular and respiratory systems.

MANAGEMENT OF TOXIC AND ALLERGIC REACTIONS

Every patient receiving a local anesthetic should undergo objective monitoring of vital signs. All team members must be familiar with toxic doses associated with different local anesthetics. In addition, the staff must be familiar with symptoms of allergic reactions and be able to recognize signs of allergic reaction. Maintaining verbal contact with the patient helps to identify symptoms. A patient report of any adverse symptom must trigger further assessment.

Resuscitative equipment *must be immediately available whenever a local anesthetic is administered.* CNS toxicity is treated in the early stage with intravenous benzodiazepines or thiopental. If respiratory arrest occurs, mechanical ventilation may be necessary. This requires emergency intubation or positive pressure ventilation through a mask.

During any emergency, the surgical technologist responds in accordance with his or her training and knowledge. Cardiopulmonary resuscitation is the minimum requirement for emergency response. Beyond this, licensed personnel usually are involved in administration of reversal drugs, establishment of an airway, and performance of more advanced life support procedures.

Methods of Regional Anesthesia
MONITORED ANESTHESIA CARE

Monitored anesthesia care or MAC is the service provided by an ACP during regional anesthesia. In some institutions this is called *anesthesia standby.* MAC is required when the patient is at high risk under even local anesthesia. The ACP performs biophysical monitoring and balanced sedation, and manages adverse or toxic reactions to drugs or other changes in the patient's condition. He or she administers oxygen and supplemental drugs to produce amnesia and sedation. If the need arises, the ACP can administer a general

anesthetic. An example of MAC is the care of a patient with cardiovascular disease who is having a pacemaker implanted under local anesthesia.

TOPICAL ANESTHESIA

Topical anesthetics are used on mucous membranes and on superficial eye tissues during ophthalmic surgery. Topical agents are used before insertion of endotracheal and LMA devices and also before laryngoscopy and bronchoscopy, in which direct insertion of the instrument causes reflexive gagging. During cystoscopic procedures, instruments that contact the delicate mucosal lining of the urethra are coated with topical anesthetic gel. Topical skin agents may be used at an intravenous site to anesthetize the area before insertion of a catheter. This is usually done for pediatric patients.

Topical agents can be absorbed readily through the mucous membranes. Although the amount of agent applied is limited, the patient must be monitored for toxic reactions. Agents used in topical anesthesia are listed in Table 12-3.

LOCAL INFILTRATION

Local infiltration is the simplest form of regional anesthesia. In this technique local anesthetic agent is injected into superficial tissues to produce a small area of analgesia and anesthesia. Local infiltration is used to produce anesthesia in removal of superficial skin lesions, suturing of a wound, or slightly more invasive surgery such as insertion of chest tubes.

When local infiltration is planned, it is a part of the sterile procedure. The surgical technologist should provide a 25-, 26-, or 30-gauge needle and 10-ml and 25-ml syringes. After the initial infiltration, larger-bore needles can be used. The surgical technologist is responsible for keeping track of the amount of anesthetic that has been used and reporting it to the circulator. The total amount infiltrated must be noted and recorded. Maximum safe dosage varies with the agent used, the concentration, and the weight of the patient. When the patient receives local anesthetic, standards of protocol are followed at all times (refer to Chapter 13). Local anesthetics have the potential to cause serious toxic complications. The surgical technologist must know these complications and the signs of toxicity.

PERIPHERAL NERVE BLOCK

A peripheral nerve block is achieved when anesthetic agent is injected around a specific large nerve such as the ulnar, median, radial, saphenous, or intercostal nerve, or in a region such as the entire arm or leg. These large nerves generally follow a major artery. Administering a peripheral block requires experience in locating the nerve without injecting the artery, because this would create a risk of anesthetic overdose. The nerve is sometimes identified with a nerve simulator. This device uses a needle to deliver small pulses of current to the tissue, which causes muscle twitching. As the pulse gets closer to the nerve, less current is required to elicit a strong twitch. Common nerve blocks are named for their

Table 12-3   LOCAL ANESTHETICS FOR TOPICAL USE

Generic Name	Trade Name	Eyes	Mucous Membranes*	Skin	Comments
Benzocaine	Americaine Dermoplast†	0	+	+	Widely used. Included in many nonprescription preparations to relieve sunburn, itching, and mild burns. Long acting and poorly absorbed.
Butamben	Dermacaine	0	+	+	Mucosal formulation includes benzocaine and tetracaine. Also available as a nonprescription ointment to relieve itching and burning.
Cocaine hydrochloride	Cocaine	+	+	0	Schedule II drug. Medically used in ear, nose, and throat procedures when vasoconstriction and shrinking of mucous membranes are desired. Ophthalmic preparations anesthetize cornea and conjunctiva.
Dibucaine hydrochloride	Nupercaine†	0	+	+	Nonprescription skin ointment or cream; also cream for relieving hemorrhoids.
Dyclonine hydrochloride	Dyclone Sucrets	0	+	+	Lozenges relieve sore throat. Topical formulations suppress gag reflex and lessen discomfort of genitourinary endoscopy. Precipitated by iodine in contrast media employed in pyelography and should not be used in this procedure.
Lidocaine	Xylocaine†	0	+	+	Widely used for topical anesthesia in ear, nose, and throat procedures; upper digestive tract procedures; and genitourinary procedures. Rapid onset and intermediate duration. Not irritating and low incidence of hypersensitivity.
Lidocaine hydrochloride	Xylocaine †	0	+	+	
Pramoxine hydrochloride	Fleet Pain-Relief Pads Tronothane†	0	+‡	+	Nonprescription cream or ointment primarily used to relieve pain of itching, burns, and hemorrhoids.
Proparacaine hydrochloride	Ophthaine†	+	0	0	Applied topically to eye to anesthetize cornea and conjunctiva.
Tetracaine hydrochloride	Pontocaine†	+	+	+	For topical administration, onset is 5 min and duration is 45 min. Usual topical dose is 20 mg; maximum is 50 mg because of toxicity and slow degradation. Ophthalmic preparations are dilute solutions for instillation.

From Clark JF and Queener SF: *Pharmacologic basis of nursing practice,* ed 6, St Louis, 1999, Mosby.
+, Site suitable for application; 0, site not suitable for application.
* Mucous membranes include the oral esophageal mucosa, the bronchotracheal mucosa, and the mucosa of the urethra, rectum, and vagina.
†Available in Canada and the United States.
‡Not for application to the bronchotracheal mucosa.

location, such as ulnar, radial, deep peroneal, saphenous, tibial, and intercostal nerve blocks.

When a nerve plexus (group of nerves in one location), such as the brachial plexus, is injected, anesthetic surrounds the nerve network and produces anesthesia throughout the tissues innervated by that plexus.

REGIONAL BLOCK

A regional block is one that affects a single nerve, a deep plexus or network of nerves, or a confined superficial area.

Nerves are classified as motor, sensory, or autonomic. Myelinated nerves (those with a myelin sheath) carry pain sensation quickly. Unmyelinated nerves conduct pain more slowly. For anesthesia to be achieved, all nerve fibers must be reached by the anesthetic agent. The goal of each type of regional block is to deposit and hold anesthetic agent in contact with the nerves. Epinephrine is used to constrict blood vessels at the site and prevent dissipation of the anesthetic. Epinephrine also facilitates the entry of the anesthetic into the nerve cell.

INTRAVENOUS ANESTHESIA (BIER BLOCK)

During intravenous anesthesia, blood is temporarily displaced from an extremity and replaced by anesthetic. This technique was first described by August Bier in the early 1900s and is sometimes called a **Bier block.** To displace the venous blood, one elevates the extremity and places a **pneumatic tourniquet** at the proximal end but does not inflate it. An elastic bandage called an **Esmarch bandage** then is wrapped the entire length of the extremity, starting at the distal end and extending to the proximal end (refer to Chapter 11). This pushes the venous blood to the proximal end. The tourniquet is then inflated and the Esmarch bandage removed. Anesthetic is injected into the major vein through a previously placed IV catheter. Double tourniquets also may be used—one proximal and one distal. Adjunct drugs are given to sedate the patient and reduce anxiety.

The risks of intravenous anesthesia are related to drug overdose. This can occur if the tourniquet suddenly loses pressure, releasing a bolus of anesthetic into the circulatory system. Signs and symptoms of overdose are discussed later in the chapter.

SPINAL ANESTHESIA
Patient Preparation
Patients undergoing regional anesthesia in the spinal area are usually fearful. They often fear spinal headache, permanent paralysis, or insufficient anesthesia, especially during major surgery. Reassure the patient by speaking in a calm voice and respond to his or her fears attentively. The patient must remain still during the spinal procedure. Your calming presence helps the patient to relax and maintain the required position. Place one hand over the shoulders and the other behind the patient's thighs to help stabilize the patient (Figure 12-15, *A*). Ensure that the patient is covered with a blanket or sheet, so that only the injection area is exposed. The patient also may sit on the edge of the operating table. The circulator should stand in front of the patient to support him or her, as shown in Figure 12-15, *B*.

Technique
During spinal anesthesia, anesthetic agent is injected into the subarachnoid space through a spinal needle inserted through a lower lumbar intervertebral space. To help facilitate the correct placement of the anesthetic in the spinal canal, dextrose sometimes is added to the agent. This makes the drug heavier than the cerebrospinal fluid. In accordance with the patient's position, the drug settles in the dependent areas and is absorbed at a specific site along the spinal cord. Nerve conduction along the nerve roots that emerge from that location is blocked. The areas of skin supplied by these nerves are called dermatomes (Figure 12-16). The anesthetic can be directed up, down, or laterally until it is fixed in the tissues. Spinal anesthesia can be used for many procedures but is most often used for gynecological, obstetrical, orthopedic, and genitourinary surgery.

After preparing the puncture site, the ACP infiltrates the area with a small amount of local anesthetic. He or she then inserts the spinal needle. When the needle enters the subarachnoid space, the spinal anesthetic is injected. The patient is then positioned in accordance with the surgery to

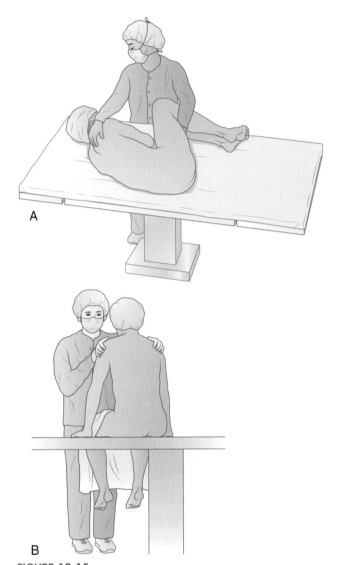

FIGURE 12-15
A and **B,** Positioning the patient for spinal anesthesia.

be performed, usually in a slight reverse Trendelenburg position.

Risks
Risks associated with spinal anesthesia include the following:

▶ **Hypotension**—A severe drop in blood pressure occurs when the spinal anesthetic blocks the conduction of sympathetic nerves that control vascular muscle tone. Adequate blood volume is no longer returned to the heart, and this results in stasis or pooling of blood in the lower extremities. To counteract a potential hypotensive event, intravenous fluid is administered before injection of spinal anesthetic.
▶ **Post–dural puncture headache**—The post–spinal anesthesia headache is related to reduced cerebrospinal pressure resulting from a leak at the puncture site in the dura mater. One treats it by hydrating the patient, administer-

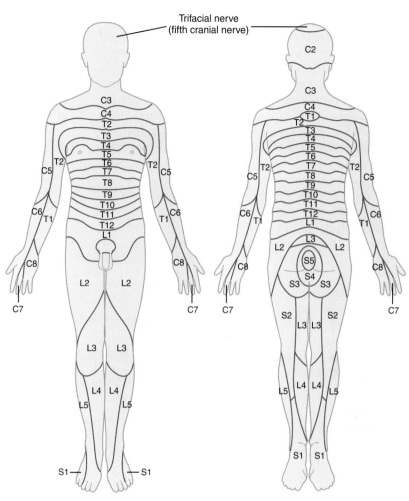

FIGURE 12-16
Dermatomes (Redrawn from Phillips N: *Berry & Kohn's operating room technique,* ed 10, St Louis, 2004, Mosby.)

ing caffeine, and having the patient lie flat. In severe cases the ACP may create a blood patch over the puncture site. One performs this procedure by epidurally injecting a small amount of blood, which coagulates over the puncture and seals the leak.

▶ **Total spinal anesthesia**—This occurs when the hyperbaric spinal anesthetic is too high and blocks the nerves controlling the diaphragm and accessory breathing muscles. Emergency intubation and ventilation are performed immediately.

EPIDURAL ANESTHESIA

Epidural anesthesia is produced when the anesthetic agent is injected into the epidural space that surrounds the dural sac (Figure 12-17). This space is closed at the foramen magnum where the spinal cord enters the cranium. Its boundaries are defined by the dura mater and the vertebral spaces. The space is filled with loose connective tissue, semiliquid fat, arteries, an extensive venous system, and the spinal nerve roots. After injection, the anesthetic agent

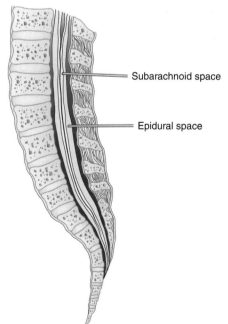

FIGURE 12-17
Area of injection for spinal anesthesia and epidural anesthesia. (Redrawn from Phillips N: *Berry & Kohn's operating room technique,* ed 10, St Louis, 2004, Mosby.)

is very slowly absorbed into the cerebrospinal fluid through the dura mater. It spreads both caudally (toward the feet) and cephalad (toward the head). For a single-shot epidural, the patient's position and the molecular weight of the anesthetic have no effect on its distribution. However, with a continuous epidural, the position of the patient does seem to affect the spread of the local anesthetic. Epidural anesthesia is often used in obstetrical, gynecological, urological, and rectal surgery. It also is used for postoperative pain control.

The patient's skin is prepared as for spinal anesthesia. The epidural needle is advanced through the ligamentum flavum until it enters the epidural space. A thoracic, lumbar, or caudal puncture site is used, depending on the target site of the anesthesia. The anesthetic agent is then injected directly into the epidural space. Lidocaine, chloroprocaine, and bupivacaine are commonly used.

Continuous or intermittent epidural anesthesia is created by the delivery of an anesthetic drug through a small indwelling catheter. This technique also is used for postopera-

Table 12-4 LOCAL ANESTHETICS FOR INJECTION

Generic Name	Trade Name	Local Infiltration or Nerve Block or Epidural Block	Spinal Block (Subarachnoid)	Duration*	Comments
Bupivacaine hydrochloride	Marcaine† Sensorcaine MPF	+	+	Long‡	Produces long-acting epidural anesthesia in labor with no reported effects on fetus. Maximum dose is 200 mg.
Chloroprocaine hydrochloride	Nesacaine	+	0	Short	Little systemic toxicity because of rapid hydrolysis in plasma. No effects reported on fetus after epidural anesthesia in mother. Maximum dose is 800 mg.
Etidocaine hydrochloride	Duranest	+	0	Long	Highly lipid soluble. Onset time for epidural block is 5 min. Profound muscle relaxation is desirable for abdominal surgery but not for labor.
Lidocaine	Xylocaine†	+	+	Intermediate	Widely used local anesthetic. Maximum dose is 300 mg (4.5 mg/kg body weight). Can cause drowsiness, fatigue, and amnesia.
Mepivacaine	Carbocaine†	+	0	Intermediate	Chemically related to lidocaine. Maximum dose is 400 mg (7 mg/kg body weight).
Prilocaine	Citanest†	+	0	Intermediate	Used for dental procedures. Maximum dose is 400 mg.
Procaine hydrochloride	Novocain†	+	0	Short	Noted for its safety because of its rapid hydrolysis in plasma. Maximum dose is 600 mg (10 mg/kg body weight). Duration of epidural block is unreliable.
Propoxycaine and procaine	Ravocaine and Novocain with Neo-Cobefri	+	0	Short to intermediate	Used for dental procedures. Dose is 4 mg propoxycaine and 20 mg procaine.
Ropivacaine	Naropin†	+	0	Long	Used for epidural, field block, and major nerve block anesthesia. Dose is 20-40 mg.
Tetracaine	Pontocaine†	0	+	Long	Most widely used drug for spinal anesthesia. Onset is 5 min. Dose for spinal anesthesia is 2-15 mg. Available in hyperbaric, isobaric, and hypobaric solutions.

From Clark JF and Queener SF: *Pharmacologic basis of nursing practice*, ed 6, St Louis, 1999, Mosby.
+, Suitable use; 0, not suitable use.
*Duration without epinephrine: short, 1 hr; intermediate, 2 hr; long, 3 hr (approximations).
†Available in Canada and the United States.
‡Duration of bupivacaine in nerve block is 6-13 hr.

tive or intractable pain in selected patients. A programmable drug reservoir and pump device are implanted in the patient. An opioid drug is then administered at the preprogrammed dose and rate.

In contrast to spinal anesthesia, epidural anesthesia requires a much larger amount of anesthetic agent. Accidental puncture of the dura mater can cause total spinal anesthesia. When this occurs, bradycardia, vasodilation, and respiratory paralysis result. The presence of an extensive network of veins in the epidural space also can lead to overdose by accidental venous injection. In such a case the patient is imme-diately intubated and ventilated. Although there is a risk of hypotension with epidural anesthesia, the onset is slower than with spinal anesthesia, and thus it is easier to control and correct.

LOCAL ANESTHETIC AGENTS

Local anesthetics are distinguished by their overall safety, specific use, duration of action, and chemical structure. Agents commonly used for infiltration, nerve block, and epidural block are listed and compared in Table 12-4.

CASE STUDIES

Case 1

You are serving as circulator on surgery to repair carpal tunnel entrapment. The anesthesiologist decides to use a Bier block. Halfway through the case, the operative site suddenly fills with blood. What does this indicate to you? What will you do? What are the specific risks to the patient?

Case 2

You are scrubbed on a case involving removal of a breast lump. You receive anesthetic agent from the circulator and label it properly. The patient is uncomfortable, and the surgeon continues to administer more local anesthetic by infiltration. You lose track of how much has been used. What will you do? How might you avoid this issue in the future? Why is it important?

Case 3

You are scrubbed on a cholecystectomy case. The circulator has left the room momentarily to check supplies for the next case. After skin closing, the surgeon announces that he wishes to perform an intercostal block to reduce postoperative pain. During the block procedure, the patient has a cardiac arrest. Only the surgeon, the anesthesiologist, and you (the scrubbed surgical technologist) are in the room. What do you think the sequence of events might be? Would you be prepared to participate in resuscitation? What would be your role as the scrubbed technologist?

Case 4

During a laparotomy, the patient begins to move. You are scrubbed, and the Mayo stand is in its normal position over the patient's knees. The patient is struggling so much that she is in danger of falling off the table. What will you do?

Case 5

You are serving as circulator on a thyroidectomy case. The patient undergoes anesthesia induction, and just before intubation he stops breathing. During the attempt to intubate the patient, he begins coughing and becomes cyanotic (skin turns blue). The circulator tells you to stand out of the way. The surgeon tells you to assist him by holding the patient's head still. What will you do?

Case 6

You are in the hallway of the operating room. A laboratory worker comes in carrying a Styrofoam container holding several units of blood. He asks you where it goes. You report that it should go in the unit secretary's office. You continue your work and later learn that the blood was not found when needed in an emergency. Later the unit secretary finds it in her office under the desk, but it is too late to use it. How could this situation have been prevented? What should you have done? Who is responsible for the lost blood bags? If you were the supervisor, how would you handle this situation?

REFERENCES

American Association of Nurse Anesthetists: *Consideration for policy guidelines for registered nurses engaged in the administration of sedation and analgesia,* June, 1993.

Barash PG, Cullen BF, and Stoelting RK, eds: *Clinical anesthesia,* ed 4, Philadelphia, 2000, Lippincott, Williams & Wilkins.

Beers MH and Berkow R, eds: *The Merck manual of diagnosis and therapy,* ed 17, 1999-2003, Merck & Co.

Graber MA and Lanternier ML: *University of Iowa: the family practice handbook,* ed 4, St Louis, 2001, Mosby.

Hata T et al.: *Guidelines, education, and testing for procedural sedation and analgesia,* University of Iowa, 1992-2003.

Joint Commission on Accreditation of Healthcare Organizations: *Comprehensive accreditation manual for hospitals: revisions to anesthesia care standards,* Jan, 2001.

Novak LC: ASA updates its position on monitored anesthesia care, *ASA Newsletter* 62, Dec, 1998.

Wenker OC: Review of currently used inhalation anesthetics: part II, *Internet Journal of Anesthesiology* 3:3, 1999.

Chapter 13

Surgical Pharmacology

Learning Objectives

After studying this chapter the reader will be able to:

- Name agencies that regulate drugs and resources for drug information
- List categories of controlled substances
- List the pregnancy categories for drugs
- Discuss the legal aspects of drug handling
- Accurately define and use terminology describing drug handling and drug administration
- Describe the process of drug prescription, transcription, dispensing, and administration
- Accurately convert values within and between measurement systems
- Perform selected drug calculations
- Briefly describe the aspects of drug action
- Discuss the difference between therapeutic and toxic or lethal doses, using correct terminology
- Correctly identify the parts of a drug label
- Explain the "six rights" of drug handling
- Describe the correct method for receiving and passing drugs to and from the sterile field
- Describe the categories of drugs used intraoperatively
- Identify the parts of a syringe and explain the importance of syringe safety features

Terminology

Adverse reactions—Unexpected reactions to a drug that are not related to dose.

Antibiotic—A drug that inhibits the growth of or kills microorganisms in living tissue.

Anticoagulant—A drug that prolongs blood clotting time.

Concentration—A measure of the quantity of a substance per a specific volume or weight.

Contrast medium—A radiopaque (not penetrated by x-rays) solution that is introduced into body cavities to outline their inside surface.

Controlled substances—Drugs that have the potential for abuse. Controlled substances are rated according to their risk potential. These ratings are called schedules.

Dosage—The regulated administration of prescribed amounts of a drug. Dosage is usually expressed as a quantity of drug per unit of time.

Dose—The quantity of a drug to be taken at one time or the stated amount of drug per unit of distribution (e.g., 0.5 mg per milliliter of solution).

Drug—Chemical substance that, when taken into the body, changes one or more of the body's functions.

Drug administration—The actual giving of a drug to a person by any route.

Dye—A drug typically administered to allow a surgeon to observe under direct visualization the patency of a tubular structure (e.g., fallopian tube, ureter).

Generic name—The formulary name of a drug.

Parenterally—Referring to administration of a drug by injection.

Terminology—cont'd

Pharmacodynamics—The biochemical and physiological effects of drugs and their mechanisms of action in the body.

Pharmacokinetics—The movement of a drug through the tissues and cells of the body, including the processes of absorption, distribution, and localization in tissues, biotransformation, and excretion by mechanical and chemical means.

Pharmacology—The study of drugs and their action on the body.

Prescription—A written order for a drug. Only licensed personnel may prescribe drugs.

Side effects—Anticipated effects of a drug other than those intended. Side effects may be uncomfortable for the patient or may have a positive consequence.

Stain—A substance that is applied directly to anatomical surfaces to differentiate normal from abnormal cells.

Topical—Referring to application of a drug to the skin or mucous membranes.

Trade name—The name given to a drug by the company that produces and sells it.

Transdermal—Referring to administration of a drug through a skin patch impregnated with the drug.

U.S. Pharmacopeia (USP)—A compendium of standards for drugs approved by the Food and Drug Administration for their labeled use. All approved drugs have been tested for consumer safety, and written information is available about their pharmacological action, use, risks, and dosage.

WHAT IS PHARMACOLOGY?

The study of **drugs** is called **pharmacology.** Pharmacology encompasses drug composition, mechanism of action, **adverse reactions** and **side effects,** and the proper methods for dispensing and administering a drug. This chapter focuses on the surgical technologist's role and the *safety* aspects of drug handling. Drugs that are dispensed to the sterile field intraoperatively are emphasized. Refer to Chapter 12 for a discussion of anesthetics, the central nervous system, and drugs administered preoperatively.

LEGAL POLICIES AND RESPONSIBILITIES FOR DRUG HANDLING

Legal Policies

The regulations affecting the handling of drugs in the medical setting are defined by each state's medical and nurse practice acts. The Joint Commission for the Accreditation of Healthcare Organizations requires health-care organizations to develop policies that agree with state laws regulating who may handle drugs and how. These policies regulate the following activities:

▶ Procurement, storage, and selection of drugs
▶ Prescription, ordering, and transcription of drug orders
▶ Preparation and dispensing of drugs
▶ Administration of drugs
▶ Monitoring of the patient after the administration of a drug

To prevent patient harm or death, all personnel who participate in these activities must be trained and specifically designated to perform them by hospital policy and individual state law. The surgical technologist is responsible for knowing and complying with these laws and regulations. Although laws among states are similar, they are not all the same. Most do not directly identify the surgical technologist but rather specify whether a *licensed* or *unlicensed* person may carry out specific tasks.

DRUG STORAGE AND SELECTION

The operating room uses a rotating supply of drugs from the hospital pharmacy. Drugs usually are stored in a restricted area on open shelves or in a computerized drug-storage device. Some operating rooms have their own pharmacy located within the operating room. **Controlled substances** always are kept in a locked cabinet or dispenser and are inventoried by licensed personnel according to hospital policy, usually once per shift.

Selecting the correct drug is a critical activity in the medication process. Trained personnel (and in some cases only licensed personnel) select necessary drugs from the operating room stock on a case-by-case basis. The selection and retrieval of controlled substances always must be performed by a licensed health-care worker. The selection of standard drugs often used during various surgical procedures is based on the surgeon's order, which is found in his or her preference sheet for each type of procedure, and is confirmed with the surgeon before use in the surgical suite.

PRESCRIPTION, ORDERING, AND TRANSCRIPTION OF DRUG ORDERS

A **prescription** is a written or verbal order for dispensing and administering a drug. Only persons licensed by law to prescribe drugs may give a prescription order. A drug transcription is a handwritten or typed transfer of a drug order. Only licensed personnel can give and take verbal orders for a drug. In the operating room, the surgeon usually gives a verbal order for the drugs to be used in a particular procedure. This order then is transcribed to his or her orders and preference sheet. The surgeon also may verbally prescribe (request) a drug during surgery.

PREPARATION AND DISPENSING OF DRUGS

Drugs usually are prepared and dispensed to the hospital departments by the pharmacy, as mentioned previously. In the operating room, the circulator dispenses drugs to the scrub. Both the person who dispenses the drug and the person who receives it are responsible for checking the drug's identity, strength, condition, and expiration date. Scrubbed personnel are required to mix and label drugs at the sterile field. As dispensing agents, scrubbed personnel also are accountable for verifying the drug's identity, strength, condition, and expiration date. If they have mixed drugs together, they have created a new drug and are responsible for ensuring the correct drug identity, correct ratio of drugs, and correct **dose** as well as verifying the other information already mentioned. These activities carry a high risk for error and injury. The approved procedures for conducting these activities are described in the next section.

DRUG ADMINISTRATION AND MONITORING

Drug administration is the physical act of giving a drug to the patient by any route. State practice acts and hospital policy determine who may administer a drug and the route by which it may be administered. Only licensed personnel can legally administer drugs, including **topical** medications. Anyone who administers a drug takes the responsibility for accurately determining the correct identity, dose, **concentration,** strength, and expiration date of the drug. He or she also must be able to monitor the patient for adverse reactions. This requires knowledge of the patient's medical history as well as of the drug's therapeutic range, safe **dosage,** time to onset of effects and peak action, rate and means of absorption, distribution, metabolism, and elimination. He or she also must be able to perform a clinical evaluation of the patient for adverse or toxic reactions and must have the training to deal with a drug-related emergency.

State Practice Acts and Legal Responsibility

The surgical technologist's role in handling medications is defined by the medical and nursing practice acts of his or her state. It is very important to use specific definitions when discussing the responsibility of the surgical technologist.

- The role of the surgical technologist in handling drugs is to serve as an intermediary between two licensed people.
- The licensed nurse is responsible for selecting the drug prescribed by the physician. This is *not* because the surgical technologist is unable to read the physician's orders or obtain a drug from the pharmacy. It is because the *licensed nurse has the responsibility to ensure that it is the correct drug.* Lawsuits that arise out of medication errors target licensed personnel. Many licensed nurses prefer to perform as many of the drug-handling tasks as possible rather than delegate them to another person. They are protecting their licenses and fulfilling their own professional responsibilities.
- The surgical technologist is responsible for knowing the name of the drug, the strength, and its use. Before any

drug is passed from the instrument table to the surgeon, the surgical technologist must identify the drug by name and must verify the strength, amount, and expiration date.

- **The surgical technologist must calculate the amount of drug administered. When asked, he or she must be able to report this immediately.**
- **The surgical technologist never administers drugs to the patient.** The scrubbed technologist sometimes must calculate the ratio or strength of a solution in surgery. In this case, the surgical technologist must be able to work with fractions and proportions easily and quickly.
- **The surgical technologist** *monitors* **the amount and strength of every drug he or she passes to the surgeon.** The surgeon administers the drug, the anesthesia care provider (ACP) monitors the patient's physiological response, and the circulator gets the drug, calculates the dosage, distributes the drug, and monitors the patient along with the ACP.
- **Anyone involved in patient care and medication handling, including the surgical technologist, must be able to perform drug calculations.** The purpose of this skill is to enable the individual to correctly mix drugs in the field and to *produce accurate reporting* both before and after a drug is administered.

ACCEPTING AND HANDLING OF MEDICATION IN THE STERILE FIELD

Standards have been developed for the handling of medication in the sterile field and should be strictly followed. These standards were developed to protect patients and prevent medication errors.

Follow this procedure for accepting medications in the sterile field:

1. The surgical technologist has a sterile medication cup (or sterile container for larger solutions) available to receive the medication.
2. The nurse *shows* the vial to the surgical technologist so that he or she can read the *name, amount, expiration date,* and where applicable the *percentage* (strength) of the drug.
3. The surgical technologist recites *aloud* to the nurse the information described in step 2 (e.g., "1% Xylocaine, with epinephrine, one to two hundred thousandths, 50 cc"). The nurse then distributes the drug to the surgical technologist.
4. The nurse shows the vial to the surgical technologist a second time. The surgical technologist mentally notes the name and amount of the drug he or she has just received, and labels drug containers (e.g., medication cups, syringes) appropriately.

In summary, the surgical technologist reads, recites, accepts, and reads again the type and amount of medication received. This routine for accepting medication is sometimes dangerously ignored when a commonly used medication is distributed (e.g., a local anesthetic). The nurse and surgical technologist must not allow supposed familiarity with bottle size and label color to interfere with the proper identification of medication. Poor technique and disregard for accepted procedure may cause severe injury to the patient.

The surgical technologist always should follow these precautions when handling medications:

1. Always use accepted procedures when receiving any drug.
2. Never accept a medication from a vial that is cracked or chipped. This might indicate the presence of bacteria or glass chips in the solution.
3. Label all medications and solutions received on the sterile field with a marking pen.
4. Monitor and record how much irrigation solution is used within the wound so that blood loss can be accurately determined.
5. Never accept a medication that appears discolored or is otherwise suspicious.
6. If you are uncertain for any reason (or have forgotten) which basins contain which medications or solutions on the back table, *discard* them all and request additional solutions to be distributed.
7. Do not accept a medication whose vial or bottle you have not read. Occasionally in a very rushed procedure, a nurse may distribute a medication to the back table without the scrub person's knowledge and may then inform the scrub person that a certain drug is in a certain basin (or in an emergency the surgical technologist may not be able to turn his or her attention to the nurse). *This is unacceptable technique.* The circulator and the surgical technologist both are responsible for making certain the correct drug in the correct amount and in the correct strength is distributed. Likewise during a shift change when one scrub person replaces another at the field, the incoming person must verify all medications and solutions.
8. Check the expiration dates of all medication and solution distributed to the sterile field during the surgical procedure. Many drugs become expired or "outdated" with time, and their composition and effect may be altered. All medications stored in the surgery pharmacy must be periodically checked for "outdates." These medications then are discarded or returned to the hospital pharmacy.

MATH SKILLS AND DRUG CALCULATIONS

Although the surgical technologist does not directly administer medications to the patient, he or she occasionally is asked to mix solutions used in surgery. The circulator may distribute several types of medications to the surgical technologist, who is then required to mix them in the proper proportions. One such case would occur when certain **antibiotics** are distributed for use as irrigants within the wound. When the surgical technologist receives any medication from the nurse, the technologist should be able to identify the drug and determine the exact amount received. This may require amounts to be converted from one system of measurement to another. Because of these challenges, every

surgical technologist must be able to perform simple arithmetic calculations and conversions.

This chapter assumes that the reader has achieved *at least high school competency in mathematics.* Any student must be comfortable performing the following basic mathematical operations before scrubbing in surgery. This ability is a prerequisite for performing the drug calculations presented in this chapter:

▶ Arithmetic of whole numbers—addition, subtraction, multiplication, division.
▶ Rounding off
▶ Computations involving fractions, including proper, improper, whole, and mixed fractions
▶ Computations involving ratios and proportions
▶ Computations involving decimals
▶ Computation of percentages and conversion of percentages to decimals, fractions to percentages, and percentages to fractions

Review of Arithmetic
FRACTIONS

A *fraction* defines a number by specifying the *division* necessary to create that number. For example, the fraction 3/4 is the number that results by dividing the top number (the numerator), 3, by the bottom number (the denominator), 4. When the numerator is smaller than the denominator, the number is less than 1; when the numerator is larger than the denominator, the number is greater than 1. When the numerator and denominator are the same, the number is 1.

ADDITION AND SUBTRACTION

For addition or subtraction of two fractions, the fractions must have the same denominator. Thus to complete 1/3 + 1/3, simply add the numerators; the answer is 2/3. Adding or subtracting fractions that have different denominators requires an extra step that requires understanding of the concept of *equivalent fractions.* That is, if both the numerator and denominator of a fraction are multiplied (or divided) by the same number, the resulting fraction is equal to the original one. Thus if both the numerator and denominator of the fraction 1/3 are multiplied by 2, the resulting fraction is 2/6. The fraction 2/6 is exactly equal to the fraction 1/3. Therefore to add or subtract fractions of different denominators, all one must do is to choose an equivalent fraction of each that has the same denominator. The denominator selected should be the *lowest common denominator* (LCD), that is, the lowest number that can be divided by the two denominators of the fraction you need to add or subtract.

Examples:

Addition

$$\frac{1}{2} + \frac{1}{3} \ (\text{LCD} = 6)$$

$$\frac{(1 \times 3)}{(2 \times 3)} = \frac{3}{6}; \frac{(1 \times 2)}{(3 \times 2)} = \frac{2}{6}$$

$$\frac{3}{6} + \frac{2}{6} = \frac{5}{6}$$

$$\frac{3}{4} + \frac{1}{5} \ (\text{LCD} = 20)$$

$$\frac{(3 \times 5)}{(4 \times 5)} = \frac{15}{20}; \ \frac{(1 \times 4)}{(5 \times 4)} = \frac{4}{20}$$

$$\frac{15}{20} + \frac{4}{20} = \frac{19}{20}$$

Subtraction
$$\frac{7}{8} - \frac{3}{16} \ (\text{LCD} = 16)$$

$$\frac{(7 \times 2)}{(8 \times 2)} = \frac{14}{16}; \ \frac{(3 \times 1)}{(16 \times 1)} = \frac{3}{16}$$

$$\frac{14}{16} - \frac{3}{16} = \frac{11}{16}$$

$$\frac{4}{7} - \frac{1}{9} \ (\text{LCD} = 63)$$

$$\frac{(4 \times 9)}{(7 \times 9)} = \frac{36}{63}; \ \frac{(1 \times 7)}{(9 \times 7)} = \frac{7}{63}$$

$$\frac{36}{63} - \frac{7}{63} = \frac{29}{63}$$

MULTIPLICATION AND DIVISION

To multiply, simply multiply the numerators of the two fractions, and then multiply the denominators. Thus:

$$\frac{2}{3} \times \frac{5}{8} = \frac{(2 \times 5)}{(3 \times 8)} = \frac{10}{24}$$

One may *reduce* (simplify) any fraction by dividing both the numerator and denominator by the same number:

$$\frac{10}{24} = \frac{(10 \div 2)}{(24 \div 2)} = \frac{5}{12}$$

The numbers 5 and 12 cannot be divided evenly by any number, so 5/12 is a fully reduced fraction.

To divide a fraction, first write the division as a big fraction. Thus:

$$\frac{2}{3} \div \frac{5}{6} = \frac{\dfrac{2}{3}}{\dfrac{5}{6}}$$

Then multiply both numerators of the fractions that make up the big fraction. Thus:

$$\frac{\dfrac{2}{3}}{\dfrac{5}{6}} = \frac{\dfrac{2}{3} \times 6}{\dfrac{5}{6} \times 6} = \frac{\dfrac{12}{3}}{\dfrac{30}{6}} = \frac{4}{5}$$

Another method is to invert the divisor and multiply. For example,

$$\frac{2}{3} \div \frac{5}{6} = \frac{2}{3} \times \frac{6}{5} = \frac{12}{15} = \frac{4}{5}$$

Examples:
Multiplication
$$\frac{1}{13} \times \frac{2}{3} = \frac{(1 \times 2)}{13 \times 3)} = \frac{2}{39}$$

$$\frac{3}{7} \times \frac{4}{5} = \frac{(3 \times 4)}{(7 \times 5)} = \frac{12}{35}$$

Division
$$\frac{1}{3} \div \frac{5}{8} = \frac{1}{3} \times \frac{8}{5} = \frac{8}{15}$$

$$\frac{1}{4} \div \frac{1}{16} = \frac{1}{4} \times \frac{16}{1} = \frac{16}{4} = 4$$

DECIMALS

The number system we use is the decimal system, which is based on powers (multiples) of 10. Each position to the left or right of the decimal point is a higher or lower power of 10.

To convert from a fraction, such as 4/5, to a decimal, simply divide the numerator by the denominator (4/5 = 0.8). Some fractions do not result in simple decimal numbers. For example, 1/3 is .33333..., and so on forever. For most purposes, one may simply round off after three figures. To round off, raise the last digit by 1 if it is 5 or more. Thus .33333... is .333, but .66666... is .667.

PERCENTAGES

A percentage is a fraction expressed as parts of 100. To convert a fraction to a percentage, convert to a decimal and multiply by 100. Thus:

$$\frac{4}{5} = 0.8 \times 100 = 80\%$$

RATIOS

A ratio is similar to a fraction. A ratio of 1 to 2 (written 1:2) means that there is 1 unit for every 2 units out of each 3 units (1 + 2) of the item being described. To convert a ratio to a fraction, add both terms to make the denominator, and use the first term as the numerator. In the above example,

$$1{:}2 = \frac{1}{3}$$

PROPORTIONS

A proportion is an expression of equality between two fractions. For example, one can write 1:3 = 2/6. This is the same as 1/4 = 2/8. The most common use of proportions is for dilutions. Dilution usually is expressed as a percentage, such as a 1% solution. A common problem is to determine how much of a chemical to add to a given quantity of liquid to produce a particular dilution. The unknown amount is written as *X*. For example, to make a 1% solution using 500 ml of water, how much chemical is needed? Written as a proportion, it is:

$$\frac{X}{500 \text{ ml}} = \frac{1}{100}$$

To solve, multiply the numerator of the first term (*X*) by the denominator of the second (100) and vice versa (500 × 1). In this case $100X = 500 \text{ ml} \times 1$. Multiplying a number by 1 gives the same number, so $100X = 500$ ml. To solve for *X*, divide both sides by 100. Thus:

$$X = \frac{500}{100} = 5 \text{ ml}$$

Adding 5 ml of the chemical will produce 505 ml of a 1% solution.

SAMPLE PROBLEMS

1. To produce 30 cc of 50% Hypaque solution, how much 100% Hypaque and how much sterile saline solution are required?
2. To prepare a 1-L solution of alcohol in water in a ratio of 1:70, how much alcohol is required?
3. To prepare a single solution in which the ratio of bacitracin to neomycin is 1:3 and the ratio of the bacitracin/neomycin mixture to sterile solution is 1:1, how much bacitracin, neomycin, and sterile saline solution do you need to make a total of 100 cc of solution?
4. To produce 30 cc of 0.5% Xylocaine, how much sterile saline solution and how much 1% Xylocaine are required?
5. To produce a 100 cc solution of Hypaque in a ratio of 1:3, how much 50% Hypaque solution and how much sterile solution should you use?

Systems of Measurements

Measurement systems allow physical properties to be quantified. In medicine the properties of concern are weight and volume:

▶ Weight is the *gravitational force* of an object or substance.
▶ Volume is the *amount of space* that a substance occupies.

The two measurement systems used most often to specify these properties are the *metric* system and the *apothecary* system. The household system (e.g., teaspoons, measuring cups) is used occasionally when a patient must measure a drug such as cough syrup or antacid liquid at home. The household system, however, is not precise enough for use in the health-care setting.

METRIC SYSTEM

The metric system is based on units or powers of 10. It is the most commonly used system in medicine. Weight measurements include the gram, kilogram, milligram, microgram, and nanogram.

The cubic centimeter (cc) often is used in measuring liquid amounts. One cubic centimeter is equal to 1 milliliter (ml).

Box 13-1 lists the units of the metric system.

APOTHECARY SYSTEM

The apothecary system uses Roman numerals to represent measurements and symbols to represent units of measure. The basic units of weight in the apothecary system are grains and ounces. Volume is expressed in drams and minims. Grains are the most common apothecary measurement unit used in drug labeling in the United States.

HOUSEHOLD SYSTEM

The household system rarely is used in the medical setting. Its measurements are too imprecise for patient safety.

Box 13-1 Metric System

Units of Mass	Units of Volume
1 kg = 1000 g	1 L = 1000 ml
1 g = 1000 mg	1 ml = 1000 µl
1 mg = 1000 mcg	1 ml = 1 cc

However, occasionally the surgical technologist must convert values from the household system to one of the other systems.

INTERNATIONAL UNITS (IU)

International Units (IU) are an internationally accepted method of measuring certain drugs. Any measure that is expressed as units describes the number of units per ml after addition of a diluent. For example, if a label states that a vial contains 400,000 IU of a drug, one can make varying concentrations of the drug by adding different amounts of diluent. Remember, however, that the same number of units is contained in the vial regardless of how much diluent is added to the vial. Only the concentration changes.

INTERNATIONAL SYSTEM OF UNITS (SI)

The General Conference on Weights and Measures accepts certain units as part of the International System of Units (SI). A standard international system of weights and measures is necessary to promote standardization in drug manufacturing, distribution, and administration.

Unit Conversion

To perform any drug calculation, you must convert all values into units of the same system. Therefore as a surgical technologist you must be competent in unit conversion. To convert values from one system to another, you must use unit conversion tables. Common conversion formulas should be memorized. Refer to Table 13-1 for common conversions.

Example: Convert a larger unit to smaller units in the metric system. Multiply the units that are needed by the equivalent value in the conversion chart.

You have a liter of saline solution. You are asked to deliver 500 ml to the surgeon. How many liters is this? Convert both numbers to the same units

1 liter = 1000 ml (from the conversion table)

The desired unit is liters. Liters are larger than ml. Your conversion will result in a fraction of a liter. There-

Table 13-1 UNIT CONVERSION BETWEEN APOTHECARY AND METRIC SYSTEMS

Apothecary		Metric
1 grain (gr)	=	0.065 g
1 dram (dr)	=	3.888 g
1 minim (m)	=	0.06 ml
1 fluid dram (fl dr)	=	3.70 ml
1 teaspoon (t)	=	5 ml
1 tablespoon (T)	=	15 ml
1 fluid ounce (oz)	=	29.57 ml
1 pint (pt)	=	473 ml
1 quart (qt)	=	946 ml
1 gallon (gal)	=	3.785 L

fore you must divide the larger amount by the smaller amount.

$$X \text{ liters} = \frac{500 \text{ ml}}{1000 \text{ ml}} = 0.5 \text{ liters or } \tfrac{1}{2} \text{ liter}$$

Example: Convert 120 grains (gr) to drams. Convert both numbers to the same units.

60 grains (gr) = 1 dram

$$X \text{ drams} = \frac{120 \text{ gr}}{60 \text{ gr}} = 2 \text{ drams}$$

Example: Convert a larger unit into a smaller one in the apothecary system. To convert a large measurement to a smaller one in the apothecary system, multiply the measurement that is needed by the equivalent value.

Convert 5 drams to grains
Convert both numbers to the same unit using the following conversion factor:

1 dram = 60 grains (gr)

Grains are smaller than drams. The desired units are grains. The answer in grains will be larger than the dram amount. You must *multiply*.

60 grains × 5 drams = 300 grains

Calculations

RATIO SYSTEM VS. FORMULAS FOR DRUG CALCULATION

Formulas are a quick way to measure and calculate drugs. However, formulas can be forgotten or misused. Another danger with formulas is that they cannot be easily validated. If the for-

mula is wrong, the answer is wrong. If you must rely on a formula, you may not fully understand the mathematics required.

Rather than relying on formulas, it is better to use ratio calculations. You can validate ratio calculations, and you do not need to memorize formulas. If you understand ratio calculations, you will understand exactly how you derived your answer. To perform ratio calculations you must understand how to cross multiply fractions.

This system of calculations uses the relationship of one value to another to solve a problem. Remember that the words *in, per, of,* and the symbols ":" and "/" denote a ratio. A ratio is a way of expressing a fraction. Study the following example.

Example: The label on a 2-ml ampule reads **50 mg/ml.**
How many mg are contained *in* 1.5 ml?

You are asked about concentration. Concentration is expressed in weight per amount of liquid, such as milligrams per milliliter.
Known ratio of mg to ml is:
50 mg **per** 1 ml, or
50 mg:1 ml, or
50 mg/1 ml

Unknown ratio is:
X mg **per** 1.5 ml, or
X mg:1.5 ml, or
X mg/1.5 ml

Set up the ratio as an equation   50 mg:1 ml = X mg:1.5 ml

A ratio is a fraction $\dfrac{50 \text{ mg}}{1 \text{ ml}}$

$\dfrac{X \text{ mg}}{1.5 \text{ ml}}$

Cross multiply $\dfrac{50 \text{ mg}}{1 \text{ ml}} \times \dfrac{X \text{ mg}}{1.5 \text{ ml}}$

Solve for X $X(1) = 50(1.5)$
Answer   **$X = 75$ mg**

CALCULATION OF SOLUTION STRENGTH

Many of the drugs used in surgery are in solution. Refer to Table 13-2 for a list of equivalent concentrations. A *solution* is a specific substance (*solute*) dissolved in a specific volume of liquid (*solvent* or *diluent*).

A solution can be described in two ways:

1. By concentration: weight per volume:

$$Concentration = \frac{\text{Mass (weight) of the drug}}{\text{Volume of solution}}$$

Table 13-2   EQUIVALENTS FOR CONCENTRATION EXPRESSIONS

%	Ratio	g/L	g/dl	mg/ml	mg/dl	mcg/ml
10	1:10	100	10	100	10,000	100,000
1	1:100	10	1	10	1000	10,000
0.1	1:1000	1	0.1	1	100	1000
0.01	1:10,000	0.1	0.01	0.1	10	100
0.001	1:100,000	0.01	0.001	0.01	1	10
0.0001	1:1,000,000	0.001	0.0001	0.001	0.1	1

From Osis MJ: *Dosage calculations in SI units,* ed 3, St Louis, 1995, Mosby.

2. **By percent solution:** volume per volume, solution, or strength. This is expressed as a *percentage* or as a *ratio.* For example, a 6% solution has 6 g of drug in each 100 ml of solution. A drug that is labeled 1:1000 means that 1 g of medication is dissolved in 1000 ml of diluent. The *strength* of the solution is 1 mg per milliliter.

Example: Prepare 1 L of a 6% solution
Known 6% = 6 g per 100 ml
1 L = 1000 ml
6 g:100 ml = *X* g:1000 ml

Cross multiply $\dfrac{6\ g}{100\ ml} \times \dfrac{X\ g}{1000\ ml}$

Solve for X   100(*X*) = 6(1000)
Answer   **X = 60 g**

Example: There are 400,000 units of antibiotic per ml.
If 1 mg equals 1600 units, what is the dose (ml) containing 200 mg?

1 mg = 1600 units
200 mg = 320,000 units
1 ml:400,000 units = *X* ml:320,000 units

Cross multiply $\dfrac{1\ ml}{400,000\ units} \times \dfrac{X\ ml}{320,000\ units}$

Solve for X   *X*(400,000) = 1(320,000)
Answer   **X = 0.8 ml**

CALCULATION OF DOSAGE BY WEIGHT

Many drugs are administered according to the weight of the patient. The patient's weight is *always* calculated for pediatric patients. The weight of an adult patient is calculated when critical drugs are being administered. The proper calculation is the *amount of drug per kilogram of body weight.* Recommended dosage for drugs is obtained from the package insert or a reliable pharmacology reference. Calculations are written out and the safe range is verified whenever licensed personnel administer drugs to pediatric patients.

Reconstitution of Drugs

Many drugs used on the sterile field are topical solutions. Many of these topical drugs are manufactured as powders and mixed with a sterile diluent (a liquid added to form a solution) by the circulating registered nurse and distributed to the surgical technologist. *The surgical technologist must never add more diluent to the drug or use it for any purpose except topical application!* The concentration specified by the surgeon's orders must not be changed. Bacitracin, topical thrombin, and heparin solution are examples.

To reconstitute a drug, the registered nurse circulator reads the physician's orders and adds the correct amount of sterile aqueous diluent.

A surgeon orders 250,000 IU of a drug per milliliter. The drug label states that 250,000 IU per milliliter is achieved by adding 35 ml of diluent. If 45 ml of diluent is added, the concentration of the drug is reduced. What information do you need to know to calculate the number of units you are passing to the surgeon?

DRUG APPROVAL AND STANDARDS

Drug Approval and Safety

A drug is a chemical that, when taken into the body, changes one or more of its functions. In the United States, drugs are approved for medical used after application to the Food and Drug Administration (FDA) and rigid testing. The FDA authorizes the sale and distribution of drugs and also is responsible for ensuring that approved drugs have met consumer safety requirements. It approves drug literature and labeling so that health-care providers and the public can know the nature, use, and risks associated with a drug.

Drug Standards

To protect the public from harm, all drugs must meet standards for quality, strength, packaging safety, and dosage. These standards are contained in the **U.S. Pharmacopeia (USP).** All drugs that meet these standards have the initials USP after their generic (noncommercial) names. Approved drugs are published in the *U.S. Pharmacopeia National Formulary.* This reference is updated every 5 years. The World Health Organization (WHO) publishes an international formulary called the *International Pharmacopeia.*

Drug Control

Drugs that have the potential for abuse (deliberate overuse of a drug) are given a ranking based on the risk of abuse or dependency, harmful effects, and other factors. Lists of drugs within particular rankings are called drug schedules. The Drug Enforcement Agency (DEA) classifies drugs on the schedules. Drugs that are proven to have a potential for abuse are called controlled substances and are classified by rank number or schedule. Schedule I drugs have no medical use and show the highest potential for abuse. Schedule III through V drugs have less potential for abuse. Schedule II drugs have an accepted medical use; however, they have a

Table 13-3 SCHEDULES OF CONTROLLED SUBSTANCES

Schedule	Examples of Substances	Description
I	Heroin, hallucinogens (LSD, marijuana, mescaline, peyote, psilocybin)	Drugs with high abuse potential. No accepted medical use. Labeled C-I.
II	Meperidine (Demerol), morphine, hydrocodone, hydromorphone, methadone, oxycodone, codeine, amphetamines, secobarbital, pentobarbital	High potential for drug abuse. Accepted medical use. Can lead to strong physical and psychological dependency. Labeled C-II.
III	Some codeine preparations, paregoric, nonnarcotic drugs (pentazocine, propoxyphene)	Medically accepted drugs. Potential abuse is less than that for schedules I and II. May cause dependence. Labeled C-III.
IV	Phenobarbital, benzodiazepines (diazepam, oxazepam, lorazepam, chlordiazepoxide), chloral hydrate, meprobamate	Medically accepted drugs. May cause dependence. Labeled C-IV.
V	Opioid controlled substances in strengths used to treat cough and diarrhea, such as cough preparations with codeine	Medically accepted drugs. Very limited potential for dependence. Labeled C-V.

From Kee JL and Hayes ER: *Pharmacology: a nursing process approach,* ed 3, Philadelphia, 2000, WB Saunders.
C, Control; *LSD,* lysergic acid diethylamide.

high potential for abuse. Schedule V drugs have the least risk for abuse or dependency. Table 13-3 lists the schedule categories of controlled substances.

Pregnancy Categories

Drugs are classified by pregnancy category to inform healthcare workers of potential risk to the fetus of a mother taking the drug. Categories are A, B, C, D, and X. Category A drugs carry no risk to the fetus, while category X drugs are proven to have a risk that outweighs the benefit of the drug.

Drug Resources

Resource books list currently available therapeutic drugs and their action, use, dosage, and other important information. Primary health-care providers often use the *Physicians' Desk Reference,* which is updated yearly and contains detailed information about most drugs. Other commonly used references include the *American Hospital Formulary Service Drug Information* and the *United States Pharmacopeia Drug Information.* Nursing drug handbooks are useful for quick reference.

PROPERTIES OF DRUGS AND DRUG ACTION

All drugs have certain pharmacologic characteristics. The *half-life* of the agent is the amount of time after which only half the amount of drug administered remains active in the body. The *onset* is the time from administration until the effects of the drug are seen. The time to *peak* effect is the time from administration until the drug is most potent in the body. The *action* of the drug is what it does and how it affects the body. The *indication* is the intended use of the drug. In

the discussion of drug groups and examples later in the chapter, only the indication and a description of the drug are included.

Pharmacodynamics

Pharmacodynamics is the physiological action of the drug on the body. The pharmacodynamic properties are onset, peak effect, duration of action, indication, and contraindication factors.

Pharmacokinetics

Pharmacokinetics is the movement of a drug in the body to achieve a change in function. Four separate processes are involved in pharmacokinetics. These are absorption, distribution, metabolism, and elimination.

Absorption occurs actively or passively, that is, it does or does not require energy. Drugs taken by mouth are absorbed through the small intestine, while those administered **parenterally** are absorbed by the tissues and carried to the bloodstream. Some drugs are taken up by the liver, which retains or metabolizes a portion, or all, of the drug for excretion.

Distribution of a drug in the body depends on the drug's ability to bind in protein, on blood flow, and on the affinity of the drug for tissue. Drugs that are highly bound to proteins are less active because they are not free to move to the target tissue.

Metabolism of drugs takes place primarily in the liver. Circulating drugs are inactivated by liver enzymes and converted into water-soluble substances that are excreted. However, the liver converts some drugs to active metabolites (byproducts of metabolism), which results in a greater pharmacologic effect. In a patient with liver disease, certain drugs cannot be broken down. Those that remain in the liver become toxic. Drugs are described by their half-life, or how fast they are metabolized.

Elimination of drugs occurs primarily through the kidneys. Those drugs that are not protein bound pass through unchanged. Protein-bound drugs cannot pass through the kidney's filtering system until they are freed. Other routes of elimination included feces, lungs, saliva, and breast milk.

The onset, peak, and duration are affected by pharmacokinetics. The therapeutic dose and lethal dose, toxic effects, side effects, and adverse reactions also are related.

ONSET, PEAK, AND DURATION OF EFFECT

As noted earlier, the onset time of a drug is the time from administration until the drug begins to show an effect and before it reaches peak (full) action in the body. The duration of effect is described in terms of the drug's half-life. Many different conditions can affect these parameters, including the presence of kidney and liver disease, and the type and amount of drug administered.

THERAPEUTIC INDEX

The therapeutic index is the ratio between the toxic or lethal dosage of a drug and the dosage producing the desired (therapeutic) effect. It describes the margin of safety in using the drug. A drug with a high therapeutic index has a margin of safety. One with a low therapeutic index is one for which the difference between the toxic or lethal dose and the therapeutic dose (the therapeutic window) is very small.

SIDE EFFECTS

Drug side effects usually are not related to the therapeutic function of the drug. Rather, they are effects that occur predictably and may not cause a problem. Some side effects are desirable, and the drug may be prescribed for its side effects rather than its labeled use.

ADVERSE REACTIONS

An adverse reaction is an undesirable or intolerable reaction to a drug administered at the normal dosage. Adverse reactions are not expected, although they may be predictable in certain individuals. Adverse reactions range from severe allergic response to circulatory failure. An adverse reaction can occur unexpectedly at any time.

TOXICITY

Toxicity occurs when the therapeutic dosage of a drug is exceeded. Patients who are prescribed drugs with a narrow therapeutic range are tested at regular intervals for blood levels of the drug. True toxicity is not the same as an adverse reaction, because toxicity is directly related to dosage, while an adverse reaction is not.

DRUG LABEL INFORMATION

All personnel handling drugs in the operating room must be able to correctly identify components of a drug label. Figure 13-1 shows the parts of a label.

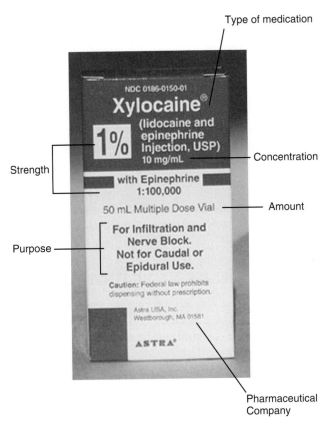

FIGURE 13-1
Parts of a drug label. (Courtesy of AstraZeneca Pharmaceuticals LP, Wilmington, Del.)

Drug Nomenclature

Every drug has three different names. These are the generic, trade, and chemical names. Only the generic and trade names are used in the health-care setting.

The **generic name** identifies a specific drug formulation. Drugs with the same generic name must have the same chemical composition regardless of which company manufactures the drug and what trade name has been assigned to that drug.

The **trade name** (commonly called the brand name) identifies a generic drug manufactured by a specific pharmaceutical company. The same generic drug manufactured by different companies can have many different trade names. For example, penicillin V potassium is the generic name for the drug with the trade names Beepen-VK, Ledercillin-VK, Pen-Vee K, Veetids, and V-Cillin K.

Drugs also are named according to an international nomenclature system that precisely describes the molecular structure of a chemical. This designation is called the *chemical name* of the drug.

Dose

The dose of a drug is the amount of drug administered at one time or the amount in a specified volume or unit of administration. *Dose is not the same as dosage.* Dosage usually refers to the therapeutic drug regimen prescribed by the physician. For example, the usual adult dosage of aspirin is two 325-mg tablets every 4 hours. The dosage changes according to the needs of the patient. The dose contained in a specific solution, tablet, or other unit of administration is fixed.

Lot Number

The lot number of a drug identifies the specific batch of drug prepared by the pharmaceutical laboratory. In the event of contamination or incorrect formulation of a batch, all drug samples included in the batch can be identified, recalled, and destroyed.

Expiration Date

Drugs must not be used beyond the specified expiration date. Over time, many drugs lose their efficacy and can become toxic.

PREVENTION OF MEDICATION ERRORS

A medication error can occur during any stage of the drug-handling process. A medication error can result in serious injury or death of the patient. The most common types of medication errors are the following:

▶ The wrong drug is administered because it is confused with a "sound-alike" drug.
▶ The drug is prescribed, dispensed, or administered in the wrong dosage.
▶ The person mixing, dispensing, or administering the drug is unable to perform the necessary drug calculations.
▶ Health personnel improperly label a drug or fail to label the drug at all.

To help prevent medication errors, the *five rights of medication administration* were defined for licensed personnel administering medications in all health-care settings. These are the following:

1. The right drug
2. The right dose
3. The right route
4. The right patient
5. The right time

A sixth right applies to medications used in the surgical field:

6. The right label

Although the surgical technologist does not administer medications, he or she directly participates with others in selecting, receiving, dispensing, mixing, and labeling drugs. By following an exact protocol for handling drugs, the surgical technologist adapts the six rights to the practice of surgical technology.

The Right Drug

"The right drug" is the drug that has been ordered by the surgeon. This means that the correct drug must be selected from the operating room pharmacy stock *before* surgery and

from among other drugs on the sterile field *during* surgery. Failure to make both selections correctly results in a medication error.

The Right Dose

"The right dose" means the right amount of drug is administered at one time and cumulatively (in the case of drugs that are given intermittently throughout the surgery, such as a local anesthetic agent). The right dose results when the drug is correctly identified and the amount ordered is correctly reflected in the dose calculation. It also means the correct strength or ratio of drugs mixed on the sterile field. One must remember that one medication often is available in different strengths. For example, epinephrine comes as a 1:1000 solution and a 1:100,000 solution. If the surgeon orders 1 cc of epinephrine, the technologist must know which of these concentrations he is requesting. Improper mixing of epinephrine solution is a fairly common drug administration error.

The Right Route

"The right route" is the one intended for that drug and prescribed by the surgeon. Drugs are labeled according to approved route (e.g., for topical use only or not for use in the eyes).

The right route also means the drug is approved for the intended route. This is especially true for drugs that are used in cardiovascular or peripheral vascular surgery, in which solutions are injected directly into blood vessels in the wound. A solution intended for wound irrigation is not used for intravenous flushing unless it is approved for that specific use. Ophthalmic drugs are specifically approved for use in the eyes only. Indiscriminate instillation of a drug in the eye can cause damage or blindness.

The Right Patient

"The right patient" means that the patient is identified as the right patient when he or she enters the surgical holding area and again when he or she is brought into the surgical suite. The circulator must use a precise protocol for patient identification.

The Right Time

Although "the right time" originally meant that drugs were administered according to a timed schedule, in surgery this right can mean preparing drugs at the correct time. Some drugs must not be allowed to remain on the back table for hours but must be prepared just before administration to preserve their physical properties.

The Right Label

When the scrubbed technologist receives a drug from the circulator, he or she must *immediately and accurately* label the drug. Improper labeling (or worse, no labeling) is a violation of standard operating room procedure and is a risk to the patient. All drugs must be labeled, even if there is only one. There is no excuse for not labeling drugs or solutions on the instrument table. Do not rely on a specific unlabeled basin or cup to indicate a drug's identity.

You must watch the drug being poured and label it then. Solutions such as irrigating saline and sterile water used in the sterile field also should be labeled.

DRUG DISTRIBUTION PROCESS

Selection

The circulator selects the correct drug as ordered by the surgeon verbally or in transcription. Many drugs are ordered verbally by the surgeon before or during surgery.

Remember that only licensed personnel can take a verbal order for a drug.

Inspection

After the drug is selected, the drug container and its contents are examined. The label is inspected to confirm that the drug and amount are correct, to verify correct dosage, and to check the expiration date. The vial or container must be intact with no signs of cracking or chipping. The seal must be unbroken, with no sign that sterility has been breached. The drug itself must appear normal. A drug that is normally clear should be clear with no sign of precipitation or cloudiness. The color of the drug may be an indication of changes in the chemical structure. Checking this requires familiarity with the normal appearance of the drug.

Delivery to the Sterile Field

When the circulator dispenses a drug to the sterile field, *both the circulator and the scrub participate.* The circulator *may not* transfer any drug without this dual participation. The reason is that, when a drug is passed from one person to another, the receiver must verify the "six rights" to prevent a drug error. These steps cannot be performed unless the scrub participates in the transfer.

The recommended protocol is as follows (Figure 13-2):

1. The circulator holds the drug container so that the scrub can easily read it.
2. The scrub reads and recites *out loud* the name, dose, amount, strength, and expiration date.
3. The circulator pours or injects the drug into a sterile basin or cup offered by the scrub. Drugs may be poured only from containers that have a safety tip, which maintains sterility during pouring. The scrub should *not* insert a needle into a vial held by the circulator. This is poor aseptic technique and places the circulator at risk for needle puncture.
4. The circulator again shows the drug container to the scrub and both verify that the information is correct.
5. The scrub immediately labels the drug. Various labeling systems are available; some are more efficient than others. Many hospitals use sterile blank self-sticking paper labels and a colored skin marker. Most skin markers bleed on

damp paper, which obscures the labeling. This is not an approved system for labeling.
6. When a container is labeled, the entire name of the drug and concentration or strength must be included on the label.
7. When any drug is passed to the surgeon, the name and concentration or strength are again repeated out loud so that he or she is aware of what has been dispensed.

Maintenance of Drugs and Solutions on the Sterile Field

Drugs and solutions are maintained in a specific manner to protect the patient and prevent medication errors.

DRUG IDENTIFICATION

After drugs have been received and labeled on the sterile field, they must be protected from contamination, and the identification must be visible at all times. Drugs should be placed in one spot on the instrument table and kept there throughout the case. If additional amounts of the drug are needed, the protocol given earlier must be followed again. If anyone has any doubt about the identification of a drug, the drug must be discarded and the correct drug redistributed to the field.

All drugs must be identified when there is a permanent change of scrubbed personnel, such as during shift changes.

TRACKING OF AMOUNT OF DRUG OR SOLUTION USED

The scrubbed technologist is responsible for keeping track of the total amount of drug or solution used during surgery. This can be tallied with a sterile marking pen. The amount of irrigation solutions used must be totaled to compute total blood loss. Contrast media amounts also are computed to ensure that safe levels are not exceeded.

When a local anesthetic is used as part of the procedure, the amount of drug used must be recorded and tallied. The scrubbed person must know at all times exactly how much anesthetic has been injected. Local anesthetics are administered in *milligrams per kilogram of body weight.* Each drug has a different therapeutic range and level of overdose.

MEASUREMENT OF DRUGS

When measuring drugs in a syringe or other measuring device, you must read the value at the meniscus. This is the bottom of the curve formed by the liquid in a container (Figure 13-3). Reading the value at the top of the curve will not give the correct measurement.

IRRIGATION SOLUTIONS

Irrigation solutions must be kept clean and separate from those used to soak instruments. Irrigation solutions should be dispensed at approximately body temperature to avoid causing hypothermia or burns in the patient. This is especially important for pediatric, elderly, or very thin patients. Sterile saline and water for irrigation can be kept at a

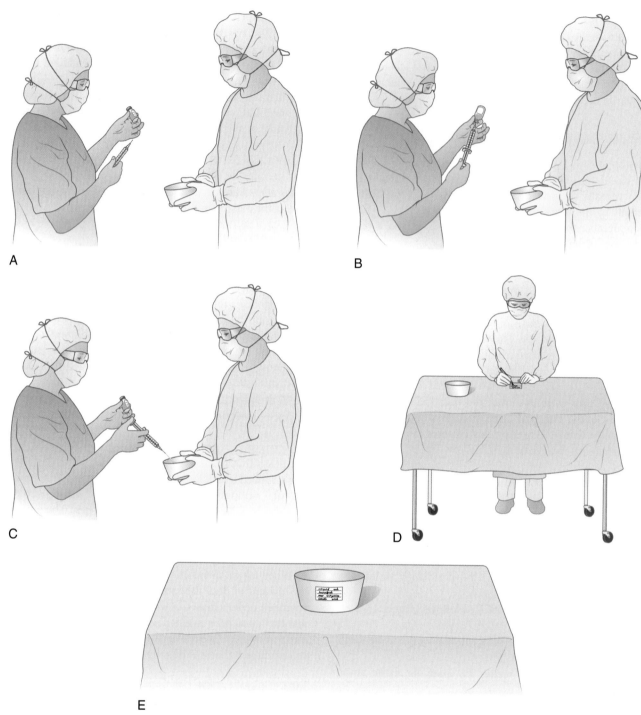

FIGURE 13-2
A through **E,** Delivery of drugs to the sterile field.

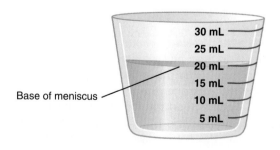

FIGURE 13-3
Meniscus.

controlled temperature in a solution warmer until ready for use. Always calculate the amount of irrigation solutions used during the procedure to help the ACP calculate the patient's blood loss.

MEDICATION DEVICES

Syringes

The syringe is used for dispensing, measuring, and parenterally administering drugs. Two-part syringes consist of a *bar-* *rel*, which is the tubular portion that holds the liquid, and a plunger (Figure 13-4). The plunger is essentially a piston that is designed to draw in and expel liquid. Syringes are available in many sizes and types. All syringes except the insulin syringe are calibrated in milliliters (ml), which also can be expressed as cubic centimeters (cc). One cc equals 1 ml. In most ORs, syringes are calibrated in cubic centimeters. The most common sizes of syringes are 1, 3, 5, and 10 cc (Figure 13-5). Large syringes are calibrated to greater volumes than smaller syringes; smaller syringes can measure very small amounts down to 0.01 cc.

The *tuberculin syringe* is the smallest metric syringe (Figure 13-6, *A*). The total volume of this syringe is 0.5 or 1 cc. The barrel of the syringe is inscribed with measurement hashes.

The two most common types of syringe tips are the locking (Luer-Lok) and catheter tips. The syringe tip accepts a hypodermic needle or a catheter. The Luer-Lok syringe locks the needle in place, while syringes with a catheter tip are smooth and do not contain a locking mechanism, allowing the tip to slip on and off.

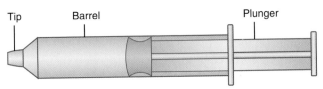

FIGURE 13-4
Parts of a syringe. (From Kee JL and Marshall SM: *Clinical calculations: with application to general and specialty areas,* ed 5, Philadelphia, 2004, WB Saunders.)

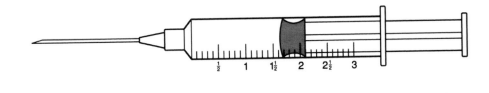

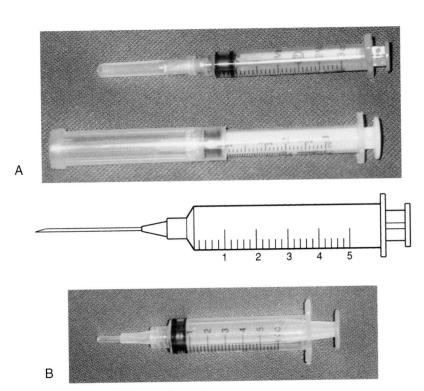

FIGURE 13-5
A, 3-ml syringe. **B,** 5-ml syringe. (From Kee JL and Marshall SM: *Clinical calculations: with application to general and specialty areas,* ed 5, Philadelphia, 2004, WB Saunders.)

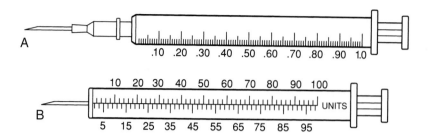

FIGURE 13-6
A, Tuberculin syringe. **B,** Insulin syringe. (Modified from Kee JL and Marshall SM: *Clinical calculations: with application to general and specialty areas,* ed 5, Philadelphia, 2004, WB Saunders.)

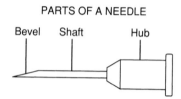

FIGURE 13-7
Parts of a hypodermic needle. (From Kee JL and Marshall SM: *Clinical calculations: with application to general and specialty areas,* ed 5, Philadelphia, 2004, WB Saunders.)

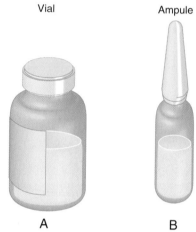

FIGURE 13-8
A, Glass vial. **B,** Glass ampule. (From Kee JL and Marshall SM: *Clinical calculations: with application to general and specialty areas,* ed 5, Philadelphia, 2004, WB Saunders.)

The insulin syringe is calibrated in insulin units rather than in metric system units (Figure 13-6, *B*). *Never* use an insulin syringe for measuring drugs on the sterile field. The calibrations are incorrect for all drugs except insulin. The insulin syringe easily can be confused with a tuberculin syringe. In the United States all insulin syringes have orange tips for identification.

Needles

Hypodermic needles are sized according to gauge (lumen or bore size) and length (Figure 13-7). The larger the gauge, the smaller the needle bore. Size 18-gauge to 26-gauge needles are commonly used.

Because of the risk of blood-borne diseases, the National Institute of Occupational Safety and Health (NIOSH) now requires that syringes have some feature that allows the needle to be retracted or protected so that personnel will not be punctured during or after use. Needleless systems are now in common use but are not available in all operating rooms. The surgical technologist handles needles and syringes often. Care must be taken to avoid puncture injuries.

Never recap a needle by hand. Place the cap on the table and scoop it up with the point of the needle or use a needle-capping device. In this device, the cap is held in a rigid container and the needle and syringe combination is pushed down into the cap.

Drug Containers

Drugs are contained in many different types of bottles, packages, and wrappers. Liquid drugs are dispensed from a glass vial or ampule (Figure 13-8). The glass vial is capped with a rubber stopper and protective metal cap. One opens glass ampules by breaking the top off the container. If you are required to open a glass ampule on the sterile field, cover the top with a sponge and snap the top *away from you. Do not distribute this sponge onto the field—it may have glass particles embedded in it.*

Some drugs are dispensed in dry form. Dry-tissue forceps are used to retrieve these from inside the container.

Petrolatum gauze and other types of sticky material should be grasped with forceps to remove them from the wrapper. Some oils can weaken surgical gloves, so try to avoid using your sterile gloved hand to grasp materials containing such oils.

Intravenous solutions or those used for continuous irrigation are packaged in flexible solution bags (Figure 13-9). Intravenous solutions that would interact with polyvinyl chloride are packaged in glass bottles.

DRUG ADMINISTRATION

Drug Routes

Drug action is in part regulated by the route of administration. Serious drug errors and death can result from delivery of a drug by the wrong route. The surgical technologist must

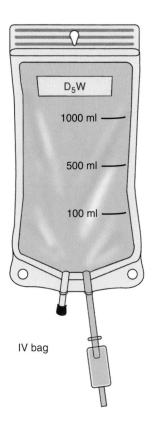

FIGURE 13-9
Flexible intravenous solution bag. (From Kee JL and Marshall SM: *Clinical calculations: with application to general and specialty areas,* ed 5, Philadelphia, 2004, WB Saunders.)

know the correct administration route for any drug passed on the sterile field.

AEROSOL SPRAY
An aerosol drug is delivered in fine droplets or particles, which the patient inhales.

BUCCAL
A buccal drug is placed between the cheek and gum and is absorbed through the highly vascular oral mucous membrane.

INHALED
Inhaled drugs, such as some anesthetics, are volatile (convert to a gaseous state) at room temperature or slightly higher. The patient breathes the gas, which is absorbed through the alveoli in the lungs.

PARENTERAL
Injection of a liquid drug via a hollow needle is called parenteral administration. Intravenous injections are administered directly into a blood vessel. This is the fastest route of administration. Intramuscular injections are administered into a muscle. Subcutaneous administration is injection into the adipose or fat tissue. In intradermal injections the needle is placed between the dermis and epidermis.

ORAL
Oral administration is by mouth, abbreviated as PO (per os). Tablets, capsules, and liquids often are administered by mouth.

SUBLINGUAL
Sublingual tablets are placed under the tongue for rapid absorption into the vascular system. Nitroglycerin, a cardiac drug, is administered sublingually.

TRANSDERMAL
Transdermal medication is absorbed systemically through an adhesive skin patch impregnated with drug.

TOPICAL
Topical medications are applied directly to the skin or mucous membrane. These are produced in the form of gels, liquids, foams, pastes, and semisolid adhesives.

Drug Forms and Packaging
The form of a drug determines how it is administered and the part of the body in which it is administered. During manufacturing, the drug itself is mixed with other substances to create the form needed. The nontherapeutic substance is called the vehicle. This vehicle is the substance added to a drug to give the drug bulk or suitable consistency, which may be a liquid, gel, tablet (compressed solid), or capsule.

Table 13-4 lists commonly used drug forms and types of packaging.

INTRAVENOUS DRUGS AND FLUIDS USED

Only certain distinct categories of drugs are used in surgery. This chapter focuses on those drug categories. This discussion excludes central nervous system agents and those used as preoperative medications, such as gastric acid reduction agents, which are discussed in Chapter 12.

Table 13-5 lists types and specific names of IV drugs and fluids and their uses.

Intravenous Fluids
Intravenous fluids are given during surgery for the following purposes:

▶ To create immediate venous access for the administration of drugs
▶ To maintain and manipulate intravascular fluid volume
▶ To maintain electrolyte balance as needed

Recall that body fluids are balanced in the intracellular (inside the cell) and extracellular (outside the cell) spaces. The extracellular fluid normally is found in the tissue spaces and within the vascular system. The fluid balance in these spaces is controlled by electrolyte distribution (positive and negative ions), and by solutes such as dextrose, sodium

Table 13-4   DRUG FORMS, ROUTES, AND PACKAGING

Drug Form	Route	Packaging
Liquid	Parenteral administration—single-dose injection	Glass vial, ampule
	Intravenous infusion	Glass bottle or plastic pouch
	Intermittent wound irrigation	Plastic bottle
	Instillation	Dropper bottle
	Oral administration	Single-dose or multiple-dose container
	Continuous irrigation	Plastic pouch
Tablet	Oral administration	Blister pack
	Sublingual administration	Glass or metal bottle
Suppository	Rectal, vaginal insertion	Blister pack
Ointment, cream	Topical administration—skin	Pouch or tube
Ointment	Instillation administration—eye	
Water-based gel	Application to mucous membrane–lined tubular organ	
Skin patch	Transdermal administration	Dry package
Wax	Topical administration—bone	Sterile aluminum pouch
Powder	Topical administration—capillary bed	Plastic or glass jar
Absorbable collagen fiber, mesh	Topical administration—capillary bed	Glass jar
Gelatin sponge	Topical administration—capillary bed	Dry paper envelope
Gas	Inhalation via mask, endotracheal tube, laryngeal mask airway, nasal cannula	Tank or in-line supply
Aerosol droplet	Inhalation	Nebulizer or mask
Volatile liquid	Inhalation	Anesthesia machine

chloride, and serum albumin. Fluid follows solutes, moving from areas of lesser concentration to those of greater concentration across the cell membrane. Manipulation of intravascular solutes is one method of maintaining the correct balance of fluids in the body spaces. Refer to Table 13-6 for a list of intravenous fluids.

CRYSTALLOIDS

Solutions that are *hypertonic* contain more solutes than does plasma. Hypotonic solutions contain less solute than plasma, and *isotonic* solutions are equal to plasma in osmolality. As a group, these solutions are called *crystalloids*. When these solutions are administered intravenously, they create osmotic pressure that controls the movement of water into and out of the intravascular space. Examples of crystalloids are lactated Ringer's solution, dextrose, and saline.

COLLOIDS

Colloids are vascular volume expanders. As large proteins, they cannot cross the cell membrane and thus cannot draw fluid from the extravascular space. Dextran solutions have properties similar to those of human albumin. Hetastarch is a hypertonic synthetic starch. Plasma protein fraction is a 5% protein solution obtained from pooled human blood, serum, or plasma.

Blood and Blood Products

Whole blood and blood products are infused during surgery when the patient's blood loss is excessive or when the oxygen-carrying capacity of the blood is significantly reduced. When blood products are used, an exact protocol must be followed for typing and cross matching (ensuring compatibility) of donor blood. Before donor blood is infused, *two licensed professionals* must match all patient identification information with that on the blood unit. Patient identification number, name, and type must match exactly. If they do not, the blood must be returned to the blood bank immediately.

Blood products must be stored at temperatures between 33.8° F and 42.8° F (1.0° C and 6.0° C). External temperature tape may be used to monitor the temperature of individual units. Units must be used within 30 minutes in a nonmonitored environment. After that, the blood cannot be returned to the blood bank. During infusion, blood and blood products must first pass through a warming system to prevent patient hypothermia and cardiac arrest. The temperature must not exceed 98.6° F.

Transfusion reaction can be a life-threatening event. The most common causes of transfusion reaction are failure to accurately verify the patient's blood type and cross match, and improper blood storage conditions. Allergic reaction to

Table 13-5 COMMON SURGICAL MEDICATIONS

Generic (Brand) Names	Uses	Action
Anticoagulants		
Heparin	To prolong the clotting time of blood; to prevent and treat deep venous thrombosis (DVT) and pulmonary embolism; as an irrigant in cardiovascular surgery to prevent formation of clots within the wound.	Inhibits thrombosis by inactivating factor X and inhibiting conversion of prothrombin to thrombin.
Coagulants (Hemostatics)		
Avitene (microfibrillar collagen hemostat)	As a direct topical application to areas of active bleeding to control the bleeding.	When it comes in contact with a bleeding surface, it attracts platelets, which adhere to the fibrils. The platelets then aggregate, beginning the clotting cascade. Available as a loose fibrous form or a compact nonwoven web form.
Gelfoam (absorbable gelatin sponge)	Same as Avitene.	A pliable gelatin sponge that absorbs fluid, expands, and exerts pressure on adjacent structures.
Surgicel (oxidized regenerated cellulose)	Same as Avitene.	An absorbable, white, knitted fabric that when saturated with blood, swells into a dark gelatinous mass, which aids in the formation of clots.
Protamine	To neutralize the effects of heparin (1 mg of protamine neutralizes 100 units of heparin).	Protamine by itself is an anticoagulant and will cause an increase in clotting time. When mixed with heparin, the drugs are attracted to each other and form a stable salt that neutralizes the effects of heparin.
Thrombin	As a topical hemostatic agent, usually used in combination with an absorbable gelatin sponge (gelatin).	Induces clotting on bleeding surfaces where conventional methods of hemostasis are contraindicated, such as friable and delicate tissue.
Oxytocics		
Oxytocin (Pitocin)	To induce and maintain labor; to prevent or control hemorrhage postpartum.	Stimulates contractions of uterine smooth muscles.
Methylergonovine (Methergine)	To prevent postpartum bleeding.	Same as Oxytocin.
Corticosteroids		
Betamethasone sodium phosphate (Celestone)	As a treatment of many inflammatory diseases and conditions.	Mostly used for their antiinflammatory properties, both systemic and local.
Betamethasone sodium phosphate (Celestone phosphate)	Same as betamethasone sodium phosphate.	Same as betamethasone sodium phosphate.
Dexamethasone (Decadron, Dexamethasone, Hexadrol)	Same as betamethasone sodium phosphate.	Same as betamethasone sodium phosphate.
Hydrocortisone sodium succinate (Solu-Cortef)	Same as betamethasone sodium phosphate.	Same as betamethasone sodium phosphate.
Methylprednisolone acetate (Depo-Medrol)	Same as betamethasone sodium phosphate.	Long-acting corticosteroid.
Methylprednisolone sodium succinate (Solu-Medrol)	Same as betamethasone sodium phosphate.	Same as betamethasone sodium phosphate.
Triamcinolone acetonide (Kenalog)	Same as betamethasone sodium phosphate.	Same as betamethasone sodium phosphate.
Triamcinolone diacetate (Aristocort)	Same as betamethasone sodium phosphate.	Same as betamethasone sodium phosphate.

Continued

Table 13-5 COMMON SURGICAL MEDICATIONS—cont'd

Generic (Brand) Names	Uses	Action
Antibiotic, Antimicrobial, and Anti-infective		
Cefazolin (Kefzol, Ancef)	To prevent postoperative wound infections caused by gram-negative organisms (e.g., *Staphylococcus epidermidis*); to treat respiratory, genitourinary, skin/soft-tissue, and blood infections caused by gram-positive and certain gram-negative organisms.	Inhibits bacterial cell wall synthesis (bactericidal).
Clindamycin (Cleocin)	To treat infections caused by susceptible aerobic and anaerobic gram-positive organisms.	Inhibits bacterial protein synthesis (bacteriostatic).
Gentamicin (Garamycin)	To treat respiratory, genitourinary, gastrointestinal, ophthalmic, and blood infections caused by gram-negative organisms.	Inhibits bacterial protein synthesis (bactericidal).
Vancomycin	To treat respiratory, genitourinary, bone, skin/soft-tissue, and blood infections caused by gram-positive organisms.	Inhibits bacterial cell wall synthesis (bactericidal).
Levofloxacin (Levaquin)	To treat respiratory, genitourinary, ophthalmic, skin/soft-tissue, and blood infections caused by certain gram-positive organisms (e.g. pneumococci), gram-negative organisms, and atypical organisms (e.g. *Mycoplasma*).	Inhibits bacterial DNA replication and transcription (bactericidal).
Metronidazole (Flagyl)	To treat infections caused by anaerobic organisms.	Inhibits bacterial protein synthesis (bactericidal).
Irrigation Solutions		
Bacitracin	As an irrigation solution to prevent gram-positive infections at site of the surgical procedure.	Inhibits bacterial cell wall synthesis (bactericidal).
Neomycin	As an irrigation solution to prevent gram-negative infections at site of the surgical procedure.	Inhibits bacterial protein synthesis (bactericidal).
Polymyxin B	As an irrigation solution to prevent gram-negative infections at site of the surgical procedure (urological).	Binds to phospholipids, alters permeability, and damages bacterial cytoplasm membrane, permitting leakage of its components.
Diagnostic Imaging Agents		
Renografin	For cholangiography and hysterosalpingography.	When injected, shows as white on x-ray.
Cystografin (Cysto-Conray)	To x-ray the urinary tract.	Same as Renografin.
Hypaque	To x-ray the biliary tract, kidney, and other internal structures.	Same as Renografin.
Hyskon	In hysteroscopy, as an aid in distending uterine cavity and irrigating and visualizing surfaces.	An electrolyte-free and nonconductive solution.
Dyes		
Methylene blue	To mark a specific surface or area; to color solutions; to test patency of specific organs.	Turns skin blue when used topically and turns urine a greenish color when used systemically.
Indigo carmine	Same as methylene blue.	Same as methylene blue.
Diuretic		
Mannitol	To promote diuresis and treatment of oliguric phase of acute renal failure after cardiovascular surgery; to reduce elevated intraocular and intracranial pressure.	Inhibits water/electrolyte reabsorption in kidneys and increases urinary output.
Analgesics		
Fentanyl (Sublimaze)	As a preoperative medication; as an adjunct therapy during local, regional, and general anesthesia.	Narcotic analgesic that increases pain threshold and alters pain perception. Rapid onset and short duration.
Alfenta (Sufenta)	Same as fentanyl.	Narcotic agonist analgesic with rapid onset and short duration.

Table 13-5   COMMON SURGICAL MEDICATIONS—cont'd

Generic (Brand) Names	Uses	Action
Analgesics—cont'd		
Morphine sulfate	Same as fentanyl.	Same as fentanyl, but slightly longer onset (5-15 minutes) and longer duration (4-5 hours).
Meperidine (Demerol)	Same as fentanyl.	Same as fentanyl, but slightly longer onset (5-15 minutes) and longer duration (3 hours).
Hydromorphone (Dilaudid)	To relieve moderate to severe pain (alternative to morphine).	Mechanism of action similar to fentanyl, but 8-10 times more potent analgesic effect than morphine. Onset 10-15 minutes and duration 4-5 hours.
Benzodiazepines		
Diazepam (Valium)	To provide sedation or muscle relaxation, and/or alleviate anxiety before surgery; to treat seizures.	CNS depressant. Long-acting benzodiazepine with sedative, hypnotic, and anticonvulsant properties.
Midazolam (Versed)	To provide sedation or muscle relaxation, and/or alleviate anxiety before surgery; to impair memory of perioperative events.	CNS depressant. Intermediate-acting benzodiazepine with sedative, hypnotic, and anticonvulsant properties. Also has anterograde amnestic effects.
Lorazepam (Ativan)	Same as diazepam.	Same as midazolam, except with no anterograde amnestic effects.
Emergency Drugs		
Epinephrine (Adrenalin)	To treat cardiac arrest/asystole; to treat severe bradycardia or hypotension.	Causes vasoconstriction, increases blood pressure, increases heart rate, and increases cardiac output.
Norepinephrine (Levophed)	To treat severe hypotension associated with cardiogenic or septic shock.	Causes vasoconstriction, increases blood pressure.
Dopamine	To treat severe hypotension associated with cardiogenic or septic shock; to increase urinary output (lower doses should be used).	Low dose increases urinary output; intermediate dose increases cardiac output and blood pressure; high dose decreases vasoconstriction and increases blood pressure and heart rate.
Nitroprusside (Nipride)	To treat hypertensive emergencies.	Arterial and venous vasodilator; decreases blood pressure very quickly; reflex increases heart rate and increases cardiac output.
Amiodarone	To treat severe life-threatening ventricular arrhythmias (Vfib/Vtach); in cardiac arrest with persistent Vfib; for treatment of atrial arrhythmias (atrial fibrillation).	Prolongs conduction and refractory period in ventricles (increases electrical stimulation threshold). Also decreases AV/SA node conduction, which is why it is beneficial in patients with atrial fibrillation.
Lidocaine	To treat ventricular arrhythmias (Vfib/Vtach); in cardiac arrest with persistent Vfib.	Increases electrical stimulation threshold; prolongs conduction and refractory period in ventricles during diastole.
Atropine	To treat sinus bradycardia.	Competitive antagonist of acetylcholine in smooth and cardiac muscle; increases heart rate.
Sodium bicarbonate	To treat metabolic acidosis.	Neutralizes hydrogen ion concentration and raises blood and urinary pH.
Magnesium sulfate	To treat ventricular arrhythmia, torsades de pointes.	Prolongs conduction through ventricles and slows SA node conduction.
Digoxin (Lanoxin)	To slow rate of tachyarrhythmias such as Afib/A flutter or supraventricular tachycardia; to relieve signs and symptoms of congestive heart failure (CHF).	Suppresses AV node conduction to increase refractory period and decrease conduction velocity. Inhibits Na^+/K^+ ATPase pump, which increases intracellular Ca^{++} to increase myocardial contractility.

Continued

Table 13-5 COMMON SURGICAL MEDICATIONS

Generic (Brand) Names	Uses	Action
Blood and Blood Substitutes		
Hetastarch (Hespan)	Blood volume expander used in treatment of shock or impending shock (e.g., as a result of hemorrhage) when blood or blood products are not available. *Not* a substitute for blood or plasma because it *does not* have oxygen-carrying capability.	Produces plasma volume expansion by virtue of its highly colloidal starch structure.
Albumin	To expand plasma volume and maintain cardiac output in shock or impending shock.	Produces plasma volume expansion by virtue of its structure. Increases intravascular oncotic pressure and causes mobilization of fluids into intravascular space.
Fresh frozen plasma, washed packed cells, whole blood, cryoprecipitate, and factor VIII	Blood and blood components to restore cell volume.	Maintain blood volume; improve coagulation.
Solutions		
Sodium chloride 0.9% (normal saline solution)	To restore blood volume in hemorrhage and blood pressure in shock; to compensate for fluid loss from burns, dehydration, and many similar conditions; as a means of giving needed intravenous medications.	Electrolyte solutions are given to maintain balance. The type used depends on the needs of the patient.
Lactated Ringer's solution	Same as sodium chloride 0.9%.	Same as sodium chloride 0.9%.
Dextrose solution	Same as sodium chloride 0.9% but with added nutrients/calories.	Prepared in isotonic sodium chloride, lactated Ringer's solution, and distilled water for use as patient's condition indicates.
Local Anesthetics		
Lidocaine (Xylocaine)	To reduce pain of minor or superficial procedures.	Injected into a specific area. Local anesthesia to relieve local discomfort of skin and mucous membranes.
Bupivacaine (Marcaine)	Same as lidocaine.	Same as lidocaine.
Cocaine	As a topical anesthetic.	Applied directly to the skin and mucous membrane, which readily absorb the agent.
Epinephrine (Adrenalin)	When added to a local anesthetic, to slow the absorption of the drug and to keep the anesthetic at the desired site.	Vasoconstrictor.
Miscellaneous		
Propofol (Diprivan)	Adjunct treatment for induction and maintenance of anesthesia. Adjunct treatment to reduce nausea/vomiting in postoperative setting. Sedation for mechanically ventilated patients.	General anesthesia with sedative/hypnotic properties. CNS depressant.
Granisetron (Kytril)	To prevent and treat postoperative nausea and vomiting.	Selective 5-HT3 antagonist that blocks stimulation of vagal nerve terminal and chemotherapy trigger zone.

Table 13-6 SOLUTIONS FOR INTRAVENOUS USE

Contents of Solutions	Cations (mEq/L)					Anions (mEq/L)			HCO₃⁻	Glucose
Type of Solution	Na⁺	K⁺	Ca⁺⁺	Mg⁺⁺	NH₄⁻	Cl⁻	Lactate	PO₄⁻		(g/L)
5% dextrose in water										50
10% dextrose in water										100
Normal saline (0.9%)	154					154				
Ringer's solution	147	4	4			155				
5% dextrose in Ringer's lactate	130	4	3			109	28			50
Ringer's lactate	130	4	3			109	28			
5% dextrose in 0.2% saline	34					34				50
5% dextrose in 0.45% saline	77					77				50

From Phipps WJ et al: *Medical-surgical nursing: health and illness perspectives,* ed 7, St Louis, 2003, Mosby.

transfused blood occurs when the patient is sensitive to antigens in the blood.

If a transfusion reaction occurs, surgery is halted, and the patient is treated in accordance with the severity of the reaction.

WHOLE BLOOD

Whole blood contains serum and blood cells. It is used only when the patient's blood loss exceeds 30% of total blood volume or approximately 1500 ml. A combination of packed red blood cells (RBCs) and plasma expanders is effective in increasing total intravascular volume and oxygen-carrying capacity.

PACKED RED BLOOD CELLS

PRBCs are administered to increase the oxygen-carrying capacity of the blood. Among the advantages of using PRBCs is a reduced risk of blood-borne disease transmission. Packed cells are handled and monitored in the same way as whole blood. Clinically, 1 unit of packed PRBCs raises the hemoglobin by about 1 mg/dl.

AUTOLOGOUS BLOOD

Elective-surgery patients can donate their own blood before surgery. The blood then is stored in the blood bank and is made available for use during the surgery. Autotransfusion is the mechanical recovery and transfusion of the patient's own (autologous) blood during surgery.

PLATELETS

Platelets are the blood components given to increase the patient's platelet count. Factors important in hemostasis are contained in and attached to platelets, and act together with coagulation factors.

FRESH FROZEN PLASMA

Fresh frozen plasma (FFP) is transfused as an adjunct intravascular expander. Blood typing and cross match are not required. FFP is most often administered to increase clotting factors in the blood.

Topical Hemostatic Agents

Absorbable and nonabsorbable topical hemostatic agents are used to control small vessel bleeding, especially in highly vascular areas or those that are not safe to coagulate by other means, such as brain tissue. The agents are placed directly over the bleeding site. Nonabsorbable agents are removed after several minutes.

Absorbable hemostatic agents that are packaged in films, sheets, mesh, or fibers are cut or separated into pledgets depending on the size needed. Absorbable collagen and some cellulose products may be soaked in thrombin before use. Bone wax is softened between the fingers and offered to the surgeon in small pieces. One prepares fibrin glue by mixing the two components (thrombin and fibrinogen) before use.

Examples of topical hemostatic agents are the following:

- Absorbable gelatin (Gelfilm, Gelfoam powder, and Gelfoam sponge)
- Microfibrillar collagen hemostat (Avitene)
- Oxidized cellulose (Surgicel, Oxycel)
- Absorbable collagen sponge (Gelfoam, Superstat, Helistat)
- Fibrin glue (human thrombin and fibrinogen)
- Hemostatic wax (bone wax)
- Thrombin (Thrombogen)

Thrombin is a liquid drug used to soak small cotton or foam pledgets for use in hemostasis. Thrombin is one of the chemicals of the body's normal clotting mechanism. When applied to a hemorrhaging small vessel, it causes rapid clotting. The drug must be reconstituted from a powder before distribution onto the sterile field.

Thrombin poses a high risk in the event of medication error. If accidentally injected or allowed to seep into a blood vessel, it can cause thrombosis (blood clotting), which may lead to death.

Anticoagulants

An **anticoagulant** is a liquid agent that temporarily prevents normal blood clotting. During vascular surgery *heparin sodium* solution is injected into open blood vessels to prevent platelet aggregation. It also is used to prime certain types of vascular grafts. In cardiac bypass surgery, heparin is administered to maintain blood flow through the bypass pump.

Heparin dosage is measured in *units*. When receiving heparin from the circulator, make certain that the drug order matches the number of units distributed.

The heparinized patient is at high risk for hemorrhage. *Protamine sulfate* is administered to reverse the effects of heparin.

If both *heparin* and *thrombin* are available in medicine containers, strict attention must be given to labels and identification. Injecting thrombin directly into a blood vessel causes immediate life-threatening clots.

Antibiotics

Antibiotic drugs are those that inhibit growth of or kill microorganisms in the body. Each class of antibiotics is used against a particular group of infectious organisms, and the mechanism of microbial destruction varies with the drug. Antibiotics often are administered before surgery (called *prophylactic administration*). This is common in trauma cases, in cases involving the gastrointestinal or biliary tract, and in selected orthopedic cases. If the surgical wound is contaminated, or if it becomes grossly contaminated during surgery, intravenous antimicrobial therapy begins immediately.

Allergy to antibiotics can be life threatening. No antibiotic should be dispensed without knowledge of the patient's drug allergies. This information is available on the patient's chart or on the patient's identification band.

Bacterial infections are the most common cause of surgical site infection (SSI) (see Chapter 1). Therefore antibacterial agents are usually added to solutions used for wound irrigation and prophylaxis. The most common topical antibiotic used in wound irrigation for wound management is bacitracin.

Classes of antibacterial agents and common examples are listed in Table 13-7.

Radiopaque Contrast Agents

A liquid contrast agent is one that is impenetrable by x-rays. Diagnostic surgical procedures often require indirect visualization of an anatomical structure (observation of the structure without exposing it surgically). When a tubular structure such as a blood vessel or duct is infused with a radiopaque substance, the structure is clearly visible on radiograph. This enables the surgeon or radiologist to follow the path of the structure and look for strictures (narrowing), dilation, pouching, or other anomalies that require medical or surgical intervention. Barium is a commonly used **contrast medium** for the gastrointestinal tract.

Table 13-7 ANTIBACTERIAL CLASSES AND COMMON EXAMPLES

Class	Examples
Penicillins*	Penicillin G
	Penicillin V
	Ampicillin
	Amoxicillin
	Amoxicillin/clavulanic acid (Augmentin)
	Methicillin
Cephalosporins	First generation: cefazolin, cefadroxil, cephalexin
	Second generation: cefamandole, cefuroxime, cefoxitin
	Third generation: ceftizoxime, cefoperazone, cefprozil
Aminoglycosides	Streptomycin
	Gentamicin
	Tobramycin
	Neomycin
	Kanamycin
Macrolides	Erythromycin
Tetracyclines	Topical tetracycline
	Ophthalmic tetracycline
Quinolones	Ciprofloxacin
	Norfloxacin
	Ofloxacin
Sulfonamides	Silver sulfadiazine
	Sulfisoxazole
	Sulfamethoxazole
Beta lactams	Aztreonam
	Imipenem

Diatrizoates

Diatrizoates are the water-soluble, iodinated, radiopaque, x-ray contrast media used most often. The iodinized salts are used for visualization in a wide variety of diagnostic imaging methods, including angiography, urography, cholangiography, hysterosalpingography, retrograde pyelography, and computed tomography (CT scan).

Colored **dyes** generally are used for visual identification. When a dye is infused into a duct or hollow structure, the path of the dye can be traced visually. This establishes whether the structure is patent (allows the free flow of fluid). A common use of dye is to verify patency of the fallopian tubes. Indigo carmine, gentian violet, and methylene blue are the three most common dyes. Although these have therapeutic uses, they also can be very toxic. *No drug is without side effects.*

Dye pens containing *gentian violet* dye are usually used to mark the incision site or to outline areas of remodeling in plastic surgery.

Staining Agents

Stains are used as a diagnostic tool to differentiate normal from abnormal cells. Although a variety of staining agents are used in the clinical laboratory setting, several types of stains are used in the surgical setting to enable surgeons to see areas of diseased tissue appropriate for ablation or excision. Stains typically are applied under direct visualization with a sterile sponge or cotton-tipped applicator. The stain generally is taken up (absorbed) by the abnormal cells, giving these cells an appearance different from healthy surrounding cells.

Examples of staining agents used in the surgical setting include acetic acid (vinegar), Monsel's solution (an iron-based solution), and Lugol's solution (a strong iodine-based solution). Acetic acid usually is used to identify areas of dysplasia (abnormal tissue cells) in gynecological and urogenital procedures. It is liberally applied to the skin and mucous linings of the cervix, perineum, and anus to identify condyloma. The vinegar is absorbed by these abnormal cells, causing them to appear whitish and enabling the surgeon to easily identify these areas for ablation or excision.

Lugol's solution is used in performing Schiller's test to identify dysplastic tissue on cervical tissue. This solution is absorbed by healthy cells, which causes them to appear darker than the areas of dysplasia. The use of Lugol's solution is contraindicated in patients with hypersensitivity to topical iodine.

Diuretics

Diuretics increase the flow of urine by drawing fluids from tissue. This group of drugs has two primary uses. The drugs lower blood pressure by extracting fluid from the vascular system, and they reduce peripheral and pulmonary edema in liver and kidney disease and congestive heart failure. The exact mechanism of action varies among the different classes of diuretics.

A diuretic is prescribed preoperatively for specific procedures that require reduced intraocular, vascular, or intracranial pressure. Classes of diuretics include thiazide diuretics, loop or high-ceiling diuretics, carbonic anhydrase inhibitors, and osmotic diuretics. Of these classes, only osmotic and loop diuretics are usually used intraoperatively.

Ophthalmic Drugs

Many drugs that are not used in other surgical specialties are often used in eye procedures. They are presented together here rather than in the discussion of the drug categories. Ophthalmic drugs are used in all perioperative phases: before, during, and after surgery. Drugs are dispensed in small-dose vials for administration to each individual patient. Table 13-8 lists commonly used ophthalmic drugs. For the specific use of these drugs within specific procedures, refer to Chapter 24.

Table 13-8   MEDICATIONS USED DURING OPHTHALMIC SURGERY

Drug/Name	Purpose/Description
Mydriatics	
Phenylephrine (Neo-Synephrine, Mydfrin), 2.5%, 10%	Mydriasis (dilates the pupil but permits focusing), used for objective examination of the retina, testing of refraction, easier removal of lens; used alone or with a cycloplegic
Cycloplegics	
Tropicamide (Mydriacyl), 1%	Cycloplegia (paralysis of accommodation; inhibits focusing); dilates the pupil; anticholinergic, used for examination of fundus, refraction
Atropine, 1%	Anticholinergic, dilates pupil, inhibits focusing; potent, long duration (7 to 14 days)
Cyclopentolate (Cyclogyl), 1%, 2%	Anticholinergic, dilates pupil, inhibits focusing
Scopolamine hydrobromide (Isopto Hyoscine), 0.25%	Anticholinergic, dilates pupil, inhibits focusing
Homatropine hydrobromide (Isopto Homatropine), 2%, 5%	Anticholinergic, dilates pupil, inhibits focusing
Epinephrine (1:1000) preservative free (PF)	Dilates the pupil; added to bottles of balanced salt solution for irrigation to maintain pupil dilation during cataract or vitrectomy procedure
Miotics	
Carbachol (Miostat), 0.01%	Potent cholinergic, constricts pupil, used intraocularly during anterior segment surgery
Carbachol (Isopto Carbachol), 0.75%, 1.5%, 2.25%, 3%	Potent cholinergic, constricts pupil, used topically for lowering intraocular pressure in glaucoma
Acetylcholine chloride (Miochol-E), 1%	Cholinergic, rapidly constricts pupil, used intraocularly during anterior segment surgery; reconstitute immediately before using
Pilocarpine hydrochloride, 1%, 4%	Cholinergic, constricts pupil, used topically for lowering intraocular pressure in glaucoma

From Rothrock JC: *Alexander's care of the patient in surgery,* ed 12, St Louis, 2003, Mosby.   *Continued*

Table 13-8 MEDICATIONS USED DURING OPHTHALMIC SURGERY—cont'd

Drug/Name	Purpose/Description
Topical Anesthetics	
Tetracaine hydrochloride (Pontocaine), 0.5%	Onset: 5-20 seconds; duration of action: 10-20 minutes
Proparacaine hydrochloride (Ophthaine), 0.5%	Onset: 5-20 seconds; duration of action: 10-20 minutes
Injectable Anesthetics	
Lidocaine (Xylocaine), 1%, 2%, 4%	Onset: 4-6 minutes; duration of action: 40-60 minutes, 120 minutes with epinephrine
Methylparaben free (MPF)	Preservative free; adjunct to topical anesthesia
Bupivacaine (Marcaine, Sensorcaine), 0.25%, 0.50%, 0.75%	Onset: 5-11 minutes; duration of action: 480-720 minutes with epinephrine; often used in 0.75% combination with lidocaine for blocks
Mepivacaine (Carbocaine), 1%, 2%	Onset: 3-5 minutes; duration of action: 120 minutes; duration of action greater with epinephrine
Etidocaine (Duranest), 1%	Onset: 3 minutes; duration of action: 300-600 minutes
Additives to Local Anesthetics	
Epinephrine 1:50,000 to 1:200,000	Combined with injectable local anesthetics to prolong anesthesia and reduce bleeding
Hyaluronidase	Enzyme mixed with anesthetics (75 units per 10 ml) to increase diffusion of anesthetic through tissue, improving the effectiveness of the block; contraindicated if skin inflammation or malignancy present
Viscoelastics	
Sodium hyaluronate (Healon, Amvisc, Provisc, Vitrax) in a sterile syringe assembly with blunt-tipped cannula	Lubricant and support; maintains separation between tissues to protect the endothelium and maintain the anterior chamber intraocularly; removed from anterior chamber to prevent postoperative increase in pressure; should be refrigerated (except Vitrax); allow 30 minutes to warm to room temperature
Sodium chondroitin-sodium hyaluronate (Viscoat) in a sterile syringe assembly with blunt-tipped cannula	Maintains a deep chamber for anterior segment procedures, protects epithelium of cornea, and improves visualization; may be used to coat intraocular lens before implantation; should be refrigerated
Duovisc	Packages of separate syringes of Provisc and Viscoat in the same box
Viscoadherents	
Hydroxypropylmethylcellulose 2% (Occucoat) in a sterile syringe assembly with blunt-tipped cannula	Maintains a deep chamber for anterior segment procedures, protects epithelium of cornea, and may be used to coat intraocular lens before implantation; removed from anterior chamber at end of procedure; stored at room temperature
Hydroxyethylcellulose (Gonioscopic Prism Solution)	Bonds gonioscopic prisms to the eye; stored at room temperature
Hydroxypropyl methylcellulose 2.5% (Goniosol)	Bonds gonioscopic prisms to the eye; stored at room temperature
Irrigants	
Balanced salt solution (BSS, Endosol)	Used to keep cornea moist during surgery; also used as internal irrigant into anterior or posterior segment
Balanced salt solution enriched with bicarbonate, dextrose, and glutathione (BSS Plus, Endosol Extra)	Used as internal irrigant into anterior or posterior segment; need to reconstitute immediately before use by addition of part I to part II with transfer device
Hyperosmotic Agents	
Mannitol (Osmitrol)	Intravenous osmotic diuretic; increases the osmolarity of the plasma, causing osmotic pressure gradient to pull free fluid from the eye to the plasma and reduce the intraocular pressure
Glycerin (Osmoglyn, Glyrol)	Oral osmotic diuretic given in chilled juice or cola; increases the osmolarity of the plasma, causing osmotic pressure gradient to pull free fluid from the eye to the plasma and reduce the intraocular pressure

From Rothrock JC: *Alexander's care of the patient in surgery,* ed 12, St Louis, 2003, Mosby.

Table 13-8   MEDICATIONS USED DURING OPHTHALMIC SURGERY—cont'd

Drug/Name	Purpose/Description
Antiinflammatory Agents	
Betamethasone sodium phosphate and betamethasone acetate suspension (Celestone)	Glucocorticoid; injected subconjunctivally after surgery for prophylaxis; also used to treat severe allergic and inflammatory conditions
Dexamethasone (Decadron)	Adrenocortical steroid; injected subconjunctivally after surgery for prophylaxis; also used to treat severe allergic and inflammatory conditions and intraocularly for endophthalmitis
Methylprednisolone acetate suspension (Depo-Medrol)	Glucocorticoid; injected subconjunctivally after surgery for prophylaxis; also used to treat severe allergic and inflammatory conditions
Antiinfectives	
Polymyxin B/bacitracin (Polysporin ointment)	Topically to treat superficial ocular infections of the conjunctiva or cornea; prophylactically after surgery
Polymyxin B/neomycin/bacitracin (Neosporin ointment)	Topical treatment of superficial infections of the external eye; prophylactically after surgery; potential hypersensitivity to neomycin
Neomycin and polymyxin B sulfates and dexamethasone (Maxitrol ointment or suspension)	Topical treatment of steroid-responsive inflammatory ocular conditions or bacterial infections of the external eye; potential hypersensitivity to neomycin
Tobramycin/dexamethasone (TobraDex)	Topical treatment or prevention of superficial infections of the external part of eye; also has antiinflammatory properties
Cefazolin (Ancef, Kefzol)	Prophylactically injected subconjunctivally after procedure; also topically, intraocularly, and systemically for endophthalmitis
Gentamicin sulfate (Garamycin)	Prophylactically injected subconjunctivally after procedure; also topically, subconjunctivally, and intraocularly for endophthalmitis
Ceftazidime (Fortaz, Tazicef, Tazidime)	Injected subconjunctivally and intraocularly for treatment of endophthalmitis
Miscellaneous	
Cocaine, 1% to 4%	Topical use, never injected; used on cornea to loosen epithelium before débridement and on nasal packing to reduce congestion of mucosa
5-Fluorouracil (5-FU)	Antimetabolite used topically to inhibit scar formation in glaucoma-filtering procedures; handle and discard in compliance with Occupational Safety and Health Administration (OSHA) and facility policies for safe use of antineoplastics
Mitomycin (Mutamycin)	Antimetabolite used topically to inhibit scar formation in glaucoma-filtering procedures and pterygium excision; handle and discard in compliance with OSHA and facility policies for safe use of antineoplastics
Tissue plasminogen activator (TPA) (Activase)	Thrombolytic agent; to treat fibrin formation in postvitrectomy patients; lysis of clots on retina
Fluorescein	Yellowish green fluorescence of this intravenous (IV) diagnostic aid is used in fluorescein angiography to diagnose retinal disorder; topical stain: fluorescein strip temporarily stains the cornea yellow-green in areas of denuded corneal epithelium
Timolol maleate (Timoptic)	Beta-adrenergic receptor blocking agent; treatment of elevated intraocular pressure in ocular hypertension or open-angle glaucoma
Acetazolamide sodium (Diamox)	Carbonic anhydrase inhibitor; given intravenously to reduce the secretion of aqueous humor; results in a drop in intraocular pressure; diuretic effect
Dextrose, 50%	Added to BSS, Endosol, BSS Plus, or Endosol Extra for diabetic patients during intraocular procedures

From Rothrock JC: *Alexander's care of the patient in surgery,* ed 12, St Louis, 2003, Mosby.

Miscellaneous Drugs
EPINEPHRINE

Epinephrine is produced by the adrenal gland. It is used in surgery for its ability to constrict blood vessels. It is usually mixed with local anesthetics to constrict the capillary bed and prevent dispersion of the anesthetic out of the local area. It also may be used in very small amounts in ear surgery to control capillary bleeding. Medically, this drug causes rapid heart rate (tachycardia) and bronchial dilation.

OXYTOCIN

Oxytocin is a hormone normally produced during late pregnancy, labor, and lactation. It is sometimes prescribed during labor to increase the intensity of uterine contractions. It is given after delivery to constrict the uterus and thus the blood vessels in the uterus to reduce postpartum bleeding. It usually is given only after the expulsion of the placenta. Giving it before expulsion of the placenta can cause the uterus to clamp down on the placenta and prevent its expulsion.

CASE STUDIES

Case 1

You are asked to mix two drugs together in a particular ratio and are unable to perform the calculations. What will you do?

Case 2

You are scrubbed on an orthopedic case. While you have your back turned to the circulator, she distributes antibiotic irrigation solution into a basin on your instrument table. She yells out what she gave you. What will you do?

Case 3

You are scrubbed on an eye case. You notice that one of the drugs distributed to you is probably the correct drug, but it is not labeled. What will you do?

REFERENCES

Hata T et al: *Guidelines, education, and testing for procedural sedation and Analgesia,* 1992-2003, University of Iowa, Iowa City.

Jech AO: Med errors: a new approach to preventions, *Nurse Week* website. *Mosby drug consult,* St Louis, 2004, Elsevier.

Chapter 14

Environmental Hazards

Learning Objectives

After studying this chapter the reader will be able to:

- Describe toxic substances in smoke plumes
- Identify safe use of the smoke evacuator
- Recognize international hazard communication signs
- Differentiate between latex allergy and nonallergic dermatitis
- Describe the symptoms of true latex allergy
- Identify necessary precautions to prevent latex reaction in allergic patients
- Discuss fuels and sources of ignition commonly found in the operating room
- Identify methods associated with preventing fires in the operating room
- Describe how to respond appropriately to a patient fire
- Describe how to respond appropriately to a structural fire
- Identify the practice of standard precautions
- Identify the practice for transmission-based precautions
- Describe proper body mechanics for lifting, pulling, and pushing objects
- Discuss various techniques to prevent sharps injuries
- Describe measures to safely store, transport, and use compressed gas cylinders
- Identify methods to properly handle and dispose of hazardous waste in the operating room
- Identify precautions to prevent exposure to ionizing radiation
- Identify precautions to prevent patient burns resulting from electrical equipment
- Describe methods to avoid chemical injury
- Analyze a chemical label

Terminology

Airborne transmission precautions—Precautions to prevent the transmission of airborne disease from a known carrier to others in the environment.

Blood-borne pathogens—Pathogenic microorganisms that may be present in and transmitted through human blood and body fluids. Examples are hepatitis B virus and human immunodeficiency virus.

Genetic mutation—Having the ability to cause permanent change in genetic structure.

Latex—A naturally occurring sap obtained from rubber trees and used in the manufacture of medical devices and other commercial goods.

Needleless system—A system of parenteral access that does not use needles for the collection or withdrawal of body fluids through venous puncture.

Neutral zone (no-hands) technique—A method of transferring sharp instruments on the surgical field without hand-to-hand contact. A neutral zone is identified and sharps are exchanged in this zone.

Occupational exposure—Exposure to hazards in the workplace. Examples include exposure to hazardous chemicals or contact with potentially infected blood and body fluids.

Terminology—cont'd

Personal protective equipment—Protective clothing or equipment that protects the wearer from direct contact with hazardous chemicals or potentially infectious body fluids.

Postexposure prophylaxis—Recommended procedures to help prevent the development of blood-borne diseases after an exposure incident.

Potentially infectious materials—(1) The following fluids: blood, semen, vaginal secretions, cerebrospinal fluid, synovial fluid, pleural fluid, pericardial fluid, peritoneal fluid, amniotic fluid, saliva during procedures involving the mouth, any body fluid that is visibly contaminated with blood, any body fluid in a situation in which it is difficult or impossible to differentiate among various body fluids; (2) any unfixed tissue or organ (other than intact skin) from a human (living or dead); and (3) human immunodeficiency virus (HIV)–containing cell or tissue cultures, organ cultures, and HIV-containing or hepatitis B virus–containing culture medium or other solutions.

Risk—The statistical probability of a given event based on the number of such events that have already occurred in a certain population.

Sharps—Any objects that can penetrate the skin and have the potential for causing injury and infection, including but not limited to, needles, scalpels, broken glass, broken capillary tubes, and exposed ends of dental wires.

Smoke plume—Smoke created during the use of an electrosurgical unit or laser. This smoke contains toxic chemicals, vapors, blood fragments, and viruses.

Standard Precautions—Guidelines recommended by the Centers for Disease Control and Prevention (CDC) to reduce the risk of transmission of blood-borne and other pathogens.

Transmission-based precautions—Standards and precautions to prevent the spread of infectious disease by patients *known* to be infected.

RISK, STANDARDS OF PRACTICE, AND RECOMMENDATIONS

Risk and Risk Management

Risk is the statistical probability of a harmful event. Risk is defined as the number of harmful events that occur in a given population. Risk and probability are not difficult to measure. Statistics give us information about the number of people who have been harmed (and *how* they were harmed) as a result of exposure to particular environments, participation in given activities, or work in specific occupations (such as skateboarding or working in health care). People often ignore risk factors because they believe they will somehow escape harm.

Taking risks means trying to beat the odds, *but it does not change the probability that a given event will occur.*

Within the general population are subgroups whose risk of a harmful event is higher or lower because of their occupation, lifestyle, age, and other factors. When risks are managed, there is less chance of harm. Risk management means taking specific precautions to *reduce the risk.*

Surgical personnel are at high risk for occupational and environmental injury. The risk factors include daily contact or potential contact with blood and body fluids, harmful chemicals, heat, and powerful electrical devices; the need to lift heavy objects and move patients; frequent handling of sharp objects; and stress. Although these factors cannot be changed, the risk of harm can be reduced.

Many tragic accidents and deaths could have been prevented had the individual *known the risk, accepted the real possibility of harm, and taken precautions to protect himself or herself and fellow workers.*

Safety Standards

Occupational safety guidelines established by professional and governmental organizations are designed to protect workers. Some are standards that are required. For example, hospitals must now use retractable needles or **needleless systems** for injection. Others are practices that are strongly recommended but are not required. Recommendations are created by people familiar with surgery and health care who have seen and studied the devastating effects of injury. Researchers, professionals, and field inspectors of the organizations that set occupational safety standards maintain surveillance of occupational risks—specifically those in health care. From surveillance records and study, recommendations are developed to reduce these risks.

Safety standards and recommendations evolve after rigorous examination of accident cases.

The following governmental organizations create standards and recommended practices to reduce the risk of injury to workers and the public:

▶ **OSHA**—Occupational Safety and Health Administration
▶ **NIOSH**—National Institute for Occupational Safety and Health
▶ **CDC**—Centers for Disease Control and Prevention
▶ **EPA**—Environmental Protection Agency
▶ **APIC**—Association for Professionals in Infection Control and Epidemiology
▶ **AORN**—Association of periOperative Registered Nurses
▶ **ACS**—American College of Surgeons

The risk categories considered in this chapter do not cover all possible harm. This chapter focuses on the potential risks to surgical personnel. Most hazards involving electrosurgical and laser technology are discussed in Chapter 17. For further information on occupational risks in surgery, contact the organizations listed above. Standards are periodically updated and renewed; it is important to remain current as practices and standards evolve.

Hazards and risks change as new technologies develop.

FIRE

Fire Triangle

All fires require three components: fuel (combustible material), a source of ignition (an energy source capable of producing sufficient heat to ignite the fuel), and oxygen, which supports combustion (Figure 14-1). Abundant sources of all three components are present in the operating room. The surgical environment is unlike other environments, in which many materials normally would not ignite. Because of the high concentration of oxygen, oxidation is rapid and intense, which makes the operating room a high-risk environment for fire.

Oxygen and Oxidizers

Fuel can burn in a gaseous state, when the fuel vapor combines with sufficient oxygen. Heat is necessary to produce the vapor, either by evaporating liquids or by vaporizing a solid such as plastic. In surgery, high concentrations of oxygen are associated with anesthesia delivery, in-line supply, and tanks. Oxygen is heavier than air and settles under drapes and within confined areas such as body cavities, where it remains trapped. In the presence of sufficient heat (ignition) and fuel, oxygen supports a fire. When nitrous oxide decomposes in the presence of heat, it becomes another source of oxygen. As the concentration of oxygen increases, so does the speed of ignition, duration, and temperature of the fire. Thus items that normally would not burn in atmospheric air are highly flammable in the surgical environment.

The normal oxygen content of air is about 21%. An area that contains a higher concentration of oxygen is considered to have an oxygen-enriched atmosphere (OEA). Operating rooms by their very nature are considered to have an OEA. Therefore the risk of fire in the operating room is greater than other areas of the health-care setting.

Fuel

Any material that is capable of burning is potential fuel. Substances that burn are described as flammable. These include materials used in and around the patient, and the patient himself or herself. Note that the words *flammable* and *inflammable* are identical in meaning. Both indicate combustibility. Sources of fuel commonly found in the operating

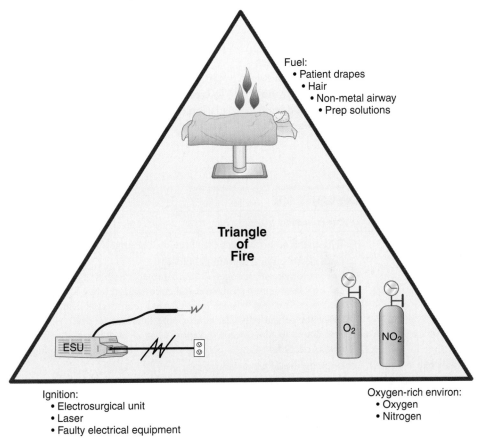

Fuel:
• Patient drapes
• Hair
• Non-metal airway
• Prep solutions

Triangle of Fire

O₂   NO₂

Ignition:
• Electrosurgical unit
• Laser
• Faulty electrical equipment

Oxygen-rich environ:
• Oxygen
• Nitrogen

FIGURE 14-1
The three components required for fire: fuel, source of ignition, and oxygen.

room are listed in Table 14-1. Although many items used in the surgical setting are considered "flame-resistant" or "flame-retardant," when exposed to the OEA present in the operating room they may readily catch fire in the presence of a heat (ignition) source.

PREPARATION SOLUTIONS AND OTHER FLAMMABLE CHEMICALS

Preparation solutions, particularly those containing alcohol, are the most common source of fuel in surgical fires. Alcohol at greater than 20% concentration is flammable and highly volatile. Most skin preparation solutions contain 70% alcohol, which ignites at 900° C. Vapor from volatile preparation solutions such as alcohol can be trapped under drapes. When the vapor is ignited, the fire may not be immediately noticeable and may produce second-degree or third-degree burns within moments. Povidone iodine solution (Betadine) also is flammable and explosive in the presence of high concentrations of oxygen and nitrous oxide. Chemicals such as cyanoacrylates (fibrin glue), used as tissue glue and for taking tissue grafts, and methyl methacrylate (bone cement) are volatile and flammable.

MEDICAL DEVICES

All rubber, plastic, Silastic, and vinyl materials are flammable. Use of these materials is common in nearly every surgical procedure. Disposable anesthesia equipment, such as endotracheal tubes, airways, masks, cannulas, and corrugated tubing, is combustible. Endotracheal tubes, except those specifically designed for use during laser surgery and electrosurgery, are frequently cited as the cause of patient fires during neck and head procedures. An endotracheal fire can begin as an explosion, causing extensive burns within moments. The operating table mattress and positioning devices made of foam and liquid gels also are potential sources of

fuel. In addition, as these items burn, they release toxic gases that can be fatal if inhaled.

WOVEN AND NONWOVEN MATERIAL

Surgical drapes are a common source of fuel in surgical fires. Both woven (fabric) and most nonwoven (disposable) drapes ignite and burn easily. Similar materials used in surgical gowns, caps, and shoe covers also are combustible. Surgical draping materials and surgical gowns are considered flame-resistant; however, in an OEA they may readily ignite.

PATIENT HAIR

Although hair is not an obvious source of fuel, it is readily combustible. Lanugo, which is the fine hair found on the face and other body surfaces, burns at the rate of 2 to 10 ft per second.

INTESTINAL GASES

The human intestine produces up to 200 ml per day of hydrogen and methane gas. Intestinal gas is composed of oxygen, nitrogen, carbon dioxide, hydrogen, and methane. Oxygen, nitrogen, and carbon dioxide are ingested (swallowed), and hydrogen and methane are produced by bacteria in the gastrointestinal tract acting on food residue. Forty percent of these gases are contained in the large bowel. Human flatus contains approximately 44% hydrogen and 30% methane.

In an environment of at least 5% oxygen, hydrogen is explosive at concentrations of 4% to 72%. Methane also is explosive at concentrations of 5% to 15%. In the event of bowel perforation during surgery, intraabdominal fire is a risk.

Ignition

To create fire, a source of heat is necessary to increase the oxidation rate of a fuel. Any heat-producing device has the potential to cause a fire. The more intense the heat, the more

Table 14-1 FUEL SOURCES AT THE OPERATIVE SITE	
Fuel Source	Fire Prevention
OEA—Oxygen-rich environment	Tent drapes away from patient's head during surgery.
Dry sponges and drapes	Place electrosurgical unit tip in holder.
	Use wet towels, wet sponges, or nonflammable drapes at operative site.
Endotracheal tube and other flammable anesthesia equipment	Use only laser-approved airways and endotracheal tubes.
	Use reflective shield between patient's head and surgical field.
Volatile prep solutions	Drape the patient only after all prepping solutions are dry.
	Tent drapes to allow escape of vapors when alcohol-based prep is used.
	Always check for solution pooling under the patient before draping.
Lanugo (fine patient body hair)	Use water-based gel on lanugo near laser or ESU sites.
Petroleum-based products	Do not use around laser or ESU sites.
Suction catheter and other PVC devices	Do not use around ESU or laser sites.
Smoke plume evacuator tip	Use noncombustible evacuator tip.
	Use moist sponges around lasing area.
Gastrointestinal gas	Use suction to remove gases at operative site.

rapidly oxidation and ignition are likely to occur. In addition to laser and electrosurgical energy, other sources of heat must be considered in fire prevention.

LASER ENERGY

Laser ignition is responsible for laser-associated surgical fires, especially those that arise in the trachea and associated structures. This is because laser surgery of the trachea and adjacent structures is performed in close proximity to a high concentration of oxygen and near combustible materials such as surgical drapes, preparation solutions, and a flammable endotracheal tube. Endotracheal fires are particularly dangerous because they occur in a confined area and can be explosive. Rubber, plastic, and Silastic endotracheal tubes are flammable. Endotracheal tubes made of nonreflective metal or other noncombustible material must be used during laser surgery.

ELECTROSURGICAL ENERGY

The electrosurgical unit, which is used to cauterize and cut tissue, creates enough heat to ignite surgical drapes, sponges, plastics, and most nonmetal materials in and around the surgical wound. The tip of the active electrode frequently becomes coated with eschar (oxidized tissue residue) and holds heat in much the same way as charcoal. Even when the unit is not in active mode, the tip can remain hot enough to cause ignition. Sparking, which occurs when the active electrode tip contacts a metal instrument, can ignite tissue, manufactured materials, or flammable vapor. Table 14-1 describes fuel sources and fire prevention in the use of electrosurgical units and lasers.

UNSHIELDED HIGH-INTENSITY LIGHT SOURCES

Light sources used in surgery are, by necessity, intense and bright. Although light sources developed more recently are cooler, the risk of ignition remains high for most high-intensity light sources. Fiberoptic light, used in endoscopic instruments to illuminate target tissue, is extremely intense. When it is directed onto drapes, cloth, or other materials, it can cause ignition, especially in an oxygen-rich atmosphere. To prevent ignition of fires by unshielded high-intensity light, follow these practices:

▶ Turn the light unit to standby when it is not in use.
▶ Turn the light off before disconnecting the unit.
▶ Never place the lighted end of a fiberoptic cable on drapes while the unit is turned on.
▶ Secure connections between the light source and fiberoptic cable before activating the unit.

ELECTRICAL MALFUNCTION

Electrical short or other malfunction can cause spark or arcing, which can ignite any combustible material on the surgical field. Never use any malfunctioning instrument. If the instrument begins to malfunction during surgery, it must be removed from the field immediately *and labeled* "Needs repair." Always label malfunctioning medical devices to prevent someone else from using them. They must be sent out for repair. If

an electrical device malfunctions during a surgical procedure, the device, along with attached handpieces, must be sent to biomedical engineering for evaluation. Never attempt to repair malfunctioning electrical equipment.

OTHER HEAT SOURCES

In addition to the more common sources of ignition discussed previously, other devices can ignite combustible materials. These include power instruments, burrs, drill bits, saws, and the harmonic scalpel, which uses high-frequency sound waves to cut and coagulate tissue. Although the environmental humidity in the operating room is high, it does not prevent electrical devices from sparking. When high-speed drills are in use, irrigate the tissue at the tip of the drill bit or saw slowly to prevent the buildup of heat created by friction between the metal tip and the bone. Never place hot drill bits, saw blades, or other metal tips in contact with drapes or other combustible materials.

Response to Fire in the Operating Room
PATIENT FIRE

Patient fires are extremely serious. The surgical technologist and all other operating room personnel must know how to react. The fire occurs either inside or on the surface of the patient. *Protection of the patient is the primary concern; self-protection is secondary.* It takes less than a minute for a flash fire to engulf the patient. To stop the progression of the fire, the *triangle of fire must be broken.* That is, one or more of the required components—fuel, oxygen, or ignition—must be removed. During a fire in progress, the ignition source is the fire itself. One can quickly extinguish a very small ignition site by patting the area or covering it with wet towels.

Excellent communication among surgical team members is essential during a patient fire because time is critical. Three steps are immediately taken to protect the patient and stop the fire:

1. *Shut off* the flow of all gases to the patient's airway.
2. *Remove* any burning objects from the surgical site.
3. *Assess* the patient for injury and respond appropriately.

STRUCTURAL FIRE

If the fire extends beyond the immediate patient area, the surgical team must activate the hospital fire plan. All accredited hospitals are required to have a written fire plan for each unit. This plan explains the exact duties of personnel and the actions to be taken to protect patients and staff. This plan is based on four immediate actions, called "RACE":

▶ Rescue patients in the immediate area of the fire.
▶ Alert other people to the fire so that they can assist in patient removal and response. Activate the fire alert system.
▶ Contain the fire. Shut all doors to slow the spread of smoke and flame. Always shut off the zone valves controlling in-line gases to the room.
▶ Evacuate personnel in the areas around the fire.

If the fire is limited to a very small area, such as a trash receptacle, appropriate extinguishing agents may be used to extinguish the fire. Never let a fire get between you and the exit.

FIRE DRILLS AND FIRE EXTINGUISHERS

Fire drills are held regularly in most hospitals. All hospital employees are expected to know where fire exits, fire extinguishers, and fire hoses are located. In addition, everyone should be able to activate the fire alert system. Fire extinguishers are classified for use according to the fuel of the fire:

▶ Class A (water): wood, paper, and cloth.
▶ Class B (carbon dioxide): flammable liquids
▶ Class C (bromochlorodifluoromethane): electrical and laser fires

To activate and use the fire extinguisher, pull the ring from the handle, aim the nozzle at the base of the fire, squeeze the handle, and sweep the fire with the tank contents. These steps can be remembered by the acronym, "PASS": Pull, aim, squeeze, and sweep.

COMPRESSED GAS CYLINDERS

Gases such as oxygen, nitrous oxide, argon, and nitrogen are compressed into metal cylinders for medical use. Compressed gas is under extremely high pressure and is released through the regulator that is attached to the cylinder.

Oxygen is delivered in portable tanks when in-line systems are not available or when a patient receiving oxygen is transferred into the operating room from another unit. Compressed nitrogen is used as a power source for instruments such as drills, saws, and other high-speed tools. Argon is used in laser surgery. Nitrous oxide is an anesthetic gas that may be delivered through tanks. Carbon dioxide is used for insufflation during laparoscopy or pelviscopy. Other departments use flammable compressed gases for tasks such as welding.

The tank itself is made of heavy steel to withstand the pressure of the gas and resist puncture or breaking. The *regulator* is fitted into the cylinder by a threaded connection. The regulator contains two gauges—one displays the flow of gas from the regulator to the equipment being used, and the other shows the amount of gas in the tank (measured in pounds per square inch or psi) (Figure 14-2). The regulator is activated by a valve handle. A valve stem or handwheel is fitted into the top of the tank. Gas flows through the regulator when the tank valve is opened.

Regulators are *gas specific* and are *not* interchangeable! Do not attempt to modify a regulator gauge to fit the gas that you are using.

Handling of Gas Cylinders

Any compressed gas cylinder has the capability of exploding or rupturing. If the gas is also flammable or supports combustion, such as oxygen and nitrous oxide, the risk increases significantly. Tanks must be handled with caution. A leak in a tank or separation of the valve from the tank can propel the tank with the force of a missile, sending it through walls with tragic consequences. Regulations for the handling of compressed gases are necessarily strict. *All* surgical personnel

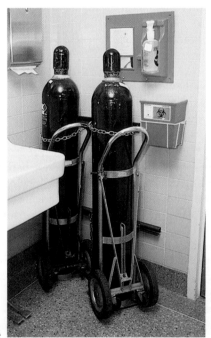
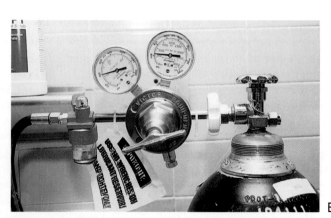

FIGURE 14-2
A, Regulators with stands. **B,** Gauges of the regulator. (From Ignatavicius DD and Workman L: *Medical-surgical nursing: critical thinking for collaborative care,* ed 4, Philadelphia, 2002, Saunders.)

using compressed gas cylinders must know how to handle them properly.

Storage and Transport

Use the following guidelines when storing and transporting gas cylinders:

▶ Label storage areas with the names of the gases being stored.
▶ Never use a gas cylinder that is not labeled properly.
▶ Keep all gas cylinders secured *at all times.*
▶ Store cylinders so that the valve is accessible at all times.
▶ Never store oxygen cylinders in the same area as flammable gases.
▶ Never use grease or oily materials on oxygen cylinders or store them near these cylinders.
▶ Always secure a gas cylinder before transporting it. Use a caged rack, chain, or other secure device designed to prevent the cylinder from falling or tipping over.
▶ Do not store cylinders of different gases together or allow one to strike another.
▶ Never store gas tanks near heat or where they might come in contact with sources of electricity.
▶ Never roll, drag, or slide a gas cylinder. Always use a handcart to transport a tank.
▶ Do not tamper with tank safety devices.
▶ *Always read the identification label of any gas cylinder. Do not rely on the color for identification.*
▶ Do not attempt to repair a cylinder or valve yourself. The tank must be returned to the bioengineering department or regulator supplier for repair.
▶ Never use pliers to open a cylinder valve. Cylinders are equipped with a wheel or stem valve to initiate the flow. Operation of stem valves requires a key, which must remain with the cylinder at all times.
▶ Make sure all compressed gas storage areas have adequate ventilation.

Use During Surgery

Many modern operating rooms have in-line gas outlets that dispense oxygen, nitrogen, and air. Gas cylinders, however, especially oxygen cylinders, are common in the hospital environment. Many hospitals use compressed gas cylinders to operate power equipment. The surgical technologist should be familiar with the following steps used to open, adjust, and connect the cylinder to a power hose.

Remember that there are two valves—one *opens the gas cylinder* and allows gas to flow to the regulator. This valve is located on *top* of the cylinder.

The second valve is located *on the regulator.* This valve controls the flow from the regulator to the power instrument. It must be adjusted according to the requirements of the instrument.

The right-hand gauge displays the pressure in the cylinder. The left-hand gauge displays the pressure in the power hose to the instrument.

The following describes the process for opening, adjusting, and regulating a valve, and attaching the power hose to a cylinder.

1. If the regulator is already attached to the cylinder, slowly *open* the tank valve to its full open position. With the valve in this position, the tank pressure will be displayed on the right-hand pressure gauge. Do not use the tank if the pressure is less than 500 psi. This means there is insufficient gas remaining in the tank. The pressure in the tank keeps particles (e.g., rust, dust) trapped at the bottom of the tank. If the pressure becomes too low, these particles may become caught up in the turbulence of the gas and be carried into the hose, where they can damage the equipment or cause injury to a patient.
2. Attach the power hose securely to the regulator outlet. Most connectors lock the hose in place when the hose is pushed and twisted into the regulator.
3. Turn the regulator wheel handle to set the pressure at the correct level. The required pressure level depends on the instrument manufacturer's specifications. For the pressure to be adjusted correctly, the sterile scrub may have to run the instrument as the circulator makes the pressure adjustments.
4. Make sure that the correct pressure is maintained throughout use.
5. After use, turn the tank pressure valve *off.* The scrub then should bleed the gas remaining in the air hose by activating the instrument.
6. Close the regulator valve by rotating the regulator dial. The pressure should now read zero.
7. Do not return a tank to storage if the pressure is below 500 psi.

ELECTRICITY

Risk

Electrical malfunctions are a *major leading cause* of hospital fires in the United States. The cause of electrical malfunction cited most often is *failure to comply with safety standards.* Accredited hospitals are required to install explosion-proof outlets and to comply with building and environmental codes designed to prevent electrical fire. However, electrical equipment also must be maintained. The probability of malfunction increases as devices become technologically more sophisticated and have greater requirements for repair and maintenance. Modern medical devices are complex. A high level of expertise is required to operate and maintain these devices properly to prevent malfunction and accidents.

Electrical malfunction can result in sparking or electrocution. Sparks can easily ignite flammable materials in an OEA. An electrical problem may be revealed yet the device may remain in use because it is in high demand or no one is available to repair the device quickly. Sometimes the problem may not be discovered until surgery is in progress. In either case, the risk remains the same. Continuing to use equipment known to be faulty is another example of an attempt to beat the odds of a serious incident, as discussed at the beginning of this chapter, and must be avoided.

Characteristics of Electrical Energy

The characteristics of electricity (the flow of electrons) are current, voltage, resistance, and grounding.

Current is the rate of flow. Direct current (DC) is low voltage and originates from a battery. Alternating current (AC) is transmitted by a 220-V or 110-V line such as that normally found in wall outlets. The available power is much higher with AC than with DC.

Voltage is the driving force behind the moving electrons.

Resistance describes the ability of a substance to stop the flow of electrons (electricity). Electricity follows a path of least resistance. Nonresistant materials include metal, water, and the human body. When electricity enters the body and is not directed back to the ground, severe burns and cardiac arrest can result. This is commonly referred to as electrocution.

Grounding is the discharge of electrical current from the source to ground, where it is dispersed and rendered harmless. As long as electrical current can travel unhindered through the body and is directed back to its source, electrocution will not occur. An improperly grounded electrical device can send electricity through the patient but does not control its dispersal to the ground (its source). Normal grounding is established by the use of a three-prong plug. Two of the prongs send the current through the device. The ground wire or third prong connects the device to the ground. If there is no ground wire, current can leak into other conductors and will follow a nonresistant path.

Prevention

Use the following guidelines to prevent electrical malfunctions:

▶ All hospital personnel must be trained in cardiopulmonary resuscitation and must know how to turn off the electrical supply in the event of life-threatening electrical shock.

▶ Equipment with frayed cords or devices with exposed wires must *never* be used.

▶ Cords must not be spliced or threaded through solid obstacles.

▶ All switches must be protected from moisture.

▶ Only devices that are intended for use around fluids should be employed.

▶ All equipment must be properly grounded.

▶ An electrical device always must be turned off before it is unplugged.

▶ Interference between electrosurgical and laser units should be avoided. The devices should be plugged into separate outlets and placed apart.

▶ All equipment used in the operating room must be inspected and must be UL approved. UL refers to Underwriters' Laboratories, which develops and maintains standards of safety for consumer electrical products. Electrical items that do not have a UL approval rating must not be used within the operating room.

The most common source of electrical injury to the surgical patient is the electrosurgical unit (ESU). To prevent electrical injury to the patient, a dispersive electrode is applied to trap electrical current and return it to the electrosurgical unit.

Electricity flows through a circuit. A circuit is essentially a circle that allows electricity to flow in a continuous loop. In the surgical patient, the greatest amount of electricity that enters the patient is from the ESU. In an isolated power system, the ESU becomes the "source" of electricity. Remember that electricity always wants to return to its source and will take the path of least resistance to return to the source. A patient circuit is created when there are an active electrode and a passive electrode touching the patient.

In the case of electrosurgery, the active electrode is the monopolar ESU (Bovie) hand piece. The passive electrode that completes the circuit is typically the dispersive electrode or grounding pad. The grounding pad serves to spread the flow of electricity over a relatively large area of the patient to prevent burns to the patient where the electricity leaves the body. In a situation in which the grounding pad is not connected properly, electricity may leave the patient at another area of the body. This results in alternate-site burns. Alternate-site burns will occur wherever electricity finds a path of least resistance back to its source (the ESU, ground).

In the case of bipolar cautery, electricity flows from the generator unit (ESU) through the cord and into the hand-piece, where it flows through one side of the hand-piece, into the tissue, and back into the other side of the hand-piece, from which it returns to its source (the ESU). Bipolar hand-pieces are shaped as grasping forceps, and as they pinch the tissue together, current flows between the two tips of the hand-piece. Bipolar cautery devices are foot-operated and deliver a lower current than monopolar devices. Because the current flows between the tips of the hand-piece, a grounding pad is not required for bipolar cautery. Certain monopolar devices have hand-pieces that grasp and pinch the tissue for greater control; however, these function when the tips (or other conductors) come into contact with each other.

The scrub and circulator must know whether a device is bipolar or monopolar. Monopolar devices require the use of dispersive electrodes (grounding pads), while bipolar devices do not. If you are not certain, a grounding pad should be applied to the patient.

DISEASE TRANSMISSION

Health-care workers are at high risk of exposure to diseases spread by airborne particles, aerosol droplets, blood, and other body fluids. To minimize the risk of disease to both workers and patients, OSHA and the CDC have developed a set of recommendations and precautions. These standards cover a wide variety of situations and are tailored to the type of disease and mode of transmission.

Standard Precautions

Standard Precautions (formerly known as universal precautions) are behaviors and methods of working in the health-care setting. When implemented properly, they significantly reduce the incidence of disease transmission. According to Standard Precautions, all patients are potential carriers of diseases. A patient's blood and other body fluids pose a risk of infection to health-care workers and others who come into contact with these substances.

The most serious risks from exposure to these potentially infectious fluids include hepatitis B, hepatitis C, and the human immunodeficiency virus (HIV). These substances also may contain other pathogenic organisms, including methicillin-resistant *Staphylococcus aureus* (MRSA) and vancomycin-resistant enterococci (VRE). Other patient tissues also may harbor infectious organisms that may cause a health-care worker, a patient's family member, or a health-care worker's family member(s) to become ill. Preventing exposure to potentially infectious material is as important as maintaining aseptic technique to prevent a patient from becoming exposed to pathogenic organisms. Therefore, Standard Precautions are used at all times and with all patients.

The following section describes standards formulated by the CDC and recommendations developed by the AORN.

HAND WASHING

▶ Wash hands after touching blood, body fluids, secretions, excretions, and contaminated items, regardless of whether gloves are worn. Wash hands immediately after gloves are removed, between patient contacts. One may need to wash hands between tasks and procedures on the same patient to prevent cross-contamination of different body sites.

▶ Use a plain (nonantimicrobial) soap for routine hand washing.

▶ Wear gloves (clean, nonsterile gloves are adequate) when touching blood, body fluids, secretions, excretions, and contaminated items. Put on clean gloves just before touching mucous membranes and nonintact skin. Change gloves between tasks and procedures on the same patient after contact with material that may contain a high concentration of microorganisms. Remove gloves immediately after use and before touching noncontaminated surfaces, and before going to another patient.

FACE, EYE, AND BODY PROTECTION

▶ Wear a mask and eye protection or a face shield to protect mucous membranes of the eyes, nose, and mouth during procedures and patient care activities that are likely to generate splashes or sprays of blood, body fluids, secretions, and excretions. Prescription eyeglasses are not considered adequate because they do not shield the sides of the eyes.

▶ Always wear gloves if there will be any direct contact with contaminated items.

▶ It is recommended, but not required, to wear a clean, nonsterile cover jacket to protect skin and prevent soiling of clothing during procedures and patient care activities that are likely to generate splashes or sprays of blood, body fluids, secretions, or excretions.

▶ Remove a soiled gown as promptly as possible and wash hands to avoid transfer of microorganisms to other patients or environments.

PATIENT CARE EQUIPMENT AND LINEN

▶ Handle used patient-care equipment soiled with blood, body fluids, secretions, and excretions in a manner that prevents skin and mucous membrane exposure, contamination of clothing, and transfer of microorganisms to other patients and environments. Single-use items should be discarded properly.

▶ Handle soiled linens with gloved hands only. Hold soiled linen away from your body and place in a biohazard laundry bag for disposal.

SHARPS

▶ Take care to prevent injuries when using needles, scalpels, and other sharp instruments or devices; when handling sharp instruments after procedures; when cleaning used instruments; and when disposing of used needles.

▶ Always keep **sharps** on a magnetic plate or in a container with a magnetic bottom. At the close of surgery, the holder should be closed and moved to the sharps container.

▶ Never recap used needles or otherwise manipulate them using both hands, or use any other technique that involves directing the point of a needle toward any part of the body; rather, use either a one-handed "scoop" technique or a mechanical device designed to hold the needle sheath.

▶ Do not remove used needles from disposable syringes by hand and do not bend, break, or otherwise manipulate used needles by hand.

▶ Place used disposable syringes and needles, scalpel blades, and other sharp items in appropriate puncture-resistant containers located as close as practical to the area in which the items were used.

Transmission-Based Precautions

Transmission-based precautions are implemented when a patient is known or suspected to have a highly infectious disease and standard precautions are insufficient to prevent transmission to others. Guidelines in this section are to be followed *in addition* to those that maintain aseptic technique and environmental safety.

AIRBORNE TRANSMISSION PRECAUTIONS

Airborne transmission precautions reduce the risk of transmission of airborne agents by droplet nuclei of 5 μm or less (discussed in Chapter 7). Because of their small size, such droplets remain suspended in air and disperse widely in the environment. Any patient with one of the diseases in the following list must wear a surgical mask during transport. Health-care personnel must wear respiratory protection when within 3 feet of such a patient. Masks must pass NIOSH-approved high-efficiency particulate air (HEPA) standards to be completely effective.

Airborne transmission precautions must be taken for the following diseases:

▶ Measles
▶ Varicella (including disseminated herpes zoster)
▶ Tuberculosis (More detailed information on tuberculosis can be obtained from the CDC publication *Guidelines for preventing the transmission of tuberculosis in health-care facilities;* see References at the end of this chapter.)

DROPLET PRECAUTIONS

Droplet precautions are implemented to reduce the risk of infectious disease transmission by large, moist, aerosol droplets. These are spread from the mouth, nose, oropharynx, and trachea to a susceptible host. The traveling distance of droplets is 3 feet or less, and they do not remain suspended in the air. Patients with one of the diseases in the following list must be separated from other patients by at least 3 feet. Workers must wear a mask when within 3 feet of the patient. The following is a partial list of the infections for which droplet precautions should be implemented:

▶ Invasive infection with *Haemophilus influenzae* type b
▶ Invasive infection with *Neisseria meningitidis*
▶ Streptococcal pharyngitis
▶ Influenza
▶ Rubella

CONTACT PRECAUTIONS

Contact precautions are used with patients known or suspected to harbor an infection transmitted by direct contact. In addition to standard precautions, the following steps also are required:

▶ Gloves must be worn, and hands must be washed before and after contact with the patient.
▶ Health-care personnel must wear protective gowns.
▶ All items that come in contact with the patient must be disinfected or sterilized.

The following are contagious conditions for which implementation of contact precautions is required:

▶ Infection with herpes simplex virus
▶ Impetigo
▶ Noncontained abscesses, cellulitis, or decubitus ulcers
▶ Disseminated herpes zoster
▶ Infection with *Clostridium difficile*
▶ Infection with any multidrug-resistant bacterium

Blood-Borne Disease Transmission

Transmission of **blood-borne pathogens** occurs when the blood or other body fluids of an infected person come into direct contact with another individual. In the operating room, frequent contact with blood and other body fluids before, during, or after surgery increases the risk of disease transmission.

Blood-borne pathogens (discussed in Chapter 7) include the following viruses that cause potentially fatal diseases:

▶ HIV
▶ Hepatitis B virus (HBV)
▶ Hepatitis C virus

SHARPS INJURY

The most common source of transmission of blood-borne pathogens to health-care workers is sharps injuries. To ensure a safe workplace, in 1999 OSHA issued its blood-borne pathogen rule affecting the handling of sharps in the workplace. The guidelines in the CDC's standard precautions are reflected in the recommendations and standards formulated by professional organizations.

Common sources of sharps injury in the operating room are:

▶ Hypodermic needles
▶ Suture needles
▶ Scalpel blades
▶ Needle-point electrosurgical tips
▶ Trocars, such as those used in performing endoscopic surgery or placing wound drains
▶ Sharp instruments such as skin hooks, rakes, and micro-point scissors
▶ Metal guide wires and stylets
▶ Orthopedic drill bits, screws, pins, wires, and cutting tips such as saw blades and burrs

Activities that result in sharps injury are:

▶ Preparing and passing sutures
▶ Passing and receiving a scalpel
▶ Colliding of two people's hands when they reach for the same sharp instrument
▶ Mounting or removing a scalpel blade from the handle
▶ Manually retracting tissue
▶ Suturing

The risk of sharps injury can be reduced when team members follow recommended guidelines and standards. This usually means changing the way a task is carried out. All health-care workers should understand that they are responsible not just for themselves but also for others on the team. Thus compliance with guidelines is an ethical as well as a safety issue.

The following practices are proven to reduce the risk of blood-borne disease transmission:

▶ Whenever possible, retractable or self-sheathing needles and scalpels should be used.

▶ If hollow-bore hypodermic needles are used, they must never be recapped by hand. One should replace the cap by grasping it with an instrument. Removable needles must be handled only with an instrument, never by hand. Self-sheathing needles have nonremovable parts.

▶ Scalpel blades must be mounted and removed with an instrument.

▶ One must dispose of all sharps in an approved puncture-proof container. The container must be removed and replaced at frequent intervals to avoid overflow—another common source of sharps injury.

▶ On the instrument table, sharps should be contained on a magnetic board or in a special holder.

▶ All health-care employees should receive immunization against HBV.

POSTEXPOSURE PROPHYLAXIS

Persons exposed to HBV should be tested for HBV surface antigen and an immunization series should be initiated. Health-care workers are at particular risk for exposure to blood-borne pathogens. All workers in the health-care setting should be vaccinated against hepatitis B. This is a series of three intramuscular injections administered in the upper arm. Health-care workers who are not previously vaccinated should be given hepatitis B immune globulin (HBIG) if they have suffered a mucous membrane exposure or penetrating exposure to a patient's blood or other body fluids.

HIV **postexposure prophylaxis** (PEP) consists of a regimen of antiviral drugs followed by regular testing. Postexposure prophylaxis must be initiated soon after exposure and has a limited effect, and additional health risks are associated with the medications used. Because PEP must be initiated within a brief period (less than 24 hours) after exposure, it is vital that health-care workers be evaluated rapidly and that the patient be screened for HIV before leaving the health-care setting. Because antibodies generally take 25 days to 3 months to appear on standard HIV tests, it is important for the physician to attempt to assess the patient's risks of exposure to HIV to help the health-care worker to make an informed decision about whether to initiate PEP. PEP includes the use of two to three antiretroviral agents to prevent the virus from attacking the immune system. These drugs are administered orally, and the regimen usually lasts for 1 month. These antiretroviral agents have a number of serious side effects that must be considered before PEP is initiated. The greatest risk of infection with HIV (in the health-care setting) appears to come from hollow-bore needles like those used to administer injections.

NEUTRAL ZONE (NO-HANDS) TECHNIQUE

The **neutral zone (no-hands) technique** is based on the fact that many sharps injuries occur when instruments are passed and received on the field. OSHA, the CDC, the AORN, and the Association of Surgical Technologists (AST) now strongly recommend that the neutral zone technique be adopted in surgical settings whenever possible. This technique is described in Chapter 15, Surgical Technique.

SPLASH CONTAMINATION

Blood-borne pathogens may gain entry into the body through the eyes, mouth, or other mucous membranes of the face. Masks, splash shields, and goggles or other protective eyewear must be worn to protect oneself from this hazard. In special circumstances, hoods that cover the entire head are used. These provide simultaneous air cooling and complete head protection, and are used during surgery on high-risk patients.

SKIN CONTACT

Contact with body fluids through cracks, sores, or other skin lesions can allow the transmission of blood-borne pathogens in the health-care setting. Gloves must be worn *whenever there is a possibility of contact with body fluids or tissue, including tissue specimens.* Many different types of gloves and glove liners are available. Double gloving is a common practice, although this may not prevent injury from sharps.

HUMAN FACTOR

Although the nature of blood-borne disease, its transmission, and prevention methods are known, the human factor must be included in the planning and implementation of any risk-reduction program. Some of the reasons why people have difficulty in risk reduction are the following:

▶ Too fast a work rate and rushing to accommodate a schedule

▶ Distraction from the task at hand

▶ Purposeful or inadvertent failure to comply with precautions and standards ("It can't happen to me")

▶ Extreme fatigue

▶ Lack of support in designing and maintaining a prevention program

▶ Difficulty in abandoning old and valued methods of working

▶ Difficulty in adapting to newer, safer medical devices

HAZARDOUS WASTE

Definition of Medical Waste

The EPA defines medical waste as "any solid waste that is generated in the diagnosis, treatment, or immunization of human beings or animals, in research pertaining thereto, or in the production or testing of biologicals, including *but not limited to:*

▶ Soiled or blood-soaked bandages

▶ Culture dishes and other glassware

▶ Discarded surgical gloves after surgery

▶ Discarded surgical instruments, scalpels

▶ Needles used to give shots or draw blood

▶ Cultures, stocks, swabs used to inoculate cultures

▶ Removed body organs—tonsils, appendices, limbs, etc."

The federal agencies associated with the regulation of various aspects of medical waste are:

▶ Environmental Protection Agency (EPA)
▶ Department of Transportation HAZMAT (DOTRSPA)
▶ Food and Drug Administration (FDA)
▶ Nuclear Regulatory Commission (NRC)
▶ Occupational Safety & Health Administration (OSHA)
▶ United States Postal Service (USPS)

In addition to the federal regulatory agencies, medical waste disposal also is regulated at the state level, and each individual state has laws specific to medical waste.

Waste Handling

Infectious waste is separated from all other waste and placed in red biohazard disposal bags. (The common term for medical waste is "red bag" waste.) The biohazard symbol (Figure 14-3) may or may not appear on the bag. The bag color and biohazard symbol are a form of hazard communication to anyone who later handles the waste material. Any person handling infectious waste, from the point of generation until its destruction, must wear **personal protective equipment.** Gloves must be worn at all times. Face shields and protective gowns guard the handler from splash hazards.

The following guidelines apply to handling and disposal of waste in the operating room environment:

▶ Always wear gloves when handling any object contaminated with blood or body fluids.
▶ Red waste bags for infectious material must be available during case cleanup.
▶ Do not place noninfectious waste in red bags. The cost of processing is 10 times higher for infectious waste than for noninfectious waste.
▶ Place all sharps in an impenetrable sharps container.
▶ Do not overload sharps containers. Container overflow is one of the major causes of blood-borne disease transmission among health workers!
▶ Handle suction canisters and other blood containers with extreme caution. The practice of opening suction canisters used during surgery and pouring the contents into an open hopper puts workers at extremely high risk for disease transmission. Blood and fluid solidifiers are available. After fluids are solidified, they can be placed in plastic bags provided the bags are tear resistant and do not also contain any item that can puncture the bag. Bags

must not be loaded beyond their tensile strength. Double bagging may be necessary.
▶ Separate soiled reusable linen from disposable paper products and nonsoiled items at the point of use.
▶ Keep all contaminated (soiled) or potentially contaminated waste separate from noncontaminated goods.
▶ Always place small disposable sharps on a magnetic pad or in a closeable container during surgery. Dispose of the container immediately after the procedure after counts have been completed. Sharps must go directly from the field to the container during surgery.
▶ Always wear gloves when receiving specimens from the surgical field. The scrub must pass specimens off in a manner that prevents splash, direct contact, and spray from the specimen. Operating room policy should require specimens to be double bagged in a container within a container.
▶ Do not compact waste contained in plastic bags. Pack loosely and secure the open end.
▶ When transporting medical waste, do not use trash chutes or dumbwaiters. Use a transport cart.

A designated area of the operating room is reserved for the disposal of infectious waste. This must be completely separated from restricted and semirestricted areas of the department. Biohazard signs should be posted in areas of waste disposal.

SMOKE PLUME

Risk

During the use of laser surgery or electrosurgery, tissue is destroyed or incised, and this process creates toxic smoke called **smoke plume.** Smoke plume contains about 95% water and 5% other products. The 5% other products include chemicals, blood cells, intact or fragmented bacteria, and viruses. The potential hazards of these substances are infectious disease transmission, toxicity from chemicals, and allergy. The size of aerosol particles ranges from 0.10 to 0.80 μm. These droplets are capable of harboring viral and bacterial particles whose sizes are much smaller.

Chemical Content

Smoke plume contains a number of toxic chemicals in concentrations that can potentially exceed those recommended by OSHA. Among the chemicals found in plume are the following:

▶ Toluene—Causes liver and kidney damage, anemia, and irritation to the respiratory tract, nose, and eyes.
▶ Acrolein—Causes irritation to the eyes, nose, throat, and respiratory system.
▶ Formaldehyde—Used to preserve tissue specimens; causes irritation to mucous membranes. Repeated exposure causes kidney damage.
▶ Hydrogen cyanide—Used commercially for pest control; causes nausea, dizziness, and headache. At high levels it leads to paralysis, seizures, and respiratory arrest.

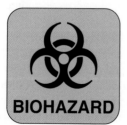

FIGURE 14-3
Biohazard symbol.

Plume collected from laser sites contains these harmful chemicals in concentrations of about 10 times the recommended exposure limit.

Viral and Bacterial Content

Both laser and electrosurgical plume contains living and dead cells, including blood cells, viruses, and bacteria. These particles are smaller than the aerosol droplets of plume. Examples are:

HBV	0.042 μm
HIV	0.180 μm
Human papilloma virus	0.045 μm
Mycobacterium tuberculosis	0.500 μm

Disease transmission through smoke plume is a known risk to surgical personnel. Other transmissible biological particles, such as cancer cells at laser and electrosurgical sites, are an additional concern.

Risk Reduction

All regulating and professional organizations now recognize the need for smoke removal during the use of lasers and electrosurgical equipment. Normal room ventilation is not sufficient to capture chemical and biological particles from smoke plume. Three methods currently are used to prevent workers from inhaling smoke plume. These are high-filtration surgical masks, in-line room suction systems, and commercial smoke-evacuation devices. Room suction is designed to carry liquids, not smoke. These devices pull at a much lower rate than commercial smoke-evacuation systems and must have in-line filters attached to be safe. The use of high-filtration surgical masks should be considered during laser or electrosurgical procedures. Only smoke-evacuation systems, however, are specifically designed to extract most smoke plume from the surgical wound.

Smoke-Evacuation System

A smoke-evacuation system contains a nozzle tip, suction hose inlet, tubing, filters, absorbers, and vacuum pump. Smoke plume is evacuated at a rate of about 100 to 150 ft per minute at the site of generation. It is then carried through high-efficiency particulate air (HEPA) filters and is trapped in absorbers. The filters are considered biohazard waste, and one should dispose of them according to hospital and government regulations. When a smoke evacuator is used, the nozzle tip must be within 2 inches of the surgical site to be effective. Fresh filters and tubing must be used for each patient. Manufacturers' recommendations for operation and maintenance must be followed to ensure safety and efficiency.

Safety considerations during the use of a smoke-evacuation system include the following:

▸ The evacuation nozzle must be fire resistant. Because the nozzle is close to the laser or electrosurgical tip, a non–fire resistant tip could possibly catch fire, causing injury to the patient and surgical personnel.

▸ The evacuation system must carry an Underwriters' Laboratories (UL) rating for electrical safety. The system must be properly grounded and unaffected by electromagnetic interference. Current leakage must be below 100 μA.

▸ The evacuation system must be designed to prevent tissue trapping or damage. When the nozzle comes into direct contact with tissue, it must be manually retracted, and this can cause severe damage. The evacuator must be turned off before one removes tissue trapped over the opening.

▸ Care must be taken when changing contaminated filters. Some filters are self-contained and prevent workers from coming in direct contact with the hazardous material.

LATEX

Sensitivity and true allergy to **latex** rubber are risks to both patients and workers in health care. True allergy is differentiated from other types of sensitivity by the immune response. Study of the immune system is beyond the scope of this text. Table 14-2 lists three types of skin reactions. Note that true allergy is only one type.

Allergy and Sensitivity

Latex is a naturally occurring sap obtained from rubber trees. It is used commercially in the manufacture of many products, including medical devices.

True allergy is an abnormal immune response to a substance. Previous exposure and sensitization are needed for the body to initiate formation of antibodies against the allergen.

Latex allergy is a very rapid local or systemic reaction mediated by the body's immune system. The reaction causes the release of histamines, which occur normally in the body. This causes edema (swelling) and redness. When histamines are released in massive amounts, the reaction can be life-threatening. The extent of the reaction depends on the exact location and nature of the contact. Allergies are a response to proteins within a substance.

Hypersensitivity is a type of delayed reaction that causes dermatitis on contact with the object. In the case of latex gloves and medical devices, this reaction generally is related to chemicals that are in the latex product rather than the latex itself. Hypersensitivity is a cell-mediated response.

Nonallergic dermatitis (skin inflammation) is caused by many irritants found in the operating room environment. Chemicals, antiseptic residue from surgical scrub or hand washing, and glove powder are known to cause irritation in some sensitive individuals.

Exposure and Symptoms

One can be exposed to latex through the skin, circulatory system, respiratory system, and mucous membranes. Gloves and glove powder containing latex molecules are a major concern. Other latex medical devices also can cause skin reactions, including sores, skin cracks, lumps, and itching.

Table 14-2 SKIN REACTIONS

Type Reaction	Symptoms/Signs	Cause	Prevention/Management
Contact dermatitis (Nonallergic)	Scaling, drying, cracks in skin. Bumps and sores, especially on the dorsal side of the hand, caused by gloves.	Skin irritation caused by gloves, powder, soaps, and detergents. Incomplete rinsing after hand washing and surgical scrub. Incomplete hand drying.	Use alternative products. Rinse hands thoroughly after exposure to detergents and antiseptics. Dry hands completely before donning gloves.
Allergic contact dermatitis (Delayed hypersensitivity or allergic contact sensitivity)	Blistering, itching, crusts, similar to a poison ivy reaction. Cracks that occur on hands or arms after skin exposure caused by gloves.	Chemicals used in latex processing. These include accelerators (thiurams, carbamates, and benzothiazoles).	Correctly identify cause. Use gloves that do not contain these chemicals.
Natural rubber latex (NRL) allergy (IgE/histamine mediated) (Type I immediate hypersensitivity)	Hives in the area of contact with NRL. Generalized redness (urticaria), nasal irritation (rhinitis), wheezing, swelling of the mouth, and shortness of breath. Can progress to anaphylactic shock.	Direct contact with or breathing of natural latex proteins, including those contained in glove powder or found in the environment.	Eliminate or drastically reduce exposure to NLR protein. Use nonlatex, powder-free gloves.

Circulatory system contact results from intravenous catheters, tubing, and other intravascular devices. If the latex reaches the bloodstream, large amounts of chemical mediators are released. These can cause severe bronchial obstruction, pulmonary edema, and death. Respiratory and anesthesia equipment causes inhalation exposure leading to bronchial spasm and laryngeal edema.

Individuals at Risk

Certain populations are at particular risk for latex allergy. These include anyone:

▶ Who has had repeated surgeries or frequent contact with medical devices, especially in early childhood. Remember that true allergy depends on previous contact.
▶ Known to have a positive reaction to a serum latex antibody test.
▶ Who has a history of an immunologically mediated allergy, such as an individual with asthma or allergies to particular foods such as bananas.
▶ Who has experienced undiagnosed allergic symptoms after contact with medical devices.

Sources of Latex in the Operating Room

There are many potential sources of latex in the operating room environment. The most common concern among surgical personnel is latex gloves. Because of the strength and resilience of latex, most surgical and examination gloves contain it. However, many nonlatex gloves are on the market. These should be made available to workers.

Latex is found in other sources in addition to gloves. Latex-free medical devices must be available to patients and healthcare workers. Common sources of latex are listed in Box 14-1.

Box 14-1 Common Sources of Latex

▶ Blood and tubing
▶ Blood pressure cuffs
▶ Blood pressure tubing
▶ Bulb syringe
▶ Catheters, internal and external
▶ Esmarch bandages (used with pneumatic tourniquet)
▶ Gloves, sterile and nonsterile
▶ Glove powder containing latex protein
▶ IV catheters
▶ Medical tape
▶ Needles
▶ Oxygen delivery systems
▶ Pneumatic tourniquet
▶ Rebreathing bag for anesthesia machine
▶ Respiratory tubing and all connectors
▶ Stethoscope
▶ Stopcocks
▶ Syringes
▶ Urinary drainage systems
▶ Wound drains

Prevention

Preventing latex reaction among patients and workers requires identification of those who are at risk and avoidance of latex contact. When a latex-sensitive patient is about to arrive in surgery, all equipment and devices containing latex must be replaced with nonlatex products. A supply area containing latex-free devices should be maintained. If the patient is known to be latex sensitive, a sticker or stamp stating this will appear on the patient's chart. The information also is included within the chart. Failure to check patient allergies before surgery can result in serious injury or death.

Workers who believe they are sensitive or allergic to latex should be tested. The use of low-allergen latex and powder-free gloves is recommended by NIOSH and other organizations concerned with the health risks of latex in the health-care setting.

IONIZING RADIATION

Risk

Ionizing radiation in quantities high enough to cause tissue damage emanates from x-ray machines, fluoroscopes, and unshielded radioactive implants. Exposure occurs when workers are not protected during procedures that use radiography or fluoroscopy. Hazard warnings should be posted whenever radiographic or fluoroscopic studies are in progress (Figure 14-4).

Tissue damage depends on the duration of exposure, the distance from the source of radiation, and the tissue exposed. Repeated exposures have cumulative effects. Among the risks of overexposure to radiation are **genetic mutation**, cancer, cataract, burns, and spontaneous abortion. Certain areas of the body are more vulnerable than others. These are the areas in which cell reproduction is the most rapid, including the ovaries, testes, lymphatic tissue, and bone marrow.

Prevention

Radiography and fluoroscopy are used in diagnostic areas and in the operating room, where surgical personnel assist in procedures. Lead shields are the most effective method of stopping radiation. These guidelines should be followed:

▶ Although lead aprons are uncomfortable and heavy, team members should wear them under their sterile gowns during any procedure that requires radiation. Many lead aprons shield only the front of the body, so workers should face the radiation source during exposure.
▶ Remember that a lead apron protects only the areas of the body that are covered by the apron. The eyes and hands are not protected.
▶ Lead glasses should be worn during exposure to a fluoroscope.
▶ Neck shields are available to protect the thyroid, which is sensitive to radiation, during fluoroscopy.
▶ Sterile team members should stand at least 6 feet from the source of the radiation. Lead screens are available in some hospitals.
▶ Nonsterile workers should step outside the range of exposure, either behind a lead screen or outside the room.
▶ In the radiology department, the walls are lined with lead to protect workers when diagnostic studies are performed. In this circumstance, one may be able to step behind the lead wall while the equipment is in operation.

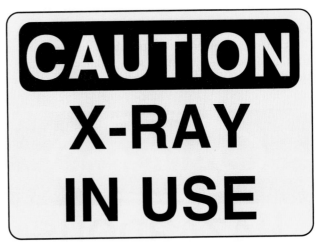

FIGURE 14-4
Radiation hazard warning sign.

▶ Whenever possible, a mechanical holding device should be used to support x-ray cassettes to avoid exposure to the hands.
▶ If a team member is required to hold a cassette during exposure, he or she should wear sterile leaded gloves.
▶ Dosimeters are available to measure cumulative radiation dose for those who are often exposed to radiation.

TOXIC CHEMICALS

Risk

Operating room workers are exposed to many different types of chemicals. Many of these are hazardous and can produce serious long-term effects, such as respiratory or skin problems, genetic changes, and fetal injury. One must remember that, although exposure to a particular chemical may be brief, constant exposure to chemicals in a variety of work situations has a cumulative effect. For example, it is conceivable that, in a given day, a surgical technologist or nurse might be exposed to glutaraldehyde disinfectant, vapor from methyl methacrylate cement, small amounts of unscavenged anesthetic gases, formaldehyde used as a specimen preserver, a phenolic agent using during environmental cleaning, and peracetic acid used as a sterilizing agent. Although the effects of any single exposure event may be limited, the cumulative and synergistic effects can be much greater.

Standards and guidelines for handling chemicals are designed to reduce the risk of **occupational exposure** and associated injuries. The use of Material Safety Data Sheets (MSDSs) can alert staff members to proper handling techniques for each chemical encountered in the health-care setting. Each department must have MSDSs for chemicals used within the department, and the emergency department (ED) must maintain a master copy of all MSDSs used within the health-care facility. The MSDS describes the chemical, precautions for handling the chemical, hazards associated with the chemical, and fire-fighting techniques and first-aid for exposure. The MSDS is prepared by the manufacturer of the chemical.

Exposure

Toxic chemicals can enter the body through the respiratory tract, by direct skin contact, by splash contact, or by ingestion. Personal protective equipment protects personnel against high concentrations of chemicals. However, such equipment works only when it is worn!

Exposure to an airborne chemical (vapor) is measured by concentration, in parts per million or milligrams of substance per cubic meter of air. Every chemical used in the health-care setting has a safe limit of exposure, which is determined by government agencies.

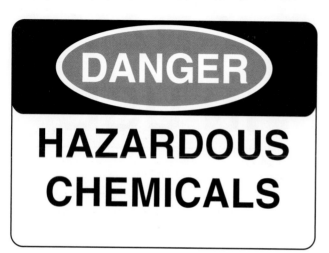

FIGURE 14-5
Chemical hazard warning sign.

Prevention

Chemicals used in the health-care setting must carry a label containing information about the chemical, including its intended safe use, toxicity, and postexposure precautions in the event of poisoning. All personnel must be familiar with chemical labels and know how to interpret them (Box 14-2). When working with any chemical, you must know and use the appropriate concentration and the proper procedure (e.g., glutaraldehyde must be used under a hood to prevent respiratory irritation). Hazard warning labels are posted on the container and in storage areas (Figure 14-5). Chemicals that are transferred from larger containers to smaller containers must be labeled with the exact information found on the original container.

Box 14-2   How to Read a Chemical Label

A chemical labeling system developed by the National Fire Protection Association (NFPA) gives important information about the safety of a chemical. All health-care workers should be familiar with this system. The label is divided in four colored sections. Each colored-coded section covers a type of hazard. A series of numbers is assigned to each color-coded section that corresponds with a specific risk.

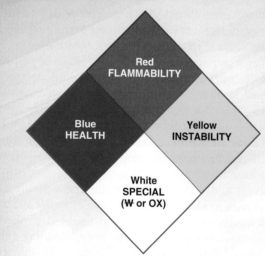

BLUE = HEALTH HAZARD

4 Danger	May cause death with short exposure. Special protective equipment necessary.
3 Warning	Corrosive or toxic; can cause serious temporary or permanent injury. Avoid skin contact or inhalation.
2 Caution	Can cause temporary incapacitation—may be harmful if inhaled or absorbed.
1	No health hazard.

RED = FLAMMABILITY

4 Danger	Flammable gas or extremely flammable liquid.
3 Warning	Flammable liquid flash point; readily ignites below 100° F.
2 Caution	Combustible liquid; flash point of 100° to 200° F.
1	Combustible if heated.
0	Not combustible.

YELLOW = INSTABILITY

4 Danger	Explosive at room temperature.
3 Danger	Can be explosive if heated, shocked, confined, or mixed with water.
2 Warning	Unstable or may react violently with water.
1 Caution	May react if heated or mixed with water.
0 Stable	Not reactive when mixed with water.

WHITE = SPECIAL HAZARD

Oxy = Oxidizing Agent
W = Water reactive
ACID = Acid
ALK = Alkali
COR = Corrosive

Toxic Substances Commonly Found in the Operating Room

Toxic substances have many different uses. Table 14-3 lists those commonly found in the operating room environment.

MUSCULOSKELETAL INJURY

Risk

Musculoskeletal injury is a risk to all personnel working in the operating room. The lumbosacral area, wrist, shoulder, and neck are particularly vulnerable. The causes of musculoskeletal injury are classified in different ways.

EXERTION

Exertion is the amount of physical effort needed to perform a task, such as moving an object. The amount of physical exertion required for a task can be modified by changing one's posture or grip, and varies with the duration and nature of the task.

AWKWARD POSTURE

Posture is a critical component of musculoskeletal stress. Twisting or turning the body disrupts normal balance. Other high-risk positions include bending, kneeling, reaching overhead, and holding a fixed position for a long time.

Retracting during surgery, although a somewhat passive activity, also can cause injury. This is because the person retracting often must twist his or her body to maintain a grip on the retractor handle. This puts the patient *and* the team member at risk, because the retractor may not be well controlled.

REPETITION

Repeating the same motions places stress on tendons and muscles. Factors that affect the risk are the speed of the movement, the required exertional force, and the number of muscles needed to complete the action.

CONTACT STRESS

Contact stress is excessive direct pressure against a sharp edge or hard surface. Increasing the pressure increases the risk of damage to nerves, tendons, and blood vessels.

In the operating room, musculoskeletal injuries occur most often during the following tasks:

- Lifting, positioning, transporting, and transferring the patient (discussed in Chapter 10)
- Retrieving and shelving heavy instrument trays overhead or near the floor
- Moving heavy equipment such as the operating table, operating microscope, or video tower
- Catching items that are falling
- Tripping over tubing or electrical cords
- Balancing a heavy instrument tray in the hand while distributing it onto the sterile field
- Attaching cords to wall sockets or overhead in-line connectors
- Climbing over operating room clutter or trying to retrieve a heavy item from a cluttered environment

Prevention

One can prevent musculoskeletal injury by creating a safe working environment and using good body mechanics. Several factors increase the risk of injury.

Table 14-3 HAZARDOUS CHEMICALS COMMON IN THE OPERATING ROOM ENVIRONMENT

Substance	Use	Precaution
Anesthetic gases	General anesthesia	Must be scavenged by anesthesia machine. Be wary of possible fetal injury.
Ethylene oxide	Sterilization	Objects must be aerated in chamber. Personnel should wear dosimeters to measure exposure. Do not handle objects until aeration is complete.
Peracetic acid	Sterilization	Use goggles, face shield, and gloves when operating sterilizer.
Glutaraldehyde	Disinfection	Use only under hood. Wear gloves, mask, and goggles.
Phenolic compounds	Decontamination (environmental)	Use proper dilution. Wear gloves and goggles.
Sodium hypochlorite (1 ppm)	Decontamination (environmental)	Use proper dilution. Wear gloves and goggles.
Formaldehyde	Tissue preservative	Wear masks, gloves, and goggles.
Methyl methacrylate	Bone cement	Do not wear soft contact lenses around this substance. Causes corneal burns and melts contact lenses. Wear mask, gloves, and goggles.
Fibrin glue	Tissue glue	Wear goggles, gloves, and mask.

CLUTTER

When the surgical suite is crowded with equipment, workers are inclined to shift their weight off balance to move around. In the presence of multiple tubing and electrical lines, extra attention is required just to cross the room. When an individual carries a heavy weight in a cluttered room, he or she faces an additional risk of falling. Clutter in hallways and equipment rooms usually leads to extra exertion and awkward positioning.

To ensure a safer work environment, alternate storage systems must be created. Clutter in the surgical suite results when large equipment is brought into a room that is too small to accommodate everything needed. Staff can reduce their own risk in such situations by being conscious of the risk and moving slowly and deliberately around equipment.

FATIGUE

Fatigue and stress result in a lack of accurate muscle control, which can lead to injury. Standing and walking for long periods of time stress muscles, tendons, and joints.

One can reduce muscle fatigue while standing by placing the feet a shoulder width apart. If a lift (raised platform) is used, it should be wide enough to accommodate a wide stance and should not require the scrub to step up and down while working between the instrument table (back table) and the patient. Shifting the weight back and forth on a level surface can reduce muscle strain. Standing on one foot for long periods, however, increases stress and puts the body off balance. Elevating the feet during breaks helps increase circulation to the legs.

Special support stockings and leggings *significantly* reduce muscle ache. These can be purchased in medical supply stores. Supportive shoes distribute pressure on the foot to avoid heel spurs and arch problems. The use of clogs or other backless shoes is discouraged because they make running difficult in an emergency.

POORLY DESIGNED STORAGE SYSTEMS

Heavy items such as large instrument trays must be stored at elbow height, never above the head or at floor level. If they must be stored at floor level, attention to good body mechanics in retrieving these items helps to prevent lower-back injury. The appropriate way to shelve equipment is to place the heaviest items even with the elbows and smaller items on shelves above and below this height.

INSUFFICIENT HELP

When workers attempt to move a patient with insufficient help, both the patient and the team members are at risk for injury. Help must be summoned before the patient is moved. Never begin a move or patient transfer if you cannot complete the action.

Body Mechanics

All workers should make a habit of using work methods that conform to good body mechanics. Students and new employees should learn these methods before entering the clinical area for work. If you are injured on the job, obtain medical care as soon as possible.

LIFTING

▶ When lifting an object, keep it as close to your body as possible. This reduces the force of exertion (Figure 14-6).
▶ Always bend at the knees when raising or lowering a heavy object. This takes pressure off the lower back and uses the body's heaviest muscles to do the work (Figure

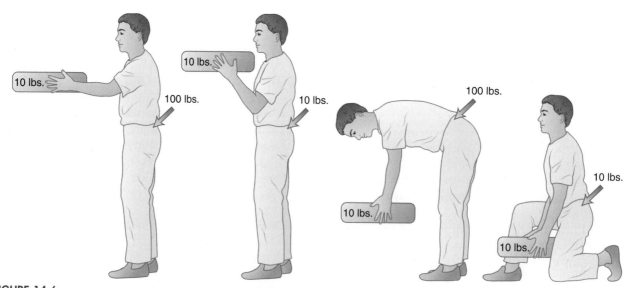

FIGURE 14-6
Lifting properly reduces the force of exertion. (Modified from Saunders DH and Saunders R: *Evaluation, treatment, and prevention of musculoskeletal disorders,* vol 1, ed 3, Chaska, Minn, 1995, Saunders Group.)

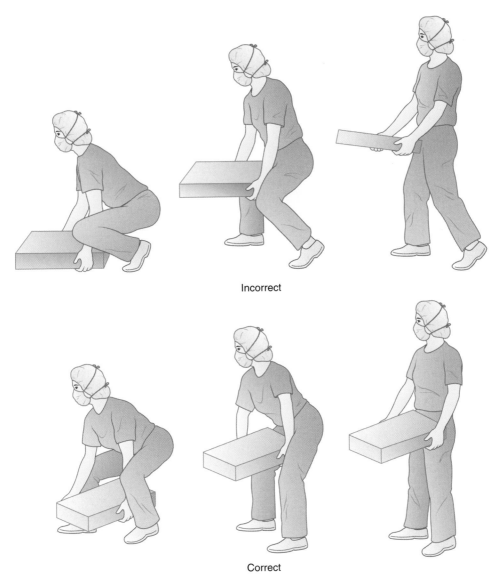

Incorrect

Correct

FIGURE 14-7
Always bend at the knees when lifting or lowering a heavy object. (Redrawn from Saunders DH and Saunders R: *Evaluation, treatment, and prevention of musculoskeletal disorders,* vol 1, ed 3, Chaska, Minn, 1995, Saunders Group.)

14-7). Remember to *keep your back straight* and legs wide apart with both feet flat on the floor for balance.

▶ Never lock the knees and bend over to pick up an object (Figure 14-8). This puts stress on the lower back and does not permit use of the thigh muscles to help lift the body.

PUSHING AND PULLING

▶ When pushing a cart ahead of you from a standstill, place one foot behind the other. The back foot should be braced comfortably as shown in Figure 14-9. Use the back foot to push off while transferring your weight to the front foot. Pushing is the preferred method of transporting objects rather than pulling. Make certain you can adequately see any obstacles in your path.

▶ When pulling a cart toward you, use the same stance as in pushing. Use your front leg to exert backward pull while the back foot maintains balance and support.

▶ When performing a horizontal transfer (straight across from one surface to another), use abdominal and arm muscles actively. Do not simply lean back and pull.

BENDING

▶ When you must bend or reach upward to connect an electrical outlet or in-line gas connection, *never* twist your body or balance on one foot (Figure 14-10). This combination not only places the body off balance, it also increases the risk of back injury because the standing leg is locked in position.

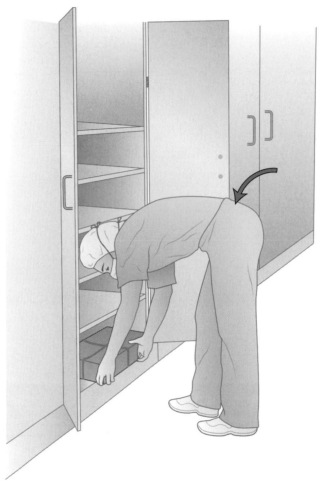

FIGURE 14-8
Locking your knees and bending straight over puts extra stress on the lower back.

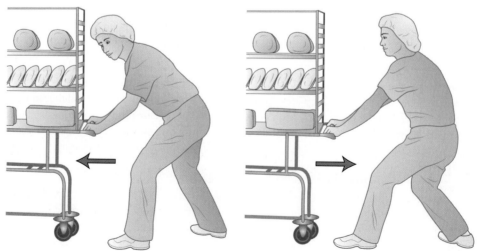

FIGURE 14-9
The proper stance for pulling or pushing a cart.

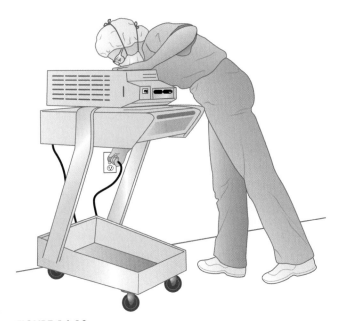

FIGURE 14-10
Twisting your body and balancing on one foot increases risk of injury when reaching.

▶ To lift or transfer a patient, use your abdominal muscles to hold the weight of your upper body. When the abdominal muscles are not engaged in exertion, the back muscles, especially those in the sacral and lumbar region, must support the entire trunk—a common cause of back injury. Tighten your abdominal muscles as you lift and notice that your back feels much more supported.

CASE STUDIES

Case 1
You are scrubbed on a radical mastectomy case. The electrosurgical unit has been in operation for nearly an hour, and the wound is filled with smoke. You mention to the surgeon that the team might remove smoke plume with the wall suction device. He tells you, "Don't worry about it. Everyone overrates the danger. It won't hurt you." What will you do, and how will you respond?

Case 2
You are cleaning up after a case and notice that someone has thrown a used razor into the linen hamper. Do you have a responsibility to report this? Will you do anything?

Case 3
You are asked to scrub on a thoracic case involving a patient known to be HIV positive. What precautions will you take?

Case 4
You have just handed the surgeon a suture. He suddenly sticks himself and throws the suture with the needle attached onto the Mayo stand. What will you do?

Case 5
You have been hired to work in a hospital that disposes of blood and body fluids in a large flushing hopper located in the workroom. To pour the blood into the tank, you must first remove the suction canister lid. There is considerable splash during the transfer. How will you protect yourself, considering that you must remove your gown, gloves, and mask before leaving the surgical suite? Is it your responsibility to request a safer system for disposal of blood and body fluids?

Case 6
You are scrubbed on a liver biopsy procedure involving a patient known to be carrying HBV. When the surgeon passes you the biopsy needle, you are accidentally punctured. How do you think you would react? What will you do? Is this a critical incident requiring a written report? How could this have been prevented?

Case 7
You would like your hospital to institute a no-hands passing technique. How will you gain the backing of others? What kinds of obstacles are you likely to encounter if your idea is approved? How will you research products that are needed?

REFERENCES

Centers for Disease Control/National Institute for Occupational Safety and Health: *Guidelines for protecting the safety and health of health care workers,* DHHS (NIOSH) publication no 88-119, Sept, 1988.

ECRI: Patient burn caused by excessive illumination during surgical microscopy, *Health Devices* 23:8-9, Aug-Sep, 1994.

ECRI: The patient is on fire! A surgical fires primer, *Health Devices* 21:1, Jan, 1992.

Goodner B: *The OSHA handbook: interpretive guidelines for the bloodborne pathogen standard,* El Paso, 1993, Skidmore-Roth Publishing.

Joyce FS and Rasmussen TN: Gas explosion during diathermy gastrotomy, *Gastroenterology,* Feb, 1996.

Kern B: Preventive instrument maintenance: a prudent investment with many dividends, *Infection Control Today,* Sept, 2000.

Moyer P: Operating room fires: how to prevent and minimize spread, *Today's Surgical Nurse,* Nov/Dec, 1998.

National Institute for Occupational Safety and Health (NIOSH): *NIOSH alert: preventing needlestick injuries in health care settings,* Nov, 1999, National Institute for Occupational Safety and Health, Cincinnati.

Occupational Safety and Health Administration: *OSHA regulations, occupational and safety health standards, bloodborne pathogens,* standard no 1910.1030.

Occupational Safety and Health Administration (OSHA): *Revision to OSHA's bloodborne pathogens standard technical background and summary,* April, 2001.

Podnos YD and Williams RA: Fires in the operating room, *Bulletin of the American College of Surgeons* 82:8, August, 1997.

Rockwell RJ: *The laser safety officer,* Rockwell Laser Industries website.

Sehulster L and Chinn RYW: Guidelines for preventing the transmission of tuberculosis in health-care facilities, *Morbidity and Mortality Weekly Report,* The Centers for Disease Control and Preventions, June 6, 2003.

Thompson JT et al: Fire in the operating room during tracheostomy, *Southern Medical Journal* 91:3, March, 1998.

University of California, San Diego Medical Center website: *Appendix E—other workplace ergonomics. Ergonomic healthcare guidelines.*

Chapter 15

Surgical Technique

Learning Objectives

After studying this chapter the reader will be able to:

- Identify the correct set-up of a surgical case
- Identify methods to open surgical supplies correctly
- Describe the process to perform sponge, needle, instrument, and sharp counts correctly
- Demonstrate neutral zone (no-hands) technique
- Demonstrate passing instruments so they are properly oriented for use
- Identify methods to care for specimens correctly
- Discuss methods of wound irrigation
- Identify methods to achieve hemostasis during surgery
- Discuss the selection and preparation of wound drains
- Demonstrate preparation of the surgical wound dressing
- Describe safe techniques for handling tissues

Terminology

Biopsy—Removal of a sample of tissue for pathological analysis.

Bleeder—A bleeding vessel.

Blunt dissection—The technique of separating tissue layers by teasing them apart with a rough sponge dissector.

Case planning—The process of organizing the tasks and equipment required for a surgical procedure. Case planning requires the ability to prioritize, organizational skills, and knowledge about the procedure.

Count—A systematic method of accounting for all sponges, needles, instruments, and other items that can be retained in the patient. Counts are performed on all cases in which there is a possibility of leaving an item in the surgical wound.

Culture—A process in which a sample of exudate, pus, or fluid is grown in culture media and analyzed for the presence of infectious microorganisms. When the microorganisms have colonized, they are examined for type and sensitivity to specific antibiotics. This procedure is called a C and S (culture and sensitivity).

Eschar—Tissue that is burned to the point of carbonization.

Frozen section—A microscopic slice of frozen anatomic tissue that is evaluated for the presence of abnormal cells. Frozen section analysis is performed during surgery to diagnose malignancy.

Implant—A synthetic or metal replacement for an anatomical structure such as a joint or cranial bone.

Sharp dissection—The technique of cutting tissue with sharp or electronic instruments such as a knife, scissors, or electrosurgical unit tip.

Sharps—Any objects that can penetrate the skin and have the potential for causing injury and infection, including but not limited to, needles, scalpels, broken glass, broken capillary tubes, and exposed ends of dental wires.

Stent dressing—A type of dressing in which a molded pressure dressing is sutured to the wound site.

CASE PLANNING (PREOPERATIVE PLANNING AND SETUP)

After receiving a case assignment, both the circulator and the scrub must plan for the case. **Case planning** is a process in which the scrub and circulator prioritize tasks, organize and gather materials, and carry out preparations in an orderly manner. Case planning requires knowledge about the procedure to be performed as well as efficient use of time, space, and efforts. Successful case planning is a learned skill. Attention to detail, neatness, and organizational skills improve case planning.

Types of Surgery

Surgical procedures can be classified into five categories. Knowledge of these categories can aid in case planning because different surgical procedures within a specific category require common skills and techniques.

▶ Diagnosis
▶ Reconstruction
▶ Repair
▶ Removal
▶ Replacement or implantation

DIAGNOSIS

The goal of a diagnostic procedure is to investigate the *cause* of the patient's signs and symptoms. The results of a diagnostic procedure produce information about the nature of a medical problem and the options available to correct it. Diagnostic procedures can be performed as a part of surgery to address the problem or as a separate procedure.

A case plan for diagnostic procedures must address the following issues:

▶ What is the target structure or tissue (e.g., biliary tree, esophagus)
▶ What technique will be used to perform the diagnosis (e.g., radiography, **biopsy,** dye study)?
▶ If a biopsy is to be performed, what instruments are required?
▶ What special equipment is needed for the planned technique (e.g., endoscope and accessories, dye catheters, syringes)?
▶ How will the information be documented (e.g., radiograph, pathologist's report, video record, fluoroscopic image)?
▶ Is the procedure scheduled to take place in a procedure room or in the operating room (OR)? Have radiologic staff been notified that they will be needed (if the procedure takes place in the OR)?
▶ Will the surgeon need other diagnostic films or reports during surgery, and are these available in the room?
▶ What kind of anesthesia will be required?

RECONSTRUCTION

Reconstruction is the change of an anatomical structure for functional or aesthetic reasons. A reconstructive procedure may be performed in a single stage or multiple stages. Re-

construction often requires specialty instruments. For example, a cranioplasty requires neurological and orthopedic instruments, **implants,** and possibly tissue cement. A procedure to reconstruct the nose requires plastic surgery and nasal instruments.

In reconstructive procedures, extensive radiographs, photographs, or computer images often are needed in the planning of the surgery. Extensive reconstruction might require intraoperative dye studies to determine the patency of a structure that will be remodeled.

A case plan for reconstructive procedures must address the following issues:

▶ What specialty instruments are needed for the surgery?
▶ What is the patient position to be used?
▶ Will grafts be taken, and if so, what tissue will be selected?
▶ Does the procedure require more than one operative site?
▶ What is the age of the patient? Congenital defects often are corrected during infancy or childhood. These procedures require pediatric-size instruments.
▶ Does the reconstruction require external support, such as special dressings, a rigid cast, or traction?
▶ If implants are to be used, are they available in different sizes and types?

REPAIR

Repair aims to produce *restoration of function* to a particular anatomical area. Repair implies that a part of the body has been injured, by either disease or trauma. The goals of surgical repair are to restore tissues to their original anatomical position (as much as possible) and secure the repair internally or externally.

Repair can involve any type of tissue. Most orthopedic procedures are performed for *repair.* Although there are a bewildering number of different orthopedic procedures, all are based on the same principle—to restore function and secure the repair until healing is complete. Another type of repair involves soft tissue, such as a hernia repair or repair of a liver laceration. These procedures require the materials for the actual repair and the special instruments needed to gain access to the target tissue.

A case plan for repair procedures must address the following issues:

▶ What is to be repaired?
▶ What special instruments are needed for the type of tissue being repaired?
▶ What materials will be used to make the repair (e.g., sutures, plates, synthetic mesh)?
▶ How will the repair be held in place (e.g., sutures, screws, fibrin glue)?
▶ Does the patient have recent injuries and movement limitations?
▶ Will radiographs be required? Many orthopedic cases require radiographic or fluoroscopic imaging.
▶ Is the repair area particularly vascular (will additional hemostasis be required)?

REMOVAL

Removal refers to removal of *tissue* or a *foreign body* such as a tumor, bullet, or debris (e.g., penetrating objects from a car accident). Consider the process involved in removal. First, the surgeon must gain access to the target tissue. This means dissection.

When tumor tissue is to be removed, a need for extra hemostasis can be anticipated. The reason is that tumors grow randomly (without an anatomically correct pattern) and usually have their own blood supply. This means unpredictable hemorrhage and perhaps undiagnosed involvement of tissues near the tumor. These *unknowns* are cues to ensure extra hemostatic control, excellent lighting, and meticulous dissection, that is, the use of sharp, well-functioning instruments, extra sponges, suction, and sutures.

Removal of a foreign body requires access (dissection). After removal, *repair* of the entry tissues is needed.

A case plan for removal procedures must address the following issues:

▶ What is being removed, and what tissue is involved?
▶ What is the surgical approach (e.g., abdominal, thoracic)? What retractors are needed for that approach?
▶ If a foreign body is being removed, is there an exit wound?
▶ If a portion of the intestine is to be removed, will an ostomy be constructed?
▶ How large is the tissue to be removed? Removal of more extensive tissue structures requires additional clamps and perhaps different kinds and lengths of dissecting instruments.
▶ Will a specimen be taken for **frozen section** analysis (immediate tissue analysis to determine malignancy)?
▶ Is heavy blood loss expected?
▶ Is the wound heavily contaminated? Many trauma cases require extraction of metal, glass, or wood. In these cases the wound is contaminated, and antibiotic irrigation solutions are used.

REPLACEMENT OR IMPLANTATION

Tissue replacement refers to replacement of an organ or other anatomical structure that has lost function. An implant is usually a metal or synthetic prosthesis. Replacement tissue is usually a skin graft or donated organ. In some procedures, diseased or damaged tissue is removed. During insertion of a pacemaker or intraaortic balloon pump, implantation of the medical device is the goal of the surgery and no tissue is removed.

A case plan for replacement or implantation procedures must address the following issues:

▶ What is being replaced or implanted (e.g., heart valve, joint, pacemaker)?
▶ What organ system or tissue is involved (e.g., bone, ligament, blood vessel, heart muscle)?
▶ How will the target tissue be accessed (through what type of incision)?

▶ What is the nature of the implant? Does it require sizing?
▶ If nonfunctioning tissue is to be removed, how will the removal be performed (e.g., dissection, bone cutting, laser)?
▶ How will the implant be held in place (e.g., sutures, orthopedic devices)?
▶ What is the procedure for maintaining the graft or tissue before placement? Tissue grafts require special handling.

General Case Planning

Although most of the needed instruments and supplies are listed in the surgeon's preference notes, the scrub and circulator need information that may not be documented. This information includes the following:

▶ Preoperative diagnosis
▶ Procedure planned
▶ Previous surgery in the same area (extensive dissection through old scar tissue may be required)
▶ Radiographs available or needed during the case
▶ Patient position to be used
▶ Draping required
▶ Age and general condition of the patient
▶ Size of the patient (a large table or additional help with transfer may be required)
▶ Level of consciousness and sensory alterations
▶ Incision to be used
▶ Special equipment required
▶ Particular drugs needed
▶ Wound classification
▶ Infection status of the patient (e.g., positive test for hepatitis B virus)
▶ Presence of drug or latex allergy

OPENING A CASE

Preparing Nonsterile Equipment

Nonsterile equipment is prepared by both the scrub (before performing the surgical hand and arm scrub) and the circulator.

1. Arrange room furniture so that the head of the OR table is in a proper position to accommodate the surgery (Figure 15-1). The head of the table is sometimes removed and the patient positioned with the feet at the head end. The table may require rotation to accommodate large equipment such as an x-ray machine or C-arm fluoroscope. Always make sure that the OR table is directly under the overhead surgical lights.
2. Place furniture so that draped tables are no closer than 18 inches from a nonsterile surface.
3. Place clean linen on the OR table and ensure that arm boards and other attachments are available *in the room*. Secure one end of the patient safety strap to the table.
4. Connect suction tubing to canisters, ensuring that the connections are tight. Pretest the suction lines for adequate pressure.

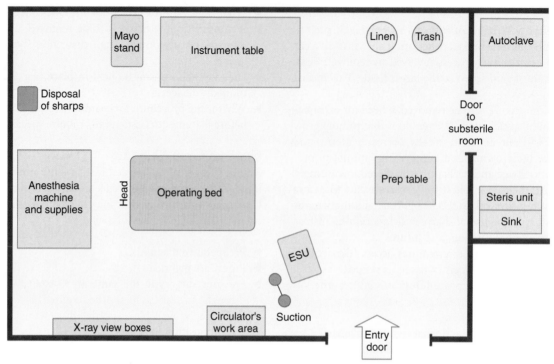

FIGURE 15-1
Proper setup of the OR. (Modified from Phillips N: *Berry & Kohn's operating room technique,* ed 10, St Louis, 2004, Mosby.)

5. Gather needed diagnostic studies, such as radiographs, magnetic resonance images, or other data the surgeon needs during the case.

6. If an anesthesia aide is unavailable, the circulator assists by assembling monitoring equipment and other accessories such as cardiac leads, airway equipment, compression devices, and warming or cooling blankets.

7. If power equipment is to be used during surgery, the in-line or tank gas sources must be tested and gauges set to the manufacturer's recommendations.

Opening Sterile Supplies

Sterile supplies are opened in a logical manner: Heavy items are opened first, and smaller items are placed over them. (Refer to Chapter 9 to review the aseptic technique for opening sterile items.) Many hospitals require that an exact sequence be followed for opening goods. The following sequence is often employed:

1. First open the case pack or large linen pack onto the back table. This establishes the sterile area. This area expands as the Mayo stand and tables are draped.

2. After the tables are draped, place goods solidly on the sterile surface. Try to avoid balancing items precariously.

3. Always open sterile packages in the same way. Lightweight items are gently projected onto the sterile table. Maintain a safe distance to avoid contaminating the table, but stand close enough to accurately project the item you are opening.

4. When opening packages, break the tape seal rather than tearing it. This prevents the outer wrap from ripping and possibly allowing contamination.

5. When opening double-wrapped packs, open the wrappers sequentially to expose the item.

6. Packages wrapped in sealed pouches usually contain an inner wrapper. Open only the pouch and distribute the item with its inner wrapper intact.

7. Never open a large instrument tray by unwrapping it while holding it in midair and then placing it on the sterile field. This puts excess strain on the median nerve, tendons, and wrist joints. Rather, place the instrument tray on a small table and open it in place. This exposes the inner sterile side of the wrapper and instruments.

8. When opening instruments in closed sterilization trays, break the seal and lift the top straight up and away from the tray. Remember that the edges of the tray are *not sterile.* Do not open any sterile goods into this tray.

9. While opening sterile goods, place clean wrappers in clean trash receptacles. Do not use kick buckets or biohazard bags for clean waste.

10. Open knife blades and other **sharps** onto a *conspicuous area* on the sterile field. Verbally warn the scrub if the sharps become inadvertently hidden by other items. Sterile blades can easily cut through the table cover as items are moved during setup.

11. Do not open any items that may not be needed. Extra sutures, special equipment, and implants should be held unopened until the surgeon asks for them. This prevents waste.

12. Open the scrub's gown and gloves onto a surface other than the back table. This avoids contamination of the back table with water drops.

SETUP OF STERILE WORK AREAS AND SUPPLIES

Organization of Equipment

After the scrub has been gowned and gloved, he or she must organize the sterile items on the back table and Mayo stand. This is called *setup* or *setting up a case.* Students and even experienced surgical technologists in a new service can be overwhelmed by the amount of equipment that must be organized and ready by the time the surgeons arrive to start a case. Using a methodical approach to all setups improves efficiency, but randomly performing tasks usually results in lost time and extra movement.

As you first approach the pile of sterile equipment, do not move anything until you have a plan. The following are *general guidelines* that are efficient and time saving.

▶ *Increase the size of the sterile working area.* Before organizing and preparing supplies, increase the size of the sterile area. Drape the Mayo stand and preparation stand first (Figure 15-2). If you need additional workspace, you may ask for additional small tables and drapes for power equipment or other specialty items, but all tables should be placed in one location—close to the back table.

▶ *Avoid shifting items around from one place to another.* Shifting items from one place to another increases the chance of contamination and is not productive. Rather than aimlessly sorting equipment, retrieve the items you need and place them in their proper location. When placing these items, do not move the other equipment unless necessary to make room. One of the most efficient ways to do this is to ask yourself, "If the case were an emergency, which items would need to be immediately available?" Prepare those items first. Place other items in their locations when the case is under way.

▶ *Try to avoid doing several things at once. Perform one task and then proceed to the next.* During setup, surgical technologists new to the profession often are distracted from the task at hand. A typical scenario is the following: You begin to prepare the suction tubing and realize you will need a clamp to secure it to the top drape. To retrieve the clamp, you have to make space for the other trays. You place the other instrument trays on the preparation table, from which they will have to be moved to set up the preparation supplies, and so on. Try to avoid this. Set your mind to one task in order of (time and use) priority, and complete that task. In the scenario just described, wait until you are ready to open the instrument tray before looking for the draping clamp. It is not a priority at that moment.

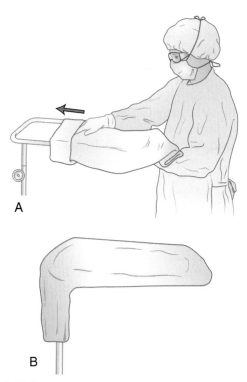

FIGURE 15-2
A and **B,** Draping the Mayo stand. (**A** redrawn from Phillips N: *Berry & Kohn's operating room technique,* ed 10, St Louis, 2004, Mosby.)

Priority Setup

Before you begin to set up any equipment, ask yourself, "What are the preliminary steps of the procedure?" For most procedures follow this sequence of events:

1. Towels are distributed to team members, and they are gowned and gloved.
2. The patient is prepared.
3. The patient is draped.
4. Suction tubing and the electrosurgical pencil are set up.
5. Sterile light handles are attached.
6. Two sponges are placed on the field.
7. The incision is made.

Knowing this sequence, retrieve and prepare the following items *in this order:*

1. *Distribute towels, gowns, gloves, drapes.* Arrange towels, gowns, and gloves in order of use. Pull the drapes out from the pile and stack them in order of use from the top down. If you plan to place the drapes, gowns, and gloves on the back table, you may have to shift things over to make room. If you do, just move them slightly, but do not start arranging other things.
2. *Prepare light handles, suction tubing, and electrosurgical pencil and holder.* You might place these in a dry instrument basin. These will be placed on the field as soon as the patient is draped. Do not place them on the Mayo

stand, or you will have to move them again when you set up the instruments.

3. *Prepare knife and basic instruments.* These consist of clamps, scissors, shallow retractors, and nonpenetrating towel clamp. Put the tray of general surgical instruments in place. Locate knife handles, dissecting scissors, forceps, and retractors. Mount and remove knife blades while using an instrument, never with the bare hand (Figure 15-3). Place these along with a few necessary instruments on the Mayo stand. Place all other sharps together on a magnetic board or in a sharps holder (Figure 15-4).

4. *Organize sponges, sutures, and small counted items.* Put all sponges in one location organized by type, so you are ready to count when the circulator is free to do so. Place suture packets and other small items together in one or more small basins.

5. *Stack remaining linen and drapes.* At this point you might need to make some space on the back table by stacking towels and extra drapes at the rear of the table.

You now have all the "priority" equipment you need to start a case. All other equipment can be set up as "secondary preparation." This concept is very important during an emergency, when there may not be time to organize any equipment. For example, if a trauma victim is brought into surgery, the most important priority may be to stop a major hemorrhage. You must be able to start the case with the minimum but correct equipment. The priority of the setup is to find exactly what is needed to locate the hemorrhage and stop the hemorrhage.

Secondary Preparation
SUTURE

The selection of suture material is almost always prescriptive, that is, written on the surgeon's case plan or information card ahead of time. Although there are many different types of suture materials and needles, actual preparation is not difficult. After working in a particular specialty, you will become familiar with the types of sutures used during those procedures. Few people memorize every single suture-needle combination.

Refer to Chapter 16 for a complete discussion of the preparation, physical characteristics, and absorption properties of chemical and natural fiber sutures.

Suture ties (strands) may be needed shortly after the surgery begins. Many scrubs place free ties on the Mayo stand between two towels, under the instruments. This system allows ready access to the ties but also requires instruments to be moved as new suture ties are added. When free ties are available in labyrinth packages or reels (see Chapter 16), the package can remain on the Mayo stand and individual ties removed as needed. An alternative method is to make a "suture book" with towels. Suture ties can be put between sections of a fan-folded towel and placed on the Mayo stand. Each fold can accommodate a different size or type of suture. Swaged sutures (suture material commercially attached to needle) can be placed in a small basin on the back table until needed.

INSTRUMENTS

You may have up to 10 trays on a complex case. This is why it is important to think about what you need, locate it among all the supplies, and then *put it in a specific place.*

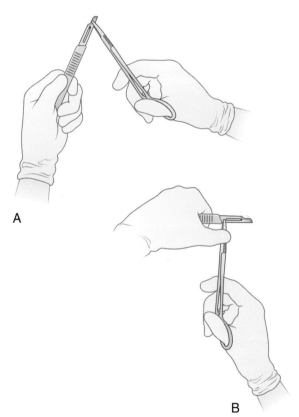

FIGURE 15-3
Mounting and removing knife blades.

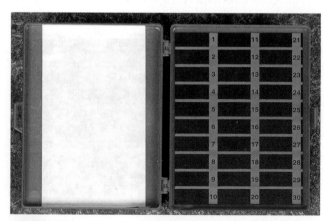

FIGURE 15-4
A sharps holder. (Courtesy of DeRoyal Industries, Powell, Tenn.)

Remember that space is valuable, so use it wisely. If you must stack instrument trays, place heavier ones on the bottom of the stack. Place the most important instrument tray (the one that has most of the instruments you will need) in a convenient place. Do not stack any other trays on top of this one. There are many ways to arrange instruments on the back table. Regardless of the method you use, make sure that you know each instrument's specific or general location.

Except on very simple cases, you will not have enough room to place every instrument out on the table. Most instruments remain in the trays. Place the most frequently used instruments in the most accessible areas of the instrument table. Place those that are used at the beginning and throughout the case on the Mayo stand. Arrange the others neatly in their trays or place them in a convenient location on the back table. Figure 15-5 illustrates a classic Mayo setup.

During the case you will transfer instruments from the Mayo stand to the back table. Every surgical specialty requires different instruments. Knowing which ones to have ready is a matter of experience *and* tips from helpful preceptors.

Many hospitals require a strict setup, so that when staff members relieve each other, the setup is familiar. Most people prefer to use their own individual setups. It is quite frustrating, however, to replace a scrub in the middle of a case and not know where items are located. Honor the hospital system if one is in place.

DELICATE INSTRUMENTS

Endoscopic, microsurgical, ear, and eye instruments are extremely delicate. These are retained in their racks. The rack can be placed on the Mayo stand or on a separate table.

SOLUTIONS AND DRUGS

Irrigation and soaking solutions usually are distributed after the case is underway or just before the case begins. These are distributed into basins in a ring stand, a solution warmer, or a slush basin (Figure 15-6). Medications are distributed into labeled containers on the back table. The procedure for receiving medications is detailed in Chapter 13.

MICROSCOPE DRAPING

When the operating microscope is to be used right away during a case, it is draped during the setup. If it will not be used for an hour or more after the case begins, it can be draped during the procedure.

The microscope drape is a single-use disposable plastic drape. As with all drapes, place your hands under the wide cuff, which is clearly marked on the drape itself. The drape resembles a Mayo stand cover in structure except that it has "pockets" that cover the protruding parts of the scope. The scrub starts the draping and, if the circulator is available, he or she assists by pulling the drape down by holding the bottom portion, which will be outside the sterile field after the drape is in place. The ocular portions and optics of the microscope are not covered. The drape is secured over the

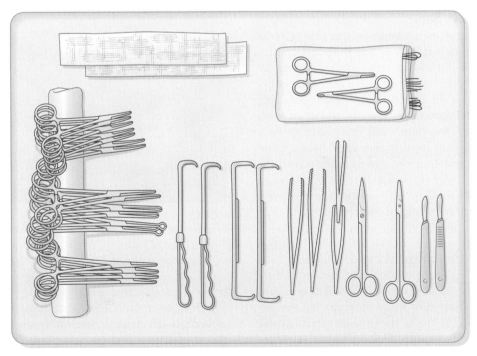

FIGURE 15-5
Traditional Mayo stand setup. (Redrawn from Phillips N: *Berry & Kohn's operating room technique,* ed 10, St Louis, 2004, Mosby.)

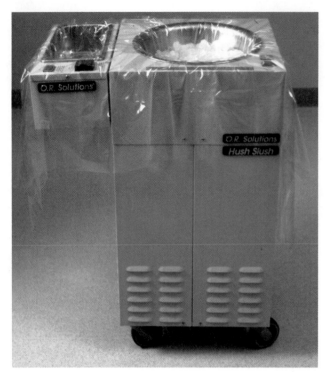

FIGURE 15-6
A slush basin. (Courtesy of DeRoyal Industries, Powell, Tenn.)

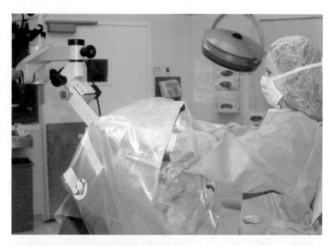

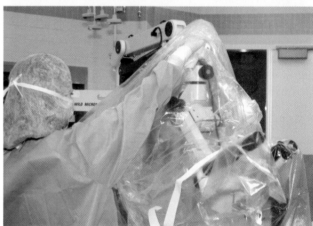

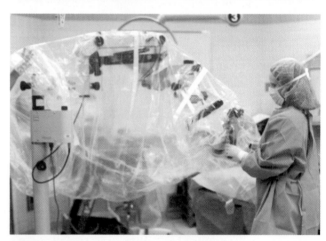

FIGURE 15-7
Proper procedure for draping a microscope.

lenses with sterile caps. After the drape is in place, it is loosely bound to the body of the microscope with adherent tapes that are an integral part of the drape itself. Figure 15-7 illustrates the procedure for draping the microscope.

Completion of the Setup

After you have set up all the equipment you need to start the case, you can begin to sort the remaining supplies and instruments. If you do not have enough time to complete the setup, at least you will be ready to begin the case. Arrange extra instrument trays in logical order. Small dissecting sponges, small vessel retractors, stopcocks, and other small items can be easily lost. Place small items together in a square basin, or contain them in individual basins. Extra towels, gloves, and drapes can be stacked at the rear of the back table. Try to arrange supplies so they are within reach. Key instruments that will be used as the case progresses should be laid out prominently on the table or within their trays.

Preparation of the Surgical Field

The patient is usually brought into the surgical suite during the latter part of the setup. The anesthesia care provider and circulator then focus on preparing the patient for anesthesia. The role of the circulator during these activities is detailed in Chapter 10 and Chapter 12. Anesthesia begins only after the surgeon has arrived and is ready to scrub.

The surgeon and assistant(s) perform their surgical hand scrub and enter the surgical suite to be gowned and gloved by the surgical technologist.

While the surgeon and assistants are being gowned and gloved, the circulator performs the surgical preparation. If the surgeon performs the skin preparation, he or she requires regloving. Draping follows immediately (detailed in Chapter 11).

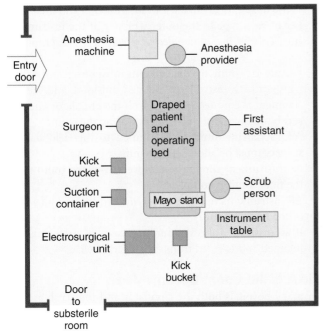

FIGURE 15-8
The surgical field. (Modified from Phillips N: *Berry & Kohn's operating room technique,* ed 10, St Louis, 2004, Mosby.)

As soon as the drapes are secured, the instrument tables are brought into position at the surgical field (Figure 15-8). The patient is now the *center* of the surgical field.

Sterile light handle covers are attached while the scrub secures suction and irrigation tubing, electrosurgical unit (ESU) tip, light cords, and hoses to the top (procedure) drape. When securing these instruments, make sure that there is enough slack between the instruments and the edge of the sterile field. After tubing and cords are in place, the ends cannot be brought back up to the field. The scrub passes the ends of the attachments to the circulator or drops them over the edge of the operating table on the *appropriate side,* where they will be connected.

The scrub places two sponges on the field and offers the surgeon the scalpel or marking pen as needed.

Incision

The first incision marks the surgical start time and is noted on the patient's operative record. Some surgeons use separate scalpels on the skin (skin knife) and in deep tissue (deep knives).

SURGICAL COUNT

Why Is the Count Performed?

Retained items in the surgical wound cause infection and tissue damage and can be lethal. Retained items are the major cause of lawsuits arising from surgery. To protect the patient from injury, all items that *could* be retained in the surgical wound are counted in a prescribed manner. Policies directing

sponge, sharps, and instrument counts (called simply a **count**) have been established by the Joint Commission for the Accreditation of Healthcare Organizations (JCAHO), the Association of periOperative Registered Nurses (AORN), and the Association of Surgical Technologists (AST). Hospitals create their own policies based on those of the accrediting and professional organizations. A retained item is grounds for a negligence charge against members of the surgical team.

Who Is Responsible for Tracking Items?

All team members are responsible for ensuring that no item is left in a patient. Performing counts is one method of reducing the risk of retained items. Other precautions require that the scrub know at all times how many sponges and other items are *inside* the patient. He or she must know at all times *where* all suture needles are. In addition, it is good practice to exchange new sponges or needles for used items. The surgeon and the scrub must track the number and type of instruments that are *inside the wound.*

When Is a Count Performed?

A count is performed at the following times:

▶ Before surgery begins to establish a baseline count
▶ Before the closure of a hollow organ
▶ Before closure of a cavity, such as the thoracic cavity or peritoneum
▶ Before skin closure
▶ Whenever there is suspicion of a retained item
▶ Whenever there is a permanent change in personnel, such as during a change of shift or when relief personnel come into a case

How Is a Count Performed?

The count is performed by *two people.* The *law* does not specify the qualifications of those who perform the count (licensed or unlicensed) or the manner in which it is performed. However, the professional standard for counts as published by AORN requires a licensed registered nurse and another health-care worker such as the surgical technologist to perform the count. One person must be in the scrub role. Most institutions honor this standard.

The count is performed in a systematic manner. Items should be counted according to their type. For example, count all laparotomy sponges, and then count all Raytec sponges; continue to count all other types of sponges on the field according to their classifications. Count suture needles, blades, and instruments (and their loose parts) as separate groups. Written hospital policy identifies the preferred method for counting. The initial count is similar among institutions and is typically performed before the patient is brought into the operating room suite. The items being counted should be grouped together and readily accessible for the initial count.

During the procedure, one must account for all of the items used in the procedure. The method for counting during the procedure also is determined by written hospital policy. Some institutions count items (by type or group) in the following order: items on the sterile field, items on the Mayo stand, items on the instrument table, and items that have been discarded from the field. Other institutions begin by first counting the items on the back table, and then items on the Mayo stand, items that have been discarded from the field, and items in the sterile field. The important point is to follow the same routine for each type of item counted.

What Is Counted?

Any item that can be retained within the surgical wound is included in a count. This includes all sponges, sharps, instruments, retraction devices (e.g., umbilical tapes, elastic vessel loops), instrument bolsters, suture reels, Bovie cleaners, and any other small items that are used on the sterile field. Hospital policy dictates exactly what items are included in the count. The accepted practice is to count any item that could be lost in the surgical wound.

SPONGES

▶ Each sponge is separated fully from the others in a stack or group.
▶ Sponges are counted *audibly* and viewed by *both* people performing the count.
▶ Sponges are commercially prepared. Never assume that the number of sponges *stated* on a commercial package matches the *actual* number of sponges in the package.
▶ If a package contains more or fewer than the number of sponges that are supposed to be in the pack, the package should be isolated and removed from the room.
▶ All sponges used in a surgical procedure must be radiopaque (radiographically detectable).
▶ Never cut a surgical sponge for any reason. Do not use surgical sponges as dressings.
▶ All counted sponges must remain in the room during the entire procedure. Do not remove any linen or waste from the room until after the last count of the procedure.

SHARPS

▶ All sharps should be mounted on an instrument or medical device, or contained on a magnetic board or other sharps holder. Sharps should never be loose on the field.
▶ Sharps counts are performed at the same time and in the same manner as sponge counts, audibly and visually.
▶ If a sharp breaks during surgery, all parts must be retained and isolated from the surgical field.
▶ A counted sharp must never be removed from the room until the after the final count.
▶ One must dispose of sharps in a designated sharps container at the close of surgery.

INSTRUMENTS

▶ Instruments are counted in a systematic manner. That is, always count instruments in the same order for each count and each case.

▶ Some hospitals attach a list of instruments and the number of each type to the outer wrapper of the instrument tray. This list is *not intended to replace a physical count in surgery.*
▶ During the count, the instruments must be *separated.* The name of each instrument is stated out loud, and the instrument is counted audibly. Both the circulator and the scrub must see each instrument during the count.
▶ Additional instruments distributed to the field during surgery must be added to the count.
▶ No instrument should be removed from the room until the final count is complete.
▶ All instruments must be *removed* from the room as part of the final cleanup.
▶ If an instrument breaks during a case, all parts must be retained and isolated from the surgical field.

How Is the Count Documented?

In many hospitals both the circulator and the scrub are required to sign the count on the patient's operative record. This is a legal document and attests to the outcome of the count. Anyone who performs a count, including relief personnel, must sign their count.

What Happens in an Emergency?

In an extreme emergency, performing a count before the start of surgery may not be possible. Subsequent counts must be performed. If a count is omitted or not performed according to hospital policy, this must be documented in writing. Generally, in an emergency the circulator will save the empty sponge containers, suture packets, and containers from other items opened so that they can be counted after the patient is stabilized. This is to assist in achieving a proper closing count.

LOST AND RETAINED ITEMS

Loss of sponges, needles, instruments, or other surgical equipment extends anesthesia time, increases risk to the patient, raises costs, and increases stress on the surgical team. The best way to deal with loss or retention of items is to prevent such incidents from occurring.

How Items Are Lost

Sponges often are retained when they are placed in the wound and not found. When small sponges are separated from the field, back table, or counting area, they can easily be lost. Because of their small size, they are often found in the folds of drapes, under basins, or among preparation sponges. Small needles are lost when they snag on drapes or other linen and spring off the field. Small items such as instrument parts can easily drop into the wound.

How to Search for a Lost Item

When an item is missing, a search is begun immediately. All trash and waste receptacles are emptied on an impervious drape, and each piece is searched. As each bag is searched, the contents are rebagged systematically. Equipment on the back table must be shifted to allow a search under instrument trays and basins. The floor around the operating table is thoroughly examined, and team members are asked to step away from the field. Sponges often are found between the team member and the table or patient. A rolling needle magnet is used to search all floor spaces. Team members must show the bottoms of their shoes for inspection, as this is another place where lost needles often are found. Very small needles are not visualized by x-ray or the naked eye, and often are never found.

If a sponge or needle is not found, an intraoperative radiograph is ordered. If the item is lost during closure, the procedure may be halted until the resulting radiograph is read. Not all retained items are easily seen on radiograph. When a lost item is neither found in the room nor revealed on radiograph, it may possibly be retained in the wound. In such an instance, all layers of the surgical wound may be reopened and searched. If the item is still not recovered, radiography may be repeated. If the item is not located, an incident report must be filed.

MAINTAINING THE SURGICAL FIELD

Keeping an Orderly Surgical Field

One of the responsibilities of the scrub is to maintain a clean and orderly instrument table and sterile field. Remove all cut suture ends and place them in a trash receptacle (a small sterile paper bag can be attached to the Mayo stand for suture wrappers and other small trash items). Small bits of tissue also should be removed from the drapes. If the drapes become soaked around the incision, a small impervious drape can be placed over the site.

Instruments should be kept off the patient when not in use. As instruments are passed back from the field, they should be wiped clean to prevent blood and body fluids from drying on the surface. One must periodically clear suction tips and tubing of blood clots and debris by running small amounts of water through them. An extra suction tip should be available for use while another is being cleared. A metal stylet is used to remove solidified clots that cannot be rinsed off with water.

A sterile basin of water is placed near the back table to soak soiled instruments during surgery. *Do not use this water for irrigation.* Only sterile normal saline should be used for wound irrigation.

Try not to overmanage the sterile field. Too much movement and rearranging of instruments can be a distraction to the surgeons. Do remove instruments that are not in use and replace sponges when they become soiled. However, use as little movement as possible. When replacing a sponge, pick up the soiled sponge and lay the clean one on the field at the same time. Try not to pull sponges out from under instruments or the surgeon's hand. This disrupts concentration and displaces instruments on the field. If instruments begin to pile up out of reach, wait for a pause in the surgery before asking the surgeon or assistant to return the instruments to you. Remove instruments that are not in use and always replace the ESU tip in its holder.

Surgery requires extreme concentration. If the surgeon asks for an instrument that is already on the field, *pick it up and pass it to him or her.* Do not simply state where it is (unless it is out of your reach).

Maintaining Adequate Light

Inadequate lighting increases the risk of mistakes on the field and creates frustration and stress. The surgical technologist must adjust lights as needed. Overhead lights produce a small, shadowless beam that spreads peripherally to focus on a large or small area as needed. If the surgeon is working high in the abdominal cavity or low in the pelvis, the light must be *lowered vertically* and *directed horizontally* to angle the beam correctly. It is the surgical technologist's responsibility to respond to lighting needs if instructed to do so by the surgeon. Some surgeons prefer to adjust their own lights and will not allow the lights to be adjusted by anyone but themselves.

HANDLING AND MAINTAINING SPONGES

Surgical sponges are available in a variety of sizes, shapes, and materials. Because of their compactibility and pliability when wet, sponges can become lodged in the surgical wound and become difficult to differentiate from tissue. Therefore every surgical sponge is sewn or impregnated with a radiopaque strip that helps identify its location in the wound in case it is retained or lost.

Sponges have a number of uses in surgery:

▶ Blotting and absorbing blood and fluids
▶ Protecting tissue such as bowel and mesentery before a retractor is placed in the wound
▶ Performing **blunt dissection**
▶ Serving as a filter between delicate tissue and the suction tip to prevent injury to the tissue

Standards for Handling Sponges

Follow these guidelines when handling sponges:

▶ Use standard precautions in handling sponges.
▶ Never handle soiled sponges with bare hands.
▶ Handle wet sponges gently to avoid splash. Even when dry, soiled sponges can be a source of pathogenic droplet nuclei.
▶ Never remove a surgical sponge from the surgical suite.

Types of Sponges
RAY-TEC

The RAY-TEC sponge is commonly referred to as a "4 × 4" sponge because of its size. It is a large square of loosely woven gauze, folded into a 4-inch-square pad with a radiopaque-detectable strip impregnated in the sponge. A sponge of this size is ideal for superficial surgery of the skin but too large for microsurgery. Its rough surface makes it an ideal instrument for blunt dissection (manual separation of tissue planes). In this dissection technique, the surgeon wraps the sponge around one finger and uses it to tease tissue layers apart, an alternative to cutting them. When used in a deep incision, the RAY-TEC is always mounted on a sponge forceps, commonly called a "sponge stick" or "sponge on a stick." To mount a RAY-TEC, fold it in equal thirds in one direction and in half in the other direction. The folded edge should face outward.

LAPAROTOMY SPONGES

Laparotomy sponges or "laps" (Figure 15-9, *A*) are used in major surgery, in procedures in which the abdominal or thoracic cavity is opened, during major orthopedic surgery, or in procedures in which large blood vessels are encountered or the surgical wound is large. They are used to blot and absorb blood and fluids. Laparotomy sponges also may serve as padding beneath the blades of large retractors. This helps to prevent injury resulting from direct contact of the retractor blade with the wound edges during extended periods of retraction. Moistened lap sponges prevent tissue from drying. Abdominal sponges may be moistened with normal saline or used dry depending on the surgeon's preference.

DISSECTORS

Dissectors (Figure 15-9, *B*) (commonly called "peanuts" and "pushers") are small, round or oval sponges that are overwrapped with gauze. These sponges vary in size from 0.5 to 1.5 inches. Dissectors *always* are mounted on clamps. The type of clamp varies with the depth of the incision and the size of the sponge. These sponges are used for blunt dissec-

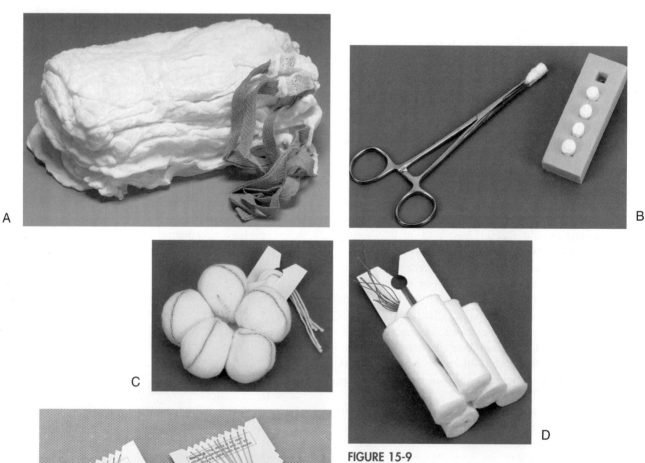

FIGURE 15-9
A, Laparotomy sponges. **B,** Dissectors. **C,** Round sponges. **D,** Surgical cotton balls. **E,** Flat sponges. (Courtesy of DeRoyal Industries, Powell, Tenn.)

tion (discussed earlier) and also for blotting blood or fluid in narrow, deep areas of the wound.

ROUND SPONGES

Round sponges (commonly called "tonsil sponges") are covered with gauze and attached to a retrieval string (Figure 15-9, *C*). This type of sponge is commonly employed in throat surgery and is often used to control bleeding in the tonsillar fossa after tonsillectomy. The string is draped outside the patient's mouth for easy sponge removal. The use of round sponges *without* strings is extremely dangerous in throat surgery. Such sponges can easily drop into the trachea and cause complete airway blockage. Asphyxia and death can occur very quickly, especially in the pediatric patient. When the round sponge is returned after use, always make sure the complete string and sponge are returned, because the surgeon occasionally may cut the string while working.

COTTON BALLS

The surgical cotton ball (Figure 15-9, *D*) is specially manufactured to resist shredding and is commonly used in neurosurgical procedures, especially around fragile brain and spinal cord tissue. Cotton balls may be dipped in normal saline before use to help achieve hemostasis. Cotton balls also may be dipped in topical thrombin to enhance coagulation.

FLAT NEUROSURGICAL SPONGES

The flat sponge, also called a "cottonoid" or "patty" (Figure 15-9, *E*) is a compressed square of synthetic or cotton material with a string attached at one end. Flat sponges are available in many different sizes for use during neurosurgical, ear, and vascular procedures. They may be dipped in normal saline to achieve hemostasis, and may be dipped in thrombin to achieve hemostasis when direct pressure or other techniques cannot be used. The flat sponge often is used as a filter during suctioning. The sponge is placed in the area to be suctioned, and the suction tip is applied to the sponge rather than held directly over the tissue. This technique protects the tissue from trauma but removes fluid from only a small area. As with the round sponge, when the flat sponge is returned after use, always be sure to account for the complete string and sponge, because occasionally the string may be cut during surgery.

Maintenance of Sponges

Used laparotomy and RAY-TEC sponges are dropped into a kick bucket. The circulator retrieves the sponges with *gloved hands* or an instrument and isolates them within a sponge holder or impervious container. Used dissection sponges are retained in their holders on the sterile field. Neurosurgical sponges are placed on a small container or towel on the back table, or on a separate prep table near the back table. Regardless of the type of sponge to be counted, the circulator places used sponges where the scrub can see them so that both can participate in the counts. As additional sponges are needed

during surgery, these are counted as soon as the scrub receives them. The circulator adds these to the count on the operative record. When blood loss must be estimated, the circulator may be required to weigh each sponge. The amount of irrigation fluid used is factored into this calculation.

Sponges are used to apply direct pressure and to pack the wound during surgery. Packing aids in clotting small bleeding vessels in the absence of external pressure. When assisting the surgeon with hemostasis, always *blot* bleeding tissue rather than wipe it. Wiping removes fibrin from the bleeding surface and increases rather than reduces bleeding. Blotting provides momentary pressure and better absorption of blood into the sponge.

Postsurgical packing is performed in body cavities such as the nose, vagina, or septic surgical wound. Packing material is available in the form of long, tapelike gauze strips or large absorbent gauze dressings.

PASSING AND HANDLING INSTRUMENTS

Handling and passing instruments are two of the primary tasks of the scrub. As with all manual skills, time is needed to develop speed and coordination in these tasks. Surgical instruments are finely balanced tools that are designed to be handled in a particular way. As you gain coordination, speed will *follow naturally*. Do not attempt to increase speed until coordination is secure. Rushing results in dropped instruments, mistakes on the field, and injury. Work at a pace that feels safe and comfortable.

All instruments are passed in their closed (locked) position unless the surgeon requests otherwise. Instruments must be oriented spatially so that the person using the instrument does not have to reposition it or look away from the operative site to receive it (Figure 15-10). General surgical and medium-weight to heavy instruments are passed firmly. When delicate instruments are passed, they are placed lightly in the surgeon's hand. When a specific instrument is

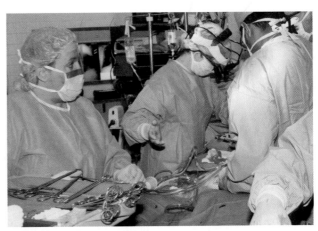

FIGURE 15-10
Passing instruments properly.

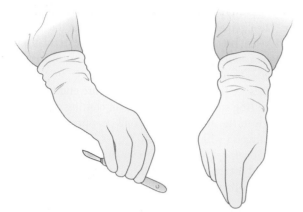

FIGURE 15-11
Hand signal for scalpel.

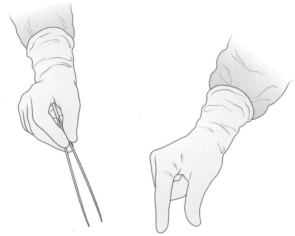

FIGURE 15-12
Hand signal for forceps.

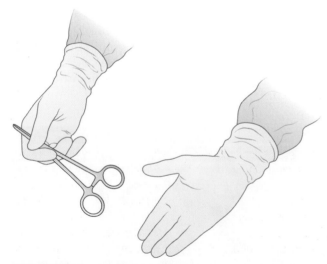

FIGURE 15-13
Hand signal for hemostat.

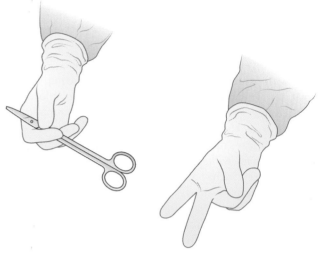

FIGURE 15-14
Hand signal for scissors.

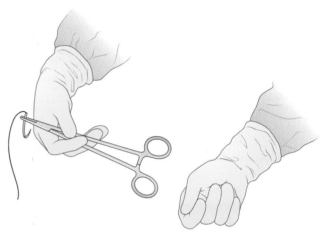

FIGURE 15-15
Hand signal for suture.

Long Instruments

When the surgical wound is deep, replace short instruments on the Mayo stand with longer clamps, dissecting scissors, forceps, needle holders, and sponge clamps. Some instruments are passed with tips facing downward. Examples are ligation clips and mounted sponge clamps. If you see the surgeon repositioning an instrument each time you pass it, adjust your passing technique to match.

Microsurgical Instruments

When receiving microsurgical instruments, the surgeon does not remove his or her eyes from the microscope. The scrub must place the instrument in the surgeon's hand in exactly the correct position without touching the microscope.

Do not jar the microscope or the surgeon's hand when passing microsurgical instruments—the patient may be severely injured by an instrument in the surgeon's opposite hand or by sudden movement of the microscope.

Because the instrument must be oriented according to its intended target, the surgeon rotates the receiving hand into

required, the surgeon positions his or her hand as if using the instrument. Some surgeons use specific hand motions to indicate whether forceps, scissors, suture, or knife is needed. These hand motions are illustrated in Figures 15-11 through 15-16.

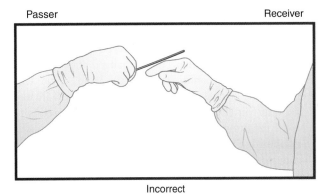

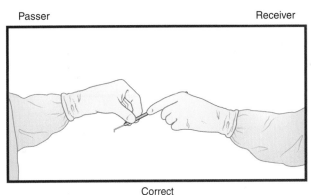

FIGURE 15-18
Incorrect and correct way to pass microinstruments.

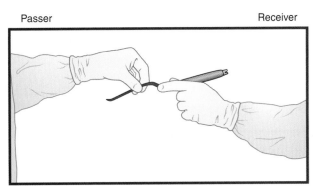

FIGURE 15-19
Passing bayonet forceps correctly.

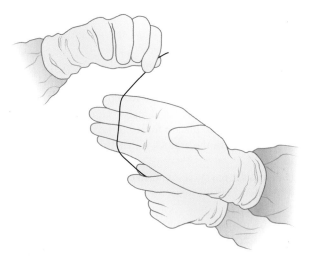

FIGURE 15-16
Hand signal for a free tie.

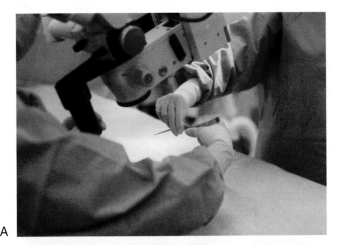

A

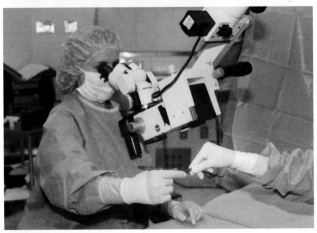

B

FIGURE 15-17
A and **B,** Passing instruments at the proper orientation.

various positions. This requires the scrub to adjust the instrument to complement the hand position. To determine the correct orientation, imagine yourself in the surgeon's place looking through the microscope. If the surgeon wants to use the instrument at the 12 o'clock position from the location in which he or she is working, he or she must reach *around the*

front of the microscope to receive it (Figure 15-17, *A*). Using the instrument at the 3 o'clock position requires that the instrument be pointed into the side of the microscope head (Figure 15-17, *B*). The surgeon indicates the correct position of the instrument by the position of his or her hand.

When passing microinstruments, do not handle the tips. Grasp the midportion of the instrument as shown in Figure 15-18. Bayonet forceps are oriented with the middle break of the instrument curved upward (Figure 15-19).

Sharps

All sharps should be passed with a neutral zone (no-hands) technique. If hospital policy or an individual surgeon has not implemented this technique, the scrub must pass sharps in the traditional manner.

In the neutral zone technique, a designated area is established on the surgical field near the surgical wound. The site must be easily accessible to both the scrub and the surgeon. Whenever sharp instruments are exchanged, they are placed in this zone rather than directly into the hands of the team members. The neutral zone can be a magnetic pad with a recessed reservoir (Figure 15-20) or a shallow basin used to receive the instruments. This eliminates hand-to-hand contact.

Establishing the practice of neutral zone instrument exchange requires collaborative teamwork. Good communication among team members is essential. For the technique to be effective, everyone must agree that it is worthwhile. This is because use of the technique requires changing time-honored practices. The procedure for establishing and using a neutral zone is described in Box 15-1.

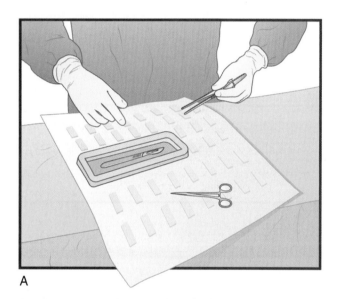

A

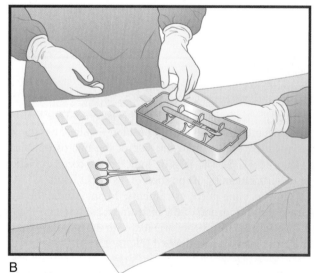

B

FIGURE 15-20
A and **B,** The neutral zone can be a magnetic pad with a recessed reservoir. (Courtesy of Tyco/Healthcare/Kendall-LTP Devon OR Products, Chicopee, Mass.)

SCALPELS

If operating room policy has *not* specified a neutral zone (no-hands) technique, the scrub passes the scalpel (commonly called *knife*) by grasping the handle in the middle with the cutting side of the blade down. The scalpel should not be released until the surgeon has complete control of the handle. To receive the returned scalpel from the surgeon, the safest technique is to place a folded towel or square basin on the field to receive the scalpel, rather than taking it back by hand.

If sharps are passed in the traditional manner without regard to a neutral zone, extreme caution should be exercised. The surgical scalpel blade is a precision instrument, designed to cut smoothly and easily through tissue. A truly sharp scalpel should glide through tissue with minimal pressure. The blade of the surgical scalpel loses its "buttery" feel after several passes through tissue, especially through skin and fibrous tissue such as cartilage and periosteum. Surgeons who favor the scalpel over other cutting instruments may need many fresh blades during surgery. The surgical technologist knows this in advance by working with a particular surgeon or by reading the surgeon's written preference sheets.

Whenever you pass a scalpel with a new blade to the surgeon, you must announce, "new blade." This alerts the surgeon to exactly how much pressure is required to make a cut. There is almost no circumstance in which a dull blade is advantageous. Anticipate when a blade is getting dull and replace it. If you see the surgeon "sawing" through tissue with a scalpel blade, it is probably dull (or will be after it is used in this manner).

Box 15-1　Procedure Using Neutral Zone Technique

▸ The location of the neutral zone is established by agreement between the surgeon and scrub.

▸ Do not use a kidney basin or other small receptacle as a neutral zone. A small space with steep sides increases the risk of injury because the hand must reach into the container for the instrument.

▸ Only sharps are to be placed in the neutral zone.

▸ The neutral zone should contain only one item at a time.

▸ Suture-needle combinations are exchanged one to one but never hand to hand. The prepared suture is placed in the neutral zone; the surgeon uses it and returns it to the zone.

▸ The scrub then replaces it with a fresh suture.

▸ Mounted suture needles and rakes should be turned downward but oriented correctly for use. The surgeon should not have to look away from the wound to pick up the instrument.

▸ When a sharp is placed in the zone, the person placing it calls it out, as in, "suture" or "scalpel up" (i.e., up on the sterile field). A means of communication must be established by team members so there is no confusion.

SHARP RETRACTORS

Skin hooks and rakes can easily puncture a glove or sleeve. When passing a sharp retractor, always keep the tips facing downward. Do not grasp the retractor near the sharp end. Remove the retractor from the field as soon as the surgeon extracts it from the wound.

SUTURE NEEDLES

Many needle-stick injuries occur during suturing. To prevent injury, pass the needle holder to the surgeon on an exchange basis. That is, when he or she returns the needle holder and needle, pass another. Do not use more than two needle sutures on the field at one time unless two surgeons are suturing. If double-armed sutures are used (sutures with a needle at each end), make sure the second needle does not snag on the surgeon's sleeve, drapes, or sponges. Refer to Chapter 16 for a complete discussion of sutures and needles.

HANDLING AND CARING FOR SPECIMENS

Responsibility for Specimens

During surgery tissue is often removed for pathological analysis. Critical medical decisions are based on specimen analysis. Every person who handles a specimen carries responsibility for its protection, preservation, and accurate identification. Damage to or loss of specimens can result in misdiagnosis, the need for additional surgery, and increased emotional stress among the patient and family. In addition to the medical accountability for specimens, there is legal responsibility. The serious consequences of loss of or damage to specimens can rapidly result in litigation. Safety control measures are necessary to reduce the potential for errors involving specimens.

Care of Specimens

All specimens are handled with standard precautions. In addition, special procedures are necessary to protect and preserve specimens.

Use the following precautions and guidelines in handling specimens:

▶ Never allow a specimen to dry out.
▶ Do not wrap specimens in radiologically detectable sponges. Use a moist Teflon pad to protect a bone or tissue specimen.
▶ Never send a specimen to the pathology department in a radiologically detectable sponge.
▶ Never remove a specimen from the sterile field without the surgeon's specific permission to do so.
▶ Never bury a specimen under trays, drapes, or other materials.
▶ Protect the specimen in a basin. Examination of a very small piece of tissue sometimes determines the need for radical surgery.

▶ Do not soak a specimen unless the surgeon requests it.
▶ Never discard any tissue unless the surgeon requests it.
▶ Do not use bone clamps, hemostats, or other crushing instruments on specimens. This can destroy cells.
▶ All specimen containers must be labeled and accompanied by a written document that states the patient's name, identification number, location, and type of specimen.

Types of Specimens
TISSUE

Biopsy is the removal of tissue or cells for analysis by a pathologist. Microscopic analysis results in a definitive diagnosis such as malignancy, or is used to determine the nature of an abnormality. The surgeon performs a biopsy during endoscopic or guided imagery surgery, or as a part of an open procedure. Types of biopsy are the following:

▶ *Excisional (incisional)* biopsy is used when a large, deep section of tissue is required for analysis. The tissue is removed with a cutting instrument.
▶ *Fine-needle aspiration (FNA)* uses a long, fine needle to aspirate (suction) small pieces of tissue from a tumor.
▶ *Needle biopsy* is similar to FNA, but a large-bore hollow trocar or needle is used to collect tissue. The needle is inserted into an organ such as the liver, and tissue is aspirated for analysis.
▶ *Brush biopsy* is performed during flexible endoscopic procedures. A fine brush is used to collect cells on the surface of mucous membrane tissue.

FLUID

Fluid *specimens* include blood, urine, semen, and other body fluids. These are collected only occasionally during surgery.

STONES

Stones are removed from the urinary tract, salivary ducts, and gallbladder. These are not cellular tissue but are treated as pathological specimens.

FOREIGN BODIES

Any nontissue item removed from the body is considered a specimen. Some specimens, such as bullets and knife blades, are critical as forensic evidence and may be used for legal purposes. A retained item from a previous surgery has obvious legal importance. Other items such as implants and fragments of metal, glass, wood, or any other foreign material also are retained as specimens.

FROZEN SECTION SPECIMENS

The specimen is passed to the scrub after removal. If an *immediate* diagnosis is required, the tissue is prepared for frozen section analysis. In frozen section analysis, the pathologist divides the frozen specimen into microscope slices for immediate examination. He or she then returns the diagnosis by intercom or by face-to-face consultation with the surgeon in the operating room. The surgeon identifies potentially malignant margins on a specimen with a suture. A suture should never be cut or removed from a specimen. Frozen section specimens are never placed in formalin but are kept moist.

OTHER TISSUE

Tissue for routine analysis is transferred from the back table directly into a sealable specimen container. Depending on the type of tissue, the specimen may be preserved in 10% formalin or normal saline. When transferring the specimen, always confirm with the circulator the exact location and type of tissue removed. Stones are kept in a dry container to prevent disintegration. Cytologic specimens that are received during brush biopsy are collected in normal saline. Laboratory policy determines whether tissues are preserved in aqueous formalin or normal saline.

Foreign bodies are kept in dry containers properly identified with the patient's name and the source.

AMPUTATIONS

When an amputation is performed, the body part is usually draped and contained before removal. Many patients undergo amputation during regional anesthesia. Do not allow the patient to view the amputated part. Transfer it directly to the back table. It should be secured in a small drape and passed off the field. The disposition of the body part depends on the patient's wishes, which may be influenced by **culture** or religious faith.

SPECIMENS FOR CULTURE

A culture is the propagation of microorganisms from a small amount of exudate or other potentially infectious fluid or tissue. The sample is cultured in the laboratory, and any microorganisms grown are analyzed for type and sensitivity to specific antibiotics, a procedure called a *C and S* (culture and sensitivity). Table 15-1 lists types of specimens, the site from which they are obtained, and the types of infectious organisms to be examined.

Culture specimens are taken during surgery when an infection is present or suspected. Sampling is performed with a culture tube, dry container, or liquid medium (Figure 15-21). A culture tube contains one or two cotton-tipped swabs, which are swiped across the suspect tissue and replaced in the tube. For a pure culture to be grown, the tip of the swab must not touch any other surface. Some culture tubes contain a preservative at the bottom, which is released when the tube is squeezed.

Two very common cultures taken during surgery are aerobic and anaerobic cultures. *Aerobic* culture specimens require oxygen for the growth of microorganisms. *Anaerobic* culture specimens require the absence of oxygen (air) for growth of microorganisms.

Never transfer suspect material directly from a syringe into a handheld vial or hand-cap a syringe containing the material. Use special transfer devices intended to protect the handler from needle-stick injury. When transferring culture specimens off the field, take care not to contaminate the outside of the tube. The circulator should always wear gloves when handling specimens.

CARE AND HANDLING OF TISSUE

Surgery is intentional *traumatization* of tissue. The manner in which the surgical team and postsurgical caregivers manage this traumatized tissue contributes to the success or failure of the surgery. Never forget that tissues are alive, functioning, and very much subject to unintentional physiological and physical injury. Wound management is the process the entire surgical team uses to care for tissues during surgery. A favorable outcome in wound management reflects strict surgical technique.

The tissues within and around the surgical wound are at risk for injury during surgery. The surgical technologist contributes directly to tissue care by doing the following:

▶ Understanding the nature of body tissues and how they can be injured during surgery
▶ Providing correct instrumentation
▶ Observing tissues for desiccation (local dehydration)
▶ Assessing the potential for patient injury by devices and instruments
▶ Preventing incidents that interrupt the flow of the procedure
▶ Preparing sutures, medications, and irrigation solutions precisely
▶ Offering wound management assistance and materials at the appropriate time
▶ Participating directly in a procedure (such as tissue retraction) as permitted by hospital policy and state practice codes
▶ Preventing team members from leaning onto the patient or placing heavy instruments on the patient's body

Controllable factors that contribute to tissue injury include the following:

▶ Excessive bruising from too much handling or rough handling
▶ Tissue dehydration from heat and exposure to the environment
▶ Hemorrhage
▶ Pooling of serous fluid as a result of inflammation and edema
▶ Unintentional blunt, sharp, or burn injury

Rough or Excessive Handling of Tissues

Rough handling of deep tissues such as the bowel, blood vessels, and other delicate structures can cause extensive bruising, tissue swelling, and ischemia. This results in increased inflammatory response and delayed healing. Gentle handling of tissues and prevention of drying, heating, hemorrhage, and trauma reduce inflammation and lead to faster recovery.

Table 15-1   IMPORTANT SPECIMENS FROM VARIOUS SITES AND TYPES OF INFECTIONS

Site/Type of Infection	Type of Specimen			
	Fluid	Tissue	Swab	Other
Urinary tract				
Bladder	Urine			
Kidney	Urine	Renal biopsy		
Gastrointestinal Tract				
Intestine			Rectal swab	Feces
Mouth	Washings			
Liver		Liver biopsy		
Biliary tract	Bile			
Abdomen	Pus Peritoneal aspirate Ascitic fluid			
Respiratory Tract				
Nose			Nasal swab	
Ear			Ear swab	
Eye			Eye swab	
Nasopharynx Throat	Washings (V)			"Cough plate"—patient coughs directly onto agar plate Direct inoculation of culture plates at bedside
Lung	Sputum Alveolar lavage			
Pleural space	Pleural fluid	Lung biopsy		
Central Nervous System				
Meninges encephalitis (herpes)	Cerebrospinal fluid (CSF)	Brain biopsy		
Brain abscess	Pus; CSF			
Genital Tract				
Urethra			Urethral swab	Direct microscopy and culture in clinic
Vagina			High vaginal swab	
Cervix			Cervical swab	
Endometrium		Endometrial biopsy		
Skin and Soft Tissue				
Skin	Vesicle fluid (V)	Skin biopsy (M)	Skin swab (carriage)	Impression plates
Wound	Pus	Scrapings (F)	Wound swab	
Bone and Joint				
Osteomyelitis	Pus	Bone*		
Joint	Aspirate			
Septicemia	Blood			
Pyrexia of Unknown Origin	Blood			Blood films for malarial parasites
Endocarditis	Blood	Heart valve*		

* Collected at operation
(V) specimens for virology
(F) specimens for fungi
(M) specimens for mycobacteria
From Mims C et al: *Medical microbiology,* ed 2, London, 1998, Mosby.

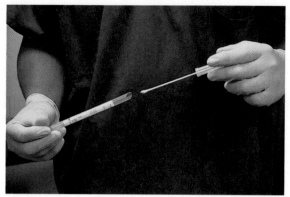

FIGURE 15-21
A culture tube. (From Elkin MK, Perry AG, Potter PA: *Nursing interventions and clinical skills,* ed 3, St Louis, 2004, Mosby.)

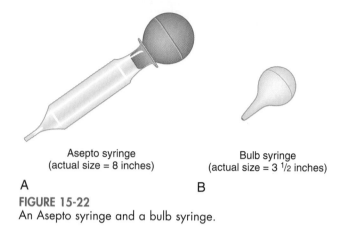

Asepto syringe
(actual size = 8 inches)

Bulb syringe
(actual size = 3 ½ inches)

A

B

FIGURE 15-22
An Asepto syringe and a bulb syringe.

During surgery, tissue must be handled as little as possible. Any physiological stress on the body, including surgery, causes increased release of catecholamines such as epinephrine. This produces an increase in intravascular (*intra* means "inside" and *vascular* means "blood vessels") volume, swelling, and fluid accumulation at the site of surgically injured tissues. This stagnant fluid can become a reservoir for microorganisms in the postoperative period.

Excessive or rough handling of bowel tissue can cause a sympathetic nerve response called *paralytic ileus* in which the intestine becomes paralyzed.

Although actual tissue handling is the task of the surgeon, the surgical technologist contributes to safe surgery by providing the correct instruments and by being prepared for bleeding during dissection. The less tissues are manipulated, the less trauma results. The surgical technologist can prevent the need for excessive manipulation by responding quickly to events such as hemorrhage and inadvertent tissue tearing. These events can be caused by use of the wrong needle-suture combination or the wrong size suture, or by accidental trauma. If the surgeon is preparing to tie a **bleeder** (hemorrhaging blood vessel) and receives the wrong suture, he or she may have to stop, reposition the hands, and wait for the correct suture. Single events may not be consequential. A series of such events has cumulative effects.

Tissue Dehydration

Tissues must not be allowed to dry out during surgery. Extremely dry tissues cannot withstand handling and may slough during the healing phase. Wound edges, bowel tissue, muscle, and subcutaneous tissue are particularly subject to dehydration and bruising. To protect delicate tissues, intermittent irrigation is necessary, or tissues may be covered with a sponge moistened in normal saline. During eye surgery, the surgical technologist must irrigate the cornea with a balanced salt solution (BSS), as directed by the surgeon.

In open surgery, irrigation fluid is offered both when the surgeon asks for it and whenever tissues appear to be dehydrated. Signs of dehydration in internal tissues are dullness, loss of surface elasticity, and tissue fraying. The surgical wound is irrigated periodically to remove tissue debris and blood clots. Irrigation solutions are warm normal saline or topical aqueous antibacterial solution.

Solution is distributed to the surgeon with an Asepto or a bulb syringe (Figure 15-22). Two syringes may be required; while one is in use, another is being filled. Irrigation solution is removed from the wound with the suction tip. A suction guard must be used whenever delicate tissues are exposed. This guard is a perforated sleeve that distributes the total suction pressure over many openings and prevents tissue trauma.

Antibiotic irrigation solutions often are used in a final irrigation before wound closure as a prophylactic measure against postoperative infection.

The surgical technologist must keep track of the amount of irrigation fluid used in the wound so that estimated blood loss can be calculated.

DISSECTION

Tissues of the body occur in *planes* and *layers*. These are distinct layers that are bound together with collagen fibers, loose areolar tissue, or connective tissue. Some tissue layers are adhered so close together that they cannot be separated without tearing the tissues. Others are easily separated manually. Organs are contained in body cavities such as the peritoneal or thoracic cavity. In these areas there are no distinct layers between the organ and the cavity wall. However, the tissues of the organs and the lining of the cavity are layered. Muscle and fascia are examples of distinct layers. It is important for the scrub to recognize tissue layers, because he or she must anticipate both the separation and the closing (suturing) of certain layers.

When a body cavity must be entered or the skin penetrated, ideally the surgeon can separate the layers without cutting them. However, this is not possible in all situations.

Sharp Dissection

Sharp dissection is the cutting of tissue with a scalpel, scissors, electrosurgical unit (ESU) tip, laser, or other device. Always anticipate bleeding when tissue is dissected with a sharp instrument. Muscle tissue is particularly vascular. The omentum contains many fine blood vessels that cause brisk bleeding when cut. Other highly vascular tissues include the scalp, facial skin, outer ear, structures of the mouth, and organs such as the spleen, kidney, liver, and pancreas.

When bleeding occurs, anticipate the need for ESU tip, clamps (of appropriate length and weight depending on the depth and type of tissue), sutures, suture ties, vessel clamps, or topical hemostatic agents.

Blunt Dissection

Blunt dissection is the process of separating tissue planes without cutting them. This is performed manually or with a sponge dissector mounted on a clamp. The surgeon uses the sponge to tease apart the tissue layers rather than cutting them. Countertraction is needed during blunt dissection so that the layers can be pulled away. A nontraumatic clamp such as an Allis clamp or the surgeon's hand is used to apply traction. Blunt dissection often is used during hernia repair and rectocele-cystocele repair.

When a dissection sponge becomes bloody, the surface is no longer rough enough to separate the tissue layers. Anticipate the need for additional dissector sponges during blunt dissection. Blunt dissection can cause small hemorrhages. These are usually coagulated with the ESU.

RETRACTION
Purpose

When tissue is dissected, the surgical wound become increasingly deep. Retractors are placed at the wound edge to protect underlying tissues from injury during dissection.

As the wound gets deeper, anticipate the need for deeper retraction. Sharp-tipped retractors are used only on skin and subcutaneous tissue, never in deep tissues. Retractors may be self-retaining or handheld. Pass a retractor in the same position it will lay in the surgical wound. Occasionally the scrub is asked to perform retraction, depending on hospital policy. Retraction almost always involves delicate tissues such as internal organs, tendons, muscle, and skin. Serious tissue damage can occur during retraction. Nerve damage resulting from excess pressure or inattention to the retractor blade or tip can result in patient loss of mobility and sensation. Excess pressure on tissue can cause local ischemia (loss of blood supply) and necrosis.

Technique

Retraction does not require exertional force. The blade of the retractor is used as a backstop to prevent tissue from obstructing the open incision. The proper method of retracting is to allow the surgeon to place the retractor, and then hold it in place *without toeing the blade inward* (Figure 15-23). The blade should be maintained in a constant right-angle position to prevent tissue damage. If the surgeon repositions the retractor, let go of it momentarily and then resume holding it. *Never look away from the wound if you are retracting.* You must remain alert to prevent the retractor from shifting or putting downward or angled pressure on the tissue. Retraction requires a balance between gentle tissue displace-

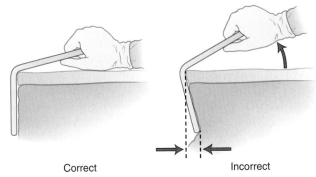

Correct   Incorrect

FIGURE 15-23
Proper and improper technique for retracting.

ment and minimization of fatigue, so that the tissue does not slip back and obscure the surgeon's view. If the retractor begins to slip, let the surgeon know. He must reposition it appropriately.

Blood vessels, tubular organs such as the esophagus, and other elongated structures are retracted with a length of narrow rubber tubing or plastic. *Vessel loops* or cotton *umbilical tapes* are used on blood vessels. The spermatic cord is retracted during herniorrhaphies with a Penrose drain. Generally when these types of retraction are necessary, the surgeon secures the ends with a small clamp to hold them in place.

Traction sutures are sutures placed in the patient to retract skin or tissue flaps, such as in eye or cardiac surgery. These do not remain in the wound but are removed at the close of the procedure. A small clamp is placed over the ends of the sutures to hold them in place.

Preventing Intraoperative Tissue Trauma

Tissue can be severely bruised or damaged by direct pressure during surgery (as discussed earlier). Trauma results in increased inflammatory response and increased risk of surgical site infection. Retraction often is implicated as a cause of local nerve damage and ischemia, which can result from excessive or inward pressure on retractors. Whenever possible, nontraumatic rake retractors should be offered. When a sharp skin hook or rake is used for retraction, maintaining the most delicate, precise tension is critical to prevent the retractor from ripping through the tissue.

HEMOSTASIS
Surgical Goals

Maintaining the body's total blood volume and controlling bleeding is called hemostasis. Hemostasis within the surgical wound is necessary to conserve the body's total blood volume, preserve a clean wound, and prevent infection. Blood is a perfect medium for bacterial growth. Clots left in the wound can become a source of bacterial growth and retard healing, because the body must break down and absorb clots as part of the healing process.

Autotransfusion

Autotransfusion is defined as the reinfusion of blood or blood products derived from the patient's own circulation. When a patient is scheduled for elective surgery and a large amount of blood loss is anticipated, many patients choose to have blood drawn several weeks before surgery. This blood is then stored in the blood bank and returned intravenously as needed during surgery.

An alternative method of autotransfusion is to collect the patient's blood from the surgical site intraoperatively (during surgery) and return it (reinfuse) intravenously. In this method special equipment, such as a "cell saver" device, is required to collect, rinse, anticoagulate, and filter the blood, and separate the blood cells from unwanted components. In this procedure, blood is collected through a special Yankauer tip and routed through tubing directly attached to the "cell saver." "Cell saver" units are made by different manufacturers and are very beneficial in vascular thoracic and orthopedic procedures, when a large blood loss is anticipated.

Autotransfusion is acceptable to those patients who, for religious, cultural, or other reasons, decline transfusion of blood from another person.

Coagulation

ELECTROSURGICAL COAGULATION

Surgeons use the electrosurgical unit (ESU) extensively to cut and coagulate tissue. Continuous use of the ESU causes **eschar** (carbonized tissue) to build up on the ESU tip. The appearance of a flame or a glow on the tip of the ESU means that eschar is present and is overheated. This causes a wider burn area and unnecessary tissue trauma. In addition, the eschar retains heat (in the same way as charcoal) long after the ESU is deactivated and *must* be removed to prevent flame and ignition. The scrub must remove this eschar using a scratch pad, or if a Teflon tip is used, it may be wiped clean with a damp sponge.

Never use a scalpel blade or other sharp blade to remove eschar. This produces microabrasions on the tip, which trap eschar and cause it to build up more quickly. The abrasions lead to high tip temperatures, sparking, and flame.

The ESU tip must be replaced in its holder when not in use. When one is ready to place the ESU tip back in the holder, this is the best time to examine the tip and clean it if necessary.

FULGURATION

Fulguration is the use of high-frequency electrical current to coagulate surface tissue. This current is higher in frequency than the ESU current and creates an arc. When fulgurating, the electrode does not touch the tissue. The process is called *spray coagulation*. Fulguration is useful for sealing small, hidden bleeders or large bleeders. Patient grounding is required to prevent stray voltage and severe burns.

COAGULATION WITH THE ULTRASONIC (HARMONIC) SCALPEL

The ultrasonic scalpel delivers ultrasonic energy through a grasping instrument capable of coagulating (and dividing) tissue by low-temperature cavitation or implosion. The tip of the instrument contains a blade that closes against a flat anvil. The blade portion of the instrument is used to separate tissue planes, and the flat plate is used to coagulate. While the ESU and laser actually burn through the tissue, the harmonic scalpel does not use heat, and no eschar is produced. The harmonic scalpel cuts most efficiently through fibrous tissue and is used in the morselization (fragmentation) of myometrial myomas (fibrous muscle tumors of the uterine wall). Blood and tissue can build up on the tip of the instrument, as in electrosurgery. The surgical technologist must periodically remove this tissue.

ARGON PLASMA COAGULATION

Argon plasma coagulation instruments use a combination of argon gas and monopolar electrical energy to coagulate tissue. Argon is supplied to the instrument and ionized by electricity. This makes the gas electrically conductive. The current flowing between the probe and the tissue coagulates the tissue without actual contact with the instrument. The beam seeks the least-resistant path to complete the electrical circuit and coagulates active bleeders within a 2-mm to 10-mm range of the tip. Because the tip does not actually touch the tissue, there is no tissue adherence, little smoke plume, and less charring than with ESU coagulation. Because the ionized argon seeks a nonresistant electrical path, the current flows toward active bleeding.

LASER COAGULATION

Laser energy is used to control bleeding by thermal coagulation. Refer to Chapter 17 for a complete discussion of laser technology and safety considerations.

Ligation and Occlusion

Suture ligation is used to occlude large blood vessels. After a blood vessel is located, the surgeon clamps it and secures it with a free tie or a suture ligature (ligature applied by a suture-and-needle combination). Absorbable or nonabsorbable sutures are used to ligate vessels. Metal ligation clips, called vessel clips, are contained in a cartridge and are used in both open and endoscopic surgery. These ligation techniques are described in Chapter 16.

Pneumatic Tourniquet

The pneumatic tourniquet (Figure 15-24) is a surgical device used to control venous and arterial circulation to create a bloodless surgical site in limb surgery. Pressure is applied circumferentially upon the skin and underlying tissues of a limb; the pressure is transferred to the walls of the vessels, causing them to become temporarily occluded. The tourniquet cuff is a non-latex air bladder encased in a nylon cuff much like a blood pressure cuff, except that it is narrower and the bladder completely encircles the limb. Compressed gas from a tourniquet instrument connected to the cuff is used to inflate the bladder after preparation of the limb.

Tourniquet cuffs are manufactured in a variety of sizes and widths, and are designed for specific use on different areas of the extremities. The portion of the limb that will lie under the cuff may be covered with a premanufactured sleeve or stockinette to help protect the skin and prevent folds or pinching. The tourniquet cuff then is placed over the protective sleeve or stockinette. Before tourniquet inflation, the limb is exsanguinated (blood is forced out of the limb) with an Esmarch bandage or elastic wrap such as an Ace bandage as described in Chapter 11 or less effectively by elevation of the limb. The Esmarch bandage is a 3-inch to 4-inch–wide rubber bandage that is wrapped tightly around the limb from distal to proximal end. This pushes the blood toward the trunk of the body. The tourniquet cuff is then inflated by the tourniquet instrument, and the Esmarch bandage is removed.

Follow these safety precautions when using a pneumatic tourniquet:

▶ When the pneumatic tourniquet is inflated, the period from cuff inflation to deflation is called *tourniquet time* and is measured precisely. Both inflation and deflation times are documented on the patient's intraoperative chart.

▶ The tourniquet may remain inflated for up to 1 hour on an upper extremity and 1½ to 2 hours on a lower extremity. After that period the patient is at risk for nerve, vascular, and tissue necrosis related to ischemia.

▶ The surgeon or registered nurse circulator applies the tourniquet and Esmarch bandage.

▶ The tourniquet pressure must not exceed 50 to 75 mm Hg over the patient's systolic blood pressure for an upper extremity on adult patients, 100 to 150 mm Hg systolic blood pressure for a lower extremity on adult patients, and 100 mm Hg systolic blood pressure for pediatric patients.

▶ Strict policies regarding the use of tourniquets are enforced in all hospitals.

▶ Preparation solutions and moisture should be prevented from seeping under the tourniquet cuff, because this can cause severe burns or tissue injury.

▶ The pressure gauge must be tested before cuff inflation.

▶ If surgery continues beyond the recommended inflation time, the tourniquet is deflated for 10 minutes and reinflated. As soon as it is deflated, the field will fill with blood. The surgical technologist must be prepared with sponges, ESU tip, and other hemostatic means appropriate to the tissues involved.

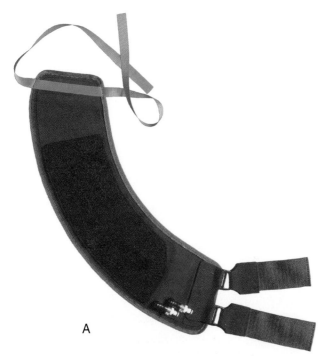
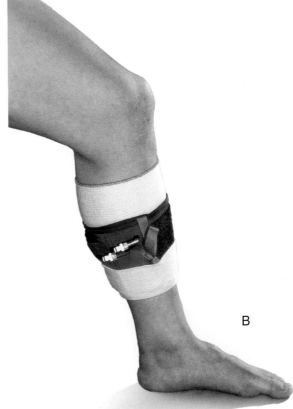

FIGURE 15-24
A, A pneumatic tourniquet. **B,** A pneumatic tourniquet placed on a lower limb. (**A** and **B** courtesy of Delfi Medical Innovations, Vancouver, British Columbia, Canada.)

▶ The surgical technologist always should reroll the Esmarch bandage after it is removed because it may be needed again.

▶ The circulator assesses the limb and selects the site for the tourniquet before it is applied. The site is assessed a second time and charted when the tourniquet is removed.

▶ Always follow the manufacturer's recommendations for maintaining and cleaning the tourniquet to prevent malfunction.

Topical Hemostatic Agents

PLATELET CONCENTRATES

A platelet concentrate is a hemostatic agent made from autologous plasma (from the patient). Platelet gel is mixed with bovine thrombin and calcium chloride. Platelet concentrate differs from fibrin adhesive in its composition. Platelet concentrate is autologous, while fibrin adhesive is manufactured from pooled plasma. Platelet concentrate is acceptable for use in surgery on individuals whose faith does not permit the use of transfused blood.

TOPICAL THROMBIN

Topical thrombin (of bovine origin) is mixed with saline solution. Small pieces of gelatin sponge (Gelfoam) or sponge patties are soaked in this solution and placed over delicate bleeding capillaries such as those in the brain, ear, or spinal cord area. Gelatin sponges also can be used alone to encourage the formation of fibrin on oozing surfaces.

OXIDIZED CELLULOSE

Oxidized cellulose is a USP (United States Pharmacopeia) product that adheres to bleeding tissue and promotes coagulation. Its primary use is in vascular, neurological, liver, and spleen surgery to control capillary bleeding. It is available in mesh, fiber, and power form. Oxidized cellulose is always applied dry and may be left in the wound, where it is later digested during the process of healing. Trade names are Oxycel and Avitene.

WOUND DRAINS

A drain is a device used to continuously or intermittently remove serous fluid from a healing wound. Tissue that has been traumatized or is edematous (swollen) or infected produces serous or serosanguineous (bloody serous) fluid. To prevent infection, this fluid must be drained. Two basic types of wound drains are used in tissue. These are passive drains and suction drains.

Passive Drains

Passive drains create a passage from the tissue inside the wound to the outside of the body. These usually are placed when drainage is minimal. The *Penrose* drain (Figure 15-25) is a simple tubular length of nonlatex material similar to surgical glove material. Before closing, the surgeon places the drain loosely in the wound and secures sutures around it. The drain itself may be secured with one or two skin sutures to prevent it from being pulled out. A sponge dressing is placed over the drain to collect fluid from the wound. The gravity drain is a tube that is placed in the wound, such as the T-tube, usually after surgery of the biliary tract. This tube is connected to a closed gravity drainage bag. Other gravity drainage devices include the urinary drainage system attached to a retention catheter.

Suction Drains

Suction drains are placed either in areas that produce a large amount of fluid or in areas that cannot tolerate the presence of any fluid, such as the chest cavity. Commonly used suction drains are the *spring action* drainage system, or Hemovac (Figure 15-26), and the *Jackson-Pratt* drain (Figure 15-27).

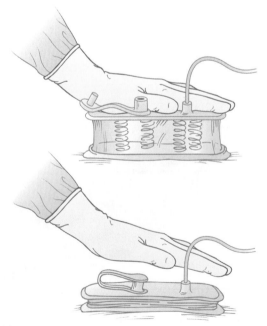

FIGURE 15-26
The Hemovac drain. (Redrawn from Phillips N: *Berry & Kohn's operating room technique*, ed 10, St Louis, 2004, Mosby.)

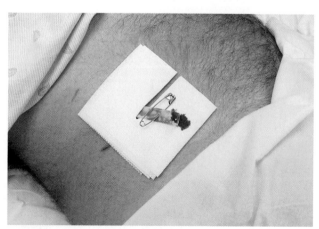

FIGURE 15-25
The Penrose drain. (From Elkin MK, Perry AG, Potter PA: *Nursing interventions and clinical skills*, ed 3, St Louis, 2004, Mosby.)

Water-Sealed Drainage System

The water-sealed drainage system is used to pull fluid or air from the thoracic cavity after thoracic surgery or trauma to the thorax. The thoracic cavity is under negative pressure. The difference between atmospheric pressure and thoracic pressure allows the lungs to expand normally. When this negative pressure is lost, such as during accidental or surgical trauma to the thoracic cavity, negative pressure must be restored. The underwater drainage system performs this task. The drainage system contains three separate water chambers sealed in a plastic unit. One or more chest drainage tubes are placed in the thorax and connected to the drainage system. When suction is applied to one of the chambers, air or fluids are pulled into the collection system. Each of the remaining chambers contains a small amount of water, which prevents the loss of negative pressure in the thoracic cavity (Figure 15-28).

When any drainage system is in use, the collection unit must remain *below the level of the insertion tube*. This prevents the reentry of fluids into the drainage space. Chest drainage systems must never be allowed to back up into the thorax. This can cause immediate collapse of a lung. When

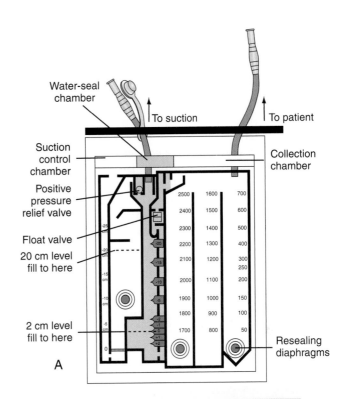

A

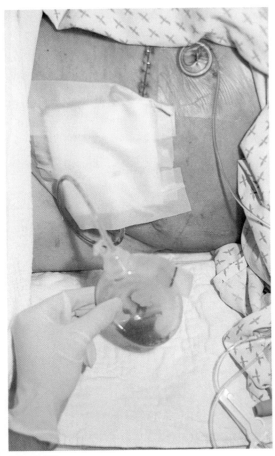

FIGURE 15-27
The Jackson-Pratt drain. (From Elkin MK, Perry AG, Potter PA: *Nursing interventions and clinical skills*, ed 3, St Louis, 2004, Mosby.)

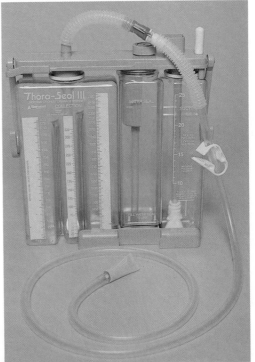

B

FIGURE 15-28
A, Pleur-evac disposable chest suction system. **B,** Disposable chest drainage system. (**A** from Lewis SM, Heitkemper MM, and Dirksen SR: *Medical-surgical nursing: assessment and management of clinical problems,* ed 6, St Louis, 2004, Mosby; **B** from Elkin MK, Perry AG, Potter PA: *Nursing interventions and clinical skills,* ed 3, St Louis, 2004, Mosby.)

transferring a patient with an underwater chest drainage system, keep the system upright. If the collection system falls over, place the system upright and check it for cracks. Make sure all tubes and connections are tight. If there is any doubt about the integrity of the system, seek help immediately.

WOUND DRESSINGS

Sterile wound dressings are placed over the incision site at the close of surgery. Many types of wound dressings are available. Those that are applied to the surgical wound immediately after surgery have a specific purpose. All dressings protect the wound from environmental contamination. Other purposes are to provide pressure, support, skin closure, absorption, and débridement (removal of necrotic or devitalized tissue). Wound dressings do not have a radiopaque-detectable strip and should never be opened for use until the wound is closed and the final count has been completed.

Skin Closure

Small superficial wounds may be closed with thin adhesive strips (Steri-Strips) (Figure 15-29, *A*). These are available

in different widths and lengths. To increase their sticking ability, a small amount of biological adhesive may be applied to the skin before the strips are applied. Benzoin usually is used for this purpose.

Other types of skin-closure dressings include transparent adhesive patches and biological films that occlude the wound but allow air to flow to it (Figure 15-29, *B*).

Barrier Protection and Absorption

During the first 48 hours of healing, the wound is particularly susceptible to bacterial growth. Therefore, any dressing that is placed directly over the incision or wound must be *sterile*. An uncomplicated wound that is clean and dry usually is covered with one to four layers of square gauze secured with tape. Teflon-coated gauze squares also may be used to prevent the gauze from sticking to the wound.

A wound that is draining or contaminated often requires additional dressings to absorb fluid. Fluffed gauze or a thick absorbent pad (also called a combine pad, abdominal pad, or ABD pad) is used (Figure 15-30). If a drain has been put in the incision, additional gauze is placed around the area where it emerges from the skin.

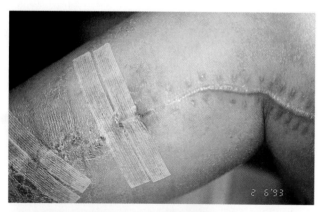

A

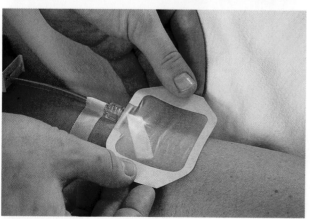

B

FIGURE 15-29
A, Steri-strips. **B,** Transparent adhesive patch. (From Elkin MK, Perry AG, Potter PA: *Nursing interventions and clinical skills,* ed 3, St Louis, 2004, Mosby.)

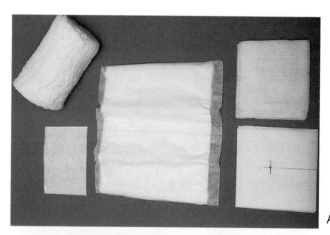

A

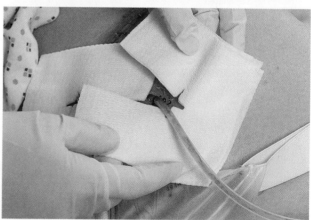

B

FIGURE 15-30
A, Types of wound dressings. **B,** Gauze dressing placed around a drain. (From Elkin MK, Perry AG, Potter PA: *Nursing interventions and clinical skills,* ed 3, St Louis, 2004, Mosby.)

Pressure

A pressure dressing is used most often over a skin graft. The graft must remain in close contact with the underlying tissue to retain its vitality and become integrated into the new site. Slight pressure on the graft site prevents serous fluid from lifting the skin graft away from the recipient site.

A **stent dressing** is a type of pressure dressing in which gauze or other material is molded into a thick pad that fits the graft area. Sutures are placed around the graft site. The long suture ends are then tied over the pad to secure it in place (Figure 15-31).

Nonadherent Barrier

Gauze squares or strips (gauze tape) impregnated with plain or antibacterial ointment are used when barrier protection is necessary for a moist wound, and dressing changes would disrupt the healing tissue or cause bleeding. An example of a site requiring such a barrier is a skin graft donor site or other delicate tissue such as the nasal sinuses. Trade names of non-adherent barrier dressings include Adaptic, Xeroform, and Nu Gauze dressings.

Packing

Packing is a method of filling a wound site or cavity with gauze material to absorb draining fluids or to purposely débride (remove dead tissue) during the dressing change. If a wound is packed, it is not sutured closed. The wound is filled with gauze strips or fluffed gauze squares moistened with saline (Figure 15-32). When the dressing is changed, the dry gauze is removed and lifts dried serum, necrotic tissue, and other debris from the wound. This is called a "wet-to-dry" dressing.

Support

Supportive dressings are used to prevent or limit movement of the surgical wound during healing. Orthopedic procedures often require the use of supportive dressings and appliances. One achieves soft support by wrapping a limb in thick rolled cotton, which is secured with additional wraps of elastic or stretch gauze bandages. Hard casting materials are used when complete immobility is required (Figure 15-33). Before casting materials are applied, compressed cotton is placed to protect the limb.

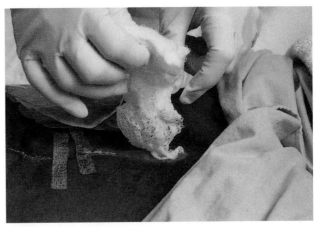

FIGURE 15-32
Packing a wound with gauze. (From Elkin MK, Perry AG, Potter PA: *Nursing interventions and clinical skills*, ed 3, St Louis, 2004, Mosby.)

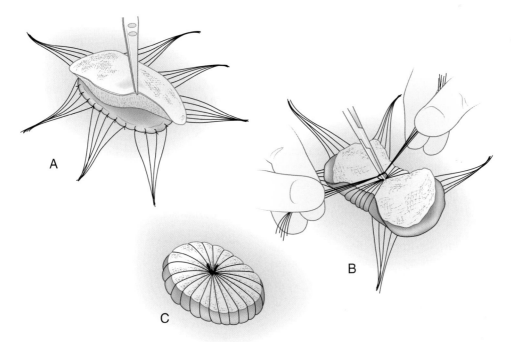

FIGURE 15-31
A through **C,** Stenting a skin graft.

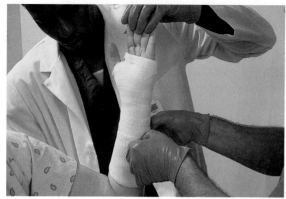

FIGURE 15-33
A hard cast. (From Elkin MK, Perry AG, Potter PA: *Nursing interventions and clinical skills,* ed 3, St Louis, 2004, Mosby.)

Tape and Binders

Flat gauze dressings are secured with nonsterile tape. Tape is made of paper, cotton, or synthetic materials. Many patients are sensitive to adhesives and tapes. It is the circulator's responsibility to check the patient's chart for tape sensitivity. Nonsterile gloves always should be worn when applying tape.

Some wounds require frequent dressing changes. To avoid the need to remove tape with each dressing change, a binder is used to hold the dressings in place. *Montgomery straps* are a common type of abdominal binder. This binder consists of two large adhesive patches with soft laces. The patches are attached on each side of the wound, and the dressing held in place with the laces. To change the dressing, the laces are untied and the dressing removed.

Procedure for Assisting with Dressing Application

Near the close of surgery, the circulator distributes sterile dressing materials to the scrub. These should be kept clean and dry. The dressings are arranged in order of their use. Before dressings are applied, the wound site is gently cleaned with a sterile damp towel or sponges. Blood, tissue debris, and preparation solutions are removed from the incision. The site must be dried before dressings are applied.

The scrub may apply a simple dressing as directed by the surgeon. Complex dressings are usually applied by the surgeon with assistance from the scrub and circulator. Remember that only sterile materials can come in direct contact with the wound. The scrub or surgeon holds the sterile dressings in place over the incision while the circulator removes the drapes. Complex or multilayer dressings are applied after the initial sterile covering is in place and drapes have been removed.

CASE STUDIES

Case 1

You have begun a sterile setup and have draped the Mayo stand. You planned to have 20 minutes for the sterile setup. You are about to arrange the drapes, gowns, gloves, and other supplies when the circulator comes in and tells you that another emergency patient will be arriving in a few minutes. The surgeons are already scrubbing. What will you do?

Case 2

Your hospital has established a policy that all surgery must use a neutral zone (no-hands) technique. As you are about to start the case, you place a neutral zone pad on the patient. The surgeon tells you he refuses to use it. You are concerned for your safety. What will you do?

Case 3

You are handed a specimen for frozen section analysis. The surgeon has placed a silk suture on one side of the specimen.

Do you need to be concerned about the orientation of this suture?

Case 4

During an abdominal procedure, you notice that the participating medical student is leaning on the patient while retracting the abdominal wall. The retractor is no longer where the surgeon placed it and is toed inward. Will you correct this situation? If so, how?

Case 5

The surgeon has placed a chest tube in the patient and attached an underwater chest drainage system. After surgery you are transferring the patient to the stretcher when the collection system falls to the floor. What do you think is the appropriate action?

REFERENCES

Association of periOperative Registered Nurses: Recommended practices for use of the pneumatic tourniquet, *AORN Journal* 75:2, February, 2002.

Nandi PL et al.: Surgical wound infection, *Hong Kong Medical Journal* 5:1, March, 1999.

Chapter 16

Sutures and Wound Healing

Learning Objectives

After studying this chapter the reader will be able to:

- Recognize suture properties and materials by observing and handling suture
- Identify sutures by package labeling, and select proper sutures
- Distinguish between inert suture materials and those that cause inflammation
- Identify and anticipate the need for specific sutures during a procedure
- Demonstrate proper preparation of sutures for use
- Properly pass suture-needle combinations
- Identify the need to maintain sutures on the sterile field in an orderly manner
- Identify safety precautions to prevent needle-stick injuries during suture use
- Identify basic needle types and their applications
- Distinguish between absorbable and nonabsorbable sutures
- Distinguish among different suture sizes
- Recognize commonly used stapling devices
- Identify the uses of fibrin glue

Terminology

Absorbable sutures—Suture materials that are rapidly or eventually digested by enzymes in the body after the wound is healed.

Anastomosis—A connection created between two vessels, spaces, or organs that normally are separated.

Approximate—To bring tissue together by sutures or other means.

Bleeder—A bleeding vessel.

Blunt needle—A curved, tapered needle with a blunt point. This type of needle is usually used in highly vascular organs such as the liver. Surgeons are encouraged to use the blunt needle for other tissue types to reduce the risk of needle-stick injury.

Bolsters—Tubing through which retention sutures are threaded to prevent them from cutting into the patient's skin.

Brown and Sharp (B & S) gauge—Sizing standard used to measure the diameter of wire or stainless steel.

Capillarity—The ability of suture material to soak up fluid along the strand from the immersed wet end into the dry nonimmersed end. Capillarity is high in braided sutures.

Chromic salt—Chemical used to treat surgical gut so it resists rapid enzymatic absorption by body tissues, reduces irritation of tissue, and increases tensile strength in the suture strand.

Control-release—Suture material with swaged needles that are designed to "pop-off" with a twist of the wrist after the suture has been passed through tissues.

Dehiscence—The separation of the layers of the surgical wound; it may be partial and superficial only, or complete, with disruption of all layers.

Double-armed sutures—Suture-needle combinations containing a needle at each end of the suture. Double-armed sutures are used to approximate tissue in a circumference, as in joining two ends of a blood vessel.

Elasticity—The amount of stretch exhibited by a suture material.

Terminology—cont'd

Evisceration—The protrusion of an internal organ through a wound or surgical incision.

First intention wound closure—Wound closure in which all layers of the wound are approximated and the collagen scar formation is minimal; sometimes called primary intention wound closure.

Inert—A type of sutures and implants that, because of their biochemical properties, provoke little or no inflammatory reaction by the body.

Interrupted suture—A technique of suturing tissues using individual sutures and tying each one separately.

Keith needle—A straight cutting needle used on superficial tissue.

Ligate—To tie or bind with a ligature.

Ligature—Any suture substance or wire used to tie a vessel or strangulate a duct.

Mattress suture—A technique of suturing in which one passes the suture material through the tissues on one side of wound, across the incision, and through the tissues on the opposite side, and then passes the suture material through the opposite-side tissues and back through the tissues of the original side.

Memory—For suture material, the recoil of the suture after it has been removed from the package. Some suture materials are more resistant to straightening than others (have high memory).

Monofilament suture—Suture composed of a single strand of material.

Multifilament suture—Suture composed of many fine strands of fiber that are twisted or braided together.

Nonabsorbable sutures—Suture materials that resist breakdown in the body.

Pliability—The flexibility of a suture material.

Purse-string—A suturing technique in which a continuous strand is passed in and out of the circumference of a lumen, and then is pulled tight like a drawstring.

Reel—A continuous strand of suture mounted on a spool for ligation purposes.

Retention suture—Heavy nonabsorbable suture placed behind the skin sutures and through all tissue layers to give added strength to the closure. Also called secondary suture line.

Reverse cutting needles—Curved surgical needles with three honed edges. One of the edges is on the outside of the curve of the needle.

Running suture—A method of suturing that uses one continuous suture strand for tissue approximation.

Second intention wound closure—Wound closure that is accomplished by leaving the wound open to heal by granulation from the inner layer to the outer surface.

Stick tie—Name given to a suture ligature or transfixion suture; a suture needle combination that is passed through a vessel or duct for ligation, commonly used in deeper cavities. Commonly called a "stitch."

Swaged needle—The fused connection of the eyeless needle and the suture strand.

Tensile strength—The amount of force or stress a suture can withstand without breaking. This term also is used to refer to the strength of tissues as they heal.

Third intention wound closure—A delayed primary wound closure. A wound that is infected or has dehisced may be left open until the infection subsides, the tissue edges heal, and the healthy granulous tissue can be approximated.

Throw—The wrapping of suture ends to form a knot.

Tie-down—The ability of a suture to lie flat when knotted.

Tie on a passer—A strand of suture material attached to the tip of an instrument (such as a right angle) for ligation of vessels and ducts.

Tissue drag—The quality that produces friction between the suture and the tissue. Tissue drag can cause microtrauma in the wound or suture fraying.

INTRODUCTION TO SUTURES

Suture materials are used to **approximate** (sew tissue together) while healing takes place and to **ligate** (tie off) blood vessels or ducts during surgery. Many types of suture materials are available. The choice of suture material to be used on a particular tissue is based on the individual characteristics of the suture material (durability, handling, and knot security), the age and condition of the patient, and the surgeon's expertise, experience, and preference.

During surgery, it is the duty of the scrub or nurse to properly prepare suture materials until the surgeon needs them and to pass the material to him or her in an acceptable manner. Suture products are extremely expensive and, in many cases, delicate. The goal of proper suture handling is to maintain the suture material's inherent strength and integrity, and to promote economical use of the materials. In addition to sutures, a number of nonsuture products (discussed later in this chapter) are available that can be used for tissue approximation.

Many students learn suture types by associating a suture with its packaging. Packaging, including design and color, is a marketing tool and therefore is subject to change. Like medications, every suture has a trade name and a chemical material name. Even natural materials like silk have trade names, such as *Sofsilk*.

Difficulties also may arise in recognizing sutures because many different types of sutures and needles are used, and identical suture materials made by different companies have different names and may be dyed different colors. This can make recognizing them difficult.

The surgeon writes orders for a specific suture to be used on specific tissue, such as "2-0 Dexon for fascia." During the surgery, however, he or she may say only, "Give me some 2-0." The surgical technologist must learn to recognize that the fascia layer is about to be closed so that he or she *knows which 2-0 suture* is needed. Many different types of 2-0 suture may be on the instrument table.

For nearly every procedure, the surgeon's preference cards or sheets include the type and size of suture required for suturing different tissue layers during the given procedure. These are not consistent among surgeons. The surgical technologist must, at first, memorize the sequence of sutures used for each surgery. Eventually, after the surgical technologist has worked repeatedly with the same surgeons, knowing which suture to pass becomes easier. During the learning process, however, this task is challenging for most people. Most surgical personnel new to the operating room find suture identification and handling to be one of the more difficult tasks to learn. It is important to learn the different principles, characteristics, and materials of suture to begin to comprehend which type of suture is used on each type of tissue.

Regulation of Sutures

The United States Pharmacopeia (USP) began, historically, as an organization whose physician members set minimum standards for medical products and substances. These standards were adopted by the federal government and now are included in the regulations of the federal Food and Drug Administration (FDA). All substances, including suture products, that bear the USP label must meet minimum standards. Included in the standards for suture materials are those for size, **tensile strength,** and sterility. Additional standards for packaging, dyes used in the suture, and integrity of **swaged needle** are also included.

Suture Sizes

The diameter of the suture or the thickness of the strand determines its numerical size (Figure 16-1, *A*). Sizes run from size 5, the largest suture size available, to size 0. The greater the diameter, the larger the designated size (e.g., size 1 is larger than 0, size 2 is larger than 1). For sutures smaller than size 0, sizes are designated by a second digit in front of the zero. The larger the number, the smaller the suture size (e.g., size 2-0 is smaller than size 0, size 3-0 is smaller than size 2-0). The smallest diameter suture available is 11-0, which is light enough to be suspended in air. The 11-0 sutures are very fine, delicate, and expensive, and must be handled with extreme care. Very fine sutures usually are used in microsurgery, and the heaviest sutures can be used to **approximate** (bring together) bone tissue. USP suture sizing is standard in the industry. Approved materials bear the USP label.

An additional method of sizing uses the **Brown and Sharp (B & S) gauge,** which is used to indicate the diameter of stainless steel wires and sutures. Stainless steel sizes (called gauges) have a numbering system different from other types

DIAMETER	U.S.P.	B and S
.0031 inch	6-0	40
.0040	6-0	38
.0056	5-0	35
.0063	4-0	34
.0080	4-0	32
.0100	3-0	30
.0126	2-0	28
.0159	0	26
.0179	1	25
.0201	2	24
.0226	3	23
.0253	4	22
.0320	5	20
.0360	6	19
.0400	7	18

A

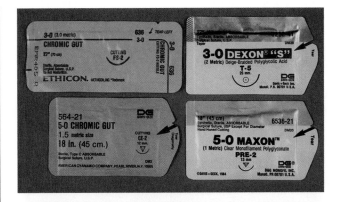
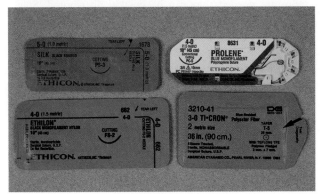

B

FIGURE 16-1
A, Diameters of various sutures. **B,** Suture packaging. (**A** from *Wound closure manual,* Ethicon, Inc, Somerville, NJ, 1999. **B** from Bonewit-West K: *Clinical procedures for medical assistants,* ed 6, Philadelphia, 2004, Saunders.)

Table 16-1	TABLE FOR STAINLESS STEEL SIZING										
B & S Gauge	#40	#35	#32	#30	#28	#26	#25	#24	#23	#22	#20
USP Size	6-0	5-0	4-0	3-0	2-0	0	1	2	3	4	5

of suture. The numbers begin at 18 gauge (the thickest gauge) and end with size 38/40 (the most delicate or smallest gauge) (Table 16-1). Note that as the number of the gauge increases, the size decreases.

Suture Packaging

Suture manufacturers have developed many methods of packaging sutures that facilitate their removal from the package and also maintain the sterility and integrity of the suture. Individual suture packages are commercially boxed and distributed on a rack in the sterile supply area. Boxes are stamped with an expiration date. Do not use any suture with an expired date, because quality and strength cannot be guaranteed beyond this date.

All sutures are double-wrapped in peel-apart envelopes. The *outer wrappers* are nonsterile on the outside but sterile on the inner surface. The *secondary sterile wrapper* is made of strong, transparent synthetic material, paper, or foil. Wrappers are notched for rapid removal.

The *inner envelope* is sterile both inside and outside. One face of the outer envelope is a transparent film that allows easy inspection of the data printed on the inner package. These data include the type, size, length, needle type and size (when applicable), date of manufacture, and expiration date of the suture. Inner packages are color coded, according to the type of suture, for quick selection (Figure 16-1, *B*). Each manufacturer uses its own color-coding system. Individual suture packets are boxed with 12 to 36 packets of sutures in each box.

The *inner wrapper* of a suture-needle combination is made of stiff paper. The swage of the needle is exposed so one can load the needle onto the needle holder without removing the entire suture. Packs of multiple needles expose each needle so needles can be easily counted and loaded.

Follow these guidelines when opening suture packages:

▶ Open the minimum number of suture packs required. As more are needed they can be quickly distributed. Stay ahead of the surgeon, however. If you are about to use the last few sutures, ask the surgeon how many more will be needed.
▶ Keep unopened suture packages clean.
▶ Most sutures are packed dry. Gut is packed in alcohol solution. This solution is highly flammable and must not be splashed onto the sterile field. When opening the inner pack of gut suture, empty the fluid onto a towel kept on the back table. Do not use this towel on the sterile field!
▶ Gut must be dipped in saline before use to soften it and prevent tissue drag. Do not soak gut sutures. Prolonged contact with saline weakens the strands.

▶ Dry-packed sutures should be stretched *slightly* to remove excess memory. Stainless steel sutures require careful handling to prevent glove puncture.

Since the adoption of swaged needles in surgery, the technique of rapid-sequence threading has been replaced by the use of multiple needle-suture packs. The manner in which the needle is packaged often determines how quickly and safely sutures can be passed to the surgeon. More paper is generated and many more needles are used than in the past, which increases the risk of needle loss or retention in the patient.

To prevent needle injury and keep pace with the surgeon, follow these guidelines:

▶ Keep suture packs organized on the Mayo stand or back table. Know where each type of suture is located.
▶ As soon as a needle is returned, immediately place it on the magnetic board or in the sharps holder.
▶ Have a loaded needle holder available at all times. Pass sutures on an exchange basis.
▶ If you are passing sutures to more than one surgeon at a time, work more slowly to avoid injury or needle loss. Safety is always more important than the schedule. For safety, use of the neutral zone (no-hands) technique is recommended. Review Chapter 15 for a discussion on neutral zone (no-hands) passing.
▶ Load the needle holder before removing the entire needle-suture combination from its package.
▶ Place suture wrappers in a sterile paper bag taped to the back table. This prevents suture wrappers from cluttering the Mayo stand. Do not use the sponge bucket for suture wrappers. A needle may be lost among the sponges, and it is extra work for the circulator to pick out the wrappers.
▶ Keep suture-needle packages organized by type. Always stay one package ahead of the surgeon.

PROPERTIES OF SUTURES

Advances in precision manufacturing and biochemical technology have produced many different kinds and configurations of suture materials. Most surgeons prefer to use the suture materials they were trained to use. Health-care institutions now enter into contracts with medical supply manufacturers, so the choice is often limited to the sutures produced by one company. Ultimately, the qualities most desired in selecting sutures are high tensile strength, ability to preserve maximum knot security, ease of handling, tendency to cause the least tissue reaction in the patient, and maintenance of high tensile strength for wound healing.

The choice of suture is based on the properties of the suture material. The selection depends on the physical properties, handling characteristics, knotting properties, tissue reaction characteristics, size of suture, and type of needle.

The mechanical and physical characteristics of the suture reflect its physical structure. These characteristics are most important for the security of the suture line.

Pliability

Pliability is flexibility. It describes the stiffness of a material. For example, cotton thread is more pliable than wire. Increased pliability allows a suture to be knotted more easily. Stiff sutures require more pulling and stretching for the knot to be fixed tightly.

Memory

Suture **memory** describes its recoil. When some materials are coiled or looped, they retain a "memory" of the coiled state and resist straightening, as does, for example, new nylon fishing line. Nylon suture has a high memory and tends to untie itself to try to return to its original state. When removed from their packages, some particular sutures are difficult to straighten for use and become tangled and knotted easily.

Tissue Drag

Friction of the suture against the tissue is called **tissue drag** and is a result of the type of coating and configuration (braided or **monofilament**) of the strand. Braided or twisted suture tends to have more drag than monofilament suture unless it is coated.

Elasticity

The amount of stretch or elongation exhibited by a suture strand when pulled is its **elasticity.** Excessive stretch can lead to suture weakening or breakage.

Tensile Strength

The strength of the suture material is important because the suture material must approximate the tissues together and be able to withstand knotting. The amount of force needed to break a strand of suture is called its tensile strength. The surgeon's choice of suture for a particular surgery depends, in part, on the amount of strength needed to hold the given tissue in place for healing to occur.

Knot Security

The knot is the weakest part of the suture. The tensile strength of the knot depends on the type of suture being used and the proper handling of the suture materials. If the suture is very slippery, the knot is more likely to slip. **Tie-down,** or tendency to resist knot slippage, is a quality that determines the extent to which a suture knot (referred to as a **throw**) will lie smooth and remain snug when tied. Increased tie-down increases the security of the knot and the suture line. Materials that are stiff *and* have strong memory

tend to untie. This can be a dangerous characteristic, especially when one is securing large blood vessels or suturing a wound that has increased internal tension.

Biological Reaction

Suture material is foreign to the body, that is, the body recognizes it as "nonself." The body's immune system reacts to suture as it would to *any* foreign material. The tissue becomes inflamed, and the body attempts to destroy the foreign material by breaking down the suture. The biological properties or reactivity of a suture determine the body's response to the material or its coating. High reactivity causes inflammation, discomfort, delayed healing or failure to heal, and possible infection. A suture that causes little or no tissue reaction is said to be very **inert.**

Inflammatory reaction is extremely important in certain tissues, such as those of the genitourinary system, where severe tissue irritation can lead to the formation of renal calculi (stones).

Sutures made of **multifilament** strands can absorb moisture or body fluids. In the presence of pathogenic bacteria, multifilament suture materials may draw more bacteria into the wound by **capillarity** (bacteria are drawn into the wound along the length of the suture), causing the suture to retain and spread infection within the suture fibers. Sutures with low capillarity (monofilament) capabilities are preferred when the risk of infection is high. Any material that causes inflammation should be avoided if the risk of postoperative infection is high or the wound is septic.

The current new generation of synthetic polymer sutures offers increased tensile strength, nonreactivity, and absorbability.

SUTURE MATERIALS

The configuration of the suture is the design of each strand:

▶ *Monofilament*—a single strand or fiber
▶ *Multifilament*—many strands or filaments twisted or braided together
▶ *Twisted*—multiple fibers twisted in the same direction
▶ *Braided*—multiple fibers that are braided (intertwined)

Suture materials are coated for ease of handling and to prevent friction (tissue drag) as they pass through tissue. A multifilament suture with a central core of multiple braided fibers may be coated with the same material to form a monofilament exterior. In the past, absorbable sutures were coated with nonabsorbable material such as beeswax, paraffin, or silicone. Newer sutures are now coated with absorbable materials consistent with the suture itself. Coatings that are similar to the suture are more biocompatible and cause less tissue reaction in the patient.

Figure 16-2 illustrates the design of monofilament and multifilament sutures.

Suture materials also are classified as being either absorbable or nonabsorbable. The surgeon chooses a category

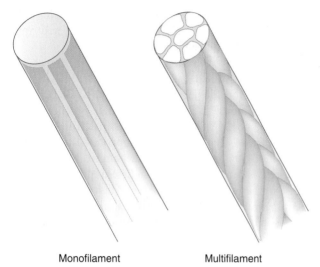

Monofilament   Multifilament

FIGURE 16-2
Monofilament and multifilament sutures. (Redrawn from Rothrock JC: *Alexander's care of the patient in surgery,* ed 12, St Louis, 2003, Mosby.)

of suture and then the type of suture within that category, depending on the type of tissue, its location in the body, the strength of the tissue, and the general condition of the patient.

The following terms typically apply to sutures:

▶ *Absorbable*—digested by the body within a short time
▶ *Nonabsorbable*—remain in the body indefinitely or for an undetermined period of time
▶ *Synthetic*—formed of manufactured materials
▶ *Natural*—made from naturally occurring tissue or plants such as cotton or collagen protein

Natural and Synthetic Absorbable Sutures

Absorbable sutures are those that the body digests or breaks down in a relatively short time. The amount of time the suture remains intact depends on the type of tissue, the size and type of absorbable suture, whether the wound is infected, and the general physical condition and age of the patient. Absorption can take from a week to several months. Absorbable suture is made of synthetic or natural materials. Synthetic absorbable sutures are those that are made of synthetic polymers. Synthetic absorbable sutures are hydrolyzed by *water,* which causes the breakdown of the polymer material. Natural absorbable sutures are made from collagen of healthy mammals. Natural absorbable sutures break down via the action of the body's *enzymes* and are absorbed.

SURGICAL GUT

Surgical gut is a naturally occurring material derived from the submucosa of sheep intestine or the serosa of beef intestine. Surgical gut is used on tissues that heal rapidly and is available in two forms: plain and chromic. *Plain* (untreated) *surgical gut* is quickly digested by the body and can cause significant inflammatory response. It retains its ten-

sile strength for 7 to 10 days. *Chromic gut* is treated with **chromic salt** to resist breakdown. Chromic gut resists digestion for up to 21 days, depending on the inflammatory response and other physiological factors. Both types of gut are absorbed rapidly in the presence of infection, and their use is contraindicated in wounds that are known to be contaminated and in debilitated patients. Under these circumstances, the use of surgical gut may lead to wound **dehiscence.**

Surgical gut is packaged in alcohol, which is a source of ignition on the surgical field. Do not open packages of surgical gut near the wound or electrosurgical unit. One prepares surgical gut for use by first dipping (not soaking) it in saline solution. This softens the strands so one can straighten them by grasping the end and pulling gently. One should be careful not to jerk the strands because this weakens them. Handling gut should be avoided as much as possible because continued contact and friction cause fraying of the suture.

Surgical gut is used in general soft-tissue approximation and ligation, including ophthalmic surgery.

Surgical gut is contraindicated for use in the following situations:

▶ When extended approximation of tissues under stress is required
▶ If the patient has known sensitivities or allergies to collagen or chromium
▶ On cardiovascular or neurological tissues

The colors of surgical gut are pale yellow (plain gut) and brown (chromic gut).

POLYGLYCOLIC ACID (BRAND NAMES: DEXON S AND DEXON II)

Polyglycolic acid was the first available synthetic absorbable suture material. It has high tensile strength compared with surgical gut and retains approximately 65% of its strength after 14 days in the wound. Dexon S is uncoated and is available braided or monofilament. Dexon II is a coated braided material. Knot security is good, and reactivity is minimal.

Polyglycolic acid suture is used in soft-tissue approximation and ligation, including ophthalmic surgery.

Polyglycolic acid suture is contraindicated for use on cardiovascular and neurological tissues.

The colors of polyglycolic acid suture are green and pale beige (undyed).

POLYGLACTIN 910 (BRAND NAMES: COATED VICRYL AND COATED VICRYL RAPIDE)

Polyglactin 910 suture is available braided or monofilament, and is coated to reduce tissue drag. It handles like polyglycolic acid suture but has greater tensile strength. At day 14 it retains 75% of its tensile strength in the wound. Complete absorption occurs between 56 and 72 days.

The uses of polyglactin 910 suture are general soft-tissue approximation, including ophthalmic procedures.

Polyglactin 910 sutures are contraindicated for use in the following situations:

▶ When extended approximation of tissue is required
▶ On cardiovascular and neurological tissues

"Rapid-absorption" polyglactin 910 is braided and absorbed more quickly than polyglactin 910. All tensile strength in the wound is gone between 10 and 14 days. It is completely absorbed within 42 days.

"Rapid absorption" polyglactin 910 is used for superficial soft-tissue approximation of the skin and mucosa only.

"Rapid absorption" polyglactin 910 is contraindicated for use in the following situations:

▶ When extended approximation of tissue under stress is required
▶ When wound support beyond 7 days is required
▶ For ligation, ophthalmic, cardiovascular, or neurological procedures

The colors of polyglactin 910 and "rapid absorption" polyglactin 910 are violet and pale beige (undyed).

LACTOMER (BRAND NAME: POLYSORB)
Lactomer is a synthetic polyester material composed of glycolide and lactide. It is a coated, braided, synthetic absorbable suture. It has excellent strength and knot security. It has good handling properties and a predictable absorption rate. Tensile strength remains at 80% at 14 days.

The uses of lactomer are soft-tissue approximation or ligation, including ophthalmic surgery.

Lactomer suture is contraindicated for use on cardiovascular and neurological tissues.

POLYDIAXANONE (BRAND NAME: PDS II)
Polydiaxanone suture is a synthetic monofilament material. It causes minimal tissue reaction and is usually used in wounds that are at risk for infection. At 14 days it has 70% of its original wound tensile strength. Absorption is complete at 6 months.

The uses of polydioxanone suture are all types of soft-tissue approximation, including pediatric, cardiovascular, and ophthalmic procedures.

Polydioxanone suture is contraindicated for use in the following situations:

▶ On adult cardiovascular tissue, microsurgery, and neurological tissue.
▶ When prolonged approximation of tissues under stress is required
▶ On prosthetic devices, such as synthetic grafts or heart valves

The colors of polydioxanone suture are violet, blue, and clear.

POLYGLYCONATE (BRAND NAME: MAXON CV)
Polyglyconate is a copolymer of glycolic acid and trimethylene carbonate. Polyglyconate suture is a monofilament, synthetic absorbable suture that causes little or no tissue reaction. It has high tensile strength and good knot tie-down. Polyglyconate retains 75% of its original tensile strength at 14 days.

The uses of polyglyconate suture are general soft-tissue approximation and ligation, including use in pediatric cardiovascular tissue, where growth is expected to occur, and in peripheral vascular surgery.

Polyglyconate sutures are contraindicated for use in adult cardiovascular tissue, ophthalmic surgery, microsurgery, and neural tissues.

The colors of polyglyconate suture are green and clear.

GLYCOMER 631 (BRAND NAME: BIOSYN)
Glycomer 631 suture is a monofilament, synthetic polyester material. It produces minimal tissue inflammation. It has excellent tensile strength and knot security, and has minimal memory. At 14 days it retains about 75% of its original strength. Absorption occurs between 90 and 110 days.

The uses of glycomer 631 suture are soft-tissue approximation and ligation, including ophthalmic surgery.

Glycomer 631 suture is contraindicated for use in cardiovascular or neurological surgery.

The colors of glycomer 631 suture are violet and pale beige (undyed).

POLIGLECAPRONE (BRAND NAME: MONOCRYL)
Poliglecaprone suture is a monofilament synthetic suture. It has excellent handling properties, good tie-down, minimal tissue drag, and high initial tensile strength. Tensile strength of the wound at 14 days is 20% to 30% for undyed suture, and 30% to 40% for dyed suture. Complete absorption takes from 90 to 120 days.

The use of poliglecaprone suture is general soft-tissue approximation and ligation.

Poliglecaprone is contraindicated for use in the following situations:

▶ When extended approximation of tissue under stress is required
▶ Because undyed suture is not indicated for use on fascia
▶ On cardiovascular and neurological tissues

The colors of poliglecaprone suture are violet and pale beige (undyed).

Natural and Synthetic Nonabsorbable Sutures
Nonabsorbable sutures are those that resist digestion by the body. Nonabsorbable sutures normally are encapsulated (enclosed in fibrous tissue) by the body. Nonabsorbable sutures also may be subdivided into those made of *natural fibers,* those made of *synthetic materials,* and those made of *metal.* Examples of natural fibers are silk and cotton.

SILK (BRAND NAMES: SOFSILK AND PERMA-HAND SILK SUTURE)
Sutures of natural silk are used today in spite of their inflammation-provoking properties. Use of silk sutures was common in the 1900s, and Halsted's original innovative

techniques in which many small interrupted silk sutures were placed remain the standard for technical excellence in wound closure. Many surgeons prefer the feel and handling qualities of silk. Because of its soft, pliable structure, silk is both supple and strong, and has good knot security. Surgical silk is braided and may be coated with silicone or wax

The uses of silk suture are general tissue approximation and ligation, including cardiovascular, ophthalmic, and neurological procedures.

Silk suture is contraindicated for use in patients with active infection or known sensitivities or allergies to silk.

The colors of silk suture are black and white.

COTTON

Surgical cotton suture is manufactured from the fibers of the cotton plant. It is a multifilament suture. Cotton sutures are used much less often than other types of suture. Cotton suture strengthens when dipped in normal saline before use. Cotton has low tensile strength, high capillary action, and inflammatory properties.

The main use of cotton suture is in gastrointestinal surgery. Cotton also is used in umbilical tapes, which are often used for retraction of delicate structures during surgical procedures.

The use of cotton suture is contraindicated in contaminated wounds.

The colors of cotton suture are white and blue.

NYLON (BRAND NAMES: ETHILON, DERMALON, MONOSOF, NUROLON, AND SURGILON)

Nylon was the first synthetic suture material available (1940) and is still widely used today. It is available in braided or monofilament strands. Dermalon, Monosof, and Ethilon are monofilament nylons. Nurolon and Surgilon are braided nylon sutures. Nylon is very inert in tissue. Monofilament nylon is very smooth and passes very easily through delicate tissues of the eye or blood vessels, and it also resists capillary action. Nylon has high tensile strength but can cut through tissue and in larger sizes is very stiff, is difficult to snug down in knots, and has low knot security. Nylon is considered a nonabsorbable suture material, but tensile strength diminishes over a period of time as a result of hydrolysis.

The uses of nylon suture include the following:

▶ Skin closure
▶ General soft-tissue approximation or ligation, including cardiovascular, ophthalmic, and neurological procedures

Nylon is contraindicated for use when permanent tensile strength is required.

The colors of nylon suture are black, blue, green, and clear.

POLYESTER (BRAND NAMES: ETHIBOND, MERSILENE, DACRON, TI-CRON, SURGIDAC, TEVDEK, NOVAFIL, AND VASCUFIL)

Polyester suture is braided or monofilament synthetic suture with high tensile strength. It causes little inflammatory reaction and is known for its minimal memory, good knot security, fray resistance, and ease of handling. Multifilament polyester is coated with silicon or Teflon to reduce tissue drag.

The uses of polyester suture include the following:

▶ Suturing in cardiac surgery
▶ Tendon repair
▶ Suturing in orthopedic surgery
▶ Vascular tissue suturing
▶ Suturing in ophthalmic surgery
▶ Suturing in neurosurgery
▶ General soft-tissue approximation and ligation

There are no known contraindications to use of polyester suture.

The colors of polyester suture are blue, green, and white (undyed).

POLYPROPYLENE (BRAND NAMES: PROLENE AND SURGIPRO)

Polypropylene suture is a synthetic monofilament suture with few or no inflammatory properties. Polypropylene is extremely smooth and is often used in skin closure and for cardiovascular surgery and microsurgery. It has high tensile strength and low memory. It retains nearly all its tensile strength over time and has good knot security.

The uses of polypropylene suture are general soft-tissue approximation or ligation, including use in cardiovascular, ophthalmic, and neurological procedures.
There are no known contraindications to use of polypropylene suture.

The colors of polypropylene suture are clear and blue.

SURGICAL STAINLESS STEEL

Stainless steel is the strongest of all suture materials. Stainless steel suture is widely used in orthopedic procedures and for approximation of the sternum and ribs in cardiothoracic surgery. Surgical stainless steel suture has minimal tissue drag and almost no inflammatory properties. It is available in monofilament and twisted multifilament configurations. Multifilament suture and strands are more flexible and resist stress breakage at flex points. When handling stainless steel suture, exercise caution to prevent puncturing your glove or a team member's glove. Always collect the suture ends and contain them as you would a sharp. Dispose of them in the sharps container at the close of surgery. Steel sutures often are passed with a hemostat clamped to the free end. This is called a tag.

The uses of stainless steel suture are abdominal wound closure, hernia repair, sternal closure, and orthopedic procedures, including cerclage and tendon repair.

Stainless steel is contraindicated for use in patients with known sensitivities or allergies to stainless steel, nickel, or chromium.

See Table 16-2 for a complete list of the types of absorbable and nonabsorbable suture materials described above.

Table 16-2   TYPES OF ABSORBABLE AND NONABSORBABLE SUTURE MATERIALS

Trade Name	Generic Name	Material	Color	Structure	Size
Absorbable Sutures					
Chromic Surgical Gut	Chromic surgical gut	Submucosa of sheep intestine or serosa of beef intestine; treated with salt solution	Brown	Monofilament	7-0 to 3
Plain Surgical Gut	Plain surgical gut	Submucosa of sheep intestine or serosa of beef intestine	Pale yellow	Monofilament	7-0 to 3
Dexon II	Polyglycolic acid (coated)	Homopolymer of glycolide	Pale beige (undyed), green	Braided	
Dexon S	Polyglycolic acid (uncoated)	Homopolymer of glycolide	Pale beige (undyed), green	Braided	
Vicryl Rapide	Polyglactin 910 (coated)	Copolymer of glycolide and lactide with polyglactin 379 and calcium stearate	Pale beige (undyed)	Braided, monofilament	5-0 to 1
Vicryl	Polyglactin 910 (coated)	Copolymer of glycolide and lactide with polyglactin 379 and calcium stearate	Violet, pale beige (undyed)	Braided	8-0 to 3
Polysorb	Lactomer (coated)	Copolymer of glycolide and lactide copolymer	Violet	Braided	8-0 to 2
PDS II	Polydioxanone	Polyester of poly (p-dioxanone)	Violet, blue, clear	Monofilament	9-0 to 2 (violet); 9-0 to 7-0 (blue)
Maxon CV	Polyglyconate	Copolymer of glycolide and trimethylene carbonate	Clear, green	Monofilament	7-0 to 1
Biosyn	Glycomer 631	Copolymer of glycolide, dioxanone, and trimethylene carbonate	Violet; pale beige (undyed)	Monofilament	7-0 to 2
Monocryl	Poliglecaprone	Copolymer of glycolide and epsilon-caprolactone	Violet, pale beige (undyed)	Monofilament	6-0 to 2
Nonabsorbable Sutures					
Sofsilk	Silk (coated with silicone or wax)	Natural fibroin silk fibers	Black	Braided	9-0 to 5 or 2
Perma-hand	Silk (coated with wax)	Natural fibroin silk fibers	Black, white	Braided	9-0 to 5
Ethilon	Nylon	Polyamide polymer	Green, black, clear (undyed)	Monofilament	11-0 to 2
Dermalon	Nylon	Polyamide polymer	Blue	Monofilament	6-0 to 1
Monosof	Nylon	Polyamide polymer	Black, clear	Monofilament	11-0 to 2
Nurolon	Nylon	Polyamide polymer	Black, clear (undyed)	Braided	6-0 to 1
Surgilon	Nylon (coated)	Polyamide polymer	Black, clear	Braided	7-0 to 2
Ethibond Excel	Polyester (coated)	Polymer of polyethylene and terephthalate	Green, white (undyed)	Braided	7-0 to 5
Mersilene	Polyester	Polymer of polyethylene and terephthalate	Green, white (undyed)	Braided, monofilament	6-0 to 5 (white, green); 10-0, 11-0 (green)
Ti-Cron	Polyester (coated or uncoated)	Polymer of polyethylene and terephthalate; coated with silicone or uncoated	Blue, white (undyed)	Braided	8-0 to 5

Data from Ethicon: *Wound closure manual*, Somerville, NJ, 1999.

Continued

Table 16-2	TYPES OF ABSORBABLE AND NONABSORBABLE SUTURE MATERIALS—cont'd				
Trade Name	Generic Name	Material	Color	Structure	Size
Nonabsorbable Sutures—cont'd					
Surgidac	Polyester (coated)	Polymer of polyethylene and terephthalate	Green, white (undyed)	Braided	5-0 to 5
Novafil	Polyester	Polymer of polyethylene and terephthalate	Green, blue, or white (undyed)	Monofilament	
Vascufil	Polyester (coated)	Polymer of polyethylene and terephthalate	Green, blue, or white (undyed)	Monofilament	
Steel	Stainless steel	Stainless steel	Steel	Monofilament	10-0 to 7
Steel	Stainless steel	Stainless steel	Steel	Multifilament	10-0 to 7

Data from Ethicon: *Wound closure manual,* Somerville, NJ, 1999.

SURGICAL NEEDLES

Surgical needles are precision made from high-quality stainless steel. The combination of metals used in the manufacturing process renders them strong and inert. Needles are available in several types according to their eye (area where suture is threaded or attached), shape or curvature, and point style.

Needle Eyes

Surgical needles have three distinct parts—the point, the body, and the eye. The eye of the needle is the point of attachment for the suture. There are three types of needle eyes: closed eye, French split or spring eye, and eyeless or swaged. The conventional closed-eye needle resembles a sewing needle, and the shape of the eye hole is rounded, rectangular, or square. True "eyed" needles are rarely used. French-eyed needles have two eyes connected by a slit from the top through the eyes with ridges that hold the sutures in place.

Most commercial needles are manufactured with the suture preattached to the needle eye area. This is called a **swage.** When eyeless or swaged suture-needle combinations were first manufactured, the suture was inserted by hand *inside* the eye end of the needle; this end was then crimped and sealed, which produced a nearly seamless connection between the needle and the suture. This innovation allowed for faster suturing, eliminated the need for individual sutures to be threaded, and minimized tissue trauma resulting from the extra loop of suture at the eye of the needle.

Today laser technology is used to drill a hole in the eye end parallel to the axis of the needle. The suture is inserted into the hole and sealed with an adhesive. A major advantage of the laser-drilled swage is that the surgeon can grasp the needle close to the back end without crushing the swage. With the traditional channel swage, the needle holder jaws must be forward of the swage by one-third the distance of the shaft.

A **control-release** suture (Figure 16-3) is one in which the surgeon releases the suture from the swage by pulling straight back sharply, rather than having to cut the suture. This allows the surgeon to quickly return the needle to the scrub and receive new sutures in rapid succession.

Double-armed sutures (Figure 16-4) are used to approximate blood vessels or other circular structures. When a dou-

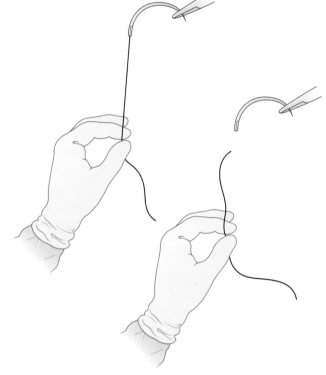

FIGURE 16-3
A control-release suture.

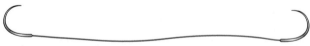

FIGURE 16-4
Double-armed suture.

ble-armed suture is passed, only one needle is mounted on the needle holder. The surgical technologist must take care during passing that the unsecured needle does not snag on drapes or other items on the surgical field.

Some surgeons prefer to use eyed needles rather than swaged ones. Eyed needles are identified by their shape and by the type of eye (Figure 16-5). Threading and passing eyed needles in rapid succession are skills that require practice.

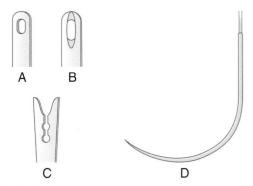

FIGURE 16-5
Eyed needles. **A** and **B,** Closed eye. **C,** French eye.
D, Swaged. (Redrawn from Phillips N: *Berry & Kohn's operating room technique,* ed 10, St Louis, 2004, Mosby.)

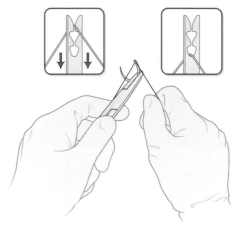

FIGURE 16-6
Threading a French eye or spring eye needle. (Redrawn from Phillips N: *Berry & Kohn's operating room technique,* ed 10, St Louis, 2004, Mosby.)

When the needle is threaded, the suture must be passed from the inside of the needle curve to the outside. The short end should extend approximately 4 inches from the eye. Both ends must be prevented from adhering to the shank of the needle holder. When the surgeon receives the suture, both the short and the long ends must be free.

The French or spring-eye needle was usually used before swaged sutures became available, and some surgeons still prefer them. When the spring-eye needle is threaded, the end of the suture is pressed down over the top of the spring, which causes it to snap into the eye (Figure 16-6). The suture should not be pulled through the eye after it is in place, because it may break.

Needle Curvature

The needle shape or curvature may vary according to its use. Curvature relates to the body and radius of the needle. Needle curvature is measured as the needle's fraction of the circumference of a complete circle. Curvatures designations are ¼, ⅜, ½, and ⅝ (Figure 16-7, *A*). Thus, a ½ curve needle is exactly one-half the distance around a circle.

In general, the deeper the tissue is in the surgical wound, the more acute the circle or curve should be. The curved needle allows the surgeon to dip beneath the surface of the tissue and retrieve the point as it emerges. The shape of the needle body determines the angle of insertion and emergence—that is, how close the insertion point is to the location where the needle resurfaces. Characteristics of a needle are illustrated in Figure 16-7, *B*.

The straight cutting needle (called a **Keith needle**) and ⅜ curve needle are usually used for skin closure. Compound needles are curved tightly at 80 degrees at the point end and decrease to 45 degrees near the back. These are used in ophthalmic surgery. The *size* of the needle is *not* related to the curvature. Size is simply another dimension of the needle. All curved needles are grasped with a needle holder.

A straight needle creates a linear path in tissue and therefore must be used in flat, superficial areas such as the skin. A straight needle is grasped between the fingers just as a normal sewing needle is.

Primary uses for needles on tissue:

▶ Straight needle: Skin, gastrointestinal tract, tendon, nerve, pharynx, oral cavity
▶ ¼ circle needle: Eye
▶ ⅜ circle needle: Skin, tendon, dura, eye, muscle, cardiovascular, gastrointestinal, urogenital, lung, periosteum, biliary tract, perichondrium, vessels
▶ ½ circle needle: Gastrointestinal, urogenital tract, muscle, fascia, pelvis, peritoneum, subcutaneous fat, skin, biliary tract, eye, oral cavity, nasal cavity, pharynx, respiratory tract
▶ ⅝ circle needle: Urogenital tract, pelvis, anal, nasal cavity, oral cavity
▶ Compound curved needle: eye

Needle Points

Many different types of needle points are available (Figure 16-8). There are, however, only three basic points, and all points are variations of these three types of points:

▶ Blunt
▶ Tapered
▶ Cutting

The **blunt needle** is a round shaft that is blunt at the tip. It *pushes tissue aside* as it moves through the tissue. It does not puncture the tissue, but slides between tissue fibers. It is the least traumatic and the safest of the needle points. It has traditionally been used only for suturing and for blunt dissection of friable tissues or organs that are soft and spongy, such as the liver, spleen, and kidney. It is gaining popularity for use in other tissues, however, because it significantly reduces the risk of needle-stick injury and transmission of blood-borne diseases.

The *tapered* needle has a round body that tapers to a sharp point. It punctures tissue, making an opening for the body of the needle to follow. Its primary use is for suturing soft tissue such as muscle, subcutaneous fat, peritoneum, dura, and gastrointestinal, genitourinary, biliary, and vascular tissue.

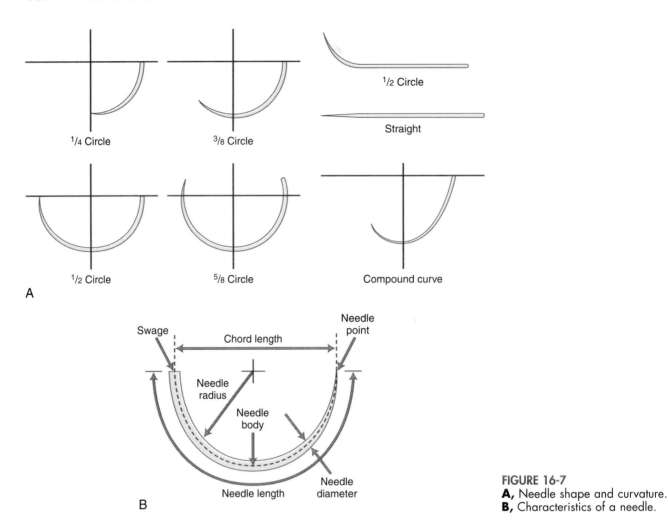

FIGURE 16-7
A, Needle shape and curvature.
B, Characteristics of a needle.

The *cutting* needle is one that is honed to form cutting edges on three sides. It has a triangular body with a sharp edge on each side and a third cutting edge on the inside or outside curve of the needle body. Needles whose third cutting edge is on the *inside* of the curve are called *conventional cutting needles.* Those with the cutting edge on the *outside or lower* edge of the curve are called **reverse cutting needles.** The cutting needle actually incises the tissue as it passes through it. Cutting needles are used on fibrous connective tissue such as the skin, joint capsule, and tendon. The regular cutting needle has the disadvantage of slicing tissue in an upward direction as the needle is drawn through the tissue. The reverse cutting needle solves this problem by locating the third, cutting edge on the outside of the curve, away from the direction of tension during suturing. It is stronger than the regular cutting needle and produces minimal scarring.

A relatively recent development is a cutting needle called the *tapercut,* which is a combination of a taper-point needle and a reverse cutting edge. The tapercut has a reverse cutting edge at the tip and a round body. Tapercut needles are used for suturing dense fibrous connective tissue, such as the fascia, tendon, and periosteum. Tapercut needle tips will not cut through these tissues as cutting sutures do, which can cause separation of the tissues.

Spatula needles are side-cutting needles that are designed flat on the top and the bottom, with side-cutting edges. This design eliminates unnecessary cutting out of tissue. These are designed and used for eye surgery to separate corneal and scleral tissue.

SUTURE TECHNIQUES

The surgical technologist should know what suturing technique is to be used so he or she can anticipate the number of suture packs needed. The surgical technologist may be required to cut sutures or perform other tasks. Suture placement is performed by the surgeon, the physician assistant, or other personnel permitted by hospital policy to assist.

The following instruments and supplies are needed for suturing:

▶ Correct suture and needle in the size specified. Do not open more than needed in advance to avoid waste.
▶ Tissue forceps. Delicate tissue requires smooth or vascular forceps. Fibrous connective tissue requires toothed forceps. The more delicate the tissue, the finer the teeth should be. Most surgeons use toothed Adson forceps for skin. Longer instruments are required for deeper tissue.

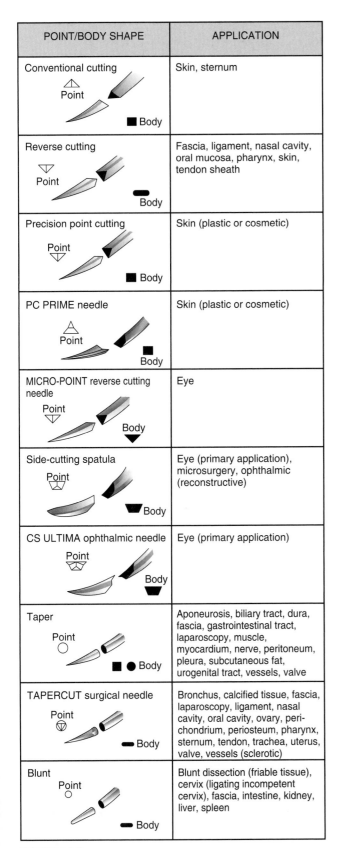

POINT/BODY SHAPE	APPLICATION
Conventional cutting	Skin, sternum
Reverse cutting	Fascia, ligament, nasal cavity, oral mucosa, pharynx, skin, tendon sheath
Precision point cutting	Skin (plastic or cosmetic)
PC PRIME needle	Skin (plastic or cosmetic)
MICRO-POINT reverse cutting needle	Eye
Side-cutting spatula	Eye (primary application), microsurgery, ophthalmic (reconstructive)
CS ULTIMA ophthalmic needle	Eye (primary application)
Taper	Aponeurosis, biliary tract, dura, fascia, gastrointestinal tract, laparoscopy, muscle, myocardium, nerve, peritoneum, pleura, subcutaneous fat, urogenital tract, vessels, valve
TAPERCUT surgical needle	Bronchus, calcified tissue, fascia, laparoscopy, ligament, nasal cavity, oral cavity, ovary, perichondrium, periosteum, pharynx, sternum, tendon, trachea, uterus, valve, vessels (sclerotic)
Blunt	Blunt dissection (friable tissue), cervix (ligating incompetent cervix), fascia, intestine, kidney, liver, spleen

FIGURE 16-8
Different types of needle points. (From *Wound closure manual*, Ethicon, Inc, Somerville, NJ, 1999.)

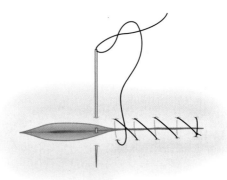

FIGURE 16-9
Continuous (running) suture.

▶ Suture scissors. Never use dissecting scissors for cutting suture. This rapidly dulls the blades and may put them out of alignment.
▶ Retractor to pull back superficial tissue layers as deeper layers are closed.

Continuous Sutures

Continuous suturing (also known as a **running suture**) uses one strand of suture to approximate tissue edges (Figure 16-9). The continuous suture can be placed rapidly, but if the suture breaks during the healing process, the wound could open along the entire length of the incision. Thus continuous sutures usually are used in areas of minimal stress.

Continuous suture is used on many different types of tissue, including peritoneum, blood vessels, muscle, fascia, joint capsule, and skin. When a continuous suture is placed, the suture is first pulled to nearly its full length at one end of the incision. The short end is secured with a hemostat or knotted in place. The surgeon then takes successive bites along the edges of the incision, pulling the suture snug but not tight with each stitch.

A subcuticular continuous suture is one in which the needle is threaded close to the surface of the skin but not through it (Figure 16-10). This type of suture is often used in plastic surgery or in pediatric procedures in which the suture must be buried. Subcuticular sutures often are sprayed with colloidal tissue adhesive to protect the wound edges. Minimal dressings are required.

A **purse-string** suture is a continuous suture used to approximate the open end of a lumen (hollow tubular structure) (Figure 16-11). The suture is threaded in and out of the edges of the lumen and drawn together like a purse-string. It is traditionally used during appendectomy to close the base of the appendix after the distal portion is removed.

Interrupted Sutures

Interrupted sutures are individually placed, knotted, and cut. Each stitch is a separate, secure unit. This technique is used when greater support is needed along the suture line (Figure 16-12). The simple interrupted suture is used in deep tissues and on skin. The *vertical* **mattress suture** (Figure 16-13, *A*) and *horizontal mattress suture* (Figure 16-13, *B*) offer increased strength to the wound.

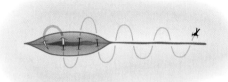

FIGURE 16-10
Subcuticular continuous suture.

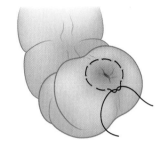

FIGURE 16-11
Purse-string suture.

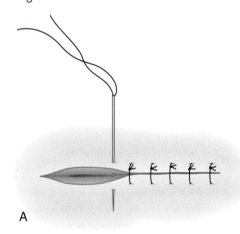

FIGURE 16-12
A, Interrupted suture. **B,** Deep interrupted suture.

Interrupted sutures are more reliable in areas that are under strain because the stress is distributed among all of the individual sutures. The surgeon's preference sometimes specifies whether the suture is to be continuous or interrupted. For example, the peritoneum or other membrane that closes a body cavity usually is closed with a continuous suture. This is because stress on the suture is minimal, and the tissue edges heal quickly. Closure of other tissues, such as fascia in the abdomen or skin tissue, may require the strength of individually tied sutures.

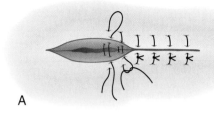

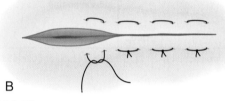

FIGURE 16-13
A, Vertical mattress suture. **B,** Horizontal mattress suture.

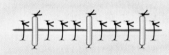

FIGURE 16-14
Retention suture.

Retention Sutures

Retention sutures are used in areas where great strength is required, such as in some abdominal incisions (Figure 16-14). They are used in conjunction with routine abdominal suture layers to add support to the closure. Heavy suture material, usually size 2 or 3 nylon or steel, is placed through the skin and carried down to the fascia or peritoneum on one side of the wound. The suture then is brought up through the layers of the opposite side, where it emerges through the skin. After the individual layers of the abdomen are closed, the two ends of the retention suture are threaded through **bolsters** (short lengths of rubber or Silastic tubing). The suture ends then are tied together. The bolsters distribute the pressure and prevent the heavy retention sutures from cutting into the patient's skin.

SELECTION AND USE OF SUTURES DURING SURGERY

Suture manufacturers identify their needles by code, usually a number or a letter-number combination. When selecting the sutures needed for a given procedure, consult the surgeon's preference information, which states the following:

▶ Name of the suture (e.g., Dexon II)
▶ Size of the suture (e.g., 3-0)
▶ Type of needle (e.g., ½ curve taper point)

Scrub tech

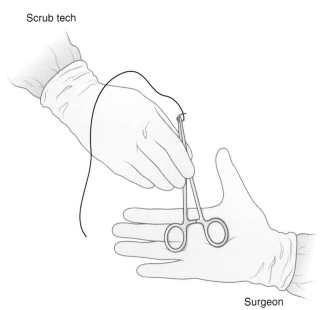

FIGURE 16-15
Passing a needle holder to the surgeon.

Surgeon

Needle type may be specified as the manufacturer's code number or as the type, such as "½ curve taper point for *sub Q*." This means that the surgeon wants a ½ curve round (rather than cutting) needle of the correct size to close the subcutaneous layer. Needles for very specific needs usually are requested by code number, such as in plastic or cardiovascular surgery.

This description does not yet supply all the information needed to select the correct needle-suture combination. The exact *size* of the needle is not stated. Many different sizes of ½ curve round needles are available. The surgeon assumes that the person selecting the materials knows the correct needle size for suturing the particular tissue layer. *One learns this by practice* and by familiarity with tissue types, anatomy, and each surgeon's preferences. Occasionally the surgeon might describe the kind of suture he or she needs, relying on the surgical technologist to list the types of needles available.

SUTURE PASSING TECHNIQUES

Needle Holder

During suturing, the surgeon pierces the flat plane of the tissue and rotates his or her wrist. This causes the needle to push through the tissue in a semicircular path and emerge a short distance from the entry site. The needle holder usually is passed to the surgeon with the point of the needle aimed toward the surgeon's chin (Figure 16-15). The positioning of the needle holder in relation to the suture needle depends on whether the surgeon is right-handed or left-handed. The long end of the suture should not come in contact with the surgeon's palm. It may be draped over the scrub's hand or allowed to hang downward.

Double-armed sutures have a needle at each end of the suture. These are passed with the second needle free.

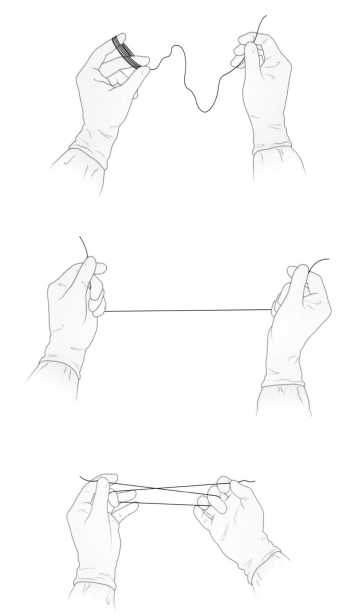

FIGURE 16-16
Cutting full-length suture strands. (Redrawn from Phillips N: *Berry & Kohn's operating room technique*, ed 10, St Louis, 2004, Mosby.)

Some surgeons prefer to receive them on a towel to prevent the needle from dragging across the drapes and snagging.

Suture Ties

Suture ties are available in precut or full-length strands. Precut ties range from 12 to 30 inches. Those that are not precut vary from 30 to 60 inches. The scrub must cut full-length sutures according to the surgeon's requirements. Long sutures are coiled. To avoid tangling the suture, place the coil over one hand and pull the free end slowly to uncoil. Pull gently at each end to remove some of the recoil (Figure 16-16, *A* and *B*).

When cutting full-length sutures into thirds, grasp each end of the strand and pull the center into thirds as shown in Figure 16-16, *C*.

Long suture strands also are available on **reels** or rolls. The reels are 54 inches long. The reel is distributed directly to the surgeon, who keeps it in his or her hand and uses it to tie **bleeders** in rapid succession.

If the wound is too deep to allow hand tying of a suture, the suture tie is placed in the tip of a long clamp. Right-angle clamps or those with a slight curve at the tip are used most often. This is called a **tie on a passer** (Figure 16-17). The surgeon might not ask for a passer; workers usually understand that one is needed because of the depth of the incision.

Ties (**ligatures**) on a large bleeding vessel must be secured into tissue to prevent them from slipping off. A suture-needle combination is passed through the middle of the vessel, and the ends of the suture are secured around the circumference. This is called a suture ligature or "**stick tie**" (Figure 16-18).

Vessel Clips

Vessel clips (often called Weck clips) are small **V**-shaped staples that close down and occlude a vessel. Small, medium, and large clips are available in small cartridges that are color-coded by size. The size of the *clip applier* must be matched to the size of the clip (Figure 16-19). To load the clip, grasp the proper size clip applier at the hinge. Press the open jaws of the applier *straight down* over the clip. This will lock the clip into the jaws. Pass the clip applier with the tip down, taking care not to squeeze the handles, which would release the clip prematurely.

SUTURE REMOVAL AND CUTTING TECHNIQUES

Removal of Old Sutures

When the surgeon needs to remove old (deep) sutures from a previous surgery, the knots usually are embedded in scar tissue and may be difficult to grasp and cut. A *straight, fine-tipped* hemostat works best for pulling out old sutures. If the sutures require cutting, fine-tipped suture scissors or even a sharp, pointed knife blade (such as a No. 11) may be used. One always should provide a towel on which the surgeon can deposit the old suture pieces so they do not drop back into the wound.

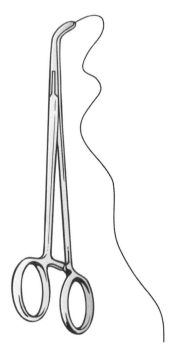

FIGURE 16-17
Tie on a passer. (Redrawn from Phillips N: *Berry & Kohn's operating room technique*, ed 10, St Louis, 2004, Mosby.)

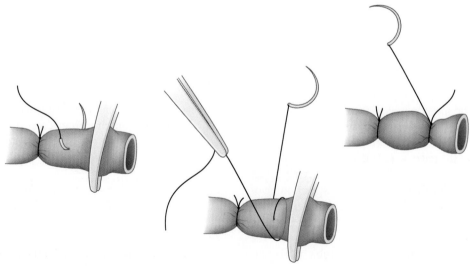

FIGURE 16-18
Suture ligature or "stick tie."

Cutting of Suture Ends

Occasionally the surgeon asks the surgical technologist to cut suture ends when tying a knot. When sutures are cut, the ends must be short to reduce the amount of foreign material in the wound, but long enough that the knot does not untie. When the suture is cut too short, the knot may actually be cut. If this happens, the surgeon replaces the suture with another. Some hospitals do not allow the surgical technologist to cut sutures, because this may be defined as *first assisting*. The institution might restrict such duties to licensed personnel only.

The proper technique for cutting sutures is as follows:

▶ Use only sharp suture scissors; *never* use tissue scissors on suture material.
▶ To cut the suture, open the scissors slightly. *Use only the tip* of the scissors to cut, never the midportion of the blades. Using the tip of the scissors allows more precise cutting.
▶ Hold the scissors as shown in Figure 16-20.
▶ Place your index finger over the top of the scissors to steady the blades. Turn the scissors at a 45-degree angle. This creates a small "whisker." Cut the suture ends while keeping the scissors at an angle.
▶ If you slide the scissors down to the knot and cut, you probably will cut too close and cause the knot to untie.

▶ The more steeply you angle the blades, the longer the whisker will be. It is desirable to leave as little foreign material in the wound as possible, while also leaving enough length to prevent the knot from slipping loose.
▶ When cutting sutures and performing other tasks at the same time, it is convenient to "palm" the scissors in one hand (Figure 16-21).
▶ Remove any cut suture ends from the wound area to prevent them from falling into the wound.

SURGICAL STAPLING DEVICES

Surgical stapling instruments have dramatically advanced the field of wound closure. This family of wound-closure products includes vessel-ligation and wound-approximation instruments as well as those that both divide and approximate or anastomose tissue. Staplers are available as single-use medical devices or stainless steel instruments. Both types use manufactured cartridges. Reusable devices that cut also must be loaded with a knife and anvil assembly. Each type of instrument holds a cartridge that contains a prescribed number and size of staples that fire individually or together in single, double, triple, or quadruple lines. Each type of instrument has specific applications. The advantages of surgical staplers are listed below:

▶ Tissue handling is greatly minimized, thus reducing trauma by manipulation and exposure.

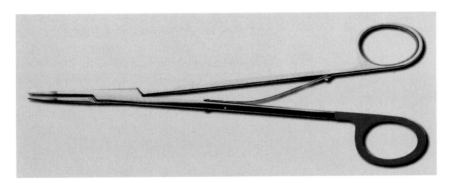

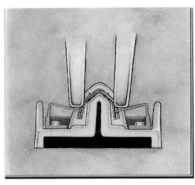

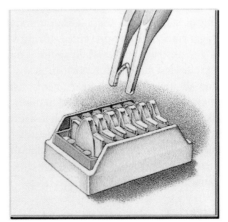

FIGURE 16-19
Loading a vessel (or Weck) clip. (Courtesy Weck Industries, Research Triangle Park, NC.)

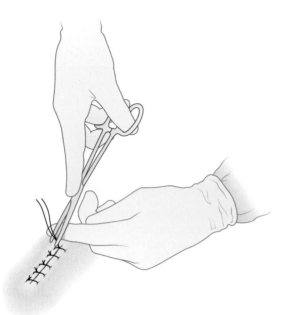

FIGURE 16-20
Proper way to hold suture scissors.

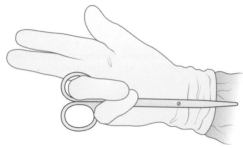

FIGURE 16-21
"Palming" suture scissors.

▶ The suture lines are strong and dependable.
▶ The staples are nonreactive in tissue.
▶ The staples are noncrushing, thereby preventing tissue necrosis resulting from compromised blood and nutrient supply to the tissue edges.

The surgical technologist must become familiar with the proper handling of staplers and the loading of staple cartridges. Much aggravation can be prevented during surgery if one studies the instruments carefully before they are needed. There are several manufacturers of surgical stapling instruments, and all are reliable. The instruments discussed in this text are available through the United States Surgical Corp. (Norwalk, Conn.), and the name of each instrument is that applied by this company only; however, the function of the instruments will be similar to those manufactured by other companies. These instruments have been chosen for discussion because of their widespread use.

Premium Surgiclip

The Premium Surgiclip is a disposable clip applier used to occlude vessels and other tubular structures, and for vagotomy, sympathectomy, and radiographic markings (Figure

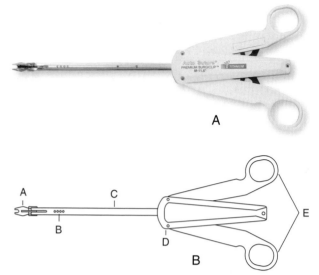

FIGURE 16-22
A, Premium Surgiclip clip applier. **B,** Schematic view of Premium Surgiclip clip applier: (A) Clip applier jaw. (B) Alert indicator window. (C) Preloaded applier shaft. (D) Palm grip. (E) Handles. (Courtesy United States Surgical Corporation, Norwalk, Conn.)

16-22). It consists of an applier shaft with attached handles and an integral cartridge containing 15 or 20 titanium clips. The clip applier jaw is placed around a vessel or other tubular structure. As the handles of the applier are released, a new clip is automatically loaded into the clip applier jaw.

Powered Disposable LDS Stapler

The Powered Disposable LDS stapler is used in abdominal, gynecological, and thoracic surgery for ligating and dividing blood vessels and other tubular structures (Figure 16-23). The instrument places two stainless steel staples to ligate the tissue within the cartridge jaw, and the knife divides the tissue between the two closed staples. One activates the instrument by squeezing the instrument handle.

Premium Multifire TA Disposable Surgical Stapler

The Premium Multifire TA Disposable Surgical Stapler is used for resection and transection in many types of surgical procedures (Figure 16-24). This instrument places a double or triple staggered row of titanium staples, depending on the model used. One activates the instrument by squeezing the handle. The choices of staple size are the V, the 3.5, and the 4.8 sizes.

Auto Suture TA 90 B and TA 90 BN Stapling Instruments

The Auto Suture TA 90 and TA 90 BN are used only in bariatric surgery (those dealing with obesity, i.e., stomach stapling procedures) (Figure 16-25). These instruments place four equidistant staggered rows of stainless steel staples. One activates each instrument by squeezing the handle. The notch in the instrument head of the TA 90 BN stapling

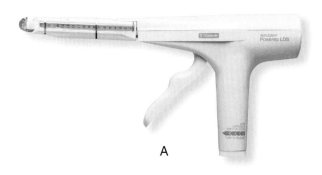

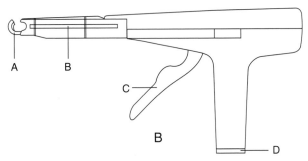

FIGURE 16-23
A, Powered Disposable LDS stapler. **B,** Schematic view of Powered Disposable LDS stapler: (A) Cartridge jaw. (B) Staple counter. (C) Moveable handle. (D) Knob. (Courtesy United States Surgical Corporation, Norwalk, Conn.)

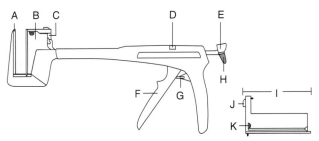

FIGURE 16-24
Schematic view of Premium Multifire TA stapler: (A) Anvil. (B) Metal cartridge housing. (C) Pin retainer (white). (D) Tissue approximation window. (E) Upper approximating button (white). (F) Handle. (G) Safety. (H) Lower approximating button (gray). (I) Single-use loading unit (SULU). (J) Pin slide (clear). (K) Finger pads. (Courtesy United States Surgical Corporation, Norwalk, Conn.)

instrument creates a channel 1 cm wide on activation of the disposable unit.

Auto Suture TA Premium 55 Surgical Stapling Instrument

The Auto Suture TA Premium 55 surgical stapling instrument is used in abdominal and thoracic surgery for resection and transection (Figure 16-26). Using a disposable loading unit, the TA Premium 55 places a row of titanium sutures. When used in conjunction with the Premium Polysorb 55 loading unit, it places a double staggered row of lactomer absorbable copolymer staplers. The size of the staple is determined by the choice of the loading unit.

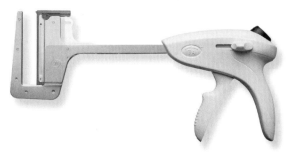

FIGURE 16-25
Auto Suture TA 90 stapler. (Courtesy United States Surgical Corporation, Norwalk, Conn.)

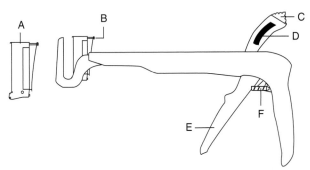

FIGURE 16-26
Schematic view of Auto Suture TA 55 Premium stapler: (A) Disposable loading unit. (B) Retaining pin. (C) Approximating lever. (D) Black markings. (E) Handle. (F) Safety. (Courtesy United States Surgical Corporation, Norwalk, Conn.)

Multifire GIA 60 or 80 Disposable Surgical Stapler

The Multifire GIA 60 or 80 disposable surgical stapler (Figure 16-27) and Multifire 60 or 80 disposable loading units are used for resection and creation of **anastomoses** in abdominal, gynecological, pediatric, and thoracic surgery. This instrument places two double-staggered rows of titanium staples and simultaneously divides the tissue between the two double rows.

Auto Suture GIA 50 Premium Surgical Stapler

The Auto Suture GIA 50 Premium surgical stapler (Figure 16-28) is used in abdominal, gynecological, pediatric, and thoracic surgery for resection, transection, and creation of anastomoses. The Auto Suture GIA 50 disposable loading unit is used in surgical procedures that require placement of four parallel staple lines. It places two double staggered rows of stainless steel staples and simultaneously divides the tissue between the two double rows.

Roticulator 30 and 30-V3 Disposable Surgical Stapler

The Roticulator 30 and 30-V3 disposable staplers (Figure 16-29) are used in many different types of surgical procedures for resection and transection. The Roticulator 30 places a double staggered row of stainless steel staples, and the 30-V3 model places a triple staggered row of staples. The

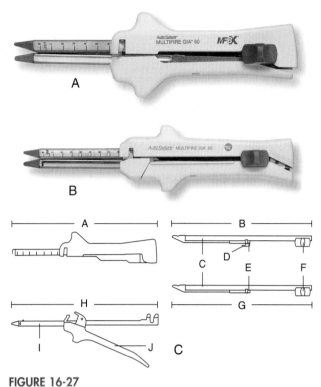

FIGURE 16-27
A, Multifire GIA 60 stapler. **B,** Multifire GIA 80 stapler.
C, Schematic view of Multifire GIA 60 stapler: (A) Cartridge half. (B) Single-use loading unit (SULU). (C) Cartridge. (D) Tissue gap control mechanism. (E) Push-bar knife assembly. (F) Plastic handle. (G) Knifeless single-use loading unit (SULU). (H) Anvil half. (I) Anvil fork. (J) Lock lever. (Courtesy United States Surgical Corporation, Norwalk, Conn.)

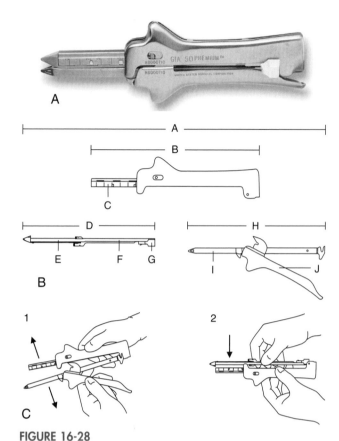

FIGURE 16-28
A, Auto Suture GIA 50 Premium stapler. **B,** Schematic view of Auto Suture GIA 50 Premium stapler: (A) GIA 50 Premium stapler. (B) Cartridge half. (C) Cartridge fork. (D) Single-use loading unit (SULU). (E) Cartridge. (F) Push-bar mechanism. (G) Plastic knob. (H) Anvil half. (I) Anvil fork. (J) Handle. **C,** Loading the Auto Suture GIA 50 Premium stapler. (Courtesy United States Surgical Corporation, Norwalk, Conn.)

size of the staples is determined by the selection of the 3.5, 4.8, or vascular staple size.

Auto Suture Premium Plus CEEA

The Auto Suture Premium CEEA disposable surgical stapler (Figure 16-30) is used in general, thoracic, and bariatric surgery for creation of end-to-end, end-to-side, and side-to side anastomoses. The instrument places a circular, double staggered row of titanium staples. Immediately after staple formation, a knife blade in the instrument resects the excess tissue, thus creating a circular anastomosis. One activates the instrument by squeezing the handles firmly as far as they will go. The Low Profile Anvil for use with the CEEA is used in procedures in which the anvil normally supplied with the CEEA is too tall for comfortable use. After the Low Profile Anvil is attached to the center shaft it is permanently affixed and cannot be removed.

Auto Suture Purse-string

The Auto Suture Purse-string (Figure 16-31) is a disposable automatic purse-string instrument. It is used in intestinal, colorectal, and esophageal surgery to place temporary purse-string closures. It places a circumferential strand of 2-0 monofilament nylon held in place by stainless steel staples.

The stainless steel staples are attached to the structure of the organ where a purse-string closure is desired.

Auto Suture Multifire Premium Disposable Skin Stapler

The Auto Suture Multifire Premium disposable skin stapler (Figure 16-32) is used for skin closure in abdominal, gynecological, orthopedic, and thoracic surgery. It also may be used to close incisions in vein stripping, thyroidectomy, and mastectomy procedures; for scalp closure or incisions; for skin grafts; and in plastic and reconstructive surgery. The instrument places one staple each time the instrument handles are activated.

TISSUE ADHESIVES

The primary use of a tissue adhesive is to seal the bleeding surface of the intestine or a highly vascular organ such as the liver or spleen. For the tissues to eventually heal, the binding material must be absorbable. This requires a biodegradable product that is liquid when applied but semisolid when cured. Tissue adhesives used in surgery are derived from bi-

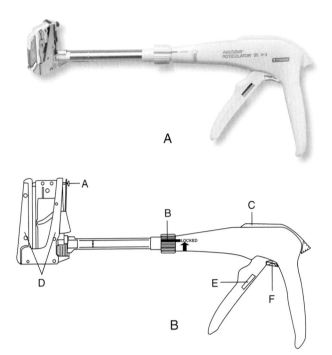

FIGURE 16-29
A, Roticulator TA 30-V3 Disposable stapler. **B,** Schematic view of Roticulator TA 30-V3 Disposable stapler: (A) Retaining pin. (B) Lock mechanism. (C) Approximating lever. (D) Instrument jaws. (E) Handle lock. (F) Safety. (Courtesy United States Surgical Corporation, Norwalk, Conn.)

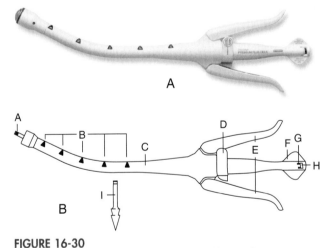

FIGURE 16-30
A, Auto Suture Premium CEEA disposable stapler. **B,** Schematic view of Auto Suture Premium CEEA disposable stapler: (A) Orange band. (B) Centimeter markings. (C) Instrument shaft. (D) Safety release. (E) Instrument handles. (F) Wing nut. (G) Black markings. (H) Approximation indicator. (I) White trocar. (Courtesy United States Surgical Corporation, Norwalk, Conn.)

ological sources like collagen and human fibrin. Tissue adhesives also are often used for skin closure.

Fibrin Glue
Fibrin glue is the most common type of tissue adhesive used in surgery. In structure and action it is similar to the body's

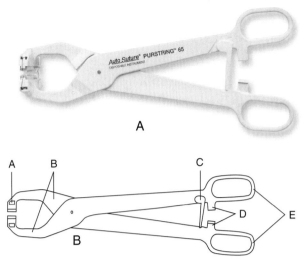

FIGURE 16-31
A, Auto Suture Purse-string stapler. **B,** Schematic view of Auto Suture Purse-string stapler: (A) Purse-string slot. (B) Jaws. (C) Safety. (D) Handle lock. (E) Ring handle. (Courtesy United States Surgical Corporation, Norwalk, Conn.)

normal clotting process. The presence of additional fibrin on the wound surface encourages increased endothelial cell growth and also hastens the development of new blood vessels at the healing site.

Because of the risk of blood-borne disease transmission, fibrin from human sources is rigidly tested and purified before manufacture. The components must be mixed just before use. The kit is stored at a temperature below 10° C and then thawed to room temperature. The order of mixing is critical. Always follow the manufacturer's directions. The aqueous solution is mixed with fibrinogen powder. A second vial of aqueous liquid is mixed into thrombin powder. The solutions are drawn up into separate syringes and loaded into a cartridge fitted with a Y connector (Figure 16-33). The surgeon then injects both components simultaneously over the tissue surface. A pressurized spray system also is available.

Synthetic Cement
The synthetic cement methyl methacrylate is frequently used to secure prosthetic implants into bone and in cranioplasty procedures during remodeling of bones. Methyl methacrylate is a highly noxious material whose fumes are damaging to mucous membranes. Therefore a system of closed mixing has been devised. The scrub must mix together the two components—a liquid and a powder—just before use. The cement must be used at a precise stage of drying to be molded to the bone tissue. The manufacturer's recommendations for proper mixing and safety precautions should be followed.

Surgical Mesh
When two incision edges have extreme tension or a tissue plane has a pathological tear, mesh products are used to bridge

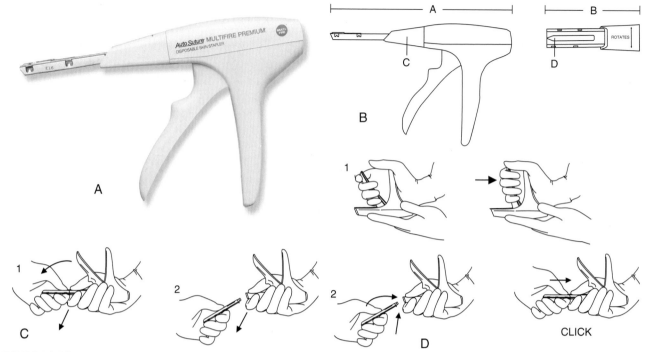

FIGURE 16-32
A, Auto Suture Multifire Premium disposable stapler. **B,** Schematic view of Auto Suture Multifire Premium disposable stapler: (A) Side view. (B) Instrument nose (top). (C) Instrument nose (rotating). (D) Locating arrow. **C,** Unloading the Auto Suture Multifire Premium disposable stapler. **D,** Reloading the Auto Suture Multifire Premium disposable stapler. (Courtesy United States Surgical Corporation, Norwalk, Conn.)

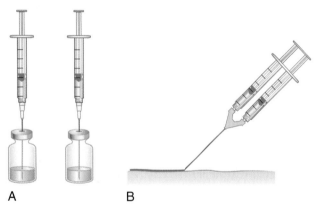

FIGURE 16-33
Loading and injecting fibrin glue.

the gap and effectively expand the available tissue. This relaxes the tension and allows healing. Mesh is used to close defects in the abdominal wall and in hernia repair to strengthen and widen the defect. Mesh is available in four materials:

▶ Stainless steel
▶ Polyester fiber
▶ Polypropylene
▶ Polyglactin 910

Stainless steel mesh causes little or no inflammatory response in tissue but is difficult to work with because of its stiffness. Polyester and polypropylene meshes are strong and relatively inert (cause little inflammation). They are

also flexible and can be easily shaped and molded to fit the defect. Polyglactin 910 mesh is absorbable and therefore supportive only during the healing phase. When mesh is used, it is cut to fit the defect and sutured directly to tissue edges. Nonabsorbable suture is used to secure the mesh patch.

PROCESS OF WOUND HEALING

Physiology of Wound Classification
Recall from Chapter 7 that wounds are classified according to the risk of contamination during surgery. This classification system is important in understanding wound healing. The classification is presented again in Box 16-1.

The human body is extremely efficient in its ability to recover from trauma. The patient's surgical wound actually starts healing as soon as the surgeon makes the skin incision. For a wound to heal, collagen and blood vessels must be generated on both sides of the wound edges.

Wound healing occurs in three stages (Figure 16-34):

Substrate phase (or inflammation)
Proliferative phase (or tissue formation)
Remodeling phase (or matrix formation)

SUBSTRATE PHASE
The first stage in wound repair is called the substrate phase, also often called *lag phase* (or inflammation phase), and usually lasts from 1 to 4 days. The substrate phase is necessary to

Box 16-1 Wound Classification

Clean Wound (1% to 5% risk of postoperative infection)

Example: total hip replacement, vitrectomy, nerve resection

▶ Uninfected

▶ Clean

▶ No inflammation

▶ Closed primarily (all tissue layers sutured closed)

▶ The respiratory, gastrointestinal, genital, or uninfected urinary tracts are not entered

▶ May contain closed drainage system

Clean-Contaminated Wound (3% to 7% risk of postoperative infection)

Example: cystoscopy, gastric bypass, and removal of oral lesion

▶ Respiratory, gastrointestinal, genital, or urinary tracts are entered without unusual contamination

▶ No evidence of infection or major break in aseptic technique

▶ Includes operations of the biliary tract, appendix, vagina, and oropharynx

Contaminated Wound (10% to 17% risk of postoperative infection)

Example: removal of perforated appendix, removal of metal fragments related to an explosion

▶ Open, fresh, accidental wound

▶ Surgical procedure in which a major break in aseptic technique has occurred

▶ Gross spillage from the gastrointestinal tract occurs

▶ Acute, nonpurulent inflammation is present

Dirty or Infected Wound (>27% risk of postoperative infection)

Example: incision and drainage of an abscess

▶ Old traumatic wounds with devitalized tissue

▶ Existing clinical infection

▶ Perforated viscera

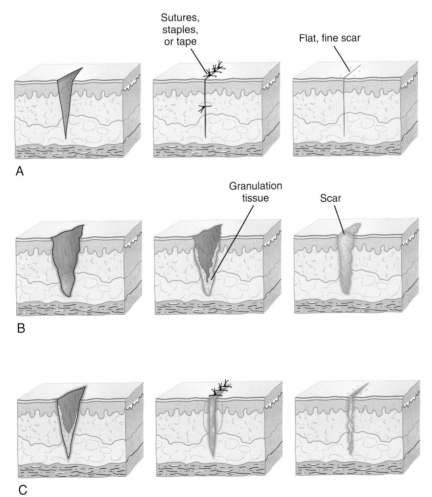

FIGURE 16-34

Stages of wound closure. **A,** First intention. **B,** Second intention. **C,** Third intention.

establish hemostasis and begin mobilization of the immune system. Initially the tissue responds to trauma with a brief period of vasoconstriction. Small blood vessels constrict, then dilate. This mechanism brings increased blood supply to the area of injury and also brings plasma protein and other agents that defend the injured tissue.

This inflammatory stage is followed by one of hemostasis. Small blood vessels contract in an attempt to control hemorrhage. Blood platelets begin to fill the lumens of the capillaries and arterioles and act as tiny "plugs." After a complex series of chemical reactions at the site of injury, the body releases a substance called fibrin to the wounded tissue, and clotting begins. The fibrin forms into networks that collect red blood cells, platelets, and white blood cells. During the *lag* phase of healing, clotted blood and fibrin cover the incision, which attracts neutrophils to the area.

About 14 hours after trauma, cellular changes appear at the wound site. Special white blood cells release substances into the tissue that help clean the wound of tissue debris, unneeded cellular components, and bacteria. In the first 2 days after surgery, the basement layer of the epidermis begins to grow rapidly, and by the third day macrophages outnumber neutrophils. Granulation tissue containing fibroblasts and newly formed capillaries increases at the wound site. Collagen synthesis is necessary to form scar tissue. During this time the strength of the wound depends on the wound closure materials.

PROLIFERATIVE PHASE

The second phase of wound healing is the proliferative stage (or tissue formation phase). This phase of wound healing lasts from 5 to 20 days. It is during this phase that tissue is actually repaired. During the proliferative phase, collagen fibers form a network or bridge between the wound edges, and this is followed by epithelial migration into the collagen network. Wound strength increases steadily, and the sutures are removed at the end of this stage. New cells form and, in some areas of the body, the wound contracts. Wound contraction occurs when a large wound closes without scarring or forming permanent fibrous tissue (cicatrization). Wound contraction takes place on the back, buttocks, and posterior neck.

REMODELING PHASE

The last stage of wound repair, the remodeling phase, begins on the twenty-first day. During this phase the wound regains the original strength that it had before trauma. During the remodeling phase, which lasts from 22 days to 1 year, the collagen is continually replaced and absorbed in stress areas. Through a complex series of cellular activities, collagen, a fibrous protein substance that gives the wound its strength, is formed. The wound regains its former strength. When proliferation of collagen is excessive, the scar is called a keloid scar. This phase of wound healing also is called the *maturation* phase.

Wound Healing Categories

Wounds are classified by the way they are repaired and heal. Wound healing is described by the technique used to close the wound. Refer to Figure 16-34, which illustrates types of wound closure.

FIRST INTENTION

The clean wound that is sutured closed and heals with minimal scarring and without incident does so by **first intention** (or primary union). It is the ideal closure for all surgical procedures. The wound edges are brought together throughout all layers in normal anatomical position. There are no gaps in closure, and edges adhere quickly after surgery. During healing there is minimal scar formation and no infection present.

SECOND INTENTION

When the wound is not closed, such as in the presence of infection, it heals by a process called granulation (healing from the bottom up) and is said to heal by **second intention** closure. Traumatic or infected wounds often are left to heal through second intention, because closing the wound with sutures would increase infection. Most sutures do not remain in the body in the presence of inflammation, phagocytes, and bacterial enzymes. During healing the wound must be protected from drying out and is packed with moist dressings. As these dry, they are removed, which at the same time removes necrotic tissue and pus that adhere to the dry dressing. Fresh moist dressings are applied, and the process is repeated. Healing may require weeks to months, because the tissue edges are constantly inflamed until the infection subsides. If there is no infection, the wound is filled slowly with granulation tissue, and the scar slowly shrinks.

THIRD INTENTION

Healing by **third intention** is usually called delayed primary closure. Delayed closure occurs when suturing must be postponed or when the wound is closed primarily, then dehisces, and is sutured at a later date. Delayed closure may be performed when the wound is infected or requires continuous irrigation. Wounds that have dehisced usually have ragged or weak edges that must heal before closure can remain secure.

Complications in Wound Healing
INFECTION

The presence of infection causes increased *collagenolysis*. This is the breakdown of collagen tissue near the incision site and is necessary to build new collagen at the incision. Collagenolysis occurs most often in bowel tissue and may result in a breakdown of tissue some distance from the original wound site. Wounds with blood or fluid pockets have a much higher incidence of postsurgical infection.

HEMATOMA OR SERUM ACCUMULATION

As previously stated, a hematoma or blood-filled pocket may become a reservoir for infection. All attempts are made to remove free fluid from the wound. If continuous production of serum or serosanguineous fluid is anticipated, a surgical drain is placed before wound closure (see Chapter 15).

DEAD SPACE

A dead space is an area in the wound that is not brought back into normal anatomical proximity. For example, when an abdominal wound is closed in routine order—peritoneum, fascia, subcutaneous layer, and skin layer, little or no space is left between tissue layers. If, however, the subcutaneous layer were to remain open while the other layers were closed, a dead space would occur between the fascia and the skin. This space is subject to infection, because blood and serous fluid flow into it, providing an excellent culture medium for bacteria.

TISSUE TRAUMA

When tissue is bruised, macerated, and dry, normal wound healing is prevented. The tissue may be ischemic or the inflammatory response may overwhelm the normal process of collagenolysis and formation of new collagen.

POOR NUTRITION

Nutrition is among the most important contributions to rapid wound healing. The body requires extra protein and carbohydrates during the proliferation phase, because metabolism is higher during this time. Protein deficiency deprives the body of nutrients needed to form new tissue.

WOUND TENSION

Excessive tension on the wound can cause destruction of tissue, a premature breakdown in the suture line, and ultimately wound dehiscence (splitting open). Infection and further delay in normal healing may follow. To prevent wound dehiscence, retention sutures usually are placed to reinforce primary suture lines and also may be placed in large or obese patients. These are sutures that pass through the skin and all other tissue layers to add strength to the suture line. Skin protectors (sometimes called "bolsters") are threaded over the retention sutures to prevent discomfort and trauma to the skin. Retention sutures are placed before individual tissue layers are sutured. After all individual layers have been closed, the retention sutures are tied.

INADEQUATE BLOOD SUPPLY

Adequate blood supply is needed to bring cell components to the wound site and remove dead cells and waste products. Areas that heal very quickly usually are those that are highly vascular, including the head, face, mouth, and mucous membranes.

CHRONIC DISEASE

Chronic diseases such as diabetes mellitus and kidney disease have a negative effect on wound healing. Normal metabolic function is needed for the removal of waste cells and the building of new tissue.

DEHISCENCE

Wound dehiscence is the separation and opening of the wound edges. This generally occurs shortly after the surgery and can be caused by one or more of the following conditions:

▶ Surgical site infection
▶ Excessive pressure on the wound site, usually related to the patient's size or weight
▶ Poor nutrition
▶ Diseases that constrict blood vessels and inhibit the healing process, such as diabetes mellitus

When dehiscence occurs, the underlying body contents may spill out of the wound. This is called **evisceration** and requires immediate surgical repair. If the wound is infected, one or two layers may be closed with inert sutures and the remaining tissues left to heal by third intention.

CASE STUDIES

Case 1

The surgeon asks you for size 2-0 silk suture. After you have given the surgeon the suture, you realize that you have mistakenly passed a 3-0 suture. The surgeon has already inserted the suture and is about to tie it. What will you do?

Case 2

You placed a package of surgical gut in a basin to rinse it and make it more pliable. You forgot that the suture was in the basin, and now it is very limp. Is it safe to use?

Case 3

While you are passing a double-armed suture, the free needle snags on the drapes and breaks. What is the next step?

Case 4

You have been working on a vascular case for 3 hours. You are completely out of silk ties. When should you have requested more ties? After you receive the ties from the circulator, you cannot take the time to place them under the Mayo stand towel. Now you have three packages of ties in three different sizes. The ties are mixed up on top of the Mayo stand in no particular order. What problems can this cause, and how should you have avoided this problem?

Case 5

At the close of the case, the surgeon's assistant leaves to attend to another patient. The surgeon asks you to cut sutures for him. When you cut the first suture, you slice through the knot and the suture comes out. What is the next step?

REFERENCES

Ethicon Endo-Surgery website: *Atlas of surgical stapling,* Somerville, NJ, 1999.

Ethicon: *Wound closure manual,* Somerville, NJ, 1999.

Terhune M: Materials for wound closure, *eMedicine Journal* 3:3, March 13, 2002.

Chapter 17

Laser Surgery and Electrosurgery

Learning Objectives

After studying this chapter the reader will be able to:

- Describe the characteristics of laser energy
- Describe the basic parts of the laser chamber
- Identify safety precautions followed in laser surgery
- Explain why safety precautions are needed for laser surgery
- Explain why personnel entering the operating room suite during laser surgery must be monitored for compliance with safety precautions
- Describe the nature of eye injury caused by laser energy
- Compare the classification of lasers
- Describe how electricity flows
- Use proper terminology when discussing electricity
- List the variables that affect the output of an electrosurgical unit (ESU)
- Describe safe use of dispersive and active electrodes
- Explain the difference between impedance and resistance
- Describe how to set modes on the ESU properly
- Describe why it is important to recognize occurrences in which settings are too high on the ESU power unit

Terminology

Ablation—Removal and destruction of tissue by erosion or vaporization, usually through intense heat.

Active electrode—An instrument or device used in surgery to deliver concentrated electrical current to tissue.

Alternate site burn—A patient burn at a site other than the target tissue. Alternate site burns have many causes.

Ampere—Unit used to measure the strength of electric current.

Amplification system—In laser technology, a series of mirrors that reflect photons or free electrons within the optical resonant chamber. This causes emission of more photons and creation of laser energy.

Amplitude—The height of an energy wave.

Circuit—The closed path through which current flows.

Coagulation—Clotting of blood.

Coherent—A characteristic of light in which all the light waves are lined up so that their peaks and troughs are matched. It is a characteristic of laser light.

Current—The flow of electrons (measured in amperes).

Dispersive electrode—The grounding pad applied to the patient that directs current flow from the patient back to the power unit.

Electromagnetic spectrum—Wave energy in the universe that is quantitatively measured. The visible waves of the spectrum appear colored to humans.

Frequency—In wave science, the number of waves per second measured in hertz.

Terminology—cont'd

Fulguration—An electrosurgical technique in which a spray of electrical energy coagulates and removes tissue. Also called *spray coagulation*

Gas—Matter in its least dense state (e.g., air at room temperature is a gas).

Infrared—The portion of the electromagnetic spectrum just below visible light. All warm objects give off infrared radiation.

Laser—Light amplification by stimulated emission of radiation.

Laser medium—The gas, liquid, or solid through which light energy is passed to create a laser beam. The medium is contained within the optical resonant chamber.

Laser safety officer—A person who is knowledgeable in laser safety and use and is assigned by the hospital to monitor and maintain safety standards for laser use.

Monochromatic—Having a single color.

Optical resonant cavity—The chamber that holds the laser medium. When light energy enters the chamber, it passes through the laser medium, and the number of photons increases.

Parallel—Denoting light in which the light waves move in narrow columns. It is a characteristic of laser light.

Photon—Particle of light that has no mass and no electric charge.

Power—The rate at which energy is used (measured in watts).

Pulsed wave—Single bursts of laser light. Q-switched lasers produce this type of wave.

Radiant exposure—The total effect of laser energy, which depends on the energy density of the laser beam, the diameter of the beam, and the exposure time.

Semiconductor—A material, such as silicon, that is neither a conductor of electricity nor an insulator. Its electrical properties can be changed by the addition of minute amounts of other elements. Semiconductors are the basis of transistors and computer chips.

Solid—Matter in a rigid state, not liquid or gaseous.

Solid-state—Using the electrical properties of solid components (such as transistors) instead of vacuum tubes.

Voltage—The electrical force that drives electrons from one point to another (measured in volts).

Wavelength—The distance from the peak of one wave to the peak of the next wave.

LASER TECHNOLOGY AND SURGERY

Laser is an acronym for light amplification by stimulated emission of radiation. Laser surgery uses an intensely hot, precisely focused beam of light to remove or vaporize tissue and control bleeding in a wide variety of procedures. Laser surgery is designed to cut or destroy diseased tissue without harming healthy normal tissues. Laser is also designed to shrink and destroy tumors, and cauterize blood vessels for control of bleeding.

Stimulated is the key word to understanding lasers. Light waves stimulate atoms to generate additional light waves; if this process is allowed to continue, millions of similar waves are generated until an intense beam of light is created. The word *laser* refers to both laser energy and the device used to create it.

Albert Einstein theorized that the stimulated emission of light could occur. According to his theory, the stimulated emission of **photons** by other photons could make light act as if it were matter. This theory was proven correct with the invention of the ruby laser. The first ruby laser was built in 1960. Since then, lasers have caused radical changes in both the methods and outcomes of modern surgery.

Importance of Laser Standards and Regulations

The laser is a powerful tool that has a variety of applications in manufacturing, engineering, biotechnology, health, and warfare. Laser technology has created a new field in medicine. However, lasers also have the capacity to cause irreparable injury and destruction. Because of this, laser standards have been developed by both governmental and private agencies. In health care, these standards are designed to protect both the patient and those who work with lasers.

▶ **American National Standards Institute (ANSI)**—An organization of expert volunteers who participate in developing the standards for various fields that use lasers. ANSI has published at least seven standards that are specific to different application areas.

▶ **Center for Devices and Radiological Health (CDRH)**—A regulatory bureau of the U.S. Food and Drug Administration (FDA) and the Department of Health and Human Services (DHHS). This governmental organization has been ordered by Congress to standardize the performance safety criteria for manufactured laser products. It has established a laser hazard classification (see Laser Hazards below).

▶ **Occupational Safety and Health Administration (OSHA)**—A government regulatory body. OSHA does not currently have a laser safety standard but uses FDA-CDRH manufacturer requirements and accepted industry laser standards.

▶ **Association of periOperative Registered Nurses (AORN)**—This organization has published a review of laser safety for operating room workers.

Understanding Lasers
ELECTROMAGNETIC SPECTRUM

To understand how lasers work, one must have some knowledge of the **electromagnetic spectrum** (Figure 17-1). This is a spectrum of wave energy that occurs naturally in the universe.

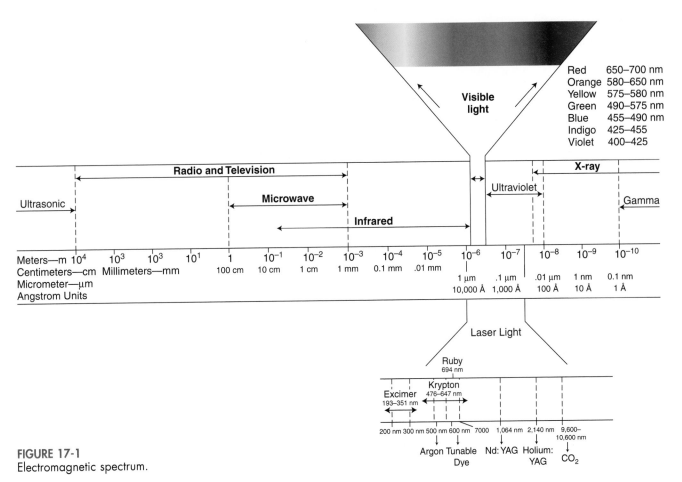

FIGURE 17-1
Electromagnetic spectrum.

When photons (light particles) exit the optical cavity of the laser, an intense stream of light is emitted. This light has three basic characteristics that make it different from any other type of light. These characteristics are illustrated in Figure 17-2. Light is also wave energy. What the eye perceives as white light actually is composed of light of many different **wavelengths** or colors.

The reaction of this light to biological tissue varies according to absorption properties, power settings, time of exposure, and size of the target tissue. The sum total of these factors is called the **radiant exposure** and is measured by the depth the laser beam will travel into the target tissue. When the laser beam touches the tissue, the cells heat to incredible temperatures, explode, and change into steam and carbon. This vaporization process allows the surgeon to treat tumors, abnormal cells, strictures, burns, and decubitus and gastrointestinal ulcers.

Waves are described according to certain characteristics:

▶ **Amplitude**—the height of the wave
▶ **Frequency**—the number of waves per second
▶ **Width**—the distance from the peak of one wave to the peak of the next wave, called the wavelength

Waves move out from their source as do the waves formed by a stone thrown into a pool of water. In this analogy, the water is energized by the force of the stone disturbing the water. This creates concentric waves. When the

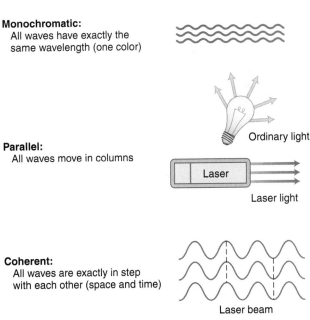

Monochromatic:
All waves have exactly the same wavelength (one color)

Parallel:
All waves move in columns

Ordinary light

Laser

Laser light

Coherent:
All waves are exactly in step with each other (space and time)

Laser beam

FIGURE 17-2
Basic characteristics of a laser.

stone sinks, the energy source is no longer present, and the waves begin to diminish in size and finally stop. Waves in the electromagnetic spectrum, including light waves, behave in very much the same way. Ordinary light diffuses in all directions.

LASER SYSTEM

Laser light is unlike any other light. All the waves in laser light have exactly the same wavelength or color—it is **monochromatic.** All the waves move in narrow columns—it is **parallel** light. All the waves are lined up so that their peaks and troughs are in exactly the same location—it is **coherent.**

The distinctive characteristics of laser energy are created when light is pumped into a sealed chamber filled with a medium—**gas, solid,** or liquid. This chamber is called the **optical resonant cavity.** When photons of a specific energy enter the chamber, they stimulate the high-energy atoms in the chamber to resonate in the same wave pattern. Mirrors in the laser system produce increased emission of light. They do this by bouncing the photons back and forth through the **laser medium** in the chamber. This increases the number (population) of resonating parallel photons and is called the **amplification system** (Figure 17-3). If a photon is not of the correct **frequency** or does not travel along the optical axis of the chamber, it is lost.

Just like the pool with the stone, the laser must have a continual *source of energy* to create continuous waves and more energy. This energy is derived from the pumping source. The pumping source balances the laser energy released from the system with the input of energy to the system. The difference between the waves caused by the stone in the pool and electromagnetic waves is that no medium is required for the propagation of an electromagnetic wave. In the stone and water example, the water is the medium. Electromagnetic waves can occur in a vacuum.

Lasers can be grouped into two categories according to the duration of the output waves:

► **Continuous wave lasers** produce a steady stream of light.
► **Q-switched lasers** contain the light in the system until it is released by a shutter that permits passage of a single intense burst or pulse of laser light. This type of laser light is called a **pulsed wave.**

Types of Lasers

Lasers are distinguished by the medium—the element or compound that is activated to emit photons. The medium can be a liquid, solid, gas, or **semiconductor.** The types of lasers are the following:

► Gas
► Solid
► Semiconductor
► Excimer
► Solid-state
► Dye

Effects of Lasers

When laser light is directed at a surface, any of the following can occur:

► Absorption
► Reflection
► Scattering
► Transmission

Lasers are distinguished by the functional or biophysical reaction of the target tissue. The tissue reaction varies with laser wavelength, power setting, and exposure time, as well as the absorption qualities and structure of the cells (e.g., density, moisture content) of the target tissue. The quality of the laser energy depends on its density, which is determined by the electrical wattage, the diameter of the beam, and the exposure time. The sum of these factors is called the radiant exposure.

When certain types of laser light contact tissue, the cells heat to extremely high temperatures, explode, and change into steam and carbon. Laser light also bonds tissue together (welding). These vaporization and **coagulation** effects are the surgical tools used in laser surgery. Of the hundreds of types of lasers available, only a few are used in medicine. The laser wavelength (color) determines tissue penetration and other biophysical effects on tissue.

Laser light produced by different lasing media is absorbed by different kinds of tissue. Energy in the form of heat and light cuts and coagulates tissues of differing moisture content and density. In surgery, a particular laser is selected because it is optimal for the target tissue. Selective absorption is an important characteristic in laser surgery because it prevents the spread of heat and tissue damage outside the target

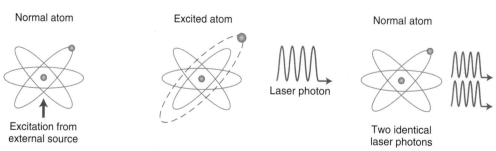

FIGURE 17-3
Amplification system.(Redrawn from Ball KA: *Lasers: the perioperative challenge,* ed 2, St Louis, 1995, Mosby.)

tissue. Table 17-1 lists different laser media, the wavelengths of light emitted, and the types of tissue by which the light is absorbed.

All of the lasers and components described in Table 17-1 are essentially similar in construction. They all have:

▶ An optical resonator or optical cavity, usually a glass tube
▶ The lasing medium
▶ Reflective mirrors, located at each end of the optical cavity
▶ A pumping source (electricity, heat, or light) that stimulates the photons to create more photons

Laser Media

ARGON (GAS)

Argon gas lasers produce a visible blue-green beam that is color specific and is absorbed by red-brown pigmented tissue such as hemoglobin. The argon beam is not absorbed by clear or translucent tissue; thus the beam can pass through the cornea, vitreous, and lens of the eye without creating a thermal effect. Biophysical uses of the argon laser include coagulation and sealing.

The beam produced by an argon laser scatters more than that produced by other laser types. It is used most often in dermatological (skin) and ophthalmic (eye) procedures. It is used in dermatology for skin disorders such as port wine stains, dark skin lesions, and cutaneous lesions. In ophthalmology it is used for treating retinal tears, glaucoma, macular degeneration, retinopathy, and retinal vein occlusion. It also is used with light-sensitive dyes to treat tumors in a procedure called photodynamic therapy (PDT).

CARBON DIOXIDE (CO_2) (GAS)

The carbon dioxide laser medium is actually a combination of helium, nitrogen, and carbon dioxide, and the beam is invisible to the human eye. A helium-neon laser beam, which produces a red light, is added to the carbon dioxide laser beam to make the beam visible. The helium-neon beam is sometimes called the "pilot light" because of its guiding function. The laser energy is delivered through an articulating arm. The carbon dioxide laser beam has a high affinity for water and is used widely in plastic surgery for resurfacing and removal of skin lesions. It is also used for cervical **ablation,** ablation of condylomata and warts, and microlaryngoscopy and stapedectomy procedures. It also is used in vascular surgery, microsurgery, and endoscopic procedures. Its biophysical uses are coagulation, incision, ablation, and vaporization. The moisture content of the tissue determines how quickly the beam is absorbed.

KRYPTON (GAS)

Krypton laser light is absorbed by hemoglobin and retinal epithelium. The krypton laser is electrically powered and water cooled. The krypton beam is highly selective for retinal tissue, and krypton lasers are used widely for retinal applications.

EXCIMER (GAS)

The excimer laser produces a cool beam by stripping electrons from the atoms of the medium in the chamber. This is a photochemical reaction and causes the energy bonds in the atom to break. The resulting "shock waves" stimulate the release of short bursts of laser light. The light is delivered to the target tissue through fiberoptic bundles.

The beam of the excimer laser creates less heat than the thermal or photothermal energy produced by other types of laser. This reduces damage to nearby tissues and also results in less carbonization of lased tissue. Specialized ultraviolet mirrors and optics are required to operate the laser safely. The gas medium used in excimer lasers is extremely toxic or lethal and can cause genetic mutations by separating the

Table 17-1	TYPES OF LASERS			
Laser Medium	Wavelength (Microns)	Significant Properties and Action	Medical Use	Delivery System
Argon	0.48	Absorbed by pigmented tissues (red-brown) Coagulation, sealing	Ophthalmology Dermatology Gastroenterology Otology	Hollow tube with mirrors or fiberoptic cable
Ruby	0.69	Pigment specific Coagulation, sealing		
Nd:YAG	1.06	Nonspecific absorption Deep coagulation	Gastroenterology Pulmonology Ophthalmology Urology Gynecology	Fiberoptic cable
CO_2	10.6	Highly absorbed by water Vaporization, coagulation, sealing, drilling	Gynecology Rhinolaryngology Neurosurgery Dermatology	Hollow tube with mirrors or fiberoptic cable

hydrogen bonds in DNA. The excimer laser is extremely precise. Its beam can remove 9 millionths of an inch of tissue in 12 billionths of a second.

HOLMIUM:YTTRIUM-ALUMINUM-GARNET (YAG) (SOLID)

The holmium:yttrium-aluminum-garnet (holmium:YAG) laser is a crystal containing holmium, thallium, and chromium. Its beam is outside the visible light range and is highly penetrating of all tissues. The holmium:YAG laser cuts, shaves, contours, smooths, ablates, and coagulates tissues and cartilage. It is extremely versatile and is capable of ablating renal calculi as well as soft tissues. It has low-depth thermal penetration to a maximum of 0.4 mm. The holmium:YAG laser is often used in urological; orthopedic; ear, nose, and throat; gynecological; gastrointestinal; and general surgery.

NEODYMIUM:YAG (SOLID)

The neodymium:YAG (Nd:YAG) laser is created from a **solid-state** crystal of neodymium, yttrium, aluminum, and garnet (Figure 17-4). As with the carbon dioxide laser, a helium-neon beam is used for visibility. The Nd:YAG laser beam has a high affinity for tissue protein but little for water. The beam is near the **infrared** region of the electromagnetic spectrum and has a penetration of 3 to 7 mm. Of all the laser types, the Nd:YAG laser has the greatest ability to coagulate blood vessels. Because of its deep penetration it can coagulate vessels up to 4 mm in diameter. This laser can be used during endoscopic or flexible fiberoptic surgery. The

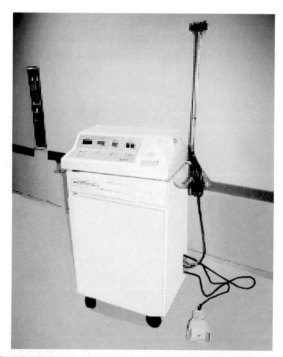

FIGURE 17-4
The neodymium:YAG (Nd:YAG) laser. (From Nagle GM: *Genitourinary surgery*, St Louis, 1997, Mosby.)

thermal energy of the Nd:YAG laser is absorbed by pigmented tissue. Because the Nd:YAG is absorbed by pigmented tissue, it is very effective for the removal of tattoos and other pigmented tissue. It is absorbed less by blood but has higher absorption in water than the argon beam. Biophysical uses of the Nd:YAG laser include coagulation, vaporization, and ablation. The Nd:YAG laser makes blood clot quickly and allows surgeons to see and work in areas or parts of the body that normally would have been reached through invasive surgery.

POTASSIUM-TITANYL-PHOSPHATE (SOLID)

The potassium-titanyl-phosphate (KTP) laser is less powerful than the carbon dioxide or Nd:YAG laser but is capable of producing a minute beam that is well suited for microscopic surgery. The laser light is readily absorbed by red and black tissue and can be delivered by a number of different methods, including an insulated fiber, scanner, or microscope. The KTP laser offers two wavelengths, which allows two separate sets of laser characteristics to be selected at any time. These dual wavelengths allow for hemostatic cutting and ablation, as well as deep coagulation. The KTP laser is used in otorhinolaryngological (ENT), urological, gynecological, and general surgery, and in dermatological procedures, including treatment of spider veins. The KTP laser is known for its precise cutting ability and is used in many different specialties. KTP crystals can be combined with neodymium to double the frequency of the Nd laser wave and boosts its effectiveness and surgical versatility.

RUBY (SOLID)

The solid ruby crystal is actually a synthetic material made of aluminum oxide and chromium atoms. These atoms are activated by flash lamps in the resonator cavity of the laser. When they are activated, the ruby laser beam is created. Ruby laser light is not absorbed by oxyhemoglobin in blood vessels and transparent substances but is strongly absorbed by blue and black pigments and by melanin. Modern ruby lasers are available as Q-switched devices with a fiberoptic cable to deliver the beam. The beam can damage bone and internal organs. The ruby laser is used in the removal of port wine stains and other dark skin lesions. The ruby laser was the first laser to be applied in the medical setting and also is used for tattoo removal.

TUNABLE DYE (SOLID)

The pulsed dye laser beam is formed when fluorescent liquid or other dyes and vapor are exposed to argon laser light. The dye absorbs the light and produces a fluorescent broad-spectrum light. The spectrum of the light is then "tuned" to produce light of a particular wavelength (color). Different wavelengths are absorbed by different types of tissue. This laser, however, is used most often for PDT. In this therapy, the patient receives a photosensitive drug about 48 hours before surgery. Both normal and malignant tissues absorb the drug. The drug is metabolized out of normal tissue but remains in the malignant tissue. When lased, the dyed tissue is destroyed. Another use of the tunable dye laser is the destruction of vascular lesions.

FREE ELECTRON LASER

The free-electron laser uses free electrons—those that are not attached to a specific atom—to produce a tunable electromagnetic beam. The beam passes through a series of magnets and reflectors before emission. The free-electron laser beam is tunable across all wavelengths between the infrared and ultraviolet regions. It is used for destruction of calculi and for precise tissue incision. Unlike other lasers that use the specific wavelengths of the atomic material from which electrons are normally bound, the free-electron laser simply uses electrons as a medium to produce an intense light that is very effective on soft tissues.

Laser Hazards

Hundreds of different types of lasers are used in medicine, engineering, and other fields. Not all lasers produce an intense thermal effect. Lasers are classified by their health risks as follows:

▶ *Class 1.* These lasers are not hazardous for continuous viewing, are considered incapable of producing damaging radiation levels, and are exempt from control measures. An example is the laser in a laser printer.
▶ *Class 2.* These lasers emit radiation in the visible range of the electromagnetic spectrum. They do not normally cause harm when viewed but may be aversive (cause blinking, turning away). When viewed for an extended time, *they can be hazardous.* An example is the laser in a laser pointer or a bar code scanner.
▶ *Class 3a.* These lasers normally do not cause injury to the eye if viewed momentarily but present a hazard if viewed with collecting optics (e.g., fiberoptic cable, magnification loupe, or microscope).
▶ *Class 3b.* These lasers *cause severe eye injury* when viewed directly or by reflection. They do not cause injury when the laser beam is diffused and do not normally present a fire hazard.
▶ *Class 4.* These lasers cause eye damage if viewed directly or if viewed indirectly by specular reflection and diffuse reflection. They also can ignite materials and produce skin burns.

Note that class 3B and class 4 lasers cause instantaneous retinal injury that may be *irreparable.* Class 4 lasers can penetrate the sclera and injure the retina. Turning one's head away or not looking directly into the laser does not ensure protection because of the risk of scatter or reflection of the beam. Most medical lasers are class 4.

TISSUE INJURY

Recall the three specific characteristics of laser energy that separate it from ordinary white light: it is coherent (peaks and troughs match), monochromatic (all waves are of the same wavelength), and parallel (waves move in one direction only). These qualities make laser light extremely hazardous. Laser light can concentrate a tremendous amount of energy in one spot.

The two most common injuries associated with unintentional laser exposure are eye injury and skin burn. Lasers in the ultraviolet and infrared areas of the spectrum are the most damaging. They can penetrate the sclera and enter the lens, cornea, and retina. Eye injury can be permanent, especially if the retina is involved. Injuries range from corneal burns to blindness caused by destruction of the retina or other eye structures. Many hospitals require their students and employees to undergo a retinal examination as a part of their health examination before allowing them to work in an operating room with lasers. This establishes the health of the retina before working with the lasers.

Heat generated by the lasing light beam medium (gas, solid, or liquid) is the major cause of tissue damage. Intentional use of the laser results in incision or dissection, tissue vaporization, and welding. Unintentional exposure can cause the same effects. Effects of the intense thermal energy can range from reddening of the skin to third-degree (full-thickness) burns. When the laser beam enters the eye, it passes through the vitreous and then the lens of the eye focuses the energy on the retina.

The following factors determine the degree of thermal damage:

▶ The sensitivity of the irradiated tissue
▶ The amount of tissue affected
▶ The wavelength of the laser beam
▶ The energy level of the laser beam
▶ The amount of time the tissue is exposed

Laser energy can cause changes in the chemistry of the cell. Because of ensuing photochemical effects, the energy continues to damage tissue even after the source is removed. This most often occurs with lasers with wavelengths shorter than 600 nm. The excimer laser is the most hazardous.

Some lasers produce a photoacoustic effect that generates rapid pulsations that blow apart the tissue. The medical use for such lasers is the destruction of renal calculi and posterior capsulotomy in eye surgery. Unintentional exposure can cause serious eye injury.

FIRE

Not only is there risk of tissue damage from unintentional exposure, but the intense heat of the laser beam can ignite patient drapes, flammable preparation solutions, polyvinyl chloride endotracheal tubes, and the patient's hair and skin. Patient fires usually are attributed to lasers and electrosurgical units (ESUs).

ELECTRICAL SHOCK

Electrical hazards associated with laser equipment require the same vigilance as hazards associated with other high-energy devices used in the operating room. Cords and connections must be checked regularly and before each procedure, and only grounded outlets are permissible. Extension cords should *not* be used with lasers. If there is any doubt about the integrity of the system, the laser *must not be used.*

Laser Injury Prevention

SYMPTOMS OF LASER EYE INJURY

The characteristic eye symptom associated with exposure to a carbon dioxide laser beam (outside the visible range) is burning pain at the site of exposure on the sclera or cornea. Eye exposure to a visible laser beam is detected as a bright flash that is the color of the emitted wavelength. This is followed by an afterimage of the complementary color. Retinal damage results in difficulty in seeing blue or green shades. Injury from a Q-switched Nd:YAG laser is insidious because the injury initially may be undetected. The reason is that the retina has no pain sensory nerves.

EYE PROTECTION

The eye is the tissue most vulnerable to accidental laser exposure. The high water content and sensitivity of eye tissue make it extremely susceptible to injury. To protect the eyes during laser use, one must shield them from specific wavelengths of light. Protective eyewear of the correct optical density is required for various types of laser. *Note that colored lenses alone do not offer any protection. The lens color of protective eyewear simply codes the optical density of the lenses.* One must consult the laser manufacturer to select the correct density of eyewear to use with a particular laser.

All patients undergoing laser surgery (except ophthalmic surgery) must wear suitable protective eye cups or be fitted with eyewear of the same specifications as that worn by staff. Window shields are available for observation rooms.

Eyewear must wrap completely around the eyes, covering the sides, top, and bottom, so that no diffuse laser energy can reach the eye. Examples of protective eyewear are illustrated in Figure 17-5. Prescription glasses may be worn under protective goggles. Contact lens wearers also must wear protective eyewear. Eye-protection devices do not work if they are not worn!

SKIN PROTECTION

Skin injuries result from direct contact with the laser beam. Environmental precautions are necessary to prevent skin injuries. In addition, anyone entering a room in which lasers are in use must remove any metallic items, as these can reflect the laser beam or absorb heat. Patient tissues also must be protected from inadvertent laser injury. Wet towels are placed around the affected area to prevent fires and prevent burns to the patient. One should periodically moisten towels with water or normal saline to maintain their effectiveness during the procedure.

AIRWAY PROTECTION

Endotracheal tubes or other anesthesia equipment can easily ignite in the presence of laser energy. Polyvinyl chloride (PVC) endotracheal tubes must not be used during laser

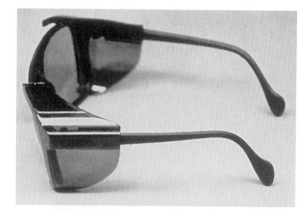

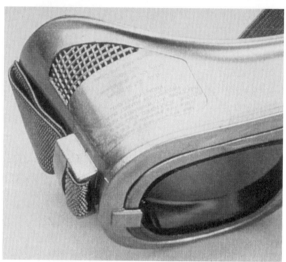

FIGURE 17-5
Examples of protective eyewear. (From Ball KA: *Lasers: the perioperative challenge,* ed 2, St Louis, 1995, Mosby.)

surgery. Most laser energy is capable of penetrating the PVC tubing and reacting with oxygen and the tubing to cause a fire. The oxygen-rich environment of the OR presents a high risk of patient fire, especially during surgery of the head and neck. Only matte-finish metal airways should be used, as medical-grade lasers do not penetrate the metal. The matte finish prevents scatter or reflection of the laser energy.

ENVIRONMENTAL SAFETY

The following guidelines are not meant to replace hospital policy or organizational standards, only to highlight important features of these documents:

▶ A laser warning sign (Figure 17-6) must be placed on all entrances to areas where laser surgery is being performed.
▶ All personnel entering a room in which lasers are in use must wear protective eyewear. Protective eyewear of the correct optical density must be available outside the door of the room.
▶ To protect staff from accidental exposure to laser energy, all reflective surfaces, including those used for the surgery

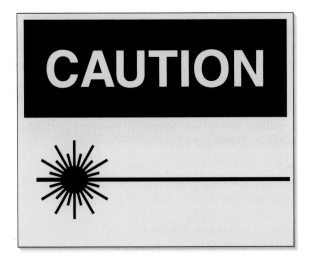

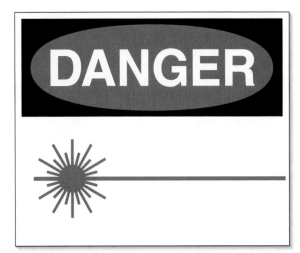

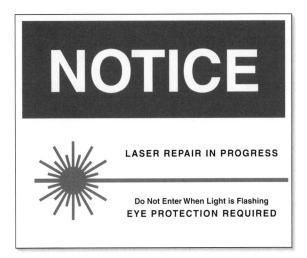

FIGURE 17-6
Laser warning signs.

itself, must be covered to be made nonreflective or be removed from the room. Ebony or matte-finish instruments must be used, and walls and other environmental surfaces must be nonreflective. No one entering the room should wear metal jewelry.

▶ Only personnel trained in and proven knowledgeable about laser use and precautions should be allowed to operate laser equipment.

▶ Fire-prevention measures must be in place at all times during laser use. The surgical field should be surrounded with wet towels, and only metal matte-finish endotracheal tubes should be used. When not in use, the laser tip should be placed on a moist towel, not a dry drape. Flammable preparation solutions should not be used before laser surgery. Oxygen should be delivered at the lowest possible concentration.

▶ The patient's head must be protected from inadvertent laser exposure with a nonreflective anesthesia screen.

▶ Prep solutions used on the skin must be allowed to dry thoroughly before the laser is used.

▶ Flame-retardant drapes always should be used during laser surgery.

▶ To prevent electrical shock, all electrical cords must be inspected for soundness before surgery. Only biomedical engineers should be allowed to access power units. Documented cases of electrocution have occurred when technical or nursing personnel came into contact with the equipment. Liquids must not be allowed to pool on the floor near the laser system or operating team.

▶ Regular staff training should be in place to provide education and reinforcement about the importance of following hazard precautions.

▶ A **laser safety officer** should be designated to monitor and enforce laser standards and precautions.

ELECTROSURGERY

Like laser energy, the energy used in electrosurgery is part of the electromagnetic spectrum. Electrosurgery uses energy to coagulate (congeal or desiccate) and cut tissue. Rapid technological advances in the last decade have improved the safety of electrosurgical devices. However, change requires a new understanding of how these devices work. They still have hazards. Patients and staff alike are involved in serious electrosurgical accidents every year. We cannot rely on the device to protect our patients or ourselves. Each person is responsible for actively seeking information on the tools used in surgery.

Elements of Electricity
CONDUCTION, CURRENT, AND VOLTAGE
Electricity is the flow of electrons through a *conductive* medium. A conductive medium is any gas, solid, or liquid that allows electrons to flow through it easily. Some materials are excellent conductors of electricity; electrolyte solutions and copper wire are good examples. Body tissue is less conductive. The flow of electricity is called the **current.** The pressure that pushes the current through a medium is called the **voltage** and is controlled by the *power source.* For example, the city power plant is a power source. High voltage produces a higher current. **Power** is the rate at which energy is used. Current flow is measured in units called **amperes.** The amount of power determines the voltage. If voltage drops, however, such as when demand for power is too high for a city's power plant, the power cannot be transmitted.

RESISTANCE
A very important concept in electricity is *resistance.* Resistance is anything that stops or impedes the flow of current. For example, some materials are resistant to electrical flow (current). The material that covers electrical wires is safe to touch because it is nonconductive. It is resistant. The electricity does not stop flowing; it simply does not flow through the resistant material. When current meets a resistant material, it seeks an alternative route that offers less resistance to flow. This is called the *path of least resistance.* Electricity always takes this path. If no alternative path is immediately available, however, some of the *electricity is transformed into heat at the site of resistance.* This is the heat that is used during electrosurgery. The amount of heat produced depends on the power source, which is the ESU.

HOUSEHOLD CURRENT
As with other energy in the electromagnetic spectrum, *electrical current is wave energy.* The electrical waveform has height (magnitude), frequency, and length. Ordinary household current is called *alternating current* (AC) because its magnitude varies over time. Frequency is the number of wave peaks (oscillations) per second and is measured in units called hertz (Hz). AC is delivered at 50 to 60 Hz.

CURRENT PATH
Electrical current travels continuously until it reaches a point of complete blockage or resistance. In electrosurgery, the current flows *through the body* and is collected at a **dispersive electrode,** which discharges it into a conductive cord

back to the ESU machine. The current does *not seek an alternate path to ground but stays within the circuit.* This is called an isolated system. The dispersive electrode is discussed in detail later.

Response of the Body to Electrical Current
The human body uses electricity to perform many vital functions. It responds to outside electrical stimulation in a number of different ways:

▶ At 10 mA* current is perceived but is not painful.
▶ At 20 mA current produces pain and strong involuntary muscle contractions. Current at this level also may cause respiratory arrest.
▶ At 75 mA cardiac fibrillation occurs.
▶ At 6 A current produces burns and severe tissue injury.

The body is very sensitive to wave frequency. The *higher the frequency, the lower the response.* The **upper limit** for stimulation of the human nervous system is 100,000 Hz. Wave energy above 100,000 Hz does not interfere with the bioelectrical activity needed to sustain life. A human can be burned by current at these frequencies, but the heart and other bioelectrical mechanisms are not affected.

The ESU operates at 300,000 to 1 million Hz. Each mode used in electrosurgery is produced by a specific combination of frequency, voltage or power, and time of exposure to the tissue. The thermal effects of the ESU and the **active electrode** (the instrument that delivers the electricity) are used to cut and coagulate tissue. The amount of heat generated depends on the density of the tissue, the amount of time the tissue is exposed, and the current density at the active electrode.

Coagulation (congealing) occurs at a relatively low temperature. During this process collagen is converted into glucose, the tissue shrinks, and hemostasis occurs. High-frequency alternating current *vaporizes* tissue—tissue vaporizes to a gaseous form. *Cutting* is achieved during vaporization.

Carbonization is the same as a fourth-degree burn. Carbonization occurs when the temperature at the electrode tip exceeds 200° C (392° F). Excessive carbonization is not desirable because it delays healing, and eschar may slough from the tissue and cause postoperative bleeding.

Monopolar Versus Bipolar Electrosurgery
In *bipolar* electrosurgery the surgeon uses double-tipped forceps to coagulate tissue. The bipolar forceps transfer the electricity from one tine of the forceps directly to the other. No dispersive electrode is required because the current does not pass through the patient's body. The energy travels from one tine of the bipolar forceps, through the tissue grasped by the forceps, and into the opposite tine of the forceps. The bipolar ESU uses a slower, lower current than the monopolar ESU. The current path is shorter, and the procedure is

---

* The rate of current flow is measured in amperes (A) and milliamperes (mA).

much safer than is monopolar electrosurgery. Because of the lower power, however, the use of a bipolar ESU is restricted to neurosurgery (surgery involving the nervous system) and surgical procedures on other delicate tissue.

In *monopolar* electrosurgery the current passes into the patient's body via the active electrode (i.e., the Bovie pencil), travels through the body, and exits through the dispersive (or passive) electrode (Figure 17-7). The dispersive electrode captures the current through its size and conductivity, attracting the electrons through the path of least resistance. From the dispersive electrode, the current returns to the power unit so that a circular path is formed.

ESU Equipment
POWER UNIT
The ESU power unit is a compact portable device that has adjustable controls for power, modes, audible alarms, and volume. The rear panel contains the power entry module, foot switch receptacle, and grounding lug. Serial ports allow a computer to be connected to the generator. All newer models can operate in either bipolar or monopolar mode and include memory recall. Newer ESUs also operate as an isolated power source to prevent accidental electrical injury.

ACTIVE ELECTRODE
The active electrode is constructed to be used as a pencil or probe. The electrode may be activated by a switch located on the pencil itself or by a foot pedal. Endoscopic procedures require long, thin electrodes that can be threaded into the cannula. These are available in several configurations, such as grasping tips, suction-coagulation combinations, and probes. Open procedures usually require a more limited selection of electrode tips (Figure 17-8). They include the following:

▶ Flat blade—useful for cutting and coagulation

▶ Teflon-coated flat blade—ease of cleaning for cases requiring a large amount of cautery
▶ Needle point—creates the highest concentration of current; used for fine cutting
▶ Ball tip—has greater surface area; excellent for coagulation and fulguration
▶ Loop—used for cutting and resection

DISPERSIVE ELECTRODE
Current density is the concentration of current at the tip of the electrosurgical instrument and is increased or decreased by adjustments to the power setting on the ESU. As current enters the tissue, it coagulates or cuts the tissue depending on the temperature or current density at the ESU tip. As current moves away from the point of contact, current density decreases in the body *but does not diminish in power.* Current must exit the body to complete the electrical **circuit.** Recall that the frequency of the electrical current is too high for the current to interfere with the bioelectrical functions of the body or to cause cardiac or respiratory failure. It may burn the patient, however, if it meets another point of resistance. This is called an **alternate site burn.** To prevent such a burn, we have the current exit the body through the highly conductive dispersive (passive) electrode (also called the *patient return electrode* or *grounding pad*). This electrode disperses the current over the width of the pad to prevent burns.

The dispersive electrode (Figure 17-9) is a flexible, insulated pad coated with conductive (electrolytic) gel. The pad is self-sticking and is placed near the surgical site. Because of the potential for severe burns if the pad is placed incorrectly, these recommendations should be followed:

▶ Place the pad in a fleshy area. Uniform contact with the skin is essential. Do not apply the pad over a bony

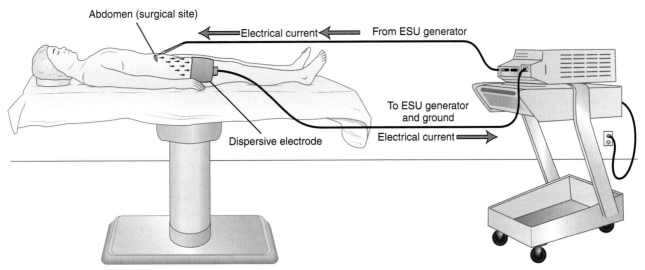

FIGURE 17-7
Monopolar electrosurgery.

prominence. Place it in an area of high vascularization to maximize current flow.

▸ Place the pad as close to the operative site as possible.

▸ Prepare the pad site by removing any lotion or other substances before applying the pad. People with extensive sun exposure have increased keratin in the skin. This can prevent good conduction. Place the pad away from sun-exposed areas.

▸ If necessary, shave hair from the pad site to promote pad adherence.

▸ Position the dispersive electrode with its long side parallel to the surgical incision.

▸ Avoid areas of skin-to-skin contact.

▸ Do not place the pad in a position that might cause the return current to cross other bioelectrical devices such as electrocardiograph leads or a cardiac pacemaker.

▸ Do not apply a pad that is dry. The conductive gel must be fresh. Topical lubricating gel is *not* conductive and never should be used to coat the pad.

▸ Do not position the dispersive electrode over an implant because excessive scar tissue impedes conduction.

The dispersive (passive) electrode can cause a burn because of two effects: the *edge* effect and the *proximity* effect. The edge effect occurs because the concentration of current is highest at the edges of the pad. If the concentration is too high, a burn can result. This might happen if the pad is not placed with equal pressure on all portions or the gel is not equally distributed across the pad. The proximity effect is caused by increased current density on the side of the active electrode (closest to the source of the current in the body).

Newer ESUs contain self-monitoring systems that register differences in current density at the pad. The safer monitoring systems shut the system down when the pad is displaced or in poor contact with the patient. In other systems, an alarm sounds when contact is lost between the patient and the return electrode. The first type is much safer because it *prevents* a burn from occurring. The second type only alerts personnel that the problem has occurred. Many surgeons request that the monitor alarms be turned off. This defeats the purpose of patient protective devices. Never switch these features off or disable them.

Variables That Affect Output

The mode of the ESU is the type and quality of power available during electrosurgery. One controls these characteristics by adjusting the output settings. The mode determines the peak voltage (power) available at the active electrode and depends on the waveform. Lower current density is required for coagulation, whereas higher density is better for cutting tissue. Most new ESU models have automatically regulated modes. Without this regulation, output voltage can fluctuate widely based on external variables such as the following:

▸ Shape and size of the active electrode—the larger the surface area of the electrode, the greater the current flow through the electrode.

▸ Tissue density—the denser the tissue, the more difficult it is to cut.

▸ Tissue resistance—increased resistance reduces current flow.

▸ Tissue vascularization—increased vascularization reduces resistance.

▸ Presence of fluid—large amounts of fluid reduce the heat of the active electrode.

▸ Surgeon's technique—the preference in settings, duration, speed, and pressure of tissue contact with the active electrode affects voltage output.

These variables affect operation in the designated mode so that cutting or coagulation is not always predictable. For example, when the surgeon cuts through dense tissue while in the coagulation mode, voltage and temperature may increase far beyond the safe level that is required to perform the task. As a consequence, tissue beneath the target tissue may be burned unintentionally. If resistance is high in certain tasks, increased voltage is required. Effective use of the modes available on the ESU prevents unnecessary trauma to adjacent tissue.

Modes available on the ESU often are inappropriately selected and used. If the surgeon repeatedly asks for increased power (voltage), the mode may be incorrectly chosen. All operating room personnel are responsible for understanding the way the ESU functions and the relationships between voltage and mode. Simply increasing the voltage beyond normal levels without investigating why a higher voltage is needed may result in severe injury to the patient.

ARCING OR SPRAY MODE

The arcing or spray mode creates the highest peak voltage available. This mode is used for **fulguration.** Fulguration is fast superficial coagulation. It is used when large areas of tissue must be coagulated.

CUTTING MODE

Cutting tissue requires sufficient voltage (power) to vaporize cells without charring the tissue. The active electrode initially is placed in contact with the tissue. After that, increased current concentration produces a vapor that allows sparking between the electrode and the tissue; this creates a clean cut by increasing vaporization.

The cutting mode is usually marked "cutting" or "pure cut" on the ESU. The current used for cutting is continuous, and the peak voltage is low at the corresponding power setting. In the continuous mode, the *duty cycle* is 100%. The duty cycle is the percentage of time during which the electrical current actually flows in the circuit. When the duty cycle is less than 100%, a diagram of current flow shows waves followed by a flat line. As the duty cycle becomes shorter, increased coagulation is possible.

BLEND MODE

Blend mode is not a combination of cutting and coagulation but rather the length of the duty cycle. The current flow for

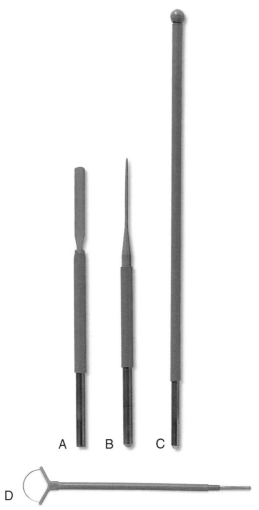

FIGURE 17-8
Active electrodes coated with a Teflon-like coating. **A,** Flat blade. **B,** Needle point. **C,** Ball tip. **D,** Loop. (Courtesy Megadyne Medical Products, Inc, Draper, Utah.)

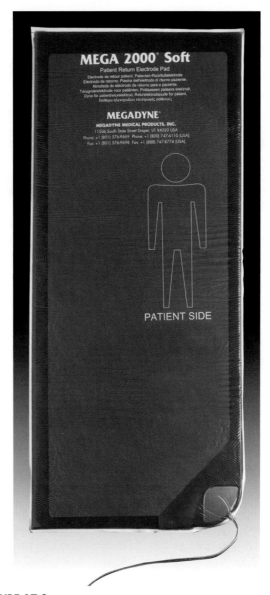

FIGURE 17-9
The dispersive electrode is a flexible, insulated, disposable pad coated with conductive gel. (Courtesy Megadyne Medical Products, Inc, Draper, Utah.)

different blends is not continuous. That is, the *duty cycle*, which is the proportion of time the current flows, is less than 100%. In blended mode, the duty cycle is about 70%.

Impedance

Impedance is probably the least understood concept in electrosurgery. Comprehending it is important, however, especially for endoscopic surgery. When AC is applied to a continuous circuit, the flow of electricity is uninterrupted. If two conductive surfaces separated by a *nonconductive material* are introduced into the circuit, however, the current will continue to flow by alternating back and forth between the power source and the conductive surfaces.

Impedance describes the flow of electrical current into structures that are not designed to be a part of the electrical circuit. It is a measurement of the reactance and resistance of structures. Certain materials tend to allow the flow of electricity through them. For example, both metal and human tissues are conductive (or react to the passage of electricity through them), but many metals are more reac-

tive to the flow of electricity than human tissues. This difference in conductivity is called resistance. In human tissues, tissue density affects the amount of resistance present in the tissues. Tissues with high liquid content (e.g., soft-tissue cells) are less resistant to the flow of electricity than tissues with less water content (e.g., bone). Both tissues are conductive, but bone has a higher impedance than soft-tissue cells.

In endoscopic surgery, impedance becomes an issue when the active electrode passes through a sheath or port. The active electrode is covered with a nonconductive insulating material. If the insulation is cracked or otherwise damaged, electrical current can flow through the break in the insulation. Because many endoscopic ports are metal, which is highly conductive, the electricity will flow through the sheath or port and cause thermal injuries to structures that are in contact with the port. Impedance occurs at the site where the active electrode tip is positioned because the metal of the sheath or port is more conductive than the tissue to which the active electrode tip is applied.

To prevent impedance and patient injury, only metal-sheathed endoscopic instruments should be used. These instruments are constructed so that the insulated portion of the instrument is sheathed in metal. This prevents contact between the insulation and the conductive endoscopy port. Metal is reactive (conductive) and does not resist the flow of electricity. Impedance is the difference between an object's reactivity (conductivity) and its resistance; reactivity minus resistance equals impedance. Metal, being very conductive, would be the connection between electricity and another object that is conductive (e.g., human tissue). Disposable ports are made of plastic and demonstrate a higher impedance than metal ports.

General Safety Precautions

These safety precautions should be followed in the use of the ESU:

▶ Electrosurgery carries a high risk of patient and environmental fire, especially in the presence of flammable preparation solutions. Avoid using flammable solutions. If they must be used, make sure that the skin is completely dry before draping the patient.

▶ Check the ESU power source before use. Inspect cords and insulation for fraying and loose-fitting connections. Weakened insulation on endoscopic instruments can cause severe burns.

▶ Never disable the alarm system on an ESU.

▶ Always use a nonconductive holster for the active electrode. Do not allow it to come into contact with the patient or the drapes.

▶ When changing the active electrode tip, use an instrument, not your hand.

▶ Never loop ESU cords around instruments or metal devices.

▶ The patient must remove all metal jewelry to prevent alternate-site burns.

▶ Use a smoke evacuation system during ESU use. (See Chapter 14 for a complete discussion of smoke plume hazards.)

▶ Do not allow fluids to come into contact with the dispersive electrode.

▶ Do not allow the patient to come into contact with metal or other conductive objects such as the operating table frame.

▶ Do not allow the active electrode cable and the dispersive electrode cable to contact each other.

▶ Remove tissue and eschar from the active electrode tip with a damp cloth or Teflon scratch pad—never with a knife blade or other sharp instrument.

▶ A malfunctioning ESU must be taken out of service *immediately.*

CASE STUDIES

Case 1

During abdominal surgery, the surgeon asks you to "buzz" a hemostat. In this technique a blood vessel is grasped with a hemostat and the active electrode is placed on the shank of the instrument. This transfers electricity to the tissue and cauterizes it. Would you do this? Why or why not?

Case 2

You are serving as circulator on a pediatric laparotomy procedure. The patient is 2 weeks old. The surgeon states that he will use electrosurgery. Where will you put the dispersive electrode? Can you cut it because the patient is so small?

Case 3

You are in a hurry to pass through a surgical suite where Nd:YAG laser surgery is in progress. You do not use protective glasses even though they are hanging on the door outside. You enter the room and turn your head away from the

patient as you proceed to the other door. Just to be safe, you close your eyes for a few moments until you reach the door. Are you safe?

Case 4

You are asked to bring a 16-year-old from the holding area for a breast biopsy. When you arrive, you see that she has a metal ring through her nipple. You explain to her that it is a hazard during electrosurgery. She tells you she cannot take it out because she has no way to remove it. How will you handle this?

Case 5

You are scrubbed on an eye procedure that uses laser surgery. When the assistant arrives, you see that he is wearing a large, shiny religious medal around his neck. You know that the reflective surface is dangerous. Can he tuck it into his scrub top to reduce the risk?

REFERENCES

AORN website: *Perioperative laser safety: an overview.*

ConMed Corp website: *Electrosurgical safety* (online course).

ECRI: Electrosurgery, *Operating Room Risk Management,* January, 1999.

Moak E: Electrosurgical unit safety: the role of the perioperative nurse, *AORN Journal* 53:3, March, 1991.

Rockwell RJ Jr: *The laser safety officer,* Rockwell Laser Industries website.

Rockwell Laser Industries: *Statistical data for RLI incident database,* Rockwell Laser Industries website.

Valleylab website: Alternate site lesions, *Hotline News* 5:4, December, 2000.

Valleylab website: Electromagnetic interference, *Hotline News* 6:1, March, 2001.

Watson J and McPherson G: Lasers, 1996, http://vcs.abdn.ac.uk/ENGINEERING/lasers/lasers.html.

Chapter 18

Endoscopic Surgery and Robotics

Terminology

Adhesions—Scar tissue that binds internal tissues together. Adhesions present a technical problem during endoscopic surgery because they can cause wide variations in the anatomical locations of organs. Because the initial incisions often are made blindly, adhesions can result in trauma to tissues.

Coupling—Electrosurgical contact between two or more instruments during endoscopic surgery. This can result in serious burns.

Endoscope—The optical instrument inserted into a body cavity during endoscopic surgery.

Fiberoptic—Pertaining to a lighting system that uses bundles of flexible reflective fibers to transmit light through a cable. Fiberoptic light is extremely in-

tense. The source may be a xenon or halogen metal vapor arc lamp.

Hasson cannula—A type of blunt-tipped trocar-and-cannula assembly used in "open" laparoscopic procedures that is anchored to the body wall with sutures.

Insufflator—The device used to deliver carbon dioxide gas from the tank to the patient to achieve pneumoperitoneum. The insufflator monitors the amount and rate of flow and contains an alarm system to alert to excessive intraabdominal pressure.

Monitor—The screen used to display the camera image during endoscopy.

Morcelization—A process in which tissue is fragmented so it can be withdrawn easily through an endoscopic cannula or suction device.

Objective—The distal end of the endoscopic telescope.

Ocular—The proximal end of the endoscopic telescope.

Open procedure—A traditional surgical procedure that includes incision and wide access to the target tissue.

Pneumoperitoneum—Technique in which the peritoneal cavity is inflated with a compressed gas such as carbon dioxide (CO_2) so that endoscopic surgery can be performed with reduced risk of trauma to tissues and organs.

Ports—Cannulated incisions made in the body wall. The ports receive and stabilize the endoscopic instruments used to perform endoscopic surgery.

Terminology—cont'd

Resect—To cut through and repair a body cavity or solid tissue.

Sequential compression devices—Pneumatic devices that wrap around the patient's legs and deliver pressure sequentially. The devices are worn to prevent embolism that results from lack of blood flow from the legs to the heart.

Trocar and cannula—Instrument inserted through incision site with a sharp or blunt tip. The trocar tip is inserted through the lumen of the cannula and introduced into the incision site. The trocar then is removed and the cannula remains in the incision site for introduction of instruments for endoscopic procedures.

Uterine manipulator—A probelike instrument that is inserted into the distal cervix and used to reposition the uterus during gynecological endoscopic procedures.

Veress needle—A long, slender needle inserted through the abdominal wall to deliver carbon dioxide gas during the creation of pneumoperitoneum.

RIGID ENDOSCOPY

Most endoscopic surgery (usually called minimally invasive surgery) is performed through one or more small incisions, through which a **trocar and cannula** is inserted; the trocar tip is removed, and the lumen of the cannula remains in the incision site to provide a **port** of entry for the instrumentation that will be used to perform the surgery. An **endoscope** is inserted through one port, and specialty instruments are passed through one or more other ports. The operative site is viewed and the procedure is performed directly through the endoscope, or the image is transmitted to a video screen. Digital pictures can be made throughout the procedure, and many teaching institutions use interactive video telecasting of surgery for teaching purposes. Examples of such procedures include laparoscopy, mediastinoscopy, pelviscopy, arthroscopy, and thoracoscopy.

Certain endoscopic procedures do not require incisions because the endoscope is introduced through a natural opening (orifice) (Figure 18-1). These procedures include bronchoscopy, colonoscopy, cystoscopy, esophagoscopy, esophagogastroduodenoscopy (EGD), hysteroscopy, laryngoscopy, and ureteroscopy.

The development of endoscopic surgery is the greatest advance in surgical technique. The first practical stapler was introduced by United States Surgical Corporation (USSC) in 1964. In 1990 USSC introduced the first EndoClip applier, allowing surgeons to remove diseased gallbladders by laparoscopy. Technological advances have drastically increased the number of procedures that now may be performed through an endoscope. The benefits of endoscopic surgery over open techniques include reduced postoperative pain, earlier recovery, and reduced disability. Although an endoscopic procedure may be no shorter than an **open procedure,** tissue trauma is significantly reduced, which results in less pain, quicker healing, and earlier return to normal daily activities.

Many procedures have a steep learning curve for all members of the surgical team. One reason is the ongoing evolution of instruments and equipment and the continuing development of technique.

Many procedures cannot and should not be performed endoscopically. These remain as the mainstay of traditional surgery. This chapter describes the equipment, instrumentation, and practical application of endoscopic techniques. Discussions of specific procedures are included in the surgical specialties chapters.

The essential differences between open and closed surgery are the following:

▶ In endoscopic surgery, the operative field is viewed through an operative endoscopic lens, and its image is projected onto a video screen. In open procedures, the surgical site is immediately accessed through a large incision.

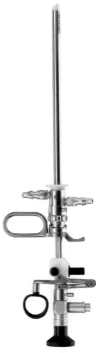

FIGURE 18-1
This type of rigid endoscope must be introduced through a natural opening (orifice). (© Karl Storz Endoscopy America, Inc.)

▶ Endoscopic surgery requires that the operative site be distended with gas or water to allow space for the instruments and prevent accidental injury to tissue.

▶ Endoscopic procedures require the use of very small instruments that can fit through the access ports.

▶ In open surgery, substantial retraction is required. In endoscopic surgery, the gaseous or aqueous environment at the site allows visualization of the target tissue. The patient is positioned intraoperatively so that gravity moves abdominal viscera away from the target tissue.

▶ Open procedures can be performed with one surgical assistant. In complex endoscopic procedures, extra hands often are needed.

▶ Video-assisted endoscopic surgery depends wholly on the proper operation of the camera and other electronic equipment. If the video equipment fails, the surgical field becomes dark and the tissues inaccessible. During open procedures, the operative field is always in view.

▶ In endoscopic procedures, extreme patient positions often are required for access to the target tissue. This causes unstable patient hemodynamics and other negative physiological events.

Preparation of the Patient
PREOPERATIVE PREPARATION TO MINIMIZE RISKS

Patients undergoing endoscopic surgery are prepared according to the anatomical location of the surgery. Laparoscopy patients are required to have minimal bowel preparation. Normal preoperative workup is performed. Surgical skin preparation is identical to the skin prep for an open procedure.

When the patient has entered the surgical suite, special precautions must be taken to minimize risks associated with laparoscopy. These include the following:

▶ Embolism related to pneumoperitoneum (inflation of the abdomen with gas).

▶ Thrombus (blood clot in the circulatory system).

▶ Nerve, vascular, and tissue damage caused by intraoperative positional changes.

▶ Alternate-site burns from electrosurgery.

▶ Rapid hypotension, which can be irreversible (related to extreme positional changes).

▶ Damage to abdominal viscera resulting from the inability to see structures or from interference between two or more surgical instruments in a small area.

▶ Trauma to the bladder wall. A Foley catheter is inserted before all pelvic procedures to prevent inadvertent trauma to the bladder wall. The surgeon may wish to keep the bladder drained for other laparoscopic procedures, and any surgery lasting longer than 6 hours requires urinary drainage.

To prevent embolism, **sequential compression devices** must be placed on the patient's legs (Figure 18-2). These wrap around the leg and sequentially inflate to push blood

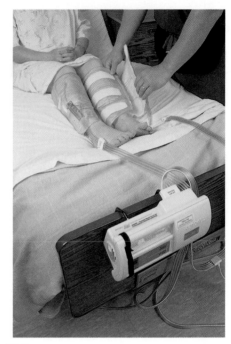

FIGURE 18-2
Sequential compression devices being placed on the patient's legs. (From deWit SC: *Fundamental concepts and skills for nursing,* Philadelphia, 2001, Saunders.)

toward the head. When the patient is to be placed in lithotomy position, thromboembolic stockings often are used.

PATIENT POSITIONING

The positions used for endoscope procedures depend on the target tissue and the patient's physiological condition. For surgery of the upper abdomen or lower esophagus, the patient must be tipped into extreme reverse Trendelenburg position. A padded footboard can be used to prevent the patient from sliding down the operating table, but the footboard must be used with caution. Substantial padding is required to prevent nerve and vascular damage.

For pelvic endoscopy, use of the Trendelenburg position relieves pressure on the pelvic contents by the abdominal viscera. This position compromises the patient's respiratory system and may result in sympathetic nerve reaction. Pressure on the vena cava can cause severe hypotension, requiring immediate attention. This procedure may require a modified lithotomy position for access.

Thoracoscopic procedures are performed with the patient in a lateral position. Cystoscopy, hysteroscopy, and ureteroscopy are performed with the patient in lithotomy position. Colonoscopy may be performed with the patient in a lateral position or in the Sims position. Laryngoscopy, bronchoscopy, esophagoscopy, and mediastinoscopy usually are performed with the patient in a supine position, although the conscious patient undergoing bronchoscopy may be in a Fowler position.

Laparoscopy is usually performed with the patient in a modified lithotomy position using low stirrups (Figure

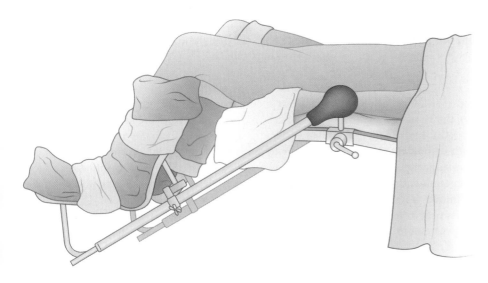

FIGURE 18-3
The modified lithotomy position using low stirrups.

18-3). Refer to Chapter 10 for precautions associated with the use of the lithotomy position.

POSITIONS OF THE SURGICAL TEAM MEMBERS

The positions of the surgical team members depend on the nature of the surgery and the patient's position. The scrub can stand at the side of the table or, in the case of pelvic laparoscopy, at the foot of the table. Other team members stand at the patient's sides.

Equipment and Setup
TECHNICAL EQUIPMENT PROBLEMS

The success of an endoscopic procedure depends heavily on the equipment. The following problems may be encountered:

▶ Poor insufflation
▶ Excessive pressure
▶ Inadequate light
▶ Overly bright light
▶ Lack of picture on the monitor
▶ Poor-quality image
▶ Inadequate suction
▶ Weak electrosurgical capability

INSTRUMENT SETUP

The scrub should keep most endoscopic instruments in a rack on the instrument table. This prevents them from falling off the table or damaging their tips. Endoscopes in particular must be prevented from rolling off the table. Many surgical technologists prefer to work without a Mayo stand during endoscopic surgery. As usual, nonpenetrating clamps must be used to secure cords and tubing on the field. With endoscopic instruments, this is particularly important to avoid injury to the electronic and **fiberoptic** bundles. Sufficient slack must be maintained on all cord attachments. Planning before the start of the procedure

avoids the need to reposition instruments after the procedure is underway.

When one passes endoscopic instruments to the surgeon and assistants, the working end of the instrument should point downward, toward the cannula or endoscope opening. The scrub may assist in positioning the working end of the instrument in the cannula opening.

One of the technical problems encountered in endoscopic procedures is lighting. The room lights often are dimmed or turned completely off. This leaves the surgical technologist with little or no light to identify instruments and prepare materials. A small light should be available for the instrument table. One of the operating lights can be positioned over the instruments and adjusted to a low setting. If a dedicated light is used for the instrument table, ensure that no light is reflected from the instruments into the eyes of the surgeon and assistants.

PREPARATION FOR CONVERSION TO AN OPEN CASE

Every endoscopic procedure has the potential to become an open case. Operative permits are signed with this consideration in mind, and the risks involved in endoscopy (hemorrhage, power problems, or severe imaging problems) increase the possibility that an unplanned open procedure will be required. Some surgeries are scheduled and planned to include both open and endoscopic components. If the endoscopic procedure might confirm a diagnosis that requires extensive open surgery, the patient is informed and preparations are made before surgery.

An emergency conversion to open surgery is very rapid. The scrub and circulator always must be prepared for this event, even in the simplest cases. Appropriate instrument sets, sponges, electrosurgical pencil, suction, and suture materials must be *immediately* available. A switchover should take no longer than 3 to 4 minutes.

When planning the endoscopic procedure, the scrub and circulator also must be thinking about how tables will be set up and what equipment will be needed to convert to an open procedure. If a switchover is required, one can save precious time by preplanning.

Access

PNEUMOPERITONEUM

To view the target tissue in the abdomen, the **Veress needle** is inserted and a **pneumoperitoneum** is created. In this technique, the abdominal cavity is filled with carbon dioxide. This creates a gaseous space that allows the surgeon to insert trocar tips and to manipulate tissues and instruments to perform a procedure. In an alternative technique, sometimes called "open laparoscopy," a **Hasson cannula** with a blunt tip is introduced to establish the pneumoperitoneum. This technique reduces the risk of visceral injury.

Carbon Dioxide

Carbon dioxide is selected for insufflation because it is readily available, stable, and absorbed naturally by the body. A lower incidence of embolism occurs with carbon dioxide than with air. Carbon dioxide does not support combustion and is odorless. The disadvantage of carbon dioxide is the potential for hypercarbia (excess carbon dioxide in the body, leading to metabolic acidosis). This can result in respiratory and cardiac disturbances. However, carbon dioxide remains the safest of all gases for abdominal insufflation. In some cases the surgeon may request the use of nitrous oxide because it does not break down to carbolic acid as carbon dioxide does in the presence of water. However, nitrous oxide is an oxidizer and will support combustion. If the use of laser or electrocautery is anticipated, the use of nitrous oxide is strongly discouraged.

Insufflator

The medical device used to deliver the carbon dioxide is the **insufflator** (Figure 18-4). This device measures both the pressure and the amount of gas flowing into the abdomen. The insufflator should have the following features:

▶ Both high-flow and low-flow pressure control settings
▶ Effective leakage compensation
▶ Gas-warming capacity (expanding carbon dioxide gas is rapidly cooling)
▶ Fluid sensor and filter guard to protect against cross-contamination

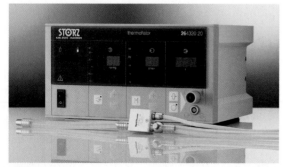

FIGURE 18-4
An insufflator. (© Karl Storz Endoscopy America, Inc.)

▶ Audible and visual warning signals to indicate when pressure exceeds the programmed amount
▶ Reserve tank capacity

Technique

To achieve pneumoperitoneum, a small-bore Veress needle is used (Figure 18-5). Veress needles are available in an assortment of lengths appropriate for patients of different sizes. The distal tip has a small hole in it to permit the flow of gas. The proximal end is fitted to the flexible insufflation tubing.

To insert the needle, the surgeon makes a small stab incision in the superficial abdominal tissues with a no. 11 knife blade (Figure 18-6). The abdominal wall is elevated with penetrating clamps or by hand. The needle is then pushed through the incision at an angle to avoid puncturing the viscera.

A saline test is used to verify the position of the needle. A 10-ml syringe filled with normal saline is attached to the hub of the Veress needle (Figure 18-7, *A*). If needle placement is correct, the saline will drain by negative pressure into the ab-

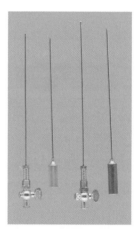

FIGURE 18-5
Veress needles and stylets (medium and long) *(left to right).* (From Tighe SM: *Instrumentation for the operating room,* ed 6, St Louis, 1999, Mosby.)

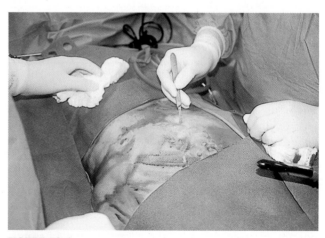

FIGURE 18-6
The Veress needle is inserted through the incision. (From Nagle GM: *Genitourinary surgery,* St Louis, 1997, Mosby.)

dominal cavity. After the Veress needle is in place, it is connected to inflow insufflator tubing (Figure 18-7, *B*). This tubing must have a filter attached and should be flushed with carbon dioxide before insufflation to remove air. A safe level of gas flow should be sustained until the abdominal pressure reaches 12 to 18 mm Hg.

In the alternative technique of using a Hasson cannula, a 1 cm incision (typically infraumbilical or supraumbilical) is made. Two heavy (#1 or #0) absorbable sutures are placed in the fascia on each side of the incision and tagged with the needles left attached. Blunt dissection is used to identify the peritoneum, which is grasped with curved hemostats. After the surgeon ensures that the abdominal viscera is protected, the peritoneum is incised and the Hasson cannula with blunt obturator is introduced. The sutures are wrapped around locking tabs on the cannula, and the insufflation tubing is connected to the insufflation port on the cannula.

Pneumoperitoneum can result in an embolism in the venous system because some venous bleeding is inevitable during the procedure. This exposes the vascular system to carbon dioxide under pressure. Complications occur when the gas blocks the right ventricle and blood cannot flow. Free gas within the vascular system can result in a fatal embolus. If the gas enters the coronary arteries, the coronary blood flow may be blocked. One cubic centimeter of air in the coronary circulatory system can result in death. Free gas also may obstruct cerebrovascular flow, resulting in a cerebrovascular accident (CVA).

TROCARS

Cutting trocars penetrate tissues of the abdominal wall by sharp trauma. A major disadvantage of the cutting trocar is the risk of slicing into unseen tissues lying in the path of the trocar. The *blunt trocar* is ideal when **adhesions** (internal scar tissue) bind the abdominal wall to the viscera. Various trocars that retract automatically after the abdomen has been penetrated also are available. The *optical trocar* allows passage of the viewing telescope as the cannula is advanced. The *screw-threaded* trocar can be twisted into tissue. Minimal gas leakage occurs with this type. The different types of trocars are shown in Figure 18-8.

CANNULAS

Cannulas are designed to accept endoscopic instruments. The most common sizes for abdominal and thoracic surgery are 5 mm and 10 mm. Larger and smaller sizes are available. To maintain pneumoperitoneum, the proximal end of the cannula must form a snug seal around the instrument that is passed through it. A number of different designs have been developed to create this seal.

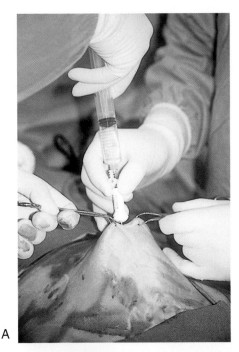

A

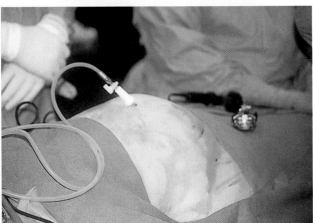

B

FIGURE 18-7
A, The saline test is performed. **B,** The Veress needle is connected to insufflator tubing. (From Nagle GM: *Genitourinary surgery,* St Louis, 1997, Mosby.)

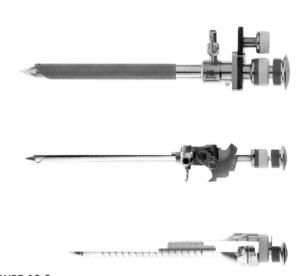

FIGURE 18-8
Optical cutting trocar, blunt-tipped trocar, screw-threaded cutting trocar *(top to bottom).* (© Karl Storz Endoscopy America, Inc.)

The *trumpet valve* is a spring-loaded piston on the cannula that allows passage of an instrument when depressed and closes securely when released. This type of valve, however, can cause scratching or actual tears in insulated housing if the piston is released prematurely. Any interruption in the insulation can result in serious electrosurgical burns. Stainless steel housing over the insulation prevents this problem.

All cannulas contain a silicone rubber seal at the proximal end. Adapters or *reducers* that fit into the proximal end of the cannula also may be used to allow a smaller-diameter instrument to be passed through a large cannula. *Variable-diameter* seals also are available.

After it is in place, the cannula must remain anchored to the body wall to prevent inadvertent withdrawal during surgery. Cannula retention is a function of design. The Hasson cannula is retained in tissue with sutures (Figure 18-9). The screw-shaped trocar also offers good retention. Cannulas with *balloon anchors* are retained in the abdominal wall by an inflatable balloon at the distal tip of the cannula.

Flexible synthetic cannulas made of Teflon, Gore-Tex, or plastic are used when tissue protection is critical, such as in neurovascular tissue.

Cannulas must remain free of tissue to maintain clean passage of instruments.

TROCAR-CANNULA SYSTEMS

Trocar-cannula systems are used to create ports into the abdomen or other body cavities for the insertion of endoscopic instruments. The trocar fits inside the cannula sleeve. The trocar-cannula combination is inserted into the abdominal wall through a small incision and advanced forward. The trocar is then withdrawn, and the hollow cannula remains. A wide variety of combinations and configurations are available, including disposable systems and reusable systems. Single-use trocar-cannula systems often are preferred because they are always sharp and do not require the complex cleaning of stainless-steel valve systems.

BALLOON DISSECTION

Balloon dissection is the separation of body planes with an inflatable balloon (Figure 18-10). The balloon is inserted into a tissue space and inflated. The air-filled sac separates the tissue planes without trauma and is used in hernia repair.

Viewing with the Laparoscope

The endoscopic laparoscope is an elongated optical instrument that is inserted into the cannula. The proximal lens of

the telescope is called the **ocular**, and the distal lens is the **objective**. The most common laparoscopes are illustrated in Figure 18-11. They are the following:

▶ Forward or *zero-degree*
▶ Forward-oblique or *30-degree*
▶ *45-degree*
▶ 2-mm *zero-degree*

The optical systems of most laparoscopes produce resolution equal to that of the human eye. Distortion, bloodstaining, and fogging remain problems. Lens fogging results from the presence of debris or blood on the objective, and from differences between air temperature and the temperature of the body. A chemical lens-defogging agent can be used inter-

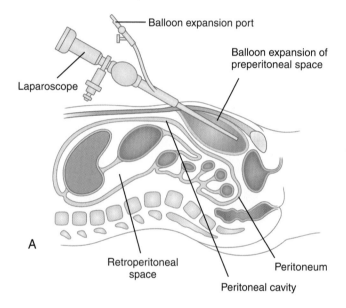

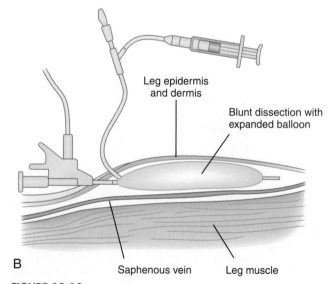

FIGURE 18-10
Balloon expansion of surgical planes. **A,** Preperitoneal expansion. **B,** Saphenous vein harvest using balloon dissection technique. (Redrawn from Rothrock JC: *Alexander's care of the patient in surgery,* ed 12, St Louis, 2003, Mosby.)

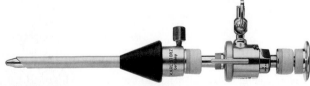

FIGURE 18-9
Hasson cannula. (© Karl Storz Endoscopy America, Inc.)

mittently during the procedure. However, the lens should be wiped with warm water and dried before the agent is applied. An alternative method of defogging is the *scope warmer*. This is equivalent to a small, open-ended thermos. The scrub retains the scope warmer on the instrument table and inserts the laparoscope to keep it at body temperature when it is not in active use. Solutions remain warm in the thermos for up to 4 hours. A disadvantage of the scope warmer is its tendency to tip over.

The laparoscope and all endoscopes must be handled with extreme care at all times. Their slender shafts and delicate lens systems can be easily damaged. One should never handle endoscopes by the tip, because the weight of the optical end will bend the shaft.

LIGHT SOURCE

Light is projected through the endoscope from a high-intensity source. The most common light source is a 300-watt xenon lamp or halogen metal vapor arc lamp (Figure 18-12, *A*). Light is transmitted through a fiberoptic or fluid cable that is attached to the endoscope. The fiberoptic cable

is composed of many minute longitudinal fibers that traverse the length of the cable (Figure 18-12, *B*). To produce fiberoptic light, light is projected through the hollow fibers and is reflected along the bodies of the fibers. This concentrates the light and also allows it to bend with the cable. Although fibers are contained in a heavy flexible cable housing, individual fibers can easily be broken if the cable strikes a hard surface or is overflexed. The quality of the cable usually degenerates slowly as more and more fibers become broken. An extra cable always should be available during surgery.

When a fiberoptic cable is in use, it must never be activated until it is attached to the system. The cable should be turned off or turned down to the lowest setting when not in use. The intense beam easily can ignite patient drapes. Other combustible materials, such as pooled preparation solutions that may not be visible from the outside of the drapes, produce vapors that can ignite and start a patient fire.

Do not allow kinks to develop in the fiberoptic cable. This breaks the fibers. Fiberoptic cables cannot be placed in an ultrasonic cleaner. Fluid cables must not be placed in endoscopic-instrument cleaning systems. Always follow the manufacturer's recommendations for processing these cable systems.

CAMERA, MONITOR, AND DOCUMENTATION

The video camera allows the surgeon to transmit the image in the endoscope's "eye" to a video **monitor** (Figure 18-13). The optical qualities of the image of a superior telescope can be reduced significantly, depending on the quality of the

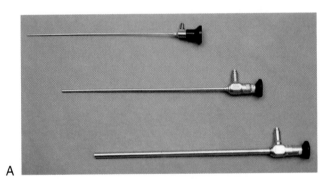

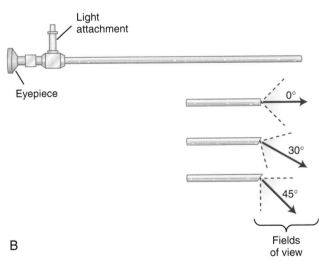

FIGURE 18-11
A, Common lengths of laparoscopes: 2 mm, 5 mm, and 10 mm (shown with 0 degree views). **B,** Common degree views of laparoscopes: 0 degrees, 30 degrees, and 45 degrees. (**A** from Goldberg JM and Falcone T: *Atlas of endoscopic techniques in gynecology*, Philadelphia, 2001, Saunders. **B** redrawn from Phillips N: *Berry & Kohn's operating room technique*, ed 10, St Louis, 2004, Mosby.)

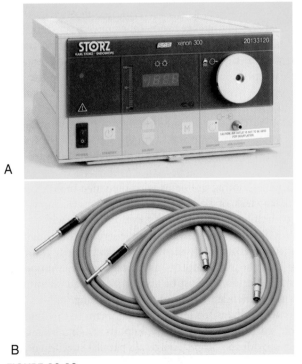

FIGURE 18-12
A, Xenon light source. **B,** Fiberoptic light cord. (© Karl Storz Endoscopy America, Inc.)

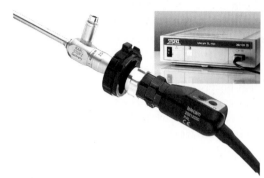

FIGURE 18-13
Endovision telecam. (© Karl Storz Endoscopy America, Inc.)

video camera. The core of the camera is a charge-coupled device. This is a solid-state silicon computer chip. It consists of light-sensitive silicon elements that produce an electrical charge when exposed to light. Because electricity can be amplified, the output of the silicon elements also can be amplified and displayed on a digital monitor. Each silicon element represents one *pixel*. The resolution of the image depends on how many pixels or silicon units the chip contains. The more units, the clearer the image appears. Thus a three-chip camera creates higher resolution than a single-chip camera. Newer camera models are *parfocal*. Because of this characteristic, they enlarge the image, which requires refocusing of the lens system of the telescope.

The endoscopic procedure is documented in still photographs or on videotape. The camera image must be captured in a camera box that translates the signal into a continuous electronic waveform. This waveform, like all others, can be distorted by interference from other energy sources. The camera box must be compatible with the video screen to maximize the capabilities of the camera. Still images are best when taken through a 35-mm camera attached to the laparoscope. Newer camera heads have hand controls that allow the surgeon to make a permanent photograph of the camera image while surgery is in progress. In other systems, the circulator must perform this procedure using the video system controls. Videotaping and remote telemedicine also are possible.

Troubleshooting problems with the video monitor is an important task of both the scrub and the circulator. The video monitor is the surgeon's eye. Problems with image quality, lighting, or blackout can have serious consequences. Most manufacturers of video systems offer on-site training. Even if the hospital employs a surgical bioengineer, operating room personnel must be able to set up equipment and perform elementary tasks and troubleshooting.

Attaching the video recording equipment to the imaging system correctly is particularly important. *Parallel attachments* provide the clearest images. In parallel attachment, the recorder and the main viewing monitor are attached to the camera. In *serial attachment,* the camera, recording unit, and monitor all are connected in a line. If the camera signal is in-

put directly into the recording box and the latter is then connected to the monitor, the image quality will be low.

The descriptions given here are general directions for imaging and documentation. Refer to the manufacturer's instructions for the setup requirements of a specific system. Hybrid systems may pose the most difficult troubleshooting problems.

Rigid Endoscopic Instruments
INSTRUMENT CARE

Endoscopic instruments represent a significant investment for any health-care institution. Because of the nature of their use, they are delicate, slender, and finely manufactured. Attention to detail is important in the handling and care of equipment and instruments. Telescopes and video instruments are particularly vulnerable to irreparable injury if bent, dented, or scratched. The best way to avoid harm to all equipment is to follow the manufacturer's recommendations for cleaning and terminal sterilization (discussed later in the chapter), and to actively protect the instruments at all times before, during, and after the procedure.

INSTRUMENT DESIGN

Because endoscopic instruments must enter deeply into the surgical incision, they are narrow. The handles of instruments are located at some distance from the working end. Hinges, springs, and valves are very small, and the success of the surgery depends on the economy and efficiency of the mechanical design. Instruments are available in reusable and disposable models. Use of disposable instruments reduces the risk of cross-contamination, and such instruments are extremely sharp.

Nondisposable instruments require a large initial investment and maintenance. Reliability is a serious consideration when selecting single-use instruments. Considering the need for consistent performance, not only must the time and cost of resterilization be compared, but the cost of repeated purchase of items that become damaged from improper use or maintenance also must be factored.

CHARACTERISTICS OF INSTRUMENTS

Endoscopic instruments are nearly as numerous and complex as their open-surgery counterparts. The design of the instrument permits the surgeon to thread the working end and shaft into the access port with minimal risk of injury to the instrument.

Endoscopic instruments perform precise surgical tasks in a confined space. They are very delicate and must be maintained carefully. It is particularly important that insulation housing on the instrument be unblemished in any way. Even a small dent in the housing can cause an unintentional electrosurgical burn. Most endoscopic instruments are capable of transmitting electrosurgical energy. The multifunction instrument design avoids insertion, removal, and reinsertion of instruments when coagulation or cutting is required. As with all electrosurgical instruments, the insulated housing on the shafts of electrosurgically capable endoscopic instruments must be inspected often for integrity.

Both disposable, nonreusable instruments and reusable instruments are employed. Although disposable instruments are expensive, their use saves the labor required to thoroughly clean and sterilize reusable instruments.

Grip mechanisms on endoscopic instruments are important to the ergonomics and precision of the tool. Long procedures require continued delicate control. This control is created by comfortable handles and balance within the design. The most common handle design is a *transaxial* design, which has two finger rings at a 90-degree angle to the long axis of the instrument. When one opens and closes the finger rings, the tips of the instrument open and close.

TYPES OF INSTRUMENTS AND THEIR USES

Retractors
Many different retractor designs are available, each using the same principle as open-surgery retractors. Because of the limited space, retractors must extend from the tip of the shaft and either flare out or curve at various angles (Figure 18-14).

Forceps and Scissors
Like their open-surgery counterparts, grasping instruments for endoscopic surgery can be purchased in hundreds of different types from various manufacturers. Many different types of tip designs are available. Some provide atraumatic grasping, while others penetrate the tissue. The working tips of endoscopic graspers match those of graspers for open surgery. The only difference is the working length between the hinge and the tip. Because of the short fulcrum and flexibility of the instruments, the amount of applied grasping force is greatly reduced in an endoscopic instrument. Endoscopic forceps and scissors are illustrated in Figure 18-15. Forceps used to perform a tissue biopsy are illustrated in Figure 18-16.

The endoscopic instrument is less resistant to force, and the metal must have memory (recover to the original shape after deformation when force is applied). Graspers now are available in hingeless designs to increase the angle of the grasping jaws (Figure 18-17). Scissors are extremely delicate and fine. Dissection is usually performed with scissors or with electrosurgical or laser instruments.

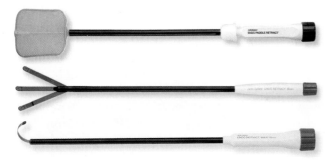

FIGURE 18-14
Retractors. (Courtesy of United States Surgical Corporation, Norwalk, Conn.)

Manipulators
A **uterine manipulator** is inserted into the cervix before gynecological endoscopy (Figure 18-18). This instrument is used to position the uterus so as to increase access to regions of the female pelvis.

Probes
The probe is used to move tissues around and usually is capable of electrosurgical hemostasis. It is a conductive rod coated with nonconductive material to within an inch or less of the distal tip.

Suction and Irrigation Devices
Irrigation is used continually or intermittently. Irrigation is needed to keep the operative field clear (see below). Because of the small size of the optical telescope, any blood or debris within the focal view is magnified on the video screen. If hemorrhage occurs, the surgeon has no way to locate and occlude the bleeding vessel without pinpoint suction. Irrigation is delivered through a single irrigation tip or a combination suction-irrigation tip. Nonconductive isotonic solution is used (i.e., normal saline or lactated Ringer solution). Continuous irrigation is required to maintain a clear surgical field during surgery of the prostate, surgery of the interior bladder wall, and intrauterine surgery. In arthroscopic surgery, aqueous solution is used to inflate the joint space.

When continuous irrigation is required, it is the circulator's responsibility to replace irrigation solutions as they are used. Solution is pumped from the supply pump through a sterile system of tubing. Two bags of solution can be loaded into the pump, one for current use and the other for reserve. As one bag is emptied, the other must be activated, and the empty one must be replaced immediately.

Figure 18-19 illustrates some common suction and irrigation instruments.

Suturing and Ligation Devices
Ligation in endoscopic procedures is performed with many different devices and techniques. Various instruments have been designed to tie knots, snug knots, and suture tissue using a straight or ski-shaped needle. Synthetic and metal clips often are used in endoscopic surgery. These are introduced through the surgical port and applied in the same way as in open surgery.

Products are constantly being developed to improve the technical capabilities of endoscopic surgery. Ligation and suturing is an area in which product designs change frequently. Figure 18-20 illustrates the design and use of a common suturing and ligation instrument.

Stapling instruments are routinely used in endoscopic surgery to **resect** tissue (divide and reconnect or seal the cut tissue edges). Endoscopic stapling instruments can be disposable or reusable. Most surgeons favor disposable instruments.

STERILIZATION AND DISINFECTION OF RIGID ENDOSCOPES
Endoscopic instruments often come in contact with *critical areas* such as sterile organs and the vascular system. These instruments must be *sterilized* between patient uses.

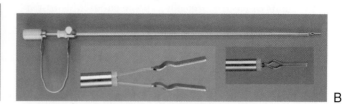

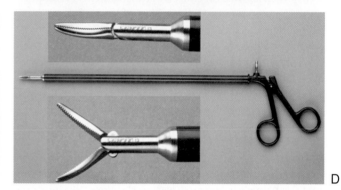

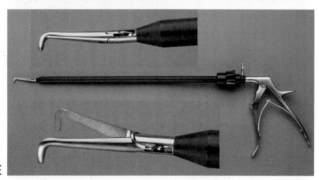

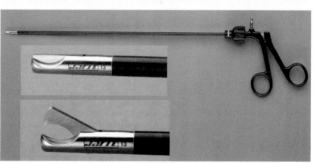

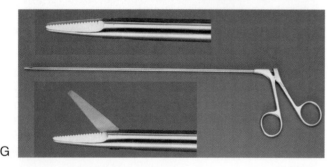

FIGURE 18-15
Endoscopic forceps and scissors. **A,** Bipolar forceps (micro). **B,** Bipolar forceps (large). **C,** Tapered Maryland forceps. **D,** Maryland dissecting forceps. **E,** Mixter-spreader forceps. **F,** Hook scissors. **G,** Jarit supercut scissors. (Courtesy of Jarit Instruments, Hawthorne, NY.)

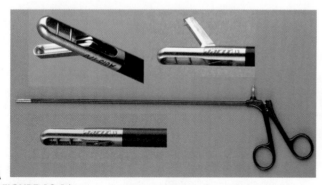

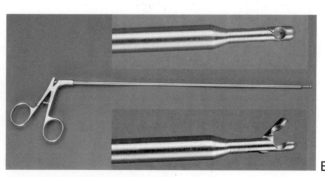

FIGURE 18-16
Biopsy forceps. **A,** Biopsy punch. **B,** Micro biopsy forceps. (Courtesy of Jarit Instruments, Hawthorne, NY.)

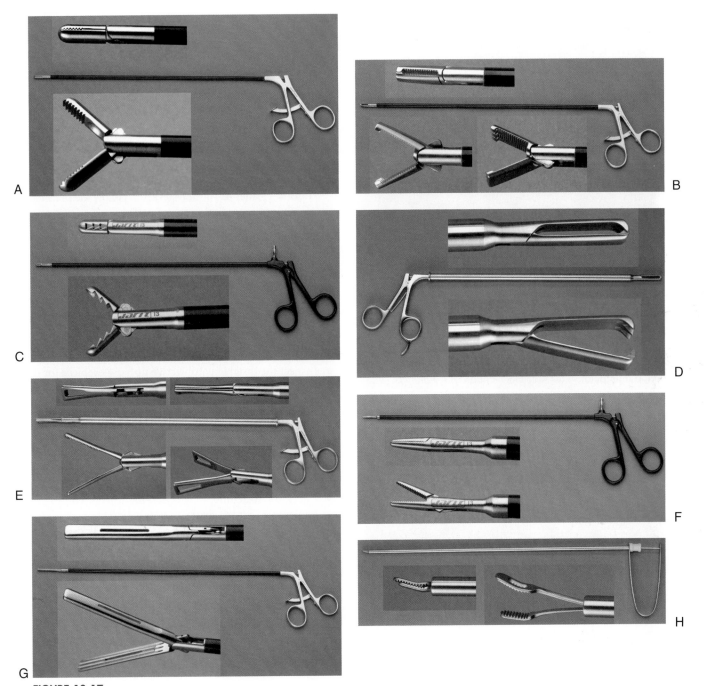

FIGURE 18-17
Graspers. **A,** Grasper forceps with ratchet. **B,** Allis grasper forceps. **C,** Toothed grasper forceps. **D,** Claw grasper and extracting forceps. **E,** Jarit-Duval grasper forceps. **F,** Micro grasper forceps. **G,** Jarit-Debakey forceps. **H,** Strong Atrau forceps. (Courtesy of Jarit Instruments, Hawthorne, NY.)

Endoscopic instruments used in *semicritical* areas require high-level disinfection.

Intraoperative Care

During surgery, rigid endoscopes and endoscopic instruments should be kept as clean as possible. Suction tips should be flushed frequently to prevent clogging. As with all delicate instruments, endoscopes and endoscopic instruments should be protected from damage by heavier instruments. Before transporting to the workroom or decon-

tamination area, disconnect the light cable from the telescope.

Cleaning and Decontamination

To clean and decontaminate the rigid endoscope:

1. First disconnect the light cable from the telescope. Remove any cable adapters.
2. Place the endoscope in an enzymatic soaking solution compatible with the instrument. Confirm the use of

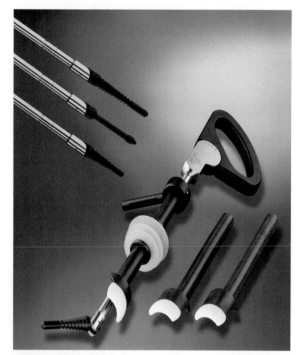

FIGURE 18-18
Uterine manipulator. (© Karl Storz Endoscopy America, Inc.)

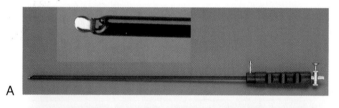

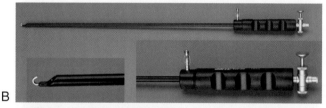

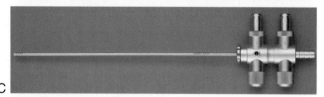

FIGURE 18-19
Suction and irrigation instruments. **A,** Suction coagulator with spatula tip. **B,** Suction coagulator with hook end. **C,** Suction/irrigation cannula. (Courtesy of Jarit Instruments, Hawthorne, NY.)

appropriate solutions as specified by the manufacturer's instructions. Using a soft cloth, clean off any tissue debris, blood, and body fluids from all surfaces of the endoscope.

3. Rinse the endoscope with *distilled water* to protect the surface from mineral stains and corrosion. Optical lenses are cleaned with 70% alcohol to remove detergent residue.

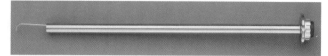

FIGURE 18-20
Suturing and ligation instrument—Elkus suture passer. (Courtesy of Jarit Instruments, Hawthorne, NY.)

4. Use a soft cloth or pressurized air hose to dry the endoscope and all ports.
5. Some rigid endoscopes may be decontaminated in an ultrasonic cleaner or washer-sterilizer. Follow the manufacturer's recommendations.

Inspection

Rigid endoscopes and are subject to bending, scratching, and cracking. When handling rigid endoscopes, *never handle the metal shaft,* or the weight of the headpiece will bend the shaft and ruin the endoscope and any instrument that passes through it. Specific guidelines apply to the inspection of endoscopes and accessories.

When inspecting endoscopes:

▶ Inspect the distal lens (objective tip) and eyepiece for debris by observing indirect light on the surfaces. Look for scratches, chips, and fingerprints.
▶ Look through the eyepiece to check for lens clarity. Rotate the endoscope shaft to check all surfaces. If any obstruction appears, the lens may be damaged. Fogging of a lens may be caused by moisture between the lens and the seal, an indication of leakage.
▶ Check for straightness by observing it from end to end. Remember that the shaft contains delicate optical parts. A bent sheath can damage the endoscope and other instruments passing through it.
▶ Stopcocks must be freely moveable.

When inspecting endoscope accessories:

▶ Check fiberoptic and liquid-light cables for continuity of light. Broken fiberoptic cables are visible as black spots on a light glassy background. If more than 15% of the fibers are broken, the cable must be repaired.
▶ Veress needles must be straight and sharp with no burrs on the ends.
▶ Trocars must be sharp and straight.
▶ Grasping instruments must be straight and hinges freely moveable.
▶ Use a magnifying glass to inspect working tips and hinges.
▶ Any instrument that is used for electrosurgery must be carefully evaluated for damage to insulated housing. Any break in the continuity of insulation such as tears, cuts, or holes can cause patient burns. These instruments must be removed from service and repaired.
▶ Electrosurgical unit (ESU) cables should be checked for any holes, abrasions, or cuts. A broken wire in the ESU cable can result in spark gap, which can cause the cable to ignite. Any cable that might be damaged must be discarded.

▶ Never attempt to repair endoscopes or any accessories yourself. This may result in patient injury or irreparable damage to the instrument.

FLEXIBLE ENDOSCOPY

Flexible endoscopes are designed for use in tubular structures such as the gastrointestinal (GI) tract, genitourinary tract, small ducts, vascular structures, ear, nasal passages, and sinuses. The endoscope houses a control head, which is contiguous with a long, flexible fiberoptic tube. The tube is passed into the body through an incision or natural opening such as the trachea. Fiberoptic bundles in the tube transmit light to the distal end, where the image is magnified. The flexible tip of the endoscope can be rotated in any direction to create a 360-degree view of the target tissue.

Channels that are open at both ends of the endoscope allow the passage of instruments for biopsy, suction, and irrigation. Many flexible endoscopic instruments are disposable to reduce the risk of blood-borne disease transmission. Biopsy brushes always are disposable. Small snares and forceps are threaded through the endoscope channels until they emerge at the tip. Very small sections of tissue can be excised and withdrawn through the channel.

Flexible endoscopy can be incorporated into a rigid endoscopic procedure. For example, during cholecystectomy or surgery of the pancreas, the flexible endoscope can be introduced into the ducts of these systems to perform biopsy or to indirectly observe pathologic tissue.

Imaging
Like the rigid endoscope, the flexible endoscope has the capability to document findings by still or video imaging. The same recommendations for compatibility and operation that apply to rigid endoscopy also apply to flexible endoscopy. The image quality of fiberoptic endoscopes is generally inferior to that of rigid endoscopes. Camera attachments are similar to those used in rigid endoscopy.

Light
The light source used in flexible endoscopy is the same as that used in rigid endoscopy. A xenon or halogen metal vapor arc lamp emits daylight-quality light. The fiberoptic light cord and light source described earlier are usually used.

Endoscopic Procedures
Many endoscopic procedures are performed in an ambulatory or outpatient setting. Patient preparation depends on the type of endoscopy planned. When fluoroscopy is required, the procedure is performed in the GI laboratory or other specialized area of the outpatient clinic.

Flexible endoscopy has been developed for virtually every surgical specialty. The principles of lighting, instrumentation, optics, and documentation remain constant. The sizes of the endoscopes and the individual instruments vary according to the needs of the procedure (Figure 18-21). The primary use of flexible endoscopy is in diagnostic proce-

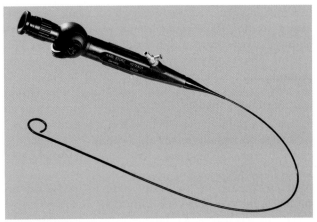

FIGURE 18-21
Flexible endoscope. (© Karl Storz Endoscopy America, Inc.)

dures, although it can be used for tissue dissection and removal. Specific endoscopic procedures associated with each specialty are described in the chapter covering that specialty.

High Level Disinfection of Flexible Endoscopes
STANDARDS FOR DISINFECTING FLEXIBLE ENDOSCOPES
Guidelines and standards for the processing of flexible endoscopes are established by the Centers for Disease Control (CDC), the Food and Drug Administration (FDA), the Society of Gastroenterology Nurses and Associates (SGNA), the Association for Practitioners in Infection Control and Epidemiology (APIC), and the Association of periOperative Room Nurses (AORN).

Safe disinfection of flexible endoscopes is a critical issue in infection control because of the risk of disease transmission. Many endoscopic procedures often are performed within a tight schedule with rapid turnover. This has led to inadequate or improper mechanical cleaning and disinfection practices. Improper hand cleaning or use of automatic cleaning devices has resulted in the transmission of infectious disease.

INTRAOPERATIVE CARE
During endoscopic surgery, telescopes, valves, and channels should be flushed to keep them moist and clean. Do not allow secretions to dry inside channels and tubes. The outside of the scopes also must be periodically wiped with a damp towel. Take special care to wipe exposed parts whenever possible during the procedure. The tips of biopsy forceps and other cutting instruments require particular attention, as tissue is easily trapped in hinges and teeth.

PRECLEANING
The flexible video endoscope contains a working head that houses the controls. These communicate with the insertion tube, which contains narrow channels and ports for suction, irrigation, viewing, and biopsy. Endoscopic instruments used in the GI and respiratory tracts carry a high bioburden

(amount of organic debris including feces, blood, and respiratory secretions). Cleaning must take place *immediately after use of the endoscope,* usually in the patient-care area. Precleaning prevents drying of secretions and tissue inside the channels and on the surface. At the end of an endoscopic procedure, remove all detachable parts. Wipe the insertion tube and all external parts with enzymatic cleaner. Purge all suction, air, and water channels with enzymatic cleaner according to the manufacturer's instructions.

LEAK TESTING

After precleaning, the endoscope must be leak-tested according to the manufacturer's instructions. In this process, a pressurized endoscope is submerged and watched for bubbles. Always protect the controls while the scope is immersed. Feel the distal tip of the scope during immersion to check for distention. Flex the tip in all directions using the controls in order to open all holes. Leaks may occur in the insertion tube, light-guide tube, connector, and control body. The presence of bubbles while working the valves and switches indicates a leak in the system.

CLEANING

During hand cleaning, fill all channels with enzymatic solution and soak *immersible* instruments according to manufacturer specifications. Usually 2 to 5 minutes are sufficient. After the instrument has soaked, use a cleaning brush to clear all debris and blood from the channels. When flushing the channels, push the brush all the way through the channel until the tip emerges so that debris is completely pushed out. Valve ports can be cleaned with a small brush or lint-free swab. A 3-cc syringe should be used to fill the elevator channel of a duodenoscope. After the soaking period, purge all channels and ports using the irrigator and adapters. Clean the outside of the scope with a lint-free cloth.

The automatic endoscope reprocessor (AER) is a mechanical washer that connects to the channels by a series of flexible tubes. During processing, enzymatic cleaner and water are injected through the tubes and channels. *This process is not intended to take the place of hand cleaning.* Precleaning by hand is necessary because the AER cannot access all channels.

Biopsy instruments, including cytology brushes and forceps, are classified as critical items because they penetrate the mucosa tissue. *They must be sterilized.* Disposable biopsy accessories are recommended.

RINSING AND DRYING

Rinse the scope with copious amounts of fresh water to remove all traces of detergent and debris. Some manufacturers recommend rinsing with distilled water to prevent mineral deposits or spotting. Detergent solutions may interact with chemical disinfectants, so meticulous rinsing is important. Do not use alcohol to clean lenses as it can weaken the cement that secures the lens. Use lens paper to clean optical parts. After thorough cleaning, dry the scope and all loose parts with a hand-held power hose. All moisture must be removed from channels.

Accessories that break the mucous-membrane barrier or enter sterile tissues, such as biopsy forceps and cytology brushes, *must be sterilized* before reuse. Disposable biopsy forceps and cytology brushes are preferred.

INSPECTION

Flexible endoscopes must be inspected routinely for lens fogging. This may be caused by leakage or loosening of the lens. Also check for lens scratches, tears, or wrinkles in the insertion-tube housing, as well as:

▶ Leakage (use leakage test to check)
▶ Broken fibers in light bundle
▶ Broken deflector
▶ Frozen valves or control switches

Endoscopes must be handled gently. Fiberoptic bundles and optical portions can be easily broken. Never place the endoscope near the edge of a table or counter. Make sure you have adequate room to process the instruments to avoid striking the insertion tube or control head on a hard surface.

DISINFECTION

Endoscopes that are classified as critical (used on a sterile field) must be sterilized using a method approved by the manufacturer. All other endoscopes require high-level disinfection with liquid chemical sterilant.

Solutions must be prepared according to the manufacturer's instructions. Particular solutions may be used multiple times as long as the instruments are thoroughly cleaned and dry. Disinfectant must be contained in a tightly covered pan that is labeled with the name of the disinfectant and the date of preparation. Hazardous chemicals such as glutaraldehyde must be prepared and used under a safety hood. Solutions must be tested with a concentration monitor strip every 10 cycles or at least daily.

Processing of the instrument begins with disassembly. The endoscope and all detachable parts must be *completely immersed* in a soaking pan with disinfectant solution. All channels must be filled with solution using adapters while the instrument is submerged. The lid is then placed tightly on the soaking pan and exposure timed according to the manufacturer's instructions.

Strict criteria that determine the efficacy of the solution include:

▶ Cleanliness of the instrument
▶ Absence of moisture on the instrument, which would dilute the disinfectant
▶ Temperature of the solution
▶ Concentration of the chemical
▶ Complexity of the instrument's structure
▶ Lumen size (smaller lumens are more difficult to process)
▶ Contact time

If an automatic reprocessor is used for disinfection, connect all tubing to channels and ports. Make sure that all tubing is well secured. Do not exceed the recommended pressure for reprocessing.

RINSING

After exposure, rinse the endoscope by submerging it completely in a fresh-water bath. Purge all disinfectant from the channels and lumens using the controls, or if an AER is used, make sure that the rinse cycle is complete.

DRYING AND FLUSHING

After rinsing the endoscope, one must thoroughly dry it and flush it with 70% alcohol to facilitate drying. Follow the alcohol flush with a forced-air infusion through all channels, and dry the outside and all other parts with a lint-free cloth.

STORAGE

Endoscopes must be stored in a ventilated storage area with the control head secured in an upright position and the distal part of the insertion tube hanging downward. Endoscopes must be terminally decontaminated (disinfected) at the end of the workday and *again the following day before use.*

ELECTROSURGERY AND LASER SURGERY

Electrosurgery is used in nearly every type of endoscopic procedure. For a detailed description of this technology, see Chapter 17. Endoscopic electrosurgery presents higher risks than open electrosurgery. This is because the surgeon does not have a complete view of the electrosurgical instrument. The shaft of the instrument can deliver cutting or coagulating energy if the insulated housing on the shaft is damaged. Recall that this covering does not have to be visibly damaged to cause severe burns and that the burn site is almost always out of the telescope's eye. For example, a burn can occur in the bowel tissue and cause leakage that may not be noticed at the time of injury.

An additional risk is inadvertent **coupling**—conduction of electricity from the active electrode to one or more other instruments. In abdominal endoscopy, as many as five or six separate ports may be created in the abdominal wall (Figure 18-22). The chance of coupling between the electrosurgical instrument and other instruments can be high in the limited space of the insufflated abdomen.

Laparoscopy carries an additional risk of ignition of gas from the bowel. The closed environment prevents the dilution of highly combustible methane. Suction always should be available to remove gases before the electrosurgical unit is activated. A fire *inside* a closed patient is a terrifying, tragic, *preventable* event.

Laser surgery, discussed in Chapter 17, is often used during endoscopic procedures. Because of its pinpoint beam, laser energy is well suited to endoscopic surgery. The usual risks and precautions for open procedures apply to endoscopic laser surgery as well. Endoscopic surgery carries the additional risk of patient ignition in a closed space. The laser is often used in endoscopic surgery of the respiratory system, and the oxygen-rich environment results in a higher incidence of patient fire at the flammable polyvinyl-chloride endotracheal tube. All risk-reducing

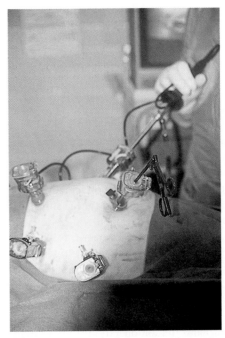

FIGURE 18-22
Several trocars being inserted into the abdominal wall. (From Nagle GM: *Genitourinary surgery,* St Louis, 1997, Mosby.)

techniques used in open procedures should be used in endoscopic surgery as well.

TISSUE REDUCTION AND RETRIEVAL

Morcelization

For tissue to be retrieved from the abdomen or other large body cavity, it must be reduced to fit through the port or cannula. If the tissue is dense, the surgeon can reduce it through a process called **morcelization** (reduction of the size of tissue by cutting it into small pieces). Tissue can be reduced using loop cauterization or a low-speed power morcelizer.

Shaving

The tissue shaver is used extensively in nasal and orthopedic procedures. In endoscopic paranasal surgery, it is used to remove large masses of polyps and redundant or diseased tissue of the paranasal sinuses. The shaver suctions soft tissue into the cutting channel, where a spiral burr shaves it into small pieces. In orthopedic arthroscopic surgery, soft tissue, cartilage, and small bone fragments may be reduced in this manner.

Retrieval Through Other Systems

Several other types of retrieval system are available. For retrieval of tissue or small organs, a retractable tissue bag (Pleatman sack) is inserted into the wound. The surgeon captures the organ into the bag and retracts the open portion to secure the contents. The bag is then withdrawn through a large port. For extremely large specimens, an 18-mm port may be required for extraction.

Calculi can be retrieved using a stone basket or similar mesh device. The stone basket is retracted inside the instrument as it is advanced into the duct or ureter. The basket is opened and the stone is manipulated inside the basket. The basket is then withdrawn, bringing the stone with it.

ROBOTICS

Electronic remote-control robotic instruments are under investigation and development. Designed primarily for use during laparoscopic surgery, the robotic arms can hold the endoscope over the target tissue or actually assist in some of the delicate procedures required for the surgery. The system can be operated from a terminal with remote handles that manipulate the endoscopic instruments. The operator can view the electronically controlled instruments through digital imaging (Figure 18-23). Although not in the mainstream of surgical techniques, this technology may be applied extensively in the future.

The primary benefits of robotic technologies include a reduction of hand tremor, operation from a distant location, increased dexterity, and the use of minimally invasive surgical techniques. Another benefit of robotic technology is the use of binocular endoscopes, which allow for three-dimensional visualization. Although the binocular endoscope is slightly larger in diameter than traditional telescopes, the binocular eyepiece produces a three-dimensional image of the operative site. Robotic technologies have been widely used in a variety of abdominal and thoracic procedures, including prostatectomy, cardiac pacing, gastric bypass, Nissen fundoplication, cholecystectomy, and wedge resection.

Hand Tremor

Occasional hand tremor is a condition that affects most people. This condition is compounded by the use of stimulants such as caffeine. Hand tremors make it difficult to operate on delicate structures. This is exacerbated when working under magnification, as with loupes or the binocular endoscope. The robotic attachments allow the computer-aided manipulation of instruments, which serves to minimize or eliminate fine tremors. This allows for precise dissection of tissues and placement of sutures in delicate structures. The reduction of hand tremor may create more opportunities to perform beating-heart bypass and precise neurosurgical intervention.

Dexterity

Traditional endoscopic procedures use instruments with rigid tips that require the surgeon to use exaggerated movements of the hand and wrist to place sutures or dissect tissues. EndoWrist devices have instrument tips that articulate in a 360-

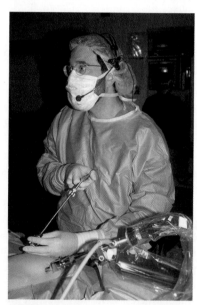
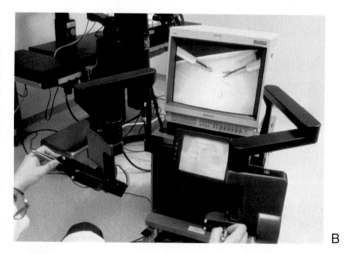

FIGURE 18-23
A, The surgeon commanding the robot. **B,** The surgeon using the robotic arms to manipulate the instruments. **C,** Positioning of the robotic arms relative to the patient. (From Goldberg JM and Falcone T: *Atlas of endoscopic techniques in gynecology*, Philadelphia, 2001, Saunders.)

degree range, which more accurately reflects the surgeon's normal hand movements during tissue dissection, suture placement, and knot tying. This advance, along with the reduction of hand tremor, allows the surgeon to work on more delicate structures through minimally invasive surgical technique.

Distant Surgical Intervention

The application of robotic technology to the performance of surgical procedures at distant locations is currently being studied. The greatest challenge associated with this is the delay from the time a surgeon makes her or his movements to the time those movements are applied to the distant surgical field. This delay occurs because the translated movement is communicated across standard telephone or fiberoptic communication lines. This problem is similar to a telephone call to a distant nation in which a minor delay occurs between the speaking of a word and the reproduction of the word on the other end of the line.

Great strides have been made in this area, and in 2001, a team of surgeons in New York removed the gall bladder of a patient in France using the da Vinci robotic system. The ability to perform a variety of surgical procedures from a great distance promises to be a significant improvement in the delivery of health care to patients in rural areas or who are otherwise unable to reach a hospital. Examples of this latter group include scientists based in remote locations, military personnel deployed in foreign units, and astronauts assigned to the international space station or other space exploration projects.

Minimally Invasive Surgery and Improved Optics

Robotic surgery incorporates the minimally invasive surgical technique that is used in traditional endoscopic procedures with binocular vision to create a three-dimensional image of the surgical field. Minimally invasive techniques serve to reduce tissue trauma and thereby may improve recovery time and reduce postoperative pain. The use of a binocular endoscope gives the surgeon an improved sense of depth perception when working on structures within the body.

CASE STUDIES

Case 1

During a laparoscopy, the surgeon decides to use two electrosurgical pencils on the field. Describe the risks involved and how you would minimize them.

Case 2

You are setting up for a laparoscopy and notice that the patient has many abdominal scars. What problems might be encountered during this endoscopic procedure, and how will you prepare for them?

Case 3

During a laparoscopy the surgeon accidentally cuts into a large mesenteric artery. He is unable to stop the hemorrhage endoscopically and tells you that he will open the patient immediately. What is your plan? What do you need initially? What are the surgical priorities?

Case 4

Explain how electrosurgical burns occur during electrical coupling between instruments.

Case 5

During endoscopic intestinal surgery, you see on the video monitor that there are sparks at the point of contact between the bowel wall and the probe. The team watches in horror as the abdominal cavity becomes engulfed in flames. What is the first response?

REFERENCES

Airan MC: *Patient preparation*, Primary Care Physician Pages, Society of American Gastrointestinal Endoscopic Surgeons, 1996-2003; www.sages.org/primarycare/chapter2.html.

Alvarado CJ and Reichelderfer M: APIC guideline for infection prevention and control in flexible endoscopy, *Am J Infect Control* 28:2, April, 2000.

Ball KA: *Endoscopic surgery: Perioperative nursing series*, St Louis, 1997, Mosby.

Ball M: How to care for your flexible endoscope in 6 easy steps, *Outpatient Surg* May, 2000.

Corwin CL: *Pneumoperitoneum*, Primary Care Physician Pages, Society of American Gastrointestinal Endoscopic Surgeons, 1996-2003; www.sages.org/primarycare/chapter5.html.

Cuschieri A and Szabo Z: *Tissue approximation in endoscopic surgery*, London, 1995, Martin Dunitz.

Holland P: How do you disinfect *that*? A look at flexible endoscope reprocessing, *Infect Control Today*, October, 2001.

Kern B: Endoscope repair issues, *Infect Control Today*, November, 2001.

Tucker RD and Voyles CR: Laparoscopic electrosurgical complications and their prevention, *AORN J* 62:1, July, 1995.

Chapter 19

Diagnostic Procedures

By Ken Warnock

Learning Objectives

After studying this chapter the reader will be able to:

- Identify basic laboratory tests and their indications
- Identify basic radiographic tests and their indications
- Identify the components of a complete blood cell count
- Recognize normal and abnormal values on a complete blood cell count
- Describe the normal electrocardiogram recording
- Describe proper precautions associated with radiation studies
- Describe proper handling of specimens

Terminology

Arterial blood gases (ABGs)—A blood test that uses an arterial blood sample to assess oxygenation and adequacy of ventilation.

Biopsy—Removal of a sample of tissue for pathological analysis.

Chemistry studies—Various tests that evaluate the presence of or levels of certain chemicals within the blood. Chemistry studies are performed to evaluate cardiac enzymes, liver function, kidney function, thyroid function, and basic metabolic function. Cholesterol, or lipid, studies are an example of a chemistry study.

Complete blood count (CBC)—A blood test that measures specific components of blood, including hemoglobin, hematocrit, red blood cells, white blood cells and types, platelets, and several red blood cell indices.

Computed tomography (CT)—A test that allows physicians to obtain cross-sectional radiographic views of the patient. The test also is called a CT scan or computed axial tomography (CAT) scan.

Culture and sensitivity (C & S)—A test used to identify the sensitivity of a microorganism to a particular antimicrobial agent. The test is used to identify the causative agent of an infection and identify the antimicrobial best suited to fight the infection.

Diagnostic agent—Pharmacologic substance used to aid in diagnostic procedures.

Differential count—Test that identifies the amount of each type of WBC in a specimen of blood; typically part of the CBC.

Doppler studies—A technique that uses ultrasound energy to measure motion within blood vessels. The test measures blood flow through a particular vessel.

Echocardiography—The use of ultrasound to diagnose conditions of the heart.

Electrocardiogram (ECG)—A noninvasive test that measures electrical activity of the heart; also abbreviated EKG.

Electrolyte levels—The measurement of levels of various minerals and elements within the blood.

Endoscopy—The use of endoscopic technology to diagnose pathology.

Fluoroscopy—A technique that uses continuous exposure of x-rays to improve the physician's view of structures or objects.

Frozen section—A microscopic slice of frozen anatomic tissue that is evaluated for the presence of abnormal cells. Frozen section analysis is performed during surgery to diagnose malignancy.

Terminology—cont'd

Hematocrit (Hct)—Test that examines the percentage of red blood cells as a part of the blood; part of the CBC or hemogram.

Hemoglobin (Hb)—Test that identifies the capacity of oxygen-carrying cells within the blood. A gram of hemoglobin (Hb) carries 1.34 ml of oxygen. Part of the CBC or hemogram.

Hemogram—A blood test similar to the CBC that is limited to hemoglobin, hematocrit, RBCs, WBCs, and platelets.

History and physical (H & P)—The process of interviewing a patient and conducting a physical examination to assess various anatomical structures and systems.

Magnetic resonance imaging (MRI)—A test that incorporates a magnetic field to identify structures within the body.

Positron emission tomography (PET)—A nuclear medicine study that involves the use of positron-emitting radionu-clides to identify areas of damaged or diseased tissue.

Red blood cell (RBC) count—A part of the CBC or hemogram that identifies the number of circulating red blood cells, or erythrocytes, in the blood.

Type and cross (T & C)—A test that specifically matches a patient's blood with a particular unit or units of blood in the blood bank. This test, also called type and cross-match, is used whenever large amounts of blood loss are expected or when a patient unexpectedly requires a blood transfusion.

Type and screen (T & S)—A test that is used to ensure that units of blood that match the patient's blood type are available if required by the patient. The test is not as sensitive as the T & C and is not used to determine whether a particular unit of blood is suitable for the patient.

Ultrasound—The use of sound waves to create a picture of structures within the patient.

Urinalysis (UA)—The study of a urine specimen to diagnose or rule out certain medical conditions.

Vital signs—Basic diagnostic indicators that help to immediately assess life-threatening situations. Vital signs include temperature, pulse, respirations, and blood pressure.

White blood cell (WBC) count—A test that identifies the absolute number of white blood cells in a specimen. The test may be combined with a differential count to identify the numbers of each specific type of white blood cell present. This may be expressed as WBC w/diff.

X-ray—Any test that uses x-rays to record a picture of structures or objects within the body. A standard x-ray often is called a flat-plate x-ray to differentiate it from fluoroscopy, which uses continuous x-ray exposure to generate a picture.

INTRODUCTION TO DIAGNOSTIC PROCEDURES

Diagnostic Procedures and the Surgical Patient

Diagnostic procedures and tests are used to give physicians the ability to determine underlying medical conditions that affect their patients. In addition to allowing the physician to identify the patient's chief complaint based on the patient's signs and symptoms, the physician also can use diagnostic tests to identify the best course of treatment for the patient. For example, a patient may present to the physician with lower abdominal pain that upon examination and diagnostic testing appears to be an inguinal hernia. However, a simple check of the patient's blood pressure reveals that this patient suffers from hypertension, which could lead to a stroke if not treated before surgery.

Certain surgical procedures can result in excessive blood loss, and underlying infections may adversely affect the patient's healing after surgery. Uncontrolled hypertension can lead to increased blood loss or stroke, and diabetes inhibits wound healing. The surgical team must recognize the patient as a whole person and not simply a surgical procedure that is easily addressed and corrected. Failure to look at the whole patient can lead to increased morbidity and mortality after surgical intervention. In this chapter we will discuss various diagnostic tools and procedures used to accurately treat the surgical patient.

Invasive and Noninvasive Testing

Diagnostic tests and procedures may be considered noninvasive, minimally invasive, or invasive. The specific tests or procedures ordered by the physician depend on the area or structures of the body that are suspected of being involved with the patient's chief, or primary, complaint. Other tests or procedures allow the surgeon to rule out or identify underlying physical or medical conditions that may potentially affect the patient's outcome after surgery.

Noninvasive tests and procedures are those that do not require an incision or perforation of intact tissues or structures. Noninvasive tests do not involve entry into an anatomical structure that is generally considered sterile. Examples of such diagnostic tools include **electrocardiogram (ECG)**, radiographic studies (without injected contrast), physical examination, **vital signs,** and certain endoscopic procedures. These tests are often performed in the physician's office or in an outpatient setting. No sedation or monitoring usually is required.

Minimally invasive tests and procedures require entry into a structure that is generally considered sterile (e.g., blood stream, urinary tract) or require a small incision or incisions (<1 cm) through the skin or mucous membranes. Examples of minimally invasive tests and procedures include venipuncture, **arterial blood gases (ABGs),** radiographic studies that involve the injection of contrast media or radioactive isotopes, and many endoscopic procedures. Although many of these procedures may be performed in the physician's office, some studies require specialized equipment, patient monitoring, or regional or general anesthesia.

Invasive procedures require entry into sterile tissues through incisions in the skin and underlying tissues. Examples of such procedures include diagnostic laparotomy or thoracotomy, and tissue biopsies.

Preoperative and Intraoperative Testing

Diagnostic tests and procedures are often ordered and completed before the patient undergoes a surgical procedure. Diagnostic tests also are conducted while the patient is on the operating table undergoing a surgical procedure. Preoperative tests allow a physician to identify a specific cause for a patient's complaint (Box 19-1). Preoperative diagnostic tools also give the surgeon a means of identifying and addressing underlying medical problems before exposing the patient to a surgical procedure. As a result of preoperative testing, the physician may order additional studies or make recommendations that may improve the patient's outcome after surgery. The results of preoperative diagnostic testing may reveal a need to delay surgical intervention or to select a different intervention to treat the patient.

During a surgical procedure the surgeon may require examination of tissue specimens to ensure the accurate placement of surgical implants before closure of the surgical incision. The surgeon also may use diagnostic radiography to verify the patency of the common bile duct or of vascular structures. Monitoring of nerve impulses can alert the surgeon to excessive strain on the spinal cord during spinal procedures. Anesthesia providers use diagnostic testing to maintain homeostasis. ECG and blood pressure readings immediately notify anesthesia providers of changes in the patient's condition. Diagnostic tests requested by anesthesia providers determine electrolyte balances, verify adequate ventilation, and create a reference for hemodynamic stability (Box 19-2).

VITAL SIGNS

Probably the most common diagnostic procedure is the obtaining of a patient's vital signs. Vital signs give a quick view of a patient's general health. The four common vital signs assess a patient's cardiac, vascular, and respiratory function, as

---

Box 19-1 Common Preoperative Tests

VITAL SIGNS*
- Temperature
- Pulse
- Respirations
- Blood pressure

COMPLETE BLOOD CELL COUNT*
- Red blood cell count
- White blood cell count
- Hemoglobin
- Hematocrit
- Red blood cell indices
  - *Mean corpuscular volume*
  - *Mean corpuscular hemoglobin concentration*
  - *Mean corpuscular hemoglobin*
- Platelet count
- Differential white blood cell count
- *Neutrophils*
  - *Eosinophils*
  - *Basophils*
  - *Lymphocytes*
  - *Monocytes*

URINALYSIS*
- pH
- Protein
- Glucose
- Ketones
- Blood
- Bilirubin
- Specific gravity

ELECTROCARDIOGRAM

RADIOLOGY
- Flat plate x-ray
  - *Chest x-ray (CXR)**
  - *Orthopedic—bone or joint*
  - *Abdominal—KUB—kidney, ureters, bladder*
  - *Dental*
- Mammography
- Contrast-enhanced x-ray
  - *Barium swallow/esophagram*
  - *Upper gastrointestinal examination (UGI)*
  - *Barium enema/lower gastrointestinal examination (LGI)*
- Computed tomography
- Magnetic resonance imaging

* Routine preoperative tests for all surgical patients

well as identifying whether a patient is febrile. Evaluating a patient's temperature, pulse, respiration, and blood pressure gives the medical team a quick and reliable baseline for later determining a patient's responses to medical or surgical treatment.

Temperature

The patient's temperature will identify the presence of fever, which often is indicative of an underlying infectious process. Normal body temperature is 98.6° F (37° C) when obtained orally with a thermometer placed under the patient's tongue. Rectal temperature generally is about 1° higher, and axillary temperature is 1° lower. In the intraoperative patient, the most reliable temperatures are obtained from bladder, esophageal, or aural (external auditory canal) readings. The temperature of cardiac patients should not be measured with rectal thermometers as vagus nerve stimuli may lead to cardiac arrhythmias.

Elevated core body temperature indicates hyperthermia, often associated with infection. A condition associated with surgical patients called malignant hyperthermia (MH) can lead to brain injury and death if not recognized and treated promptly. Reduced core body temperature is called hypothermia and if not corrected can lead to cardiac arrhythmias and clotting problems. In certain surgical procedures the patient is deliberately placed in a hypothermic state to prevent brain injury. Care is taken when re-warming these patients to prevent additional physiological stresses.

Patients who have recently consumed hot foods or beverages or who have recently exerted themselves will have a slightly elevated temperature. The health-care worker should ask the patient about these factors.

Pulse

The pulse is a measurement of heartbeat. It is the result of blood being forced from the left ventricle through the arteries of the body. A pulse usually can be palpated anywhere an artery passes near the skin. Common locations for obtaining a pulse measurement include the radial artery in the wrist, the brachial artery in the upper arm, the axillary artery in the armpit, the carotid artery in the neck, the femoral artery in the groin, the popliteal artery behind the knee, the dorsalis pedis artery at the top of the foot, and the posterior tibialis artery at the lateral aspect of the ankle.

As mentioned above, the pulse is a measurement of heart contractions. The heart normally contracts (beats) about 72 times per minute in adult males and 80 times per minute in adult females. In infants the normal heart rate is about 120 beats per minute, and children typically will have an elevated heart rate until about age 10. A heart rate of less than 60 beats per minute (bpm) in adults is called bradycardia. In well-conditioned athletes this may be normal; however, a slow heart rate can lead to thrombus formation in debilitated patients. An adult heart rate greater than 100 bpm is called tachycardia and is associated with physical exertion and stress. Tachycardia in the surgical patient also may indicate moderate to severe blood loss, particularly when associated with reduced blood pressure.

When obtaining a patient's pulse, the health-care worker should not use his or her thumb to palpate the pulse. The

---

Box 19-2 Common Intraoperative Tests

VITAL SIGNS
▶ Temperature
▶ Pulse
▶ Respirations
▶ Blood pressure

OXYGEN SATURATION

ELECTROCARDIOGRAM

HEMOGRAM
▶ Red blood cell count
▶ White blood cell count
▶ Hemoglobin
▶ Hematocrit
▶ Red blood cell indices
    ▶ *Mean corpuscular volume*
    ▶ *Mean corpuscular hemoglobin concentration*
    ▶ *Mean corpuscular hemoglobin*
▶ Platelet count

CLOTTING STUDIES
▶ Prothrombin time (PT)
▶ Partial thromboplastin time (PTT)
▶ Activated partial thromboplastin time (APTT)

ARTERIAL BLOOD GASES
▶ pHa
▶ $PaCO_2$
▶ SaO_2
▶ COHb
▶ Na^+
▶ K^+

RADIOLOGY
▶ Flat-plate x-ray
▶ Fluoroscopy

TYPE AND CROSS MATCH

END-TIDAL CO$_2$

digital artery of the health-care worker's thumb can trick the worker and cause an incorrect pulse measurement. To obtain a pulse, the health-care worker will need a watch (or clock) with a sweep-second hand. The worker palpates the pulse using the index and middle fingers of one hand and counts the number of beats for 15 seconds. The worker multiplies the count by 4 to obtain an accurate measurement. In a patient with an irregular heart rhythm, the health-care worker should count the beats of the pulse for 30 seconds and multiply the number by 2 for a more accurate measurement. Patient positioning affects heart rate, as do physical exertion and other stressors. Ideally, a patient's pulse should be obtained with the patient lying supine.

Patients with severe peripheral vascular disease or in whom a peripheral pulse cannot be palpated will require measurement of the apical pulse. The apical pulse is obtained through auscultation. Auscultation is the use of a stethoscope to listen to sounds. The apical pulse can be heard over the apex of the heart. To assess an apical pulse, the health-care worker positions the diaphragm of the stethoscope over the fifth intercostal space at the midclavicular line on the left chest (Figure 19-1).

Respirations

Patients are observed for respiratory rate and rhythm. The normal respiratory rate in adults is 12 to 20 breaths per minute. Infants have respiratory rates of 30 to 60 breaths per minute, and children under the age of 10 may have rates of 20 to 30. An adult respiratory rate of less than 12 breaths per minute is called bradypnea, and a rate of more than 20 breaths per minute indicates tachypnea.

The procedure for counting respirations is to count the number of breaths a patient takes in a 15-second period and multiply this number by four. When evaluating a patient's respirations, one also should observe respiratory effort. A patient who appears to be gasping or taking short breaths on inhalation may be suffering from pain on respiration associated with pleurisy, rib fractures, abdominal distension, or late-term pregnancy. The patient who takes rapid, deep inhalations followed by short periods of exhalation may be suffering from oxygen deprivation associated with tuberculosis or pneumonia. Rapid respirations also are associated with metabolic or lactic acidosis, and abnormally slow respirations may indicate respiratory acidosis.

Blood Pressure

Blood pressure indicates the force with which blood is expelled from the left ventricle of the heart. Blood pressure is the recording of two pressures. These are the systolic pressure, which measures the pressure of the contraction of the left ventricle, and the diastolic pressure, which measures the pressure remaining on the vascular system after the left ventricle relaxes. Blood pressure is recorded as millimeters of mercury (mm Hg). To obtain a patient's blood pressure, the health-care worker will need a stethoscope and a blood pressure cuff (sphygmomanometer).

A general rule for adults is that systolic pressure should read 100 plus the patient's age (up to age 40). Diastolic pressure should be between 60 and 80 mm Hg. A patient with a systolic blood pressure exceeding 140 mm Hg or a diastolic pressure greater than 90 mm Hg is considered hypertensive. A patient's blood pressure may be artificially inflated as a result of anxiety or stress. For this reason, a patient should have several blood pressure readings at different times to reveal the normal blood pressure. A patient with a blood pressure lower than his or her normal reading is considered to be hypotensive. In patients whose normal blood pressure is not known, hypotension typically is indicated by a systolic read-

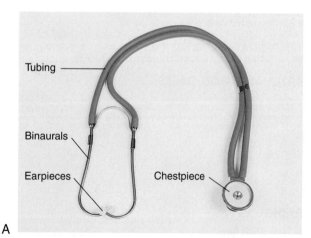

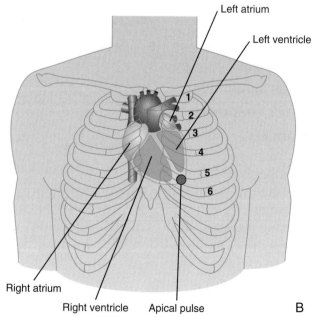

FIGURE 19-1
A, A stethoscope. **B,** Position of the apical pulse in the chest. (From Bonewit-West K: *Clinical procedures for medical assistants,* ed 6, Philadelphia, 2004, Saunders.)

ing of less than 100 mm Hg or a diastolic reading of less than 60 mm Hg.

Pulse and blood pressure will be elevated in patients who have recently exerted themselves or who are anxious or nervous. Pulse and blood pressure typically fall on relaxation. An elevated pulse with a decreased blood pressure is indicative of dehydration or moderate to severe hemorrhage, which may lead to hypovolemic shock. The surgical team should be aware of these differences and watch for changes in the patient's vital signs.

The health-care provider places a blood pressure cuff of an appropriate size around the mid-point of the patient's upper arm (Figure 19-2). The cuff should be snug but not tight. The blood pressure cuff consists of a rubber bladder wrapped in cloth. The bladder is attached to a hose with an inflation bulb that allows the health-care worker to inflate the cuff by squeezing the bulb. The health-care worker should ensure that the cuff is completely deflated before positioning it on the patient's arm. When the cuff is in place, the health-care worker should close the air-release valve on the hose (turn the valve clockwise). The worker adjusts and positions the stethoscope earpieces in his or her ears and positions the stethoscope diaphragm over the patient's brachial artery at the anteromedial aspect of the elbow. The worker should warn the patient that the cuff will become very tight as it is inflated.

The health-care worker observes the gauge on the cuff as he or she inflates the cuff to about 180 mm Hg. The worker slowly turns the valve counter-clockwise to release pressure from the cuff while simultaneously watching the gauge and listening for the first sounds, indicating systolic blood pressure. While mentally noting the measurement of mercury at the beginning of the first sound ("thud, thud, thud") the worker listens for a change in the pitch, or quality, of the sound. This change indicates the diastolic pressure.

At this point the worker opens the valve completely, which allows the cuff to deflate completely. The worker removes the stethoscope from her or his ears and then removes the cuff from the patient's arm. If an accurate blood pressure could not be recorded, the health-care worker should wait for 1 to 2 minutes before reattempting. No attempt should be made to obtain a blood pressure on the ipsilateral (same-side) arm of a female patient who has undergone a mastectomy. The mastectomy procedure frequently impairs distal lymphatic drainage. Patients who have undergone bilateral mastectomies should have blood pressure measured on the right side since the thoracic duct, which provides drainage from the head and neck, drains on the left side.

HISTORY AND PHYSICAL (H & P)

The candidate for a surgical procedure will have an appointment with the surgeon to discuss the procedure and possible outcomes. To create a plan that will produce the best possible surgical outcome, the surgeon needs to obtain the patient's medical history and surgical history. In addition, the surgeon conducts a thorough physical examination to identify any underlying conditions that may adversely affect the patient either during or after a surgical procedure.

The surgeon discusses with the patient her or his past medical conditions as well as any ongoing medical conditions currently affecting the patient. The medical history includes questions about illnesses, substance use, diet, allergies, prescription and over-the-counter (OTC) medications the patient is taking, family history of illness or disease, and other relevant medical concerns. Female patients also are questioned about their reproductive history. The patient's surgical history includes questions about past surgical

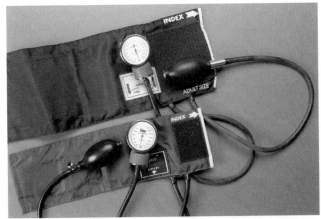

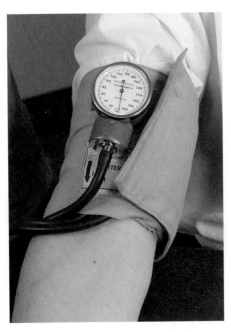

FIGURE 19-2
A, Adult blood pressure cuff *(top)* and pediatric blood pressure cuff *(bottom)*. **B,** Blood pressure cuff properly placed on a patient's arm.

procedures and dates of such procedures as well as any problems that arose as a result of the procedures.

The surgeon then conducts a head-to-toe physical examination of the patient to identify any possible underlying conditions as well as to assess the extent of the current surgical problem.

The medical and surgical history together with the physical examination allows the surgeon to identify the diagnostic tests or procedures required in preparation for surgery. Diagnostic tests and procedures fall into several broad categories: hematology, chemistry, radiology, cardiology, bacteriology, neurology, and pathology. Specific tests in these areas are discussed below.

HEMATOLOGY

Hematology is the study of blood and its cellular components. The ancient Greeks recognized the importance of blood, although it was not until the microscope was invented that scientists were able to learn that blood is actually composed of various components. Herophilus described the diagnostic importance of a pulse, or blood flowing through the artery, between 500 and 250 BCE.

Blood is responsible for the transport of substances throughout the body. Blood is essentially made up of two parts: the liquid portion, which is called plasma, and the blood cells that travel within the plasma. Hematology studies these components.

Plasma

Plasma makes up 55% of the blood by volume. It is composed of 91.5% water and 8.5% dissolved solutes. The solutes include plasma proteins, including albumin, globulin, and fibrinogen. Other solutes include dissolved nutrients, including vitamins, enzymes, hormones, and electrolytes. Hormone and electrolyte studies will be discussed later in the Chemistry section.

Red Blood Cells

Blood cells include red blood cells (RBCs), white blood cells (WBCs), and platelets. RBCs are called erythrocytes and make up almost 99% of the cells within plasma. Erythrocytes are primarily responsible for carrying oxygen throughout the body. Erythrocytes contain a substance known as **hemoglobin (Hb)**, which binds with oxygen molecules to allow the oxygen to be transported through the blood stream and into the cells, where it is released.

HEMOGLOBIN

Hemoglobin is formed by amino acids that form a protein as well as iron atoms and a reddish pigment called porphyrin. The iron atoms in hemoglobin bind with oxygen and give blood its characteristic red color. Hemoglobin also binds with carbon dioxide, which becomes carboxyhemoglobin. Carbon dioxide is a waste product of cellular activity, and the erythrocytes transport carbon dioxide to the lungs, where it is eliminated through respiration.

Reduced hemoglobin levels are associated with moderate to severe blood loss. An Hb level of less than 5.0 g/dl is considered a crisis because it will lead to heart failure. An increased Hb level (>20 g/dl) can lead to capillary obstruction resulting from hemoconcentration.

HEMATOCRIT

Hematocrit (Hct) is a measure of the percentage of blood cells that are erythrocytes. **Red blood cell (RBC) count,** hemoglobin, and hematocrit generally increase and decrease as a result of the same factors. Hematocrit readings remain stable even after moderate blood loss but rapidly decrease in the recovery phase. Hematocrit readings also are unreliable immediately after blood transfusion. A patient with iron-deficiency anemia may have a decreased hematocrit but a normal RBC count (Table 19-1).

Table 19-1 NORMAL HEMOGRAM VALUES			
	Children	Adult Males	Adult Females
Red blood cells (RBCs)	3.8-5.4 × 10⁶/mm³	4.5-5.5 × 10⁶/mm³	4.0-5.0 × 10⁶/mm³
Hemoglobin (Hb)	9.5-20.5 g/dl	14.0-17.4 g/dl	12.0-16.0 g/dl
Hematocrit (Hct)	34%-59%	42%-52%	36%-48%
White blood cells (WBCs)	<6 yrs 5000-21,000 cells/mm³ >6 yrs 4800-10,800 cells/mm³	5000-10,000 cells/mm³	5000-10,000 cells/mm³
Mean corpuscular volume (MCV)	82-98 fl (femtoliter/microliter³)	82-98 fl (femtoliter/microliter³)	82-98 fl (femtoliter/microliter³)
Mean corpuscular hemoglobin concentration (MCHC)	31-37 g/dl	31-37 g/dl	31-37 g/dl
Mean corpuscular hemoglobin (MCH)	<1 yr 24-40 pg <18 yr 25-31 pg	28-34 pg	28-34 pg
Platelets (×10³)	<2 weeks 150-450	140-400	140-400

RED BLOOD CELL INDICES

Other markers of red blood cell activity that have clinical importance include mean corpuscular volume (MCV), mean corpuscular hemoglobin volume (MCHV), and mean corpuscular hemoglobin (MCH). MCV indicates the size and shape of erythrocytes and can identify the maturity of the circulating RBCs. MCHV measures the concentration of hemoglobin in RBCs as an average. Erythrocytes vary in size and therefore will contain a larger or smaller amount of Hb per cell. One calculates MCHV by dividing Hb (g/dl) by the hematocrit (%). MCH is a measure of hemoglobin by weight; one calculates it by dividing Hb (g/dl) by the number of RBCs. These tests are used to assess the severity of certain anemias and their responses to therapies.

White Blood Cells

White blood cells (WBCs) are associated with immune responses within the body. Elevated levels of WBCs, also called leukocytes, indicate underlying stresses on the immune system. WBCs are differentiated into two groups: granulocytes and agranulocytes. These terms relate to the presence or absence of characteristic granules that appear within the cytoplasm of the cells when the cells are stained with diagnostic contrast. A differential **white blood cell (WBC) count** will identify the numbers of each of these cell types; differing results are associated with different conditions that affect the immune system (Table 19-2).

GRANULOCYTES

Granulocytes, sometimes called granular leukocytes, include the basophils, eosinophils, and neutrophils. These cells also contain a multi-lobed nucleus and often are called polymorphonuclear leukocytes or simply "PMNs." Agranulocytes do not show granules when they are stained. There are two main types of agranulocytes: lymphocytes and monocytes. Because these cells contain a nonlobed nucleus they sometimes are called mononuclear leukocytes.

The specific white blood cells known as basophils are associated with a state of chronic inflammation. Increased numbers of basophils on the **differential count** indicate certain cancers, including certain leukemias and Hodgkin's lymphoma (Table 19-3). An increased basophil count, called basophilia, sometimes is associated with sinusitis, hypothyroidism, and hemolytic anemia. A reduced basophil count,

basopenia, is found in patients with hyperthyroidism and in patients who have undergone chemotherapy, radiation, and prolonged treatment with steroids.

The eosinophil, another granulocyte, is increased with allergic reactions, parasitic infections, ulcerative colitis, and Crohn's disease. An increased eosinophil count is called eosinophilia. Eosinopenia, or a reduced eosinophil count, is associated with Cushing's syndrome, a type of adrenal insufficiency. A type of eosinophil called an eosinophilic myelocyte is found only in patients with leukemia.

Neutrophils are the most common of the white blood cells and are a primary defense against microbial infections. Neutrophilia, a condition of an increased number of neutrophils, is found with localized or general bacterial infections. Neutrophilia also is associated with uremia, chemical or drug poisoning, and hemolytic transfusion reactions. Neutrophil counts also increase in the presence of tissue necrosis and at the early phases of certain viral infections. A reduced number of neutrophils, called neutropenia, is associated with severe systemic bacterial infections, viral infections including influenza, anaphylactic shock, and exposure to drugs, chemicals, or other toxins. A type of neutropenia associated with the early death of maturing neutrophils is found in sepsis associated with *Escherichia coli*.

AGRANULOCYTES

Monocytes, along with lymphocytes, are considered agranulocytes. Monocytes are the largest of the blood cells and form the second line of defense in the body. Monocytes use the process of phagocytosis, cell digestion, to remove damaged and dead cells from the body. Monocytes also produce interferon, which is an antiviral agent. An increased number of monocytes, known as monocytosis, is found in patients with bacterial infections including tuberculosis, endocarditis, and syphilis. A reduced monocyte count is not associated with particular diseases but is found in conditions that cause neutropenia.

Lymphocytes are associated with early-stage and late-stage infectious processes. Lymphocytes produce immunoglobulins. There are two types of lymphocytes. B lymphocytes are responsible for the antigen-antibody response of immune function that is tailored to the specific antigen that causes the immune response. These cells are called "memory" cells because they bring a faster immune response

Table 19-2   NORMAL ADULT WHITE BLOOD CELL COUNT AND DIFFERENTIAL COUNT

Cell Type	Absolute Count	Differential Count
WBCs, leukocytes	5.0-$10.0 \times mm^3$	5000-10,000 cells/mm^3
Neutrophils, PMNs, segs	3000-7000 cells/mm^3	50%-60% (of total WBCs)
Eosinophils	50-250 cells/mm^3	1%-4% (of total WBCs)
Basophils	15-100 cells/mm^3	0.5%-1% (of total WBCs)
Monocytes	100-500 cells/mm^3	3%-7% (of total WBCs)
Lymphocytes	1500-4000 cells/mm^3	25%-40% (of total WBCs)

Table 19-3   ABNORMAL WBC VALUES AND ASSOCIATED CONDITIONS (ADULT VALUES)

Cell Type and Normal Values	Increased Value and Conditions	Decreased Value and Conditions
WBCs, leukocytes 5000-10,000 cells/mm³	Leukocytosis: >10,000 cells/mm³; leukemia, tissue trauma, malignancy, toxicity, bacterial infection, acute hemolysis, post-splenectomy	Leukocytopenia: <4000 cells/mm³; viral infection, severe systemic bacterial infection, splenomegaly, bone marrow disorders, anemias
Neutrophils 3000-7000 cells/mm³ or 50%-60%	Neutrophilia: >8000 cells/mm³ or >70%; acute localized or general bacterial infections, uremia, hemolytic transfusion reaction, tissue necrosis, some viral infections (early phases)	Neutropenia: <1800 cells/mm³ or <40%; overwhelming bacterial infection, viral infections, drugs, chemicals, radiation exposure, anaphylaxis
Eosinophils 50-250 cells/mm³ or 1%-4%	Eosinophilia: >500 cells/mm³ or >5%; allergies, hay fever, parasitic infection, Hodgkin's lymphoma, ulcerative colitis, Crohn's disease, adverse drug reactions, renal allograft failure	Eosinopenia: <50 cells/mm³ or <1%; Cushing's syndrome, epinephrine, ACTH or thyroxine use
Basophils 15-100 cells/mm³ or 0.5%-1%	Basophilia: >100 cells/mm³ or >1%; granulocytic leukemia, basophilic leukemia, hypothyroidism (occasionally)	Basopenia: <15 cells/mm³ or <0.5%: acute phases of infection, hyperthyroidism, prolonged steroid therapy, chemotherapy, radiation therapy, pregnancy, MI
Monocytes 100-500 cells/mm³ or 3%-7%	Monocytosis: >500 cells/mm³ or >10%; bacterial infections including tuberculosis, endocarditis, and syphilis; monocytic leukemia; carcinoma of the breast, stomach, or ovaries; lymphomas; surgical trauma; some parasitic and mycotic diseases; and recovery from neutropenia	Monocytopenia: <100 cells/mm³ or <3%; overwhelming infections, HIV infection
Lymphocytes 1500-4000 cells/mm³ or 25%-40%	Lymphocytosis: >4,000 cells/mm³ or >40%; lymphatic leukemia, lymphoma, mononucleosis, viral infections, ulcerative colitis, Crohn's disease, toxoplasmosis	Lymphocytopenia <1000 cells/mm³ or <25%; chemotherapy, radiation therapy, aplastic anemia, Hodgkin's lymphoma, inherited immune disorders, AIDS, advanced tuberculosis, CHF, renal failure

to subsequent infection. T lymphocytes are considered the master cells of the immune system. The important T lymphocytes are divided into CD4$^+$ helper cells, killer cells, and CD8$^+$ suppressor cells.

An elevated lymphocyte count, known as lymphocytosis, is associated with non-Hodgkin's lymphoma, mononucleosis, and a number of viral infections including measles, mumps, chicken pox, and hepatitis. Lymphocytopenia, a decrease in the number of lymphocytes, is associated with Hodgkin's lymphoma, immune disorders including acquired immunodeficiency syndrome (AIDS), chemotherapy or other immunosuppressive therapies, congestive heart failure (CHF), and renal failure. A severely depressed CD4 lymphocyte count indicates a great risk for the development of opportunistic infections.

Hemogram versus Complete Blood Count (CBC)

Two primary tests are performed to evaluate blood and blood cells in the surgical patient. The **hemogram** consists of an RBC count, WBC count, hemoglobin (Hb), hematocrit (Hct), RBC indices, and a platelet count. The **complete blood count (CBC)** consists of the hemogram and includes a differential WBC count. The CBC is a standard test ordered for all surgi-

cal patients. The hemogram often is used in the intraoperative setting to assess changes in a patient's hemodynamic status.

Blood and Serum Collection Tubes

Blood and serum collection tubes are available with different colored tops and may contain additives such as anticoagulants or preservatives. It is vital to ensure that the correct collection tube is used to protect the usefulness of the specimen. Using an incorrect tube to collect blood from the patient will cause a delay of diagnosis as another specimen will be required. Although the scrub typically is not involved in obtaining blood specimens, the surgeon may wish to send blood directly from an incision or exposed blood vessel. In this case it is helpful for both the scrub and circulator to have a basic understanding of appropriate collection tubes (Figure 19-3).

The different colored tops are as follows:

▶ *Red:* Contains no preservative and no anticoagulant. Used for collecting specimens for chemistry, serology, or blood bank, or any time a clotted specimen is required for diagnosis.

▶ *Pink:* Contains no preservative and no anticoagulant. Used for collecting specimens for the blood bank including **type and screen (T & S)** and **type and cross (T & C)**.

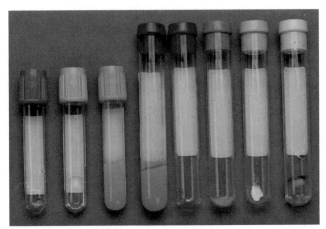

FIGURE 19-3
Blood and serum collection tubes.

▶ *Green:* Contains heparin to prevent clotting. Used for collecting arterial blood gases (ABGs) and electrolyte specimens.

▶ *Lavender:* Contains ethylene diamine tetraacetic acid (EDTA), which removes calcium to prevent clotting. Used for the collection of blood for CBCs and other hematology studies.

▶ *Light blue:* Contains sodium citrate to prevent clotting. Used for collecting specimens to test for plasma-clotting times, and to check prothrombin time (PT), partial thromboplastin time (PTT), and other clotting factor assays. To ensure accuracy, the tube must be completely filled.

▶ *Gold or red marbled:* A serum gel separator (SST) tube that allows the serum to be separated by centrifuge after collection. Used for most chemistry tests.

After collection of specimens, tubes that contain additives should be inverted several times to allow for the mixing of the blood with the additive. All specimens should be labeled with patient identification, the time it was drawn, and the initials of the person who obtained the specimen. Specimens are placed in a biohazard bag and delivered immediately to the appropriate lab (e.g., hematology, chemistry, blood bank).

CHEMISTRY

Chemistry is the study of various chemicals, hormones, and enzymes and how they interact with each other to promote homeostasis. Chemistry tests are used to determine levels of waste elements resulting from cellular metabolism. Chemistry also is used in determining therapeutic drug levels. By reviewing results from these particular tests, the physician can determine underlying cardiac, renal, and liver function to prevent intraoperative or postoperative morbidity. Specific types of **chemistry studies** include electrolyte levels, cardiac enzymes, liver function, renal function, cholesterol levels, glucose levels, thyroid function, drug levels, and fertil-

ity testing. This section will discuss electrolyte, liver function, and renal tests, as these are the tests used most often with the preoperative, intraoperative, and postoperative patient.

Biochemical Profiles

Often one must look at the results of several blood chemistry tests to evaluate a patient's condition and select proper treatment. Therefore several tests may be combined into a group to identify specific disorders and their treatment. The list below identifies some of the common individual tests that might be requested to aid in diagnosis:

▶ Albumin and globulin
▶ Alkaline phosphatase (ALP)
▶ Aspartate transaminase (AST)
▶ Blood urea nitrogen (BUN)
▶ Calcium
▶ Cholesterol
▶ Creatinine
▶ Glucose
▶ Inorganic phosphorus
▶ Sodium, potassium, and chloride
▶ Total bilirubin
▶ Total protein
▶ Triglycerides
▶ Uric acid

Tests often are grouped together to produce a profile of the patient's condition and a broad picture of underlying health problems (Table 19-4).

Electrolytes

Electrolytes are a vital component of cell function. These substances help to control water flow by osmosis, conduct electrical impulses, and maintain the acid-base balance of cells. Electrolytes are divided into *cations* and *anions.* The cations have a positive electrical charge and include sodium (Na^+), potassium (K^+), calcium (Ca^+), and magnesium (Mg^+). Anions have a negative electrical charge and include chloride (Cl^-), phosphate ($HPO_4{}^{2-}$), sulfate ($SO_4{}^{2-}$), and bicarbonate ($HCO_3{}^-$). Electrolytes are found in plasma, extracellular fluid, and intracellular fluid. Ions generally tend to move from a level of higher concentration to a level of lower concentration to create equilibrium. It is this balance, or equilibrium, that allows cells to function properly. One measures **electrolyte levels** by obtaining a blood sample and evaluating the plasma portion of the sample.

SODIUM

Sodium (Na^+) is the most abundant cation and is responsible for maintaining osmotic pressure and acid–base balance within the body. Hyponatremia, or a reduced sodium level, is found in patients with severe burns, congestive heart failure, severe diarrhea or vomiting, hypothyroidism, Addison's disease (adrenal gland insufficiency), and diabetic acidosis.

Table 19-4 COMMON BIOCHEMICAL PROFILE GROUPINGS

Biochemical Profile Panel	Specific Tests
Cardiac enzymes	CPK, AST, LDH, SGOT
Renal function	BUN, phosphorus, LDH, creatinine, creatinine clearance, uric acid, total protein, albumin, globulin, A/G ratio, calcium, glucose, cholesterol
Lipid studies	Cholesterol, triglycerides, LDL, HDL, VLDL
Liver function	Total bilirubin, alkaline phosphatase, cholesterol, GGT, total protein, albumin, globulin, A/G ratio, AST, LDH, PT, viral hepatitis panel
Thyroid function	T_2 uptake, total T_{4+}, free T_4, T_7, FTI, TSH
Basic metabolic screening	Chloride, sodium, potassium, CO_2, glucose, BUN, creatinine

A/G ratio: albumin/globulin ratio; AST: aspartate aminotransferase; BUN: blood urea nitrogen; CO_2: carbon dioxide; CPK: creatine phosphokinase; FTI: free thyroxine index; GGT: gamma glutamyl transpeptidase; HDL: high-density lipoprotein; LDH: lactic dehydrogenase; LDL: low-density lipoprotein; PT: prothrombin time; SGOT: serum glutamic-oxaloacetic transaminase; TSH: thyroid-stimulating hormone; VLDL: very low-density lipoprotein.

Hyponatremia also occurs with the use of excessive amounts of nonelectrolyte IV solutions in trauma patients. Symptoms of hyponatremia include muscle weakness, hypotension, tachycardia, and shock.

Increased levels of sodium, called hypernatremia, are found in patients with insufficient fluid replacement, diabetes insipidus, and Cushing's disease (excess cortisol production by the adrenal cortex). Symptoms include extreme thirst, fatigue, or agitation.

POTASSIUM

Potassium (K^+) is the primary cation found in intracellular fluid, with most of the body's stores of potassium being found within the cells. Potassium functions include maintenance of acid–base balances, nerve impulse conduction, muscle function, and maintenance of osmotic pressure. Potassium is vital in controlling rate and strength of cardiac contractions. Potassium works with calcium and magnesium to ensure proper cardiac output. Potassium and sodium are involved in the renal component of acid–base balances, and potassium is required for the synthesis of proteins.

Hypokalemia, a decrease in potassium, like hyponatremia, is found in patients with severe diarrhea, vomiting, or burns. It also is associated with alcoholism and respiratory alkalosis. Patients with open or draining wounds also are prone to developing hypokalemia. Symptoms of hypokalemia include cramps, nausea, increased urine output, and ECG changes. ECG changes include prolonged Q-T waves, flattened T waves, and the presence of a U wave.

Hyperkalemia is an increase in the amount of potassium and is associated with renal failure, uncontrolled diabetes, and metabolic acidosis. Hyperkalemia can present with paresthesias (abnormal sensations) and atrial or ventricular fibrillation.

CALCIUM

Most of the body's calcium is found in bone and teeth. Calcium levels are recorded as total calcium or ionized calcium. Ionized calcium is involved in the vital processes of the body.

Ionized calcium is monitored during open-heart procedures, organ transplantation, and trauma treatment. Ionized calcium is also used to assess patients with hyperparathyroidism, renal disease and pancreatitis and patients who are on dialysis or who have cancer. Hypocalcemia, a decrease in total calcium, typically is associated with albumin decreases (hypoalbuminemia). Hypercalcemia, total calcium increase, is found in patients with hyperparathyroidism and malignancy.

MAGNESIUM

Magnesium (Mg^{2+}) is required for the proper function of many enzyme-based sources of energy, including carbohydrate metabolism, protein synthesis, and nucleic-acid synthesis. It also is important in the contraction of muscle tissue. Magnesium also is involved in the clotting process. Calcium and magnesium are closely linked, and increases or decreases in either will cause an inverse response by the other. For example, a decrease in the level of serum magnesium will lead to hypercalcemia, or an elevation in the amount of calcium.

CHLORIDE

Chloride (Cl^-) is an ion that is primarily found in extracellular fluid combined with sodium as sodium chloride. Chloride affects osmotic pressure and helps to maintain cellular shape. Hypochloremia is found in burn patients, patients with severe vomiting, and patients in metabolic alkalosis. An increased chloride level, hyperchloremia, is found in metabolic acidosis as chloride levels rise when bicarbonate levels fall.

PHOSPHATE

Phosphorus is involved in generation of bone tissue. It also is involved in the metabolism of glucose. Reduced levels of phosphorus are found in patients diagnosed with diabetic coma, osteomalacia, liver disease, acute alcoholism, and malnutrition. Hyperphosphatemia, an increased phosphate level, is associated with excessive vitamin D intake, hypocal-

Table 19-5 NORMAL ELECTROLYTE VALUES AND PANIC VALUES

Electrolyte	Low Panic Value	High Panic Value
Calcium, total	<6 mg/dl	>13 mg/dl
Chloride	<70 mEq/L	>120 mEq/L
Phosphate	<1.0 mg/dl	N/A
Magnesium	<1.0 mg/dl	>5 mg/dl
		>10 mg/dl: ECG changes, respiratory arrest
		>30 mg/dl: complete heart block
		>34 mg/dl: cardiac arrest
Potassium	<2.5 mEq/L	>7 mEq/L
Sodium	<120 mEq/L	>155 mEq/L

cemia, bone tumors, and recurrence of fractures during callus formation of a fracture. Phosphate levels also are elevated during cardiac resuscitation (Table 19-5).

CLOTTING TESTS

Surgical intervention generally requires making incisions through intact structures, which leads to bleeding from capillaries or other blood vessels. Patients who have underlying blood clotting disorders or who are under anticoagulant therapy will have a prolonged bleeding time. These conditions or therapies may result in excessive blood loss during the intraoperative or postoperative phases of surgery. In certain cases, the clotting process is accelerated, which places the surgical patient at a higher risk for thrombus formation and subsequent problems including deep vein thrombosis (DVT), pulmonary embolus (PE), cerebrovascular accident (CVA), and myocardial infarction (MI). The following tests may be used to assess a patient's clotting ability: platelet count, bleeding time, prothrombin time (PT), partial thromboplastin time (PTT), activated partial thromboplastin time (APTT), and fibrinogen levels. In addition, readings of the patient's calcium level may help the surgeon in evaluating clotting disorders.

Clotting Stages

The process of forming a blood clot typically occurs in four distinct stages. Each stage is associated with specific clotting factors that are activated or deactivated as a result of trauma to a blood vessel. The tests identified above assess the clotting process at varying points in the process.

The specific clotting factors are:

▶ Factor I: fibrinogen
▶ Factor II: prothrombin
▶ Factor III: thromboplastin
▶ Factor IV: calcium
▶ Factor V: proaccelerin

▶ Factor VI: This factor no longer is considered a part of the clotting process.
▶ Factor VII: proconvertin
▶ Factor VIII: antihemophilia factor
▶ Factor IX: plasma thromboplastin (Christmas factor)
▶ Factor X: Stuart-Prower factor
▶ Factor XI: plasma thromboplastin antecedent
▶ Factor XII: Hageman factor
▶ Factor XIII: fibrin-stabilizing factor

(From Snyder K, Keegan C: *Pharmacology for the surgical technologist,* St Louis, 1999, Mosby.)

STAGE I

The first stage of the clotting process is divided into two phases. The first phase brings platelet activity and the accumulation of platelets at the site of injury. In the second phase, tissue thromboplastin is formed and released. Platelets, calcium, and factors III, V, VIII, IX, X, XI, and XII take part in this phase of clotting. Stage I of the clotting process takes approximately 3 to 5 minutes.

STAGE II

In the second stage of clotting, prothrombin is converted to thrombin in the presence of calcium. Clotting factors that take part in this stage include factors II, V, VII, and X. This stage also begins the process of converting fibrinogen to fibrin, which gives the clot its adhesive properties.

STAGE III

In the third stage of clotting, thrombin and fibrinogen interact to create the strength and security of the clot. Factor XIII is activated at the end of this stage to bring stability to the clot.

STAGE IV

The fourth stage of clot formation brings fibrinolysis, as a type of balancing process, to prevent the clot from growing and obstructing the lumen of a blood vessel.

Platelet Count

Platelets, also called thrombocytes, are measured on the hemogram and the CBC. Platelets accumulate at the site of injury to a blood vessel and temporarily obstruct the flow of blood out of the vessel. The platelet plug is a very weak and temporary method used by the body to prevent blood loss. Platelet count is simply an evaluation of the number and size of thrombocytes in a blood sample. Normal adult platelet levels are 140,000 to 400,000/mm^3. Reduced numbers indicate a diminished ability to form a blood clot, while an increased platelet count is associated with hypercoagulability.

Bleeding Time

Patients suspected of having coagulation disorders may be tested to determine the amount of time needed to form a blood clot. If a disorder is suspected, this test is conducted as part of the preoperative testing process. Bleeding time measures the ability of platelets to function normally and also reflects the ability of capillary walls to constrict as a result of trauma. Bleeding time generally should be between 3 and 10 minutes. The test is the best indicator of abnormalities associated with platelet function.

Prothrombin Time (PT)

Prothrombin time, sometimes called simply "protime," measures the functions of the clotting factors associated with part of the clotting cascade. Specifically, this test identifies abnormalities associated with the second stage of the clotting process. Normal PT is 11.0 to 13.0 seconds. Increased PT is associated with prolonged clot formation. Increased PT also may signify a vitamin K deficiency.

Partial Thromboplastin Time (PTT) and Activated Partial Thromboplastin Time (APTT)

These tests are designed to measure the overall ability of blood to clot. The tests assess the amount and function of clotting factors associated with the first two stages of clot formation. Thromboplastin is released in the presence of calcium, and a prolonged PTT or APTT may indicate inadequate calcium levels. PTT and APTT are used to monitor therapeutic heparin usage. The APTT test is more sensitive than PTT. A normal APTT reading is between 21 and 35 seconds.

Fibrinogen

Fibrinogen is associated with maturity and stability of a blood clot. Measurement of fibrinogen levels helps in determining abnormalities associated with the third stage of the clotting process. Normal levels of fibrinogen are 200 to 300 mg/dl. Because fibrinogen, along with platelets, forms the structure of a clot, reduced levels of fibrinogen are associated with weak clots that tend to break down.

URINALYSIS

Urinalysis (UA) is the process of evaluating urine for diagnosis of a patient's metabolic health. Actual urinalysis consists of three procedures. First, the physical aspects of the urine specimen are assessed. This means noting the color of the specimen, whether it is clear or cloudy, and whether it has a strong smell or odor. These results are noted in the patient's medical record.

Second, standard parameters of the urine specimen are evaluated. One performs this step by using diagnostic test-strips that are chemically impregnated to register the presence or absence of proteins, glucose, ketones, gross blood, bilirubin, urobilinogen, nitrates, and leukocytes. These test-strips also identify the pH level of urine and the specific gravity of the sample. The test-strips contain a series of small reservoir pads that absorb the urine and change color in response to contact with components in the sample. Each pad is matched to the corresponding color chart for the test strip. Results from this test also are noted in the patient's record.

Third, a microscopic examination is conducted to look for crystals or other sediment within the urine. Below is a list of normal urinalysis values.

- Color: pale yellow to amber
- Appearance: clear to slightly hazy
- Odor: none to mild
- pH: 4.5 to 8.0
- Specific gravity: 1.005 to 1.025 (weight of a substance compared with distilled water)
- Glucose: negative
- Ketones: negative
- Protein: negative
- Blood: negative
- Bilirubin: negative
- Urobilinogen: 0.2 to 1.0
- Casts: negative or occasional hyaline casts
- RBCs: negative or rare
- Nitrate: negative
- Crystals: negative
- WBCs: negative or rare

Abnormal urinalysis results may be indicative of a number of problems, including infection (presence of WBCs, RBCs, nitrate, unpleasant odor); renal insufficiency (reduced urine output, elevated pH, dark color); liver insufficiency (bilirubin, elevated urobilinogen, dark color); and diabetes (glucose, fruity odor, ketones).

Urinalysis is a standard, economical, and effective diagnostic tool.

ELECTROCARDIOGRAM (ECG/EKG)

The electrocardiogram, abbreviated ECG (sometimes EKG), measures electrical activity of the heart. Electrical impulses are conducted through nerve fibers within the heart to cause cardiac muscle fibers to contract. Obstruction of these conduction pathways can lead to inadequate heart function and a decrease in the amount of oxygenated blood delivered throughout the body.

The ECG is a routine diagnostic procedure that is performed on anyone over the age of 40, patients under the age of 40 who have a personal or family history of cardiac disease, and anyone who has had a previous heart attack or cardiac arrhythmia. ECG monitoring is a standard procedure in the operating room because many agents used during anesthesia may affect the heart's function. Changes on an ECG often are early indicators of an impending crisis in the surgical patient. Routine cardiac monitoring consists of a 3-lead ECG. Patients who have other risk factors or fall into the categories listed above may undergo a 12-lead ECG, cardiac stress testing, or 12-hour or 24-hour Holter ECG monitoring. Any cardiac test results should be available to the anesthesia provider to help in planning the patient's course of anesthesia.

Nerve impulses normally originate at the sinoatrial (SA) node, which is located in the right atrium. The SA node, like the atrioventricular (AV) node, is simply a collection, or bundle, of nerve fibers. Impulses are transmitted to the AV node, which is found at the floor of the atrium and which conducts the electrical impulses to the interventricular septum. The AV node is also called the bundle of His. The nerve fibers in the interventricular septum divide into the right and left bundle branches, pass into the right and left ventricles, and transmit the impulses to the Purkinje fibers located within each ventricle. The Purkinje fibers transmit these impulses to the cardiac muscle fibers, causing them to contract. The cardiac muscle in contraction is described as being in depolarization. As the cardiac muscle relaxes, it enters a stage of repolarization.

When viewing the ECG, one notes that a cycle or heartbeat is composed of several waves. An ECG tracing, or reading, is created on a special strip of graph paper (Figure 19-4). The graph paper is designed to record at a specific speed; a 5-mm-wide strip of graph paper records 0.2 second of electrical activity. A 5-mm-high section of the ECG tracing indicates the electrical conduction expressed as 0.5 mV or millivolts. The distance the tracing travels in its vertical plane is called its amplitude, and the distance the tracing travels in its horizontal plane is called the interval.

The ECG tracing identifies several specific wave forms that, when evaluated, help measure the health and strength of the heart. The first normal wave is called the P wave and indicates atrial depolarization. This is the stage in which the cardiac muscle fibers of the atrium contract to push blood into the ventricles. The next wave normally observed is called the QRS complex and signifies ventricular depolarization. Ventricular depolarization is the stage in which the ventricles contract to force blood out of the heart. The next normal wave to appear usually is the T wave and identifies ventricular repolarization, or a relaxation phase of the ventricles. The normal interval between the peak of "R" in the QRS complex and the next "R" peak is about 0.83 second at a heart rate of 72 beats per minute (BPM).

When viewing the ECG tracing, the health-care provider should attempt to determine the rate, rhythm, axis, hypertrophy, and infarction. For the surgical technologist, looking at the cardiac rate and rhythm can help to determine whether the cardiac activity is within acceptable parameters.

At the top of the ECG paper strip you will note thin vertical lines or small dots at regular intervals. Each of these intervals represents 3 seconds. To determine the patient's cardiac rate, select a piece of the strip with five of these 3-second intervals (a total of 15 seconds). Next, find the peak of the QRS complex, or the "R" wave, that falls closest to the beginning of the 15-second strip. Count all of the R waves that fall within that 15-second segment of the strip. Multiply this number by four to get a good idea of the patient's heart rate.

Next, one must note the patient's cardiac rhythm. To determine the patient's rhythm, one compares each wave or complex with the other waves or complexes to determine whether the rhythm is normal or there are differences to be noted. For example, is there a single P wave preceding each QRS complex? Is the distance between each P wave and the QRS complex consistent? Are the height and width of all waves equal? Differences in the number of waves or in the height or width of waves, or the absence of certain waves, may indicate a blockage in the normal electrical conductive pathways of the heart. Subtle changes in the cardiac rhythm may indicate ischemia of the heart muscle, which may be a result of a prior heart attack or an impending heart attack.

Interpreting the results of an ECG requires a great deal of practice. The ECG, however, remains one of the most common and cost-effective tools for evaluating a patient's heart. Changes in heart function as noted on the ECG reading can indicate impending disaster or can be an indicator of hypovolemia, electrolyte imbalances, response to external stimuli, or other factors that the surgical team can readily address.

CARDIAC CATHETERIZATION

The use of cardiac catheterization as a diagnostic tool enables physicians to diagnose disorders of the heart chambers, cardiac valves, and coronary blood vessels. Cardiac catheterization takes place in a suite specially equipped to perform such procedures. The suite is equipped to perform **fluoroscopy**, a type of radiographic study, and the procedure table is designed to allow radiographic examination of the entire length of the body.

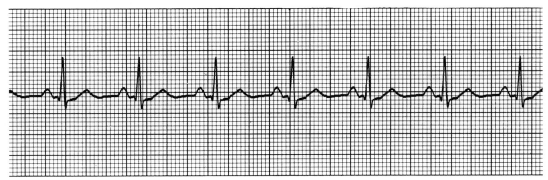

FIGURE 19-4
Example of a normal ECG tracing. (From Tait C: *EZ ECG's booklet*, ed 2, St Louis, 2001, Mosby.)

To evaluate the structure or function of the right atrium or right ventricle, one inserts a catheter through the brachial vein of the upper arm or the femoral vein of the groin and threads it through the vena cava and into the right atrium. The catheter is passed through the tricuspid valve and into the right ventricle, and is advanced to the pulmonary valve.

To allow assessment of the structures associated with the left side of the heart, the patient is heparinized. The catheter is introduced into the brachial artery of the arm, or more often, through the femoral artery. It then enters the aorta, where it passes through the aortic valve and into the left ventricle.

In the evaluation of the left side or the right side of the heart, contrast media often is used to illustrate the contours of the heart chambers, proper closure of heart valves, or patency of the coronary vessels. Contrast media is a **diagnostic agent** that sharpens the appearance of structures when radiography is used. Cardiac catheterization is performed under local anesthesia and sedation may be administered.

After the catheter is removed, direct pressure is applied to the incision site for 15 to 20 minutes. If an arterial incision has been made, pressure may be applied for a longer time. The patient is generally maintained on bed rest for 6 to 12 hours after the procedure to prevent hematoma formation.

ECHOCARDIOGRAPHY

Echocardiography uses ultrasound waves to illustrate the contours and structures of the heart. Transthoracic echocardiography is a noninvasive procedure that uses ultrasound energy to pass through the chest wall and evaluate the heart wall, heart valves, and great vessels of the heart. In transesophageal echocardiography (TEE), a small ultrasonic probe is passed down the esophagus to illustrate these same structures. TEE is used when a transthoracic approach does not produce an adequate picture of cardiac structures.

These procedures can be used to identify prosthetic heart valves, enlarged heart chambers, intracardiac tumors, thoracic aneurysms, and congenital abnormalities, including atrial-septal defect (ASD) and ventricular-septal defects (VSD). Transthoracic echocardiography and TEE both are used as part of the diagnostic process before hospital admission. TEE also is used during surgery.

ULTRASOUND STUDIES

The use of **ultrasound** technology enables physicians to use noninvasive techniques to assess many different structures. Ultrasound is inexpensive and painless, and can be used in almost any area of the health-care setting, including the physician's office. Ultrasound technology does not use ionizing radiation and therefore is safe for health-care workers and patients. The term *sonogram* describes procedures that

use ultrasound technology. Ultrasound may be used as a diagnostic tool in these areas:

▶ Obstetrics: To assess the health of a fetus, size and number of fetuses, amniotic fluid levels, fetal positioning, and abnormalities of the placenta.
▶ Gynecology: To evaluate the urinary bladder, uterus, cystoceles, or rectoceles; and during oocyte retrieval for infertility treatment.
▶ Male reproductive structures: To evaluate scrotal masses; transrectal ultrasound is a standard tool for evaluation of the prostate.
▶ Abdominal: To assess the structures of the abdomen including the:
  ▶ Hepatobiliary tract: To evaluate size, presence of masses or calculi
  ▶ Pancreas: To evaluate presence of tumors, cysts, or abscesses
  ▶ Spleen: To evaluate size and spread of lymphomas or metastatic disease
  ▶ Kidneys: To diagnose cysts, tumors, hydronephrosis, and calculi
  ▶ Aorta and other vessels: To diagnose aneurysms or thromboembolic conditions
  ▶ Gastrointestinal (GI): To confirm appendicitis; useful in diagnosing Crohn's disease and Meckel's diverticulum
▶ Head and neck: To assess thyroid and parathyroid masses, remove foreign bodies from the eye, and diagnose neonatal cerebral hemorrhage.
▶ Breast: To differentiate solid breast masses from cystic masses and also to aid in needle aspiration or biopsy.

A special type of ultrasound technique known as Doppler enables physicians to assess the flow of fluid, generally blood, through a structure. Doppler, named after Austrian scientist Johann Christian Doppler, measures the frequency of a sound wave and notes changes as the distance to the transmitted wave increases or decreases. This study can assess blood flow where no palpable pulse is found. A conductive gel is applied to the extremity of the patient and a hand-held transducer is moved up and down the extremity to evaluate the flow of blood through the extremity. **Doppler studies** can be used to assess blood flow through solid and hollow abdominal organs, including the kidneys, liver, intestine, and spleen. Doppler also may be used to assess blood flow in an ovary or testicle after trauma, including torsion.

RADIOGRAPHIC STUDIES

The use of radiation as a diagnostic tool was discovered accidentally in the 1890s. Radiographs, also called roentgenograms or **x-rays,** have become a very common method of diagnosis. In the preoperative patient, x-rays are used to diagnose pathology of solid and hollow structures. Surgeons may request x-rays in the intraoperative setting to ensure proper reduction of fractures, correct positioning of implantable devices, or patency of tubular structures, including the common bile duct, ureters, and blood vessels. In this section, we will discuss conventional radiographs, contrast-enhanced radiographs, and **computed tomography (CT)**.

X-rays are particles of radiation with a relatively short wavelength. An x-ray image is created when radiation passes through structures and strikes a medium (e.g., an x-ray film) positioned behind the body. As these rays enter the body, some of the x-rays pass all the way through the body without being absorbed or blocked by tissues. Some rays are almost completely absorbed by tissues within the body, and other rays are partially absorbed by tissues. On a conventional x-ray, dense tissues such as bone block or absorb almost all of the radiation that passes through the body. On the x-ray image, these structures will appear nearly white. Air-filled and fluid-filled structures will not block or absorb as many rays and the image will, therefore, appear darker. For this reason, x-rays are a valuable diagnostic tool when assessing bony structures and semi-solid structures, including tumor masses.

The use of contrast agents (contrast media) can assist with x-ray studies of air-filled or fluid-filled structures, including the GI tract and cardiovascular system. Contrast agents act to absorb or block x-rays as they pass through these structures, thus creating definition and allowing physicians to evaluate these structures.

Radiation Safety
Although newer technologies have reduced the amount of free, or scattered, radiation, that is emitted, the use of radiation has the potential of damaging cells in the body. Structures or organs that are particularly susceptible to injury from radiation include the thyroid gland, gonads, eyes, and blood components. During the first trimester of fetal development, the fetus also is prone to damage from radiation. Three factors contribute to the effect of radiation on the body: time, distance, and shielding.

TIME
Workers should limit the amount of time they are exposed to radiation-emitting sources. Much of the effect of radiation is cumulative, that is, the effects build up over time. Exposure to conventional x-ray machines, fluoroscopy (image-intensifier) units, and CT scanners while in operation increases the amount of radiation exposure a person experiences. Patients who have undergone nuclear medicine scans with radioactive isotopes also emit radiation. Patients who have undergone radioisotope scans should have surgery delayed for at least 24 to 48 hours to reduce staff exposure to any radioactivity. A patient who has received a radioisotope may emit up to 2 mrad per hour.

In addition to medical and dental exposure to radiation, each of us is exposed to normal background radiation in our daily activities. Microwave ovens, televisions, smoke detectors, and cellular phones all emit radiation. These levels are not dangerous, but the cumulative effect of this exposure carries the risk for injury. Excessive exposure to radiation has been linked to cancers, particularly leukemias, cataracts,

anemia, abnormalities of the thyroid gland, and genetic mutations. A woman who is in the first trimester has a slightly increased risk of spontaneous abortion. Children who were exposed in utero during the first trimester have a significantly greater risk of developing childhood leukemia and a slightly greater risk of having congenital defects.

DISTANCE
The amount of radiation, particularly x-rays, that one absorbs can be greatly reduced by increasing one's distance from the source of the radiation. For conventional x-rays, staff members should be no closer than 6 feet from the x-ray machine. Staff members should stand at right angles to the direction of the x-ray beam to further reduce exposure to scatter. Radiation exposure and distance operate on the inverse square law of distance. Twice the distance (from the source) equals one-quarter of the previous exposure.

SHIELDING
Appropriate shielding materials should be available to protect workers and patients from unnecessary exposure to radiation. Staff members who work near an active radiation source should wear lead aprons. Lead aprons should have a minimum of 0.5 mm of lead throughout the apron. Aprons should extend from the base of the neck to the knee for adequate protection from radiation exposure. Lead aprons should be handled carefully to prevent cracks in the lead shielding. Aprons should be placed on appropriate hangers when not in use, and the aprons should never be folded.

Aprons should be x-rayed annually (or more often with heavy use) to ensure that there are no cracks in the shielding material. Damaged aprons must be replaced. Staff members who are within 3 feet of an active x-ray unit also should wear thyroid shields, as the thyroid gland is particularly susceptible to radiation injury. Workers who are not wearing aprons should leave the area when x-rays are being taken or, if scrubbed, must stand behind a full-length lead screen for protection. Standing behind a person who is wearing a lead apron is not considered adequate protection. Standing behind equipment such as an anesthesia machine or the fluoroscopy monitor stand also is not appropriate protection.

Whenever possible, one should place lead shielding over the patient's lower abdomen and thighs to protect the reproductive structures (testicles or ovaries). Patients also should wear a lead thyroid shield if such placement does not impede the surgical procedure. Female patients who are in the first trimester of pregnancy should delay radiographic studies if possible. Women who are concerned about being pregnant should have a pregnancy test before undergoing any x-rays, particularly x-rays of the abdomen or pelvis.

RADIATION MONITORING
Staff members who regularly work with radiation-emitting equipment should be monitored for exposure levels. The use of a dosimeter allows the radiation safety officer to determine the level of radiation a health-care worker has received.

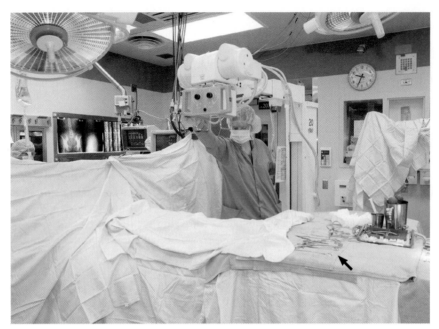

FIGURE 19-5
Proper draping of patient for obtaining x-rays. (From Ballinger PW and Frank ED: *Merrill's atlas of radiographic positions and radiologic procedures,* vol 3, ed 10, St Louis, 2003, Mosby.)

In the surgical setting, workers will be assigned one or two dosimeter badges to measure their exposure to radiation. The first dosimeter is worn at the level of the waist under the x-ray apron and measures the whole-body dose of radiation.

The second dosimeter, if assigned, measures the dose of radiation to the thyroid gland. This badge should be worn at the collar on the outside of the apron. Dosimeter badges are reviewed weekly or monthly, depending on the type of badge used. Those who work in the radiology department may wear additional dosimeters for monitoring of other tissues.

RADIOLOGY AND THE STERILE FIELD

In addition to these steps to protect patients and workers from the harmful effects of ionizing radiation, the sterile surgical fields also must be protected from accidental contamination by x-ray technologists or x-ray equipment. When intraoperative x-rays are required, the x-ray tech will need to position the portable x-ray machine near the patient and manipulate the arm into position alongside or over the patient. This poses a risk of accidental contamination either by the x-ray technologist or from contact with the x-ray machine. The scrub person is responsible for ensuring that all sterile fields remain sterile.

If conventional A/P or lateral films are expected to be needed during the surgical procedure (e.g., intraoperative cholangiogram), the circulator and scrub should ensure that the table has Bucky platforms attached. The Bucky platforms are Plexiglas or carbon platforms with posts that are mounted onto the OR table frame. Mattress pads for the OR table attach to the Bucky platforms with Velcro. The Bucky platform allows the x-ray technologist to slide a film from the head or the foot of the table under the patient without contaminating the sterile drapes. When the film is positioned, the scrub person should open a medium or three-quarter sheet over the site where the x-ray is to be obtained. Most of the overhang of this drape should be to the side of the table where the x-ray technologist and x-ray machine are positioned to protect the field (Figure 19-5). A cuff should be left in the drape remaining over the patient to allow the circulator to remove the drape after the x-ray.

A cross-table lateral film will require the use of an x-ray stand with the cassette and the stand covered with a standard x-ray cassette cover. Cross-table films will require the x-ray technologist to move into the area between the sterile back tables and the patient to position the stand (Figure 19-6). The scrub should make certain that there is adequate room to prevent the x-ray technologist from accidentally bumping into a back table or ring stand.

Conventional (Standard) X-ray

Conventional x-rays are essentially radiographic pictures of the body. Common standard-technique x-rays include mammography, chest x-ray (CXR), x-rays of bone, dental films, and abdominal x-rays. With modern techniques and proper shielding methods, conventional radiography is a safe and cost-effective diagnostic process. Portable x-ray machines allow films to be obtained in almost any area of the health-care facility (Figure 19-7).

ANTERIOR/POSTERIOR (A/P) AND POSTERIOR/ANTERIOR (P/A) FILMS

These procedures allow for visualization of structures by directing x-rays straight through the body from front to back or from back to front. The physician can use this film to

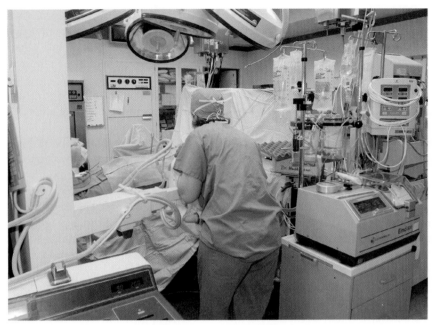

FIGURE 19-6
X-ray technologist positioning the mobile x-ray machine for cross-table lateral lumbar spine procedure. (From Ballinger PW and Frank ED: *Merrill's atlas of radiographic positions and radiologic procedures,* vol 3, ed 10, St Louis, 2003, Mosby.)

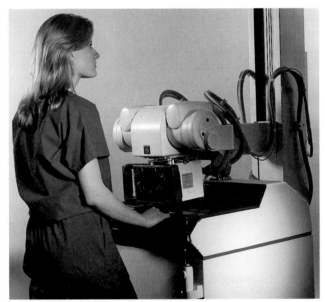

FIGURE 19-7
Portable x-ray machine. (From Ballinger PW and Frank ED: *Merrill's atlas of radiographic positions and radiologic procedures,* vol 3, ed 10, St Louis, 2003, Mosby.)

identify abnormalities, including fractures and masses within the body area, that are exposed to x-rays. Conventional A/P or P/A views usually are used to evaluate the chest, abdomen, and extremities.

LATERAL FILMS
Because x-ray images produce a single-dimension view of structures, physicians who identify abnormalities on A/P or P/A films will need to obtain a lateral film of the structure to accurately determine the extent of the abnormal finding. In suspected dislocations or fractures, a lateral film is automatically ordered to determine whether a bone or bone fragment is displaced from its normal alignment.

OBLIQUE FILMS
In certain situations a physician may order an oblique x-ray to determine the location or size of an abnormality. An oblique film is taken at a 45-degree angle to the structure. If one pictures an A/P or P/A film as being directed at 0 degrees (or 360 degrees), a lateral film is directed 90 degrees in relation to an A/P or P/A film. An oblique film is directed halfway between the A/P (or P/A) and the lateral film. This type of radiograph is helpful when dense tissues may prevent adequate assessment of an abnormality, such as cases of suspected masses of the upper lung fields where the scapula may cause obstruction, pelvic views where the iliac bones prevent adequate visualization of pelvic structures, and oblique views of the carpals and tarsals where these bones may appear to overlap.

Contrast-enhanced Radiography
Certain structures lack enough density to sufficiently appear during conventional radiography. Blood vessels, ducts, and the hollow viscera of the abdominal cavity are not readily visualized during conventional x-ray examination. For this reason radiopaque solutions often are used to assist in diagnosis of defects or abnormalities of the peripheral vascular, digestive, and urinary systems. Radiopaque solutions are called contrast media. Contrast media are not radioactive and do not contain radioactive isotopes as are used in nuclear

medicine scans. Contrast media have the ability to block or absorb x-rays to allow structures to be viewed during radiography. Examples of contrast agents include barium sulfate, used in examinations of the GI tract, water-soluble agents, and ionic or nonionic iodinated contrast agents.

BARIUM SULFATE (BaSO₄)
Barium is a water-insoluble contrast agent that is used in radiographic examination of the GI tract. Barium may be swallowed to allow physicians to determine the patency of upper GI structures, including the esophagus, stomach, duodenum, jejunum, and ileum, as well as to improve visualization of diverticula or other masses within these structures. Barium is not to be used if there is suspicion of a perforation of any structure because barium will enter the peritoneum, which will complicate surgical intervention.

Barium also may be administered via enema (barium enema; BE) to allow physicians to diagnose masses and conditions of the lower GI tract, including the rectum, sigmoid colon, descending colon, transverse colon, ascending colon, and hepatic and splenic flexures of the large intestine. A lower GI exam also may identify defects of the ileocecal valve.

Because barium may interfere with other radiographic examinations, other x-ray studies should be completed before a patient undergoes barium studies. Barium tends to cause constipation or impaction (obstruction of the GI tract), and patients are advised to take a laxative after barium studies to prevent these effects. The risk of these effects is higher among the elderly because of their decreased motility of the GI tract. The presence of barium also will alter the color of stool, and patients should be advised of this.

OTHER WATER-SOLUBLE AGENTS
When barium cannot be used for radiographic examination of the GI tract, other water-soluble agents may be employed. Such agents include oral diatrizoate meglumine 60% (Hypaque) or Gastrografin. These agents generally contain iodine and therefore are contraindicated in patients with a known hypersensitivity to iodine or shellfish. Hypaque and Gastrografin lack the viscosity of barium and are less likely to lead to constipation or impaction. Because both are clear liquids, neither will complicate subsequent laparotomy to repair a perforation in the hollow viscous structures. These agents are not intended for intravascular use but are often used intraoperatively for cholangiography.

IONIC AND NONIONIC CONTRAST AGENTS
Iohexol (Omnipaque), Optiray, Isovue, Ioxilan (Oxilan), Renografin, and Conray are used to diagnose strictures of ducts or blood vessels and to assess renal perfusion. These agents may be administered intravascularly and are used for preoperative diagnosis as well as for confirming that flow has been restored during surgery. Common uses of these agents include angiography, cholangiography, pyelography, and assessment of the ureters. Because these contrast agents contain iodine, the patient must be evaluated for potential hy-

persensitivity before administration. Although most of these allergic reactions are minor and may be managed medically, one should determine whether other diagnostic procedures may serve as an alternative to the use of contrast media.

CHOLANGIOGRAM
An intraoperative cholangiogram may be requested to rule out the presence of stones within the common bile duct during cholecystectomy (Box 19-3). In preparation for intraoperative cholangiography, the surgeon will identify the cystic artery, cystic duct, and common bile duct. After ligating the cystic duct and cystic artery, the surgeon will loosely place two silk ties around the common bile duct. These ties will serve to secure the cholangiogram catheter during the procedure. The duct is incised to allow the cholangiogram catheter to be introduced, and the ties are pulled snug to prevent leakage of the contrast agent. At this point a portable x-ray machine should be present in the room and is positioned as for a cholangiogram.

The surgeon injects 10 to 20 cc of normal saline through the catheter to clear any bile in the duct. The surgeon then injects several cubic centimeters of contrast media and has an x-ray taken. It is vital that the scrub person correctly identify the syringes containing the normal saline and the contrast solution. While injecting the contrast media first will not harm the patient, flushing the contrast out with the saline before the x-ray is taken will negate the film, causing the patient to be exposed to more radiation.

PYELOGRAM
Antegrade and retrograde pyelography are designed to assess different aspects of kidney function. Antegrade pyelography is used to assess renal function from the glomeruli. Antegrade pyelography allows the physician to determine whether a patient has adequate perfusion of the kidney and whether the glomeruli of the kidney are producing urine. Antegrade pyelography requires the injection of a contrast

---

Box 19-3 Supplies for Intraoperative Cholangiogram

▶ 20 or 30 cc syringe x 2
▶ Cholangiogram catheter
▶ 3-way stopcock (optional)
▶ 2-0 or 3-0 silk ties
▶ Contrast media (e.g., Gastrografin, Hypaque, Omnipaque, Renografin)
▶ Normal saline, does not need to be for injectable use
▶ Medicine cup or small basin
▶ Labels, to identify solutions and syringes
▶ Sterile marker, to prepare labels
▶ Lead shield, for staff members
▶ Sterile drape(s), to protect surgical field

agent into a peripheral intravenous (IV) line and viewing of x-ray images to determine the time required for the contrast agent to be excreted into the renal pelvis. Retrograde pyelography assesses the normal flow of urine from the kidney to the bladder. In a retrograde pyelogram (RP), a contrast agent is injected through a cystoscope that has been positioned in the urinary bladder to evaluate the renal pelvis and ureter for obstructions. A cystogram is performed in a similar fashion but is used to assess the urinary bladder.

ANGIOGRAPHY

Contrast-enhanced x-rays of blood vessels enable surgeons to locate obstruction or stenosis (narrowing) of the vessels. Angiography often is performed to assess peripheral vascular disease as part of the preoperative diagnostic process. In the surgical setting, angiography may be used to evaluate whether adequate blood flow has been restored to distal structures after embolectomy, thrombectomy, or vascular bypass. To perform an intraoperative angiogram, the surgeon inserts an IV catheter into the blood vessel and injects contrast media distally into the vessel, after which fluoroscopic or conventional x-ray images are obtained. Specific types of angiography include arteriography, aortography, lymphangiography, and venography; their use depends on the vessels being assessed.

Fluoroscopy

Fluoroscopy is the use of continuous x-ray to evaluate structures. Images produced by fluoroscopy are presented on video monitors connected to the fluoroscope. An example of the fluoroscope is the C-arm device commonly used in the surgical setting. The C-arm also is called an *image intensifier* (Figure 19-8). A benefit of fluoroscopy over conventional or contrast-enhanced x-rays is that the image is immediately displayed for the surgeon to view. Conventional x-ray techniques require the radiographic film to be developed before it can be viewed. Because the C-arm can be easily manipulated, multiple views of the same structure can be assessed rapidly, thus reducing the amount of time a patient must be on the operating table. This technique also allows the surgeon to quickly identify correct placement of surgical implants, including central venous lines and orthopedic implants such as intramedullary nails and dynamic compression plates and screws. When extensive use of the fluoroscope is anticipated, all scrubbed team members should don protective lead aprons before scrubbing for the procedure.

Computed Tomography (CT)

Computed tomography (CT), sometimes called computed *axial* tomography (CAT), scans are useful in diagnosing many conditions and abnormalities. While conventional x-rays simply capture the amount of radiation that passes through the body to produce an image of the structures through which the radiation has passed, CT applies computerized calculations to determine how much radiation has passed through specific structures. This produces greater visualization of specific structures. CT scans produce cross-sectional images of the tissues being assessed. CT techniques allow for imaging of different tissue thicknesses, which allows for better diagnosis of smaller masses. CT techniques can be employed to evaluate almost any anatomical structure. Common uses include:

▶ Abdominal: includes liver, gall bladder, pancreas, spleen, kidneys, adrenal glands, abdominal vessels, stomach, and intestines
▶ Pelvis: includes urinary bladder, rectum, sigmoid colon, female reproductive structures, and prostate
▶ Chest: includes mediastinum, great vessels, heart, thymus gland, and lungs
▶ Spine
▶ Extremities
▶ Head and neck: includes cranial and facial bones, sinuses, thyroid, and parathyroid glands

CT images usually are transverse "cuts" through the body. One views these images by imagining looking through the patient from the patient's feet up toward the patient's head. This allows the learner to appreciate the normal location of structures found within the particular "slice" or "cut" of tissue (Figure 19-9).

Another type of CT scanner, called a spiral, or helical, CT scanner produces a continuous corkscrew image of the body. This type of scan produces a three-dimensional view of structures and is helpful in assessing blood vessels.

Magnetic Resonance Imaging (MRI)

Magnetic resonance imaging (MRI) uses radio-frequency (RF) signals and powerful magnets to produce images of

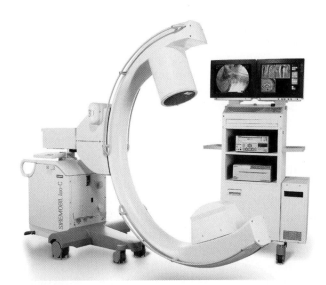

FIGURE 19-8
The C-arm, also referred to as an image-intensifier, is used in fluoroscopy. (From Ballinger PW and Frank ED: *Merrill's atlas of radiographic positions and radiologic procedures,* vol 3, ed 10, St Louis, 2003, Mosby.)

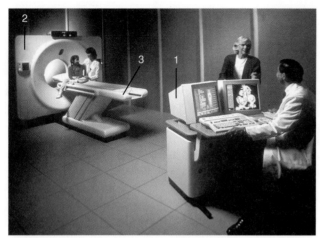

FIGURE 19-9
Components of a CT scanner: (1) Computer and operator's console. (2) Gantry. (3) Patient table. (From Ballinger PW and Frank ED: *Merrill's atlas of radiographic positions and radiologic procedures,* vol 3, ed 10, St Louis, 2003, Mosby.)

anatomical structures. Unlike CT techniques, MRI does not use ionizing radiation. MRI is typically used to evaluate structures of the brain, muscles, and other connective tissues, and the spine. MRI is not as useful as CT for assessing bony structures but may be more helpful in evaluation of soft tissues. In the rare instance where surgical intervention is performed with the aid of MRI in the MRI unit, extreme care must be taken to protect the patient and staff members from injury caused by metallic items that become projectiles when the magnets are active.

Nuclear Medicine Scans

Radionuclides can help in the diagnosis of conditions or disease processes during preoperative preparation. While radiographic studies help in assessing the anatomical structure of tissues, nuclear medicine helps in assessing the functionality of tissues. Nuclear medicine uses radioactive isotopes that are bound to specific agents that are targeted for uptake by specific cells or tissues. Nuclear medicine scans often are used to evaluate tumor function and growth. It is important to note that a patient who has undergone radionuclide imaging may emit up to 2 mrad/h. Therefore surgical procedures on these patients should be deferred for 24 to 48 hours after such imaging.

Positron Emission Tomography (PET)

Positron emission tomography (PET) uses radionuclides that emit positrons (positively charged particles) to evaluate patterns of metabolism and blood flow within tissues. PET scans are very useful in determining the location, size, and metabolism of tumors. PET imaging also is used to assess neurological and cardiac function by measuring blood flow (perfusion) and oxygen and glucose metabolism in these structures. Images presented on PET scans help in presurgical planning to minimize the trauma to surrounding healthy tissues.

Electroneurodiagnostic Testing

Occasionally the surgeon will request neurological monitoring during a surgical procedure. Somatosensory evoked potentials (SSEP), also called somatosensory evoked responses (SSER), allow the surgeon to identify potential injury to the spinal cord or specific nerve roots. In this type of monitoring, passive electrodes are inserted into the subcutaneous layer of tissue in the extremities and an active electrode is inserted that will generate impulses through the spinal cord. A monitor allows a trained electroneurodiagnostic technician to visualize feedback from the various passive electrodes to determine whether abnormal strain or injury has affected a particular segment of the spinal cord or a specific nerve root. In the preoperative phase, the patient will have undergone a similar procedure to obtain a baseline for comparison. This type of procedure is used during removal of spinal tumors, correction of cauda equina syndrome, and placement of spinal instrumentation. A surgeon occasionally uses SSEP during vertebral fusion without instrumentation.

TISSUE AND CELL DIAGNOSIS

Surgical procedures often involve the removal of cells, tissues, fluid, or other materials for diagnostic evaluation. Anatomical material and foreign bodies removed from a patient are called specimens, and each must be handled properly to ensure adequate preservation for diagnosis or other purposes. Depending on the specimen, different laboratory studies may be required. Generally, gross anatomical tissues are evaluated through anatomical pathology, cell cultures are assessed through cytology, and purulent or infected specimens are reviewed via microbiology.

Pathology is the study of disease and disease processes. Cytology is the study of cells, and microbiology is the study of microscopic life forms, including bacteria, viruses, fungi, protozoa, and other microscopic organisms. Microbiology may be further broken down into bacteriology, virology, and mycology. Most surgical specimens are referred to anatomical pathology professionals, although tissues or fluids thought to contain infectious agents may be referred to microbiology professionals for examination and diagnosis. In certain procedures, fluids may be sent to cytology professionals to determine the presence of specific cells.

Pathology

As mentioned, pathology is the study of disease. During surgery, samples of tissue often will be obtained and evaluated to determine the cause or type of the patient's disease process, with the goal of helping to plan a course of treatment for the patient. These tissue specimens are sent to the division of pathology known as anatomical pathology. The pathologist evaluates the structure and type of cells found within the tissue to produce a diagnosis for the surgeon. Depending on the nature of the tissue and the examination required, different preservation and preparation techniques are used.

SPECIMEN HANDLING

Specimens must be handled correctly from the moment they are removed from the patient. Correct handling requires excellent communication among the scrub, circulator, and surgeon. When the surgeon removes tissue from the patient, the scrub must verify what the tissue (specimen) is and what, if any, fixative is to be used. The surgeon sometimes requests an immediate assessment of the specimen. In this case, the circulator would need to contact a pathologist to come to the OR to examine the specimen. The surgeon occasionally will identify a particular margin of the tissue to note its location within the body. The surgeon will do this with a nonabsorbable suture. After the surgeon ties the knot, he or she cuts the ends of the suture, leaving them long. No specimen should be passed off of the sterile field before the surgeon gives permission to do so.

The scrub, after receiving a specimen from the surgeon, should ask the surgeon three questions:

▶ What is the specimen?
▶ How should this specimen be preserved/fixed?
▶ May I pass the specimen off the field?

The scrub person must relay the name of the specimen and the way the specimen is to be fixed to the circulator. If there are any questions, the circulator must confirm with the scrub and/or surgeon information about the specimen. Improper handling of a specimen may prevent correct diagnosis.

Any tissue removed from a patient is assumed to be a specimen unless the surgeon states otherwise.

TISSUE PRESERVATION

To ensure proper diagnosis, tissues must be carefully handled in the surgical setting. Tissues may be sent to pathology in a particular fixative (preservative), or they may be sent for fresh or fresh-frozen examination. Most tissue specimens referred to the pathology department for diagnosis will be preserved in a 10% formalin (formaldehyde) solution to prevent the breakdown of cells in the tissue.

Frozen-section Specimens

A surgeon often will request immediate pathological evaluation of a tissue specimen. This type of examination is called a **frozen section** and is usually used to rule out cancer or to determine whether adequate tumor margins have been resected. A surgeon who has requested a frozen section calls a pathologist to the room as soon as the specimen is removed. The pathologist takes the specimen to the lab, where it is frozen with liquid nitrogen. The pathologist then uses a high-speed cutter to slice single-cell layers of the tissue, which are mounted on a microscope slide and immediately assessed for the presence of abnormal cells. The pathologist also can determine the distance from the edge

of the specimen to the nearest layer of malignant cells. This information is reported back to the surgeon, and the surgeon uses the diagnosis to determine whether additional surgical intervention is required or the incision may be closed and dressed.

A surgeon may, with prior patient consent, modify the surgical procedure from a breast **biopsy** to a mastectomy, depending on his or her determination based on the pathologist's report. In some cases, the data in the pathologist's report may preclude further tissue resection if the surgeon determines that a tumor cannot be resected.

A specimen for frozen section is placed in a dry specimen container after the surgeon has given permission for the specimen to be removed from the surgical field. If tumor margin is being assessed, the surgeon may place a nonabsorbable suture into one or more of the margins for identification. This allows the pathologist to report what, if any, tumor margin is insufficient.

Fresh Specimens

Certain specimens, such as muscle tissue obtained for diagnosis of neuromuscular conditions, must not be preserved in formalin but instead kept moistened with normal (0.9%) saline. These specimens are called "fresh" specimens and must be evaluated before tissue can break down. An example of such a case is a muscle biopsy. Muscle biopsies often are obtained with the use of a special biopsy clamp. These specimens are sent to the pathology department with the clamp left in place and moistened with normal saline.

GENETIC STUDIES

Some specimens may be used for genetic studies. An example is the products of conception resulting from a tubal pregnancy or a miscarriage (spontaneous abortion). This type of specimen is fixed in a lactated Ringer (LR) solution.

NONFIXED SPECIMENS

Certain specimens do not require any type of fixative. These include foreign bodies, renal calculi, and gall stones. These are simply placed in a dry specimen container and delivered to pathology.

Microbiology

The microscopic study of organisms is called microbiology. In the health-care setting, microbiologists study infectious agents and help in identifying the antimicrobial agents that are useful in destroying infectious microorganisms. In the treatment of a surgical patient with a suspected infection, samples of tissue or body fluids may be sent to the microbiology department to determine the specific type of infectious organisms present in the tissue or fluid.

Culture and Sensitivity (C & S)

When the presence of an infectious organism is suspected, a sample of the material is obtained and a culture is prepared. One prepares a culture by placing cells from the specimen on a plate containing growth medium. The cells are allowed to grow and then compared with known microorganisms to determine the strain of infection. If no growth appears, then the culture is presumed to be negative. If growth appears, the culture is considered positive. Culture cells then are combined with appropriate antimicrobial agents to determine the level of sensitivity of each cell culture. Cell cultures that are completely destroyed are said to be highly sensitive to the antimicrobial agent. Cell cultures that are only partially destroyed are considered to have a low sensitivity to the antimicrobial agent. Cultures that are not destroyed are considered to be resistant. The level of sensitivity determines the appropriate drug therapies.

Cytology

The study of cells is called cytology. Occasionally the surgeon obtains fluid or very small tissue samples from the patient. Fluid samples are taken from free fluid in the cavity or from cell washings. The surgeon obtains cell washings by introducing normal saline into an area and aspirating the fluid into a collection trap. Other fluid samples include sputum, urine, ascitic fluid, pleural fluid, cerebrospinal fluid (CSF), pericardial fluid, and peritoneal fluid.

Small tissues are obtained on biopsy during flexible endoscopic procedures. Such biopsies may be collected with biopsy forceps or soft endoscopic brushes. These cells are sent to the cytology department for microscopic examination and diagnosis. Fluids sent to cytology are sent in the collection trap, and cell brushings and tissue biopsies obtained during flexible endoscopy are sent in a specimen container with a small amount of normal saline to keep the cells viable for examination. Cytology studies look for the presence of blood cells, tumor cells, protein, and glucose.

ENDOSCOPY

Diagnostic **endoscopy** is a valuable modality for visualizing internal structures with minimal trauma to surrounding tissues. The techniques of specific endoscopic procedures are discussed in the applicable chapters. Endoscopy is classified as noninvasive or minimally invasive. In noninvasive endoscopy, the endoscope is introduced through a natural orifice or opening into the body. Examples of noninvasive endoscopic techniques are laryngoscopy, bronchoscopy, esophagoscopy, gastroscopy, colonoscopy, hysteroscopy, and cystoscopy. Minimally invasive endoscopic techniques use small incisions for the introduction of the endoscope and biopsy instruments. Examples of minimally invasive endoscopy include thoracoscopy, mediastinoscopy, laparoscopy, pelviscopy, and arthroscopy.

Endoscopic procedures usually are used for diagnostic purposes but also may be used for operative purposes. When performing minimally invasive endoscopic procedures, the surgical team should be immediately prepared to convert to an open surgical procedure.

IMPORTANCE OF DIAGNOSTIC PROCEDURES

Diagnostic procedures and techniques are designed to evaluate the entire patient to enable the caregiver to develop an appropriate plan of care for the patient. Certain procedures are designed to assess the patient's ability to withstand the stresses of surgery, and other procedures are designed to determine whether medical or surgical intervention is considered successful. Accurate diagnosis of a patient's presenting condition as well as prompt identification of occult (hidden) medical or surgical conditions greatly improves the prognosis and care of the patient.

CASE STUDIES

Case 1
The patient is a 50-year-old male complaining of shortness of breath, chest pain on inspiration, and profuse sweating (diaphoresis). What diagnostic tests may be requested by the physician?

Case 2
The patient is a 28-year-old female complaining of right-lower-quadrant (RLQ) pain, rebound tenderness, nausea, and constipation. What is the diagnosis? What diagnostic tests confirm this diagnosis? What other diagnostic tests may be performed?

Case 3
You have just completed an abdominal aortic aneurysmectomy (AAA) with insertion of a bifurcated graft. The surgeon is unable to palpate pulses in either foot or ankle. What diagnostic tool would the surgeon most likely request?

Case 4
You have recently been informed that you are pregnant and you are in the first trimester. You are assigned to an orthopedic procedure site where x-ray is scheduled to be used. How do you handle this situation?

REFERENCES

Dubin D: *Rapid interpretation of EKGs,* ed 6, Tampa, 2000, Cover Publishing.

Cheitlin MD and Sokolow M: *Clinical cardiology,* ed 6, Los Altos, Ca, 1996, Appleton & Lange.

Fischbach FT: *Manual of laboratory and diagnostic tests,* ed 6, Philadelphia, 2003, Lippincott Williams & Wilkins.

Forbes BA, Sahm DF, and Weissfeld A: *Bailey and Scott's diagnostic microbiology,* ed 11, St Louis, 2002, Mosby.

Lacy CF, Armstrong LL, et al: *Drug information handbook,* ed 9, Hudson, Ohio, 2001, Lexi-Comp.

Selman J: *Fundamentals of x-ray and radium physics,* ed 7, Springfield, Ill, 1985, Charles C Thomas Publisher.

Thompson TT: *Cahoon's formulating x-ray techniques,* ed 9, Durham, NC, 1979, Duke University Press.

Smith AL: *Principles of microbiology,* ed 10, St Louis, 1985, Mosby.

Snyder K and Keegan C: *Pharmacology for the surgical technologist,* Philadelphia, 1999, WB Saunders.

Venes D and Thomas CL, eds: *Taber's cyclopedic medical dictionary,* ed 19, Philadelphia, 2001, FA Davis.

Chapter 20

The Selection of Surgical Instruments

Learning Objectives

After studying this chapter the reader will be able to:

- Describe the characteristics of tissue
- Identify classifications of instruments
- Differentiate types of instruments by their function
- Identify the different types of finishes on surgical instruments
- Describe the care and handling of instruments
- Describe several methods of learning about instruments
- Develop a personal plan for learning instruments

Terminology

Boggy—A characteristic of diseased tissue that makes it soft and doughy.

Box lock—The hinge point of many surgical instruments.

Chisel—An orthopedic instrument used to slice bone; one side is straight and the other is beveled.

Clamp—Instrument that is designed to occlude or hold tissue, objects, or fabric between its jaws.

Cross-clamp—To place one or more clamps at a right angle to an elongated or tubular structure such as the aorta.

Curettage—To remove tissue by scraping with a surgical curette.

Cutting instrument—An instrument with a sharp edge used to cut and dissect tissue. This group includes scissors, scalpels, osteotomes, curettes, chisels, biopsy punches, saws, drills, and needles.

Dilator—Graduated smooth instrument used to increase the diameter of an anatomical opening in tissue.

Double-action instrument—An instrument with two hinges in the middle. This provides greater leverage and cutting strength than a single-action instrument. Usually used to describe an orthopedic rongeur.

Elevator—A non-hinged sharp or dull tipped instrument. An elevator is used to separate tissues or to bluntly remodel tissue.

Friable—Condition in which tissue tears or fragments easily when handled.

Fulcrum—The area on an instrument at which the lever moves.

Hemostat—A surgical clamp used most often to occlude a blood vessel.

Histology—Study of the structure of tissue.

Honed—Sharpened.

Mixter—A type of hemostat with a straight shank and a right-angle tip.

Points—The tips of a surgical instrument.

Probe—An instrument placed within a natural lumen or fistula to determine its length and direction.

Rongeur—A hinged instrument with sharp, cup-shaped tips used to extract pieces of bone or other connective tissue.

Semi-occluding clamp—A nontraumatic clamp with jaws that either do not contact each other when closed, or exert very little pressure on tissue when closed.

Serosa—The delicate outer layer of tissue of most organs.

Shank—The area of a surgical instrument between the box lock and finger ring.

Transect—To surgically divide an organ by sharp dissection.

Undermine—To separate tissues layers on a vertical plane using dissecting scissors.

LEARNING SURGICAL INSTRUMENTATION

Learning Requirements

Learning surgical instruments is *much more* than simply matching a name with an instrument and producing that instrument when it is requested. Surgical instrumentation requires technical knowledge about:

▶ How the design of an instrument relates to its function

▶ Gross histology (the study of tissue types); knowing the characteristics of tissue types

▶ Structural anatomy; knowledge of anatomical structures and ability to visualize the structures

▶ Care and handling of instruments

▶ Ability to recognize high-quality instruments over those that malfunction, are a hazard by design, require repair, or are poorly manufactured

One of the challenges that scrubs face is to acquire knowledge about instruments without having any experience with the actual use of the instrument. The scrub must watch and learn which instrument works best for a task and, more importantly, *why*. For example, the surgeon uses a *Babcock* **clamp** to pick up the fallopian tube. This is because the Babcock exerts very little pressure, even when the clamp is closed. Using critical thinking, one can apply this knowledge to bowel tissue, which has similar histological aspects. Its surface also is delicate and requires gentle handling.

Learning Methods

UNDERSTANDING THE DESIGN

One should learn instrumentation on a basic level by associating function with design. The following are some important design features:

▶ Heavy or delicate

▶ Long or short

▶ Cutting or blunt-tipped

▶ Narrow or wide

▶ Angled or straight

▶ Completely or partially occluding

▶ Traumatic or nontraumatic to tissue (with teeth or smooth)

When applying these designs to tissue, the scrub must learn by associating which types of tissue require a particular design. For example, blood vessels are never handled with an instrument that might puncture or bruise the tissue. However, fibrous tissue is very resilient and requires toothed instruments to maintain grasping pressure.

Although each instrument has a specific name, many surgeons ask for the instrument by its function rather than its name. For example, rather than ask for a "*Weitlaner* self-retaining retractor" the surgeon more often asks for a "self retainer." When the surgeon asks for a "clamp," he or she expects to receive the appropriate type of clamp used for that particular tissue. There are hundreds of types of clamps, and it may seem an impossible task to anticipate which instrument is needed. Rather than learning *just the name* of an instrument, learn the tissue. Of course, learning the name of the instrument is important, but always associate a particular instrument with the tissue associated with it.

When anticipating needs, observe the tissue and *think about the options based on the tissue.* You will be able to narrow down the choices to one or two instruments; then it is a matter of having those ready before the surgeon asks for them.

WORKING WITH THE INSTRUMENTS

Instrument trays are assembled according to the particular surgical specialty (Figure 20-1). One of the best ways to learn the names of instruments is to assemble instrument trays by specialty. This creates an association of one instrument with others in the same specialty and permits examination of the

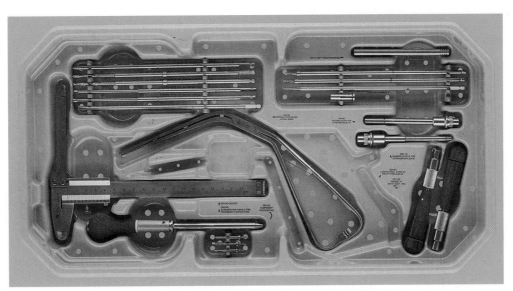

FIGURE 20-1
Example of an instrument tray. (From Tighe SM: *Instrumentation for the operating room*, ed 6, St Louis, 1999, Mosby.)

instrument. Above all, associating one instrument with others in a group cues the brain to categorize them. This is a valuable learning device.

As you set up a case and work with a preceptor, ask the name and function of any instrument you do not know. You may not remember all the names, but you will have established an association between that instrument and a specific situation. As you pass the instrument, think of its name at the same time. This creates another associative cue.

One of the *slowest* ways to memorize instruments is simply to look at pictures or flash cards of instruments. Without some associative cue, memorization is tedious and difficult. *Memory is built through association.* The neural pathway to memory is linked with other information and events that occurred with the memory. Repetition offers no specific cue. That is why simply reading study material repeatedly does not ensure recall. To remember a picture, design, or object such as an instrument, you must *associate* it with something that becomes a *cue.* The cue might be some structural aspect of the instrument or a particular case on which you scrubbed. The name may remind you of some object or person. Memorization is personal because association is personal. Cues are a powerful tool for any kind of memorization. Speed of recall comes only *after* the cue is in place.

INSTRUMENT CONSTRUCTION

Surgical instruments represent a large investment for every operating room. There are two different grades of instruments: surgical grade and floor grade. *Surgical grade* instruments are high-quality instruments that are constructed of stainless steel and other metal alloys, such as carbon and chromium, that resist marring, pitting, scratching, and dulling. Instruments discussed in this chapter and textbook that are used in surgery are surgical-grade instruments. Surgical-grade instruments are made by hand by specially trained instrument makers.

Floor-grade instruments are made from inferior metals and are not manufactured with the precision of the surgical-grade instruments. Floor-grade instruments are much less expensive than surgical-grade instruments, but they must be replaced more often because they become damaged from rust after two or three sterilization cycles. Floor-grade instruments are intended for use in less critical applications, such as suture and suture-removal kits in the emergency room. In some areas of the country, floor-grade instruments are categorized as "single-use" instruments and are not sterilized for use again. When assembling surgical instrument trays for sterilization, one must take care to select the properly manufactured surgical instruments for the trays, and not include floor-grade instruments.

Three different types of finishes are used on metal instruments. Bright or mirror finish is highly polished, reflects light, and may cause glare in the surgical field, affecting the surgeon's vision. A satin or dull finish on instruments is preferable for its reduced glare and light reflection. Ebony is a black chromium finish used for laser surgery. The dull black finish prevents laser beams from reflecting or bouncing off the instruments, which could injure or destroy nearby tissues.

Many instruments now have expensive tungsten carbide inserts to increase sharpness in scissors and gripping ability in needle holders. Instruments with tungsten carbide inserts are usually manufactured with gold-plated handles (Figure 20-2). Eye scalpels contain diamond cutting edges for precision and hardness. The care of instruments is described in Chapter 8. The operating team must understand the high level of quality materials and precision work required to create instruments.

All instruments are balanced to fit the surgeon's hand. The distribution of weight between the handle (and finger rings) and the **fulcrum** is measured and tested for optimal performance. The hinges are perfectly **honed** to create a seamless surface when the instrument is closed. Ratchets are calculated to create the correct amount of spring and ease of opening without sticking or forcing (Figure 20-3).

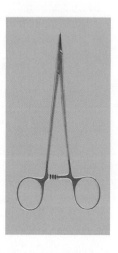

FIGURE 20-2
Instruments with tungsten carbide inserts are commonly manufactured with gold-plated handles. (From Tighe SM: *Instrumentation for the operating room,* ed 6, St Louis, 1999, Mosby.)

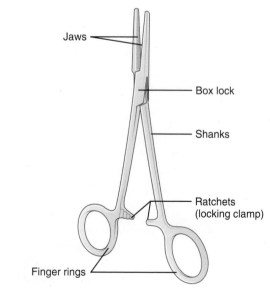

Jaws

Box lock

Shanks

Ratchets (locking clamp)

Finger rings

FIGURE 20-3
Basic parts of an instrument.

Scissors must be particularly well balanced and precise. The blades are designed to slide over each other with an exact amount of width between the blades. **Points** often are honed by hand to ensure that they have no burrs and that the tips come together perfectly.

All these design features can be destroyed by mishandling of an instrument. A microsurgical instrument used on the eye costs hundreds of dollars, and one can ruin it instantly by dropping it or placing a heavy object on top of it. Using **hemostats** to pry open metal caps or to grasp metal sutures puts the jaws out of alignment, often permanently. Cheaper instruments are less resilient to damage and can be severely compromised in their precision. The entire surgical team is responsible for handling instruments correctly.

CHARACTERISTICS OF TISSUE

Every surgical instrument used in the modern operating room was developed to overcome a technical problem in surgery arising from the characteristics of tissues. The scrub can anticipate and assist in instrumentation (selecting the correct instrument for the task at hand) by becoming familiar with tissue types and learning which instruments are used on a particular tissue. This approach to learning is different from *learning instruments by rote* according to their procedural step. This approach is based not only on knowledge of the procedure, but also on specific knowledge of anatomy and **histology**.

Normal tissues differ in texture, strength, elasticity, water, fat content, and permeability. If all body tissues were the same, there would be far fewer instruments. Normal tissue changes when diseased. Infection has a liquefying or fragmenting effect. Some tumors are extremely fibrous and tough. This information is important to both the surgeon and the scrub. The scrub must use critical thinking to apply knowledge of the procedure and the tissue type when anticipating the surgeon's need.

Fibrous

Fibrous tissue is strong and resilient. Connective tissue, muscle, tendon, fascia, and bone normally are very fibrous. This tissue requires holding and clamping instruments that grip tightly by pressure or by actually puncturing the tissue in order to maintain the grip. Fascia often is grasped with Kocher clamps, which have one or two teeth at the tip. Toothed tissue forceps are required for this tissue. **Cutting instruments** such as curved Mayo scissors must be sharp and strong. Tendons and ligaments require serrated grasping instruments.

Friable

Friable tissue is very delicate, tears easily, and has little resilience. Infection or advanced age can cause normally strong tissue to become friable. Tissues such as the liver, spleen, and lung normally are friable. A strong membrane covers and protects these organs. However, these tissues must be handled with nontraumatic instruments. Clamps must be non-occluding and forceps non-toothed. Friable tissue tends to bleed easily and fragment when compressed.

Elastic

Elastic tissue is resilient and able to withstand a limited amount of stretching without injury. The peritoneal lining of body cavities, although elastic, can tear with extreme or repeated pressure. The vaginal vault and some glandular tissue, such as the tonsils, are elastic. These tissues can tolerate the amount of pressure exerted by a hemostat or low-compression biting clamps such as an Allis. Elastic tissue tends to heal rapidly unless diseased or infected.

Boggy

Tissue is described as **boggy** when it is heavy with fluid, inflamed, or diseased. Its normal resiliency is lost and the organ becomes soft and doughy.

Semi-Solid

Semi-solid tissue has a high fat content. It does not compress well and tends to fragment into small pieces when clamped. Adipose tissue has few blood vessels compared with other types of tissue and may require a penetrating retractor such as a sharp rake. The Allis clamp, which has fine serrations at the tip, often is used to clamp or grasp adipose tissue. The high fat content of this tissue may cause instruments to become slippery and difficult to handle. Forceps with teeth are required for suturing.

Bone

Bone tissue is resilient and somewhat springy when healthy. Large bones usually are manipulated through traction or leverage rather than direct pulling pressure. Notice that most bone retractors such as the *Bennett* and *Scoville* have a toothed tip or a reverse curve that can be inserted under another bone for leverage (Figure 20-4).

Serosa (Visceral)

The viscera, organs of the body, are covered by a fine membrane. This membrane is easily punctured, and the underlying tissue layers can bleed profusely. Nontraumatic instruments are needed when handling this tissue. When the spleen, liver, and intestines are retracted, the surface area of the retractor must be sufficiently wide to distribute the pressure. Edges must be protected with sponges to prevent the retractor edge from cutting into the tissue. Intestinal clamps are only partially occluding and have longitudinal striations to intersect the bowel at a right angle. Examples of gastrointestinal clamps are the *Bainbridge* and *Doyen* clamps. The toothed *Kocher* clamp may be used to **cross-clamp** (clamp at a right angle to the tissue) the bowel, but only when that portion will be **transected** (cut across and removed).

BODY PLANES

Technical difficulties may arise during surgery because of the angles of tissue planes. Instruments are needed that can reach in all directions. The instruments' design and function allow the surgeon to penetrate, suture, extract, and ligate

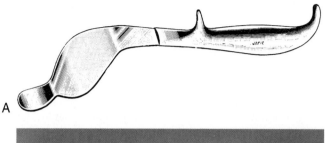

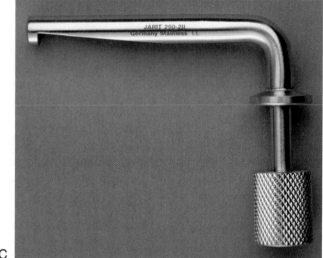

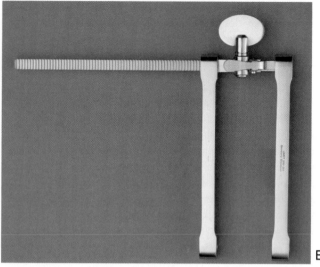

FIGURE 20-4
Bone retractors. **A,** Bennet tibia retractor. **B** and **C,** Scoville retractor frame and blade. (Courtesy of Jarit Instruments, Hawthorne, NY.)

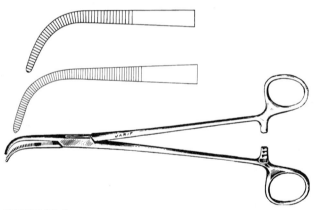

FIGURE 20-5
Mixter clamp (right angle). (Courtesy of Jarit Instruments, Hawthorne, NY.)

tissue in a variety of levels, planes, and spatial relationships. If the surgeon could flatten the body and work on a flat plane, the procedure would be much easier. However, except in superficial surgery, this is not the case. Most procedures require the surgeon to work in a limited space in a small cavity. Some procedures require access to areas that are deep, restricted, and oblique (angled). An example is an abdominal approach to the esophagus or sigmoid colon. Familiarity with the body's tissue planes gives the scrub a greater appreciation of the surgical techniques required. More important, the scrub can see how the *design* of the instrument is critical in the performance of each step of the surgery.

An angled instrument is one whose tip is curved or right-angled. The function of this clamp is to reach *underneath* or around a structure. For example, blood vessels cannot be lifted out, so the instrument must accommodate the structure. The *Mixter* or right-angle clamp is used along vertical planes of tissue, such as the sides of an incision (Figure 20-5). If the clamp were completely straight, it would have to be turned horizontally to clamp tissue along the wall of the incision. The right-angle clamp is perfectly suited for deep incisions because it is used in its vertical position.

Right-angle scissors such as *Potts scissors* allow the surgeon to insert the scissor tip inside a vessel (Figure 20-6). He or she can aim the scissors straight down into the wound, but the tips follow the horizontal plane of the vessel.

The curves and bifurcations (areas where a tubular structure forms a Y) of hollow structures also present technical challenges. Flexible instruments have been developed to overcome this difficulty. Before the refinement of flexible endoscopes, lighted rigid scopes were used exclusively. Few areas of the body follow a straight path. A rigid, straight instrument is useful only when it can be manipulated at the tip. The technical advantage of the flexible endoscope is that the surgeon can directly view areas of the body that previously were not seen except through a surgical incision (Figure 20-7). The fiberoptic bundle can curve light and magnify the focal point at the tip of the scope.

When offering the surgeon instruments, the scrub should consider the body planes, as well as wound depth. The depth of the wound is one of the most important fea-

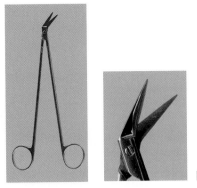

FIGURE 20-6
A, Potts-Smith scissors (right angle). **B,** Close-up of tip. (From Tighe SM: *Instrumentation for the operating room,* ed 6, St Louis, 1999, Mosby.)

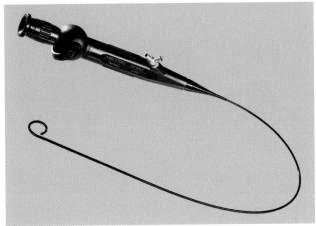

FIGURE 20-7
Flexible endoscope. (© Karl Storz Endoscopy America, Inc.)

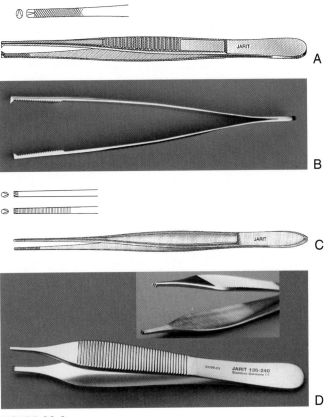

FIGURE 20-8
Toothed forceps. **A,** Tissue thumb forceps. **B,** Bonney tissue forceps. **C,** Cushing forceps. **D,** Adson tissue forceps. (Courtesy of Jarit Instruments, Hawthorne, NY.)

tures when deciding whether long instruments or extra-long instruments will be needed. Recall from Chapter 16 that one of the technical goals of surgery is to handle tissue as little as possible. Surgical instruments are extensions of the surgeon's hands and allow the surgeon to manipulate tissue with minimal manual contact, which may cause unnecessary damage to the tissue. Long instruments allow the surgeon to place his or her hands at the margin of the wound while the tips of the instruments work deep inside. It is the scrub's responsibility to watch and anticipate the need for long instruments as the procedure progresses.

TYPES OF INSTRUMENTS BY FUNCTION

Grasping and Holding

LOCKING CLAMP

The locking clamp (also called a **box lock** instrument) contains one or more ratchets, which remain closed after they are set (see Figure 20-3). The locking clamp is a design used in many instruments.

THUMB FORCEPS

Thumb forceps are used to grasp tissue. For example, during suturing, the surgeon holds the forceps in one hand and the needle holder in the other. Thumb forceps often are called "pickups." Toothed forceps have one or more teeth in the jaws. These are used to grasp skin or other connective tissue. Toothed forceps are named according to the number and type of teeth. For example, 1 × 2 forceps have one tooth and two slots, and 2 × 3 forceps have two teeth and three slots. Examples of toothed forceps include *Adson* with teeth, thumb tissue forceps with teeth, *Bonney* tissue forceps, and *Cushing* forceps (Figure 20-8).

Smooth or nontoothed forceps are used on delicate tissue such as **serosa,** bowel, blood vessels, or ducts. Examples include smooth thumb forceps, smooth *Adson* forceps, *DeBakey* forceps, and smooth *Cushing* forceps (Figure 20-9). Some forceps are serrated or have small rounded teeth. Examples include *Martin* forceps and *Russian* forceps (Figure 20-10). *Bayonet* forceps are angled and typically used in neurosurgical and nasal procedures (Figure 20-11).

BITING CLAMP

The biting clamp has teeth, cutting edges, or serrations in the jaws. An example of this type of instrument would be the *Kocher* clamp. *Kocher* clamps are used on avascular (having

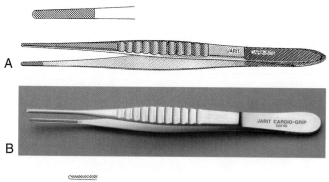

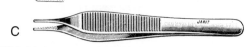

FIGURE 20-9
Smooth or nontoothed forceps. **A,** General tissue forceps. **B,** DeBakey vascular tissue forceps. **C,** Adson dressing forceps. (Courtesy of Jarit Instruments, Hawthorne, NY.)

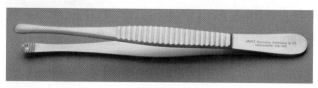

FIGURE 20-10
Russian tissue forceps.(Courtesy of Jarit Instruments, Hawthorne, NY.)

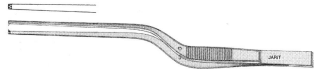

FIGURE 20-11
Bayonet tissue forceps. (Courtesy of Jarit Instruments, Hawthorne, NY.)

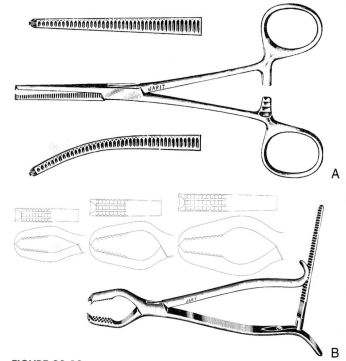

FIGURE 20-12
A, Kocher biting clamp. **B,** Lane bone clamp. (Courtesy of Jarit Instruments, Hawthorne, NY.)

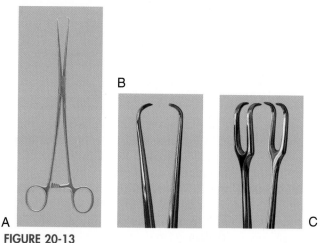

FIGURE 20-13
A, Tenaculum. **B,** Close-up of single tooth tenaculum. **C,** Close-up of double tooth tenaculum. (From Tighe SM: *Instrumentation for the operating room,* ed 6, St Louis, 1999, Mosby.)

little blood supply) fibrous tissue or tissue that will be removed as part of the procedure (Figure 20-12, *A*). The bone clamp is serrated and designed to hold large bone fragments together. An example of a bone clamp is the *Lane* bone-holding clamp (Figure 20-12, *B*).

Holding and Manipulating

The *tenaculum* contains one or more teeth in jaws that can be delicate or heavy (Figure 20-13). This instrument penetrates the tissue rather than just holding it with pressure on the outside surface. It is generally used in fibrous tissue such as the cervix. Like the biting clamp, it is used to hold tissue during dissection and removal.

Clamping and Occluding
ATRAUMATIC CLAMP

The atraumatic clamp usually has locking ratchets, but the tips do not close tightly over the tissue (Figure 20-14). This type of clamp is used on delicate tissue that is highly vascular or easily injured. An example is the *Duval* lung clamp. The *Babcock* clamp is an atraumatic, noncrushing clamp usually used on the bowel or fallopian tubes. Other types of

atraumatic bowel clamps have different kinds of jaw patterns. The jaws have flexible blades that occlude but do not crush the tissue. Examples include the *Bainbridge* intestinal clamp and *Doyen* intestinal clamp.

OCCLUDING CLAMP

An occluding clamp is one that blocks blood flow. The hemostat is the most common example. The *Kelly, Crile,* and mosquito hemostats are used to completely occlude a blood vessel while it is tied or sealed with the electrosurgical unit (ESU) (Figure 20-15). Right-angled clamps such as the *Mix-*

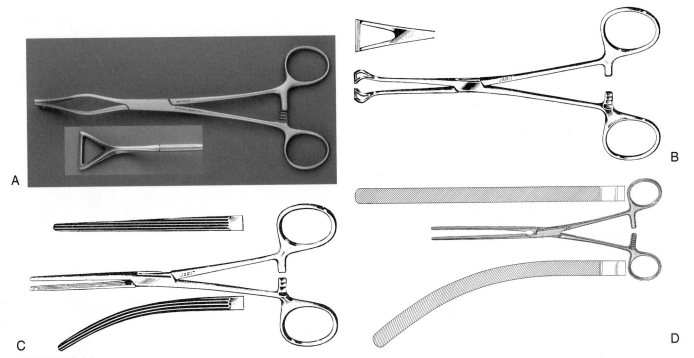

FIGURE 20-14
Atraumatic clamps. **A,** Duval lung clamp. **B,** Babcock clamp. **C,** Bainbridge intestinal clamp. **D,** Doyen intestinal clamp. (Courtesy of Jarit Instruments, Hawthorne, NY.)

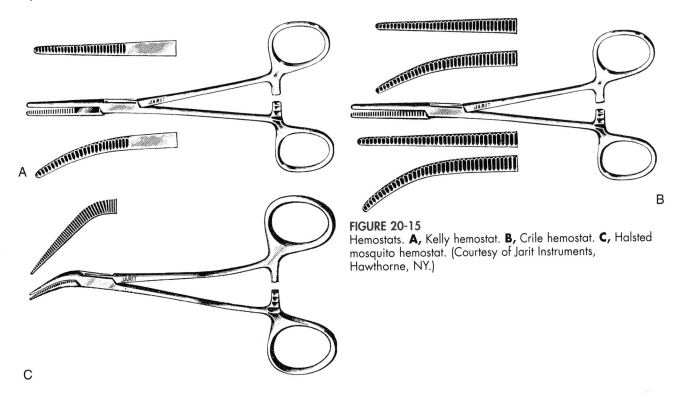

FIGURE 20-15
Hemostats. **A,** Kelly hemostat. **B,** Crile hemostat. **C,** Halsted mosquito hemostat. (Courtesy of Jarit Instruments, Hawthorne, NY.)

ter are used for dissection and occlusion in deep wounds (see Figure 20-5).

VASCULAR CLAMP

The **semi-occluding** vascular clamp is capable of varying low levels of compression between its jaws. These clamps are angled to allow access to blood vessels. Examples of vascular clamps include *bulldog, Satinsky, Fogarty,* and *Cooley* clamps (Figure 20-16).

Cutting and Dissecting
SCALPEL

The common surgical scalpel (commonly called the knife) is used whenever razor-sharp cutting is required for tissue

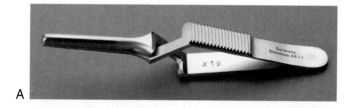

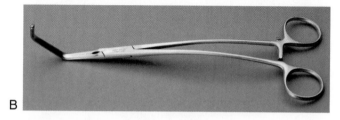

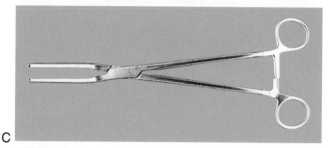

FIGURE 20-16
Semi-occluding vascular clamps. **A,** DeBakey bulldog clamp. **B,** Satinsky vena cava clamp. **C,** Fogarty clamp. (**A** and **C** Courtesy of Jarit Instruments, Hawthorne, NY.; **B** courtesy of Codman & Shurtleff, Inc, Raynham, Mass.)

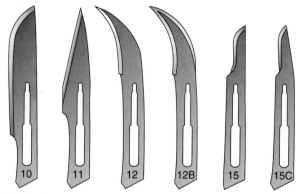

FIGURE 20-17
Scalpel blades #10, 11, 12, 12B, 15, and 15C. (Courtesy of Miltex, Inc, York, Pa.)

dissection. A scalpel blade is detachable from the knife handle. Scalpel blades are numbered consistently among manufacturers, and the number indicates the shape and size (Figure 20-17).

Scalpel blades fit specific handles as follows (Figure 20-18):

Scalpel handles: 3, 3L, 7, 9   Blades: 10, 11, 12, 15
Scalpel handles: 4, 4L   Blades: 18-25

In some areas of the country, OSHA has regulated the use of single-use disposable knife blades with safety shields during surgical procedures (Figure 20-19).

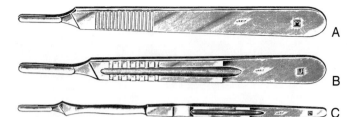

FIGURE 20-18
Scalpel handles. **A,** #3 handle. **B,** #4 handle. **C,** #7 handle. (Courtesy of Jarit Instruments, Hawthorne, NY.)

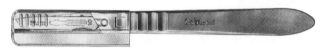

FIGURE 20-19
Disposable knife blade with safety shield. (Courtesy of Miltex, Inc, York, Pa.)

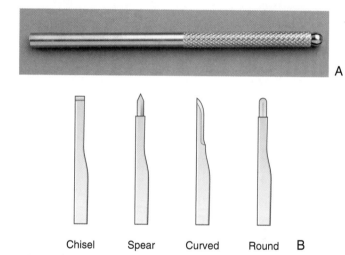

Chisel   Spear   Curved   Round   **B**

FIGURE 20-20
A, Beaver blade handle. **B,** Beaver blades. (**A** courtesy of Jarit Instruments, Hawthorne, NY.)

Another type of scalpel handle with interchangeable disposable blades is called a *Beaver blade* handle and *Beaver blades* (Figure 20-20). These are usually used in surgery of the eye and ear.

The amputation knife is a heavy, one-piece knife used to cut through soft tissue during amputation. Other types of one-piece specialty knives are meniscus knives (*Smillie* knives) and those used in ear surgery (*sickle* knives) and eye surgery (Figure 20-21).

SCISSORS

Surgical scissors are available in a wide variety of sizes and types (Figure 20-22). Small sharp-tipped scissors such as the tenotomy scissor are used for extremely fine dissection in plastic surgery. *Castroviejo* scissors may be used in microsurgery. Round-tipped, light dissecting scissors such as the *Metzenbaum* scissors are used extensively on delicate tissue in general surgery. Fibrous connective tissue requires heavier scissors, such as the curved *Mayo* scissors. Dissecting scissors often are used to **undermine** tissue. In this technique, the

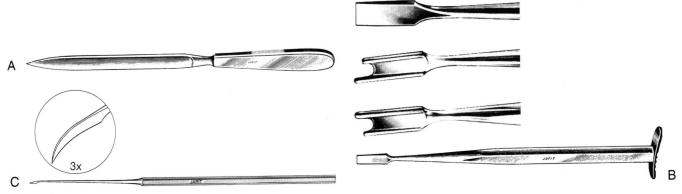

FIGURE 20-21
A, Liston amputation knife. **B,** Smillie meniscus knife. **C,** House sickle knife. (Courtesy of Jarit Instruments, Hawthorne, NY.)

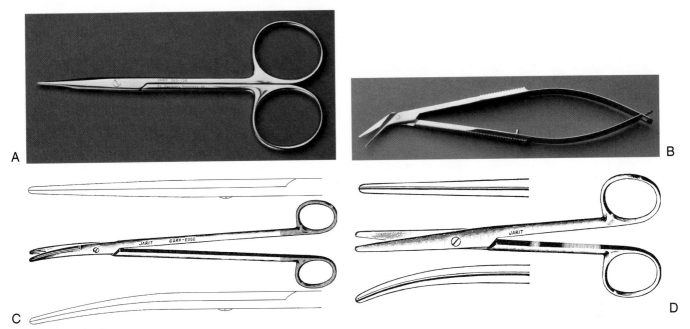

FIGURE 20-22
Surgical scissors. **A,** Stevens tenotomy scissors. **B,** Castroviejo scissors. **C,** Metzenbaum scissors. **D,** Mayo scissors (straight and curved shown). (Courtesy of Jarit Instruments, Hawthorne, NY.)

scissors are inserted between two tissue planes and opened. The outside (dull) edge of the scissor separates the layers, rather than cutting them apart, which would cause bleeding. Straight *Mayo* scissors are used for cutting suture. Scissors designed to cut tissue should never be used to cut suture. Cutting suture causes the scissor blades to become dull and not work properly on tissue.

RONGEUR
The **rongeur** is used to cut and extract tissue (Figure 20-23, *A-C*). The tips are cupped, and the edges of the "cup" are sharp. Rongeurs may contain finger rings or resemble the shape of household pliers. The rongeur has a single hinge-like scissors (called a single-action rongeur) or two hinges (called a **double-action** rongeur). The double-action rongeur creates twice the leverage of a single-action rongeur. A heavier rongeur used in orthopedic and neurosurgical procedures is called a *Stille* rongeur. The long-handled

rongeur, such as the *Kerrison* rongeur, often is used in spinal surgery. Long fine-tipped rongeurs like the *pituitary* rongeur are used to remove tissue in difficult-to-reach areas, such as the vertebral column and nasal sinus.

Many *rongeurs* are categorized by the angle of their tips and described as either *upbiting* or *downbiting* (Figure 20-23, *D*). The angle of the rongeur tips allows the surgeon to cut and remove tissue in areas that may be difficult to reach. As the surgeon is removing the tissue or bone with the rongeur, he or she will point the tip of the instrument to the scrub so that the scrub may remove the tissue from the tips of the rongeur with a moistened sponge. The surgeon does *not* look away from the surgical wound.

When the surgeon is using a rongeur, it is important to use a damp sponge to grab the tissue from the jaws of the instrument. Do not pull the rongeur out of the surgeon's hand while cleaning the tip. Watch the field carefully whenever a rongeur is used in order to keep up with the surgeon.

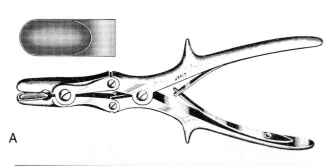

A

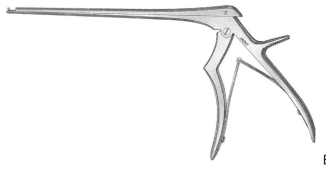

B

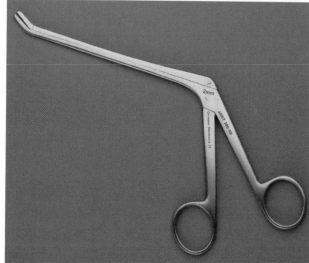

C

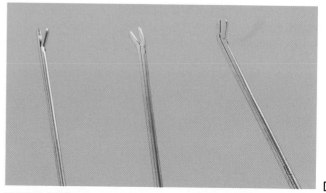

D

FIGURE 20-23
Rongeurs. **A,** Stille-Luer rongeur. **B,** Kerrison rongeur. **C,** Cushing (pituitary) rongeur. **D,** Close-up of straight, downbiting, and upbiting rongeur tips. (**A** to **C** courtesy of Jarit Instruments, Hawthorne, NY; **D** from Tighe SM: *Instrumentation for the operating room,* ed 6, St Louis, 1999, Mosby.)

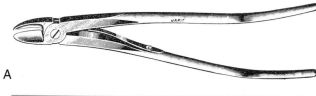

A

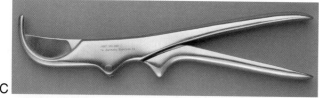

C

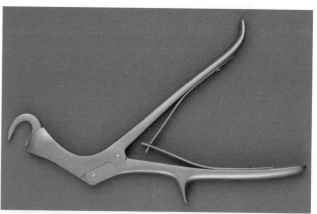

B

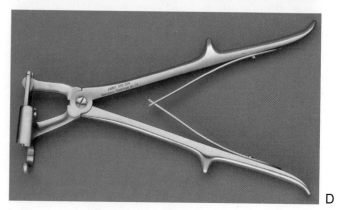

D

FIGURE 20-24
Bone shears. **A,** Bethune rib shears. **B,** Stille-Giertz rib shears. **C,** Gluck rib shears. **D,** Sauerbruch rib shears. (Courtesy of Jarit Instruments, Hawthorne, NY.)

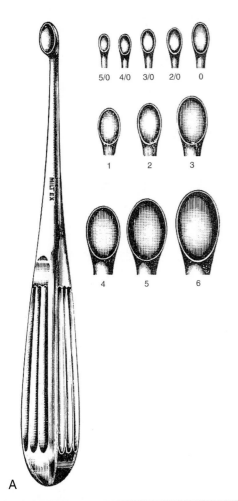

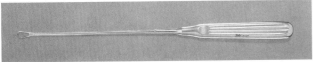

FIGURE 20-25
A, Bone curette. **B,** Sims uterine curette. (Courtesy of Miltex, Inc, York, Pa.)

Retain all tissue in a small basin as you would any tissue specimen.

SHEARS

Shears are large cutting instruments used to cut bone. Some shears are designed so the cutting edge is left or right of the hinge. Side cutting shears, as the name implies, are designed to cut to the left or the right. Examples of shears include *Bethune, Stille-Giertz, Shoemaker, Gluck,* and *Sauerbruch* rib shears (Figure 20-24).

CURETTE

The curette is used in many different specialties for scraping out tissue (Figure 20-25). Very fine curettes are used in ear, paranasal, and spinal surgery. Larger, heavier curettes are used in orthopedic procedures. Sharp and blunt curettes are used in gynecological surgery.

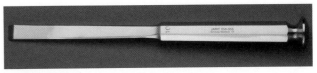

FIGURE 20-26
Chisel. (Courtesy of Jarit Instruments, Hawthorne, NY.)

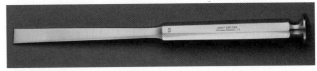

FIGURE 20-27
Osteotome. (Courtesy of Jarit Instruments, Hawthorne, NY.)

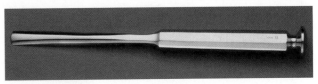

FIGURE 20-28
Gouge. (Courtesy of Jarit Instruments, Hawthorne, NY.)

OSTEOTOME AND CHISEL

The **chisel** is an orthopedic cutting instrument that is used with a mallet (similarly used in sculpting or carpentry). The chisel is available in many different widths and sizes that fit the specialty (Figure 20-26). For example, a chisel used on paranasal surgery is much more delicate than one designed for the tibia. People often confuse chisels and osteotomes. The osteotome has *two* beveled sides, while the chisel blade is sloped on one side only (Figure 20-27). The large osteotome is typically used to remove bone from the iliac crest to be used as a graft elsewhere in the body. The chisel produces a straight-sided cut, similar to a notch. Both instruments' tips must be protected from damage. When the blade becomes pitted or chipped, it loses its precision and becomes a hazard. Both types of instruments should be kept in a metal rack where their blades cannot come in contact with each other.

GOUGE

The gouge is a **V**-shaped bone chisel. Its cut looks like a small trough (Figure 20-28).

ELEVATOR

The **elevator** is used to separate or "elevate" a tissue layer (Figure 20-29). The heavy, round-shaped cutting elevator such as the *Lambott* slices tissue as it elevates. The small, square-tipped *Key* elevator also has a sharp edge but is much more delicate. Very finely balanced elevators such as the *Penfield* or *Freer* elevators are used in soft-tissue surgery. In vascular surgery, the *Penfield* or *Freer* elevators are used to separate atherosclerotic plaque from the inside of a blood vessel. The elevator must be well balanced and light enough to convey feeling from the working end (the tip) to the surgeon's hand. The *joker* is a very commonly used elevator. Its short

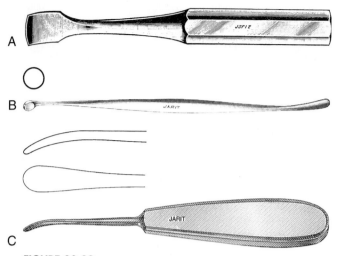

FIGURE 20-29
Elevators. **A,** Key elevator. **B,** Penfield elevator. **C,** Cushing joker. (Courtesy of Jarit Instruments, Hawthorne, NY.)

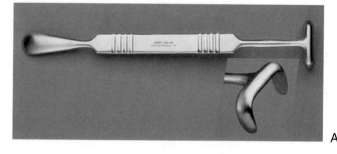

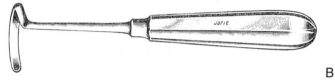

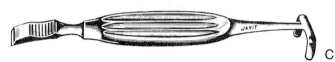

FIGURE 20-30
Rib strippers. **A,** Matson rib stripper. **B,** Doyen rib stripper. **C,** Matson-Alexander elevator and rib stripper. (Courtesy of Jarit Instruments, Hawthorne, NY.)

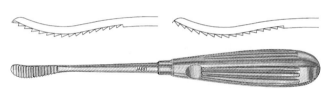

FIGURE 20-31
Aufricht rasp. (Courtesy of Jarit Instruments, Hawthorne, NY.)

handle and strong tip make it ideal for separating connective tissue planes without causing bleeding. The rib stripper is a type of elevator used to scrape tough connective tissue from the surface of a rib before it is cut with rib shears. Examples of rib strippers include *Matson, Doyen rib raspatory,* and *Alexander* (Figure 20-30).

RASP

The rasp is used to remodel bone (Figure 20-31). Many different shapes and surfaces are available. The finer the serrations or teeth, the less tissue that is removed with each stroke of the rasp. When the surgeon uses a rasp during a procedure, the blade must be cleaned. When tissue builds up among the teeth of the rasp, it becomes dull. One should not use a brush to clean the rasp because this can cause a spray of tissue and violate standard precautions. The rasp should be momentarily soaked in water and the tissue wiped from the rasp with a sponge. Avoid allowing tissue embedded in the rasp to dry out, as the tissue then will be difficult to remove.

Retracting (Exposing)

As the surgical wound is made deeper, tissue layers and other structures such as blood vessels, nerves, organs, and other tissue must be gently moved away from the focal point of the operation. The retractor is used to perform this task. Retractors are described as:

▶ Hand-held or self-retaining
▶ Deep or superficial
▶ Right-angle or curved
▶ Wide or narrow
▶ Malleable (bendable into any angle)
▶ Sharp or dull

Hand-held retractors range in size from the very fragile skin hook used in plastic surgery to the large, 4-inch-wide *Deaver* retractor used in abdominal procedures. Other common retractors are the U.S. Army retractor, the vein retractor, the Goelet retractor, the Richardson retractor, the ribbon retractor, and the Harrington retractor (Figure 20-32).

The self-retaining retractor holds tissue against the walls of the surgical wound by mechanical action. Self-retaining retractors can have many attachments suited to the needs of the surgery. The *Thompson self-retaining, Bookwalter,* and *Balfour* retractors are examples. Blades of various sizes and shapes can be attached to the frame to accommodate the specific needs of the procedure. Other examples include the *Finochetto* self-retaining retractor, which is used in cardiothoracic surgery, and the smaller *Gelpi* and *Weitlaner* retractors, which are used for superficial incisions such as in the groin. The *McPherson* self-retaining lid speculum holds the eye open during ophthalmic surgery (Figure 20-33).

The depth of the retractor blade matches the depth of the incision. At the beginning of a procedure, superficial retractors are used, and as the incision is deepened, a longer blade or deeper retractor is required to create exposure. The width of the retractor blade is determined by the size of the incision and the tissue to be retracted. The shape of the retractor blade can be curved, right-angled, or malleable (bendable to any angle).

The sharp retractor generally is used for adipose tissue only. Sharp *rakes* or *hooks* are designed to grasp the undersur-

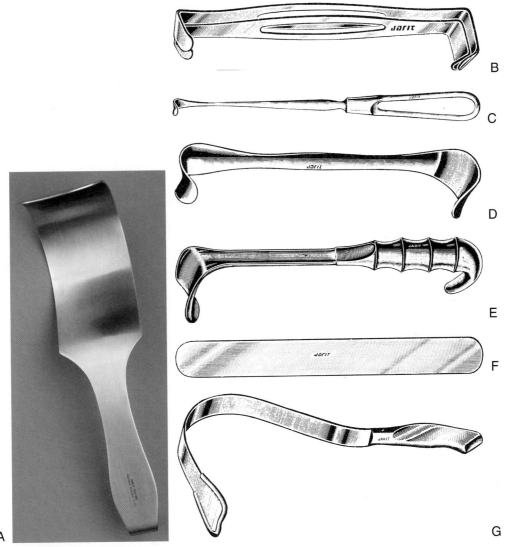

FIGURE 20-32
Hand-held retractors. **A,** Deaver retractor. **B,** U.S. Army retractor. **C,** Vein retractor. **D,** Goelet retractor. **E,** Richardson retractor. **F,** Ribbon retractor. **G,** Harrington retractor. (Courtesy of Jarit Instruments, Hawthorne, NY.)

face of superficial tissues. Dull hooks and rakes are used in areas close to viable nerves or near blood vessels (Figure 20-34).

Dilating and Probing

Dilators are used to widen or stretch the inside diameter of a lumen (hollow tissue) (Figure 20-35). Cervical dilators are used at the beginning of a dilation and **curettage** (D & C) to dilate the cervix in order to pass a curette inside the uterus. Urethral dilators are used to open strictures of the urethra. The **probe** also is used on hollow tissue but is used to *detect* an obstruction or to follow a hollow tract.

Measuring

Tissue and hollow structures are measured for many purposes (Figure 20-36). For example, the *uterine sound* is inserted into the cervix to measure the depth of the uterus from the cervix to the fundus. This is done to prevent perforation during curettage. Orthopedic *calipers* are used to measure the angle of

a joint or cut edge to match prostheses. *Depth gauges* are used in orthopedic surgery to determine the length of screws to be implanted into bone. *Sizers* are trial, reusable replicas of an implantable prosthesis. Rather than opening and contaminating many expensive implants, the sizer allows the surgeon to test a replica first. For example, before a cardiac valve is inserted, a sizer is used first to determine the correct size. A surgeon may use a basic sterile *ruler* to measure tissue or specimen removed from the patient.

Suturing

The needle holder is used to grasp a curved needle during suturing (Figure 20-37). The length, weight, and type of tip must be matched to the suture and tissue. Using a heavy needle holder such as a *Heaney* or *Mayo-Hegar* to suture a small blood vessel is similar to manipulating a straight pin with a pipe wrench. Very fine sutures require fine needle holders. If the needle holder is too heavy, the surgeon will

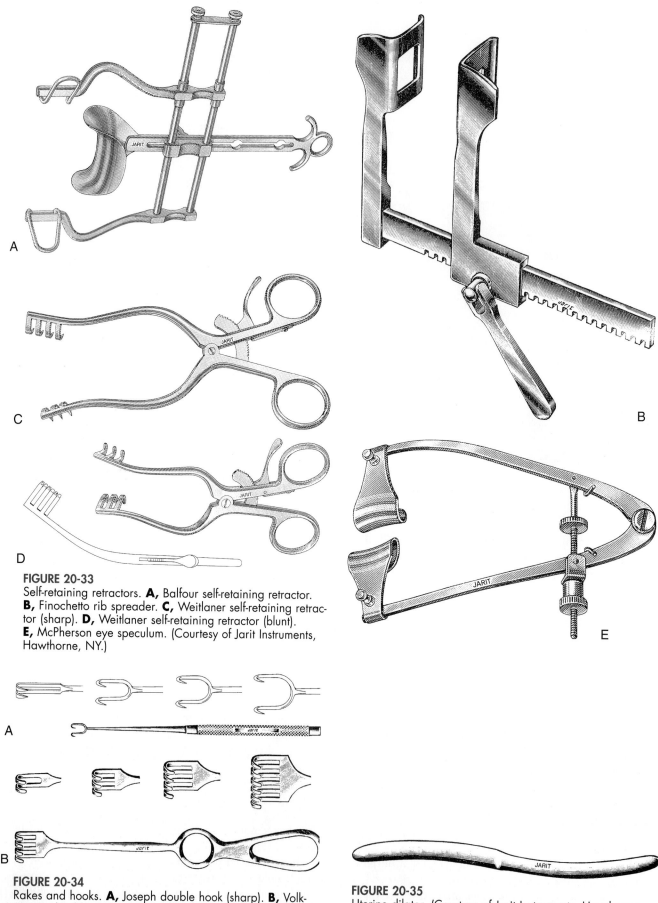

FIGURE 20-33
Self-retaining retractors. **A,** Balfour self-retaining retractor.
B, Finochetto rib spreader. **C,** Weitlaner self-retaining retractor (sharp). **D,** Weitlaner self-retaining retractor (blunt).
E, McPherson eye speculum. (Courtesy of Jarit Instruments, Hawthorne, NY.)

FIGURE 20-34
Rakes and hooks. **A,** Joseph double hook (sharp). **B,** Volkmann rake (blunt). (Courtesy of Jarit Instruments, Hawthorne, NY.)

FIGURE 20-35
Uterine dilator. (Courtesy of Jarit Instruments, Hawthorne, NY.)

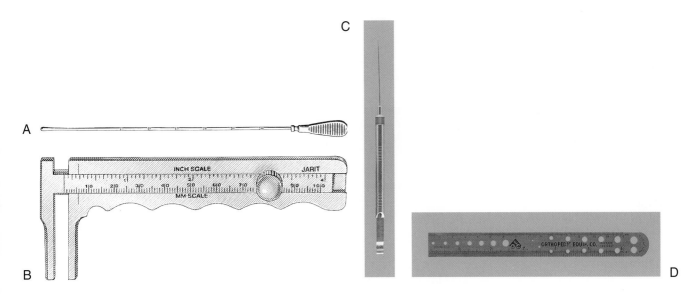

FIGURE 20-36
Measuring instruments. **A,** Sims uterine sound. **B,** Towney femur caliper. **C,** Depth gauge. **D,** Metal ruler. (**A** and **B** courtesy of Jarit Instruments, Hawthorne, NY; **C** and **D** from Tighe SM: *Instrumentation for the operating room,* ed 6, St Louis, 1999, Mosby.)

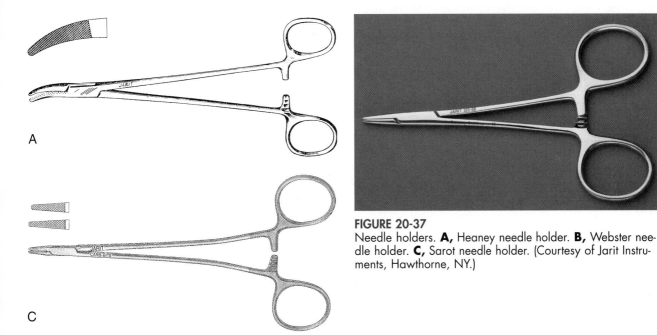

FIGURE 20-37
Needle holders. **A,** Heaney needle holder. **B,** Webster needle holder. **C,** Sarot needle holder. (Courtesy of Jarit Instruments, Hawthorne, NY.)

lose the "feel" of the needle. On the other hand, a lightweight or fine-tipped needle holder such as a *Webster* does not have enough surface area at the tip to grasp a heavy needle. A sharp-tipped needle holder such as the *Sarot* is used for fine sutures, 4-0 and smaller. Many needle holders are serrated or slotted, or contain tungsten carbon inserts in the jaws for added durability and grip.

One should use a needle holder when removing a scalpel blade from its handle; a heavy needle holder provides the grip needed to prevent the blade from slipping through the jaws. A hemostat never should be used to grasp a needle or other metal object, as this will damage the tips of the instrument.

Most needle holders are ratchet or spring locked. Always test the ratchets before using the needle holder. If they do not mesh correctly, the needle holder may spring open unexpectedly. The smallest needle holders, such as the *Castroviejo* used in eye surgery and microsurgery, have a spring catch and may be locking or nonlocking (Figure 20-38). These are easily damaged if handled inappropriately. Only gentle pressure is needed to open and close a spring catch.

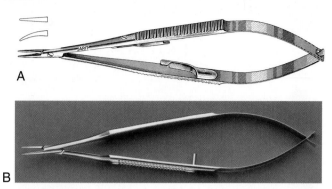

FIGURE 20-38
Castroviejo needle holder. **A,** With lock. **B,** Without lock. (Courtesy of Jarit Instruments, Hawthorne, NY.)

Suctioning

Suctioning instruments are used to suction blood and fluids from the surgical field (Figure 20-39). They are designed for specific anatomical areas based on function. *Poole* suctions are designed to work in the abdominal cavity. The Poole suction has a guard that protects bowel and intestinal organs from injury. The *Yankauer* or tonsil suction is designed to suction in the chest cavity and throat. *Frazier* suction is designed to suction in superficial areas in the face, neck, and ear, and in neurological and some peripheral vascular procedures. Depending on the diameter of the lumen of the suction tip, the scrub may need to clean the lumen if it becomes clogged with blood during use. The scrub can do this by flushing the lumen with a syringe of water or inserting a stylet into the lumen of the suction.

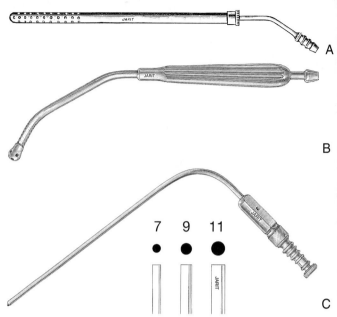

FIGURE 20-39
Suctioning instruments. **A,** Poole suction tube. **B,** Yankauer suction tip. **C,** Frazier suction tube. (Courtesy of Jarit Instruments, Hawthorne, NY.)

INSTRUMENTS BY SURGICAL SPECIALTY

Specialty instruments are discussed within each specialty surgery chapter (Chapters 21 through 31).

CASE STUDIES

Case 1

As a student you are scrubbed on a large case. Your preceptor has shown you which instruments will be needed during the case. As the preceptor names the instruments, you only remember a few of the names. To make matters more difficult, the preceptor does not tell you the technical name of the instrument, but refers to them by "nicknames" used at this hospital. How will you scrub on this case? What strategy might you use to pass the correct instrument even though you do not know the name?

Case 2

You are scrubbed on a large case. The surgeon has the radio playing, and it is difficult to hear the surgeon's requests for instruments. You know the instruments, but have not had much experience with them. You make many mistakes, and the surgeon becomes irritated. What will you do?

REFERENCES

Kern B: Preventive instrument maintenance: a prudent investment with many dividends, *Infect Control Today,* Sept, 2000.

Tighe SM: *Instrumentation for the operating room,* St Louis, 2003, Mosby.

Unit 2

Surgical Procedures

Chapter 21

General Surgery

INTRODUCTION TO GENERAL SURGERY

General surgery encompasses operations of the gastrointestinal tract, biliary system, spleen, pancreas, liver, and hernias of the abdominal wall, and procedures of the rectum and breast. A general surgeon usually performs these types of surgery and may specialize in one of these areas, such as colorectal surgery.

Most general surgery procedures require similar instrumentation, whereas procedures of the breast and rectum may require additional special items. The gastrointestinal instruments are used interchangeably for various procedures of the stomach and intestine.

SECTION I
Incisions

Behavioral Objectives

After studying this section the reader will be able to:

- Recognize specific abdominal incisions
- Associate specific abdominal incisions with access to specific organs of the abdominal cavity
- Differentiate between muscle-splitting and muscle-cutting incisions
- Describe the tissue layers of the anterior abdominal wall

Terminology

Abdominal peritoneum—Serous membrane lining the walls of the abdominal cavity.

Adipose tissue—Layer of tissue containing fat cells.

Epigastric—Region of the abdomen above the umbilicus, following the upper edge of the stomach.

Fascia—A fibrous band or membrane lying deep to the skin and supporting muscles.

Hypogastric—Below the level of the stomach.

Linea alba—A tendinous median line on the anterior abdominal wall; separates the rectus muscles.

McBurney incision—An oblique *right* muscle-splitting incision used for exploration and removal of the appendix.

Muscle-splitting incision—Incision that separates muscle tissues along the length of their fibers. The muscle is not cut. This results in little or no bleeding and prevents the moderate to severe postoperative pain associated with muscle cutting.

Paramedian—An incision of the vertical abdominal wall lateral to the midline.

Pfannenstiel—A transverse incision of the lower abdomen below the umbilicus and just above the pubis in a natural crease or fold.

Subcostal—Literally "under the rib." Describes an incision or area of the abdominal wall that follows the oblique slope of the tenth costal cartilage.

Subcutaneous tissue—The superficial fascia layer that covers the abdominal wall. Fatty tissue that attaches to this tissue can range from several millimeters to 7 or 8 inches thick.

Transverse incision—An incision that follows a line perpendicular to the midline of the body.

SURFACE ANATOMY OF THE ABDOMEN

Regions

The ventral abdomen is described by four quadrants. These are the right upper, left upper, right lower, and left lower quadrants, separated by the umbilicus and the **midline** (vertical line dividing the body into right and left portions) (Figure 21-1). Nine regions also are identified by an imaginary grid that divides the ventral abdomen by two vertical lines and two horizontal lines:

- Left hypochondriac: costal area
- Left lumbar: flank
- Left iliac: inguinal
- **Epigastric:** above the level of the stomach
- **Umbilical:** immediately around the umbilicus
- **Hypogastric:** below the level of the stomach
- Right hypochondriac: costal area
- Right lumbar: flank
- Right iliac: inguinal

Tissue Layers of the Ventral Abdominal Wall

The scrub must be familiar with the types of tissue layers in the ventral wall and their locations.. Each layer is distinct and may require separate types of grasping, retracting, and cutting instruments. The layers often are sutured separately. Suture materials for each layer are strong enough to **approximate** (bring together) the sides of the layer after it has been surgically cut, but fine enough to cause as little trauma as possible. These are technical points that contribute to wound management and a successful surgical outcome.

Directly under the skin is the superficial fascia, which is often called **subcutaneous tissue** (Figure 21-2). This layer contains loose adipose tissue, which varies in thickness from a quarter inch to more than 8 inches. Two longitudinal rectus muscles attach from the pubis to the fifth, sixth, and seventh costal cartilages. Lateral to the rectus muscles are the three flanking muscles—the transverse external oblique, internal oblique, and transverse abdominis (Figure 21-3). These muscles are encompassed by deep fascia, subserous fascia, and the abdominal peritoneum. The subserous fascia is tightly bound to the peritoneum, which is barely one cell thick. It reflects (folds back) on itself in some areas to cover the organs of the abdomen.

INCISIONS

Incisions in the ventral abdominal wall are named according to their anatomical location. The scrub must know each of

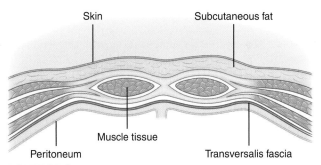

FIGURE 21-2
Tissue layers of the abdominal wall. (Redrawn from Ethicon: *Wound closure manual,* Somerville, NJ, 2002, Ethicon, Inc.)

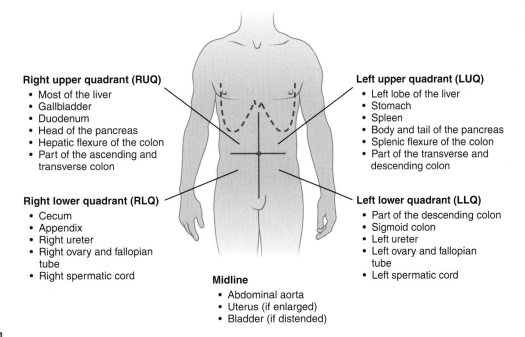

FIGURE 21-1
Four quadrants of the abdomen. (Redrawn from Ignatavicius DD and Workman ML: *Medical-surgical nursing: critical thinking for collaborative care,* ed 4, Philadelphia, 2002, Saunders.)

these incisions and the abdominal structures that can be accessed through the incisions. The incisions are illustrated in Figure 21-4. They include:

▶ Midline
▶ **Paramedian**
▶ Subcostal
▶ **Flank**

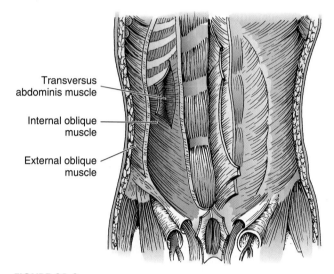

FIGURE 21-3
The muscles of the anterior abdominal wall. (Modified from Rothrock JC: *Alexander's care of the patient in surgery*, ed 12, St Louis, 2003, Mosby.)

▶ **Inguinal**
▶ **McBurney**
▶ **Transverse**
▶ **Pfannenstiel** (Used almost exclusively for gynecologic surgery and discussed in Chapter 22.)

Midline

The midline incision is the simplest and most common abdominal incision used by the general surgeon. It offers a nearly bloodless field and adequate exposure of nearly all structures of the abdominal cavity. The layers of the midline incision from ventral to dorsal sides of the body are as follows:

1. Skin
2. Subcutaneous fat
3. Fascia
4. Abdominal peritoneum

The midline incision lies directly over the *linea alba* ("white line") of the abdominal wall. There are no muscle fibers in the path of this incision, thus the nearly bloodless field. However, if the surgeon makes the incision slightly left or right of this line, the rectus abdominis muscles are encountered.

Upper Paramedian

This incision is used primarily to expose the stomach, duodenum, and pancreas. It allows the surgeon to enter the abdominal cavity with a minimum of bleeding, and the incision can be extended in a superior or inferior direction to

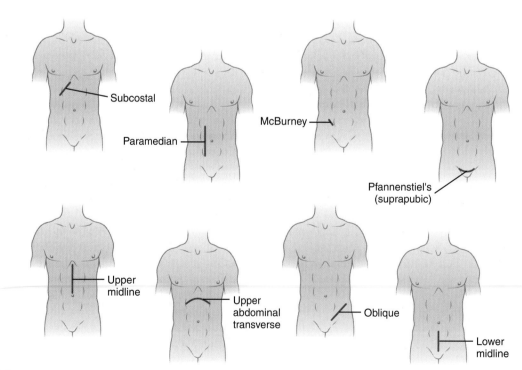

FIGURE 21-4
Abdominal incisions. (Modified from Rothrock JC: *Alexander's care of the patient in surgery*, ed 12, St Louis, 2003, Mosby.)

meet the needs of the procedure. The tissue layers include the following:

1. Skin
2. Subcutaneous fat
3. Anterior rectus muscles (retracted laterally, not severed) (Figure 21-5, *A*)
4. Rectus fascia
5. Abdominal peritoneum

Subcostal

The right subcostal incision is used to expose the gallbladder and its associated structures. It is used occasionally for operations of the pancreas. The left subcostal incision may be used to expose the spleen, but its limited exposure precludes its use in splenic trauma cases in which a midline incision would allow the surgeon to perform a more complete exploration of the abdominal cavity.

This incision follows the lower costal (rib) margin in a semi-curved shape. Because the rectus muscles are severed, this incision is more painful postoperatively than the midline incision (Figure 21-5, *B*). The tissues encountered are as follows:

1. Skin
2. Subcutaneous fat
3. Rectus muscles
4. Fascia
5. Abdominal peritoneum

McBurney

The McBurney incision is used for exploration and removal of the appendix. It is made on the right side, at an oblique angle below the umbilicus, across the flank. This incision is called a *muscle-splitting incision* because the muscle fibers are split manually, not severed. The exposure offered is very limited, and the incision cannot be lengthened easily. The tissue layers of this incision include the following:

1. Skin
2. Subcutaneous fat
3. Fascia
4. Oblique and transversalis muscle
5. Abdominal peritoneum

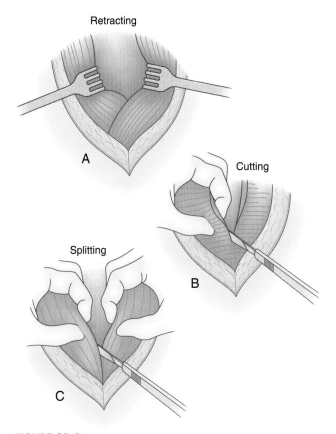

FIGURE 21-5
Surgical options for muscle. **A,** Retracting. **B,** Cutting. **C,** Splitting. (Redrawn from Ethicon: *Wound closure manual,* Somerville, NJ, 2002, Ethicon, Inc.)

Inguinal (Oblique)

The right and left oblique inguinal incision is used for inguinal hernia repair. This incision gives excellent exposure of the two common types of inguinal hernias: the direct hernia and the indirect hernia. The muscle layers of this incision converge at the hernia.

When sutured, the skin, superficial fascia, deep fascia, muscle, and peritoneum often are closed as separate layers (the subserous fascia is closed with the peritoneum). **Muscle-splitting incisions** are those that follow the length of the muscle fibers, and the muscle fibers are not cut but manually separated (Figure 21-5, *C*). These usually do not require sutures at closure.

SECTION II
Hernias

Behavioral Objectives

After studying this section the reader will be able to:

- Differentiate between types of common hernias
- Identify the anatomy involved in inguinal hernias
- Identify the anatomy involved in an incisional hernia
- Describe necessary equipment and preparation for a simple abdominal or inguinal hernia
- Describe the TEP and TAPP laparoscopic approaches to hernia repair
- Define the purpose of mesh used for hernia repair

Terminology

Direct inguinal hernia—An acquired weakness in the inguinal floor that leads to protrusion of the abdominal contents. The characteristic bulging usually follows activity that produces increased intraabdominal pressure or "bearing down," and it causes pain. The area of weakness can become larger over time, and the contents of the hernia can become trapped or strangulated (see *strangulated hernia*).

Incarcerated hernia—Herniated tissue that is trapped outside its normal location by a defect in the abdominal wall. Incarcerated tissue requires emergency surgery to prevent a tourniquet effect on the incarcerated tissue, leading to necrosis.

Incisional hernia—Occurs along the incision of a previous abdominal surgery. Incisional hernia, also called a ventral hernia, is caused by infection, obesity, excess tension on the original suture line, or any other process that breaks down the tissues. The incisional hernia may start as a small break in tissue con-

tinuity and progress to the full length of the incision. Evisceration and infection can result if the incision fully ruptures. More often, incarceration and strangulation require emergency surgery.

Indirect inguinal hernia—A hernia that protrudes across the membranous sac of the spermatic cord. The weakness in this sac usually is present at birth and may require surgery early in life. If the defect enlarges, the intraabdominal contents can slide through the deep and superficial inguinal rings and enter the scrotum, causing pain and trauma to the trapped tissue.

Mesh—Soft, pliable, synthetic material that resembles a screen. Mesh is used in hernia repair to bridge the tissue edges of the hernia. Nontension patching or plugging gives strength to the weak abdominal wall but allows normal activities and mobility after surgery. Many different mesh systems are available, and choices are based on the type of hernia and compatibility with the patient's tissues.

Reduce—To replace herniated tissue; the tissue may reduce without manipulation when the patient lies down or ceases to strain or bear down.

Strangulated hernia—Herniated tissue that is strangulated and has a compromised or absent blood supply. This is a surgical emergency, especially if the bowel is involved.

Total extraperitoneal (TEP) approach—A laparoscopic hernia repair approached from the extraperitoneal space. A pneumoperitoneum is unnecessary, because the peritoneum is not entered. Rather, the inguinal area is insufflated with a balloon dissector, and the defect is repaired from within this space.

Transperitoneal (TAP) approach—A traditional method of laparoscopic hernia repair. A pneumoperitoneum is created, and the inguinal space is entered via the lower abdominal cavity.

Ventral hernia—See *incisional hernia*.

ANATOMY OF THE SUPRAPUBIC AND INGUINAL REGION

As the fascia layers continue into the suprapubic or subumbilical region, they pass in front of the two rectus muscles. Here the inguinal canal appears as a split between the mus-

cle layers of the abdominal wall near the inguinal ligament. The inguinal canal begins as a defect or split in the transversalis fascia at the deep inguinal ring and continues to the superficial inguinal ring. This space is larger in the male than in the female, corresponding to the higher incidence of inguinal hernias in males.

The spermatic cord, which follows the inguinal canal, contains the following structures:

- Spermatic fascia
- Cremaster muscle
- Genitofemoral nerve
- Ductus deferens
- Lymph vessels
- Pampiniform veins, which form the testicular vein
- Testicular artery

SURGICAL PROCEDURES

Open Repair of Indirect Inguinal Hernia (Herniorrhaphy)

SURGICAL GOAL

An open repair of an indirect inguinal hernia is performed to restore strength to the inguinal floor and prevent abdominal tissue from extruding into the inguinal canal.

PATHOLOGY

A defect (actual tear or enlarged opening) or weakened area in the abdominal wall can occur at birth or be acquired later in life. When tissue from within the abdomen pushes out through the defect, the tissue may emerge between the layers. This is called a **hernia.** Tissue that becomes entrapped in the defect is called **incarcerated hernia.** If one does not relieve pressure on the incarcerated tissue by **reducing** the hernia (replacing tissue to its correct anatomical location), its vascular supply can be stopped. This is called a **strangulated hernia.** When tissue is strangulated, a tourniquet effect occurs at the site of the protrusion. This can lead to tissue necrosis. Strangulated bowel tissue can result in bowel obstruction—a surgical emergency. Inguinal hernias carry a high risk for incarceration and strangulation.

An **indirect** inguinal hernia is a protrusion of abdominal viscera that traverses the inguinal canal from the deep inguinal ring and may extend through the superficial inguinal ring into the scrotum (or labia majorus of the female). In the male, the hernia extends along the length of the membrane covering the spermatic cord and can emerge though the superficial ring, causing a bulge under the skin.

Many different methods are used to repair inguinal hernias. The two main surgical techniques are the closed laparoscopic technique and open surgery. Using either technique, one can perform the repair with sutures, or with synthetic **mesh** in a technique called a *nonstress* closure. The mesh closure results in a lower rate of recurrence.

Technique

- A right or left inguinal incision is made.
- Layers of the abdominal wall are incised, and the edges are retracted.
- The spermatic cord is dissected away from preperitoneal fat and other surrounding tissues.
- The spermatic cord is retracted laterally with a small Penrose drain.
- The indirect hernia sac is dissected from the cord and opened, and its contents are pushed back into the abdomen.
- The hernia sac is ligated with ties or a purse-string suture.
- A synthetic mesh patch or plug is sutured into place over the defect.
- The abdominal wall is closed in layers.

DISCUSSION

The surgeon incises the skin over the groin using the scalpel. Metzenbaum scissors, an electrosurgical unit (ESU), or a deep knife is used to continue the dissection and separate the tissue layers (Figure 21-6, *A*). Small bleeders are controlled with the ESU. Both blunt and sharp dissection is used to gain access to the hernia. After incising the fascia that lies off the spermatic cord, the surgeon places several hemostats on the edge of the incised fascia. These are used to retract the fascia, exposing the spermatic cord.

When the cord has been identified, the surgeon carefully separates it from the hernia sac (Figure 21-6, *B*). Blunt dissection with a dry Raytec sponge can help tease tissue from the surface of the cord. The scrub should moisten a small Penrose drain and pass it to the surgeon with a hemostat. The Penrose drain is then used as a retractor for the spermatic vessels and vas deferens (commonly referred to as the *spermatic cord*). Dissection is continued proximally to the defect in the abdominal wall. The surgeon dissects the indirect hernia sac away from the cord using Metzenbaum scissors.

When the sac has been isolated and freed, the scrub should moisten a small Penrose drain and pass it with a hemostat. The drain is then used as a retractor. The sac is opened, and the edges are grasped with hemostats (Figure 21-6, *C*). The surgeon then pushes the contents of the sac back into the abdomen with his finger or a small sponge. If the defect is very small, the surgeon may simply ligate it. For large sacs, a purse-string suture of 2-0 synthetic absorbable material is placed around the neck of the sac, which is then removed as a specimen (Figure 21-6, *D*).

Various types of synthetic mesh are often used to cover the defect. The mesh is cut to match the size of the inguinal canal floor, and a small hole is made to allow the spermatic cord to emerge in its normal anatomical position. The edges of the mesh are then secured with synthetic sutures or staples (Figure 21-6, *E*). Absorbable collagen materials also might be used. After the mesh has been secured, the incision is closed in multiple layers as follows:

- Fascia: 2-0 nonabsorbable or absorbable synthetic suture
- Subcutaneous tissue: 2-0 or 3-0 absorbable
- Skin: staples or 3-0 or 4-0 nonabsorbable suture for adults or 3-0 or 4-0 subcutaneous absorbable suture

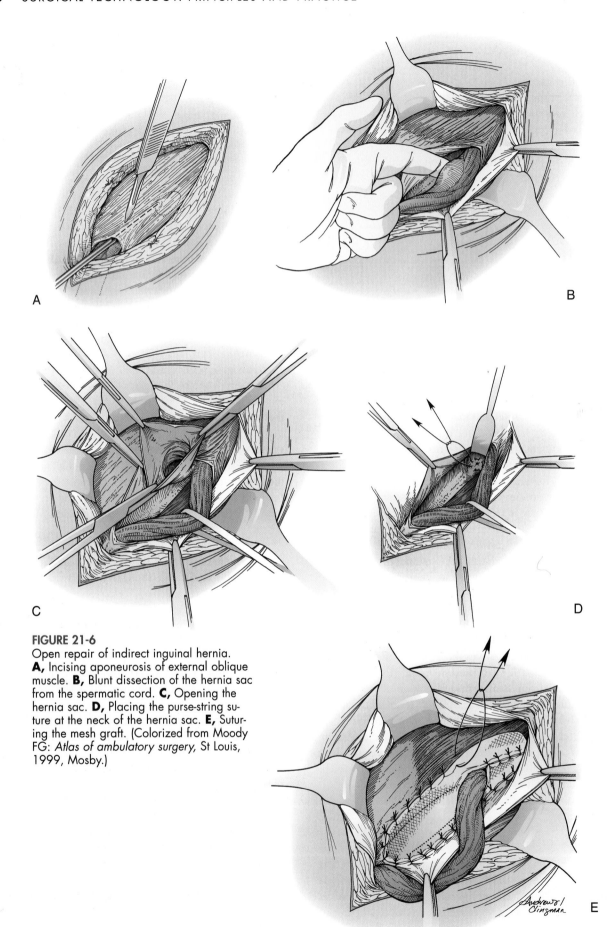

FIGURE 21-6
Open repair of indirect inguinal hernia.
A, Incising aponeurosis of external oblique
muscle. **B,** Blunt dissection of the hernia sac
from the spermatic cord. **C,** Opening the
hernia sac. **D,** Placing the purse-string suture at the neck of the hernia sac. **E,** Suturing the mesh graft. (Colorized from Moody
FG: *Atlas of ambulatory surgery*, St Louis,
1999, Mosby.)

Laparoscopic Direct Hernia Repair

Surgical exposure during the laparoscopic approach is gained through *transabdominal preperitoneal laparoscopy* (**TAPP**) or by *total extraperitoneal* (**TEP**) surgery. In the TAPP approach, a pneumoperitoneum is created and the inguinal canal is entered via the abdominal cavity. The TEP approach avoids a pneumoperitoneum by inflating and entering the preperitoneal space with a balloon dissector, which functions as a tissue expander.

SURGICAL GOAL

Laparoscopic direct hernia repair uses the laparoscopic technique to reduce herniated tissue and strengthen the inguinal floor.

PATHOLOGY

A **direct hernia** is one in which the herniated tissue bulges through a weakened area from behind the superficial inguinal ring in the inguinal floor. This is an acquired hernia, occurring most often in older men. Unlike the indirect hernia, the protruding tissue rarely descends into the scrotum. The defect may begin as a very small area of weakness but gradually becomes larger with increased age and weight. Increased intraabdominal pressure ("bearing down"), such as during lifting, often can precipitate a large, painful hernia. Like other hernias, direct hernia can become strangulated and incarcerated.

Direct hernia repair is performed through the laparoscope or as an open procedure. The laparoscopic procedure is described here.

Technique — TRANSABDOMINAL PREPERITONEAL (TAPP)

1. Pneumoperitoneum is established, and ports are inserted in the abdomen.
2. A small **transverse incision** is made above the direct hernia space.
3. The weakened area in the pelvic floor is covered with a synthetic patch or other mesh system.
4. The mesh is secured with endoscopic staples or sutures without tension.
5. The peritoneum is closed.
6. The pneumoperitoneum is released, and port incisions are closed.

DISCUSSION

Transabdominal Preperitoneal (TAPP)

The patient is placed in a supine position, prepped, and draped for a laparotomy. Because a pneumoperitoneum is required, general anesthesia is used. A urinary catheter may be inserted to remove the bladder from the operative area. Drapes should extend inferiorly to the pubis. The surgeon normally stands opposite the affected side. Pneumoperitoneum is established (described in Chapter 18). A primary port is placed in the umbilicus, and secondary ports are placed lateral to the rectus muscles (Figure 21-7, *A*).

The size of ports depends on the instrumentation and type of repair; 5-mm ports are preferable if they can accommodate the stapling instruments. The laparoscope is placed through the primary port at the umbilicus.

When the hernia has been identified, the surgeon grasps the sac with endoscopic forceps or an atraumatic grasper. The surgeon then makes a **transverse** (horizontal) incision in the peritoneum above the direct space with scissors or an ESU (Figure 21-7, *B*). The peritoneum is then retracted back to expose the pelvic floor. A piece of polypropylene mesh is introduced through the largest port and placed horizontally over the pelvic floor (Figure 21-7, *C*). Conventional 4-mm or 5-mm screw-type staples are used to tack the mesh to Cooper's ligament. The peritoneum also may be closed with regular staples (Figure 21-7, *D*). After removing carbon dioxide from the peritoneum, the surgeon closes the fascia and skin with size 2-0 sutures on a small, heavy curved needle or with skin staples.

The technique for a *direct hernia* follows the dissection technique of the indirect hernia. However, the hernia sac is grasped, and a circumferential incision made around the neck. The sac also may be dissected from the spermatic cord and inguinal canal using a blunt dissector sponge or a dry Raytec gauze sponge. Unlike many open surgical repairs, in this technique, the sac is not ligated. Polypropylene mesh is then placed over the defect and stapled into place as for an indirect hernia. Carbon dioxide is released from the peritoneal cavity, and the wounds are closed with synthetic absorbable sutures and skin staples.

Technique — TRANSABDOMINAL EXTRAPERITONEAL (TEP)

1. A small periumbilical incision is made through the rectus sheath.
2. Tissues are manually dissected and then retracted.
3. A balloon tissue expander is introduced.
4. The preperitoneal space is inflated, and the expander is removed. A balloon trocar may be inserted to seal the space and hold the trocar.
5. Two additional 5-mm ports are created.
6. The direct or indirect hernia is **reduced** and polypropylene mesh is secured over the defect.
7. The wounds are closed as for TAPP.

DISCUSSION

Transabdominal Extraperitoneal (TEP)

Preparation of the patient is the same as for the TAPP procedure. However, in the TEP approach no pneumoperitoneum is used. The surgeon makes a small incision lateral to the midline, exposing the rectus muscle sheath. The surgeon expands this opening using blunt digital dissection. A **balloon expander** is then inserted into the incision and inflated with air or normal saline (Figure 21-8, *A* and *B*). This pushes the tissues outward to create more space. The balloon

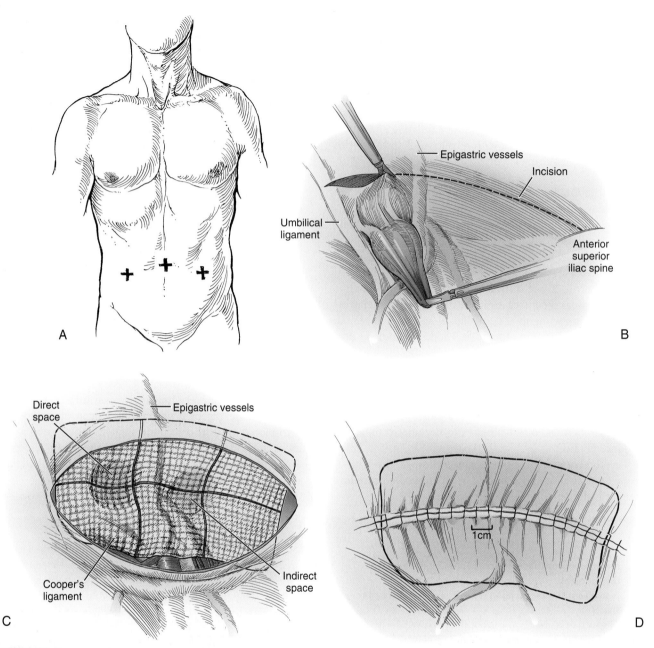

FIGURE 21-7
Laparoscopic direct hernia repair. **A,** Placement of ports. **B,** Incising the peritoneum. **C,** Placing the polypropylene mesh over the defect. **D,** Closing the peritoneum. (**A** from Economou SG and Economou TS: *Atlas of surgical technique,* ed 2, Philadelphia, 1996, Saunders; **B** to **D** colorized from Ballantyne GH: *Atlas of laparoscopic surgery,* Philadelphia, 2000, Saunders.)

dissector is removed, and the space is maintained with gas insufflation. Specially designed ports are available to seal the preperitoneal space.

Two 5-mm trocars then are placed into the preperitoneal space either laterally or in the patient's midline. A complication of this procedure can arise when the trocars are inadvertently placed into the peritoneal cavity, causing the preperitoneum to leak.

When all trocars are in place, the hernia is repaired as described above.

Open Repair of Femoral Hernia
SURGICAL GOAL

An open repair of a femoral hernia is performed to restore strength to the inguinal floor and prevent abdominal tissue from protruding into the inguinal canal.

PATHOLOGY

The femoral hernia occurs most often in the female. The abdominal-wall defect allows abdominal tissue to descend

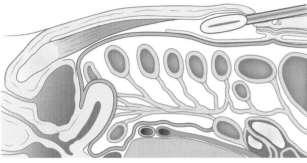

A

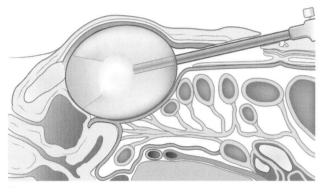

B

FIGURE 21-8
A and **B,** A balloon expander inserted into the incision and inflated with air or normal saline.

into the femoral canal inferior to the inguinal ligament. The femoral hernia is more likely to become strangulated than the inguinal hernia. It appears as a bulge below the crease line of the leg and inguinal ligament.

> ### Technique
> 1. The groin is incised on the affected side.
> 2. The hernia sac is identified and opened.
> 3. The sac is ligated and removed.
> 4. Synthetic mesh is secured over the defect.
> 5. The wound is closed in layers as for inguinal hernia.

DISCUSSION

The patient is placed in a supine position, prepped, and draped with the inguinal area exposed. The surgeon incises the groin area with the skin knife and uses the ESU to continue the incision and control bleeding. Right-angle retractors are placed at each end of the wound and held by the assistant. When the fascia layer has been incised, the outer membrane of the sac is elevated with curved hemostats and a small incision is made with the scalpel or ESU. The incision then can be opened fully, as the surgeon's hand protects the contents. A thorough digital exam of the sac reveals whether intestinal tissue is entrapped in the defect.

When the sac contents have been reduced and known to be viable, the edges of the sac are grasped with small hemostats and a purse-string suture is placed at the neck. The

edges are trimmed and passed off the field as specimens. The purse-string suture is then tightened. At this point, mesh may be sutured in place over the defect. All tissue layers are closed as described above.

Incisional or Ventral Hernia
SURGICAL GOAL

To remodel a previous scar of the abdominal wall and create sufficient strength to prevent a recurring hernia.

PATHOLOGY

A **ventral** or **incisional hernia** usually, but not always, occurs at the incisional site of a previous surgery. Weakness in the tissue layers can result from several different causes:

▶ Previous or concurrent surgical-site infection
▶ Extensive strain on the incision caused by obesity
▶ Poor tissue healing resulting from metabolic disease such as diabetes or alcoholism
▶ Repeated surgeries in the same location

If the tissue is infected at the time of closure, macrophages and other white blood cells prevent normal healing, including the formation of scar tissue. When the incision does heal, the edges are not well integrated into the peripheral tissue and the area becomes weak. Morbid obesity or excessive strain on the incisional line pulls the already-weakened tissue apart, and it becomes thinner and less resistant to stress from the abdominal side. As abdominal tissue begins to enter the defect, increasing strain pushes the defect wider.

Tissue that has been previously infected develops thin fibrous adhesions (strands of scar tissue that adhere to the abdominal wall and viscera). These are painful and may tear with pressure. The new network of mixed tissue types in the abdominal wall increases the risk of herniation, because with the normal tissue planes no longer intact, there are gaps and tracts leading into the abdominal cavity.

The condition in which abdominal contents rupture to the outside of the body is called an evisceration. This may occur during active postoperative infection. Hernia, however, is more common. In this case, the skin layer heals over the defects in the abdominal wall, but the abdominal contents protrude and slide through the nonintact layers. Any hernia may become incarcerated or strangulated, requiring emergency surgery.

> ### Technique
> 1. The old scar is removed, and the edges of the previous incision are trimmed.
> 2. If nonabsorbable suture was used in previous surgery, the knots are located and removed.
> 3. Abdominal adhesions are carefully separated from the viscera and the interior abdominal wall.
> 4. Synthetic mesh is secured over the abdominal defect.
> 5. All layers of the abdominal wall are closed.

DISCUSSION

The patient is placed in a supine position, prepped, and draped for access to the abdominal defect. Allis clamps are used to grasp the edges of the existing scar and elevate it. This places counter traction on the scar while it is incised, first with the scalpel used for skin (skin knife), then the ESU. The scrub retains the scar as a specimen, which may be sent to the pathology department, as determined by policy of individual hospitals.

If nonabsorbable sutures have been placed in the deeper tissue layers during the previous surgery, the surgeon removes them using a straight hemostat and scissors. A folded towel placed near the incision is convenient for the surgeon to wipe the hemostat and remove the old sutures from the hemostat. Because the knots constitute a foreign body, they must not be allowed to fall back into the surgical wound.

After old sutures are removed, the surgeon may attempt to reestablish normal tissue planes by trimming and reducing superficial fascia and fatty tissue. Scar tissue lacks the organized blood supply of normal tissue and heals more slowly than normal tissue. The goal is to expose the edges of **viable tissue**—tissue that is healthy and does not contain scar tissue. The surgeon remodels the edges of the incision, which usually are ragged. It is usually not necessary to enter the abdominal cavity to repair an incisional hernia unless the patient experiences pain from adhesions.

Adhesions between tissue layers prevent the abdominal-wall layers from being closed anatomically. Small tracts (passageways) containing fat and scar tissue are the result of previous infection or inflammation in the abdominal wall. These bands must be removed to close each layer securely and prevent recurrence of hernia.

Before closing the abdominal layers, the surgeon reduces tension on the skin edges by securing a synthetic mesh bridge from one edge of the abdominal wall to the other (Figure 21-9, *A*). If the patient is grossly obese, protruding abdominal viscera can make closure difficult. Mesh is sutured or stapled along the opposing edges of deep fascia (Figure 21-9, *B*). If mesh is used, it is secured with nonabsorbable or nonabsorbable **inert** (nonreactive) sutures. Individual layers are then closed with synthetic sutures and skin staples. The surgeon can reduce remaining tension at the wound edges by suturing them with a heavy continuous suture such as PDS through all layers or by using retention sutures with synthetic bolsters (see Chapter 16).

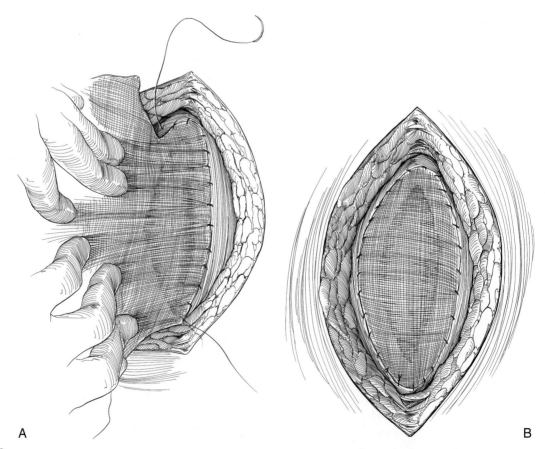

A   B

FIGURE 21-9
Incisional (or ventral) hernia. **A,** Synthetic mesh bridge is secured from one edge of the abdominal wall to the other. **B,** Mesh is sutured or stapled. (From Economou SG and Economou TS: *Atlas of surgical technique,* ed 2, Philadelphia, 1996, Saunders.)

Umbilical Hernia Repair
SURGICAL GOAL
This procedure is performed to repair a weakening of the abdominal wall around or under the umbilicus.

PATHOLOGY
Umbilical hernias are common in children and often disappear spontaneously by age 2. In adults, these types of hernias appear more often in obese people, thus making diagnosis more difficult. Umbilical hernias are potentially dangerous because they have small necks and frequently incarcerate. Surgical intervention is indicated in *all* adult asymptomatic umbilical hernias.

Technique
1. A small incision of approximately 2 to 3 inches is made just above the umbilicus.
2. The linea alba defect is identified.
3. The defect is dissected free of any tissue, and the musculofascial margins are identified.
4. The defect is repaired.
5. The repair is checked for open spaces or weakness in the suture line.

DISCUSSION
A small self-retaining retractor, such as a Jameson hinged retractor, is ideal for use on umbilical hernia repairs.

At smaller institutions, the scrub will be working double duty, holding retractors and passing instruments.

Spigelian Hernia Repair
SURGICAL GOAL
This procedure is performed to reduce a protrusion of a peritoneal sac, preperitoneal fat, or other abdominal viscera through the congenital or acquired defect in the muscle wall called the "spigelian zone."

PATHOLOGY
The "spigelian zone" is defined as the area of aponeurosis that lies between the linea semilunaris of the transverse abdominis muscle and the lateral edge of the rectus muscle. Spigelian hernias are relatively uncommon and generally difficult to diagnose. Ultrasonic scanning has improved the diagnosis. CT imaging, however, can better image the hernia orifice when ultrasonic scanning is inconclusive. Diagnosis is often made during an exploratory laparotomy for symptoms of intestinal obstruction.

Technique
1. A skin incision is made.
2. The hernia sac is identified.
3. The sac contents are closely examined for ischemia, the sac is resected, and the contents are reduced into the peritoneal cavity.
4. The defect is repaired following the same technique as for strangulated hernias.
5. Marlex or Gore-Tex mesh may be required for support of larger defects.

DISCUSSION
A spigelian hernia is located between the different abdominal layers. For this reason, it also may be called an "interparietal," "interstitial," or "intramuscular hernia."

The patient is placed in a supine position. A skin incision is made 2 cm above the symphysis pubis and extended through the external and internal oblique muscles and the transversalis muscle. The hernia sac is identified. The sac contents are closely examined for ischemia, the sac is resected, and the contents are reduced into the peritoneal cavity. The defect is repaired following the same technique as for strangulated hernias. During resection and reduction, the surgeon must identify a direct or indirect hernia. This will affect the type of repair material the scrub will require. During repair, the hernia between the muscle layers is incorporated into the suture line. Marlex or Gore-Tex mesh may be required for support of larger defects.

SECTION III
Gastrointestinal Surgery

Behavioral Objectives

After studying this chapter the reader will be able to:

- Define the procedures for gastrointestinal (GI) endoscopy
- Identify the set-up and equipment needed for a simple laparotomy
- Identify common gastric catheters
- Define GI mobilization
- Identify the tissue involved in a two-layer intestinal closure
- Identify and describe basic anastomosis and resection of the GI system
- Identify preparation of instrumentation and define techniques used in laparoscopic GI surgery

Terminology

Anastomosis—Surgical procedure in which two hollow organs are joined together. See Table 21-1.

Billroth I procedure—A gastroduodenostomy or surgical anastomosis of the stomach and the duodenum.

Billroth II procedure—A gastroduodenostomy or surgical anastomosis of the stomach and the jejunum.

Decompression—A technique or process in which the stomach contents are continually drained into a collection device. Decompression is required after gastric surgery or disease.

Duodenostomy—A surgical opening of the duodenum leading to the outside of the body via a tube, or from another hollow anatomical structure such as the stomach.

Dysphagia—Difficulty in swallowing.

Esophageal varices—Varicose veins of the esophagus resulting from advanced liver disease. The portal vein becomes engorged because fibrous tissue in the liver occludes the circulatory system. Blood then backs into esophageal veins, which become grossly distended and may burst, causing extensive hemorrhage.

Exploratory laparotomy—A laparotomy performed to examine the abdominal cavity when less invasive measures fail to confirm a diagnosis.

Gastrostomy—A surgical opening through the stomach wall connecting to the outside of the body or another hollow anatomical structure.

GERD—Gastroesophageal reflux disease. A condition in which the gastroesophageal sphincter allows gastric contents to reflux into the esophagus, causing irritation and mucosal burning, possibly leading to cancer of the esophagus.

Hiatus—An opening in tissue. For example, the esophagus passes through the hiatus of the diaphragm.

Laparotomy—A procedure in which the abdominal cavity is surgically opened. The techniques used for laparotomy are used for all open surgical procedures of the abdomen.

Mobilize—To surgically free up tissue. Most tissues of the body are attached by serous membranes or connective tissue. Whenever tissue is removed or remodeled, these attachments must be freed up. This often includes dividing and ligating blood vessels that are attached. This is called tissue mobilization. See Table 21-1.

Morbid obesity—A condition in which the patient's body mass index is 40 or greater and weight is at least 100 pounds more than the ideal weight in spite of aggressive attempts to lose weight.

Nasogastric (NG) tube—A flexible tube inserted into the patient's nose and advanced into the stomach. The NG tube is used to decompress the stomach or to create a means of feeding the patient liquid nutrients and oral medication.

Percutaneous enterostomy gastrostomy tube (PEG)—A tube inserted in the stomach for enteral feedings or gastric decompression.

Resection—Surgical removal of an organ. See Table 21-1.

Stoma—A surgically created opening between a portion of the GI tract and the outside of the body. A stoma is created when a section of the GI system is removed and the remaining limbs of the tract cannot be rejoined because of disease or anatomical limitations.

Stoma appliance—A two-piece or three-piece medical device used to collect contents of the GI system through a stoma. One part of the appliance is attached to the patient's skin over the stoma, allowing free drainage into a collection device.

INTRODUCTION TO GASTROINTESTINAL SURGERY

The GI system is a continuous hollow tube, and because of this, many surgeries follow the same techniques. A surgical vocabulary has developed that describes these common techniques. The scrub must be familiar with these terms to follow the surgeon's plan for a specific surgery. Study the terms defined in Table 21-1 before proceeding.

ANATOMY OF THE ABDOMINAL CAVITY

Esophagus

The esophagus is a tubular structure that extends from the pharynx to the stomach. It conveys food throughout its length by a combination of voluntary and involuntary muscle fibers. The esophagus enters the abdominal cavity at the level of the diaphragm. In the adult, it measures approximately 10 inches.

Stomach

The stomach lies just under the diaphragm in the upper abdomen. This organ serves to mix and liquefy food material so that it can be broken down into usable nutrients by the intestines. The stomach is composed of three major sections: the *fundus* (upper portion), *body* (central area), and *antrum* (lower portion, closest to the duodenum) (Figure 21-10). These portions are continuous with one another, and the terms are used only as landmarks, not as distinct anatomical sections.

The wall of the stomach contains an outer layer of delicate tissue called the *serosa*, two inner layers of smooth (involuntary) muscles, and an inner layer called the *submucosa*. The two orifices (openings) of the stomach, one located at each end, are the *cardia* (superior or upper end) and the

Table 21-1   SURGICAL TECHNIQUES OF THE GASTROINTESTINAL SYSTEM

Term or Technique	Definition	Example
Resection (n) **Resect (v)**	(n) Procedure in which a section of organ is cut apart or removed.	The intestine is resected when a portion is removed, leaving two "free" ends. If one of the free ends is surgically closed as a blind end, it is called a *stump*.
Anastomosis (n) **Anastomose (v)**	(n) Procedure in which two hollow organs are joined together surgically.	Placing sutures around the circumference of the two cut edges can join two hollow structures. This applies to portions of the GI system and other hollow systems, such as blood vessels and organ ducts.
Division (n) **Divide (v)**	(n) In surgery, procedure in which one section of tissue is cut away from another. This differs from resection, in which a portion of the organ is *removed*.	Recall that the small intestine is attached to the mesentery, a loose connective tissue containing many major blood vessels. When removing a section of small intestine, one must *divide* the mesentery from the intestine to free up the section.
Cross clamp (v)	To place one or more clamps at a *right angle* to a tube or vessel.	The "cross" simply refers to the angle of the clamp in relation to the organ or tissue.
Double clamp (v)	To place two clamps over a section of tissue to divide the two sections.	Double clamping is performed before dividing or cutting tissue that might bleed profusely. In the case of the GI structures, one must double clamp a section of intestine or stomach before cutting. This prevents hemorrhage and release of fluids from the intestine or stomach.
Mobilize (v) **Mobilization (n)**	(v) To free up tissue from its attachments before anastomosis or resection.	No tissues in the body are free floating. Blood and lymph vessels, connective tissue, and membranes nourish and protect tissue. To remove tissue or to reconstruct the anatomy, the tissue must be removed from its normal attachments. This is called *mobilization*. Mobilization requires *dissection* or *division*.
Clamp and divide (v)	To both double clamp and divide tissue. Because the purpose of the clamps is to prevent bleeding, the tissue inside the jaws of the clamp must be sealed with the ESU or with suture ties.	During mobilization of the intestine, the surgeon repeatedly applies two hemostatic clamps, divides the tissue, and seals the tissue with the ESU or ties the cut ends. For the technologist the tools needed are: 1. Two hemostats (e.g., Kelly, Mayo, Crile) 2. ESU or tissue scissors 3. Two ties (none are needed if the ESU is used) 4. Suture scissors if ties are used

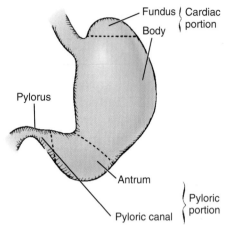

FIGURE 21-10
The stomach. (Colorized from Rothrock JC: *Alexander's care of the patient in surgery*, ed 12, St Louis, 2003, Mosby.)

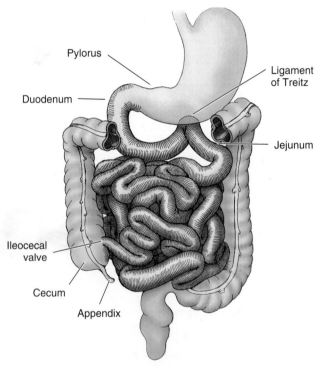

FIGURE 21-11
The small intestine. (Colorized from Rothrock JC: *Alexander's care of the patient in surgery*, ed 12, St Louis, 2003, Mosby.)

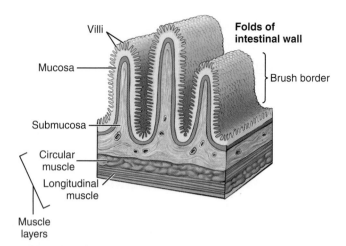

FIGURE 21-12
Tissue layers of the small intestine. (Modified from Herlihy B and Maebius NK: *The human body in health and illness*, ed 2, Philadelphia, 2003, Saunders.)

pylorus (inferior or lower end). The cardia is located between the esophagus and the stomach, and the pylorus is located between the stomach and the duodenum, the first section of small intestine.

The *omentum* is an extension of the abdominal peritoneum that lines the inner wall of the abdominal cavity. The omentum is a sheet of connective and vascular tissue that attaches to the lesser and greater curvatures of the stomach. Whenever a portion of the stomach is removed or remodeled, the omentum must be divided from its attachments.

Small Intestine

The small intestine is the first or most proximal portion of the entire intestine. It extends from the pylorus of the stomach to the cecum or proximal end of the large intestine (Figure 21-11).

The *duodenum*, the first section of small intestine, is an important anatomical structure because the pancreatic duct (duct of Wirsung) and the common bile duct from the liver drain their contents into this section of intestine. The duodenum is approximately 20.3 to 25.4 cm (8 to 10 inches) long.

The *jejunum* and *ileum* are the second and third sections of the small intestine. The jejunum is approximately 2.8 meters (9 feet) long and connects with the ileum, which is approximately 4.2 meters (13.7 feet) long. These sections are suspended from the abdominal wall by a sheet of vascular tissue called the *mesentery*, which supplies blood and lymph to the lower sections of the small intestine. It is this sheet of tissue that must be resected, and each vessel must be clamped and ligated any time portions of the jejunum or ileum are removed.

The tissue layers of the small intestine are similar to those of the stomach and the large intestine (Figure 21-12). The inner surface of the small intestine contains small fingerlike projections called *villi*. These increase the surface area of the lumen and contain blood and lymphatic vessels.

The small intestine terminates at the *cecum*, the first portion of the large intestine.

Large Intestine

The large intestine extends from the distal end of the small intestine (the ileum) to the rectum and is divided into five distinct sections. These sections are the *ascending colon, transverse colon, descending colon, sigmoid colon*, and *rectum* (Figure 21-13). The entire large intestine measures about 1.5 meters (5 feet) in the adult.

The first portion of the large intestine, called the *cecum*, is actually a long pouch where a small, thin, hollow tube called

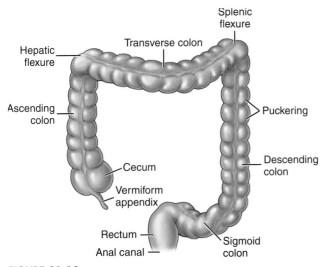

FIGURE 21-13
Structure and segments of the large intestine. (Modified from Herlihy B and Maebius NK: *The human body in health and illness,* ed 2, Philadelphia, 2003, Saunders.)

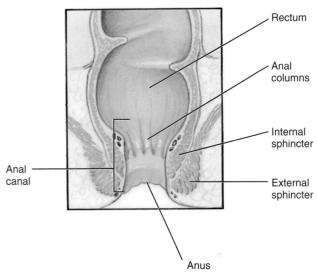

FIGURE 21-14
Anal canal and rectum. (Modified from Applegate EJ: *The anatomy and physiology learning system,* ed 2, Philadelphia, 2000, Saunders.)

the *appendix* lies. The appendix occasionally becomes infectious because its blind end becomes the site of obstruction. The ascending colon extends upward toward the liver and lies just behind the right lobe of this organ. The transverse colon then crosses the abdomen to the left, below the stomach. The descending colon extends downward on the left side of the abdomen and terminates at the sigmoid colon, which lies in the pelvic cavity. The sigmoid colon ends at the rectum, which rests near the sacrum and coccyx.

Rectum and Anus

The rectum is continuous with the anal canal and anus. The rectum is approximately 10.2 to 12.7 cm (4 to 5 inches) long. The anal canal extends from the rectum to the outside of the body. Near the anus, the muscular fibers form both internal and external sphincters that control the release of feces to the outside of the body. These sphincters contain large veins that may become engorged and enlarged, a condition called *hemorrhoids.* A complex of muscles, connective tissue, glands, and mucosa form the anus (Figure 21-14).

FLEXIBLE ENDOSCOPIC PROCEDURES

Flexible endoscopy provides complete visualization of the inner GI tract for both diagnostic and therapeutic procedures. As a diagnostic tool, the flexible endoscope enables the surgeon to examine very small structures of the mucosa and take tissue biopsies with forceps.

The flexible endoscope is a long tube that contains fiber optic bundles and a lens. These bundles carry light from a light source through a light cable and through the endoscope itself. The lighted, lensed end of the tube is inserted into the patient's GI tract (either orally or through the anal canal). The head of the instrument contains optics and controls, which direct the distal angle of the endoscopic tube and magnify the focal point observed through the optical system.

Open channels that begin at the head of the instrument and emerge at the tip allow long flexible instruments to be passed to the distal end for biopsy, coagulation, irrigation, and suction. Modern flexible endoscopes are capable of producing video or still photographic documentation.

Patients having endoscopic procedures usually are given intravenous sedation. Monitoring of anesthesia care may be required for high-risk patients. Bowel preparation is required for endoscopy of the lower intestinal tract. This may include a cleansing enema performed 1 to 2 consecutive days before the procedure. See Chapter 18 for a complete discussion of endoscopic surgery.

The following endoscopic procedures—esophagogastroscopy, duodenoscopy, colonoscopy, and sigmoidoscopy—are usually performed in an outpatient facility or GI lab.

Esophagogastroscopy

Esophagogastroscopy is endoscopic inspection of the esophagus and stomach.

ASSESSMENT

▶ Upper GI bleeding or esophageal varices (distended veins in the esophagus that may rupture and cause fatal hemorrhage)
▶ Dysphagia (difficulty swallowing)
▶ Chest pain (after myocardial disease has been ruled out)
▶ Peptic ulcer

THERAPEUTIC PROCEDURES

▶ Removal of foreign body
▶ Emergency treatment such as direct balloon pressure on esophageal varices
▶ Removal of benign or cancerous lesions
▶ Coagulation of bleeding vessels
▶ Sclerotherapy of esophageal varices

▶ Dilation of esophageal stricture

▶ Percutaneous endoscopic gastrostomy for insertion of feeding tube

Duodenoscopy

Duodenoscopy is endoscopic inspection of the duodenum.

ASSESSMENT

▶ Biopsy

▶ Ulcerative disease

▶ Inflammatory disease

▶ Examine previous surgical anastomosis

THERAPEUTIC PROCEDURES

▶ Polypectomy

▶ Removal of cancerous or benign lesions

▶ Percutaneous endoscopic duodenostomy for insertion of a feeding tube

Colonoscopy

Colonoscopy is endoscopic inspection of the colon.

ASSESSMENT

▶ Bloody stools

▶ Trauma

▶ Sudden unexplained rectal bleeding

▶ Inflammatory disease

▶ Examination of previous surgical anastomosis

▶ Persistent abdominal pain

THERAPEUTIC PROCEDURES

▶ Polypectomy

▶ Removal of small lesions that do not require resection

▶ Coagulation and treatment of small bleeding diverticula

Sigmoidoscopy

This procedure is performed to examine tissue and/or obtain a biopsy specimen of the sigmoid colon and rectum. The patient is placed in the jackknife position, and the scope is introduced into the patient's rectum. Biopsy tissue can be obtained or rectal polyps removed with the aid of a rectal snare. Because this procedure is embarrassing and uncomfortable for the patient, the scrub should offer constant emotional support during the procedure. Unlike the gastroscope, the sigmoidoscope does not have a built-in suction and irrigation system; the technologist therefore will be required to hold the suction tip for the operator. When suction is required, the scrub threads the suction tip into the scope. Other accessory instruments, such as the electrocautery tip, are passed in the same way.

INSTRUMENTS

Common GI and rectal instruments are shown in Figure 21-15.

SURGICAL STAPLING PROCEDURES

Because of recent technologic advances in the field of surgical stapling, the surgeon now can perform anastomoses, resections, and bypass operations in a fraction of the usual time. The instruments discussed in this chapter use cartridges containing a prescribed number of noncrushing stainless-steel or titanium staples. The staples are fired in single, double, triple, or quadruple lines and replace the traditional fine suture lines used in procedures of the GI system. Depending on the type of instrument used, a precision-made knife may simultaneously divide the tissue between staple lines. When the surgeon chooses surgical stapling instruments over traditional suture techniques, the scrub technologist or nurse is responsible for properly loading and unloading the staple cartridges at the surgical field. Complete instructions for these techniques and further information on the instruments are found in Chapter 16.

This chapter will address a variety of general surgical procedures performed with stapling techniques in addition to hand-sewn techniques.

SURGICAL PROCEDURES

Laparotomy

SURGICAL GOAL

During laparotomy a surgical incision is made into the abdominal cavity to confirm a diagnosis, make a medical diagnosis, or perform a specific surgery.

PATHOLOGY

Laparotomy is the term used to describe an incision made through the abdominal wall to allow the surgeon to perform an operation on the abdominal contents. A laparotomy performed as a diagnostic procedure, when the surgeon does not know the exact nature of the patient's condition or disease, is called an *exploratory* laparotomy. After the abdomen has been opened, a particular procedure can be initiated, depending on the specific conditions that are discovered. An exploratory laparotomy may be performed after trauma to the abdomen or when the patient has abdominal pain and the cause cannot be determined by diagnostic studies.

Routines that are followed during every abdominal procedure are discussed here to avoid repeating these steps for each separate procedure.

Technique

1. A midline abdominal skin incision is made.
2. The surgeon continues sharp dissection through the abdominal layers. Right-angle retractors are used to expose each separate layer.
3. Bleeders are coagulated with the ESU.

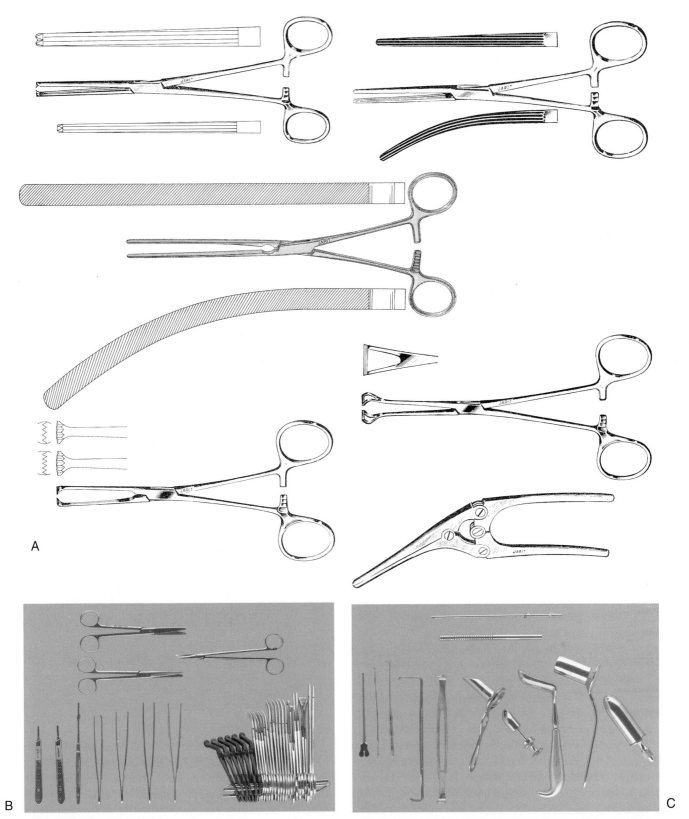

FIGURE 21-15

A, Gastrointestinal instruments. *Top, left to right,* Allen intestinal clamp; Bainbridge intestinal clamp. *Center,* Doyen intestinal clamp. *Bottom left,* Allis clamp. *Bottom right, top to bottom,* Babcock forceps; Payr gastrointestinal clamp. **B,** Rectal instruments. *Top, left to right,* two Mayo dissection scissors (straight); one Metzenbaum scissors (7 inch). *Bottom, left to right,* two Bard-Parker knife handles (no. 3); one Bard-Parker knife handle (no. 7); two thumb tissue forceps with teeth (1 × 2); two DeBakey vascular Atraugrip tissue forceps (short); two paper drape clips; two Crile hemostatic forceps (5½ inch); six Crile hemostatic forceps (6½ inch); two Allis tissue forceps; two Ochsner hemostatic forceps (short); two Pennington hemostatic forceps; two Crile-Wood needle holders (7 inch). **C,** Rectal and pilonidal cyst instruments. *Top,* one Poole abdominal suction tube and shield. *Bottom, left to right,* one grooved director; one probe dilator; one Rosser crypt hook; one Army-Navy retractor (side and front views); one Hirschman anoscope (two parts); one Hill-Ferguson rectal retractor; one anoscope (extra large) (two parts). (**A** courtesy of Jarit Instruments, Hawthorne, NY; **B** and **C** from Tighe SM: *Instrumentation for the operating room,* ed 6, St Louis, 1999, Mosby.)

4. The surgeon gently moves the bowel, omentum, and stomach aside to explore the contents of the abdominal cavity.

5. If adhesions are encountered, they are separated with the ESU pencil. Adhesions are abnormal bands of scar tissue that connect organs to each other or the abdominal peritoneum.

6. The edges of the wound are covered with a moist laparotomy sponge, and a self-retaining retractor is inserted to hold the incision open.

7. Further exploration reveals the target tissue of the procedure. All other organs and tissues are retracted back.

8. Repair, removal, remolding, or reconstruction is performed on the target tissue.

9. The wound is irrigated, and drains are inserted at this time.

10. The abdominal layers are closed individually, and dressings are applied.

DISCUSSION

The patient is placed in a supine position, prepped, and draped for a midline incision. When draping is completed, the scrub moves the Mayo stand up to the field below the wound site. The scrub usually stands opposite the surgeon with the Mayo stand positioned at the level of the patient's knees. This gives the surgeons room to work but is close enough to allow team members to comfortably pass instruments. The cautery and suction tubing are secured to the top drape by the scrub or surgeon. The scrub places two dry lap or Raytec sponges on the field. When suction, the ESU pencil, and sponges are in place on the field, the scrub passes a #20 or #10 scalpel blade to the surgeon, and the surgeon incises the skin with the scalpel (Figure 21-16, *A*). This scalpel will hereafter be called the *skin knife* and is designated for use *only on the skin*. Most surgeons believe that the skin knife carries bacteria from the skin into deeper layers, although some surgeons dispute this.

The skin incision exposes the subcutaneous or fatty layer that lies just under the skin (Figure 21-16, *B*). This layer usually is incised with the cautery pencil or scalpel. The surgeon clamps large bleeding vessels in this layer with Kelly or Crile hemostats and ligates them with absorbable suture, size 3-0, or the surgeon may simply cauterize them (Figure 21-16, *C*).

The incision is carried through to the next layer, the fascia. At this level, the scrub should have small Richardson or U.S. retractors available for the assistant. The surgeon incises the layer with a #10 or #20 scalpel blade. This scalpel then is called the *deep knife*. As lap sponges become soiled, the scrub must replace them with clean ones. The delivery of clean, moistened lap sponges and retrieval of soiled sponges continue throughout the entire procedure.

The surgeon may lengthen the fascial incision with the cautery pencil or may use curved Mayo scissors. If the incision is on the midline, no muscle tissue is encountered. If, however, the incision lies off the midline, there will be a layer of muscle tissue that the surgeon will separate manually or

with the scalpel. In preparation for entrance into the abdomen, the scrub should have available several lap sponges and a self-retaining retractor such as a Balfour retractor. The lap sponges are dipped in *warm* (not hot) saline solution and wrung as dry as possible. If small Raytec sponges have been used before the opening of the peritoneum, the scrub must remove them from the field immediately. They may not be used again (unless mounted on a sponge forcep) until the subcutaneous layer has been closed. The surgeon and assistant each pick up the peritoneum with hemostats and elevate it. The surgeon then makes a small incision in the peritoneum with the deep knife and extends the incision with Metzenbaum scissors.

The abdominal contents are then exposed. From this point on, to protect the abdominal contents from injury, *only saline-moistened sponges are allowed on the field.* The scrub passes the moistened sponges to the surgeon, who covers the tissue edges to protect them from the self-retaining retractor. The self-retaining abdominal retractor is now placed in position by the surgeon and assistant. At this time, the surgeon explores the wound for evidence of disease. When the area of disease has been located, the surgeon packs the abdominal contents away from the diseased area with several moistened lap sponges. A specific surgical procedure then can be initiated.

During the procedure, the scrub's duties are to:

1. Keep the field clear of instruments not in use.
2. Keep the cautery pencil free of tissue debris.
3. Exchange soiled sponges for clean ones.
4. Keep loose items such as needles, small dissecting sponges, and suture wrappers off the Mayo stand. Needles and sponges go on the field or Mayo tray *only* when mounted on the appropriate clamp.
5. Protect the field from contamination.
6. Anticipate the needs of the surgeon.
7. Notify the surgeon of a break in aseptic technique, if one occurs.
8. Notify the circulator if the surgeon requests a brow wipe.
9. Participate in sponge counts at the appropriate time.
10. Participate in instrument counts according to policy of your facility.

During the procedure, the surgeon may request that the patient be placed into the Trendelenburg position. As soon as this request is made, the scrub should immediately raise the Mayo stand to prevent injury to the patient's legs and feet. The Mayo stand must never be allowed to rest on the patient.

Many surgeons irrigate the wound with warm saline or antibacterial solution just before the abdomen is closed. The scrub must check the irrigation solution to be sure that it is not too hot; it should feel warm to the touch.

After irrigation, the surgeon and assistant remove all sponges and instruments from the abdomen, the first count is initiated, and the wound is closed. The incision is then

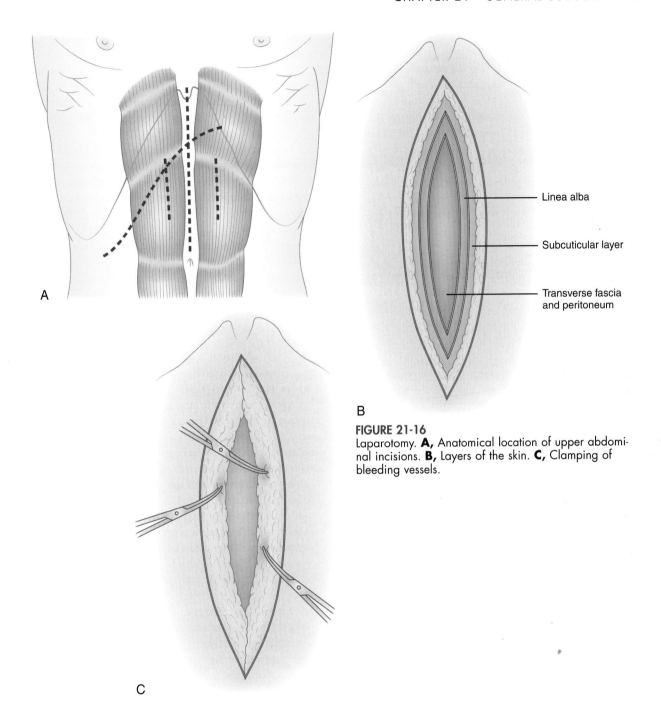

Linea alba

Subcuticular layer

Transverse fascia
and peritoneum

B

FIGURE 21-16
Laparotomy. **A,** Anatomical location of upper abdominal incisions. **B,** Layers of the skin. **C,** Clamping of bleeding vessels.

closed in layers. The choice of suture materials (absorbable, nonabsorbable, synthetic, or natural fiber) depends on the amount of tension on the incision, the wound classification, the size of the patient, and the surgeon's preference. The first count takes place before the closing of the peritoneum.

When all sponges and instruments have been removed from the abdomen, the surgeons' assistant grasps the edges of the peritoneum with several Mayo clamps. The peritoneum usually is closed with a continuous suture line, with absorbable suture swaged to a taper needle, size 0 or 2-0. Next, the fascia is closed with any of a variety of materials—silk, Dacron, Dexon, PDS II, Panacryl, Prolene, and stainless

steel are often used. Because the fascia is the strongest layer of the abdominal wall and the integrity of the closure depends on its strength, interrupted sutures are used most often to close it. Size 2-0 suture is used most often, but size 0 may be used if the patient is very large or obese. The suture may be mounted on a taper or cutting needle, according to the surgeon's preference.

During fascia closure, the assistant retracts the skin and subcutaneous layer with U.S. Army (or Navy) or Richardson retractors. The subcutaneous layer is closed next with interrupted sutures of 3-0 Dexon, Vicryl, chromic gut, or plain gut. Fine tapered needles are used. After the subcutaneous layer is closed, the assistant may choose to leave. If the assistant leaves, the scrub must step up to take his or her place and assist in skin closure by cutting the suture ends after the surgeon has tied the sutures in place.

At the completion of skin closure, the scrub or surgeon places the dressings over the wound. The drapes are then removed, and tape is applied to the dressings by the circulator or surgeon.

Anastomosis of the Small Intestine
SURGICAL GOAL
In anastomosis, a section of small intestine is removed and continuity is reestablished.

PATHOLOGY
A small section of small intestine is resected and anastomosed. The section of small intestine may be removed to treat regional diverticulosis, ulcer, obstruction, ileitis, strangulation, or volvulus (twisting of the intestine on itself).

Technique

1. A laparotomy is performed through a midline incision.
2. The surgeon explores the abdomen and selects the area of intestinal resection and anastomosis.
3. The surgeon mobilizes the intestine by surgically separating it from the mesentery. A tunnel is made in the mesentery with scissors, and small bleeding vessels are sealed with the ESU.
4. Bleeders may be double clamped with Mayo or Crile clamps, the tissue is divided with scissors, and each cut end is tied with fine suture.
5. The diseased section of duodenum is mobilized.
6. The intestine is cross clamped with two intestinal clamps, and the tissue is divided into two sections.
7. A surgical stapling device may used to simultaneously clamp and divide the intestine. The intestine is double clamped and divided.
8. The intestine is reconnected with sutures, staples, or both.
9. The abdomen is irrigated with topical antibacterial solution.
10. The wound is closed in layers.

DISCUSSION
For the open procedure, the abdomen is entered through a midline incision. When retractors are in place, the surgeon gently explores the bowel, palpating (examining by feeling) the loops for irregularities and making note of large blood vessels in the mesentery. Selecting a site for anastomosis must ensure that the diseased tissue is removed but adequate blood flow is retained.

The intestine is mobilized from the omentum (refer to anatomy section) along the site of resection. The surgeon opens the mesentery with Metzenbaum scissors or the ESU. The surgeon then fans out the mesentery tissue and continues to divide it from the intestine. Clips or silk or absorbable sutures are used to ligate bleeders in the mesentery. Larger mesenteric arteries are secured with suture ligatures.

Just as in the example of GI anastomosis, the bowel is cross-clamped with two intestinal clamps placed close together at each incision site. The intestine is incised between the clamps, and the freed portion of intestine is removed as a specimen.

When resecting the small intestine, the surgeon has several methods for performing an anastomosis and reestablishing continuity. In end-to-end anastomosis, the two cut ends are sutured circumferentially. Side-to-end or side-to-side anastomosis results in a longitudinal suture line on one or both of the intestinal limbs (Figure 21-17, A-D). In open surgery, the technique is the same as that described for open gastric resection.

If surgical stapling instruments are used, resection and anastomosis are completed simultaneously. The surgeon performs a hand-sutured anastomosis by aligning the two ends of the intestine and rotating them outward. The inner layer is closed with a continous or interrupted stitch of absorbable suture, such as chromic or Vicryl, and the outer serosa with interrupted absorbable or non-absorbable sutures such as Vicryl or silk, size 4-0 or 3-0. Most surgeons prefer this two-layered closure technique for hand-sutured anastomoses. The inner layer of the bowel is generally closed with continuous or interrupted stitch of absorbable suture because it is very vascular and heals quickly. The outer layer of the bowel is sutured with interrupted absorbable or nonabsorbable sutures because of the possibility of infection. If infection or breakdown of a suture occurs with the interrupted sutures, only an individual suture will be affected, not the entire suture line. The mesentery is repaired with interrupted absorbable sutures.

The wound is irrigated with topical antibiotic solution, all bleeders are controlled, and the incision is closed in layers.

Colon Resection and Anastomosis
Note: In all procedures involving the large intestine, special precautions are taken to prevent contamination of the field by the bowel contents. When the bowel has been opened, all contaminated instruments, sponges, and other equipment are kept separate from equipment that is used for closure. Many scrubs set up a separate closure stand with the needed suture materials and instruments. This equipment is not touched until the bowel has been closed and the team has been regloved and regowned according to the operating room policy manual.

SURGICAL GOAL
In this procedure a section of the large intestine is removed and its continuity is restored.

PATHOLOGY
This procedure is performed to remove cancerous lesions or to correct other conditions, such as ulcerative colitis or diverticula of the colon.

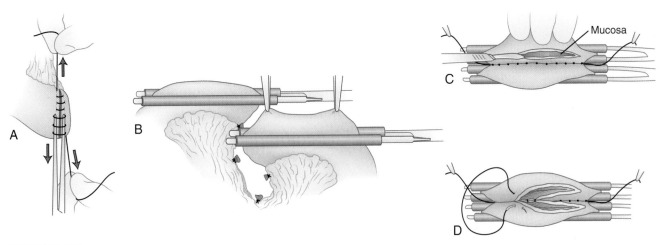

FIGURE 21-17
Side-to-side anastomosis. **A,** The two intestinal stumps are closed. **B,** The two bowel segments are aligned side-to-side. **C,** Two incisions are made, one on each side of the suture line. This exposes the intestinal mucosa, which is then approximated. **D,** A final layer of sutures joins the two intestinal limbs.

Technique

1. The abdomen is entered.
2. The diseased portion of the bowel is identified and isolated.
3. The bowel is cross clamped and divided.
4. An end-to-end anastomosis is performed.
5. The wound is closed.

DISCUSSION

The surgeon enters the abdomen through an incision determined by the location of the lesion. A midline incision, however, usually is chosen to give the best exposure to all segments of the bowel. When the abdomen has been entered, the surgeon explores loops of intestine to identify the portion to be removed. A wide margin of intestine on each side of the lesion also is removed if the lesion is cancerous.

To free the bowel from its peritoneal and mesenteric attachments, the surgeon dissects them with an ESU or Metzenbaum scissors (Figure 21-18, *A-C*). The scrub should have available an ample supply of Mayo clamps and ties of the surgeon's choice. Silk in sizes 2-0 and 3-0 usually is used. Portions of mesentery are double clamped, divided, and ligated. Large vessels are controlled with suture ligatures. The surgeon completes the mobilization procedure along the full length of bowel to be resected. Many surgeons use a soft rubber Penrose drain looped around the bowel for retraction.

When the bowel is isolated, the segment is double clamped at each end with intestinal clamps (Figure 21-18, *D* and *E*). Using the cautery pencil or scalpel, the surgeon divides the bowel between each set of clamps and passes the specimen to the scrub. The scrub should have a basin ready to accept the specimen. At this point the bowel is open and

the potential for fecal contamination is present. To help prevent this, the surgeon may place two lap sponges around the base of the intestinal stumps or use rubber bands to seal the openings of the stumps.

The anastomosis begins as the assistant places the two bowel ends in close approximation. The first layer of interrupted sutures is placed. Fine silk or Vicryl suture-release needles are typically used. The scrub should take care to place *returned* needles on a magnetic needle board or other such device *as soon as* the surgeon discards the needle. These needles are very small and may be easily lost in the rapid exchange between the surgeon and the technologist. The first and last sutures of the initial suture layer are left long to be used in traction.

After making double incisions in the bowel, the surgeon places a second layer of interrupted chromic gut sutures, size 3-0, swaged to a fine GI needle. The surgeon continues the interrupted sutures until the two intestinal lumens are joined.

The intestinal clamps then are removed, and a final reinforcing suture layer of interrupted silk or Vicryl is placed.

The final step in the procedure is closure of the mesentery. Interrupted sutures of silk or chromic gut, size 3-0, are used.

Following accepted bowel technique, the scrub is now responsible for directing the changeover from a possibly contaminated field to a sterile one. The surgeon should remove all lap sponges from the wound, remove the suction and cautery pencil from the field, and pull the "dirty" Mayo stand away from the field. The circulator removes each team member's gloves and gown and opens clean gowns and gloves for

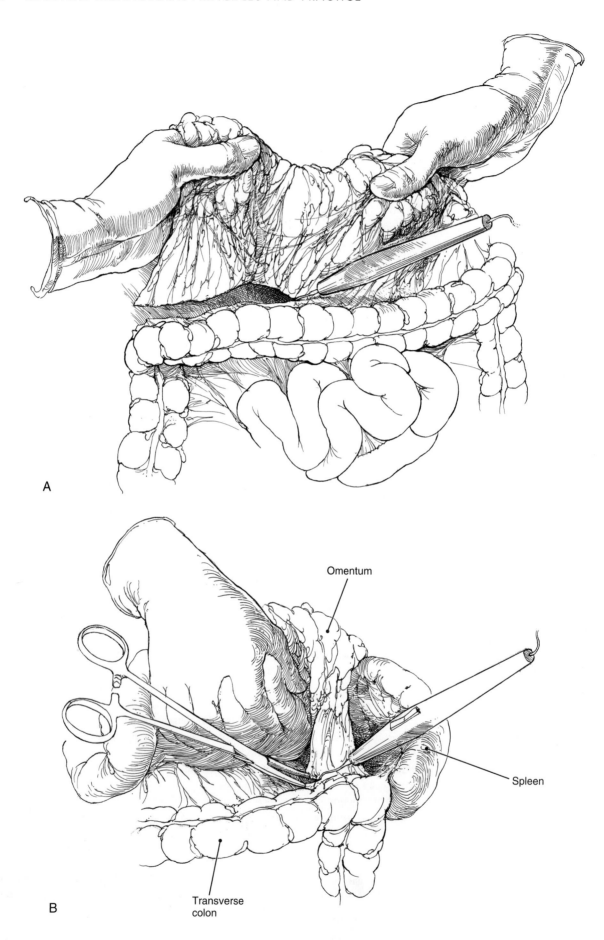

A

Omentum

Spleen

Transverse
colon

B

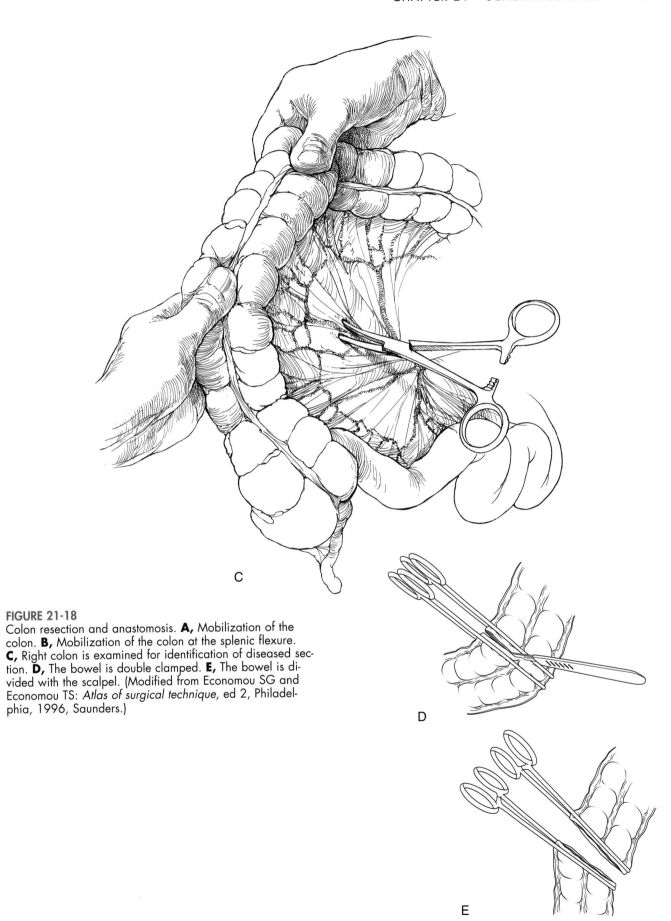

C

D

E

FIGURE 21-18
Colon resection and anastomosis. **A,** Mobilization of the colon. **B,** Mobilization of the colon at the splenic flexure. **C,** Right colon is examined for identification of diseased section. **D,** The bowel is double clamped. **E,** The bowel is divided with the scalpel. (Modified from Economou SG and Economou TS: *Atlas of surgical technique,* ed 2, Philadelphia, 1996, Saunders.)

the scrub. The scrub dons the new sterile gown and gloves and proceeds to gown and glove the surgeons. A sterile procedure (laparotomy) drape is placed directly over the contaminated one on the patient, and new suction tubing and an electrocautery pencil are clamped to it. To save time, the surgeon usually assists the scrub in these tasks. Some hospitals and surgeons are stricter than others in the extent to which they perform the changeover. Some surgeons simply change gloves, while others order a complete changeover. Occasionally the decision is left to the scrub. The relative cost of a complete changeover is minimal and will not *harm* the patient; therefore the changeover is recommended..

The scrub distributes fresh lap sponges on the field, and the wound is irrigated (in some operating rooms this is done *before* the changeover) and closed in routine fashion.

RELATED PROCEDURE
Total colectomy

Loop Colostomy
GASTROINTESTINAL STOMA
An ostomy is a procedure in which a portion of the intestine is surgically severed and the end brought to the outside of the body. The edges of the intestine are secured to the full thickness of the abdominal wall. This opening, called a **stoma,** provides a passage to the outside of the body for intestinal contents. A disposable **ostomy appliance** is used to collect intestinal fluid. The appliance system consists of an adherent skin wafer with an opening for the stoma and a collection reservoir that fits tightly into the skin wafer. The patient drains the collection reservoir as needed and changes the appliance as needed. The appliance fits tightly over the stoma and adheres to the contours of the body to limit leakage and odor. After the disruption of the GI tract, the remaining part of the intestinal system becomes nonfunctional for digestion but is left intact. A small-intestine stoma is called an **ileostomy,** while a stoma of the large intestine is

a **colostomy.** Variations on the surgical procedure are described below.

Before surgery, the surgeon discusses the exact location of the ostomy, considering lifestyle, age, and protection of the ostomy from beltline or other clothing pressure. The site is usually outlined on the skin with gentian violet dye after this consultation and assessment. Often a stoma nurse meets with the patient before surgery to relieve anxiety and educate the patient.

The location of an ostomy depends on the section of the intestine to be removed. An end colostomy is formed when the proximal end of the resected intestine is brought through the abdominal wall and sutured in place as described above (Figure 21-19). A **double-barreled** colostomy is one in which both sections of cut bowel are brought out through the abdominal wall (Figure 21-20). The double-barreled colostomy allows the bowel to remain nonfunctional for a period of healing. The two ends then are reconnected as a separate surgery. The **loop colostomy** does not require resection and anastomosis. A loop of bowel is brought out and held in place with a plastic rod or tubal appliance that prevents the loop from slipping back into the abdominal cavity (see Figure 21-21 on the following pages).

The patient's adjustment to an ostomy procedure depends on many factors. Body image, developmental age, level of debilitation before the procedure, and family and professional support affect the patient's ability to accept the change. Professional organizations are available to offer support and education to help the patient adjust.

SURGICAL GOAL
A loop of large intestine is brought out through a small abdominal incision, sutured to the skin, and opened. The resulting *colostomy* serves as a temporary channel for the evacuation of fecal material.

PATHOLOGY
A colostomy is performed to give the bowel a rest after colon resection. The procedure also may be performed in the treatment of inflammatory disease or obstruction of the colon. The loop colostomy is closed when fecal diversion is no longer needed.

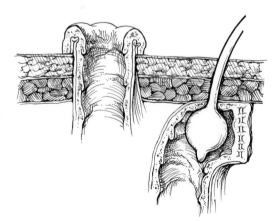

FIGURE 21-19
An end colostomy. (From Economou SG and Economou TS: *Atlas of surgical technique*, ed 2, Philadelphia, 1996, Saunders.)

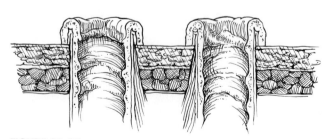

FIGURE 21-20
Double-barreled loop colostomy. (From Economou SG and Economou TS: *Atlas of surgical technique*, ed 2, Philadelphia, 1996, Saunders.)

Technique

OPENING

1. The abdomen is entered.
2. A small portion of transverse colon is mobilized.
3. The mobilized bowel is brought out through the incision.
4. A colostomy butterfly anchor or rod is inserted under the loop.
5. If a butterfly anchor is used, it is anchored through the needle ports.
6. The wound is closed.
7. The loop is incised 24 to 48 hours after the procedure.

CLOSING

1. The skin edges around the colostomy are incised.
2. Dissection is carried to the peritoneum.
3. The colostomy edges are trimmed and sutured together.
4. The loop is allowed to retract into the abdomen.
5. The wound is closed.

DISCUSSION

Opening

The abdomen is entered through a short, transverse upper-paramedian incision. The assistant retracts the abdominal wall with a medium Richardson retractor. Using one or more Babcock clamps, the surgeon grasps a loop of transverse colon and brings it forward into the wound.

The surgeon begins to free the bowel from its attachments to the omentum with Metzenbaum scissors. An avascular area of the omentum is chosen for the mobilization. However, if blood vessels are encountered, the surgeon grasps the tissue with Mayo clamps, divides the tissue between the clamps, and ligates it with 3-0 silk or Dexon ties.

When mobilization is complete, the loop of intestine is brought out of the abdomen and a butterfly anchor or plastic colostomy rod is placed under the loop to prevent it from retracting into the abdomen. If a butterfly anchor is used, it is anchored through the needle ports with suture. The wound then is closed in standard fashion around the loop.

The opening for the loop colostomy is illustrated in Figure 21-21, *A-I.*

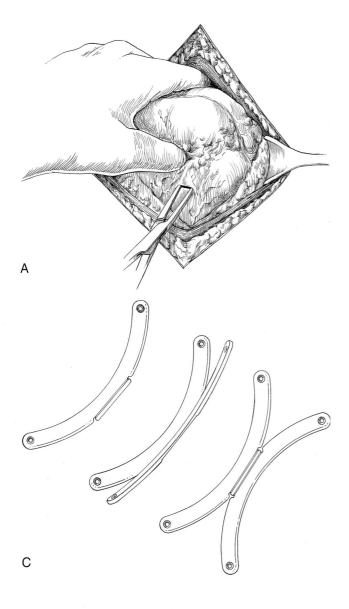

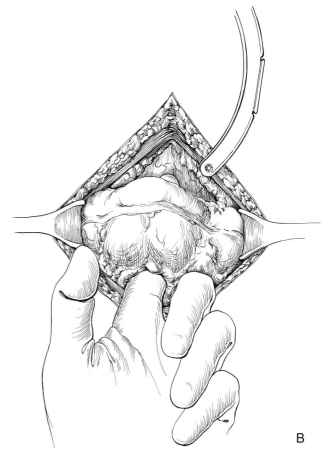

FIGURE 21-21
Opening for the loop colostomy. **A,** The distal colon is grasped and delivered through the incision. **B,** The surgeon inserts a finger under the colon for passage of the butterfly anchor. **C,** Butterfly anchor shown in closed, partially open, and open positions *(left to right).*

Continued

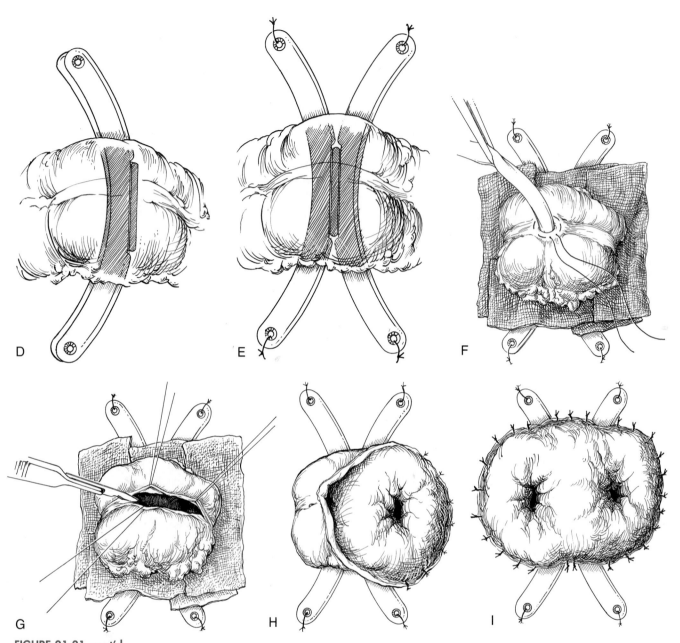

FIGURE 21-21, cont'd
Opening for the loop colostomy. **D,** Placement of the butterfly anchor in the closed position under the colon. **E,** Butterfly anchor under the colon in the open position, anchored at four ports. **F,** Insertion of catheter in colon to evacuate air and feces. **G,** Longitudinal incision into colon. **H,** Anastomosis of the colon and skin. **I,** Completion of the anastomosis. (From Economou SG and Economou TS: *Atlas of surgical technique,* ed 2, Philadelphia, 1996, Saunders.)

Closing
After prepping and draping of the patient, the surgeon initiates the procedure by placing a gauze sponge at the opening of the colostomy. This prevents gross contamination of the wound by fecal material. The surgeon then incises the skin around the edges of the colostomy. The incision is carried through the subcutaneous and fascial layers. The peritoneum is dissected free of the colostomy with Metzenbaum scissors. To prevent contamination of the peritoneal cavity, the colostomy is surrounded with one or two lap sponges. The surgeon then trims the skin from the edges of the colostomy.

The surgeon closes the colostomy by inserting two layers of suture through the colostomy edges. The first layer is closed with running or interrupted chromic gut, size 3-0, swaged to a fine needle. A second layer of interrupted silk, size 3-0 or 4-0, is placed over the chromic suture line.

The bowel is then allowed to slide back into position in the peritoneal cavity, and the wound is closed in routine fashion.

The closing for the loop colostomy is illustrated in Figure 21-22, *A-F.*

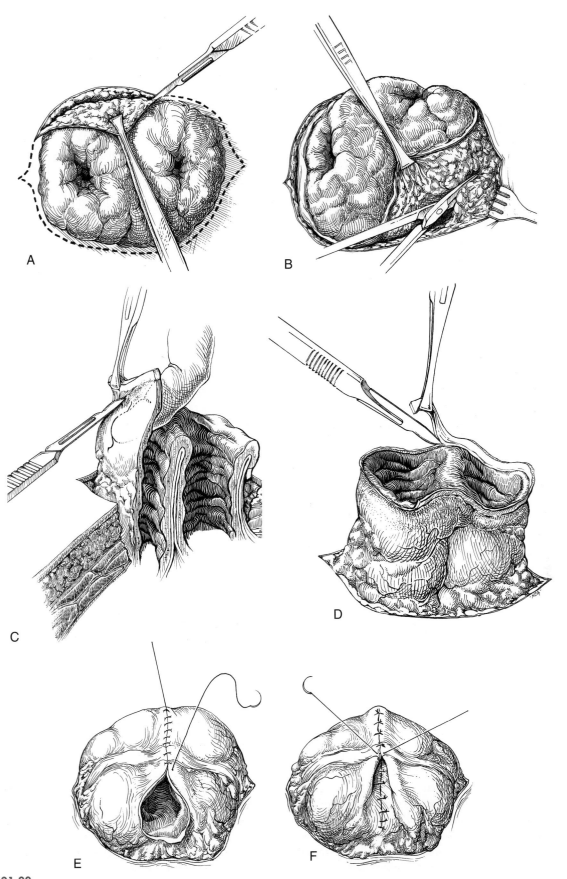

FIGURE 21-22
Closing for the loop colostomy. **A,** Skin incision is made within 5 mm of mucosa. **B,** Dissection of adipose tissue to the colon serosa. **C,** Separation of serosal layers. **D,** The skin is removed from the colon serosa. **E,** The mucosal edges are approximated with running stitch of 3-0 chromic. **F,** Inversion and closure of serosa with a 3-0 interrupted silk suture. (From Economou SG and Economou TS: *Atlas of surgical technique,* ed 2, Philadelphia, 1996, Saunders.)

Partial Colectomy with Ileostomy (Open)
SURGICAL GOAL
This procedure is performed to remove a section of diseased colon and restore continuity to the intestine.

PATHOLOGY
Colectomy is removal of part or all of the large intestine. The colon is removed to treat ulcerative colitis, diverticulitis, cancer, and intestinal obstruction. An ileostomy may be required if a large section of colon is removed.

Technique

1. A laparotomy is performed through a midline or left paramedian incision.
2. The exact position of the resection is determined.
3. The right colon is retracted, and the colon is freed from the retroperitoneal structures.
4. The mesentery between the duodenum and right colon is dissected.
5. The omentum is separated between clamps, and vessels are tied or sealed with the ESU.
6. The remaining mesentery, colon, and distal ileum are dissected free. This completely mobilizes the area of resection.
7. Atraumatic clamps are placed across the bowel at each end of the area to be resected.
8. An end-to-end anastomosis between the distal right colon and proximal ileum is performed using a two-layer suturing technique or surgical staples.
9. If a colostomy is required, it is sited well away from the abdominal incision. An incision is made through the abdominal wall at the colostomy site.
10. The proximal end of the resected colon is brought through the abdominal wall, and its edges are turned out (everted). Fine sutures are placed around the bowel opening, securing it to the skin.
11. The intestinal stump is closed with surgical staples or by hand suturing.
12. The abdomen is irrigated with warm saline and antibacterial solution. The wound is closed in layers.

DISCUSSION
Colectomy is the general term applied to removal of the large intestine. More specific terms identify the section of the intestine that is resected. Recall that the large intestine is composed of three sections: the ascending, transverse, and descending colon. Colectomy can refer to complete removal or segmental resection. In this description, the sigmoid colon and rectum are not removed.

The surgeon performs a laparotomy through a midline or paramedian incision. If a colostomy or ileostomy is planned, the paramedian incision on the *opposite side of the ostomy* often is preferred because it separates the stoma from the surgical wound, which might become contaminated and infected. The area of resection is completely mobilized as described above. Atraumatic Babcock and Allis clamps are used to grasp the bowel tissue. Systematic dissection of the mesentery, major arteries, and peritoneal reflections is performed until all attachments are eliminated. An anastomosis then is performed as described previously.

Colostomy

If a colostomy is performed, the distal intestinal stump is closed in two or three layers. Surgical staples or sutures are used. The surgeon creates the stoma by making a circular incision through the skin and abdominal wall at the stoma site (Figure 21-23, *A*). The incision is dissected down to peritoneum (Figure 21-23, *B-D*), and the proximal stump is brought through the abdominal wall. Small right-angle retractors are used to retract the wound edges. The edges are then everted, and two layers of sutures are placed; the deeper layer penetrates the full thickness of the severed ileum, and a more superficial layer is placed at the level of the skin. The epidermis itself is not sutured to the stoma (Figure 21-23, *E-G*). Sutures are usually synthetic absorbable material or fine silk, size 3-0 or 4-0.

All instruments and supplies that have come in contact with the inside surface of the bowel are considered contaminated and should not be used during the abdominal closure. A change of gloves and new closure instruments are required. Some surgeons prefer two complete set-ups, one for use when the bowel is open and a second for closure.

The wound is irrigated with antibacterial solution before closure.

Ileotransverse Colostomy
SURGICAL GOAL
This procedure is the surgical removal of a portion of the ileum and transverse colon and a side-to-side anastomosis of the ileum and colon.

PATHOLOGY
This procedure is performed in the treatment of lesions such as those caused by cancer, diverticulosis, or obstruction of the large intestine in an area close to the cecum.

Technique

1. The abdomen is entered.
2. The lesion is identified.
3. The portion of bowel to be resected is mobilized.
4. The bowel is cross clamped and divided.
5. The blind stump of the ileum is closed.
6. The ileum is anastomosed to the transverse colon.
7. The wound is closed.

DISCUSSION
After routine prepping and draping, the surgeon enters the abdomen through a right paramedian or median incision. After the wound is open, the surgeon examines loops of intestine to locate the exact position of the bowel lesion. The surgeon begins the procedure by isolating this bowel segment from the mesentery. Using Metzenbaum scissors, the surgeon locates an avascular area in the mesentery and incises a small portion. As in most intestinal procedures, Mayo

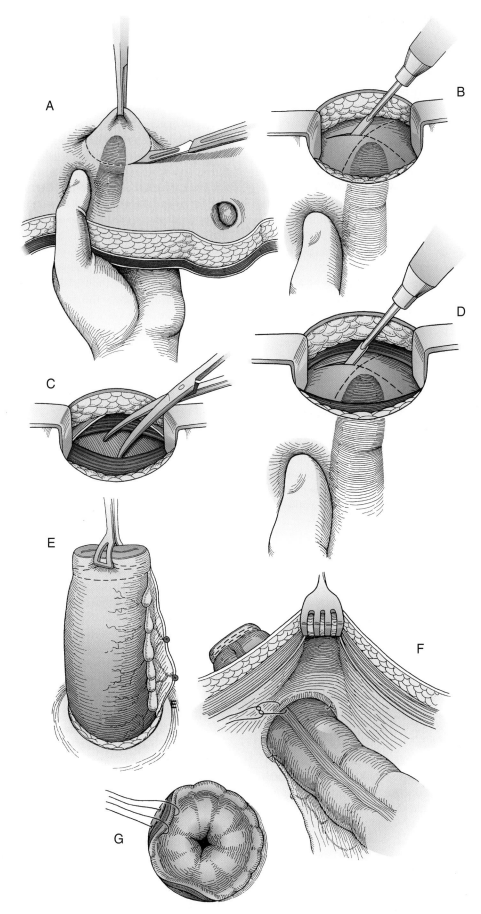

FIGURE 21-23
Partial colectomy with ileostomy (open). **A,** Circular incision through the skin at the stoma site. **B,** Muscle fibers are incised. **C,** The tissues are dissected to posterior layers. **D,** The peritoneum is incised. **E,** The bowel is delivered through the abdominal wall. **F,** The bowel is tacked internally to the peritoneal defect. **G,** The stoma is sutured. (Colorized from Bauer JJ: *Colorectal surgery illustrated,* St Louis, 1993, Mosby.)

clamps are used to double clamp sections of mesentery. The surgeon divides the tissue between the two clamps with the scalpel, scissors, or cautery pencil. The tissue sections are then ligated with silk, Vicryl, or Dexon ties. Large mesenteric vessels are ligated with suture ligatures as described for previous intestinal procedures.

When the bowel is completely free of its mesenteric attachments, the surgeon cross clamps the ileum at the proposed site of anastomosis with two intestinal clamps. The ileum then is divided between the two clamps with the knife or cautery pencil. The surgeon closes the blind (distal) stump of the ileum in two layers. The first layer is a running gut suture, size 3-0, swaged to a fine GI needle. The second layer is composed of interrupted silk sutures of the same size or smaller. Suture-release (pop-off) needles may be used for this layer.

The surgeon prepares the colon for anastomosis by grasping the area of proposed anastomosis with one or two Allis clamps. A Kocher, Allen, or similar intestinal clamp is placed in a longitudinal plane beside the Allis clamp. The colon is then incised with the cautery pencil. The excised portion of colon is passed to the scrub, who isolates it in a sterile basin separate from sterile instruments or equipment. (Proper bowel technique must be observed, because the large intestine is now open and the field may be contaminated.)

The surgeon begins the anastomosis by placing interrupted sutures of 3-0 or 4-0 silk to join the two bowel segments. The assistant holds the two Kocher clamps close together as the surgeon places the sutures. As soon as the first layer is completed, the surgeon places the second layer, using interrupted sutures of chromic gut on a fine needle. The layer is continued around the two structures until they are joined. A final layer of interrupted silk is placed through the outer tissue layers, completing the anastomosis. The mesentery is sutured to the posterior peritoneum using 3-0 interrupted silk sutures. The wound is irrigated and closed in routine fashion.

End-to-End Bowel Anastomosis
SURGICAL GOAL
The goal of this technique is the reestablishment of continuity in the large intestine after resection.

PATHOLOGY
Colectomy is removal of part or all of the large intestine. The colon is removed to treat ulcerative colitis, diverticulitis, cancer, and intestinal obstruction. An ileostomy may be required if a large section of colon is removed.

Technique
1. The abdomen is entered.
2. The large intestine is mobilized.
3. The anastomosis is created.
4. The wound is closed.

DISCUSSION
The patient is positioned, prepped, and draped for an abdominal incision. After the abdomen is entered, the surgeon locates the diseased bowel and determines the area of resection. The ligation and division stapler (LDS) is used to mobilize the bowel along the area of resection. The surgeon then resects the bowel in the usual fashion as described in the section "Colon Resection and Anastomosis" in this chapter. The surgeon then positions the serosal layers of the severed bowel ends face to face with traction sutures. The Roticulator 55 stapler is used to join one side of the anastomosis. The margin of tissue remaining outside the instrument then is removed with the knife. A second set of staples is fired over the anastomosis, and excess tissue is removed to complete the anastomosis. Note the location of the traction sutures, which are used to elevate the tissue margins during the anastomosis. The surgeon completes the anastomosis. The wound is irrigated and closed in routine fashion.

Right Hemicolectomy and Ileocolostomy
SURGICAL GOAL
The goal of this procedure is the removal of a diseased portion of the right colon. Bowel continuity is reestablished by an anastomosis between the colon and the ileum.

Technique
1. The abdomen is entered.
2. The right colon is mobilized.
3. An ileocolostomy is performed.
4. The wound is closed.

DISCUSSION
The patient is positioned, prepped, and draped for an abdominal incision. After the abdomen is entered, the surgeon mobilizes the right colon in the area of disease and transects it in the usual manner, and bowel continuity is reestablished by an anastomosis between the transverse colon and ileum (see "Colon Resection and Anastomosis" section in this chapter). An end-to-end, end-to-side, or side-to-side anastomosis may be performed.

After the removal of the diseased portion of the colon, the surgeon may use the circular end-to-end anastomosis (EEA) stapler to perform the ileocolostomy. The terminal ileum first is prepared with a purse-string suture, and the diameter of the lumen is determined. The instrument is introduced into the severed end of the colon, without the anvil. The center rod is advanced through the colon through a stab wound, around which a purse-string suture has been placed. The surgeon then ties the rod suture, places the anvil on the center rod, and introduces the anvil into the ileum. The purse-string suture is closed, and the EEA staples are fired. The stump of the colon is then closed with the transverse anastomosis (TA) 55 linear stapler. The surgeon completes the anastomosis. The wound is closed in routine fashion. The stapling procedure for side-to-side anastomoses is illustrated in Figure 21-24.

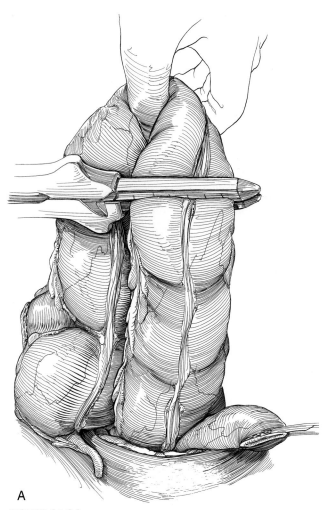

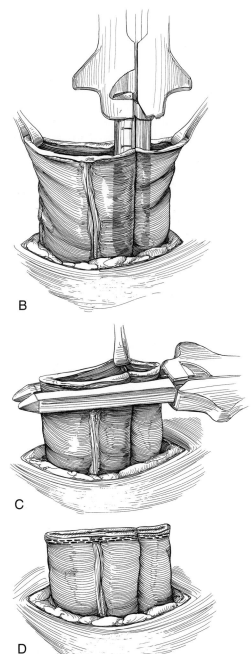

FIGURE 21-24
Right hemicolectomy. **A,** The colon is divided with the GIA stapler to the right of the midcolic artery. **B,** The ileum and transverse colon are aligned, and the GIA stapler is inserted in each intestinal lumen and fired, connecting the lumens. **C,** The openings of the ileum and transverse colon are held up and closed with the TA stapler, and excess tissues are removed with a scalpel. **D,** Completion of the anastomosis. (From Economou SG and Economou TS: *Atlas of surgical technique,* ed 2, Philadelphia, 1996, Saunders.)

Abdominoperineal Resection of the Rectum
SURGICAL GOAL
Through combined abdominal and perineal incisions, the anus, rectum, and sigmoid colon are removed en bloc.

PATHOLOGY
This procedure is performed to treat cancer of the rectum. The obliteration of the rectum necessitates the formation of a permanent colostomy in the abdominal wall for drainage of bowel contents.

Technique

1. The abdomen is entered.
2. The lesion is located and the bowel is mobilized.
3. The colon is divided in an area proximal to the lesion.
4. A colostomy is performed, and the abdomen is closed.
5. Through a perineal incision, the lower sigmoid colon, rectum, and anus are mobilized and removed.
6. The perineal incision is closed.

DISCUSSION

Abdominoperineal resection often is performed as two simultaneous procedures, with one team operating on the abdominal region and a second on the perineal portion. When the operation is performed in this manner, the patient is placed in the lithotomy position. Because the abdominal team has restricted space in which to work, the scrub on this team must stand slightly behind the assistant rather than next to him or her, as would be the usual practice during abdominal procedures. The scrub must take special care to avoid contamination while standing in this awkward position. During simultaneous procedures, the technologist on the lower team stands next to the surgeon, as for vaginal procedures. The surgeon usually performs the procedure while sitting. Both scrubs must remember that there is usually only one circulator to assist both teams. The scrubs must take care to be prepared and organized, and to anticipate needed equipment before the procedure begins. This will avoid confusion when the two surgical teams are working with one circulator between them.

To avoid confusion, the procedure is discussed here as if performed by one team. The surgeon enters the abdomen through a long midline incision. The surgeon examines the intestine and determines the line of resection.

Mobilization of the colon includes isolation of the mesenteric tissue and omentum that contain diseased lymph nodes. The surgeon frees the colon from its attachments by double clamping the tissue with Mayo clamps. The tissue between the clamps then is divided with Metzenbaum scissors or a cautery pencil, and the sections are ligated with silk, Vicryl, or Dexon ties. As mobilization continues, longer instruments are needed. The scrub must have an ample supply of Péan clamps, long right-angle clamps, and small sponge dissectors. Both smooth and toothed long tissue forceps also are required. Large blood vessels are clamped with right-angle or Péan clamps and ligated with suture ligatures. The scrub should have one or two suture ligatures ready at all times during the dissection.

Dissection and mobilization are continued through the pelvic floor to the level of the levator muscles (Figure 21-25, A). At this point the abdominal dissection is halted, because the depth of the incision is too great to allow the surgeon to work comfortably. The surgeon places two intestinal clamps across the bowel at the proximal end of the mobilized area. The bowel between the clamps is divided, and the distal end is placed in the pelvis. The proximal end of the divided bowel may be temporarily ligated with heavy silk (Figure 21-25, B). To reconstruct the pelvic floor, a portion of the omentum may be sutured to it.

To prepare a site for the colostomy, the surgeon incises a small circle in the abdomen using the skin knife. The incision is deepened to the inner abdomen with cautery. The small disk of tissue is then passed to the scrub as a specimen. The proximal end of the bowel is brought through the circular incision and temporarily clamped in place while the abdominal incision is closed in routine fashion.

To create the colostomy, the surgeon everts the edges of the bowel stoma and sutures the edges of the skin using interrupted sutures of 3-0 chromic gut on a fine cutting needle.

Surgery from the perineal end begins as the surgeon places a heavy silk purse-string suture through the anus to occlude it and incises the perineum (Figure 21-25, C). The incision is deepened with the cautery pencil. Large bleeding vessels are double clamped and ligated with silk or Dexon. As the incision becomes deeper, Péan clamps are used to grasp the bowel attachments, as described in the abdominal portion of the procedure. Raytec sponges mounted on a ring forcep (stick sponges) and suction should be available at all times during the mobilization and dissection.

Dissection is continued until the surgeon reaches the previously mobilized area of the bowel (Figure 21-25, D). The entire specimen is delivered through the perineal incision (Figure 21-25, E). The surgeon then irrigates the wound, using an Asepto syringe.

In the past, surgeons packed the wound with a large sheet of rubber (rubber dam) rather than closing it with sutures. The current trend, however, is to obliterate the "dead space" with many interrupted sutures. One or two Penrose drains are placed in the wound, which is then closed with size 0 chromic gut, Vicryl, or Dexon. The skin is approximated with the surgeon's choice of nonabsorbable material and dressed with a bulky abdominal pad and gauze sponges.

Low Anterior Resection (End-to-End Anastomosis)
SURGICAL GOAL

The goal of this procedure is the removal of a portion of the distal large intestine. Continuity of the bowel is reestablished through an anastomosis of the rectum and healthy colon tissue.

Technique

1. The abdomen is entered.
2. The area of resection is mobilized.
3. The proximal colon is resected and closed.
4. The proximal rectum is resected.
5. An anastomosis is created between the proximal rectum and the distal colon.
6. The wounds are closed.

DISCUSSION

In this procedure, the colon is mobilized through an abdominal incision. After this is accomplished, the patient is repositioned into the lithotomy position and the procedure is completed transanally (through the anus). When only one team is available for the surgery, a complete change of instruments, drapes, gowns, and gloves is necessary between the two phases, or two separate isolated set-ups are used.

When two teams are used, two separate operative set-ups must be used, and each team's equipment must be kept separated from the other. A complete discussion of a double set-up is presented in the section on Abdominoperineal Resec-

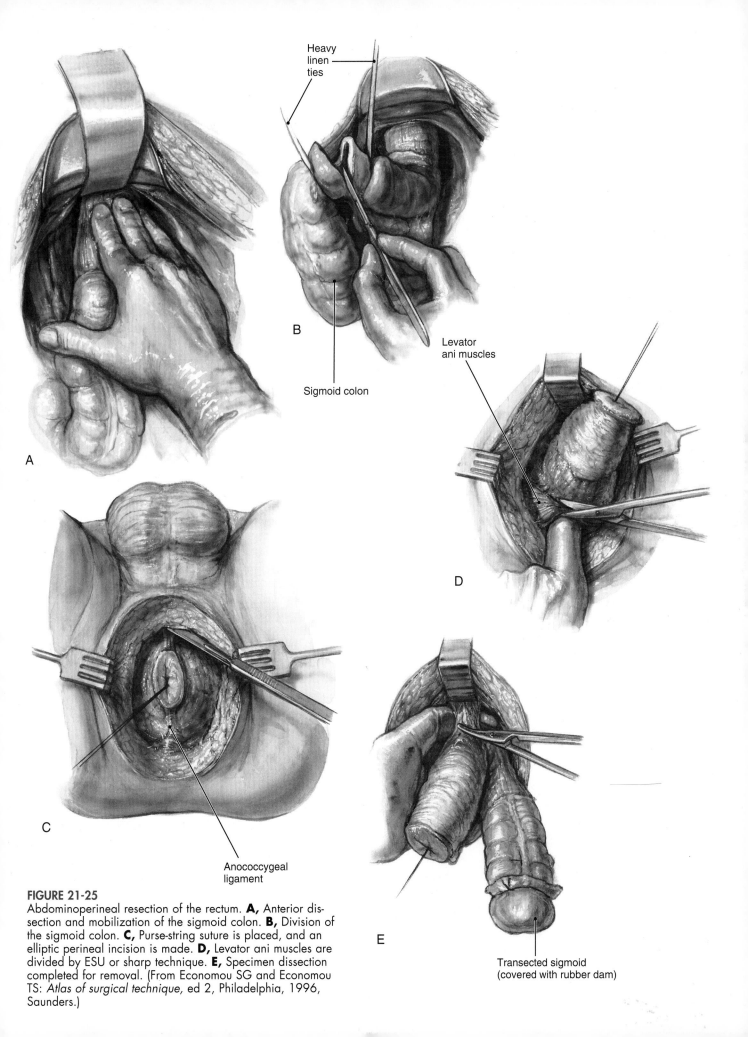

Heavy
linen
ties

Sigmoid colon

Levator
ani muscles

A

B

D

Anococcygeal
ligament

C

E

Transected sigmoid
(covered with rubber dam)

FIGURE 21-25
Abdominoperineal resection of the rectum. **A,** Anterior dissection and mobilization of the sigmoid colon. **B,** Division of the sigmoid colon. **C,** Purse-string suture is placed, and an elliptic perineal incision is made. **D,** Levator ani muscles are divided by ESU or sharp technique. **E,** Specimen dissection completed for removal. (From Economou SG and Economou TS: *Atlas of surgical technique,* ed 2, Philadelphia, 1996, Saunders.)

tion of the Rectum. The procedure described here is performed by one team.

The patient is positioned, prepped, and draped for an abdominal procedure. After the abdomen is entered, the surgeon determines the area of resection and mobilizes the colon with the LDS. The GI anastomosis (GIA) stapler is then used to close and transect the proximal colon. A purse-string instrument is applied around the proximal rectum, and the specimen is resected. Purse-string sutures are then placed around the proximal rectum. The operating team now changes its entire setup to operate transanally. The patient is placed in lithotomy position, prepped, and draped. The Premium circular end-to-end anastomosis (CEEA) stapler is used to perform the anastomosis. The instrument is introduced transanally and advanced to the level of the purse-string instrument. The purse-string instrument is removed, and the CEEA is allowed to protrude from the proximal rectum. The purse-string suture is tied, and the purse-string instrument is placed around the previously stapled closure line in the colon. Excess tissue protruding from the purse-string suture is excised with a knife.

The purse-string instrument is removed, and the tissue edges are grasped with Allis or Babcock clamps. The anvil of the CEEA is introduced into the proximal colon, and the purse-string suture is tied. The stapling instrument then is closed, and the staples are fired, creating a new stoma. The surgeon completes the anastomosis.

This stapling procedure is illustrated in Figure 21-26.

Appendectomy
SURGICAL GOAL
This procedure is removal of the appendix, which is a blind, narrow, elongated pouch attached to the cecum.

PATHOLOGY
The appendix is removed when acutely infected to prevent peritonitis, which will occur if it ruptures. Many surgeons perform an appendectomy as a prophylactic (preventive) procedure when operating in the abdomen for other reasons. The procedure then is called an *incidental appendectomy.*

Technique

1. The abdomen is entered.
2. The appendix is isolated from the mesoappendix.
3. The appendix is ligated and removed.
4. A purse-string suture is placed around the stump of the appendix.
5. The wound is closed.

DISCUSSION
The abdomen is entered through a McBurney's incision. The surgeon's assistant retracts the wound edges with a Richardson or similar retractor (Figure 21-27, *A*). The surgeon grasps the appendix with Babcock clamps and delivers it into

the wound site. The surgeon then may grasp and hold up the tip of the appendix with a Babcock, Mayo, or Kelly clamp. A moist lap sponge is placed around the base of the appendix to prevent contamination of the wound with bowel contents, in case any spill out during the procedure.

During an appendectomy or other bowel procedure, all instruments that come into contact with the inner surface of the bowel must be isolated from other clean instruments, drapes, and equipment. The scrub must have a square pan or kidney basin designated as "dirty" to receive the contaminated instruments and specimen. This pan can be kept on the back table and brought up to the Mayo stand when needed.

The surgeon isolates the appendix from its attachments to the bowel (mesoappendix) (Figure 21-27, *B*). Using Metzenbaum scissors, the surgeon makes a small hole in a vascular area of the mesoappendix near its base. The surgeon double clamps the mesoappendix and ligates it with free ties of 3-0 silk or absorbable suture and continues this process until the appendix is completely mobilized.

The surgeon grasps the base of the appendix with a straight Kelly clamp. The scrub should have a free tie for the base and a purse-string suture available. The base tie usually is size 0 and can be any of a variety of materials, depending on the surgeon's preference. The purse-string suture should be silk or cotton, size 3-0 or 4-0, on a fine taper needle. The surgeon ligates the base of the appendix. The assistant then places a straight Kelly clamp close to the knot, and the surgeon cuts the suture ends directly above the clamp.

The appendix is now ready for amputation, and the scrub should bring up the "dirty" pan. The purse-string suture is placed around the appendix stump. Using the knife, the surgeon amputates the appendix and delivers it into the "dirty" pan (Figure 21-27, *C*). The assistant then pushes the appendix stump against the cecum while the surgeon ties the purse-string suture. The stump is thus buried (Figure 21-27, *D*). The straight clamp is withdrawn and discarded into the dirty pan. The wound is irrigated with warm saline solution, and the abdomen is closed in routine fashion.

Laparoscopic Appendectomy
SURGICAL GOAL
To remove an inflamed appendix via laparoscopic technique to prevent its rupture in the abdominal cavity.

PATHOLOGY
The appendix is a small, blind pouch arising from the cecum near the junction of the terminal ileum (small intestine) and the proximal large intestine (cecum). Acute *confirmed* inflammation of the appendix is treated surgically by removal.

Technique

1. Pneumoperitoneum is established.
2. Trocars and cannulas are placed.
3. The appendix is divided from the mesoappendix.

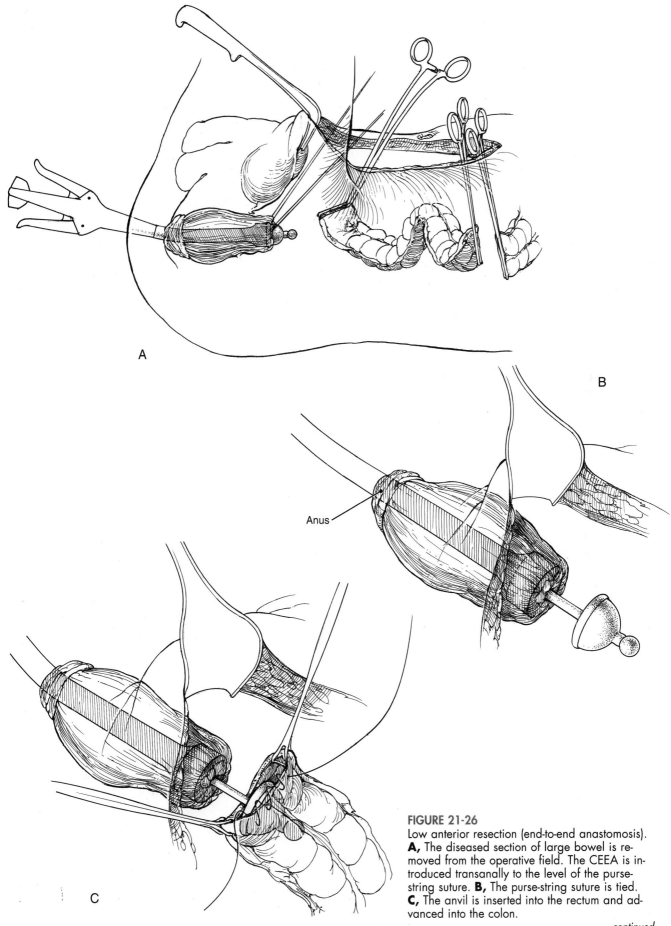

Anus

FIGURE 21-26
Low anterior resection (end-to-end anastomosis).
A, The diseased section of large bowel is removed from the operative field. The CEEA is introduced transanally to the level of the purse-string suture. **B,** The purse-string suture is tied.
C, The anvil is inserted into the rectum and advanced into the colon.

continued

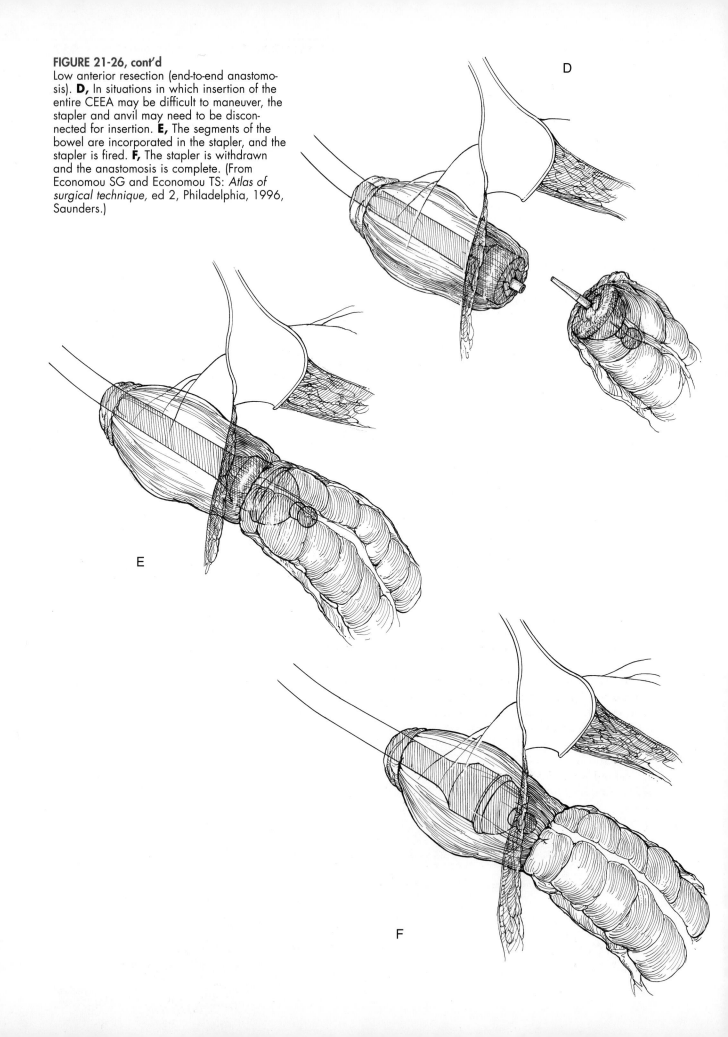

FIGURE 21-26, cont'd
Low anterior resection (end-to-end anastomosis). **D,** In situations in which insertion of the entire CEEA may be difficult to maneuver, the stapler and anvil may need to be disconnected for insertion. **E,** The segments of the bowel are incorporated in the stapler, and the stapler is fired. **F,** The stapler is withdrawn and the anastomosis is complete. (From Economou SG and Economou TS: *Atlas of surgical technique,* ed 2, Philadelphia, 1996, Saunders.)

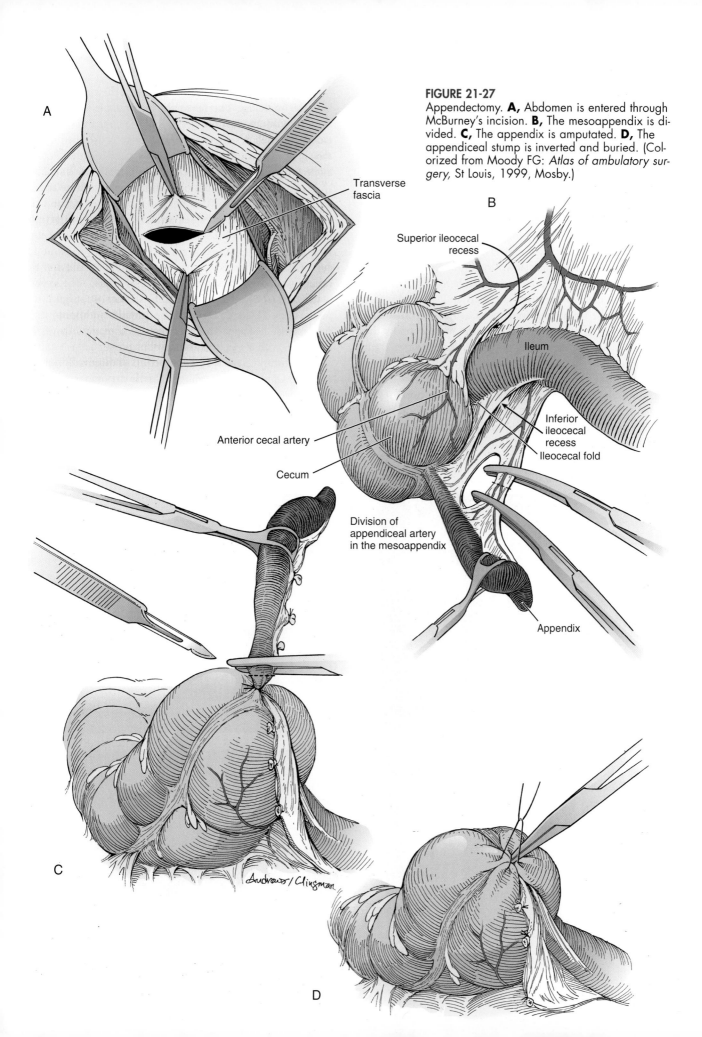

A

Transverse
fascia

FIGURE 21-27
Appendectomy. **A,** Abdomen is entered through
McBurney's incision. **B,** The mesoappendix is divided. **C,** The appendix is amputated. **D,** The
appendiceal stump is inverted and buried. (Colorized from Moody FG: *Atlas of ambulatory surgery,* St Louis, 1999, Mosby.)

B

Superior ileocecal
recess

Ileum

Inferior
ileocecal
recess
Ileocecal fold

Anterior cecal artery

Cecum

Division of
appendiceal artery
in the mesoappendix

Appendix

Andrews/Clingman

C

D

4. A ligature is placed at the base of the appendix.
5. The appendix is severed and removed through a 10-mm cannula.
6. The appendix stump is sealed.
7. Pneumoperitoneum is released, and cannulas are removed.
8. The wounds are closed.

DISCUSSION

Appendectomy is usually performed laparoscopically. Open appendectomy as discussed above is performed through a muscle-splitting McBurney (lower right quadrant) incision. The laparoscopic procedure is presented here.

A pneumoperitoneum is established and 10-mm trocar placed near the umbilicus. In cases of acute appendicitis, a second, larger trocar is inserted into the midline below the suprapubic line. A third port is placed in the upper right quadrant.

The patient is placed in Trendelenburg position so the intestines are displaced caudally (toward the head). The surgeon then locates the appendix by systematically moving aside the large intestine with an atraumatic endoscopic grasper such as a Babcock clamp until the cecum is found.

After inspecting the abdominal cavity, the surgeon mobilizes the appendix. The tip of the appendix is retracted upward to produce traction. Recall that the large intestine is attached to the mesentery. The appendix is attached to the *mesoappendix*, which is divided with scissors or the ESU and ligated with vessel clips or a surgical stapler (Figure 21-28, *A*).

When the appendix has been mobilized, it can be amputated from the cecum. Two ties must be placed around the appendix between the lines of amputation. One of the technical goals is to prevent spillage of bowel or appendiceal contents when the appendix is severed, so the ties must be secure. One tie is placed at the base of the appendix and the other just above (distal) to it (Figure 21-28, *B*). The appendix then is transected with the ESU, scissors, or surgical stapler (Figure 21-28, *C*). The stapler provides additional security against leakage. The specimen is brought out of the abdomen with a specimen retrieval bag.

The stump of the severed appendix traditionally was always inverted into the cecum. This is no longer routinely performed unless the appendix is extremely engorged or gangrenous. If necessary, the stump is pushed down into the cecum and a purse-string suture is placed around the invagination (area of inversion). This is done to contain the stump and prevent contamination in the abdominal cavity.

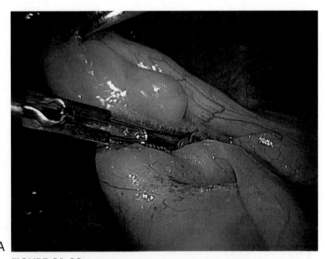

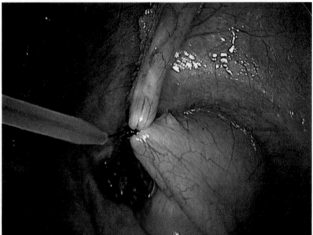

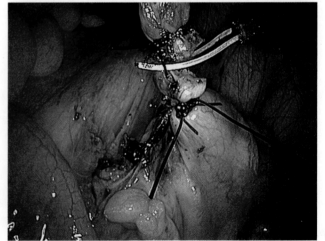

FIGURE 21-28
Laparoscopic appendectomy. **A,** The base of the mesoappendix is coagulated using the endocoagulator. **B,** The endo-loop is tightened at the base of the appendix. **C,** The appendix is excised with scissors. (From Goldberg JM and Falcone T: *Atlas of endoscopic techniques in gynecology,* Philadelphia, 2001, Saunders.)

If there are signs of contamination, the surgeon cultures free abdominal fluid.

The abdomen is irrigated with antibacterial solution, and the pneumoperitoneum is released. A soft rubber drain may be placed if there is a risk of postoperative infection or excessive drainage.

Subtotal Gastrectomy (Open Procedure)

SURGICAL GOAL
In subtotal gastrectomy, a diseased portion of the stomach is removed and the remaining portion anastomosed to a portion of the intestinal tract.

PATHOLOGY
Subtotal gastrectomy usually is performed to treat a malignant gastric tumor or chronic ulceration.

Technique

1. A laparotomy is performed through an upper right or midline incision.
2. The surgeon explores the abdomen for signs of metastasis and selects the area of gastric resection and intestinal anastomosis.
3. The surgeon mobilizes the stomach by surgically separating it from the omentum. A tunnel is made in the omentum with scissors, and small bleeding vessels are sealed with the ESU.
4. Bleeders may be double clamped with Mayo or Crile clamps; the tissue is divided with scissors, and each cut end of the vessel is tied with fine suture.
5. The gastrohepatic ligament is identified and divided. Bleeding is controlled with the ESU. Large vessels of the stomach are transected and secured with silk ties or ligation clamps.
6. Two common options for establishing GI continuity are gastroduodenostomy (further described in the Billroth I procedure) and gastrojejunostomy (further described in the Billroth II procedure). In both cases a section of the stomach is reattached (anastomosed) to the intestine.
7. The duodenum or jejunum is mobilized from the omentum.
8. The intestine is cross-clamped with two intestinal clamps, and the tissue is divided into two sections. The surgeon performs a two-layer closure on the intestinal stump.
9. A surgical stapling device may used to simultaneously clamp and divide the intestine.
10. The stomach is double clamped and divided. The open stomach edges are sutured or stapled together if surgical staples are used; the anastomosis is over-sewn with fine sutures.
11. The stomach is anastomosed to the duodenum or jejunum. Sutures, staples, or both may be used.
12. The abdomen is irrigated with topical antibacterial solution.
13. The wound is closed in layers.

DISCUSSION
Subtotal gastrectomy requires reconstruction of the GI tract. Many different methods can be used to anastomose the stomach to the intestine. The gastric pouch (remainder of the stomach after resection) can be attached along the longitudinal axis of the intestine, or the cut end of the intestine can be attached directly into the stomach. Billroth I and Billroth II techniques are very similar regardless of the site of anastomosis.

A laparotomy is performed through an upper midline or paramedian incision. The surgeon examines the abdominal contents to determine the extent of disease and to select a site for anastomosis. After the exact lines of resection are determined, the surgeon mobilizes the stomach from the ligaments, vessels, and omentum that attach to the greater and lesser curvature of the stomach. The scrub should be prepared with many Mayo, Crile, or Kelly clamps; vessel clips; and silk ties for double clamping and dividing of the omentum. Additional ties of 2-0 or 3-0 absorbable sutures usually are required. Suture ligatures are used on the major vessels of the stomach and omentum.

The surgeon begins mobilization by grasping the surface of the stomach with Allis or Babcock clamps. The assistant offers traction on these instruments. The surgeon begins dissecting the attachments to the greater curvature of the stomach. After double clamping the segments of omentum, the surgeon divides the tissue with dissecting scissors or the ESU.

A surgical stapling instrument can be used to simultaneously staple and sever the tissue. The surgeon then ties, clamps, or seals each section. The lesser curvature of the stomach is mobilized in the same manner (Figure 21-29, *A*).

When the stomach has been mobilized, the surgeon places two intestinal cross-clamps (Kocher or Allen type) side by side across the duodenum (or jejunum for Billroth II). The surgeon divides the duodenum from the stomach by cutting between the two clamps with the knife or ESU. The duodenal or jejunal stump is closed with a stapling instrument or fine running sutures. The stomach is double cross clamped with Payr clamps and divided. This results in resection of a portion of the stomach and part or most of the duodenum (Figure 21-29, *A*). A stapling instrument also can be used to cut and seal the sections.

Two techniques commonly used are to anastomose the remaining stomach on a longitudinal axis with the intestine, or to insert the severed portion of the intestine directly into the distal stomach (Figure 21-29, *B*). Although stapling instruments usually are used, the scrub should be familiar with traditional two-layer closure of the intestine and stomach using sutures. This technique is used to anastomose stomach to intestine or intestine to intestine.

Suture Technique for Gastrointestinal Anastomosis
Recall that the intestine and stomach are made up of separate tissue layers, including the outer serosa, smooth muscle, submucosa, and mucosa. To join two sections of intestine or stomach together with sutures, one must create the anastomosis with two lines of suture. The inside suture line picks up the mucosa, submucosa, and muscle layers. The serosa layers of both structures are joined separately. An absorbable suture traditionally has been used for the inner closure, and fine absorbable or nonabsorbable interrupted sutures have been used for the mucosa. Intestinal anastomosis suture techniques are based on the preferences and training of individual surgeons.

To begin the anastomosis, the surgeon brings the cross-clamped sections close together. A traction suture is placed

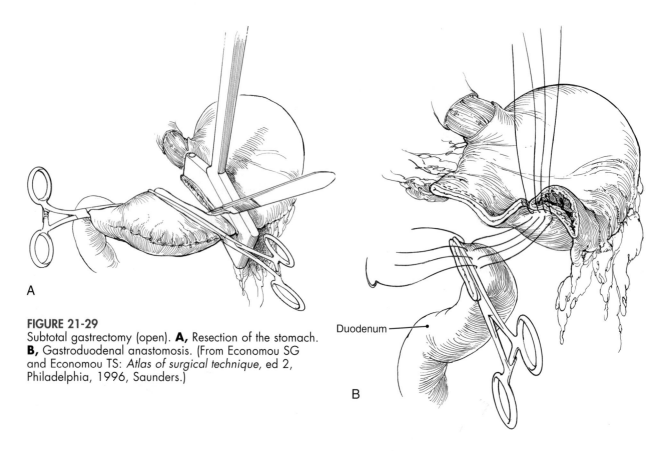

A

FIGURE 21-29
Subtotal gastrectomy (open). **A,** Resection of the stomach. **B,** Gastroduodenal anastomosis. (From Economou SG and Economou TS: *Atlas of surgical technique,* ed 2, Philadelphia, 1996, Saunders.)

Duodenum

B

at each end. An outer row of sutures is placed, joining the two tissue sections together. Next the surgeon makes two cuts, one on each side of the suture line. This exposes the inner lumen of the intestine (or stomach). The surgeon brings the inner layers together with continuous running or interrupted sutures. Finally the outer layer is completed circumferentially with interrupted sutures. The double layer of sutures prevents leakage, which is a postoperative difficulty after anastomosis. Refer to Figure 21-17, *A-D.*

Before closing of the surgical wound, the abdomen is irrigated with antibacterial solution. A wound drain may be placed in the abdomen if there is risk of postoperative infection or leaking from the anastomosis sites. A nasogastric tube may be placed by anesthesia, and air may be delivered through the tube to check for air bubbles, which would suggest leakage.

Gastroduodenostomy (Billroth II Operation)
SURGICAL GOAL
In this procedure, a portion of the stomach is removed and a new opening is created between the stomach and jejunum. The name "Billroth II" refers to the anastomosis sites.

Technique
1. The abdomen is entered.
2. The stomach is mobilized.
3. The duodenum is closed and divided.
4. The stomach is divided.
5. The gastrojejunostomy is created.
6. The wound is closed.

DISCUSSION
The patient is positioned, prepped, and draped for an abdominal incision. After the abdomen is entered, the surgeon mobilizes the stomach using the LDS instrument. Two staples automatically ligate the tissue, and the instrument's knife blade divides the tissue between the staples.

The duodenum is closed with the TA 55 instrument stapler. Before removing the instrument, the surgeon places a bowel clamp across the specimen side of the duodenum. The surgeon then divides the duodenum with the knife. The gastric pouch (the portion of the stomach that will remain functional after the surgery) is closed with the TA 90 stapler. The surgeon places a clamp across the stomach on the specimen side. The surgeon then divides the stomach between the TA 90 stapler and the clamp.

In preparation for the gastrojejunostomy, the surgeon makes two stab wounds (small incisions), one in the stomach and one in the jejunum. These wounds will be the sites of entry for the GIA instrument forks. The GIA is inserted into the stab wounds, and the staples are fired. Two double-staggered rows of staples join the two organs simultaneously, and the knife blade in the instrument cuts between the two double staple lines. This creates the new opening between the two organs. To close the stab wounds, the surgeon places several traction sutures at the edges of the wounds and trims away excess tissue. The stab wounds are then closed with the TA 55 instrument. The surgeon completes the anastomosis.

This stapling procedure is illustrated in Figure 21-30.

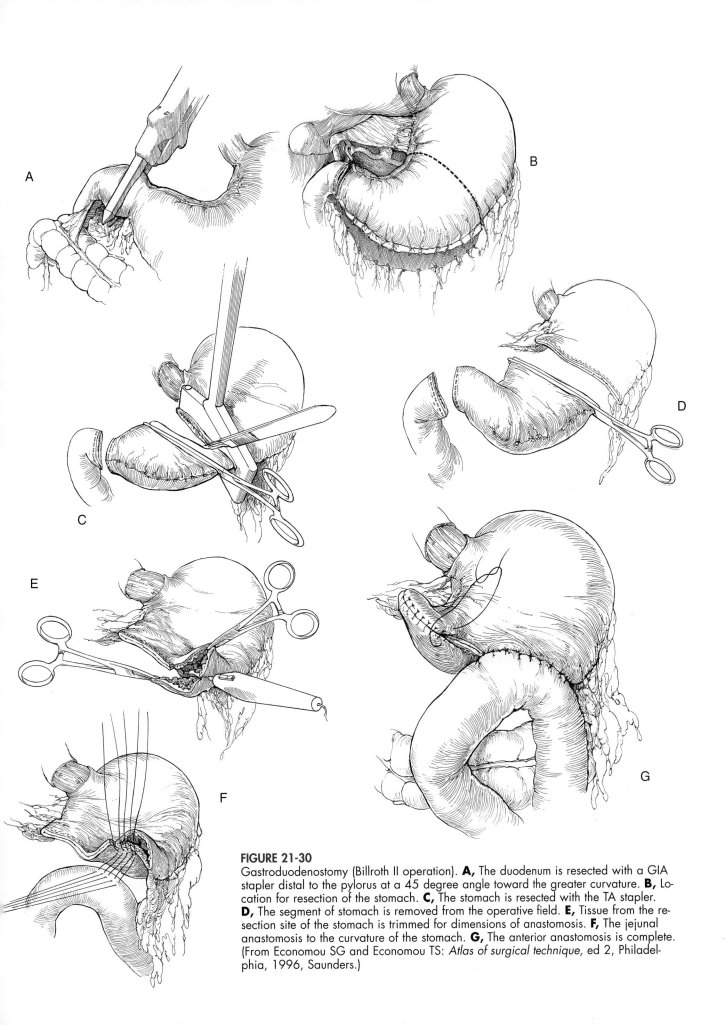

FIGURE 21-30
Gastroduodenostomy (Billroth II operation). **A,** The duodenum is resected with a GIA stapler distal to the pylorus at a 45 degree angle toward the greater curvature. **B,** Location for resection of the stomach. **C,** The stomach is resected with the TA stapler. **D,** The segment of stomach is removed from the operative field. **E,** Tissue from the resection site of the stomach is trimmed for dimensions of anastomosis. **F,** The jejunal anastomosis to the curvature of the stomach. **G,** The anterior anastomosis is complete. (From Economou SG and Economou TS: *Atlas of surgical technique,* ed 2, Philadelphia, 1996, Saunders.)

Partial Gastrectomy with Gastroduodenostomy

SURGICAL GOAL

In this procedure, part of the stomach is removed and a new opening is created between the stomach and duodenum.

PATHOLOGY

Partial gastrectomy is performed for chronic gastric ulcer, perforating ulcer, and tumor.

Technique

1. The abdomen is entered.
2. The stomach is mobilized.
3. The duodenum is mobilized.
4. The duodenum is divided and closed.
5. The stomach is anastomosed to the duodenum.
6. The wound is closed.

DISCUSSION

The surgeon enters the abdomen through an upper midline incision and examines the abdominal contents to determine the extent of disease and to choose a site for anastomosis. After determining the exact line of anastomosis, the surgeon mobilizes the stomach from the ligaments, vessels, and omentum that attach to the greater and lesser curvature of the stomach. The scrub must be ready with many Mayo clamps, Metzenbaum scissors, and silk ties, sizes 2-0 and 3-0. Additional ties of absorbable suture such as 2-0 and 3-0 Vicryl or Dexon and one or two suture ligatures of silk mounted on fine tapered needles also should be available. The suture ligatures will be used to ligate the large vessels of the stomach.

The surgeon begins mobilization by grasping the surface of the stomach with Allis or Babcock clamps. The assistant offers traction on these instruments. The surgeon begins dissecting the attachments to the greater curvature. The surgeon places two Mayo clamps for each small segment of tissue to be divided. After double clamping the segments, the surgeon divides the tissue between the clamps with Metzenbaum scissors or the cautery pencil. Each section is then tied with silk or Dexon sutures. The lesser curvature of the stomach is divided from its attachments in a similar fashion.

When the stomach has been mobilized, the surgeon resects the duodenum from the stomach. The surgeon places two intestinal clamps, such as Kocher or Allen-Kocher clamps, across the duodenum. The surgeon divides the duodenum from the stomach by cutting between the two clamps with a scalpel or cautery pencil.

The duodenal stump next is closed. A running suture of silk, chromic gut, Vicryl, or Dexon on a fine tapered needle is used to close the stump.

To begin the gastroduodenal anastomosis, the surgeon aligns the stomach and duodenum at the proposed junction site. Silk traction sutures are placed at each end of the site to hold the stomach and duodenum in alignment. The surgeon uses a continuous or interrupted suture swaged on a fine tapered needle, size 3-0 or 4-0, to form the first row of sutures.

At the completion of this row, the surgeon makes two incisions, one on each side of the suture line. This exposes the inner surfaces of the stomach and duodenum; they are then joined with fine interrupted sutures. The wound is then irrigated and closed in routine fashion.

RELATED PROCEDURES

▶ Gastrojejunostomy
▶ Esophagogastrostomy

Esophagogastrectomy

SURGICAL GOAL

In this procedure, the lower esophagus and upper stomach (fundus) are resected.

Technique

1. The abdomen is entered.
2. The distal esophagus is mobilized.
3. The fundus is stapled.
4. A gastrotomy is performed.
5. The distal esophagus and stomach are anastomosed.
6. The wound is closed.

DISCUSSION

The patient is prepped and draped for an abdominal incision. After incising the abdomen, the surgeon mobilizes the distal esophagus and proximal stomach using the LDS stapler to ligate and divide the omental vessels. The gastric fundus is stapled with two applications of the TA 90. The surgeon then divides the stomach between the two double staple lines with the scalpel.

The GIA stapler is used to incise the stomach and produce hemostasis of the cut edges. To do this, the surgeon makes a stab wound in the gastric wall at the level of the gastrotomy. He or she inserts the anvil fork of the GIA stapler into the lumen of the stomach and places the cartridge fork on the serosal surface. The instrument is then closed, and the staples are fired.

To begin the anastomosis between the stomach and esophagus, the surgeon grasps the proximal stomach with Allis clamps. He or she then applies a purse-string suture to this area, using the purse-string instrument. The EEA stapler is used to create the anastomosis. This is introduced, without the anvil, into the gastric incision. The purse-string instrument is removed, and the center rod is passed through the gastric wall. The surgeon then ties the purse-string suture and places the anvil on the center rod.

The purse-string instrument is placed around the esophagus just above the areas of transection. A purse-string suture is placed here, and the esophagus is incised. The purse-string instrument is removed, and the anvil is introduced into the esophagus. The surgeon then ties the purse-string suture and divides the esophagus, which releases the specimen.

To complete the anastomosis, the surgeon approximates the EEA stapler and fires the staples. The gastrotomy incision then may be closed with the TA 90. The surgeon completes the anastomosis. The wound is irrigated and closed in routine fashion.

This stapling procedure is illustrated in Figure 21-31.

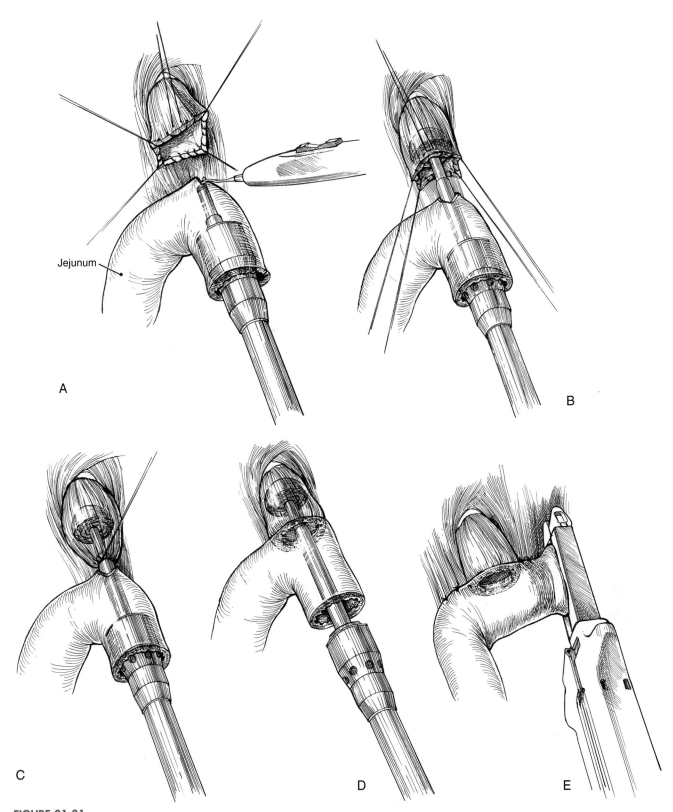

FIGURE 21-31
Esophagogastrectomy. **A,** Insertion of the EEA stapler (without the anvil) into the jejunum. **B,** The anvil is reattached and placed inside the esophagus. **C,** A purse-string suture is placed on the esophagus. The anvil and stapler are approximated and stapled. **D,** The stapler is disengaged and withdrawn. **E,** Closure of the jejunum, and the anastomosis is complete. (From Economou SG and Economou TS: *Atlas of surgical technique,* ed 2, Philadelphia, 1996, Saunders.)

Esophagectomy with Esophagogastrotomy

SURGICAL GOAL

In this procedure, a diseased portion of the esophagus and/or proximal stomach is surgically removed.

PATHOLOGY

These procedures are performed to remove portions of the esophagus that are cancerous or to remove strictures found in the esophagus. Strictures may form after trauma or infection.

Technique

1. This procedure can be performed with the patient in either a supine or lateral position. This example will use the supine position. The differences in the lateral position will be noted in the discussion.
2. This procedure uses two incision sites. The first is a midline incision from the base of the xyphoid process to 2 cm below the umbilicus. The second is over the inner border of the sternocleidomastoid muscle. The second incision is made after all the abdominal dissection is complete.
3. Upon entering the peritoneal cavity, the surgeon examines the internal contents and organs for any abnormalities and then begins dissection of the stomach and esophagus.
4. The surgeon carries the dissection through the omentum and around the stomach proximally to the diaphragm using scissors, clamps, ties, and suture ligatures. The surgeon ensures that the epigastric blood vessels are not taken during dissection.
5. After the stomach and distal esophagus have been mobilized, the surgeon performs a pyloromyotomy.
6. The surgeon performs blunt, digital dissection through the diaphragm to mobilize as much as possible of the esophagus in the pleural cavity.
7. The abdominal wound is packed and covered, and the neck incision is performed.
8. Blunt and sharp dissection is performed to mobilize the proximal esophagus in the neck, and a 3/4-inch Penrose drain is passed to isolate the esophagus.
9. A GIA stapler is used to incise the esophagus in the neck, and the esophagus then is pulled through the chest down into the abdominal wound. The neck is packed.
10. The esophagus and stomach are examined for tumor, and a margin is identified.
11. The GIA stapler is used to transect the diseased portion of the stomach and esophagus from the healthy stomach. This may take several loads. The staple line is oversewn with 4-0 polypropylene.
12. The remaining portion of stomach is attached to a large Penrose drain to retain proper orientation and prevent twisting. The stomach is pulled through the chest to the neck incision.
13. The stomach is tacked into place with 3-0 silk to hold proper positioning.
14. A hole is made in the proximal end of the stomach to match the esophageal stump.
15. The surgeon performs the anastomosis using 3-0 interrupted Vicryl sutures.
16. The anastomosis is examined for leaks, and the abdomen and neck are closed in layers.

DISCUSSION

The abdominal incision is maintained with two retraction systems. A standard Balfour retractor is used for the wound edges (a deep-blade Balfour should be available for larger patients). The second is an upper–self-retaining retractor system for the liver and diaphragm. The liver will require a narrow to broad malleable blade and a Balfour abdominal-wall blade for the left side of the abdominal wall.

Most of the dissection in the abdomen is performed with clamps, suture ties, suture ligatures, electrocautery, and scissors under direct visualization. When the surgeon dissects the esophagus in the pleural cavity, however, it is performed by blind, blunt sweep and feel, maintaining a vigilant eye for excess blood loss.

After the esophagus is passed to the abdomen, a "Saratoga sump drain" is passed into the pleural cavity through the neck incision and attached to a field suction line. This drain will be monitored for blood loss. The amount of blood loss will determine whether the surgeon places a left chest tube for postoperative drainage.

The Saratoga sump also will be used to bring the large Penrose drain through the chest cavity to help with orientation of the stomach as it is passed to the neck.

The resection of the stomach using the GIA stapler usually takes three to four loads. The staple line is then oversewn with 4-0 polypropylene suture to reinforce the staple line and prevent leaks.

After the pyloromyotomy release, the surgeon determines whether the patient will require a feeding tube after surgery. If so, the tube is placed and brought out through a stab wound to the left of the abdominal incision.

Any mesenteric defects are closed with 2-0 silk sutures. If necessary, the surgeon can reinforce the diaphragm with #1 silk sutures, making sure *not* to cause obstruction.

The abdomen is closed before the anastomosis is performed in the neck and after the surgeon performs a final inspection of the internal organs and tissues. The surgeon uses #1 interrupted Vicryl, followed by skin staples. The scrub should perform a count at this time.

After the abdomen is closed, the upper hand retractor arms are disconnected and removed from the field, as well as the brackets holding them to the table. The abdomen is covered with a towel.

The anastomosis is started in the neck. The surgeon prepares the proximal stomach by making a hole that closely matches the esophageal stump. The surgeon uses 3-0 interrupted Vicryl sutures for the anastomosis. Each stitch is tagged with a mosquito hemostat until tied to avoid rotation of the anastomosis.

Lateral Position

Both approaches require longer instruments.

Both positions require measures to maintain the patient's body temperature. This can be achieved with fluid warmers and warming blankets.

The lateral approach uses a thoracoabdominal incision in the left side of the chest. This approach includes a resection of the seventh, eighth, or ninth rib or the separation of the two appropriate ribs.

Sponge sticks, both straight and curved, are used in both procedures.

The diaphragm is opened in the lateral approach, and traction sutures are placed to improve visualization. The diaphragm is reapproximated after the lesion has been removed and the anastomosis has been finished. Interrupted, nonabsorbable 3-0 or 2-0 sutures are used.

The lateral approach allows for complete and direct visualization of the esophagus during the procedure. This enables the surgeon to deal with any blood loss immediately and directly. Compared with the midline incision, however, the thoracoabdominal incision is very painful for the patient.

Banded Gastroplasty
SURGICAL GOAL
During banded gastroplasty, most of the stomach and a portion of the small intestine are bypassed to reduce nutrient absorption and cause severe weight loss.

PATHOLOGY
Morbid obesity is a condition in which the patient is at least 100 pounds above his or her normal weight, in spite of efforts to reduce. Obesity is a major health problem in the United States and contributes to cardiovascular disease, cancers of the breast and large intestine, diabetes, stroke, urinary stress incontinence, and depression.

Society regards morbid obesity as a moral failure in the patient and does not recognize the genetic causes of the disease. The social stigma of morbid obesity prevents the patient from enjoying the freedom and full life available to others. Two effective and relatively safe surgical procedures for morbid obesity are *vertical gastric banding* and *Roux-en-Y gastric bypass*.

Technique

1. The tissues overlying the gastroesophageal junction are dissected.
2. A space is created between the stomach and the bands of tissue surrounding the esophagus at the diaphragm (the crus).
3. A 3-mm space is mobilized along the lesser curve of the stomach.
4. A small incision is made in the anterior gastric wall, and a circular stapling device is inserted through the stomach. A stapled hole is then made in the stomach.
5. A gastric bougie is passed into the stomach via the esophagus.
6. A linear surgical stapler is placed through the gastric window, creating a separation between the lesser curvature of the stomach and the fundus, near the cardioesophageal junction.
7. A strip of polypropylene is brought through the circular stapled hole and wrapped around the stomach. Interrupted sutures secure the strip to the stomach and connect the two ends of the strip.
8. The staple lines may be tested with an infusion of methylene blue dye into the esophagus.
9. Pneumoperitoneum is released, and the incisions are closed with synthetic absorbable sutures and skin staples or suture.

DISCUSSION
Banded pyloroplasty creates a 5-mm pouch that holds a small amount of food. The stomach remains functional, but the patient experiences gastric fullness after eating very little food. An adjustable polypropylene band also may be used in place of the polypropylene strip.

A pneumoperitoneum is established, with trocars placed at the xyphoid, periumbilicus, and bilateral subcostal regions. The surgeon retracts the liver upward and uses an ESU hook and tissue scissors to dissect the attachments to the esophagus free. The surgeon mobilizes the esophagus to identify the cardioesophageal junction (Figure 21-32, *A*).

A 3-mm section of the lesser curvature of the stomach is mobilized, and an esophageal bougie (flexible rod) is inserted into the stomach by mouth. A 28-mm surgical stapling anvil is inserted through the left abdominal cannula. The surgeon pushes the anvil through the stomach, creating a hole. The circular stapling device is attached to the handle and fired. This creates a stapled hole through the stomach wall (Figure 21-32, *B*).

The surgeon creates the stomach pouch with a linear surgical stapler (Figure 21-32, *C*). The device is inserted through the stapled hole and placed across the fundus of the stomach. This places a double row of staples without cutting through the fundus.

A 1.5-mm to 6-mm polypropylene band is then inserted into the abdomen and placed through the stapled circle, encircling the stomach (Figure 21-32, D). The esophageal bougie is withdrawn. The surgeon may test the staple lines by instilling methylene blue dye into the stomach pouch.

The wound is irrigated with warm saline solution, the pneumoperitoneum is released, and the incisions are closed.

Roux-en-Y Gastric Bypass
SURGICAL GOAL
The Roux-en-Y procedure is performed to bypass the stomach and reestablish continuity from the stomach to the jejunum. In this procedure, a large portion of the stomach is bypassed and a new gastric pouch is created. The anastomosis between the pouch and the jejunum substantially reduces the amount of food absorbed by the patient's GI system.

PATHOLOGY
This procedure traditionally has been performed to treat gastric ulcer, dumping syndrome, and tumor. It also is currently used to treat morbid obesity.

Technique

1. The abdomen is entered.
2. The gastric pouch is created.
3. The jejunum is transected.
4. A gastrojejunostomy is created.
5. A jejunojejunostomy (Roux-en-Y anastomosis) is performed.
6. The wound is closed.

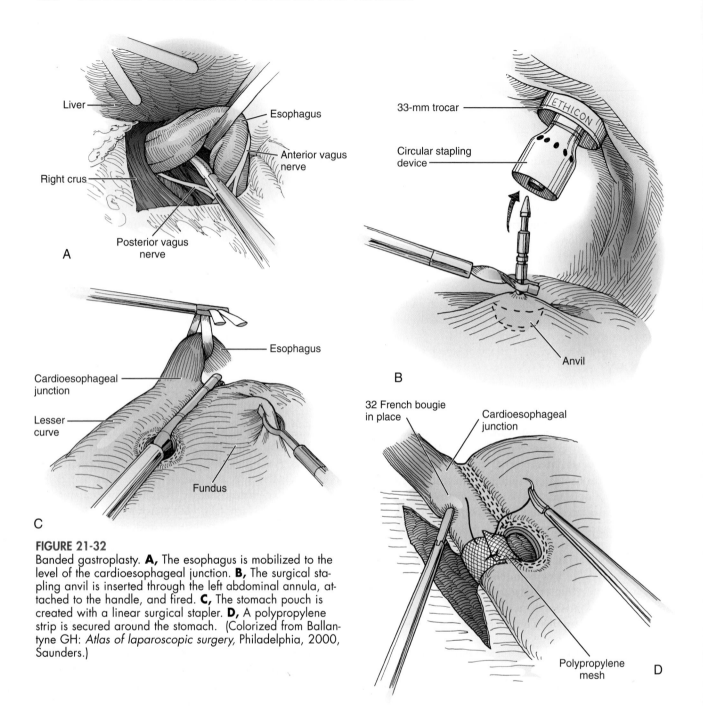

FIGURE 21-32
Banded gastroplasty. **A,** The esophagus is mobilized to the level of the cardioesophageal junction. **B,** The surgical stapling anvil is inserted through the left abdominal annula, attached to the handle, and fired. **C,** The stomach pouch is created with a linear surgical stapler. **D,** A polypropylene strip is secured around the stomach. (Colorized from Ballantyne GH: *Atlas of laparoscopic surgery,* Philadelphia, 2000, Saunders.)

DISCUSSION

The patient is positioned, prepped, and draped for an abdominal incision. After entering the abdomen, the surgeon makes a small hole in the lesser omentum at the level of the proposed partition. The TA 90 stapler is placed across the stomach at the partition site, and the staples are fired. The GIA is used to close and transect the jejunum.

To create a new opening between the jejunum and the stomach, the surgeon makes two stab wounds to accommodate the forks of the GIA. The GIA is inserted into the stab wounds, and the staples are fired. Silk sutures may be used to close the stab wounds. The Roux-en-Y (jejunojejunostomy) anastomosis is performed with the GIA instrument. The common opening between the two portions of jejunum is then closed with the TA 55. The wound is irrigated and closed in routine fashion.

This stapling procedure is illustrated in Figure 21-33.

Gastrostomy
SURGICAL GOAL

To insert a catheter or tube through the outer abdominal wall into the stomach.

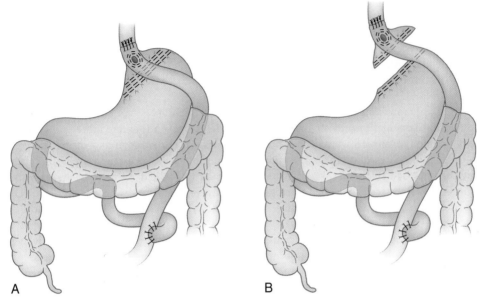

FIGURE 21-33
Roux-en-Y gastric bypass. **A,** The proximal gastric pouch and distal stomach are stapled in continuity. **B,** The proximal gastric pouch and distal stomach are stapled and divided. (Colorized from Townsend CM: *Sabiston textbook of surgery,* ed 16, Philadelphia, 2001, Saunders.)

PATHOLOGY

Gastrostomy is usually performed in patients:

▶ With esophageal disease, trauma, stricture, or esophagectomy (surgical removal of the esophagus).
▶ Who require continuous gastric decompression (removal of stomach contents).
▶ Who are at high risk for aspiration of food into the upper respiratory tract because of alteration in consciousness or loss of protective gag and cough reflexes.

Tube feeding is possible with a **nasogastric (NG)** tube (a flexible tube inserted through the nare and into the stomach to drain it or for feeding purposes). The NG tube is uncomfortable and even painful. Long-term direct GI feeding or decompression (deflation and constant suction) requires a more humane approach to feeding. The enterostomy tube provides an alternative.

Technique

1. A small (5-mm) upper midline or left upper paramedian incision is made through all layers of the abdominal wall. Bleeding is controlled with sponges and the ESU.
2. The anterior fundus of the stomach is picked up with two more atraumatic grasping clamps (Babcock or Allis). Traction sutures may be inserted through the stomach wall to replace the clamps.
3. A purse-string suture is placed in the stomach wall at the location where the tube will be inserted.
4. The stomach is perforated with the ESU within the purse-string suture.
5. The stomach contents are immediately suctioned.
6. Small bleeding vessels in the stomach mucosa are coagulated with the ESU.

7. The stomach catheter is inserted into the perforation, the pursestring suture is tied, and a second purse-string suture is placed around the catheter.
8. The abdominal wall is secured to the stomach wall with sutures.
9. A second incision is made in the abdominal wall, and the catheter tip is brought out through this incision.
10. The catheter is secured to the skin, and dressings are applied.

DISCUSSION

Open gastrostomy often is performed at the patient's bedside or in an endoscopic clinic with local filtration anesthetic. When performed with endoscopic assistance, the procedure usually takes place in the GI clinic and is called a PEG or percutaneous (through the skin) endoscopic gastrostomy. Duodenostomy and jejunostomy are similar procedures in which the feeding tube is inserted directly into these portions of the small intestine. When performed in the operating room, gastrostomy is usually part of a more complex procedure of the GI system.

Tubes used for open gastrostomy include the Malecot, Pezzer (also called mushroom catheters), or balloon catheter similar to the Foley catheter.

The surgeon enters the abdomen through a short, left upper paramedian incision. The assistant retracts the wound edges with right-angle retractors while the surgeon identifies and grasps the stomach with two Babcock or Allis clamps. The surgeon brings a portion of the stomach into view through the incision.

If used, traction sutures are placed at this time. Two separate nonabsorbable sutures are placed through the stomach wall, and the ends are used to hold up (elevate) the stomach wall and hold it taut. When traction sutures are used, the clamps are removed.

A purse-string suture is placed through all layers of the stomach where the tube will be inserted. The surgeon makes a small perforation in the center of the purse-string suture with the ESU (Figure 21-34, *A*).

The scrub should have suction immediately available as soon as the gastric incision is made, to prevent the highly acidic fluid from spilling into the surgical wound.

The feeding tube is then placed through the perforation, and the purse-string suture is tied (Figure 21-34, *B*). A second purse-string suture may be placed for added strength. The stomach is then sutured to the abdominal wall at the entry site.

The catheter tip is grasped with a large clamp such as a Péan and pulled to the outside of the body through a second small incision. The tube is secured to the skin with sutures, and dressings are applied.

Pyloromyotomy

SURGICAL GOAL
This procedure is an incision made into the pylorus to release a stenosis. Pyloromyotomy is performed to allow ingested food to pass easily into the duodenum.

PATHOLOGY
Pyloric stenosis is a congenital defect in which the muscle fibers of the structure are hypertrophied (enlarged) and form fibrous bands, causing a stricture (stenosis) within the pylorus.

DISCUSSION
The abdomen is entered through a right upper paramedian incision. The surgeon may insert a baby Balfour retractor or may have the assistant retract the abdominal walls with small hand-held retractors. The pylorus is identified. The surgeon then makes an incision into the pylorus, over the defect, with a #10 or #15 scalpel blade. The surgeon maintains hemostasis with the electrocautery pencil on a very low setting. The incision is deepened with a fine Kelly clamp. Using Metzenbaum scissors, the surgeon incises the circular muscle fibers to the depth of the inner mucosa, thus releasing the stricture. The incisions are not sutured but are left to heal in their newly released position.

The wound is closed in routine fashion with fine sutures.

Vagotomy
SURGICAL GOAL
Vagotomy is performed to reduce the release of gastric juices by severing the nerves that control their release.

PATHOLOGY
Vagotomy is selective occlusion of portions of the vagus nerve as it branches over the stomach. This interrupts nerve transmission and reduces acidic secretions. Selective disruption of the vagus nerve traditionally has been used to halt the

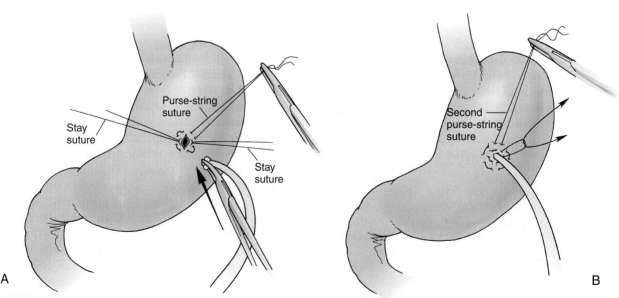

FIGURE 21-34
Gastrostomy. **A,** A purse-string suture is placed in the stomach with traction sutures. A small incision is made in the stomach wall, and the catheter is inserted. **B,** A second purse-string suture is applied and tied. (Colorized from Moody FG: *Atlas of ambulatory surgery*, St Louis, 1999, Mosby.)

release of stomach acid and treat peptic ulcer disease. Current knowledge about the mechanism of peptic ulcer and the relationship between ulcers and *Helicobacter pylori* as a causative factor has significantly reduced the number of vagotomy operations. If the procedure is performed through a small laparotomy incision or by laparoscopy, the nerve is ligated with surgical metal clips at one or more locations as it branches from the esophagus distally. This procedure is performed in conjunction with gastric resection.

Technique

1. The abdomen is entered.
2. The esophagus is mobilized.
3. The left (posterior) and right (anterior) vagus nerves are resected.
4. The wound is closed.

DISCUSSION

The abdomen already has been entered for gastric resection. The assistant exposes the esophagus as he or she retracts the liver upward using a Weinberg retractor ("Joe's hoe") or other large abdominal retractor. The operating lights are aimed upward into the wound. Using long Metzenbaum scissors and long, fine tissue forceps, the surgeon divides the esophagus from the attached peritoneal membrane. When the esophagus has been exposed completely, the surgeon retracts the esophagus to the side with a long Penrose drain that has been dipped in saline solution by the scrub.

The surgeon then catches a portion of the vagus nerve with a long nerve hook. Two long right-angle clamps are placed over the nerve. The surgeon cuts the section of nerve lying between the clamps and passes the section of nerve to the scrub. The surgeon announces "right" or "left" because the scrub must keep each side separate. The scrub can do this by simply placing the specimens on the right and left sides of a small basin; however, it is always best to have a sterile marking pen on the back table to label specimens to avoid errors. The sections of nerve are sent to the pathologist to confirm that the specimens are nerve tissue. The severed edges of the nerve are then clamped with ligation clips or ligatures. The procedure is repeated on the other side of the esophagus.

The wound is closed in routine fashion.

Transabdominal Repair of Hiatal Hernia
SURGICAL GOAL

This procedure is performed to reduce a herniated stomach.

PATHOLOGY

This technique repairs a defect that occurs in the phrenoesophageal membrane attached to the esophagus at the level of the diaphragm. The defect causes the esophagus and upper stomach to slide upward into the thoracic cavity. The hiatal hernia may be approached from the thoracic cavity or the abdomen.

Technique

1. The abdomen is entered.
2. The esophagus is mobilized.
3. The hernia is reduced.
4. The hernia defect is sutured.
5. The wound is closed.

DISCUSSION

The surgeon enters the abdomen through an upper midline or left subcostal incision, with the patient in the supine position. Before beginning the hernia repair, the surgeon examines the abdominal contents for disease or conditions other than a hernia. Sometimes the patient's complaints are due not only to the hernia but also to another condition, such as cancer. When the surgeon is satisfied that the hernia is the only cause of the patient's discomfort, the procedure begins.

The assistant retracts the liver upward using a Weinberg or other large abdominal retractor, while the surgeon carefully dissects the esophagus free from its attachments to the liver. The scrub must have long right-angle clamps and small sponge dissectors available. The surgeon performs the dissection very cautiously, because the large vessels nearby could be damaged, which would cause severe bleeding that is difficult to control. Exposure of the hernia is a major technical difficulty in this procedure. As the dissection is continued, the patient may be tipped into the Trendelenburg position so that the overhead operating lights can be directed up into the wound.

When the esophagus has been mobilized, the scrub passes a long Penrose drain mounted on a right-angle clamp to the surgeon. The scrub should dip the drain in saline solution before passing it to the surgeon. The surgeon places the drain around the esophagus and clamps the ends with a Mayo clamp. The assistant then can use the drain to retract the esophagus. The surgeon pulls the herniated stomach and adherent fatty tissue downward, thus reducing the hernia. When it is reduced, the surgeon repairs the hernia defect using nonabsorbable sutures of size 2-0 on a small taper needle (Figure 21-35, *A*). Interrupted sutures are used to close the defect around the esophagus and diaphragm (Figure 21-35, *B*). The wound may be irrigated with saline before it is closed in routine fashion.

Laparoscopic Nissen Fundoplication
SURGICAL GOAL

Laparoscopic Nissen fundoplication is performed to reduce the opening into the stomach fundus for treatment of persistent gastroesophageal reflux disease (GERD).

PATHOLOGY

GERD is a condition of abnormal gastric regurgitation of gastric contents into the esophagus. Gastric juices normally are prevented from entering the esophagus because the lower esophageal sphincter has sufficient pressure to prevent

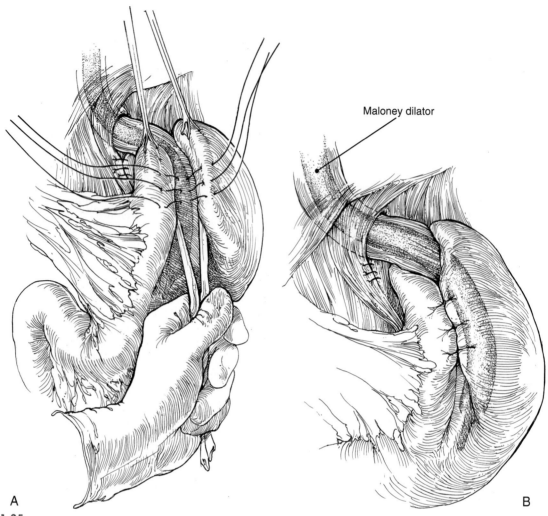

Maloney dilator

A   B

FIGURE 21-35
Transabdominal repair of hiatal hernia. **A,** The stomach is sutured around the esophagus with three to four 2-0 silk sutures.
B, Stabilization sutures are placed in the longitudinal fibers of the esophagus. (From Economou SG and Economou TS: *Atlas of surgical technique,* ed 2, Philadelphia, 1996, Saunders.)

regurgitation. In addition, the location of the lower esophageal junction as it enters the abdominal cavity creates a sphincter by the crura (bands of tissue that form a collar around the esophagus at the level of the diaphragm). Saliva clears any acidic fluids from the esophagus *as long as it can relax between episodes of swallowing.* This is called *esophageal clearing* and may not function in the patient who experiences spasmodic sphincter contractions.

A patient with GERD experiences loss of these functions because of one or a combination of factors, including hiatal hernia (herniation of the esophagus into the thoracic cavity), loss of sphincter pressure, sufficient relaxation of the sphincter, or increased abdominal pressure resulting from obesity. Improper stomach emptying and some medications also can contribute to the pathology.

GERD can result in dysphagia (difficulty in swallowing), chest pain, esophageal erosion, lung damage resulting from aspiration of stomach contents, otitis media, tooth decay, laryngitis, and esophageal cancer.

Nissen fundoplication can be performed as an open or an endoscopic procedure. The basic techniques are the same. In this procedure a portion of the stomach is wrapped around the esophagus as a collar valve to prevent reflux. This technique is called a *fundoplication.* The endoscopic procedure is described here.

Technique

1. Pneumoperitoneum is established.
2. 5-mm and 10-mm cannulas are placed.
3. If a hiatal hernia is present, the liver is retracted upward and the membrane attachment between the esophagus and liver is incised.
4. The crura (circular muscles of the diaphragm) are divided from the esophagus, and the hiatal hernia is reduced.
5. The crura are sutured near the esophagus to close the opening of the diaphragm.

6. The stomach is mobilized from the gastrosplenic ligament and gastric vessels. This creates a gastric sleeve.
7. The gastric pouch is pulled around the esophagus to form a tube and sutured in place.
8. The wound is irrigated, and the gastric tube is removed.
9. The cannulas are removed, and the pneumoperitoneum is released.
10. All trocar wounds are sutured.

DISCUSSION

The surgery is performed with the patient in low lithotomy position. This allows one of the surgeons to stand at the foot of the table for better access to the abdomen. The technologist should stand at the foot of the table at the side.

A pneumoperitoneum is established, and cannulas placed as shown in Figure 21-36, *A*. The surgeon uses 5-mm and 10-mm cannulas.

To begin the procedure, one must elevate the liver to expose the lower esophagus as it passes through the diaphragm. A liver retractor or atraumatic forceps is used to lift the liver. Next, the phrenoesophageal membrane and ligament, which adhere to the esophagus under the liver, are divided with an ESU or fine scissors (Figure 21-36, *B*). Bleeding can be controlled with the ESU. After this membrane is removed, the crura are visible. These are bands of diaphragmatic tissue that encircle the esophagus. This tissue is divided, and the esophagus is retracted downward with Babcock forceps.

The hiatus (opening in the diaphragm through which the esophagus passes) is now sutured together. Nonabsorbable sutures on a curved needle are usually used (Figure 21-36, *C*).

The surgeon next constructs a 2-cm sleeve by freeing the stomach and securing it around the esophagus. The stomach must first be mobilized from its attachments to the gastric vessels and ligaments that attach to the spleen. The tissues are ligated with surgical clips and severed with the ESU or scissors. The mobilized portion of stomach is then grasped with an atraumatic forceps and wrapped around the esophagus as shown in Figure 21-36, *D*.

The gastric tube or bougie is now passed through the esophagus and into the stomach to gauge the tightness of the gastric sleeve. With the tube in place, the stomach wrap is secured with interrupted sutures through the seromuscular layer of the esophagus and through the seromuscular layer of the stomach. This sleeve creates a valve, preventing reflux.

The sleeve is approximated with interrupted sutures on a curved needle. The gastric tube is removed, and the abdomen is irrigated with warm saline. All cannulas are removed, pneumoperitoneum is released, and wounds are closed with absorbable sutures and skin staples or sutures.

Excision of Zenker's Diverticulum
SURGICAL GOAL

Excision of an esophageal diverticulum is the removal of a weakening in the wall of the esophagus.

PATHOLOGY

The diverticulum causes small amounts of food to become trapped and causes a sensation of fullness in the neck. The diverticulum occurs primarily in the cervical region of the esophagus. Resection or excision gives complete relief of symptoms.

Technique

1. The patient is placed in a supine position with the head and neck turned and hyperextended to the patient's right.
2. The incision is made over the inner border of the sternocleidomastoid muscle, extending from the level of the hyoid bone to a point 2 cm above the clavicle.
3. A self-retaining retractor is placed to retract the thyroid medially and to retract the carotid sheath with the sternocleidomastoid muscle laterally. This exposes the diverticulum.
4. The surgeon grasps the diverticulum with a Pennington clamp to maintain control and dissects it free of surrounding tissue down to the neck.
5. The true neck of the diverticulum sac is dissected free of the surrounding muscles of the posterior wall of the pharynx.
6. The neck of the sac is ligated with chromic sutures, and the stump is invaginated into the pharyngeal wall.
7. The pharyngeal muscle opening is closed with interrupted 2-0 absorbable sutures. The skin is closed with a 4-0 absorbable subcuticular suture.

DISCUSSION

A myotomy may be performed in conjunction with this procedure because it seems to reduce the chance of recurrence. A Babcock clamp can be used if Penningtons are not available. They are less traumatic to tissue than Allis clamps.

Hemorrhoidectomy
SURGICAL GOAL

In this procedure, painful dilated veins of the anus and rectum are removed.

PATHOLOGY

Hemorrhoids are classified as *internal* (inside the rectum) or *external* (outside the rectum). Hemorrhoids are generally acquired by those whose occupations require sitting most of the day, or they may accompany pregnancy.

Technique

1. The rectum is dilated.
2. The hemorrhoid is clamped and excised.
3. The base of the vein is ligated.

DISCUSSION

The patient is placed in either the Kraske (jackknife) or the lithotomy position. Before beginning the scrub prep of the patient, the circulator tapes the patient's buttocks apart by placing 4-inch adhesive tape on each side of the anus and attaching the ends to the operating table frame. Only a

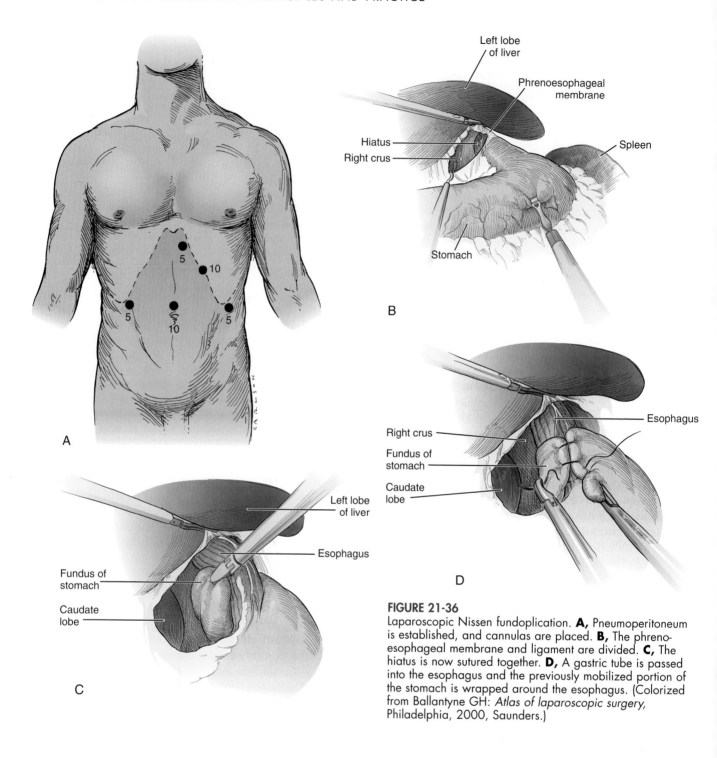

FIGURE 21-36
Laparoscopic Nissen fundoplication. **A,** Pneumoperitoneum is established, and cannulas are placed. **B,** The phreno-esophageal membrane and ligament are divided. **C,** The hiatus is now sutured together. **D,** A gastric tube is passed into the esophagus and the previously mobilized portion of the stomach is wrapped around the esophagus. (Colorized from Ballantyne GH: *Atlas of laparoscopic surgery,* Philadelphia, 2000, Saunders.)

minimal scrub prep is performed. No alcohol-based prep solution should be used if the ESU will be used.

Before beginning the operative procedure, many surgeons perform a sigmoidoscopy. After the internal examination, the surgeon dilates the rectum with his fingers and places a rectal dilator (Figure 21-37, *A*). This step is performed slowly because the musculature can be severely damaged if the dilation is hurried. After satisfactory dilation, the surgeon inserts a rectal speculum. The scrub may be required to hold the speculum in place. The hemorrhoid

is then grasped with a Pennington, Allison, or Kocher clamp, according to the surgeon's preference. Using the scalpel or cautery pencil, the surgeon amputates the vessel, excising a small amount of rectal mucosa at the same time (Figure 21-37, *B*). To ligate the vein, the surgeon uses a suture ligature of 2-0 or 3-0 chromic suture on a fine needle. The mucosa may be loosely approximated or left open. The mucosa is not sutured tightly because this would cause an abscess to form. Each hemorrhoid is removed in a similar manner.

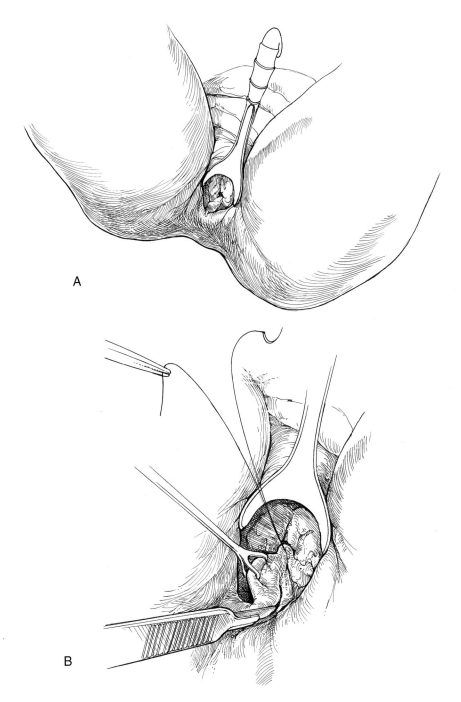

FIGURE 21-37
Hemorrhoidectomy. **A,** Anoscope is inserted in the rectum. **B,** Elliptical excision of the hemorrhoid. (From Economou SG and Economou TS: *Atlas of surgical technique,* ed 2, Philadelphia, 1996, Saunders.)

At the close of the procedure, the surgeon may examine the rectum digitally to be sure that the sutures have not constricted the rectal lumen. The anus is then dressed with packing impregnated with an antibiotic or antiseptic, such as Adaptic packing.

RELATED PROCEDURES
▶ Excision of venereal warts
▶ Rectal polypectomy

Excision of Pilonidal Cyst
SURGICAL GOAL
This procedure is performed to remove a pilonidal cyst.

PATHOLOGY
A pilonidal cyst is a congenital defect that allows epithelial tissue to be trapped below the surface of the skin in the area of the sacrum and coccyx. The cyst is removed when it

causes recurrent infection of the area. A sinus tract (channel leading to an abscess) often is present.

1. The skin is incised in a circle around the sinus.
2. The incision is carried to the sacrum, and the tissue is removed en bloc.
3. The wound is closed.

DISCUSSION

The patient is placed in the Kraske (jackknife) position, and the buttocks are taped apart as for a hemorrhoidectomy (Figure 21-38, *A*).

If there is a sinus tract, the surgeon begins the procedure by placing a probe into the tract.. The probe identifies the exact location of the sinus and the cyst itself. The surgeon may wish to inject dye into the sinus tract. If so, the scrub should have a blunt needle, syringe, and methylene blue dye available.

The area around the sinus is then incised with the skin knife (Figure 21-38, *B*). The scrub must retract the skin with rake retractors as the surgeon deepens the incision. Using the cautery pencil or a deep knife, the surgeon incises the subcutaneous layer. The incised tissue mass then is grasped with a Kocher or Allis clamp for traction. The dissection continues until the sacrum is exposed and the mass is re-

moved (Figure 21-38, *C*). Bleeding vessels are controlled with cautery or ties of 3-0 Vicryl, Dexon, or gut.

The wound is then closed. Some surgeons prefer to place a very loose closure, while others close in routine fashion. The subcutaneous tissue is closed with absorbable suture, size 3-0. The skin is closed according to the surgeon's preference. When active infection is present, the wound is not sutured but is left open. If the wound is not sutured, it may be packed with iodophor-impregnated packing. Otherwise it is dressed with gauze and tape.

Excision of Anal Fistula
SURGICAL GOAL

This procedure is performed to expose healthy tissue around the fistula so that the tract can heal.

PATHOLOGY

This is excision of tissue surrounding a draining sinus tract in the area of the anus. The fistula is continuous from the anus to the skin.

1. The extent of the fistula is determined.
2. The tract is incised around its circumference.

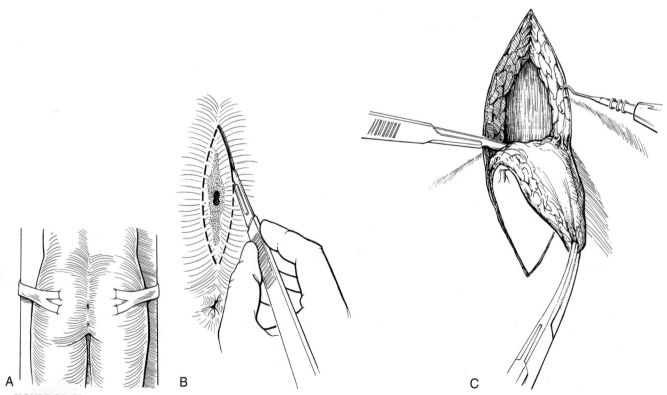

FIGURE 21-38
Excision of pilonidal cyst. **A,** The buttocks are spread with tape. **B,** An incision is made around the sinus tract. **C,** The tract is dissected to the sacrum, the excision is continued, and the tract is removed. (From Economou SG and Economou TS: *Atlas of surgical technique,* ed 2, Philadelphia, 1996, Saunders.)

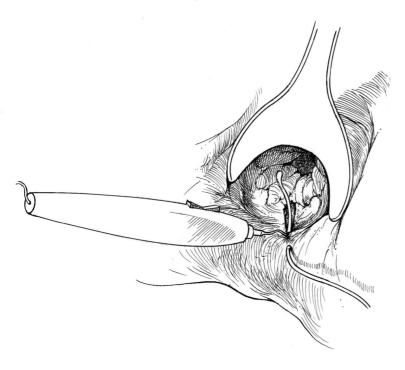

FIGURE 21-39
Excision of anal fistula. A probe is inserted into the tract and the fistula is removed by cautery. (From Economou SG and Economou TS: *Atlas of surgical technique,* ed 2, Philadelphia, 1996, Saunders.)

DISCUSSION

The patient is placed in the Kraske (jackknife) position and prepared as for a hemorrhoidectomy. The surgeon dilates the rectum and inserts a rectal retractor. A malleable probe is then inserted into the fistula to determine its exact location and depth (Figure 21-39). Because the fistula may have more than one passageway, the surgeon also identifies these.

When the extent of the fistula has been determined, the surgeon makes a circular incision around the fistula where it communicates with the skin. The incision is deepened with the cautery pencil and carried along the full length of the fistula. The incised tissue is removed as a specimen.

The wound is not sutured but is dressed with Adaptic packing or a similar material.

SECTION IV
Surgery of the Biliary System, Liver, Pancreas, and Spleen

Behavioral Objectives

After studying this section the reader will be able to:

- Describe the structures of the biliary system, liver, pancreas, and spleen
- Recognize and identify instruments required for biliary, hepatic, pancreatic, and splenic surgery
- Describe the pancreas and its communication with other accessory organs
- Identify resection techniques used to secure deep vascular and biliary structures
- Discuss techniques required for handling of dry specimens (e.g., gallstones)
- Identify the need for insertion of a T-tube (biliary system)
- Identify uses of the argon beam coagulator and ultrasonic scalpel
- Identify how to properly maintain multiple endoscopic instruments on the field
- Describe the scheme for a radical resection
- Identify and describe priorities for an emergency procedure (splenectomy)

Terminology

Anatomical resection—In liver surgery, refers to the removal of a segment by locating and ligating the biliary and vascular structures that drain into it.

Bifurcation—An anatomical term that describes a single tubular or hollow structure that leads to a Y or split in the same structure.

Bile—The digestive substance that is produced by the liver. Its main function is to emulsify (break into small particles) fats so that the body can digest them. When the diet contains excess cholesterol, the bile becomes supersaturated and releases bile salts that are irritating to the gallbladder and cause stones.

Biliary—Refers to the gallbladder and its ducts and blood vessels.

Cholecystectomy—Surgical removal of the gallbladder.

Choledochojejunostomy—A surgical anastomosis of the common bile duct and the jejunostomy.

Cholelithiasis—Condition in which calculi or bilestones are present in the bile duct or gallbladder.

Cirrhosis—Disease of the liver in which the tissue becomes hardened and its venous drainage blocked. It is usually caused by chronic alcoholism but also may result from other disease conditions.

Exteriorized—Surgical term describing any organ or object that has been "brought out" of a cavity or organ, or the abdominal wall.

Friable—Term describing tissue that is fragile and easily torn, and that may bleed profusely. Some disease states produce friable tissue. The liver and spleen normally are friable.

Glisson's capsule—A firm connective tissue that covers and protects the liver surface.

Lobectomy (liver)—The surgical removal of one or more anatomical sections of the liver.

Marginal tissue—Tissue that surrounds a tumor. During tumor surgery, it is important to include a wide margin around the tumor to prevent recurrence of the tumor.

Metastatic—Condition in which cancer spreads from a primary (original) site to other areas of the body.

Mobilize—To "free up" an organ or tissue. All tissues in the body communicate by the vascular system, connective tissue, and other organs. To remove or resect an organ or part of the structure, these connections must be divided, and all bleeding must be controlled. This is the process of mobilization.

Nonanatomical resection—Removal of a section without regard to its segmental boundaries. A wedge resection is nonanatomical.

Pancreatojejunostomy—A surgical anastomosis of the pancreas and the jejunum.

Parenchyma—Tissue that makes up an organ. For example, the liver parenchyma is the body of the liver itself. Pancreatic parenchyma is pancreatic tissue. This term is used to differentiate organ tissue from its covering or capsule.

Portal—The portal vein, which traverses the liver. Its branches form complex extensions into the liver.

Primary tumor—In oncology (the study and treatment of cancer), the original site of a cancer that spreads to other locations called secondary sites via metastasis.

Segmental resection—The anatomical resection of the liver. This procedure removes segments that are divided by specific blood vessels and biliary ducts. Although not visible from the outside of the liver, these segments are differentiated and can be removed separately after the associated structures have been managed.

Subphrenic—An anatomical description meaning "under or below the liver."

Transect—To surgically divide or cut into sections.

Trisegmentectomy—In hepatic surgery, the removal of the right lobe of the liver and a portion of the left. In practice, it is a multiple segmental resection.

Visualization—A surgical term that means to "see directly."

Wedge resection—The surgical removal of a small, sometimes pie-shaped portion of the liver. See *nonanatomical resection*.

ANATOMY OF THE BILIARY SYSTEM, LIVER, PANCREAS, AND SPLEEN

Liver

The liver, gallbladder, spleen, and pancreas are situated in the mid-abdominal cavity (Figure 21-40). The spleen (not shown in Figure 21-40) lies in the upper left quadrant beneath the diaphragm posterior to the stomach. The liver occupies most of the upper right abdominal space and a portion of the left upper quadrant.

The liver is a large, vascular organ that aids in digestion and filtration of toxic substances from the body (Figure 21-41). It is divided into two major sections or *lobes*: the right and left, which are separated by the *falciform liga-*

ment. These sections are identified by the **bifurcation** (Y-shaped division of a hollow anatomical structure) of the portal vein with right and left bile ducts. Its vascular supply is derived from the hepatic artery and hepatic portal vein. It is drained by the hepatic veins, which connect to the inferior vena cava.

These two lobes are further divided into eight separate subsections according to their blood supply. The blood supply to each section is carried in a pedicle containing a bile duct, hepatic artery, and branch of the portal vein.

Because each section is connected to its own pedicle, resection of an entire lobe requires dissection of the pedicle from the lobe and secure ligation of the pedicle, including the specific portion of the hepatic vein.

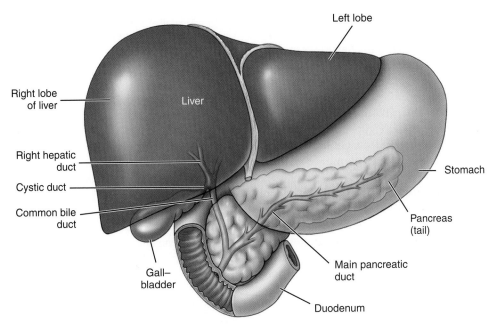

FIGURE 21-40
Locations of the liver, gallbladder, and pancreas. (Modified from Herlihy B and Maebius NK: *The human body in health and illness,* ed 2, Philadelphia, 2003, Saunders.)

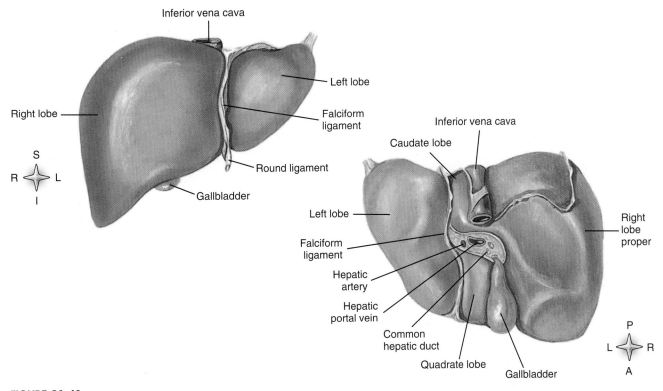

FIGURE 21-41
Anterior view *(left)* and inferior view *(right)* of the liver. (From Thibodeau GA and Patton KT: *Anatomy and physiology,* ed 5, St Louis, 2003, Mosby.)

The liver is encapsulated with a thick fibrous sheath called **Glisson's capsule.** Fibrous sheaths cover and protect the blood vessels and **biliary** (pertaining to the gallbladder) vessels. These sheaths are continuous with the abdominal fascia and must be carefully dissected and mobilized before

liver resection or anastomosis of the biliary system to another abdominal structure.

The anterior surface of the liver is in contact with the diaphragm and is called the right and left subphrenic spaces. The subhepatic space lies between the peritoneal covering on the liver and the right kidney. These spaces are clinically significant. The subphrenic spaces are a common site of abscess, and the subhepatic space can trap contents of the intestine after a rupture of the appendix and become infected.

Biliary System

The biliary system includes the gallbladder, hepatic ducts, common bile duct, and cystic duct (Figure 21-42). The gallbladder is a small sac located under the right lobe (ventral side) of the liver. It is composed of smooth muscle and has an inner surface of absorptive cells.

The function of the biliary system is to produce, store, and release **bile.** This substance is necessary for the breakdown of cholesterol and helps stimulate peristalsis in the small intestine during digestion. Bile is formed in the liver and stored in the gallbladder. Bile is composed of bile salts, pigments, cholesterol, lecithin, mucin (a glycoprotein), and other organic substances.

Bile formed in the liver is released from the right and left hepatic ducts. These ducts converge to form the common hepatic duct. From the common hepatic duct, bile then flows into the gallbladder through the cystic duct. When food enters the stomach, the gallbladder contracts, releasing stored bile into the common bile duct. Bile then enters the duodenum through an opening called the ampulla of Vater. This opening into the duodenum is shared by the pancreatic duct, which allows the release of pancreatic enzymes. The release of both bile and pancreatic enzymes is controlled by a sphincter at the ampulla called the sphincter of Oddi.

Pancreas

The pancreas is a lobulated gland that is elongated and lies inferior to the liver, behind the stomach (Figure 21-43). This organ has two landmarks: the head and the tail. The head, which is the broader portion of the gland, lies in the curve of the duodenum and is connected to the duodenal portion of the small intestine. The pancreatic duct, or *duct of Wirsung,* which is the central duct of the pancreas, communicates with the duodenum at the *ampulla of Vater,* a location shared with the common bile duct. The tail of the pancreas lies near the hilus of the spleen. The pancreas produces *insulin* and *glucagon,* which aid in the digestion of carbohydrates.

Spleen

The spleen is a kidney-shaped organ that is extremely vascular and relatively soft (Figure 21-44). It lies under the diaphragm in the left upper abdomen. This organ destroys aged red blood cells, stores blood, filters microorganisms from the blood, and plays a major role in the immune system of the body. The spleen is supplied by two major blood vessels: the splenic vein and the splenic artery. Because of its vascularity and location, the spleen is subject to trauma by

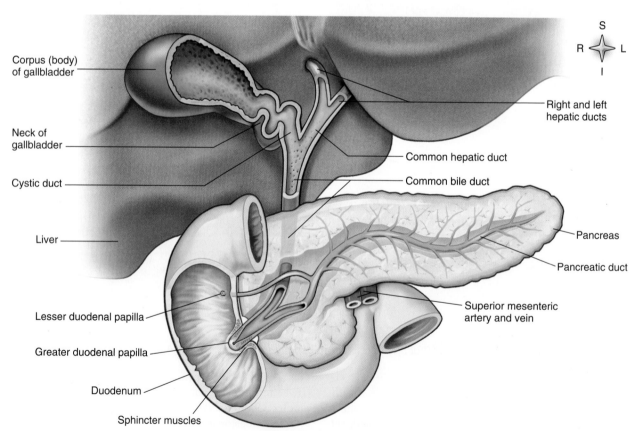

FIGURE 21-42

The biliary system. (From Thibodeau GA and Patton KT: *Anatomy and physiology,* ed 5, St Louis, 2003, Mosby.)

direct blow during vehicular and other accidents. The spleen can be safely removed without harm to body function; this procedure is indicated whenever splenic hemorrhage becomes life threatening.

INSTRUMENTS AND EQUIPMENT

Instruments

Procedures of the liver, biliary system, pancreas, and spleen require basic laparotomy instruments; biliary surgery may require a set of gallbladder-specific instruments as well (Figure 21-45). Vascular instruments are needed for major resection procedures (e.g., the Whipple procedure) and for major hepatic surgery. Vascular instruments are illustrated in Chapter 28.

Because these accessory organs contain many ducts and blood vessels, right-angle clamps should be immediately available on all procedures. These clamps allow the surgeon to reach underneath and around the blood vessels, ducts, and connective-tissue attachments of the organs.

Retraction of delicate tubular structures requires Silastic or cotton-vessel loops. Recall from Chapter 15 that whenever a tubular structure is retracted with a loop, the surgeon passes the loop under the vessel or duct with a right-angle clamp and secures it with a hemostat or ties the suture immediately.

Special Equipment and Intraoperative Procedures

Procedures of the biliary system and pancreas, including choledochoscopy and endoscopic retrograde cholangiopancreatography, sometimes require the intraoperative use of flexible *fiberoptic endoscopy*. These scopes are inserted into the small ducts of the accessory organs to locate stones, tumors, or benign lesions.

Hemostasis is a major technical concern during liver surgery. The liver **parenchyma** (organ tissue) is extremely vascular and bleeds easily. Therefore hemostatic techniques must include not only individual blood vessels but also the liver surface. The ultrasonic scalpel, argon beam coagulator, Cavitron ultrasonic surgical aspirator (CUSA), and ESU are used to cut and coagulate the tissue. The ultrasonic scalpel is particularly useful in liver surgery because it creates a "spray" of coagulation. This is discussed in Chapter 16.

SURGICAL PROCEDURES

Laparoscopic Cholecystectomy with Cholangiography

SURGICAL GOAL

Cholecystectomy is complete surgical removal of the gallbladder and the reconstruction of the biliary ducts so bile can empty directly into the intestine. This procedure is performed to prevent or treat acute inflammation and obstruction.

Operative cholangiography is the injection of radiopaque dye into the ducts of the biliary system. This procedure de-

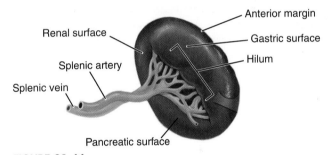

FIGURE 21-44
The spleen. (Colorized from *Mosby's medical, nursing, and allied health dictionary*, ed 6, St Louis, 2002, Mosby.)

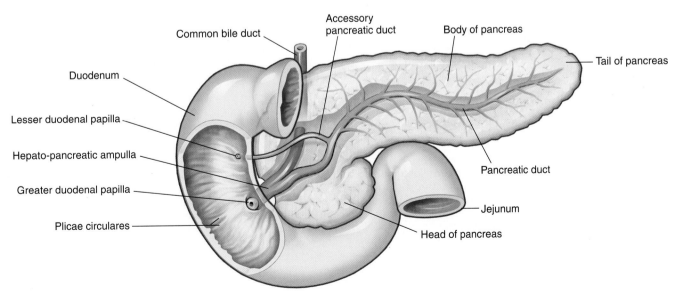

FIGURE 21-43
The pancreas. (Modified from Thibodeau GA and Patton KT: *Anatomy and physiology*, ed 5, St Louis, 2003, Mosby.)

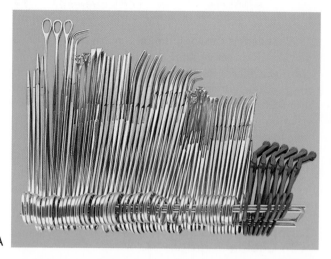

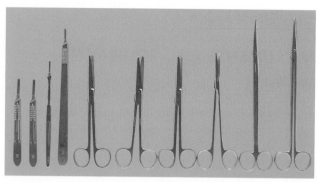

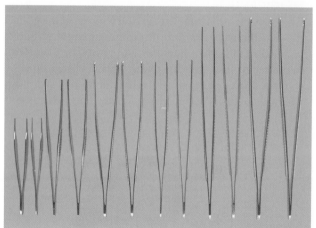

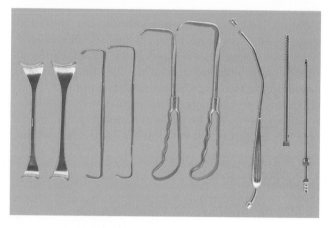

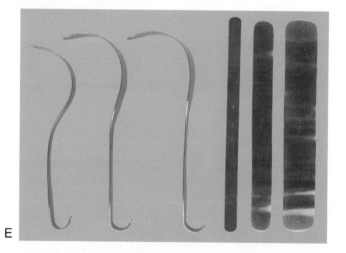

FIGURE 21-45

Laparotomy instruments. **A,** *Left to right,* two Mayo-Hegar needle holders; two Ayer needle holders (8 inch); three Foerster sponge forceps; two Mixter hemostatic forceps (long, fine point); two Babcock tissue forceps (long); two Allis tissue forceps (long); six Ochsner hemostatic forceps (long, straight); four Mayo-Péan hemostatic forceps (long, curved); six hemostatic tonsil forceps; two Westphal hemostatic forceps; four Babcock tissue forceps (short); Allis tissue forceps (short); eight Crile hemostatic forceps (curved, 6½ inch); one Halsted mosquito hemostatic forceps (straight); six paper drape clips. **B,** *Left to right,* two Bard-Parker knife handles (no. 4); one Bard-Parker knife handle (no. 7); one Bard-Parker knife handle (no. 3, long); one Mayo dissecting scissors (curved); two Mayo dissection scissors (straight); one Metzenbaum dissecting scissors (7 inch); one Snowden Pencer dissecting scissors (curved); one Snowden Pencer dissecting scissors (straight). **C,** *Left to right,* two Adson tissue forceps with teeth (1 × 2); two Ferris-Smith tissue forceps; two Russian tissue forceps (medium); two DeBakey vascular Atraugrip tissue forceps (medium); two DeBakey vascular Atraugrip tissue forceps (long); two Russian tissue forceps (long). **D,** *Left to right,* two Goelet retractors; two Army-Navy retractors; one Richardson retractor (medium); one Richardson retractor (large); one Yankauer suction tube and tip; one Poole abdominal shield and suction tube. **E,** *Left to right,* Deaver retractors (small, medium, and large); Ochsner malleable retractors (narrow, medium, and wide).

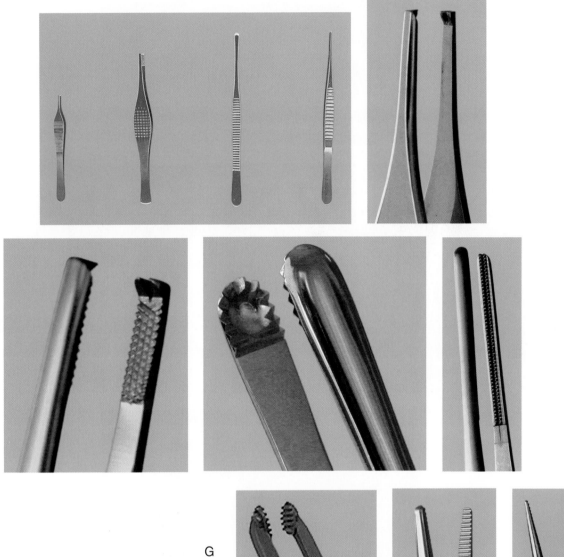

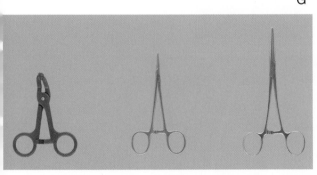

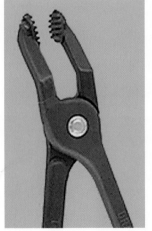

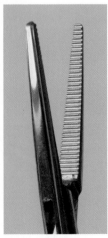

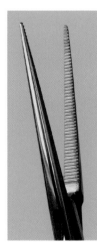

FIGURE 21-45, cont'd
F, *Top left,* Adson tissue forceps; Ferris-Smith tissue forceps; Russian tissue forceps; DeBakey vascular Atraugrip tissue forceps. *Top right,* tip of Adson tissue forceps. *Bottom,* tips of Ferris-Smith tissue forceps, Russian tissue forceps, and DeBakey vascular Atraugrip tissue forceps. **G,** *Left,* paper drape clip; Halsted mosquito hemostatic forceps (straight); Halsted hemostatic forceps. *Right,* tips of paper drape clip, Halsted mosquito hemostatic forceps, and Halsted hemostatic forceps.

continued

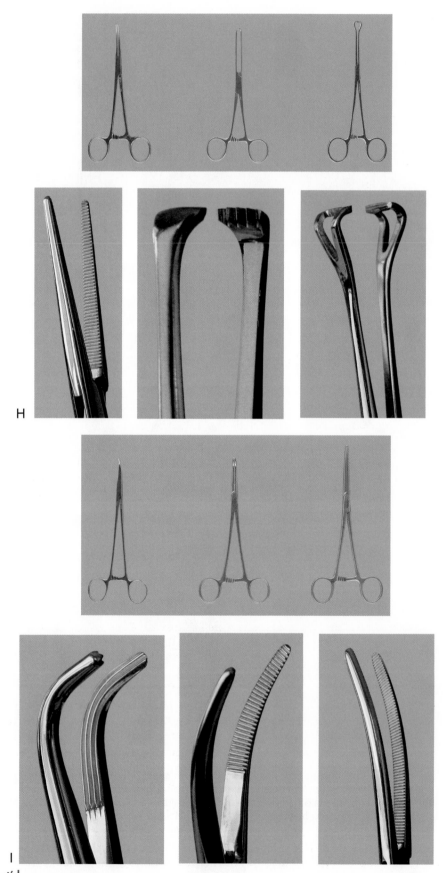

FIGURE 21-45, cont'd
H, *Top,* Crile hemostatic forceps; Allis tissue forceps; Babcock tissue forceps. *Bottom,* tips of Crile hemostatic forceps, Allis tissue forceps, and Babcock tissue forceps. **I,** *Top,* tonsil hemostatic forceps; Westphal hemostatic forceps; Mayo-Péan hemostatic forceps (curved). *Bottom,* tips of tonsil hemostatic forceps, Westphal hemostatic forceps, and Mayo-Péan hemostatic forceps.

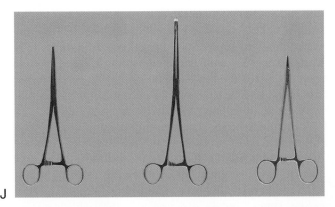
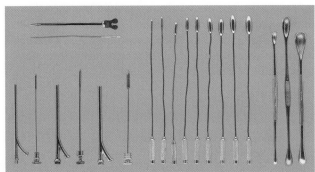

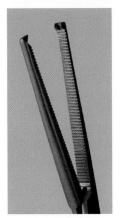
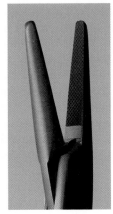
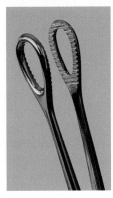

FIGURE 21-45, cont'd
J, *Top,* Ochsner hemostatic forceps; Foerster sponge forceps; Mayo-Hegar needle holder. *Bottom,* tips of Oschsner hemostatic forceps, Foerster sponge forceps, and Mayo-Hegar needle holder. **K,** Gallbladder specific instruments. *Top left,* one grooved director; one probe dilator. *Bottom, left to right,* three gallbladder trocars with inserts (small, medium, and large); nine Bakes common duct dilators, nos. 3, 4, 5, 6, 7, 8, 9, 10, 11; three Ferguson gallstone scoops (small, medium and large). (From Tighe SM: *Instrumentation for the operating room,* ed 6, St Louis, 1999, Mosby.)

termines the presence and location of gallstones or strictures so they can be removed.

PATHOLOGY

Two common diseases of the biliary system are **cholelithiasis,** the presence of gallstones, and **cholecystitis,** inflammation of the gallbladder.

Cholelithiasis

Three primary causes of gallstones are abnormal composition of bile, reduced flow of bile (stasis), and inflammation of the gallbladder (cholecystitis).

Gallstones are composed of bile salts, cholesterol, fatty acids, and other substances. Cholesterol stones typically form when the amount of cholesterol in the blood is elevated. Obesity is a primary cause of gallstones because excess cholesterol from the blood is excreted from the liver into the bile. The presence of cholesterol in bile has no function. Persons with gallstones may not experience any symptoms.

However, when stones obstruct the flow of bile, pain and jaundice can occur.

Cholecystitis

Inflammation of the gallbladder, or cholecystitis, can be acute or chronic. This condition occurs when the composition of bile is altered. A change in the balance of substances in the bile can lead to inflammation and pain. Some diseases that interfere with absorption of bile salts also lead to inflammation of the gallbladder. Acute or sudden onset of cholecystitis is usually caused by blockage of the biliary ducts by stones or stricture. Obstruction causes increased concentration of bile. The gallbladder swells, and the swelling causes local ischemia (loss of blood supply) to the gallbladder. Infection may develop. In extreme cases, the infected gallbladder can become necrotic and rupture. This releases bacteria and bile into the abdominal cavity, causing peritonitis or infection of the entire abdominal cavity.

Cancer

Cancer of the gallbladder is present in about 2% of patients undergoing surgery for biliary disease. The cancer usually is discovered during biliary surgery. Gallstones cause chronic irritation of the gallbladder and therefore may be a contributing cause of cancer.

Technique	LAPAROSCOPIC CHOLECYSTECTOMY

1. A pneumoperitoneum is established.
2. Trocars are placed in the abdomen.
3. The gallbladder is retracted upward with a toothed grasper.
4. The cystic duct, cystic artery, and common bile duct are exposed.
5. The assistant maintains gentle traction on the gallbladder.
6. The cystic artery and cystic duct are identified and exposed with sharp dissecting instruments.
7. The surgeon occludes the cystic duct and artery with endoscopic clips and divides each with sharp dissection or the ESU.
8. The surgeon performs cholangiography.

Technique	CHOLANGIOGRAPHY AND CHOLEDOCHOSCOPY

1. An incision is made into the cystic duct (choledochotomy).
2. A cholangiogram catheter is threaded into the cystic duct and secured with endoscopic clips or a cholangiography clamp.
3. Contrast media is injected into the common bile duct, and x-rays are taken.
4. If stones are present, a Fogarty balloon or similar catheter is threaded into the common duct.
5. The cystic duct is dilated.
6. The choledochoscope or ureteroscope is inserted, and stones are removed with a stone basket.
7. A second set of x-rays may be taken at this stage.

Technique	COMPLETION OF CHOLECYSTECTOMY

1. The surgeon dissects the gallbladder from the underside of the liver using the ESU probe, hook, or scissors.
2. The surgeon removes the gallbladder from the abdomen through a 10-mm trocar site using a grasper with teeth.
3. The abdominal cavity is irrigated.
4. A T-tube may be inserted for continuous postoperative drainage.
5. Individual trocar wounds are closed.
6. If used, the T-tube is attached to a drainage bag.

DISCUSSION

The patient is placed in supine position, and the abdomen is prepped and draped for a laparoscopy. In this procedure, four trocars are placed: an umbilical 10-mm trocar, an additional 10-mm trocar at the midline, and two 5-mm trocars at the axillary line. This procedure usually requires a 30-degree telescope to view the gallbladder, which lies high in the abdominal cavity.

The laparoscope is inserted through a 10-mm port. A straight locking grasper is inserted through one axillary trocar and used to apply upward traction on the gallbladder. The assistant maintains retraction on the gallbladder. Some surgeons attach the handle of the retracting grasper to the skin or drapes. The scrub may be asked to hold this clamp in place during dissection (according to hospital policy).

The patient then may be repositioned into Trendelenburg (head down) position as the dissection continues. An additional grasper may be placed on the gallbladder. The gallbladder may be drained for ease of tissue handling. The cystic duct and artery are then identified and exposed so they can be clamped and divided away from the gallbladder (Figure 21-46, *A*). Sharp dissection with scissors, an additional grasper, and an ESU hook may be used to separate the cystic duct and artery. If the gallbladder is very edematous (swollen), dissection may be more difficult. When the cystic duct and artery have been isolated from the surrounding tissue, endoscopic clips are used to double ligate both structures. An additional clip may be placed over the cystic duct at the base of the gallbladder. The duct and artery are then divided (Figure 21-46, *B*). Operative cholangiography is usually performed at this stage of the procedure.

Operative Cholangiography

In preparation for the cholangiography, the scrub should prepare contrast media according to the surgeon's written order. A 10-ml syringe is usually used to inject the dye. The surgeon makes a small incision in the cystic duct. A cholangiogram catheter or ureteral catheter is threaded into the duct through the incision. The catheter may be held in place with an endoscopic vessel clip or special cholangiography clamp. The surgeon injects the contrast media into the catheter, and x-rays are taken. All personnel must be protected by lead aprons or a lead x-ray shield during cholangiography.

If stones are located, the surgeon extends the exploration by dilating the cystic duct with a balloon catheter. The surgeon performs this procedure by threading a guide wire through the cystic duct and into the common duct. The balloon catheter is then inserted over the guide wire and slowly inflated with saline solution. The surgeon can remove single stones by slowly withdrawing the catheter (Figure 21-47). The common-duct stones also can be flushed out with a high-pressure irrigation device. Any stones that fall into the abdominal cavity are retrieved with an endoscopic grasper. Stones also may be retrieved through the fiberoptic choledochoscope or ureteroscope as described below.

Choledochoscopy for Stone Retrieval

If a choledochoscopy is to be performed, an additional camera and monitor must be available. Avoid tangling instrument cords that can cause scopes to drop off the surgical field. Secure all cords with nonpenetrating towel clamps. If fiberoptic scopes are used during laparoscopic surgery, the scrub must take care to maintain safety on the field. The scrub must make certain that the fiberoptic light is in the "off" position when the cord is not attached to the telescope. Do not allow instruments to accumulate on the patient's abdomen.

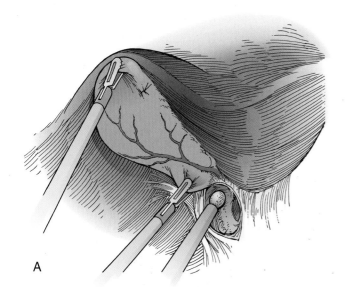

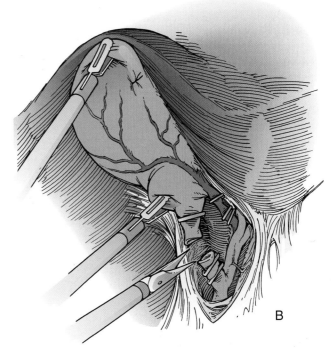

FIGURE 21-46
Laparoscopic cholecystectomy with cholangiography. **A,** The gallbladder is retracted, allowing dissection of the cystic duct and artery. **B,** The cystic artery and duct are clipped and cut. (Colorized from Moody FG: *Atlas of ambulatory surgery,* St Louis, 1999, Mosby.)

A small incision is made in the common bile duct, and the fiberoptic choledochoscope or ureteroscope can be inserted over the guide wire. Stones can be seen directly and retrieved with a stone basket (Figure 21-48, *A* and *B*).

The scrub receives all stones in a dry container. Any stones that are inadvertently dropped into the abdominal cavity are retrieved with a grasping forceps. When all stones have been removed, a second cholangiogram may be taken.

Completion of Cholecystectomy

The gallbladder is then dissected free of the underside of the liver (liver bed). Upward traction is maintained. This puts some tension on the gallbladder and the tissue plane directly underneath and facilitates dissection. The surgeon uses the ESU hook, scissors, or shears to separate the connecting tissues and free the gallbladder completely (Figure 21-49, *A*). A large grasper is inserted into the 10-mm subxyphoid (uppermost) port. The smaller graspers are used to "hand" the gallbladder to the larger grasper. The sac is then extracted through the 10-mm trocar (Figure 21-49, *B*).

The scrub should receive the gallbladder in a small basin and take care not to allow its contents to spill onto the surgical field.

A T-tube may be inserted at this time to produce continuous postoperative drainage of the common bile duct. The limbs of the T-tube are trimmed, and the tube is inserted through the uppermost trocar. The limbs of the tube are threaded into the common bile duct, and the long end is pulled through a new 5-mm trocar placed in the right upper quadrant of the abdomen. The common bile duct is closed

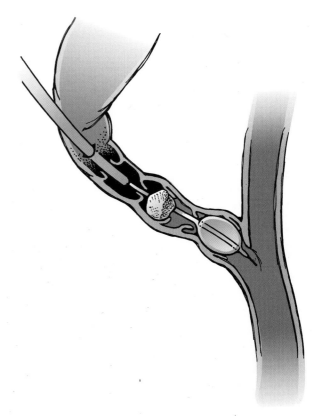

FIGURE 21-47
Extraction of a cystic duct stone using a balloon catheter. (Colorized from Moody FG: *Atlas of ambulatory surgery,* St Louis, 1999, Mosby.)

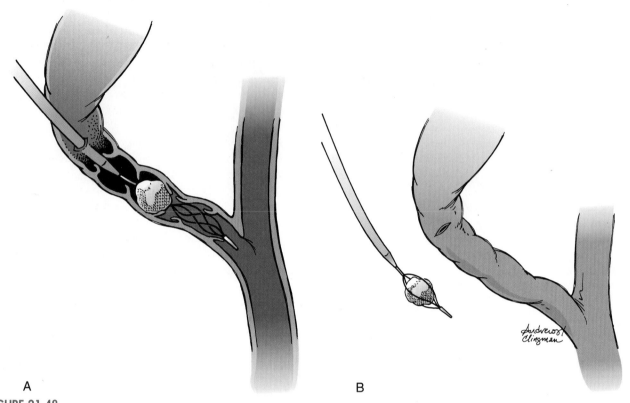

A

B

FIGURE 21-48
Extraction of a cystic duct stone using a wire basket. **A,** Insertion of the stone basket. **B,** Extraction of a stone in the basket. (Colorized from Moody FG: *Atlas of ambulatory surgery,* St Louis, 1999, Mosby.)

FIGURE 21-49
Completion of cholecystectomy.
A, The gallbladder is dissected completely. **B,** The sac is extracted through the 10-mm trocar. (**A** colorized from Moody FG: *Atlas of ambulatory surgery,* St Louis, 1999, Mosby; **B** from Economou SG and Economou TS: *Atlas of surgical technique,* ed 2, Philadelphia, 1996, Saunders.)

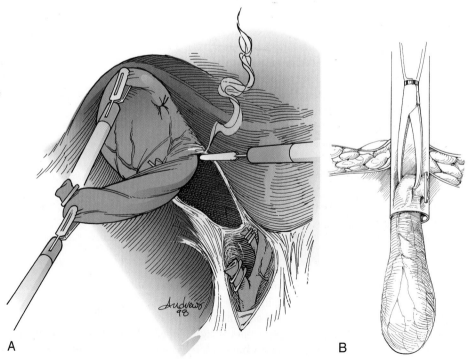

A

B

with endoscopic sutures. The abdominal cavity then is irrigated, and each trocar incision is closed with absorbable sutures and skin staples. The T-tube is secured to a drainage bag.

Cholecystectomy (Open)
SURGICAL GOAL
In this procedure, a diseased gallbladder is surgically removed.

PATHOLOGY
In acute cholecystitis, the normally bluish green gallbladder becomes distended and inflamed as a result of obstruction by one or more gallstones. In removing the gallbladder, the surgeon leaves the common bile duct unimpaired so that it becomes a functional passageway through which bile can enter the duodenum.

Technique
1. The surgeon enters the abdomen.
2. The bile ducts are identified and isolated.
3. The cystic artery is identified and ligated.
4. The cystic duct is ligated.
5. The gallbladder is dissected from the liver bed.
6. The wound is closed.

DISCUSSION
The patient is placed in the supine position with a small pad or gallbladder lift placed under the right upper quadrant. This facilitates exposure of the gallbladder and associated structures. The surgeon enters the abdomen through a right subcostal or right paramedian incision. If the patient is very obese, an upper midline incision may be used. When the abdomen is entered, the liver is covered with moist lap sponges and retracted gently upward by the assistant. A Deaver or Harrington retractor is used.

If the gallbladder is greatly distended, the surgeon may drain it of bile. The scrub passes a gallbladder trocar to the surgeon. The trocar is fitted to the suction, and the trocar tip is positioned into the gallbladder, allowing it to drain. A Mayo clamp is then placed over the hole made by the trocar. The trocar should be handed off the field to the circulator.

To identify the cystic duct, cystic artery, and common bile duct, the surgeon removes a thin peritoneal layer from these structures. The surgeon performs this procedure with both blunt and sharp dissection, using Metzenbaum scissors; long, fine-toothed forceps, and small sponge dissectors. The surgeon then identifies the vessels. Using right-angle clamps, the surgeon double clamps the cystic duct, then divides and ligates it with a long 2-0 silk tie on a passer (Figure 21-50, A). The cystic artery is clamped and ligated similarly (Figure 21-50, B).

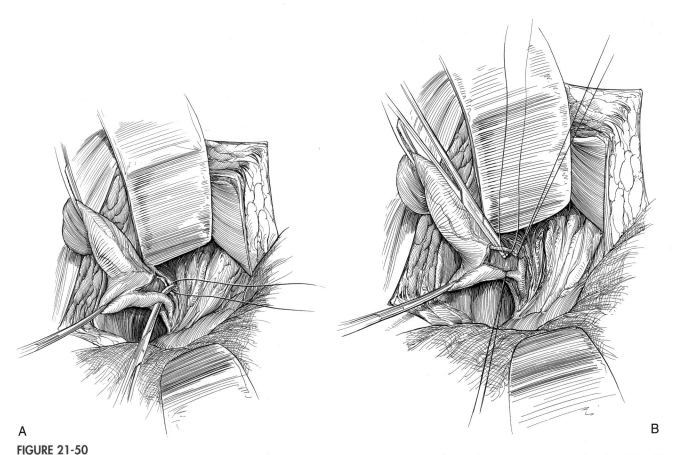

FIGURE 21-50
Cholecystectomy (open). **A,** Cystic duct is tied close to the gallbladder with a 2-0 silk. **B,** The cystic artery is tied with a 2-0 silk and ligated. (From Economou SG and Economou TS: *Atlas of surgical technique,* ed 2, Philadelphia, 1996, Saunders.)

The dissection of the gallbladder from the undersurface of the liver is performed with Metzenbaum scissors and right-angle clamps. The surgeon continues the dissection until the gallbladder is completely mobilized. The specimen is then passed to the technologist. The removal of the gallbladder leaves a raw surface on the liver. This surface may be sewn over with 3-0 or 4-0 chromic gut swaged to a fine needle, but many surgeons believe that the surface heals just as well without sutures.

The wound is irrigated with warm saline solution, and the operative site is examined for small bleeders. The surgeon lays one or two Penrose drains into the wound and brings them to the outside of the abdomen through a stab incision near the original abdominal incision. The wound is then closed in routine fashion.

Operative Cholangiography: Exploration of the Common Bile Duct

SURGICAL GOAL

The biliary vessels are injected with dye, and radiographs are taken.

PATHOLOGY

Operative cholangiography is performed to determine the presence of stones or stricture. When a stone or group of stones is located on the radiograph, the stones are removed and the ducts are dilated. These procedures usually are performed in conjunction with a cholecystectomy. Many surgeons perform cholangiography routinely with a cholecystectomy.

Technique

1. The surgeon enters the abdomen.
2. The gallbladder is drained of bile.
3. An incision is made in the common bile duct, and a biliary catheter is introduced.
4. Radiographs are taken.
5. The ducts are explored.
6. A T-tube is inserted.
7. The wound is closed.

DISCUSSION

The patient is prepped, draped, and positioned as for a cholecystectomy. The abdomen is entered through a right subcostal or upper midline incision. The assistant retracts the liver upward with a Deaver or Harrington retractor. In many cases the gallbladder is distended and must be drained; this is performed as previously described for a cholecystectomy. When the gallbladder has been drained, the trocar is passed back to the scrub, who places it in a basin. During the case, this basin receives all instruments that have been contaminated with bile.

The surgeon explores the base of the gallbladder using Metzenbaum scissors, right-angle clamps, and small sponge dissectors. The surgeon separates the common bile duct from nearby structures. If there is doubt as to whether the

common duct has been identified correctly, the surgeon may wish to aspirate the vessel with a needle. A 30-ml syringe and 18-gauge needle are suitable for this test. When the surgeon has identified the common duct, two traction sutures of 3-0 silk are placed through the wall of the duct. An incision then is made between the sutures with a #15 or #11 scalpel blade or Potts scissors.

The scrub should have a catheter for insertion into the duct, radiopaque dye, and a 30-ml or 50-ml syringe available. The scrub should prepare the dye *before* the surgeon actually needs it to avoid delay. The scrub prepares the dye using the following guidelines:

1. According to the surgeon's preference card or verbal orders, the circulator distributes dye in the surgeon's desired strength to the scrub. Many surgeons prefer the dye to be diluted with saline solution. If so, the scrub receives injectable saline from the circulator and mixes it with a proper amount of dye. At least 30 ml of solution should be prepared. The solution then is aspirated into the syringe, which then is attached to the biliary catheter.
2. *All air bubbles must be removed* from both the syringe and catheter. To do this, the scrub holds the syringe upright and injects a tiny amount of dye solution through the catheter. Tapping the syringe gently should cause the bubbles to rise to the top of the syringe, where they can be ejected from the catheter.
3. The scrub places a Kelly clamp across the catheter, near its tip, to prevent air from backing up into the syringe. If any air bubbles remain, they will appear as stones on the radiograph. The syringe, catheter, and its attaching clamp are then passed to the surgeon.

The surgeon threads the tips of the catheter through the incision in the cystic duct and advances into the common bile duct (Figure 21-51, *A*). He or she may wish to tie it in place with a strand of 0 or 2-0 silk. Before radiographs are taken, a towel should be used to protect the wound from contamination by the overhead x-ray machine. All team members except the surgeon leave the field to stand behind a lead x-ray shield brought into the room by the circulator (unless all team members are wearing lead x-ray aprons). The surgeon remains at the surgical field to inject the dye.

When the radiographs have been taken and returned and the stones are identified on the films, the exploration of the common duct may proceed. During exploration, the specific instruments and the order in which they are used will vary according to the size and location of the stones. Randall stone forceps, toothed forceps, and gallbladder scoops are used to remove the stones. The surgeon also may elect to use a special biliary irrigation catheter. Special biliary probes also are available for stone removal. The catheter probe is advanced beyond the level of the stone, the balloon is inflated, and the catheter is withdrawn, bringing the stone with it. As the stones are removed, the scrub should retrieve them as specimens. Additional films may be taken to ensure that the

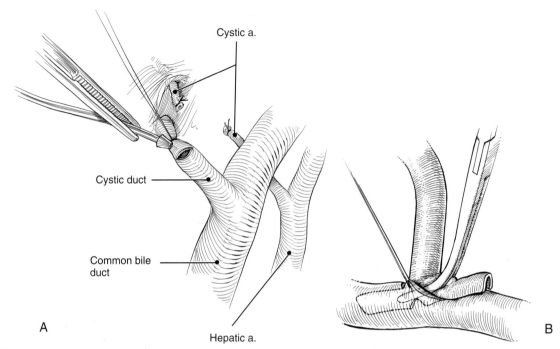

Cystic a.

Cystic duct

Common bile
duct

Hepatic a.

A

B

FIGURE 21-51
Operative cholangiography. **A,** The catheter is inserted into the cystic duct and advanced into the common bile duct. **B,** Insertion of the T-tube into the common duct. (From Economou SG and Economou TS: *Atlas of surgical technique,* ed 2, Philadelphia, 1996, Saunders.)

bile ducts are patent (open). If a cholecystectomy is planned, it is performed at this time.

After exploration, the surgeon may wish to dilate the biliary ducts using Bakes dilators. The scrub assistant should hand the dilators to the surgeon one at a time, starting with a small one and progressing to larger ones.

At the close of the procedure, a T-tube is inserted into the common duct (Figure 21-51, *B*). The surgeon will state the size of tube he or she prefers. The tube is inserted using fine tissue forceps such as Cushing forceps. The ductal incision then is closed with size 3-0 or 4-0 silk on a fine tapered needle. The long end of the T-tube is brought out from the wound and later attached to a special "bile bag," which collects bile while the wound heals. The wound is irrigated with warm saline solution and is closed in standard fashion.

Open Common-Bile-Duct Exploration (CBDE)
SURGICAL GOAL
Exploration of the common bile duct is performed to identify blockages, to search for gallstones, and to remove them.

PATHOLOGY
Because of the technological advances in endoscopic, percutaneous, and laparoscopic techniques to remove gallstones, open exploration of the common bile duct is rarely performed today. When these new techniques are not available or are prevented by previous surgery, or when an open procedure is required, open common-bile-duct exploration (CBDE) becomes necessary.

Technique

1. A subcostal or midline incision is used for CBDE.
2. If the gallbladder is intact, it is exposed and removed or retracted through the use of laparotomy packs and retractors.
3. After identifying the duct, the surgeon places two fine traction sutures below the entrance of the cystic duct.
4. A discard basin for contaminated instruments is placed at the lower end of the field.
5. The common duct is isolated with packs and narrow-blade retractors. The surgeon then opens the duct, between the traction sutures, using a #11 blade on a long #3 handle.
6. Constant suction must be maintained to keep the field free of bile. The incision into the duct is lengthened with angled Potts scissors.
7. Additional stay sutures may be required.
8. The surgeon inspects the duct visually, with probes, and using both the rigid and flexible choledochoscopes. All visible stones are removed.
9. A T-tube is placed in the common bile duct, and the choledochotomy is closed around it.
10. A final cholangiogram is performed to be certain all stones have been removed.
11. The wound is closed in layers. The T-tube is anchored to the skin, and sterile dressings are applied. Sterile tubing is used to connect the T-tube to a small drainage bag.

DISCUSSION

In a CBDE, the following items are essential:

▶ Flexible and rigid choledochoscopes with accessories: biopsy forceps, grasping forceps, and sheaths
▶ 1000-ml bag of 0.9% normal saline for irrigation of the scopes
▶ Sterile IV tubing to connect the scope to the saline bag
▶ Light source for the scopes
▶ A camera and video stack for surgeons who prefer them; some surgeons use their naked eye on the scopes
▶ Biliary scoops

Cholangiograms of the duct can be taken before, during, and after exploration to locate, identify, and confirm the presence of gallstones and ensure that none remain.

Embolectomy-type, balloon-tipped catheters can be inserted into the duct to help remove smaller stones and debris. They also can be used to demonstrate patency of the common bile duct completely through to the duodenum.

Better visualization of the duct is obtained by distending the duct via irrigation with large amounts of sterile saline. One delivers the saline through the scope by attaching sterile pressure tubing to the stopcock of the scope and then to a pressure bag off the field.

Choledochoduodenostomy
SURGICAL GOAL

Choledochoduodenostomy is a procedure that establishes a new connection between the common bile duct and the duodenum.

PATHOLOGY

This procedure is performed in conjunction with a cholecystectomy when the normal opening into the duodenum can be completely bypassed when the common bile duct is anastomosed to the jejunum (choledochojejunostomy).

Technique

1. The abdomen is entered.
2. The common bile duct and duodenum are identified and exposed.
3. The duodenum is mobilized.
4. The common bile duct and duodenum are anastomosed.
5. The wound is closed.

DISCUSSION

The patient is prepped and draped as for a cholecystectomy. The surgeon enters the abdomen through a right subcostal or upper right paramedian incision. The surgeon examines the biliary structures and determines the area of anastomosis on the duodenum (Figure 21-52, A). The assistant retracts the liver upward with a larger retractor, such as a Deaver or Harrington retractor. The surgeon dissects the common duct free of surrounding structures using Metzen-baum scissors and long, fine tissue forceps. There may be bands of scar tissue over the duct, which are removed with sharp and blunt dissection.

A small area of duodenum is mobilized. The surgeon places one row of fine sutures to connect the duodenum and common duct. The surgeon then makes two small incisions, one on each side of the suture line. The anastomosis is completed with an additional layer of fine silk (Figure 21-52, B). The abdomen is irrigated and closed as for a cholecystectomy.

Choledochojejunostomy
SURGICAL GOAL

Surgery required to reestablish the flow of bile into the intestinal tract via an anastomosis between the common bile duct and the jejunum.

PATHOLOGY

These procedures may be necessary in postcholecystectomy patients to circumvent an obstructive lesion.

Technique

1. The surgeon opens the abdomen through a midline incision.
2. The common bile duct and jejunum are identified and mobilized.
3. The common bile duct is opened.
4. The transected jejunum and common duct are approximated and anastomosed. The anastomosis may be side-to-side, or the end of the common bile duct may be anastomosed to the side of the jejunum.
5. A catheter is introduced as for cholecystoduodenostomy.
6. Jejunal continuity is reestablished by jejunojejunostomy.
7. The abdomen is closed in layers.

DISCUSSION

The abdominal midline incision is maintained with a standard Bookwalter retractor.

The jejunum is clamped with atraumatic bowel clamps and transected with a linear stapler. The divided end of the jejunum is closed and oversewn to prevent leakage, and then an end-to-side anastomosis is performed in two layers. Fine monofilament suture of size 4-0 or 5-0 should be used.

As an alternative, the anastomosis may be fashioned from the end of the severed duct to the side of a loop of jejunum, with a side-to-side jejunal anastomosis.

T-tubes may be placed for drainage, so the scrub should have varying sizes available. Gallbladder specialty instruments should be available in case they are needed. Fluoroscopy should be anticipated to check patency.

Splenectomy
SURGICAL GOAL

This procedure is performed to remove the spleen completely.

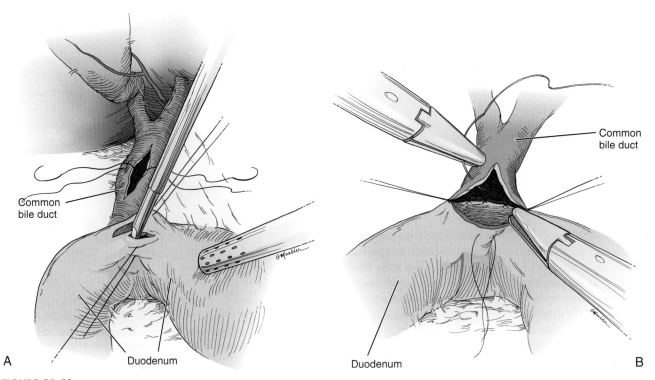

FIGURE 21-52
Choledochoduodenostomy. **A,** Determination of the anastomosis site on the duodenum. **B,** Anastomosis of the duodenum and the common duct. (Colorized from Ballantyne GH: *Atlas of laparoscopic surgery*, Philadelphia, 2000, Saunders.)

PATHOLOGY

The spleen can be safely removed to treat tumor, cysts, or diseases of the red blood cells. In these cases, splenectomy is an elective procedure. A common indication for splenectomy, however, is abdominal trauma and splenic laceration. Its **friable** (delicate and easily torn) structure makes it vulnerable to tearing and extensive hemorrhage during motor-vehicle accidents and other traumatic injury. The spleen also may be inadvertently injured during abdominal surgery.

Technique

1. A laparotomy is performed.
2. Blood and clots are immediately removed from the abdomen.
3. The splenic artery and vein are digitally compressed to control bleeding.
4. An intestinal or vascular clamp is placed across the major vessels.
5. The extent of injury is assessed.
6. If total splenectomy is to be performed, the splenic artery and vein are cross clamped, occluded, and divided to stop the hemorrhage.
7. If a partial splenectomy is to be performed, bleeding is controlled with an ESU and with hemostatic agents. Extensive bleeding, however, usually indicates the need for total splenectomy.
8. The lienorenal ligament is divided by sharp dissection.

9. The peritoneum is dissected away from the spleen with sharp and blunt dissection.
10. The gastric vessels are divided, clamped, and ligated.
11. The gastrosplenic ligament is divided.
12. A suction drain is placed in the wound.
13. Hemostasis is secured, and the wound is closed in layers.

DISCUSSION

Trauma to the spleen is a life-threatening condition that requires immediate operative intervention. Because of its highly vascular structure, the spleen can suffer extensive blood loss in a short time. In preparation for the surgery, the scrub should have a major laparotomy set. Additional instruments include vascular clamps and kidney pedicle clamps, according to the surgeon's usual procedure for splenectomy.

Sutures will be specified but usually include silk or synthetic nonabsorbable sutures to ligate the splenic artery and vein and the gastrosplenic vessels. Surgical clips are used throughout the procedure to secure small bleeders as they are encountered during the dissection.

Remember that during emergency surgery for acute hemorrhage, four steps are required to stop the bleeding:

1. **Access:** The surgeon must have access to the hemorrhage site. This starts with a rapid laparotomy.
2. **Visualization (ability to see structures directly):** Retraction, either manual or self-retaining, must be quickly

established. Suction must be *immediately available in the wound* to clear blood and clots out of the way. The technologist may be required to assist in suctioning and evacuating blood clots while passing other needed instruments.

3. **Good lighting:** Excellent lighting is required to locate and stop the hemorrhage. This is the collaborative duty of the scrub and the circulator. Remember to angle the surgical light toward the head of the wound.

4. **Clamps** are required to occlude the bleeding vessels. The scrub must have vascular, pedicle, and other hemostatic clamps immediately available on the field.

Two suctions must be available as soon as the laparotomy is performed. These are used to evacuate the blood and clots from the abdomen so the splenic vessels can be located and digitally compressed. The scrub should have a large basin available to evacuate and remove large blood clots from the abdominal cavity as soon as the laparotomy is completed. Laparotomy sponges are used in rapid succession as the bleeding is controlled.

The surgeon's assistant evacuates the blood clots and places a self-retaining retractor while the surgeon locates the splenic artery and vein. Even though the procedure moves quickly, safety techniques are still observed. The scrub must watch the wound, have equipment available, and use methodical, smooth movements in assisting.

A blood recovery system such as the Cell Saver may be used immediately to replace blood. Multiple transfusions may be performed during surgery if blood loss has been extensive.

As soon as the splenic vessels are located, they are clamped with a pedicle or vascular clamp. When the vascular supply to the spleen has been controlled, the wound can be more carefully cleared of blood and the extent of damage ascertained. The splenic artery and vein may be ligated at this time. Heavy silk or synthetic suture ligatures are used to secure the vessels. Two or more ligatures may be used (Figure 21-53).

The wound is explored for other areas of trauma. The abdominal retractors may be repositioned at this time. Sharp and blunt dissection with Metzenbaum scissors and sponge dissectors is used to separate the lienorenal ligament from the body of the spleen. The gastric vessels are clamped or clipped and divided in the usual manner. The gastrosplenic ligament is then separated with the Metzenbaum scissors, and the spleen is delivered from the wound.

If the spleen is to be repaired rather than removed, absorbable sutures are used to oversew the tear. Hemostatic agents such as Gelfoam, Avitene, and Surgicel are used to coagulate areas of capillary bleeding.

The surgeon examines the abdominal cavity again to ensure that all hemorrhage has been controlled. He or she again examines the abdominal cavity for signs of additional traumatic injury. The wound is then irrigated with antibacterial solution such as Bacitracin. One or two suction drains

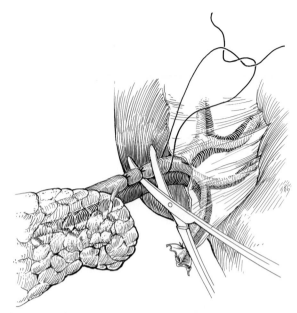

FIGURE 21-53
Splenectomy—division of the splenic artery. (From Economou SG and Economou TS: *Atlas of surgical technique*, ed 2, Philadelphia, 1996, Saunders.)

are placed in the vicinity of the splenic pedicle, and the wound is closed in layers.

Pancreatojejunostomy (Whipple Procedure)
SURGICAL GOAL
In this procedure, the head of the pancreas and duodenum, and a portion of the jejunum, distal stomach, and distal section of the common bile duct are removed. The biliary system, pancreatic system, and GI tract are reconstructed.

PATHOLOGY
A Whipple procedure is performed to treat pancreatic cancer.

Technique

1. A laparotomy is performed through a bilateral or inverted V (bilateral subcostal) incision.
2. The duodenum is mobilized with blunt and sharp dissection. All vessels in the area of the proposed anastomosis are double clamped, ligated, and divided.
3. The gastrocolic ligament and omentum are mobilized as in step 2.
4. Major arteries in the resection area are secured.
5. The distal portion of the stomach is mobilized and transected.
6. The common bile duct is clamped and separated from the duodenum.
7. Vascular attachments to the jejunum are divided.
8. The jejunum is cross clamped and divided.
9. The pancreas is transected.
10. The specimen is removed.
11. The GI, biliary, and pancreatic systems are reconstructed.

Table 21-2 WHIPPLE PROCEDURE RECONSTRUCTION

Normal Anatomical Structure	Post-Reconstruction Configuration
The **duodenum** is continuous from the distal stomach to the jejunum.	The duodenum and a portion of the jejunum are removed. A portion of the proximal jejunum is removed.
The **distal stomach** is continuous with the duodenum.	The gastric omentum attachments are divided, and the distal (lower) third of the stomach is removed. The remaining gastric section is attached to the jejunum with a side-to-side technique.
The **common bile duct** is an extension of the common hepatic duct and communicates directly into the duodenum at the ampilla of Vater.	The common bile duct is divided just below the Y junction of the cystic and hepatic ducts. The common bile duct is anastomosed to the jejunum with an end-to-side technique.
The **pancreatic duct** communicates with the duodenum at the ampilla of Vater	The head of the pancreas is removed, and the remaining portion is anastomosed to the jejunum with an end-to-end or side-to-side technique.

DISCUSSION

The pancreatojejunostomy is a radical operation requiring 5 to 8 hours to complete. Because the procedure includes elements of pancreatic, biliary, intestinal, and gastric procedures, the technologist should prepare all instruments normally used in these specialties. Most are included in a major laparotomy set. Vascular instruments should be added to the sterile set-up in case vessel repair is required. Extra suction and two ESU sets sometimes are needed. Long instruments and wide retractors, such as wide Deaver and Harrington retractors, should be available. Right-angle clamps are used throughout the procedure. A variety of types of right-angle clamps should be available; those with sharp tips typically are not used around the major blood vessels and their branches. The length of the angled portion of the tip must be matched to the amount of space in the recesses of the wound. If the scrub cannot see directly, the surgeon notifies the scrub of his or her preference.

If extreme blood loss is anticipated, the surgeon or anesthesia care provider (ACP) may request that a blood-recovery system be made available. Many sponges, needles, and sutures will be used. The circulator must provide an efficient system for tracking all discarded sponges. The scrub and circulator work together to avoid loss of any item. Two or more magnetic sharps (needle) containers should be available.

Much of the procedure includes meticulous dissection, management of bleeding, and anastomosis of the hollow accessory organs. The surgeon's preferred sutures are made available but should be distributed to the sterile field economically. Additional sutures and other equipment such as sponges, vessel loops, and scalpel blades should be held in reserve. Extra towels and half-sheet drapes should be available to keep the operative site orderly and clean. The risk of infection increases with the duration of the procedure. Recall that increased handling of instruments and equipment also increases the risk of contamination.

Sterile irrigation and water to soak instruments must be kept fresh during a long procedure. The scrub should attempt to keep instruments clean and free of tissue debris. Extra gloves for the team should be readily available but not opened onto the sterile field.

To understand the techniques used in this procedure, one should review procedures learned previously. These resection procedures are performed in succession, and the essential ducts and hollow organs are reconnected to restore function. The reconstruction (anastomosis) phase of the procedure can be performed with surgical staples, sutures, or a combination of both techniques. The following techniques are part of the radical pancreatojejunostomy (Whipple procedure):

▶ Gastric resection and **gastrojejunostomy**
▶ Intestinal resection and anastomosis
▶ **Choledochojejunostomy**
▶ **Pancreatojejunostomy**

Table 21-2 compares the normal relationships of anatomical structures with their relationships after reconstruction.

A large part of the procedure is dissection of the involved organs from their connective tissue and vascular attachments. When a vessel is encountered, it must be occluded in two locations and divided between the vessels. Each vessel stump must be ligated or coagulated with the ESU. The techniques and supplies used for vessel management are:

▶ Two to four right-angle or other clamps are used, according to the surgeon's preference and depth of the wound. Suture ties or suture ligatures are placed over each end of the vessel. Size 3-0 and 2-0 silk is typically used.
▶ A surgical stapling device is used to both cut and staple the vascular area.
▶ Surgical V clips are used to stop blood flow through the vessel. The vascular area is severed with the ESU or Metzenbaum scissors.

The patient is placed in supine position, prepped from nipple line to mid thigh, and draped for a laparotomy. The abdomen is entered through a long midline incision. The surgeon explores the bowel and other organs for evidence of metastasis. The wound is packed with moistened lap sponges, and a self-retaining retractor is placed in the usual manner. Accessory retractors or a self-retaining retractor fitted with attachments (Thompson or Bookwalter) is used.

The procedure begins with mobilization of the duodenum, which is attached to the peritoneal reflection (extension of the abdominal peritoneum). The surgeon separates loose connective tissue from the duodenum with the ESU. Hemostasis is maintained as described above. The lower third of the stomach is separated from the omentum in the area of resection.

The stomach then is resected and anastomosed to the jejunum by a side-to-side anastomosis. The surgeon performs this step using a surgical stapling instrument or by clamping the stomach with Payr or Allen clamps and performing a traditional two-layer closure. Absorbable and silk sutures, sizes 2-0 and 3-0, are used for the anastomosis.

The duodenum is retracted, and the common bile duct is exposed and divided. Major vessels connecting the pancreas to the duodenum are divided. The common bile duct is anastomosed to the jejunum.

Anastomosis of the GI tract is performed as described in Table 21-2. The cystic duct is attached to the jejunum (**choledochojejunostomy**) later in the procedure. The junction of the duodenum and jejunum (duodenojejunal flexure) is divided.

The pancreas next must be resected. The surgeon performs this step with both sharp and blunt dissection, taking care to maintain hemostasis. The pancreatic duct must be identified and preserved for attachment to the jejunum. When all bleeding is controlled and attachments have been severed between the accessory organs, the specimen is removed. The scrub should receive it in a basin. The scrub should not remove it from the sterile table until the surgeon has given permission.

Reconstruction of the GI tract continues with an end-to-end pancreatojejunostomy. An end-to-side, single-layer choledochojejunostomy is then performed (Figure 21-54).

During anastomosis, the scrub has many suture needles on the field. These must be carefully managed to avoid loss. Remember that sponge and needle counts must be made whenever a hollow organ is closed. Before the anastomosis of the stomach and intestine, individual sponge counts must be performed and recorded.

After the reconstruction is complete, the surgeon irrigates the wound with antibacterial solution and inspects each anastomosis for evidence of leakage. When hemostasis is completely secured, one or more abdominal drains are placed in the abdomen. These may be **exteriorized** (brought out through another location in the abdominal wall). The wound is then closed in individual layers.

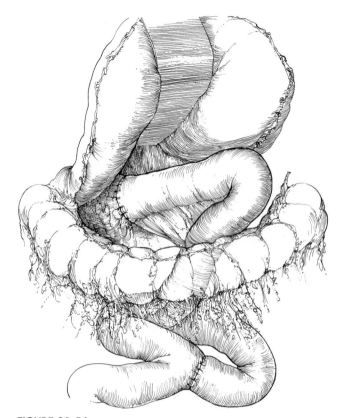

FIGURE 21-54
Completion of the pancreaticojejunostomy (Whipple procedure). (From Economou SG and Economou TS: *Atlas of surgical technique*, ed 2, Philadelphia, 1996, Saunders.)

RELATED PROCEDURE
Excision of pancreatic cyst

Endoscopic Distal Pancreatectomy
SURGICAL GOAL
In this procedure, a portion of the pancreas is removed for palliative treatment of a malignant tumor or to remove a benign lesion. Splenectomy may be performed during the procedure.

PATHOLOGY
Cancer of the pancreas is usually well advanced at the time of diagnosis. The survival rate is less than 3% in 5 years. Although not well understood, the risk is higher among smokers and those whose diet is high in fat and meat. Chronic pancreatitis is associated with pancreatic cancer. Alcoholism and biliary reflux are common causes of pancreatitis. Pancreatic resection may be performed if the tumor is localized in one area. Partial pancreatectomy offers palliative treatment for metastasis.

Technique

1. The patient is placed in supine position.
2. A pneumoperitoneum is established.
3. Four abdominal ports are created.

4. The gastric arteries and branches are coagulated.
5. The splenocolic ligament is incised.
6. The spleen is mobilized from the retroperitoneum.
7. The pancreas is retracted upward so that it may be identified.
8. The splenic artery and vein are exposed and ligated.
9. A linear surgical stapler is used to transect the tail of the pancreas.
10. The specimen is removed with a specimen retrieval bag.
11. A 15-mm port is extended by at least 2 mm.
12. The spleen is divided into sections and brought out of the abdominal cavity through the retrieval bag.
13. An abdominal drain is placed.
14. Cannulated ports are removed, and the pneumoperitoneum is released.
15. The wounds are closed.

DISCUSSION

The patient is placed on the operating table in supine position. The patient is prepped and draped for a laparoscopy. Slight reverse Trendelenburg position is used during the procedure.

A pneumoperitoneum is established, and four ports are placed in the abdomen. A 12-mm port is placed above the umbilicus under direct visualization. This port is used for the laparoscope. A 15-mm port is inserted below the left costal margin. A 5-mm port is placed at the left costal margin. The fourth port is inserted into the subxyphoid area.

After examining the abdominal cavity, the surgeon incises the gastrocolic ligament using blunt dissection. This creates access to the gastric arteries and branches. These vessels are clipped and divided or coagulated with the ESU. The splenocolic ligament and peritoneal attachment to the spleen are then incised with scissors and a dissecting probe.

The pancreas is freed from the retroperitoneum with dissecting scissors. The pancreas must be elevated with an atraumatic retractor to gain access to the splenic vein. The vein is ligated with surgical clips and divided. The splenic artery is identified, clipped, and divided. When the spleen has been freed from its vascular attachments, the pancreas is transected with a linear stapler, such as the Endo GIA II (United States Surgical Corporation). Bleeding from the severed surface of the pancreas is controlled with the ESU. The pancreas is placed in a specimen retrieval bag. The spleen is then divided into small pieces and delivered from the wound through the 15-mm port.

A small abdominal drain may be placed in the wound, which is then irrigated. All instruments are removed from the abdomen, and the pneumoperitoneum is released.

Individual ports are sutured with absorbable suture and skin staples.

Surgical Resection of the Liver
TYPES OF RESECTIONS
The goal of liver resection is to remove a portion of the liver. The structure of the liver allows the removal of a segment or an entire lobe. Three resections are typically performed. These are the **wedge resection, segmental resection,** and **lobectomy.**

Wedge resection describes the shape of a section removed from the edge of the liver to eradicate a small tumor for diagnostic purposes. Segmental resection is an anatomical removal of one of the segments.

Segments may be removed after all attachments, including ligaments, ducts, and vessels, have been identified. These structures are called the portal pedicles. **Portal** refers to the portal vein, which traverses the liver and drains it. The origin of the pedicles differs according to the individual segment. Recall from the anatomy discussion that the liver is divided into two major lobes and eight segments.

Lobectomy is the removal of one or more of the major lobes of the liver—right, left, or all of the right lobe and a portion of the left (called **right hepatic trisegmentectomy**).

The decision to perform major hepatic resection is based on the size, type of tumor, nutritional state of the patient, and function of the liver at the time of surgery. The patient with liver disease who does not have a history of acute or chronic liver disease can tolerate removal of six to eight segments. Benign liver tumors also may require resection. Marginal tissue also is removed during resection. Marginal tissue is the tissue around the tumor. During pathological examination, the goal is to ensure that none of the marginal tissue contains tumor cells. If pathological examination (frozen section) is performed during surgery, the pathologist reports to the surgeon whether the margins need to be enlarged.

Although the size of the resection varies, the techniques used are very similar. The gallbladder is attached to the ventral surface of the right lobe. Bile ducts draining from these anatomical areas must be occluded during resection.

An anatomical resection is one in which the blood supply, drainage, and bile ducts of a segment can be occluded and then the entire segment is removed. However, not all resections can be performed in this manner. If this is the case, individual blood vessels and ducts are divided and occluded as they are encountered. Wedge resection is an example of this type of hepatic procedure.

PATHOLOGY

The most common indication for liver resection is a malignant liver tumor. The tumor may be **primary** (the original source of the cancer) or **metastatic** (cancer that has spread from another location in the body). The most common type of liver tumor is metastatic, especially those that arise from primary tumors whose blood supply is drained by the portal vein. Primary liver tumors are rare.

Three conditions appear to cause liver cancer. These are chronic hepatitis B infection, cirrhosis of the liver, and carcinogens in food. Cancer of the liver usually is well advanced by the time it is diagnosed. **Cirrhosis** is caused most often by chronic, excessive alcohol use. However, it also can be caused by other conditions. Cirrhosis results in liver fibrosis and changes in the vascular structure that cause portal hypertension. Refer to surgery for portal hypertension in Chapter 29 for a discussion of this disease. Less common indications for liver resection include parasitic disease, infection, and laceration or trauma to the liver.

EQUIPMENT

Hepatic resection requires basic laparotomy instruments, drapes, and equipment. Other equipment is added according to the surgeon's preference. Common additions include the following:

▶ Long general surgery instruments
▶ Vascular clamps (for extensive resection)
▶ Gallbladder (biliary) instruments
▶ Self-retaining retractor with multiple attachments, such as the Thompson or Bookwalter retractor
▶ Vessel clips
▶ Vessel loops
▶ Absorbable collagen
▶ Hemostatic agents such as Surgicel gauze or Avitene powder
▶ Harmonic scalpel
▶ Cavitron ultrasonic surgical aspirator (CUSA)
▶ Argon beam coagulator
▶ Smoke evacuator (cutting equipment creates heavy smoke plume during hepatic surgery; be sure to use a smoke evacuator during surgery)
▶ Blunt suture needles (the blunt needle pushes tissue aside as it enters rather than puncturing or tearing it during suturing).
▶ Sponge dissectors

Wedge Resection
SURGICAL GOAL

The goal of wedge resection is to remove a marginal section of the liver. The wedge resection does not follow anatomical dissection. The incision margins include the tumor itself and an additional space outside the tumor to ensure that no part of the lesion remains outside the dissection. The technique for the segmental resection is similar to the technique for wedge resection.

Technique

1. A laparotomy is performed through a midline or paramedian incision.
2. The surgeon explores the abdominal cavity to determine the exact area to be excised.
3. Moist laparotomy sponges are used to pack abdominal viscera away from the liver.
4. A self-retaining retractor is placed in the wound.
5. Glisson's capsule is scored at the periphery of the lesion with the ESU.
6. The wedge is incised and hemostasis is maintained with the ESU, argon beam coagulator, CUSA, or harmonic scalpel.
7. Larger blood vessels may be clipped or ligated with absorbable suture.

8. The surgeon may use a hemostatic agent such as gelatin sponge, Surgicel, or Avitene to control capillary bleeding on the liver surface.
9. The incision is closed.

DISCUSSION

The surgeon selects an abdominal incision (laparotomy) that gives the best exposure to the wedge of liver to be resected. Common exposures include a midline, paramedian, or flank incision.

After performing the laparotomy, the surgeon examines the body cavity for signs of metastasis or benign disease. He then places a self-retaining retractor in the wound, using moist laparotomy sponges to protect the abdominal viscera and wound edges.

After the surgeon has determined the line of resection, he or she uses the ESU to cut a shallow trough into Glisson's capsule outside the margins of the tumor. This cut is then carried deeper with the ESU, CUSA, or harmonic scalpel. Bleeding is controlled by these devices or with the argon beam coagulator.

As the resection progresses, individual blood vessels and bile ducts are managed as they are encountered. Small vessels can be coagulated. Large blood vessels are clamped with right-angle clamps and clipped or ligated with suture ties or suture ligatures. Size 2-0 or 3-0 absorbable sutures or silk sutures are typically used. The scrub should have these available at all times during the dissection.

Larger vessels and ducts are deep within the wound, close to the vena cava, and require right-angle or vascular clamps and small suture needles to fit into the narrow space. When ligaments are encountered, these also must be included in the dissection. The surgeon may cut them by sharp dissection or strip them away from the segment with blunt dissection using sponge dissectors.

Large blood vessels, branches of the vena cava, and ducts that are *not* included in the resection are retracted with Silastic vessel loops, or a small Penrose drain.

Dissection continues until the wedge of tissue is freed. The liver segment is passed to the scrub. The specimen may require immediate examination by the pathologist to ensure that the margins are free of abnormal cells. The raw surface of the resected liver may be coagulated with the argon beam coagulator or the ESU.

When the lines of resection are dry (no hemorrhaging), the tissue is released. The wound is irrigated and checked again for bleeders. A small abdominal drain such as a Penrose may be placed in the wound, which is then closed in layers. Wedge resection is illustrated in Figure 21-55.

Segmental Resection
SURGICAL GOAL

The goal of segmental resection is to remove one or more defined segments of the liver. The primary difference between wedge resection and segmental resection is that in seg-

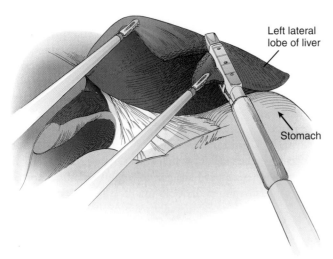

Left lateral
lobe of liver

Stomach

FIGURE 21-55
Wedge resection of the left lateral lobe of the liver using a linear stapler. (Colorized from Ballantyne GH: *Atlas of laparoscopic surgery,* Philadelphia, 2000, Saunders.)

mental resection, specific veins, arteries, and the biliary duct (pedicle structures) define the anatomical boundaries of the resection. The entire segment containing smaller branches of the pedicle is removed. This is called an **anatomical resection.** This additional surgical goal reduces the risk of metastasis via the hepatic vessels and ducts. In wedge resection, the area of resection is not defined by biliary or vascular branches (**nonanatomical resection**). If multiple segments are resected (**lobar resection**), a cholecystectomy may be performed as described above.

1. A laparotomy is performed through a midline, paramedian, or subcostal incision.
2. The surgeon explores the abdominal cavity to evaluate the extent and location of diseased tissue. Intraoperative ultrasound may be used to identify segments associated with the diseased tissue.
3. Moist laparotomy sponges are used to pack abdominal viscera away from the liver. Additional laparotomy sponges are placed between the diaphragm and liver.
4. A self-retaining retractor is placed in the abdomen.
5. The surgeon examines the abdominal cavity for evidence of disease.
6. The pedicle segment is identified, and individual vessels and ducts (bile duct, hepatic artery, and portal vein branch) are dissected free.
7. Ultrasound may be used, or methylene blue dye may be injected into the pedicle to stain the segment and identify the exact anatomical boundaries.
8. The pedicle structures are clamped and ligated.
9. The liver segment is resected.
10. Hemostasis is secured.

11. An abdominal drain is placed in the wound.
12. The wound is closed in layers.

DISCUSSION

A laparotomy is performed through a midline, paramedian, or flank incision. After entering the abdomen, the surgeon examines the liver and adjacent viscera to determine the presence of diseased tissue. This may be performed before or after a self-retaining retractor is placed in the wound. Because of the size of the liver and the wide exposure required, a self-retaining retractor with accessory attachments is often used. Before placing the retractor, the surgeon places moist laparotomy sponges over accessory organs surrounding the liver and between the liver and the diaphragm.

One of the areas in which sponges often are retained is the **subphrenic** area (under the diaphragm). The scrub counts all sponges placed in the wound, taking *special* care to note those placed in this area of the abdomen.

After all retractors have been placed, the surgeon examines the disease segment. A sterile ultrasound Doppler probe may be needed to determine the segmental location of the tumor. The ultrasound measures tissue density and identifies precise areas of disease.

Removal of liver segments requires identification and dissection of veins, arteries, and ducts that branch into each segment. The scrub must watch the field and observe the progress of the dissection, passing the appropriate instruments to the surgeon as needed.

To begin the resection, the surgeon begins by dissecting the adhesions that attach the liver to the abdominal wall, such as the falciform ligament. To perform a segmental resection, the surgeon must locate the correct segment pedicle. These two steps of the procedure are performed with the ESU, Metzenbaum scissors, and blunt sponge dissectors. The surgeon may need to place an additional retractor superiorly (at the top of the incision) to displace the liver upward. The Harrington ("sweetheart") retractor or wide Deaver retractor may be used here. The surgeon protects the liver with a moist laparotomy sponge and uses his or her hand to expose the ligaments that attach the liver to the posterior wall of the abdomen. The ultrasonic scalpel and aspirator (CUSA) is used to expose the pedicle where it branches into the parenchyma.

At this stage, the surgeon must identify the exact borders of the segment. As mentioned in the surgical goal, all branches of the pedicle must be identified and included in the resection to prevent metastasis. If the multiple segments are to be removed, all ligament attachments are transected during the procedure.

A common method is to begin dissection at the pedicle (at the hilum of the liver) and follow the structures into the parenchyma, using the ultrasonic scalpel or ESU to resect the liver tissue. If this approach is used, the surgeon temporarily stops the vascular supply to the segment by applying vascular clamps across the vessels that supply that segment. This prevents excess bleeding during the dissection.

An alternative method is to first identify the pedicle structures and then inject methylene blue dye into the pedicle. The methylene blue dye enters the pedicle structures and stains the segment that includes the tumor. If this technique is used, the scrub should have methylene blue dye, a 10-ml syringe, and the surgeon's preferred needle for injection. A small Silastic catheter may be attached to the hub of the needle and syringe for easier injection.

When the portal (branches of the portal vein) and pedicle structures and appropriate segment have been identified, the pedicle structures are individually clamped, ligated, and **transected** (divided). The pedicle and portal structures are ligated with silk, synthetic nonabsorbable suture, or surgical staples.

The liver segment next may be resected. The surgeon scores the segment using the technique described in Wedge Resection. Complete resection is performed with the ESU, CUSA, or harmonic scalpel, or by finger fracture (the surgeon uses his hand to "break" the parenchyma along the lines of resection). At the completion of the resection, the liver bed and raw surfaces must be free of hemorrhage. The argon beam coagulator and ESU are typically used to secure hemostasis. An abdominal drain, such as a Jackson-Pratt or Penrose drain, is placed in the wound, which is then closed in layers as for a laparotomy.

Biopsy of the Liver
SURGICAL GOAL
This procedure entails removal of a small wedge of liver tissue for biopsy.

PATHOLOGY
This procedure often is performed to identify the presence of metastatic carcinoma. It may be performed in conjunction with other abdominal procedures.

Technique
1. The abdomen is entered.
2. A wedge is cut from the edge of the liver.
3. The incised edges are closed.
4. The wound is closed.

DISCUSSION
The surgeon enters the abdomen through an upper midline incision. The surgeon then incises a wedge from the liver edge using the deep knife or cautery pencil (Figure 21-56). The specimen is passed to the scrub.

The edges of the liver may be approximated with chromic gut, size 2-0 or 3-0, swaged to a blunt needle. To control bleeding on the surfaces of the liver, a small strip of Surgicel gauze or a small amount of Avitene may be placed over the suture line. Some surgeons avoid suturing the liver

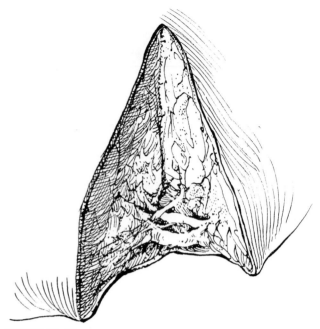

FIGURE 21-56
Excision of lesion with a 1-cm margin. (From Economou SG and Economou TS: *Atlas of surgical technique*, ed 2, Philadelphia, 1996, Saunders.)

and prefer to use the coagulating current of the cautery pencil to control bleeding from the raw edges of the liver. When oozing has stopped, the wound is closed in routine fashion.

Liver Transplantation
Liver transplantation is one of the most successful transplant procedures under current investigation. Potential recipients in end-stage liver disease are screened for the following criteria:

▶ Whether the disease is life threatening or reversible
▶ Whether the disease is correctable by transplant
▶ Age
▶ Previous abdominal surgery (kind and type)
▶ Psychological and psychosocial considerations
▶ Physical status

Organs are procured through the United Network for Organ Sharing (Richmond, Virginia), which matches recipients and donors when an organ becomes available. Liver transplants are very tedious because of the complexity of the anatomy, friable nature, and vascularity of the liver. Extensive dissection is required as well as ligation of vessels to avoid postoperative hemorrhage. Implanting a donor liver requires reanastomosis of the suprahepatic vena cava, infrahepatic vena cava, portal vein, and hepatic artery, along with biliary reconstruction with end-to-end anastomosis of donor and recipient common bile ducts.

SECTION V
Breast Surgery

Behavioral Objectives

After studying this section the reader will be able to:

- Describe the structure of the breast
- Discuss the task of providing supportive communication to the patient undergoing breast surgery
- Identify the set-up for bilateral breast biopsy
- Describe the scheme for the removal of a breast mass
- Recognize and identify instruments required for breast surgery
- Identify the anatomy of the chest wall
- Describe the process for conversion to a radical procedure after biopsy and frozen section
- Explain the surgeon's requirements for hemostatic control during breast surgery
- Describe the preparation and maintenance needed to ensure an orderly instrument table and field during a long procedure

Terminology

Areola—The darkened area surrounding the nipple, which contains sebaceous glands. The areola becomes more deeply pigmented under the influence of hormones, especially during pregnancy.

De-epithelialization—Removal of skin from a tissue flap.

Excisional biopsy—Removal of a tissue mass for pathological examination.

Frozen section—A technique used to examine biopsy tissue in which the tissue is frozen in liquid nitrogen and processed through a microtome. The microtome cuts the mass into microscopic slices for examination under the microscope. Frozen section is performed during surgery to determine the need for immediate radical surgery.

Hook wire—A device used to pinpoint the exact location of a nonpalpable mass detected during a mammogram. A fine needle is inserted into the mass during the examination, and the tissue around the needle is removed for pathological examination and definitive diagnosis.

Lumpectomy—The wide excision of a malignant mass of breast tissue. Also known as a segmental biopsy or tylectomy.

Mastectomy (simple)—Procedure that removes breast tissue, including the skin, areola, and nipple. Lymph nodes are not removed.

Modified radical mastectomy—Removal of the entire breast, the nipple, and areolar region. The lymph nodes also are usually removed. This is the most common procedure for malignant breast tumor.

Needle localization biopsy—Procedure in which tissue surrounding a hook wire device is removed.

Palpable—A quality of tissue that allows an examiner to describe and differentiate the tissue by feeling it. Palpation applies to any form of physical examination in which the examiner uses his or her hand to locate and describe tissue.

Pedicle flap—A section of tissue that is partially removed from one area of the body and transferred to a nearby location. The purpose is to retain blood supply within the flap so the reconstructed area remains viable.

Segmental mastectomy—See lumpectomy.

Sentinel lymph node biopsy—Procedure in which one or more lymph nodes are removed to determine whether malig-

nancy has spread. Other lymph nodes may be periodically removed to determine whether metastasis has occurred.

Skin flap—A flap created by incising the skin and cutting it away from the underlying tissue to which it is attached. The flap can be increased in size or "raised" as the flap is made larger by dissection.

Staging—A complex method of determining the severity of a malignant tumor. Lymph node involvement, size of the tumor, location, and type are considered.

Subcutaneous mastectomy—Procedure that removes the breast while leaving the skin, nipple, and areola intact.

Total mastectomy—Also called a simple mastectomy; procedure that removes the breast, including skin and nipple. Lymph-node dissection is not performed.

Tylectomy—Procedure of localized removal of a lesion; synonymous with lumpectomy.

Undermine—A surgical technique in which tissue planes are separated by blunt or sharp dissection. The separation of the two layers results in a "pocket" between the two layers.

ANATOMY OF THE BREAST

The breasts are a functional part of the female reproductive system. Even though they are not a contiguous anatomical part of that system, they do provide milk for the infant. They respond to hormonal changes of the reproductive system and in many cultures have an important effect on sexual identification and body image.

The two breasts are located on the anterior chest wall between the third and seventh ribs. Support is provided by the pectoral muscles, and the breasts directly adhere to the superficial fascia. Histologically, the breast is made up of glandular, connective, and fat tissue (Figure 21-57). This tissue is contained within extensions of fibrous ligaments that radiate out from the nipple to the periphery of the breast. Membranes or septal ligaments separate each of these radial sections. Each breast has about 15 to 25 separate sections. The glandular tissue forms clusters or small lobes, which are interspersed with alveoli that contain the secretory cells that form milk.

The intralobar ducts communicate from the glandular lobes. These ducts lead to the lactiferous ducts and reservoir, and then to the nipple. The release of breast milk and other secretions from the nipple is controlled by complex hormonal changes.

The *nipple* contains glandular, erectile, nerve, and epithelial tissue. The **areola** is defined as the darkened area around the nipple. Small nodes called Montgomery's tubercles contain sebaceous glands. Estrogen and progesterone secreted cyclically and during pregnancy cause the areola to become darker.

The breast tissue changes with development of the individual, hormonal changes, pregnancy status, and nutritional state.

INTRODUCTION TO SURGERY OF THE BREAST

Psychological Considerations

For most women, the breast reflects reproductive ability, affects body image, and secures feminine identity. Surgery of the breast threatens these images and can produce anxiety and depression. Public awareness about breast cancer and advanced technology for early detection have increased women's ability to take an active part in breast health. Breast tumors also may occur in men, but the incidence is very low.

Although early detection is an important advance in breast medicine, the prospect of surgery remains an emotional and difficult process for the patient. The patient's need for emotional support requires health-care workers to listen to the patient and support and acknowledge her feelings. Offering appropriate psychosocial support means that the health-care worker does not offer false hope. The worker's most important role is to provide a calm presence and to convey respect for the patient's feelings.

Reconstructive breast surgery (discussed in Chapter 26) may take place immediately after mastectomy or as a separate procedure scheduled for a later date. Postmastectomy patients may enter a deep grieving period after such radical

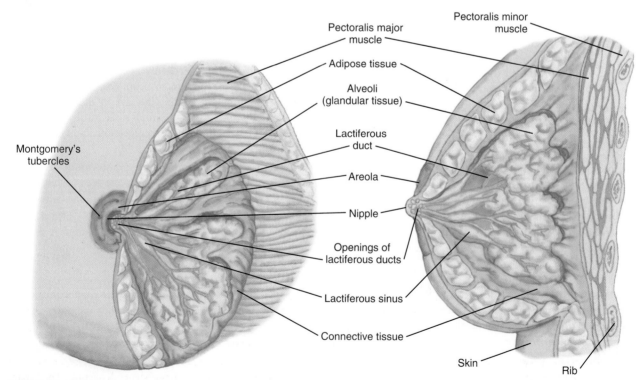

FIGURE 21-57
Anatomy of the breast. (From Murray SS, McKinney ES, and Gorrie TM: *Foundations of maternal-newborn nursing,* ed 3, Philadelphia, 2002, Saunders.)

surgery. Psychological support at this time is critical in restoring the patient's positive self-image.

Patients undergoing any type of breast surgery are given the same considerations as the mastectomy patient. Radical changes to the breast often cause anxiety about sexual identity and reproductive functions. Respect and *presence* are critical components of patient care.

Instruments and Supplies

Surgery of the breast requires general surgery instruments and a plastic surgery set (Figure 21-58). Senn, vein, and other small retractors are needed for breast biopsy and for more radical procedures. Surgical clips, absorbable and nonabsorbable sutures, and an ESU are used for hemostasis. Vessel loops are needed for retraction of deep veins, arteries, and nerves. A small Penrose drain also should be available for retraction. Wound drains include the Jackson Pratt, Hemovac, and simpler gravity drains such as the Penrose.

Skin marking is performed for all breast procedures, especially reconstructive surgery. Skin marks may be made before admission or at the time of surgery. Gentian violet skin markers or brilliant green dye are used to mark the areas of incision.

The ESU is used extensively in radical breast surgery. Two ESU units may be required. The scrub is reminded to keep

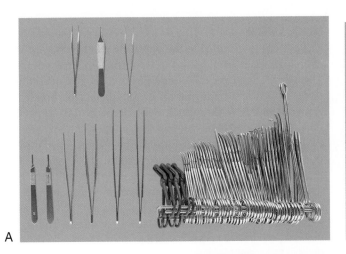
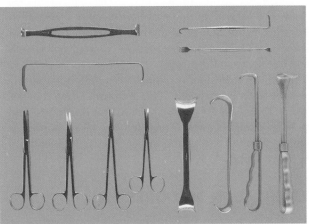
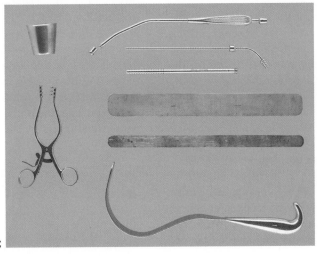

FIGURE 21-58
Basic instrumentation for breast surgery. **A,** *Top,* two Adson tissue forceps with teeth (1 × 2) (front and side views); one Brown-Adson tissue forceps with teeth (9 × 9) (front view). *Bottom,* two Bard-Parker knife handles (no. 3); two DeBakey vascular Atraugrip tissue forceps (short); two Cushing tissue forceps with teeth (1 × 2); four paper drape clips; two Halsted mosquito hemostatic forceps (curved); one Halsted mosquito hemostatic forceps (straight); eight Crile hemostatic forceps (curved, 5½ inch); one Halsted hemostatic forceps (straight); six Crile hemostatic forceps (curved, 6½ inch); four Allis tissue forceps; four Babcock tissue forceps; four Ochsner hemostatic forceps (straight); one Westphal hemostatic forceps; two tonsil hemostatic forceps; one Foerster sponge forceps; one Johnson needle holder (6 inch); two Crile-Wood needle holders (6 inch). **B,** *Top left,* two Army-Navy retractors (front and side views). *Top right,* two Miller-Senn retractors (side and front views). *Bottom,* one Mayo dissecting scissors (straight); one Mayo dissecting scissors (curved); one Metzenbaum scissors (7 inch); one Metzenbaum scissors (5 inch); two Goelet retractors (front and side views); two Richardson retractors (small) (side and front views). **C,** *Top left,* one metal medicine cup (2 oz). *Bottom left,* one Weitlaner retractor (small). *Left, top to bottom,* one Yankauer suction tube with tip; one Poole abdominal suction tube with shield; one Ochsner malleable retractor (medium); one Ochsner malleable retractor (narrow); one Deaver retractor (medium). (From Tighe SM: *Instrumentation for the operating room,* ed 6, St Louis, 1999, Mosby.)

the ESU tips clean with a Teflon pad or moist sponge. Recall that scraping the ESU tip with a sharp instrument or blade causes scratches in the tip. Eschar builds up quickly in these scratches and can cause overheating and a "charcoal effect." This buildup of eschar can easily ignite drapes in the presence of oxygen or alcohol.

The surgeon may require a nerve stimulator to differentiate blood vessels from small nerves. The nerve stimulator is an intraoperative device that delivers a small amount of current when applied over the nerve, causing the nerve to retract.

NOTE: If biopsies are to be performed on both of the patients' breasts, there must be two different sterile set-ups, with separate instruments, supplies, and equipment on each set-up. The surgical team members also must change their gloves before continuing to the next breast to avoid cross-contamination of breasts by possibly carrying cancer cells from one breast to the other.

NOTE: If a breast biopsy has just been performed during the same larger procedure (i.e., mastectomy), all instruments used on the biopsy are removed, the patient is redraped, and the team changes gloves. These steps are taken to prevent contamination of the wound by cancer cells released from the biopsy tissue.

SURGICAL PROCEDURES

Needle Localization Biopsy
SURGICAL GOAL

Needle localization biopsy is the insertion of a fine needle into a nonpalpable abnormal breast mass observed during mammography. The purpose of the needle is to identify the exact location of the mass for subsequent biopsy and microscopic examination. A definitive diagnosis then can be made.

PATHOLOGY

Breast cancer is the most common cancer among females in the United States. Risk factors include family history, gender (breast cancer in males makes up less than 1% of all cases), history of benign breast disease, and hormonal conditions that result in late menarche or late menopause. Early-detection procedures include fine needle biopsy and aspiration biopsy, which are performed without anesthesia. Tumors are classified by tissue characteristics and by **staging**. This is a complex method used to classify the severity of a cancer. The size of the tumor, affected lymph nodes, and presence of metastasis determine the stage.

Technique

1. During mammography, the patient is prepped and a local anesthetic is administered in the area of the mass.
2. A hook wire assembly is inserted into the mass.
3. The wire is secured to the patient's skin with tape.
4. The patient is transferred to the operating room.
5. Additional prep solution may be applied gently around the site of the needle

6. The patient is draped for an excisional biopsy of the breast.
7. The surgeon locates the needle and makes an elliptical incision that includes the needle and a margin of skin.
8. The incision is continued through the subcutaneous and breast tissue, including a 1-cm to 2-cm margin. Small rake retractors are placed in the wound edge.
9. The needle and tissue are removed, and the tissue is examined by the pathologist for clear margins.
10. Additional tissue may be removed if the margins are not clear.
11. The breast tissue is closed with size 3-0 absorbable suture. The skin is closed with sterile adhesive strips.

DISCUSSION

The patient is admitted to the operating room immediately after placement of a hook needle during mammography. The patient is placed in supine position on the operating table. After the administration of anesthetic, the breast is gently prepped. A fenestrated body drape is then applied. One must take extreme care not to dislodge the hook wire!

The surgeon begins the procedure by making an elliptical skin incision around the hook wire (Figure 21-59). He or she then uses Metzenbaum scissors to increase the depth of the incision. Senn retractors or small rakes are placed at the periphery of the wound. Scissors rather than an ESU are used to complete the dissection to avoid distorting the margins of the mass. Allis clamps may be used to grasp the tissue during dissection. Small bleeders can be controlled with fine suture or a needle-point ESU. The identification needle is retained in the specimen. The specimen is delivered to the pathologist, who examines it for clear margins (no tumor cells present). If the margins are not clear, additional tissue is removed and examined. When the margins include a clear area of 1 cm to 2 cm, the wound is closed.

The excision site is irrigated with warm saline and closed with several subcutaneous interrupted sutures of absorbable

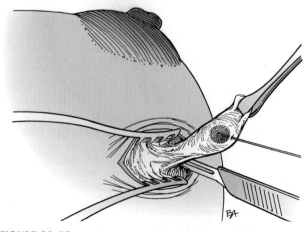

FIGURE 21-59
Needle localization biopsy—elliptical excision of breast tissue around the tip of the wire. (Colorized from Moody FG: *Atlas of ambulatory surgery*, St Louis, 1999, Mosby.)

synthetic material. The skin is usually closed with sterile strips or a subcuticular running suture.

Excision of a Palpable Breast Mass
SURGICAL GOAL

A **palpable** breast mass is one that can be felt. Palpable masses are excised for pathological examination. Excision allows for a confirmation of a diagnosis of malignancy.

PATHOLOGY
Refer to the section on Needle Localization Biopsy.

Technique

1. A short incision is made over the breast mass.
2. The surgeon explores the wound to locate the periphery of the mass.
3. The surgeon excises the mass with the ESU and dissecting scissors.
4. The mass may be immediately examined and a mastectomy initiated upon confirmation of malignancy.
5. If the mass is benign or if further surgery is to be delayed, the wound is closed in layers.

DISCUSSION
Breast biopsy for a palpable mass may be performed as the first stage of a mastectomy. If the patient is prepared for the possibility of malignancy, the case is scheduled as an excisional biopsy with a possible mastectomy. In this case, the pathologist performs a frozen section. This is a method of examining tissue. The tissue is frozen in nitrogen, and microscopic slices are taken. These are examined, and the cells are determined to be malignant or benign.

This procedure may be performed under local anesthetic if a radical procedure will be delayed. If there is a possibility of mastectomy, a general anesthetic is used.

The patient is placed in the supine position, prepped, and draped with the affected breast exposed. The surgeon makes a small incision over the area of the mass with the scalpel. The connective, fat, and breast tissues are exposed. A needle or flat-tip ESU is used to coagulate bleeders. Small rake retractors may be placed at the wound edges. The surgeon deepens the wound with the ESU, Metzenbaum scissors, or curved Mayo scissors. When the mass is partially exposed, the surgeon can grasp it with Allis or Kocher clamps. The clamps are then used to elevate the tissue as dissection continues. Some surgeons do not use the ESU but rather clamp and ligate small bleeders with fine absorbable suture.

The surgeon completes the dissection and passes the specimen to the technologist. Because the tissue may determine the need for mastectomy, the scrub must take particular care in handling it.

The breast tissue is approximated with interrupted 3-0 absorbable sutures. The skin is closed with a size 4-0 subcuticular suture followed by sterile adhesive strips.

A **sentinel lymph node** may be removed at this time. A small incision is made in the axilla, and a single node is removed by sharp dissection. The node is examined for malignancy. A sentinel node may be removed for examination at any time during the course of disease or recovery. If a frozen section is performed, the pathologist consults with the surgeon during surgery. If a mastectomy is planned, a second set-up is used.

Breast-Conserving Surgery (Lumpectomy, Segmental Mastectomy, Tylectomy)
SURGICAL GOAL
The goal of this procedure is to remove a small malignant tumor and wide marginal area while leaving the subcutaneous tissue and skin tissue intact. Axillary lymph-node biopsy is included in the procedure. Lymph-node dissection determines the extent of the cancer and also prevents recurrence in the axillary area.

PATHOLOGY
Indications for lumpectomy are a small malignant mass, fibrocystic tissue, cyst, or breast nodule. The survival rate for lumpectomy and axillary lymph node removal followed by radiation therapy has shown to be similar to the rate of survival for patients at the same stage of cancer who have had a mastectomy.

Technique

1. The skin is incised, leaving a wide margin around the tumor.
2. The excision is extended into the subcutaneous layer and parenchyma.
3. The mass and marginal tissue are excised.
4. The axilla is incised below the upper axillary fold, and the incision is extended laterally.
5. The upper axillary flap is raised.
6. The lower skin flap is developed to expose the pectoralis muscles.
7. The axillary vein is divided.
8. The axillary tissue is freed up laterally, and the lymph nodes are dissected from the subscapular muscle.
9. The wounds are irrigated and closed.

DISCUSSION
Breast-conserving surgery for cancer is a procedure that removes up to 50% of the breast tissue. The procedure usually includes removal of axillary lymph nodes. The amount of tissue removed depends on the stage of the cancer.

The patient is prepped and draped for a breast excision. The arm on the affected side also is prepped. The lower arm or hand is draped separately with stockinet so that the surgeon can manipulate it for the axillary portion of the procedure.

The surgeon draws the incision area on the breast with a surgical skin marker. The incision encloses the area of the mass and includes a wide margin. He or she begins the procedure by incising the skin with the scalpel (Figure 21-60, *A-C*). This incision is carried through the subcutaneous and parenchymal (breast) tissue with Metzenbaum or Mayo

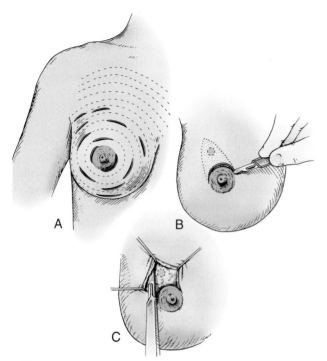

FIGURE 21-60
Breast-conserving surgery. **A,** Recommended incision sites for performing breast-conserving surgery. **B,** Technique for dissection of breast masses by the areolar margin. **C,** Skin flaps are created around the areola to provide tissue for cosmetic closure. (From Bland KI and Copeland EM: *The breast: comprehensive management of benign and malignant disorders,* ed 3, Philadelphia, 2004, Saunders.)

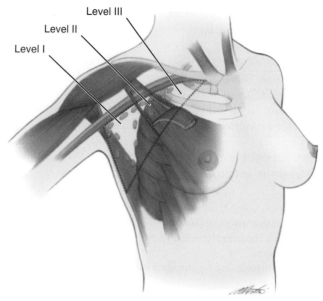

FIGURE 21-61
Axillary dissection—levels of axillary nodes. (From Donegan WL and Spratt JS: *Cancer of the breast,* ed 5, Philadelphia, 2002, Saunders.)

scissors. Small bleeders are coagulated with the ESU. A needle-point ESU tip may be used for more precise coagulation.

The surgeon grasps the subcutaneous and breast tissue with two or more Allis clamps, which can hold the tissue without tearing it. The scrub should have retractors available as the incision is carried into deeper layers. Small rake or Senn retractors can be used for shallow retraction. Small right-angle retractors or dull rakes are needed as the excision is carried deeper. If large bleeders are encountered, they can be clamped with hemostats and ligated with fine absorbable or silk sutures.

As the excision is extended, Raytec sponges should be removed from the field and replaced with laparotomy sponges. A Raytec sponge can be easily lost inside the breast wound, especially if the excision is wide.

When the surgeon has excised the tumor with a wide margin, the specimen is removed. Before removing it from the wound, the surgeon may place one or more sutures on the periphery for identification of the margins. These must be carefully preserved.

The breast wound may be closed at this time, or closure may be delayed until axillary dissection is complete.

Axillary Dissection

Axillary lymph nodes, which drain the breast and can include cancer cells, are divided into three separate anatomical levels. The extent of lymph-node dissection for cancer surgery is based on staging. Staging considers the presence of cancer in the lymph nodes. Axillary lymph nodes are located deep within the axillary fascia. The axillary nodes are identified by their relationship to the pectoralis minor muscle. Level-I nodes are lateral to the muscle, level-II nodes are behind the muscle, and level-III nodes are medial to the muscle (Figure 21-61). Advanced cancer requires more extensive axillary-node excision.

Level-II lymph-node dissections are performed in association with breast-conserving surgery. To gain access to the axillary nodes, the surgeon makes an incision just below the upper axillary fold that encompasses the lower axillary line. This tissue plane includes the subcutaneous and fascia layers. The lower flap is tapered toward the chest wall.

After the flaps have been created, right-angle retractors are placed along the edges. The pectoralis muscles are then retracted to expose the axillary vein and its small branches. These are clamped and divided. The axillary vein is ligated with silk sutures. Small branches may be clipped and divided. The surgeon continues to dissect the axillary tissue to expose the two major nerves in this area (thoracic and intercostobrachial). These nerves must be preserved during node dissection. Vessel loops are placed under the nerves with a right-angle clamp. Axillary tissue containing the nodes is then dissected away from the underlying muscle.

Before closing the axilla, the surgeon may place a Jackson-Pratt or Penrose drain in the wound. If a closed suction drain is used, the end is brought out through a small stab incision near the main incision. The drain is secured with one or two nonabsorbable sutures. The wounds are closed in two layers. The axilla and subcutaneous breast tissue are closed with interrupted absorbable sutures. The skin is closed with a running subcuticular suture of the surgeon's choice.

Total Mastectomy with Axillary Lymph-Node Dissection
SURGICAL GOAL
The goal of total mastectomy is to remove the breast and axillary lymph nodes. The extent of axillary dissection depends on the cancer stage. Invasive carcinoma requires level-I and level-II lymph-node dissection. If the lymph nodes are involved, level-III dissection is necessary.

In a skin-sparing mastectomy, overlying skin tissue, the areola, and the nipple are not removed. This produces a more pleasing cosmetic result. An implant may be placed immediately after the procedure.

PATHOLOGY
Subcutaneous mastectomy is performed for primary tumors with clear margins. The procedure is followed by radiation therapy. Patients who have a high risk for breast cancer may elect to have total bilateral mastectomy.

Technique

1. The patient is prepped and draped for a mastectomy; preparation includes the arm on the affected side.
2. The surgeon traces the incision line and area of the skin flaps with a marking pen.
3. The surgeon incises the skin to the level of the subcutaneous fat.
4. The skin flaps are raised to the previously marked areas and retracted with skin hooks.
5. Lateral edges of the flaps are carried to the edge of the latissimus dorsi muscle.
6. Large perforating blood vessels are ligated and secured.
7. The breast and deep fascia are dissected away from the pectoralis muscle.
8. If an axillary dissection is not included in the dissection, the specimen is dissected free from the lateral chest wall and axilla.
9. If axillary dissection is planned, the axillary vein and branches are exposed and divided.
10. The pectoralis minor muscle is divided for level-III axillary dissection.
11. The apex of the axillary tissues is marked with a suture for identification.
12. The axillary tissues are further dissected from the surrounding muscles.
13. Two suction drains are placed in the axilla.
14. The ends of the pectoralis minor muscle are sutured together.
15. The flaps are closed with skin staples, subcuticular suture, and sterile adhesive strips.

DISCUSSION
The total mastectomy with axillary lymph-node dissection is a long procedure that requires meticulous dissection.

The patient is placed in a supine position. A pad may be placed under the affected side at the level of the back to el-

evate the affected area. The patient is prepped for a mastectomy, with the affected arm prepped and draped free as previously described. The arm may be placed on a draped armboard.

Care must be taken not to allow the arm to drop off the armboard during surgery. Unless it is positioned for axillary exposure, it must be secured at all times.

To begin the procedure, the surgeon marks both the incision and the extent of the **skin flaps** (Figure 21-62, *A*). Incising the skin and creating a space between the skin and the underlying tissue creates a skin flap (Figure 21-62, *B*). This is called *raising a skin flap*. In some procedures the skin flap includes subcutaneous tissue. In this procedure the skin flaps do contain some fatty subcutaneous tissue. The superior and anterior flaps are extended to the previously marked lines on the skin (see Figure 21-62, *A*). Skin hooks are used to elevate the flaps as the surgeon extends them.

The surgeon uses the ESU and scalpel to carry the flaps deeper to the edge of the latissimus dorsi muscle. The technologist should have two ESU units available so that one can be cleaned while the other is in use.

As large blood vessels are encountered, they are clipped and divided or clamped and secured with silk ties. Be sure to remove all cut suture ends from the field to prevent them from entering the wound.

Sharp dissection continues with the knife, dissecting scissors, or ESU. The surgeon separates the breast and fascia tissue from the pectoralis major muscle (Figure 21-62, *C*). The skin flaps are retracted gently to preserve their blood supply and prevent bruising and ischemia at the edges.

Axillary dissection is a continuous part of this procedure. Rake or Richardson retractors are placed over the axillary edge of the incision. Blunt rakes are preferred to avoid puncturing the skin in this area. An additional right-angle retractor or narrow Deaver retractor may be needed for the medial side of the incision. Small or medium Richardson retractors are usually used.

The axillary vein is exposed during dissection (Figure 21-62, *D*). This vein is cross clamped with right-angle clamps, divided, and clipped or ligated. To perform level-III node dissection, the surgeon must sever the pectoralis minor muscle with the ESU (Figure 21-62, *E*). Retracting the pectoralis muscles with right-angle retractors exposes the axillary tissues. The specimen is dissected from the chest wall and muscles. The apex may be marked with a suture for pathological identification.

The surgeon then may pass the specimen to the scrub, who receives it in a small basin. Before closing the wound, the surgeon places two suction drains in the axilla and brings the ends out at the lateral chest wall. The ends of the pectoralis minor muscle are sutured together with absorbable sutures (Figure 21-62, *F*).

The wound is then irrigated with antibacterial solution and closed in layers. Absorbable subcutaneous sutures are placed. Skin is closed with a running subcuticular suture or skin staples, according to the surgeon's preference.

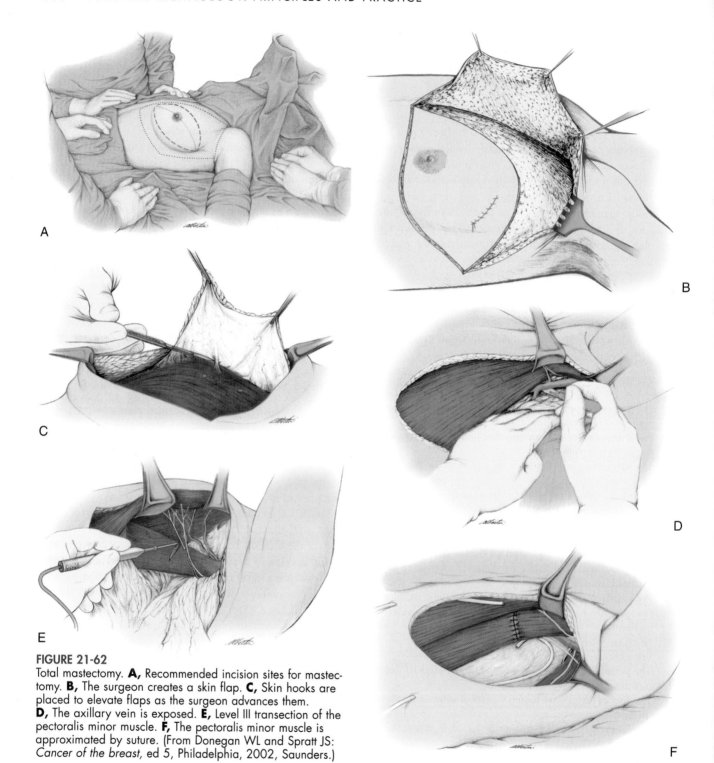

FIGURE 21-62
Total mastectomy. **A,** Recommended incision sites for mastectomy. **B,** The surgeon creates a skin flap. **C,** Skin hooks are placed to elevate flaps as the surgeon advances them. **D,** The axillary vein is exposed. **E,** Level III transection of the pectoralis minor muscle. **F,** The pectoralis minor muscle is approximated by suture. (From Donegan WL and Spratt JS: *Cancer of the breast,* ed 5, Philadelphia, 2002, Saunders.)

REFERENCES

Ballantyne GH: *Atlas of laparoscopic surgery,* Philadelphia, 2000, Saunders.

Bland KI and Copeland EM: *The breast: comprehensive management of benign and malignant disorders,* ed 3, Philadelphia, 2004, Saunders.

Donegan WL and Spratt JS: *Cancer of the breast,* ed 5, Philadelphia, 2002, Saunders.

Economou SG and Economou TS: *Atlas of surgical technique,* ed 2, Philadelphia, 1996, Saunders.

Ethicon: *Wound closure manual,* Somerville, NJ, 2002, Ethicon, Inc.

Ignatavicius DD and Workman ML: *Medical-surgical nursing: critical thinking for collaborative care,* ed 4, St Louis, 2002, Mosby.

Moody FG: *Atlas of ambulatory surgery,* St Louis, 1999, Mosby.

Murray SS, McKinney ES, and Gorrie TM: *Foundations of maternal-newborn nursing,* ed 3, Philadelphia, 2002, Saunders.

Rothrock JC: *Alexander's care of the patient in surgery,* ed 12, St Louis, 2003, Mosby.

Chapter 22

Gynecological and Obstetrical Surgery

Behavioral Objectives

After studying this chapter the reader will be able to:

- Identify instruments and equipment required in a hysteroscopic procedure
- Describe the preparation of solutions for intrauterine continuous drainage or distension
- Identify the method used for draping the patient for perineal surgery
- Describe the role of the assistant in vaginal procedures
- Explain the importance of maintaining aseptic technique during vaginal procedures
- Differentiate electrolytic and nonelectrolytic fluids used during intrauterine procedures
- Identify obstetrical and gynecological complications and procedural considerations

Terminology

Ablate—To remove or destroy tissue.

Adnexa—A collective term for the ovaries, fallopian tubes, and their connective and vascular attachments.

Cerclage—A procedure in which a suture ligature is placed around the incompetent cervix and tightened to prevent spontaneous abortion.

Cystocele—A bulging of the bladder into the vagina. The condition is related to weakness in the anterior vaginal wall.

Dermoid cyst—A primitive disorganized mass of cells and tissues that often contains teeth, hair, and skin.

Electrolytic media—Any solution that conducts electricity. During surgeries that require continuous irrigation for distension of a hollow organ, the media used must *not* be electrolytic. The use of electrolytic media would allow the current to travel through the media, causing a burn or an electrical shock.

En bloc—In one piece; describing a removal.

Endometriosis—Endometrial tissue growth outside of the uterine cavity.

Fibroid—See Leiomyoma.

Fulguration—An electrosurgical technique in which a spray of electrical energy coagulates and removes tissue. Also called *spray coagulation.*

Glycine—See Sorbitol.

Hyperplasia—Abnormal overgrowth of tissue anywhere in the body.

Hysteroscopy—A diagnostic and surgical method of performing intrauterine surgery. The hysteroscope is inserted through the cervix and surgery is conducted through the scope.

Incompetent cervix—A cervix that is unable to tolerate the weight of a growing fetus and allows it to be expelled during gestation.

Incomplete abortion—Demise of the embryo or fetus and expulsion of the tissue.

LEEP—Loop electrode excision procedure. In this technique, an electrosurgical loop is used to remove a core of tissue from the cervical canal.

Leiomyoma—A fibrous benign tumor of the uterus that usually arises from the myometrium.

Missed abortion—An abortion in which the products of conception are no longer viable but are retained in the uterus.

Nonelectrolytic media—A solution that does not conduct electrical current.

Obturator—A blunt-nosed tube inserted through the sheath of a rigid endoscope or hysteroscope to protect the tissue as the instrument is advanced.

Patency—The condition of being wide open; describes an unobstructed passageway.

Terminology

Perineum—Anatomical area between the posterior vestibule and the anus.

Photothermal ablation—Electrosurgical destruction or laser vaporization for removal of tissue.

PID—Pelvic inflammatory disease. Caused by sexually transmitted disease or other infection source. Causes scarring of the fallopian tubes and adhesions in the abdominal and pelvic cavity. PID is one of the leading causes of infertility in the United States.

Rectocele—A bulging of intestinal tissue into the posterior vaginal wall.

Reflection—A condition of turning or bending back upon its course, for example the peritoneum attached to the body wall covering an organ with a reattachment to the body wall.

Retrograde—A backward movement of fluid or an anatomical approach from back to front.

Shirodkar's procedure—See Cerclage.

Sorbitol—A nonelectrolytic solution used for distension of a hollow cavity during use of any electrosurgical device.

Transcervically—Literally, "through the cervix."

ANATOMY OF THE FEMALE REPRODUCTIVE SYSTEM

Internal Organs

UTERUS

The uterus and associated reproductive organs of the female reproductive system lie in the anterior portion of the female pelvic cavity (Figure 22-1). The uterus is a pear-shaped organ approximately 3 inches long and 2 inches deep. It is composed of thick muscular tissue and is suspended in the pelvic cavity by a series of ligaments that enclose the organ. On both sides of the uterus lie the fallopian tubes, which communicate directly with the interior of the uterus. The superior or upper portion of the organ, which lies above the insertion of the fallopian tubes, is called the *fundus*. The middle portion is called the *body,* and the lower portion is the *cervix.* The most common position of the uterus is tilted forward, toward the front of the pelvis.

The wall of the uterus is composed of several layers. These are the *endometrium, myometrium,* and *perimetrium.* The endometrium lines the uterus and changes under hormonal influence and pregnancy. It is continuous with the lining of the fallopian tubes and the vagina. The myometrium is the thick muscular layer, which is continuous with the muscles of the vagina and fallopian tubes. The muscle is capable of contraction, which occurs during childbirth and during menses. The perimetrium or outer serous layer of the uterus is a **reflection** of the abdominal peritoneum

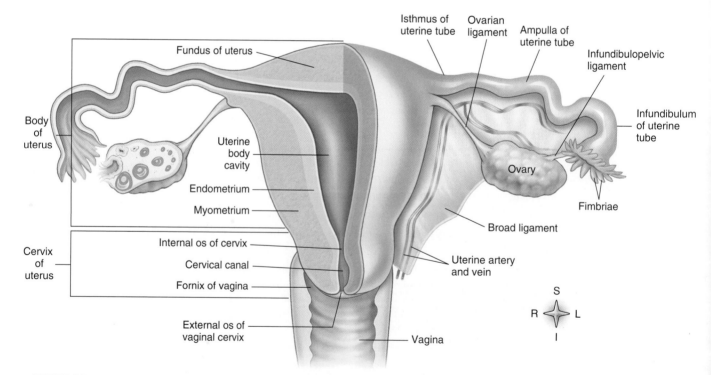

FIGURE 22-1

The uterus and associated reproductive organs of the female reproductive system. (From Thibodeau GA and Patton KT: *Anatomy and physiology,* ed 5. St Louis, 2003, Mosby.)

that is reflected over the bladder. This forms a pouch called the *cul-de-sac*. During surgery of the uterus, this portion of peritoneum may be incised and then re-sutured, and often is called the "bladder flap."

The *cervix* is the inferior neck of the uterus, which extends into the vaginal vault. The cervical *os* is the opening that may be surgically dilated or may dilate naturally under hormonal influence. The os has two anatomical sections, the external os and the internal opening. These two openings communicate by a short canal.

The *uterine ligaments* are sometimes difficult to differentiate and understand. The scrub must have a good understanding of the location and attachments to anticipate technical phases of pelvic procedures. The ligaments will be mentioned throughout this chapter. One should have a good understanding of their anatomical location before learning a procedure (Figure 22-2).

The ligaments that surround the uterus and are suspended from the pelvic cavity are called the *broad ligaments*. Above the broad ligaments, near the fallopian tubes, lie the *round ligaments*. These help to suspend the uterus anteriorly. The *cardinal ligaments* lie below the broad ligaments and provide the primary support for the uterus. The *uterosacral* ligaments curve along the bottom of the uterus to suspend the cervix and uterine body to the sacrum.

VAGINA

The vagina, which is sometimes called the *vaginal vault,* is a muscular tube that is bounded by the rectum on the posterior side and the bladder anteriorly. It connects the uterus with the *vestibule* (opening to the outside of the body). The vaginal lining has many folds of skin called *rugae* that are capable of distension during childbirth. The cervix and the Bartholin's glands provide mucous secretion into the vagina.

FALLOPIAN TUBES

The fallopian tubes communicate directly with the uterus, one on each side. Each fallopian tube has four sections: the interstitial section, which connects to the uterus, the narrow *isthmus* in the mid portion, the *ampulla*, which is the widened portion of the tube, and the *infundibulum,* which lies at the terminal end. The *fimbriae* are small projections that extend from the end of the tube. These undulate and direct the ovum toward the infundibulum at ovulation. The

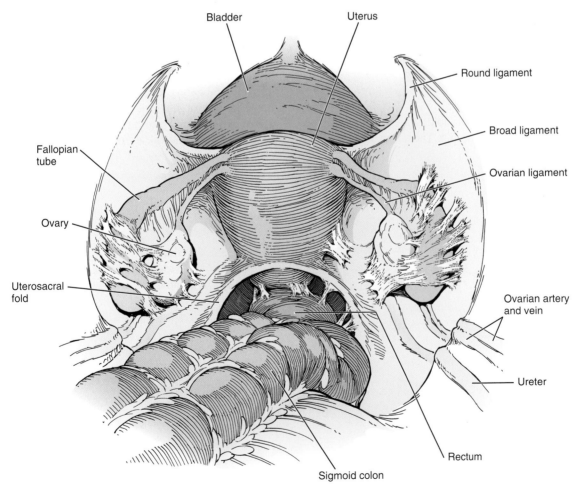

FIGURE 22-2
The uterine ligaments. (Adapted from Moody FG: *Atlas of ambulatory surgery,* St Louis, 1999, Mosby.)

fallopian tube is very narrow, 3 to 5 mm wide. It is not connected to the ovary but is suspended from the upper margin of the pelvis by the infundibulopelvic ligament. The lower margin is suspended by the mesosalpinx. The fallopian tube, the ovaries, and their ligaments are collectively called the **adnexa.**

OVARIES

The ovary is the female gonad or sex gland. The two ovaries, the organs of female reproduction and those responsible for the production of female hormones, lie on each side of the uterus in the upper portion of the pelvic cavity. The ovaries are suspended by the *mesovarium*—peritoneal tissue attached to the uterus by ovarian ligaments. Each ovary is approximately 1½ inches long and is oval. Each ovum contains approximately 1 million eggs, which are present at birth. The fibrous surface of the gland is uneven, containing follicles, which hold ova in different stages of maturity.

External Genitalia

The external genital structures of the female are collectively called the *vulva* (Figure 22-3). These structures include the mons pubis, labia majora, labia minora, clitoris, vestibular glands, and hymen.

MONS PUBIS

The mons pubis is a raised structure that covers the symphysis pubis. It contains connective and fatty tissue and forms the border of the reproductive tract.

LABIA MAJORA

The labia majora are two external folds (bisectional) of adipose tissue that envelop the perineal area. They are extensions of the mons pubis toward the anterior portion of the vulva and encircle the vestibule to protect the external genitalia.

LABIA MINORA

The labia minora are also bisectional and lie directly beneath the labia majora. These pigmented folds of tissue are delicate and are attached anteriorly by the frenulum. These folds extend from the clitoris to the posterior opening of the vagina, merging with the vaginal mucosa. Anteriorly, they meet just in front of the clitoris and form the prepuce (hood) of that structure.

CLITORIS

The clitoris is a highly vascular and sensitive organ that contains erectile tissue. It projects slightly from the anterior folds of the labia minora. The prepuce or covering of the clitoris is formed by the juncture of the labia majora. This organ is protected by the folds of the labia majora and is homologous to the penis in the male.

VESTIBULE

The vestibule is a term that refers collectively to all the structures located within the labia minora. One such structure is the distal urethra, including the meatus or opening. Within the vestibule lie the vestibular glands, so called because they lie within the vestibule of the external genitalia. Vestibular glands include Skene's glands (paraurethral glands) and Bartholin's glands. Skene's glands are two small, paired glands that lie beneath the floor of the urethra. These glands are the rudimentary homologue of the prostate gland in the male. Bartholin's glands lie on both sides of the vestibule and secrete mucus during coitus. These glands are homologous to the bulbourethral glands in the male.

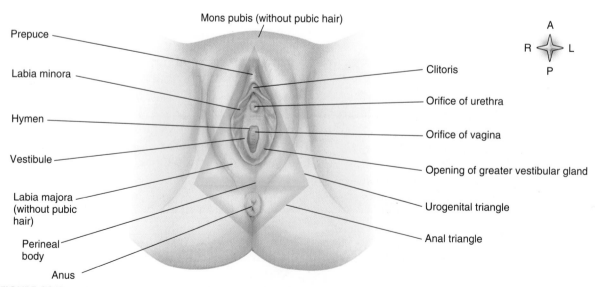

FIGURE 22-3
External genital structures of the female. (From Thibodeau GA and Patton KT: *Anatomy and physiology,* ed 5, St Louis, 2003, Mosby.)

HYMEN

The hymen is a thin vascular fold of tissue that attaches around the entrance of the vagina. The hymen separates the vagina from the vestibule. In the young female, the membrane is usually but not always intact, and its orifice may vary from pinpoint size to several centimeters. The membrane is generally broken during coitus and then remains as a notched tissue, which may be further reduced during childbearing.

PERINEUM

The perineum is located between the posterior vaginal wall and the anus. Beneath the perineal skin, connective tissue and muscles support the pelvic floor and internal reproductive structures.

INTRODUCTION TO OBSTETRICAL AND GYNECOLOGICAL SURGERY

Obstetric and gynecologic surgery involves the female reproductive structures, including the uterus, two ovaries, fallopian tubes, vagina, external mons pubis, labia major, labia minor, and clitoris. The procedures are categorized as open, abdominal, laparoscopic, and vaginal. The urinary system is in close anatomical proximity to the pelvic and external genitalia, and all procedures require technical considerations of these structures.

Psychosocial Considerations

Psychosocial considerations for the obstetrical and gynecological patient concern reproductive ability, which includes her social, cultural, family, and community expectations. Self-image and identity are closely linked with the patient's physical ability to reproduce and care for her children. When caring for the patient, the scrub should remember that developmental age is an important component. Gynecology requires the caregiver to understand how the *patient interprets* her surgery and what it means to her. Respect for the patient's modesty is extremely important in all cases.

Patient and Team Position

Most gynecology procedures are performed with the patient in supine or lithotomy position. The surgical team may operate from either side of the patient during open procedures. During abdominal procedures, the right-handed surgeon stands at the patient's left side. This creates the best access to the pelvis. The scrub should stand to the patient's right unless otherwise directed. During laparoscopic procedures, the patient is placed in low lithotomy position and one assistant is positioned at the foot of the table. The pregnant patient is usually positioned in modified left lateral position to prevent hypotension resulting from fetal pressure on the vena cava.

During vaginal procedures, the scrub is in an awkward position, with the back table placed at the foot of the patient *behind* the surgeon or at the side. This requires the scrub to either reach across the front of the surgeon and assistants or pass equipment between them. Neither option is entirely satisfactory, but one must be used to preserve aseptic technique. The only other option is for the scrub to work from an overhead table and pass instruments down to the surgeons.

Aseptic Technique during Vaginal Procedures

Many surgical team members consider vaginal procedures to be contaminated or "dirty" procedures. This belief leads to poor aseptic technique because staff members do not feel compelled to exercise care ("it's a dirty area anyway"). This belief is not valid for the following reasons:

▶ When the patient is properly prepped and draped, the perineum, which is the skin between the anus and the vagina, is excluded from the vestibule.
▶ The vestibule and external genitalia contain permanent flora, just as other areas of the body. Care is taken not to introduce these bacteria into the urethra or through the peritoneal incision during invasive vaginal procedures. Aseptic technique includes barrier practices to prevent this.
▶ *Any pathogenic bacteria can cause an infection,* including bacteria from sources on objects, in the air, and on dust particles. The vestibule, uterus, cervix, or any other perineal structure is not immune to bacterial invasion from random sources. Consider a scenario in which antibiotic-resistant *Staphylococcus aureus* bacteria (MRSA) are transferred to the patient's cervix by direct contact with a contaminated glove during surgery. Although it is true that the vagina is not "sterile," it does not harbor MRSA. Contamination can lead to devastating infection.

Remember that an infection from any source is a cause of grave concern for the surgical patient. The gynecological patient deserves the same considerations as all other patients with regard to technique.

Instruments

Special equipment includes the laparoscope, hysteroscope, and laser. The microscope and microsurgical instruments are used for reconstructive microsurgery.

Gynecological and hysteroscopic instruments are illustrated in Figures 22-4 through Figure 22-8. Table 22-1 describes the laparoscopic instruments used most often during gynecological procedures.

Laparoscopy

Laparoscopic gynecological surgery has replaced many open procedures for the following reasons:

▶ Patients are able to leave the hospital shortly after the procedure.
▶ Less pain is associated with laparoscopic procedures than with open procedures.
▶ The procedures are effective.

Text continued on page 519.

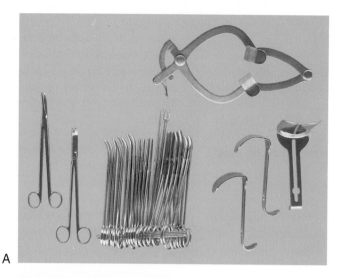

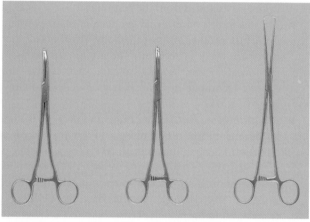

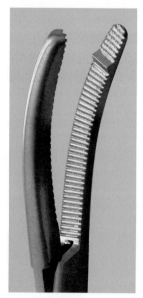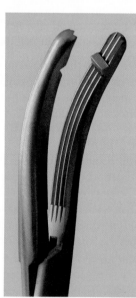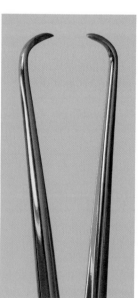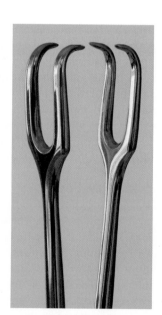

FIGURE 22-4

Hysterectomy instruments. **A**, *Top,* O'Sullivan-O'Connor retractor body. *Bottom, left to right,* Mayo dissecting scissors, curved, 9 inch; Jorgenson dissecting scissors, curved, 9 inch; four Ochsner hemostatic forceps, 8 inch; two Heaney hysterectomy forceps, single-tooth; two Heaney-Ballentine hysterectomy forceps, single-tooth; four Ochsner hemostatic forceps, 8 inch; Schroeder uterine tenaculum forceps, single-tooth; Skene uterine vulsellum forceps, straight, double-tooth; two Jarit hysterectomy forceps, straight, 8½ inch; two Jarit hysterectomy forceps, curved, 8½ inch; two Heaney needle holders; two medium blades to O'Sullivan-O'Connor retractor, side view; large blade, front view. **B**, *Top,* Heaney hysterectomy forceps, single-tooth; Heaney-Ballentine hysterectomy forceps, single-tooth; Schroeder uterine tenaculum forceps, straight, single-tooth. *Bottom,* tips of Heaney hysterectomy forceps, single-tooth; Heaney-Ballentine hysterectomy forceps, single-tooth; Schroeder uterine tenaculum forceps, straight, single-tooth; and Schroeder uterine vulsellum forceps, double-tooth. (From Tighe SM: *Instrumentation for the operating room,* ed 6, St Louis, 1999, Mosby.)

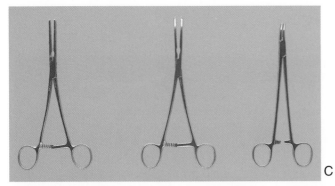

FIGURE 22-4, cont'd
Hysterectomy instruments. **C,** *Top, left to right,* Jarit hysterectomy forceps, straight, 8½ inch; Jarit hysterectomy forceps, curved, 8½ inch; Heaney needle holder, curved, 8½ inch. *Bottom,* tips of Jarit hysterectomy forceps, straight, 8½ inch; Jarit hysterectomy forceps, curved, 8½ inch; Heaney needle holder, curved, 8½ inch; and Jorgenson dissecting scissors, front and side views.

C

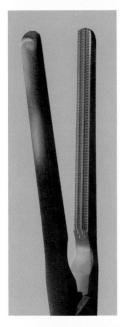
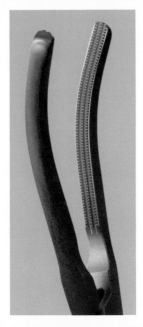
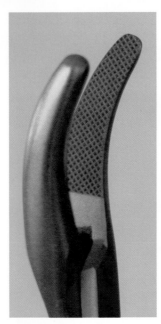
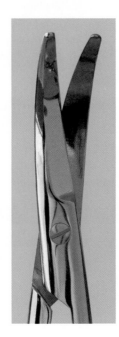
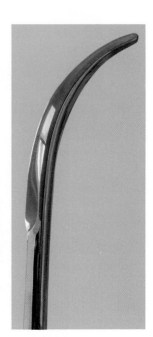

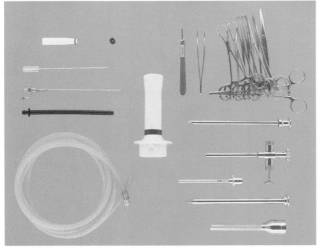

A

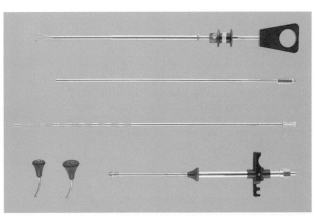

B

FIGURE 22-5
Laparoscopic tubal ligation set. **A**, *Left, top to bottom,* Fallopian ring pusher (with black ring); black nipple; Veress needle, medium; Veress needle stylet, medium; reducer cannula, 5 mm, black; insufflation tubing with Luer-Lok on one end. *Middle,* light handle. *Right, top,* Bard-Parker knife handle, no. 3; Adson tissue forceps with teeth (1 × 2); two Backhaus towel clips, large; two Allis tissue forceps; two Crile hemostatic forceps, curved; Mayo dissecting scissors, straight; Crile-Wood needle holder, 7 inch. *Lower right, top to bottom,* 8-mm trocar and trumpet-valve cannula (for Fallopian ring applier); Applied cannula, 5 mm; Applied trocar, 10/11 mm; Applied cannula, 10/11 mm. **B**, *Top to bottom,* Fallopian ring applicator, 7 mm; suction or irrigation cannula; manipulation probe; Cohen cannula with two black tips. **C,** Tip of Fallopian ring applicator, 7 mm. (From Tighe SM: *Instrumentation for the operating room,* ed 6, St Louis, 1999, Mosby.)

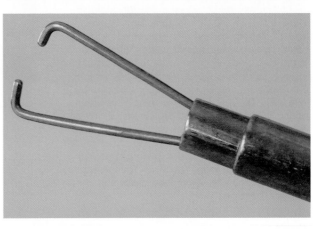

C

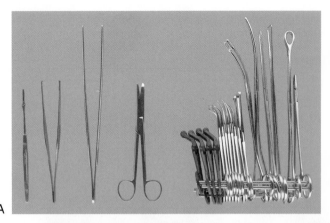
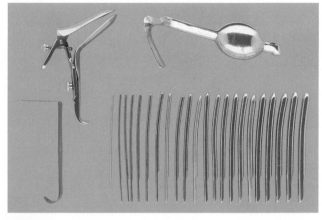

A

B

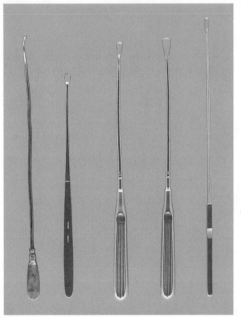
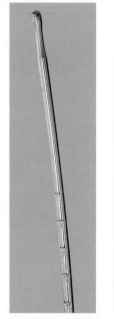
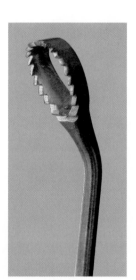
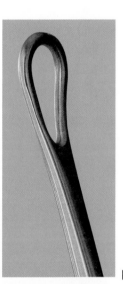

C

D

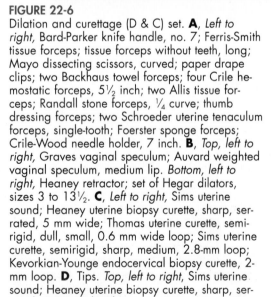
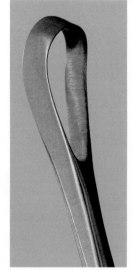
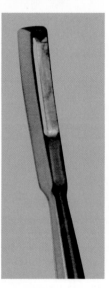
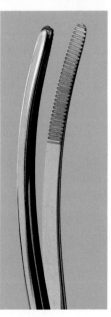

FIGURE 22-6

Dilation and curettage (D & C) set. **A**, *Left to right,* Bard-Parker knife handle, no. 7; Ferris-Smith tissue forceps; tissue forceps without teeth, long; Mayo dissecting scissors, curved; paper drape clips; two Backhaus towel forceps; four Crile hemostatic forceps, 5½ inch; two Allis tissue forceps; Randall stone forceps, ¼ curve; thumb dressing forceps; two Schroeder uterine tenaculum forceps, single-tooth; Foerster sponge forceps; Crile-Wood needle holder, 7 inch. **B**, *Top, left to right,* Graves vaginal speculum; Auvard weighted vaginal speculum, medium lip. *Bottom, left to right,* Heaney retractor; set of Hegar dilators, sizes 3 to 13½. **C**, *Left to right,* Sims uterine sound; Heaney uterine biopsy curette, sharp, serrated, 5 mm wide; Thomas uterine curette, semirigid, dull, small, 0.6 mm wide loop; Sims uterine curette, semirigid, sharp, medium, 2.8-mm loop; Kevorkian-Younge endocervical biopsy curette, 2-mm loop. **D**, Tips. *Top, left to right,* Sims uterine sound; Heaney uterine biopsy curette, sharp, serrated, 5 mm wide; Thomas uterine curette, semirigid, dull, small, 0.6 mm wide loop. *Bottom, left to right,* Sims uterine curette, semirigid, sharp, medium, 2.8-mm loop; Kevorkian-Younge endocervical biopsy curette, 2-mm loop; Bozeman uterine forceps, S-shaped.

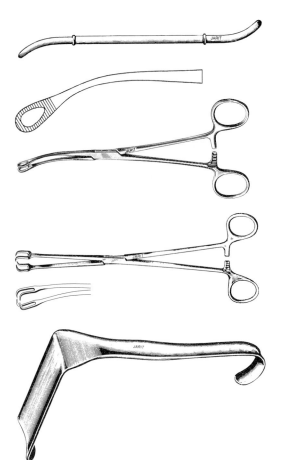

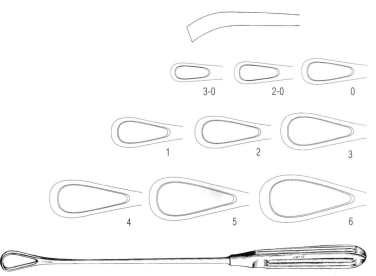

FIGURE 22-6, cont'd
E, *Left, top to bottom,* Hank uterine dilator; Laufe uterine polyp forceps; Schroeder vulsellum forceps; Eastman vaginal retractor. *Right,* Sims uterine curette. (**A** through **D** from Tighe SM: *Instrumentation for the operating room,* ed 6, St Louis, 1999, Mosby; **E** courtesy of Jarit Instruments, Hawthorne, NY.)

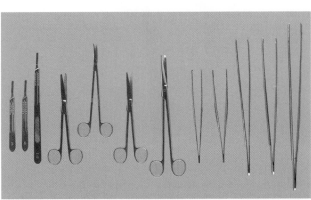

A

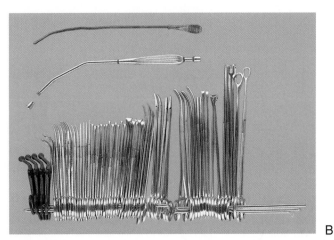

B

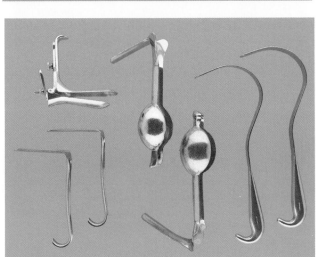

C

FIGURE 22-7
Vaginal set. **A,** *Left to right,* two Bard-Parker knife handles, no. 4; Bard-Parker knife handle, no. 4, long; Mayo dissecting scissors, straight; Metzenbaum scissors, 7 inch; Mayo dissecting scissors, curved; Mayo dissecting scissors, long, curved; two Ferris-Smith tissue forceps; two Russian tissue forceps; tissue forceps without teeth, long. **B,** *Top,* uterine sound. *Center,* Yankauer suction tube with tip. *Bottom, left to right,* four paper drape clips; two Backhaus towel clips; eight Crile hemostatic forceps, 6½ inch; four Halsted hemostatic forceps; 12 Allis tissue forceps; six Allis-Adair tissue forceps; four tonsil hemostatic forceps; two Heaney needle holders; two Crile-Wood needle holders, 8 inch; two Heaney hysterectomy forceps, single-tooth, curved; two Heaney-Ballentine hysterectomy forceps, single-tooth, curved; two Ochsner hemostatic forceps, 8 inch; two Allis tissue forceps, long; two Babcock tissue forceps, medium; two Schroeder uterine tenaculum forceps, single-tooth; Schroeder uterine vulsellum forceps, double-tooth, straight; two Foerster sponge forceps. **C,** *Top, left,* Graves vaginal speculum. *Bottom, left,* two Heaney retractors. *Center, top to bottom,* Auvard weighted vaginal speculum, medium lip and long lip. *Right,* two Deaver retractors, narrow.

continued

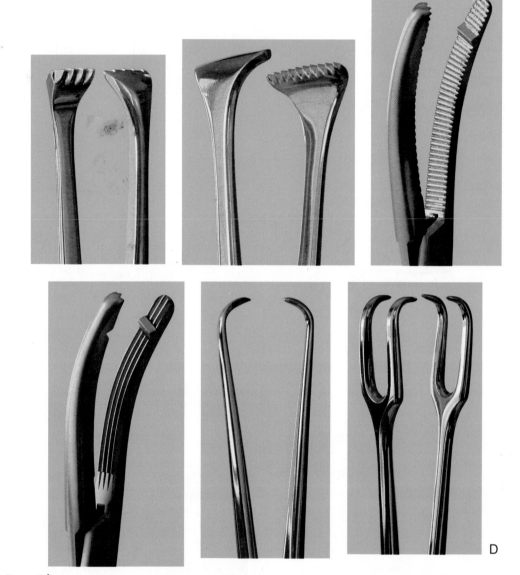

FIGURE 22-7, cont'd
Vaginal set. **D**, *Top, left to right,* Allis tissue forceps; Allis-Adair tissue forceps; Heaney hysterectomy forceps, single-tooth, curved. *Bottom, left to right,* Heaney-Ballentine hysterectomy forceps, single-tooth, curved; Schroeder uterine tenaculum forceps, single-tooth; Schroeder uterine vulsellum forceps, double-tooth, straight. (From Tighe SM: *Instrumentation for the operating room,* ed 6, St Louis, 1999, Mosby.)

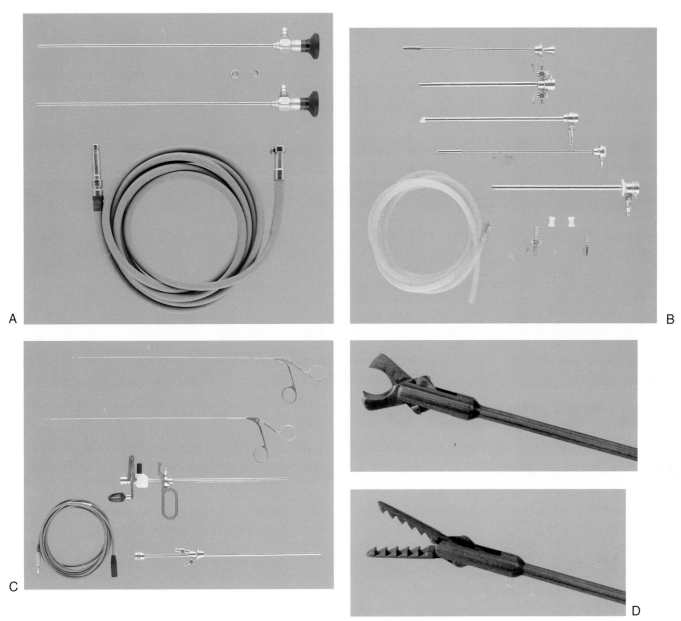

FIGURE 22-8

Hysteroscopic operative instruments. **A**, *Top to bottom,* hysteroscopic operative set: hysteroscopic lens, 4 mm, 0 degree; hysteroscopic lens, 4 mm, 30 degree; two sealing caps; fiberoptic cord. **B**, *Top to bottom, right,* for continuous-flow operative hysteroscopy: obturator, 21 Fr; operative sheath, 21 Fr. For continuous-flow resecting hysteroscopy: inner sheath, 26 Fr; obturator, 26 Fr. *Left bottom,* outflow tubing with Luer-Lok connector on one end, 17 inch. *Right bottom, left to right,* water connector with stopcock; gray nipples; male Luer-Lok connector. **C**, *Left bottom,* monopolar cord, pin type. *Top to bottom,* for continuous-flow operative hysteroscopy: semirigid hook scissors, 7 Fr, 2.33 mm; semirigid grasping forceps, 7 Fr, 2.33 mm. For continuous-flow resecting hysteroscopy: resecting working element. For continuous-flow resecting operative hysteroscopy (used with the operative sheath, 21 Fr): continuous-flow bridge with instrument channel. **D**, Tips. *Top,* semirigid hook scissors, 7 Fr, 2.33 mm. *Bottom,* semirigid grasping forceps, 7 Fr, 2.33 mm. (From Tighe SM: *Instrumentation for the operating room,* ed 6, St Louis, 1999, Mosby.)

▶ Advanced techniques and instruments allow the surgeon to perform complex procedures, such as those associated with fertility.

▶ Patient satisfaction is greater.

▶ The procedure is minimally invasive.

In the preparation for abdominal laparoscopy for gynecological procedures, the patient is placed in low lithotomy position and prepped and draped for an abdominal and vaginal approach. An indwelling catheter is inserted for continuous drainage, and the abdomen and vagina are prepped. A sterile uterine manipulator is inserted into the cervix with the aid of a cervical tenaculum and a vaginal speculum.

A small intraumbilical incision is made, and pneumoperitoneum is created with the Veress needle or trocar.

Table 22-1 LAPAROSCOPIC GYNECOLOGICAL INSTRUMENTS

Instrument	Use
10-mm Allis clamp	▶ Grasping the myometrium, large leiomyomas, and large ovarian cysts after drainage ▶ Removing specimens from the abdominal cavity
Hook scissors	▶ Cutting through very dense tissue
Metzenbaum scissors with monopolar capability	▶ Dissection ▶ Cutting ▶ Simultaneous coagulation and cutting
Bowel grasper	▶ Manipulation of bowel ▶ Retraction
Monopolar hook	▶ Incising and coagulating
Biopsy forceps	▶ Removing peritoneal or ovarian specimens
Maryland dissector	▶ Blunt dissection
Standard grasper	▶ Tissue handling ▶ Manipulation
Suction-irrigation probe with Poole sleeve. The probe connects to a handle with trumpet valves for separate suction and irrigation. Irrigation is introduced through a plastic tube connected to irrigation fluid.	▶ Hydrodissection ▶ Aspiration of fluids and clots ▶ Irrigation
Aspiration needle (14 gauge)	▶ Withdrawing fluid from cysts
Alligator grasper	▶ Grasping leiomyoma tissue ▶ Retrieving specimens

Additional trocars are placed under direct vision through a straight 0-degree laparoscope, and three ports are utilized. A 5-mm or 10-mm umbilical port is used for the laparoscope, and two 5-mm ports are used at the lateral borders of the pelvis just inferior to the level of the iliac crests. These steps are illustrated in Figure 22-9, *A-D.*

In this chapter, both laparoscopic and open procedures are discussed. Many procedures can be performed through either technique. This chapter has selected one or the other technique for various procedures to offer a variety of exposures to the student.

COMPLICATIONS IN OBSTETRICAL AND GYNECOLOGICAL SURGERY

To develop a more complete understanding of gynecological and obstetrical surgery, the technologist should become familiar with complications that are often encountered in the patient's history and physical report.

Obstetrical Complications

Before birth, the fetus may abort because of disease or injury to the mother or fetus. Most abortions require that the patient have a dilation and curettage. A **missed abortion** is a condition in which the product of conception (fetus) is nonliving and is retained in the uterus for longer than 2 months. An *incomplete abortion* is one in which only part of the products of conception have aborted. An *imminent abortion* is one in which the patient is about to abort. This may be indicated by uterine bleeding.

Just before or during childbirth, the patient and fetus may suffer from complications that require an emergency cesarean section. *Dystocia* is a term that describes painful and difficult labor. During *placenta previa,* the placenta is abnormally implanted in the lower uterine segment and may completely cover the cervical os. In *abruptio placentae,* the placenta is prematurely separated from the wall of the uterus. If the mother's pelvis is too small to accommodate the head of the fetus, the complication is termed *cephalopelvic disproportion (CPD).* The manner in which the fetus is presented (positioned in relation to the cervix) also may necessitate emergency surgery. In a *breech* presentation, the buttocks are presented; in a *transverse* presentation, the fetus is presented crosswise; in a *footling,* the feet are presented; and in a *vertex,* the upper back of the head is presented. If the fetal heart tones diminish or are completely absent, cesarean section may be performed immediately. The absence of fetal heart tones often indicates that the umbilical cord has twisted on itself or is otherwise obstructed, thus preventing blood flow to the fetus.

Gynecological Complications

Functional or metabolic complications may be indications for surgery. In *metrorrhagia,* the patient suffers from active uterine bleeding at times other than during menstruation. *Amenorrhea* is the absence of menstruation. This condition may be caused by disease or physiological imbalance but also can be caused by emotional upset. Painful or difficult menstruation is called *dysmenorrhea. Menometrorrhagia* is excessive bleeding that occurs both during menstruation and at irregular intervals. *Menorrhagia* is excessive bleeding during

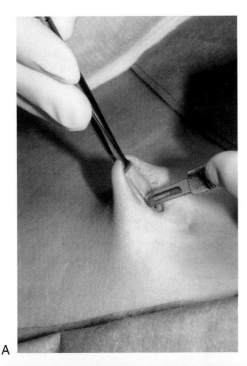

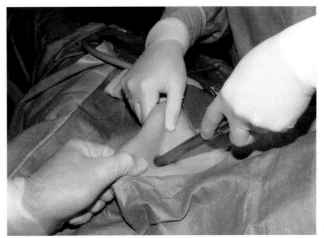

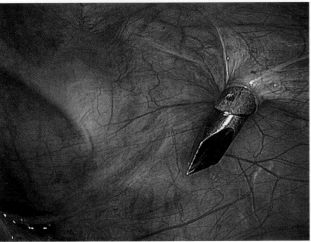

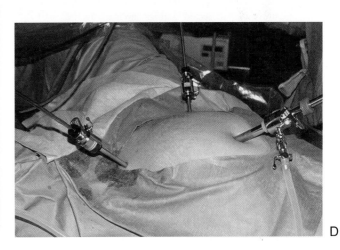

FIGURE 22-9
Preparing the patient for abdominal laparoscopy. **A**, A vertical intraumbilical incision is made. **B**, The surgeon inserts the trocar. **C**, Additional trocars are inserted under direct vision of the laparoscope. **D**, Three-port placement with 5-mm trocar placement in each lower quadrant. (From Goldberg JM and Falcone T: *Atlas of endoscopic techniques in gynecology*, Philadelphia, 2001, Saunders.)

menstruation. The surgeon may perform a dilation and curettage to determine the causes of the above conditions.

ABDOMINAL SURGICAL PROCEDURES

Abdominal Hysterectomy (Open)
SURGICAL GOAL
In this procedure, the uterus is surgically removed through an abdominal incision.

PATHOLOGY
Hysterectomy is performed for a variety of diseases. The most common indications are benign fibromas (leiomyomas), endometriosis, and cancer.

Endometrial Cancer
Cancer of the endometrium is the most common type located within the female pelvis. Among the highest risk factors for this cancer is a prolonged elevated level of estrogen. Factors that contribute to this cancer include endometrial **hyperplasia** (increased endometrial tissue) related to obesity, diabetes mellitus, hypertension, and polycystic ovary syndrome. Estrogen-secreting tumors such as ovarian cancer also increase a woman's risk for endometrial cancer. Hysterectomy is indicated as part of the treatment for this cancer.

Uterine Leiomyoma
A uterine leiomyoma (also known as a fibroid tumor or *fibroid uterus*) is a dense, benign tumor arising from the smooth

muscle tissue of the myometrium. These tumors occur in women older than 35 years and usually develop within the body of the uterus. Although not cancerous, they can cause bleeding, and when very large these tumors may impinge on other structures of the genitourinary system. The leiomyoma that arises from the submucosal layer of the uterus causes increased bleeding and may result in infection. Hysterectomy is performed to remove one or more large leiomyomas.

Technique

1. The surgeon enters the abdomen through a transverse pelvic incision.
2. The round ligament is clamped, cut, and ligated.
3. The incision is carried anteriorly to the peritoneal bladder reflection.
4. The bladder is dissected from the lower uterine segment, creating a bladder flap.
5. Dissection of the uterine ligaments and arteries is carried to the vaginal cuff.
6. The cervix is incised circumferentially and amputated from the vaginal cuff.
7. The uterus is removed, and the specimen is passed from the surgical field.
8. The vaginal cuff is grasped with clamps and sutured.
9. The previously dissected bladder flap is reattached.
10. The abdominal wound is irrigated and closed in layers.

DISCUSSION

The patient is placed in a supine position. After a routine abdominal and vaginal prep, a Foley catheter is inserted for continuous urinary drainage. Even though the lower midline incision can be used for a hysterectomy, the transverse incision (also called a "bikini" or Pfannenstiel incision) will be discussed here. Many gynecological abdominal procedures are approached through this incision. The incision traverses the lower abdomen approximately 3 to 4 inches above the symphysis pubis.

When the procedure is performed laparoscopically, surgical stapling instruments are used to mobilize the uterus, which is morcelated and brought through the abdomen with a specimen-retrieval system.

To begin the surgery, the surgeon makes a transverse skin incision and deepens it through the subcutaneous tissue with the electrosurgical unit (ESU). The next layer, the fascia, is entered with the scalpel, and the incision is lengthened with curved Mayo scissors. The surgeon then grasps one edge of the fascia margin with two or more Kocher clamps. Using blunt dissection, the surgeon separates the fascia from the underlying muscle.

This procedure is repeated on the lower fascia margin. The muscle layer is then manually divided. The peritoneum is then incised with the scalpel, and the incision is lengthened with Metzenbaum scissors.

A self-retaining retractor such as an O'Sullivan, O'Connor, or Balfour retractor is placed into the wound. The surgeon packs the bowel away from the uterus with moist lap sponges.

The surgeon isolates the uterus by severing it from the uterine ligaments, ovaries, and fallopian tubes. Beginning with the round ligaments, the surgeon double clamps, divides, and ligates each attachment with suture ligatures. Heaney, Heaney-Ballentine, or Masterson forceps are usually used for this part of the procedure. The scrub should have at least four of these clamps available on the Mayo stand.

Absorbable suture is used to ligate the ligaments. Chromic gut or absorbable synthetic suture such as Dexon II or Vicryl is used. Up to 24 sutures are needed to mobilize the ligaments from the uterus. Large tapered needles are used. To divide the ligaments, the surgeon uses curved Mayo scissors or the scalpel. Long instruments should be available if the patient has a deep pelvis.

As described earlier, the surgeon mobilizes the uterus to the level of the bladder. At this point, the bladder is continuous with the uterus, both organs being attached by a peritoneal covering. Using Metzenbaum scissors and long tissue forceps, the surgeon separates the two structures by dissecting the peritoneal covering away from the bladder. This creates the *bladder flap*, which will be reattached later. When the bladder has been separated from the uterus, mobilization is continued.

At the level of the cervix, long Allis or Kocher clamps are placed around the edge of the cervix, and it is divided from the vagina. The surgeon uses long scissors or the long scalpel to divide the tissue. This maneuver completely frees the uterus, which is passed to the scrub. All instruments that have come in contact with the cervix or vagina must be kept separate from the rest of the set-up. The specimen and isolated instruments should be received in a basin.

To close the wound, the surgeon first sutures the vaginal vault where it was separated from the cervix. Absorbable sutures of the same type used on the uterine ligaments are used. After closing the vagina, the surgeon reattaches the bladder flap. Size 2-0 or 3-0 suture on a small tapered needle is used.

The wound is irrigated with warm saline and checked for bleeders. To close the abdomen, the surgeon grasps the edges of the peritoneum with several Mayo clamps. The peritoneum is closed with a running suture of 0 absorbable suture swaged to a taper needle. The muscle tissue may be loosely approximated with 3 or 4 interrupted absorbable sutures. The fascia layer is closed with a wide variety of sutures, absorbable or nonabsorbable. Size 0 or 2-0 is usually used. The subcutaneous tissue is usually approximated with size 3-0 interrupted absorbable sutures. The skin is closed with staples or a subcuticular running suture.

Figure 22-10, *A-F,* illustrates the procedure for open abdominal hysterectomy.

SURGICAL GOAL

A radical hysterectomy is a dissection and wide removal of the uterus, tubes, ovaries, supporting ligaments, and upper vagina, along with careful removal of all recognizable lymph nodes in the pelvis.

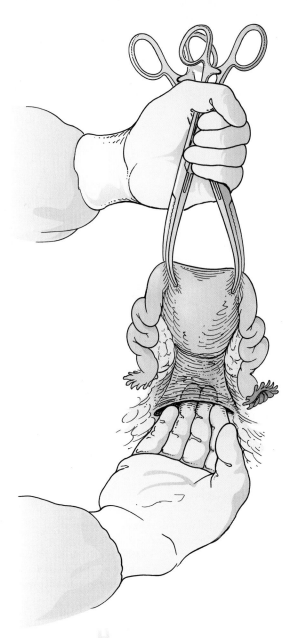

A

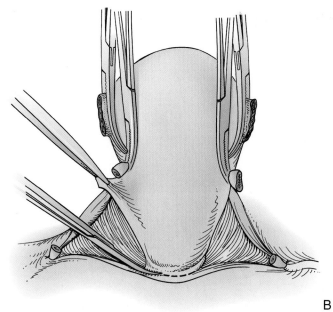

B

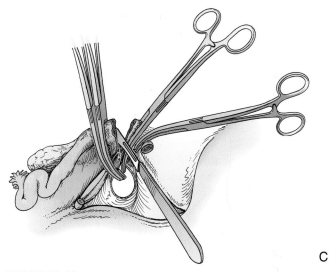

C

FIGURE 22-10
Open abdominal hysterectomy. **A**, Traction placed by clamps on the corneal region of the uterus to facilitate dissection. **B**, The anterior ligament has been clamped, cut, and tied, allowing access to the broad ligament. **C**, The tube and utero-ovarian ligament are triple clamped; the ovarian vessels are then divided. **D**, The bladder is mobilized. (Adapted from Gershenson DM, et al: *Operative gynecology,* ed 2, Philadelphia, 2001, Saunders.)

continued

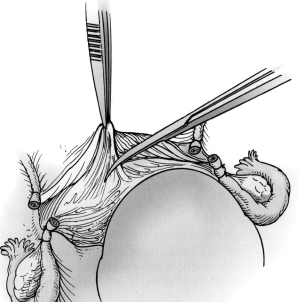

D

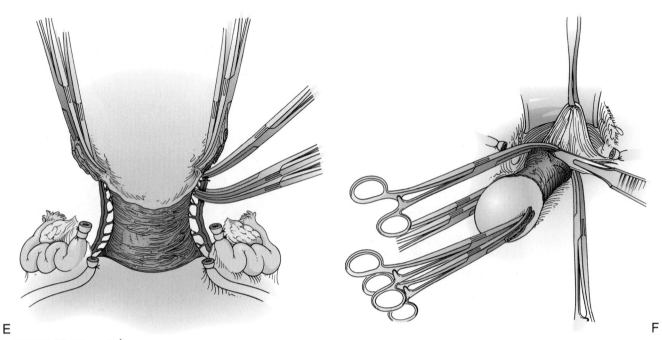

E   F

FIGURE 22-10, cont'd
Open abdominal hysterectomy. **E**, The uterine vessels are triple clamped at the level of the internal cervical os. **F**, The vagina is opened anteriorly, and a circumferential incision is made around the vagina to free the uterine specimen. (Adapted from Gershenson DM, et al: *Operative gynecology*, ed 2, Philadelphia, 2001, Saunders.)

PATHOLOGY

This procedure is performed to treat gynecological malignancy. Exploration of the abdomen determines the amount of lymph-node involvement.

Technique

1. The surgeon makes a skin incision for laparotomy and opens the abdominal layers.
2. The peritoneum is cut at its reflection.
3. The bladder surface is freed from the cervix and vagina.
4. Clamps are applied to the right round and infundibulopelvic ligaments, cut with a knife or scissors, and ligated with suture to expose the external iliac artery.
5. The ureter is identified and retracted with a vein retractor.
6. The iliac artery, obturator fossa, and ureter are dissected of lymph and other tissue.
7. A lymph-gland dissection is performed to remove tissue from the Cloquet node to the bifurcation of the iliac arteries bilaterally. The uterine artery and vein are clamped, cut, and doubly ligated.
8. The uterus is elevated, the cul-de-sac is opened, and the uterosacral and cardinal ligaments are clamped, cut with scissors, and double ligated with suture ligatures.
9. The upper vagina is skeletonized, and the paraurethral tissues are removed.
10. Heaney clamps are used to cross-clamp the upper third of the vagina. The vagina is then divided. The uterus and surrounding tissues are removed.
11. Venous oozing and bleeding is controlled with electrocautery.
12. The vagina is oversewn with a running locked stitch.
13. The pelvis is peritonealized with a continuous suture.
14. The abdominal wound is closed and dressed.
15. Vaginal packings and drains may be used.
16. An indwelling suprapubic catheter may be placed to assist in preventing postoperative bladder spasm and for bladder drainage, if the patient is unable to void after removal of the urethral catheter.
17. A perineal pad is placed.

DISCUSSION

If there is no lymph-node involvement, a wide-cuff hysterectomy is performed.

The uterus, tubes, and ovaries, together with most of the parametrial tissues and the upper portion of the vagina, are removed en bloc.

The ureters are dissected from the paracervical structures so that the ligaments supporting the uterus and vagina can be removed.

Blood loss and urinary output should be closely monitored during the procedure.

Pelvic Exenteration
SURGICAL GOAL

Pelvic exenteration is the complete removal of the rectum, the distal sigmoid colon, the urinary bladder and distal ureters, the internal iliac vessels and their lateral branches, all pelvic reproductive organs and lymph nodes, and the entire pelvic floor with the accompanying pelvic peritoneum, levator muscles, and perineum.

A partial anterior or posterior exenteration can be performed, depending on the origin and extent of the cancer.

PATHOLOGY

Exenteration is preferred for recurrent or persistent carcinoma of the cervix after radiation therapy. Advanced or recurrent vaginal, vulvar, or, occasionally, endometrial or rectal cancers also are candidates for exenteration.

Technique

1. The patient should be positioned with lithotomy stirrups and prepped for an abdominal/perianal approach. This position allows access without disruptive positioning changes.
2. The surgeon makes a long midline incision from the symphysis pubis to the umbilicus, and the abdomen is opened.
3. The surgeon makes a second incision within the perineum and encircling the vestibule and the anus.
4. The peritoneal cavity is explored for metastasis to the liver, the nodes of the celiac axis, the superior mesenteric artery, and the paraaortic tissues.
5. The surgeon explores the pelvis for lymph-node involvement. If there are negative findings, then retractors are placed, and the small bowel is packed with moist laps.
6. The sigmoid mesocolon is mobilized and sectioned with intestinal clamps, scalpel, or stapling device.
7. The proximal end of the sigmoid mesocolon is exteriorized through the left side of the abdomen; an intestinal clamp is left across the lumen for later use, when the permanent colostomy will be secured to the skin.
8. The remaining sigmoid mesentery is clamped, cut, and ligated down to and including the superior hemorrhoid vessels. Long instruments and sutures are used to reach the deep pelvic sutures.
9. The distal sigmoid colon is closed with an inverting suture. The sigmoid colon and rectum are mobilized from the sacrococcygeal area by blunt and sharp dissection.
10. The lateral pelvic peritoneum is cut, and all vessels and ligaments are clamped, cut, and double ligated.
11. The bladder is separated from the symphysis pubis down to the urethra.
12. Ureters are identified and divided; proximal ends are left open for urinary drainage, and distal ends are ligated.
13. The hypogastric artery, internal iliac vein, and superior and inferior gluteal vessels are exposed, clamped, doubly ligated, and cut. The external iliac vein is retracted to allow evacuation of the obturator fossa contents, leaving the obturator nerve intact. Care must be taken to preserve the sacral plexus and sciatic nerve.
14. Internal pudendal vessels are identified, isolated, ligated with transfixion sutures, and cut. Remaining soft-tissue attachments are clamped and cut. These steps are performed on the opposite sides of the patient.
15. The surgeon makes an elliptical perineal incision that includes the clitoris and anus, and incises the ischiorectal fat up to the area of the levator muscle.
16. The rectal coccygeal attachment is severed, as are the lateral attachments of the levator muscles. Hemostasis is maintained by pressure and traction.

17. Paravesical and paravaginal tissues are resected from the periosteum of the symphysis pubis and superior pubic rami by means of a knife. The specimen has been completely freed and is removed from the pelvis.
18. Residual bleeders are identified and controlled, and the subcutaneous tissue is closed with interrupted sutures. A drain is placed, and the skin is closed.
19. Further residual bleeding vessels in the abdomen are controlled. Packs may be left in the pelvis for removal after 48 hours.
20. The ileal segment is prepared, and the ureters are anastomosed to it. An external ileal stoma is placed on the right side of the abdomen.
21. To aid in postoperative bowel decompression, the surgeon places a jejunostomy catheter in the proximal jejunum, connects it to the bowel with a purse-string suture, brings it out through the skin, and sutures it into place.
22. In the same manner, a gastrostomy tube is placed into the stomach.
23. A final check for hemostasis is performed. Packs and retractors are removed after the small intestines and viscera are carefully repositioned into the pelvis.
24. A multi-layer abdominal wound closure is performed with interrupted sutures.
25. Finally, the surgeon prepares the colostomy stoma by removing the intestinal clamp from the sigmoid colon, opening the colon, and suturing the stoma to the skin edges.
26. The wounds are dressed, and drainage devices are applied to the colostomy and ileostomy stomas.

DISCUSSION

The bowel is cleansed preoperatively with a combination of antibiotics, enemas, and cathartics.

Antiembolic or sequential stocking devices and forced warmed-air blankets are used to maintain body temperature. *All* fluids and IV fluids should be warmed.

These are long procedures, so extremities should be positioned and padded with great care and attention.

The scrub should use a separate set-up for the abdominal and perineal approaches. Extra drapes, gowns, and gloves should be available.

The anus may be closed with a purse-string suture to help prevent contamination.

Diagnostic Laparoscopy
SURGICAL GOAL

Laparoscopy is the insertion of a laparoscope through the anterior abdominal wall to allow the visualization of the peritoneal cavity with the establishment of a pneumoperitoneum.

PATHOLOGY

Laparoscopic procedures are used to investigate, evaluate, and diagnose the causes of abdominal and pelvic pain, infertility, and pelvic masses. Secondarily, they can also be used in performing adhesiolysis, tubal fulguration, fulguration of endometriotic implants, aspiration of cysts, tissue biopsy, and aspiration of peritoneal fluid for cytological studies.

Technique

1. A small incision (large enough to accommodate the trocar and port) is made at the inferior margin of the umbilicus.
2. The surgeon elevates the skin and inserts a Veress needle.
3. The surgeon uses a 10-ml syringe, partially filled with saline, to verify position.
4. Insufflation tubing is attached, and a pneumoperitoneum is established.
5. The Veress needle is removed.
6. The trocar and sheath are inserted, and insufflation tubing is attached to maintain the peritoneal space.
7. The laparoscope is introduced into the sheath.
8. The surgeon begins visual examination of the pelvis and lower abdomen.
9. The patient is placed in Trendelenburg position to assist in visualization.
10. Some surgeons (especially recent graduates) will use a video stack and attach a camera to the laparoscope. This allows recording of the procedure for future reference and consultation with the patient.
11. If biopsy forceps or other instrumentation is needed, a second incision is placed suprapubically.
12. After the exam is completed, the laparoscope is removed and the pneumoperitoneum is reduced by allowing the gas to escape either through the scope sheath or by suction.
13. The wounds are closed with skin staples or a subcuticular stitch.
14. If a uterine manipulator has been used, it is removed, and the cervix is inspected for bleeding. Bleeding may require a suture or pressure.
15. A perineal pad is placed.

DISCUSSION

The abdomen, perineum, and vagina are prepped, and the abdomen and perineum are draped for a combined procedure. Special drapes are available for this purpose.

The bladder is emptied.

A dilation and curettage (D & C) procedure often is performed in conjunction with a laparoscopy. After the cervix has been exposed and the depth has been determined, a uterine manipulator or dilator may be inserted into the uterus. This device is used to manipulate the uterus during the procedure to aid in visibility. Most uterine manipulators incorporate a cannula that introduces dye, such as methylene blue. This assists in the evaluation of the fallopian tubes for patency.

The surgeon elevates the skin for the insertion of the Veress needle either with a towel clip or by grasping with a Raytec sponge for traction.

The surgeon can verify the position of the Veress needle using a syringe with saline. One of three things will happen. If the needle has entered a blood vessel, blood will be aspirated into the syringe. If the needle has hit a loop of bowel or possibly the stomach, bowel contents or malodorous gas is brought back. If the needle has cleared into the peritoneal cavity, it will be free of any substance when aspirated.

Approximately 2 to 3 liters of gas, carbon dioxide, or nitrous oxide is introduced into the peritoneal cavity to achieve a pneumoperitoneum. Carbon dioxide is preferred because it is nontoxic, it is highly soluble in blood, and it is rapidly absorbed from the peritoneal cavity.

Some laparoscopes may fog. There are ways to eliminate this problem; for example, commercially available products may be wiped on the distal end of the scope before insertion into the abdominal cavity. However, some old tricks may be used as well: The surgeon can lightly touch the intestine to clear the scope, or the scrub can warm the tip in saline or towels before inserting into the sheath.

Some surgeons still prefer to use the laparoscope without the camera attachment to visualize the abdomen; these surgeons will not necessitate use of the video stack.

Some possible complications of laparoscopy are:

▶ Tension pneumoperitoneum
▶ Bleeding or visceral injury from the trocar insertion
▶ Deep vein thrombosis
▶ Gas embolism

Salpingo-oophorectomy
SURGICAL GOAL

In this procedure, the ovary and fallopian tube are removed for treatment of benign ovarian tumors, endometriosis, or very large ovarian cysts, or for the potential prevention of ovarian cancer. Ovarian abscess that does not respond to antibiotic therapy also may be removed surgically.

PATHOLOGY

Benign ovarian tumors include cysts (previously discussed), cystadenoma, and mucinous cystadenoma. These tumors are rarely malignant but can be quite large, requiring oophorectomy.

Other tumors, called *functioning ovarian tumors,* secrete estrogen and androgen. These tumors can be benign or malignant. Persistent production of estrogen can cause irregular heavy bleeding, excessive endometrial tissue, and amenorrhea (absence of menses). The androgen-producing tumors inhibit ovulation and the production of estrogen. Ovarian cancer usually is far advanced when diagnosed and requires radical surgical intervention.

Technique

1. The surgeon performs a pelvic laparotomy.
2. The uterus is retracted.
3. The infundibular ligament and ureter are identified.
4. The broad ligament is separated by blunt dissection.
5. The ovarian vessels are ligated.
6. The ovary and fallopian tube are clamped and divided.
7. The surface of the uterus is oversewn.

DISCUSSION

Salpingo-oophorectomy may be performed as a laparoscopic or open procedure. The patient is placed in supine position, prepped, and draped for a laparotomy. The surgeon performs a routine laparotomy. The surgeon then examines the pelvic and abdominal contents to rule out malignancy or evidence of other disease.

To begin the procedure, the assistant grasps the uterus with a heavy tenaculum and retracts it laterally. Laparotomy sponges are placed at the boundary of the uterus to isolate it from the bowel. The patient may be tipped into Trendelenburg position to facilitate exposure. The surgeon carefully examines the fallopian tube and ovary to determine the extent of disease.

The surgeon isolates the ovarian ligament and dissects the broad ligament with his finger. The ovarian vessels may be cross-clamped with Mayo clamps and ligated separately from the pedicle.

Three Mayo clamps are placed across the pedicle structure, which contains the ovarian ligament, proximal mesosalpinx, and fallopian tube. The surgeon divides the tissue between clamps with Mayo scissors. The ESU is used to control small bleeders. Two suture ligatures of absorbable synthetic material are placed in the pedicle and tied securely.

The raw surface of the uterus is then oversewn with absorbable suture. The wound is irrigated and closed in layers.

Laparoscopic Ovarian Cystectomy
SURGICAL GOAL
In this procedure, ovarian cysts are removed to determine the pathology of the cyst. Drainage of an ovarian cyst without removal often leads to recurrence. Cysts may be painful or cause bleeding.

PATHOLOGY
Benign ovarian cysts are a common gynecological problem. When several ovarian follicles begin to mature normally, the dominant one continues to form while the others rupture spontaneously. Occasionally these form benign, fluid-filled cysts. This type of cyst usually regresses without treatment. However, it sometimes persists in causing pain.

The benign cystic ovary may be surgically removed as conservative treatment when diagnostic tests cannot determine whether the cyst is malignant or caused by **endometriosis,** a condition in which endometrial tissue is found in random locations within the abdominal cavity. Because endometrial tissue responds to hormonal stimulation, areas of endometriosis cause pain and bleeding with cyclic hormonal changes. Bleeding can sometimes be severe. Hysteroscopic ablation of endometriosis also can be performed in other areas of the abdominal cavity and pelvis.

Cystic teratomas or **dermoid** cysts develop from primordial germ cells and often contain hair and teeth. Ultrasound is not always successful in determining the nature of the cyst. These cysts must be surgically removed. Ovarian tumors require more extensive surgery, which is discussed below.

Technique

1. The patient is prepared for a three-port endoscopic laparoscopy.
2. The surgeon inserts the laparoscope and examines the abdominal contents for evidence of metastasis or other abnormalities.

3. The cyst is identified, and the outer membrane (cortex) is incised with the hook ESU dissector.
4. The edge of the cyst cortex is grasped, and the dissection is started.
5. An irrigation probe is used to continue the dissection.
6. The cortex is everted, and dissection is continued until the cyst is completely mobilized.
7. The cyst may be ruptured and suctioned or brought out through the 10-mm port or a specimen retrieval bag.
8. If the cyst is dermoid, it may be drained through an incision in the cul-de-sac of the vaginal vault, which is then closed with sutures through the vagina.
9. The surgeon examines the cystic bed and controls bleeding with the ESU.
10. If the cyst ruptures, the abdomen is irrigated with copious amounts of lactated Ringer's solution.

DISCUSSION
The patient is placed in low lithotomy position, prepped, and draped for laparoscopic surgery. This preparation includes the insertion of an indwelling Foley catheter.

A three-port approach is used, as previously described. After entry into the abdominal cavity, the surgeon examines the abdominal contents for evidence of metastasis or tumors. To begin the procedure, the surgeon incises the cyst using a monopolar ESU hook. Power settings for cutting should not exceed 20 W. The surgeon takes care not to puncture the cyst so that it may be shelled out if possible.

The cortex of the cyst is grasped with a noncrushing forcep, and a tissue plane is raised between the cortex and the cyst. Dissection is continued with a hydrodissector. As the cortex is peeled away from the cyst, it everts and the edge may be grasped with an atraumatic grasper for better traction. Dissection is completed, and the cyst body is completely mobilized. Bleeders are controlled with the ESU probe on low setting.

If the cyst is a dermoid, it may be brought out through a specimen-retrieval pouch or through an incision made in the uterine cul-de-sac. An Allis clamp is inserted through the vaginal vault, and the cyst is extracted vaginally. The cul-de-sac is closed vaginally with fine absorbable sutures.

The cystic bed is then inspected for bleeders, which are controlled with the bipolar ESU. If the cyst has ruptured, the abdominal cavity is irrigated with copious amounts of lactated Ringer's solution.

The ports are removed, and the pneumoperitoneum is released. Individual wounds are closed with absorbable sutures on a fine cutting needle, and the skin is closed with staples.

The procedure for laparoscopic ovarian cystectomy is illustrated in Figure 22-11, *A-F.*

Laparoscopic Tubal Ligation
SURGICAL GOAL
The goal of tubal ligation is to prevent pregnancy by surgically interrupting the fallopian tube. Some surgeons use techniques that preserve as much of the fallopian tube as possible in the event the patient should want to reverse the procedure and become pregnant in the future. A low failure

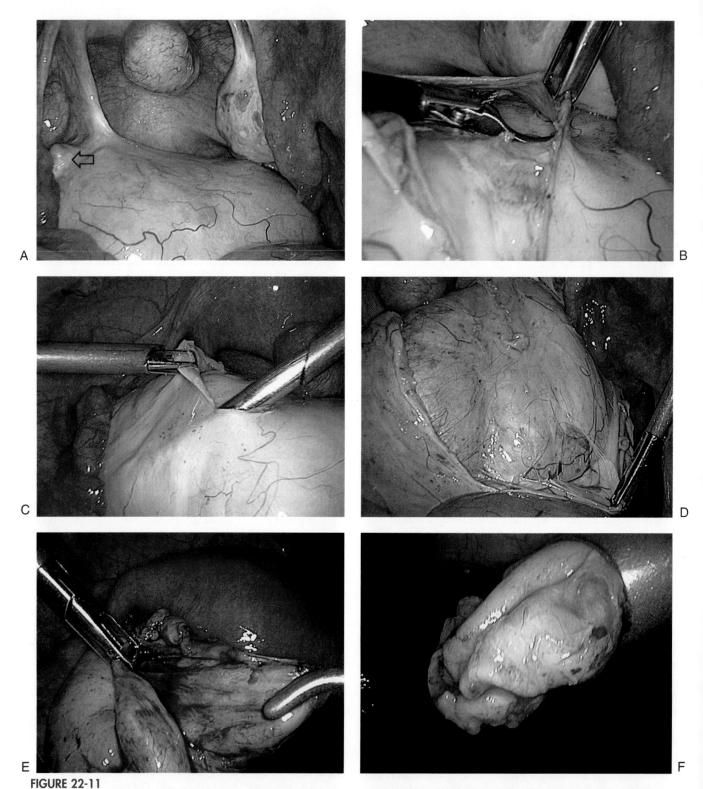

FIGURE 22-11
Laparoscopic ovarian cystectomy. **A**, Large left ovarian cyst is shown; the arrow indicates a teratoma. **B**, Graspers hold the edge of the cortex, and a plane is created between the cortex and cyst wall. **C**, Continuation with hydrodissection of the plane between the cortex and the cyst wall. **D**, The cortex is everted to expose more of the cyst. **E**, The ruptured cyst is separated from the ovary by gentle traction. **F**, The ruptured cyst is withdrawn through the 10-mm port. (From Goldberg JM and Falcone T: *Atlas of endoscopic techniques in gynecology*, Philadelphia, 2001, Saunders.)

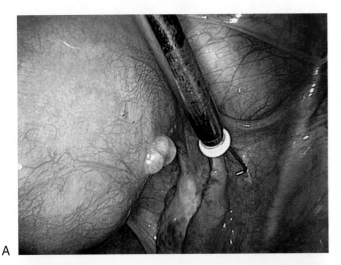

A

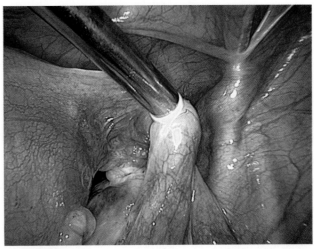

B

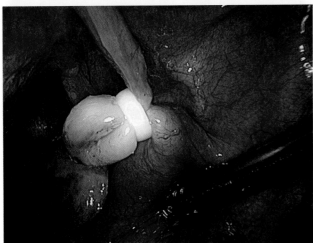

C

FIGURE 22-12
Laparoscopic tubal ligation: Fallope ring. **A**, The mid-isthmic segment of the tube is grasped with the Fallope ring applicator. **B**, The tube is elevated, and the Fallope ring is slid over the application device. **C**, Fallope ring placement is complete. (From Goldberg JM and Falcone T: *Atlas of endoscopic techniques in gynecology*, Philadelphia, 2001, Saunders.)

rate is desirable, but the procedure should not jeopardize the possibility of fertility in the future.

PATHOLOGY

The fallopian tube is the natural passageway of the female ovum when it is released from the ovary. It is also the location of normal fertilization. Interruption of the fallopian tube prevents the ovum from traveling into the uterus, where implantation normally would occur.

Technique

1. A one-port or two-port laparoscopy is performed.
2. *Method I:* Coagulation: Using a single laparoscopic port with operating channel, the surgeon can use bipolar forceps to coagulate the fallopian tube.
3. After the coagulation procedure, the fallopian tube may be transected.
4. *Method II:* Fallope ring method: Using this method, the surgeon withdraws a loop of the fallopian tube into the ring applicator. A Silastic ring is released over the loop, and the loop is then released. The ring causes necrosis of the loop.
5. *Method III:* Filshie clip: In this method, a clip is applied over the fallopian tube.
6. Ports are withdrawn, and the wounds are closed.

DISCUSSION

Tubal ligation was the first procedure to be performed with the laparoscope. The three methods outlined above are commonly used. All three procedures can be performed under general anesthesia or local anesthesia with conscious sedation.

The patient is prepped and draped for a pelvic laparoscopy, and single-port or double-port laparoscopy is performed. The uterine manipulator is inserted as previously described.

Coagulation

Through a single-port cannula, a laparoscope with operating channel is introduced. The surgeon will grasp the midsection of the tube with the bipolar forceps. The surgeon will then coagulate, and transect the tube.

Fallope Ring

The Fallope ring method uses a small Silastic ring, which the scrub loads into the ring applicator. The surgeon then inserts the applicator into the port and withdraws a loop of the fallopian tube into the applicator. The Silastic ring is ejected over the loop, which is then released back into the pelvis. The loop causes local necrosis of the loop of tissue, which interrupts the tube (Figure 22-12, *A-C*).

Filshie Clip

In this procedure, the Filshie applicator is inserted through the single port. The clip is applied over the fallopian tube

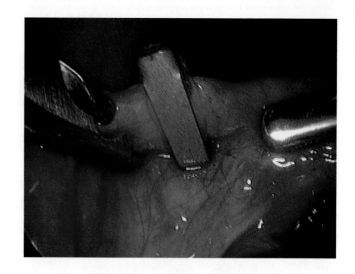

FIGURE 22-13
Laparoscopic tubal ligation: Filshie clip in place. (From Goldberg JM and Falcone T: *Atlas of endoscopic techniques in gynecology*, Philadelphia, 2001, Saunders.)

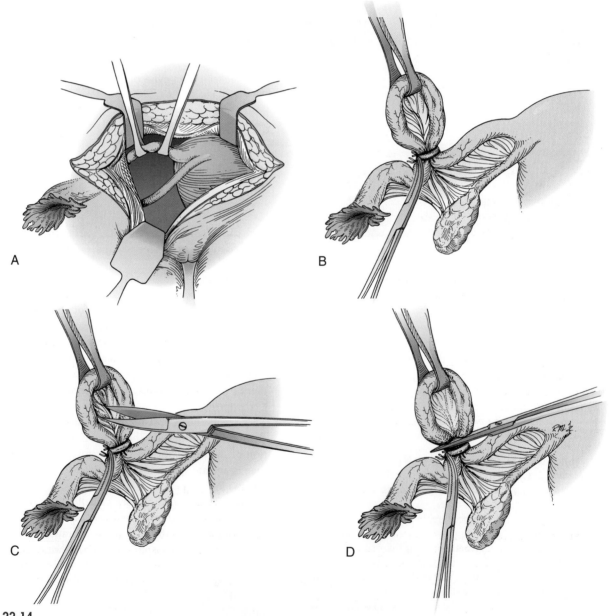

A

B

C

D

FIGURE 22-14
The Pomeroy technique. **A**, The length of the tube is exposed. **B**, A nucha of tissue is formed in the mid-portion of the tube and double tied with plain suture. **C**, A window is created in the mesosalpinx. **D**, The anterior portion of the tubal nucha is excised. (Adapted from Gershenson DM, et al: *Operative gynecology*, ed 2, Philadelphia, 2001, Saunders.)

and clamped in place. This method causes the least amount of damage to the tube but produces secure occlusion (Figure 22-13).

After the procedure, instruments are withdrawn and the pneumoperitoneum is released. One or two deep sutures are inserted, and the skin is closed with a staple.

Open tubal ligation through a mini laparotomy incision may be performed with the Irving or Pomeroy technique. Figure 22-14, *A-D,* illustrates the Pomeroy technique.

Tubal Segmental Resection for Ectopic Pregnancy

SURGICAL GOAL

In ectopic pregnancy, the egg implants and the embryo grows in the fallopian tube. The goal of surgery is to remove the embryo to prevent rupture of the fallopian tube.

PATHOLOGY

Most ectopic pregnancies occur in the ampulla of the fallopian tube. Tubal rupture, hemorrhage, and life-threatening shock can result. If rupture has already occurred at the time of admission, an emergency surgery may be required to control hemorrhage.

The surgery may be performed via laparoscopy unless the patient is in shock or other contraindications are present. The open procedure is described below. The techniques used for laparoscopy are very similar to those used in other laparoscopic procedures. Bipolar ESU and microinstruments are used.

Salpingostomy is an incision into the fallopian tube through which the products of conception (embryo and associated tissue and fluid) are removed. In this procedure, the fallopian tube is not sutured but left to close by secondary intention.

Salpingectomy (segmental resection) is the removal of a segment of the fallopian tube that includes the products of conception.

Technique SEGMENTAL RESECTION

1. Pelvic laparotomy is performed.
2. The pregnancy is identified.
3. The surgeon grasps and elevates the proximal tube.
4. Bipolar ESU is used to coagulate the proximal side of the ectopic pregnancy. The distal side is treated in the same way.
5. The fallopian tube is dissected from the mesosalpinx in the area of the pregnancy until it is completely free of all attachments.
6. The specimen is removed from the field.

DISCUSSION

The patient is placed in supine position, prepped, and draped for a pelvic laparotomy. To begin the procedure, the surgeon uses Babcock clamps to grasp the fallopian tube on the proximal side of the pregnant segment. The surgeon then uses the bipolar ESU to coagulate the tube on both sides of the tubal segment.

Using the bipolar ESU and micro scissors, the surgeon divides the mesosalpinx from the fallopian tube. This frees the segment from its attachments. It is then removed from the field. The two segments generally are not anastomosed at the time of the salpingectomy because of local swelling. Re-attachment may be attempted during a later surgery.

If the ectopic pregnancy has already ruptured when the patient is admitted, the scrub must be prepared to respond to hemorrhaging, an emergent situation. As soon as the laparotomy is performed, the scrub makes suction immediately available and, if necessary, has a blood-recovery system available.

All clots are removed manually, and the source of the bleeding is identified as quickly as possible. Remember that the bleeding cannot be controlled until it is exposed. A self-retaining retractor may or may not be inserted until the bleeding vessels have been clamped. Mayo or similar large hemostatic clamps are typically used to cross-clamp the fallopian tube and mesosalpinx. Suture ligatures must be immediately available to secure the bleeding vessels.

After the technical portion of the procedure, the wound is irrigated to remove all clots. and layers are individually closed.

Microsurgical Tubal Anastomosis

SURGICAL GOAL

Tubal anastomosis is performed to restore continuity to the fallopian tube to increase fertility. This procedure is performed to reverse tubal ligation or to re-establish continuity when obstruction is present.

PATHOLOGY

Previous pelvic inflammatory disease (**PID**) is the usual cause of tubal obstruction. PID is widespread inflammation of the uterus, fallopian tubes, and ovaries. It is most often caused by sexually transmitted diseases, such as *Neisseria gonorrhoeae* or *Chlamydia trachomatis*. Other causes include *Escherichia coli* or *Haemophilus influenzae*. Bacterial infection enters through the endocervix and spreads to the ovaries and fallopian tubes. Scarring and obstruction result in infertility. Cornual occlusion is blockage of the tube at the proximal end (closest to the uterus).

Tubal anastomosis also is performed to reverse previous tubal ligation. The following technique is used to reconstruct the fallopian tube with cornual occlusion.

Technique

1. A pelvic laparotomy is performed.
2. The proximal fallopian tube is excised.
3. The surgeon transects the proximal tube until patency can be demonstrated with indigo carmine dye.
4. The distal tube is transected and tested as in step 3.
5. Stay sutures are inserted to bring the two tube segments into exact alignment.
6. An inner layer of sutures is placed circumferentially in the tube.
7. The tubal serosa is anastomosed.
8. The mesosalpinx is sutured together.
9. The tube is again infused with dye to confirm patency.

DISCUSSION

Microscopic surgery to restore **patency** (an unobstructed passageway) to the fallopian tube is performed with the operating microscope or surgical loupes and with a fiberoptic headlight. The procedure also may be performed with the laparoscope.

The exact technique required for tubal anastomosis depends on the pathology. When the tube is diseased or there is a large disparity in size between the two segments to be joined, the procedure becomes more complex because the larger segment must be reduced to fit the smaller end.

The patient is placed in low lithotomy position for access to the cervix and intrauterine cavity during surgery. The abdomen is entered through a transverse pelvic incision. A self-retaining O'Connor or O'Sullivan retractor is placed in the wound, and the bowel is packed away from the uterus with moist laparotomy sponges. The patient may be placed in slight Trendelenburg position to allow gravity displacement of the abdominal organs.

The surgeon retracts the uterus with a tenaculum and locates the fallopian tube, mesosalpinx, ureter, and uterine ligaments. Before beginning the procedure, the surgeon may inject the fundus of the myometrium with *vasopressin* (a vasoconstrictor) to control hemorrhage. Continuous irrigation may be used to locate microscopic bleeders. A solution of glycine or lactated Ringer's is used.

The proximal end of the occluded area is grasped with toothed forceps, and the serosa of the tube is incised with a micro ESU. The incision is carried through the tube with the micro dissecting rod. Small bleeders are controlled with the microbipolar forceps.

The tube is then fully transected with iris scissors or other fine-tip scissors. The proximal side is lifted, and the peritoneal serosa is excised at the uterine body. This incision is carried deeper with scissors. If patency is not evident, the dissection is repeated proximally.

Indigo carmine dye is instilled transcervically to establish patency of the tube where it communicates with the uterus.

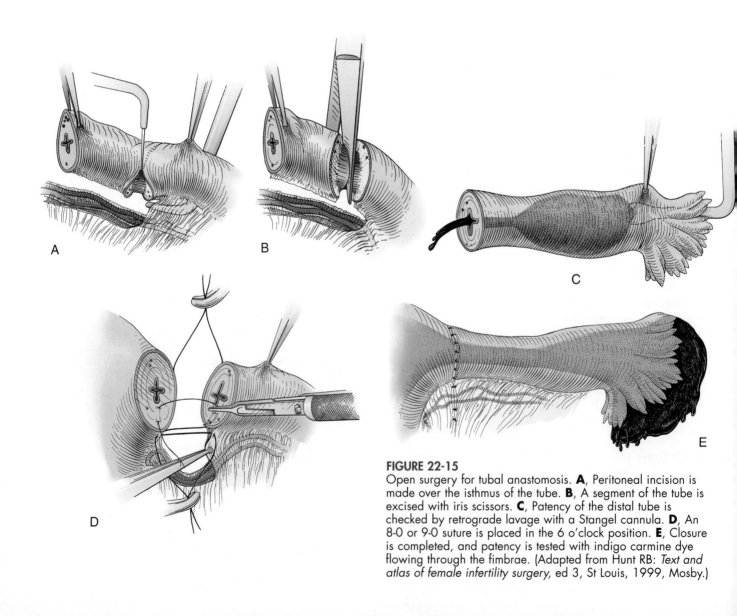

FIGURE 22-15

Open surgery for tubal anastomosis. **A**, Peritoneal incision is made over the isthmus of the tube. **B**, A segment of the tube is excised with iris scissors. **C**, Patency of the distal tube is checked by retrograde lavage with a Stangel cannula. **D**, An 8-0 or 9-0 suture is placed in the 6 o'clock position. **E**, Closure is completed, and patency is tested with indigo carmine dye flowing through the fimbrae. (Adapted from Hunt RB: *Text and atlas of female infertility surgery*, ed 3, St Louis, 1999, Mosby.)

The distal segment of the tube is then dissected from the mesosalpinx, and the outer (peritoneal) tissue of the tube is incised with the bipolar ESU. The segment is divided with iris scissors or other fine sharp-tip scissors, with the same technique as used for the proximal segment. The surgeon then irrigates the distal segment with indigo carmine dye, using a Stangel cannula. The appearance of the dye at the severed end indicates patency.

The two segments are then anastomosed. Stay sutures are placed and tagged with fine, small hemostats. Size 8-0 or 9-0 nylon or polypropylene with tapered needle is used for the anastomosis. A two-layered anastomosis is performed. If the myometrium (uterus) has been cut, a repair is made with size 6-0 sutures.

The serosa and mesosalpinx of the tube are closed with interrupted sutures in size 8-0. Indigo carmine dye is then instilled into the tube to confirm that the tube is patent. The abdominal wound is irrigated and closed in layers.

Open surgery for tubal anastomosis is illustrated in Figure 22-15, *A-E.*

Cesarean Section
SURGICAL GOAL
Cesarean section is surgical removal of the fetus through the abdomen.

PATHOLOGY
Cesarean section is medically necessary when the mother's life is in jeopardy and for obstetrical conditions that would result in fetal death. These include but are not limited to:

▶ Transverse, breech, or other malpresentation of the fetus
▶ Prolapsed umbilical cord (Figure 22-16, *A*)
▶ Ruptured placenta (abruptio placentae) (Figure 22-16, *B*)
▶ Delivery of the placenta ahead of the fetus (placenta previa) (Figure 22-16, *C*)
▶ Active genital herpes infection
▶ Previous cesarean section
▶ Cephalopelvic disproportion (CPD) (fetus cannot be delivered through the pelvis because of its shape)
▶ Failure to progress
▶ Prolapsed cord
▶ Toxemia
▶ Diabetes

Technique

1. A low transverse or midline incision is made to the level of the rectus muscles (transverse incision).
2. The surgeon manually separates the muscles.
3. The surgeon elevates the peritoneum with two hemostats and makes a small hole between the clamps.
4. The peritoneum is divided with scissors.
5. Large bleeders are clamped but not ligated or coagulated.
6. The peritoneal reflection of the bladder (bladder flap) is divided from the uterus with Metzenbaum scissors.
7. A bladder retractor is placed on the lower edge of the incision, and the bladder is displaced downward.
8. The surgeon makes a small transverse incision in the uterus with the scalpel.
9. The scrub brings the suction tube (no tip), bulb syringe, and bandage scissors near the wound.
10. The surgeon extends the uterine incision with the bandage scissors.
11. Amniotic fluid is quickly suctioned from the open uterus.
12. The assistant applies pressure to the upper abdomen while the surgeon rotates the baby's head into view.

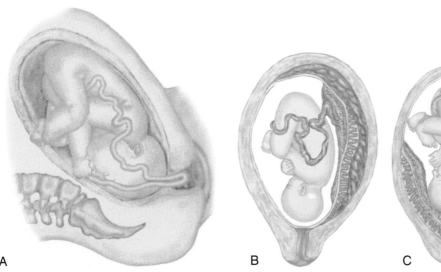

FIGURE 22-16
Reasons for cesarean section. **A,** Prolapsed umbilical cord. **B,** Ruptured placenta (abruptio placentae). **C,** Delivery of the placenta ahead of the fetus (placenta previa). (From Murray SS, McKinney ES, and Gorrie TM: *Foundations of maternal-newborn nursing,* ed 3, Philadelphia, 2002, Saunders.)

13. The nose and mouth are immediately suctioned with the bulb syringe or separate suction catheter, such as a DeLee suction catheter.
14. The baby's body is removed from the uterus.
15. The umbilical cord is double clamped and cut with bandage scissors. One clamp is released slightly to fill two blood-collection tubes.
16. The baby is handed over to the infant resuscitation team for care.
17. The placenta is delivered, and remaining fluid and blood are suctioned from the wound.
18. The uterus is closed in layers.
19. The abdomen is closed in layers.

DISCUSSION

Cesarean section can be scheduled or may occur as an emergency procedure. If the procedure is scheduled (such as for a repeat cesarean section), a spinal or epidural anesthesia is administered and a regular set-up can be performed.

An emergency delivery occurs very quickly. If a general anesthetic is given, time is extremely critical to prevent fetal anesthesia and to correct the condition that warranted the emergency.

In *emergency* surgery, there are several instruments that are used to start the procedure and safely deliver the baby. In many cases, lack of time may prevent a normal set-up.

As soon as the technologist scrubs, gowns, and gloves, he or she should prepare the following items, which are adequate to deliver the baby:

▶ Laparotomy drape
▶ Scalpel
▶ Lap sponges
▶ Mayo clamps (four to six)
▶ Metzenbaum scissors
▶ Bladder retractor (DeLee or the bladder blade from a Balfour retractor)
▶ Hemostats such as Kelly or Crile clamps
▶ Bandage scissors
▶ Suction tubing
▶ Bulb syringe

As the patient is brought into the operating room, an infant warming unit and personnel from the nursery are available to receive and care for the baby as soon as the baby is delivered. The patient is placed on the operating table in supine position. A cushioned pad may be placed under the patient's right side for elevation to prevent aortocaval compression by the fetus. Such compression can cause hypotension and fetal hypoxia.

The patient is prepped and draped quickly after administration of anesthetic, or prepping and draping may take place *before general anesthesia* is begun.

The surgeon enters the abdomen through a Pfannenstiel incision (Figure 22-17, *A*). The incision is carried to the muscles, which are divided by hand. Bleeders are clamped but are not ligated or coagulated to save time, unless the hemostats obstruct the surgeon's view or are in the way. Before entering the peritoneum, the surgeon elevates it with two Mayo clamps. The surgeon then makes a small incision between the clamps.

The peritoneal incision is lengthened with Metzenbaum or Mayo scissors. The peritoneal reflection of the bladder then must be removed from the uterus. This is performed with Metzenbaum scissors. When the bladder flap has been removed, a bladder retractor is placed over the lower edge of the incision and the bladder is retracted downward, away from the uterus.

Just before entering the uterus, the scrub must bring the suction tubing (without a tip), bulb syringe, bandage scissors, and scalpel. The surgeon makes a small incision in the uterus and deepens it with the bandage scissors. The blunt tip of the bandage scissors prevents injury to the fetus.

The scrub must remove the scalpel from the field immediately to prevent injury to the baby or a team member.

As soon as the uterus is opened, the scrub places the tip of the suction tubing at the edge of the incision to aspirate amniotic fluid. The assistant applies pressure to the upper abdomen while the surgeon grasps the baby's head and delivers it from the uterus (Figure 22-17, *B*). The bulb syringe is used immediately to suction the baby's nose and mouth (Figure 22-17, *C*). If a second suction is available, a flexible suction catheter is used to clear the baby's airway.

Extra laparotomy sponges should be available. The surgeon delivers the baby from the uterus and places him or her on the mother's abdomen. The surgeon clamps the umbilical cord with two Mayo clamps and severs it with bandage scissors. The scrub must have two blood-specimen containers in hand to receive cord blood. The surgeon releases one of the Mayo clamps slightly to fill the containers. The scrub caps these and passes them to the circulator.

The baby is handed to the resuscitation team and placed in the warming unit. The baby is again suctioned, dried, administered oxygen as needed, and assessed. The infant may be taken to the nursery or ICU.

As the baby is handed over to the resuscitation team, attention again must be directed to the mother. The scrub places a large basin on the field to receive the placenta, which is delivered from the uterus.

The surgeon grasps the edges of the uterus with sponge forceps, Duval lung clamps, or Collin tongue clamps. These are atraumatic clamps that prevent maceration of the uterine incision during closure.

A count is mandatory before the uterus is closed.

The uterine incision is closed with a two-layered running suture of size 0 absorbable suture (Figure 22-17, *D*). The surgeon then may attend to any bleeders, which are coagulated with the ESU or ligated with suture ties. When the wound is clean and dry, the remaining layers are closed.

The bladder flap is reperitonealized with a running suture of size 2-0 or 3-0 absorbable suture on a taper needle. The remaining layers are closed in routine fashion, and the wound is dressed with sterile gauze.

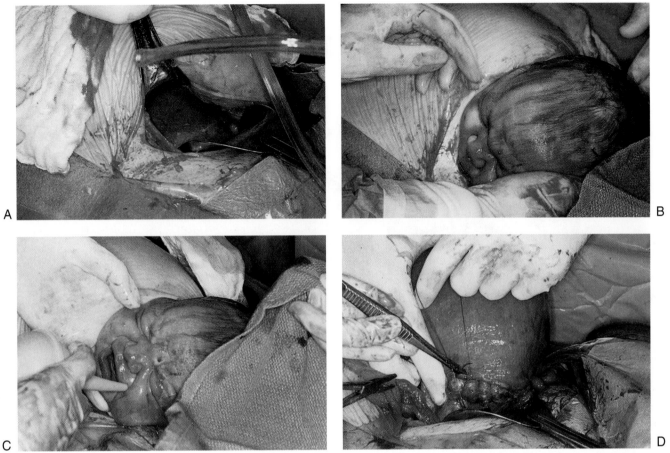

FIGURE 22-17
Cesarean section. **A**, Through a Pfannenstiel skin incision, the uterus is opened in a low transverse incision. **B**, The fetal head is brought through the incision. **C**, The mouth and nose are suctioned to remove secretions and blood before the infant takes his or her first breath. **D**, Heavy sutures are used to close the muscular layers of the lower transverse uterine incision. (From Murray SS, McKinney ES, and Gorrie TM: *Foundations of maternal-newborn nursing*, ed 3, Philadelphia, 2002, Saunders.)

VAGINAL SURGICAL PROCEDURES

Hysteroscopy

OPERATIVE USE AND PRINCIPLES

Hysteroscopy is a technique whereby a lighted fiberoptic endoscope is inserted into the uterus **transcervically** (through the cervical os) for diagnostic and operative procedures. The cavity is then infused with liquid or viscous (thick) media. Examination, biopsy, and surgical procedures are performed via the hysteroscope and operating channels in the same way that cystoscopic surgery is performed through the bladder.

Accessory equipment allows the surgeon to perform resection and to remove biopsy tissue. Laser and electrosurgical ablation is usually performed to remove uterine myomas (fibroid tumors) and endometrial tissue.

UTERINE DISTENSION

To obtain a clear view of the uterine cavity, the surgeon may distend the endometrial cavity during hysteroscopy. Two methods are used. Carbon monoxide insufflation similar to that used during laparoscopy is achieved though an insuffla-

tion device. This method is useful during clinic or office hysteroscopy. It allows thorough examination of the endocervix. This technique requires special equipment for insufflation and for measurement of intrauterine pressure. When carbon monoxide is used for insufflation, the patient is not placed in the Trendelenburg position because of the risk of gas embolism.

Fluid distension is used most often in the operating room. This method of uterine distension is used with continuous irrigation. These solutions are readily available in 1000-ml and 3000-ml bags, which can be delivered to the hysteroscope by gravity flow from an IV pole. Special pressure cuffs, pumps, or a syringe also are used (Figure 22-18).

A pouch perineal drape is used to retrieve the fluid that escapes during the procedure. The amount of inflow and returned outflow must be reported at regular, short intervals.

Nonelectrolytic solution containing 32% Dextran is a viscous fluid that retains optical clarity after infusion. Its viscosity prevents **retrograde** (backward) outflow from the uterine cavity. This technique is preferred for hysteroscopic procedures in the operating room.

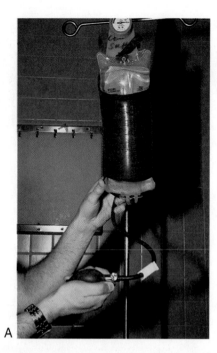

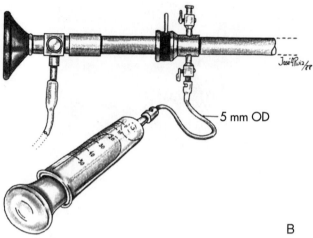

FIGURE 22-18
A, Solution is delivered to the hysteroscope from an IV pole. **B**, Solution is delivered from a syringe. (From Baggish MS, Barbot J, and Valle RF: *Diagnostic and operative hysteroscopy, a text and atlas,* ed 2, St Louis, 1999, Mosby.)

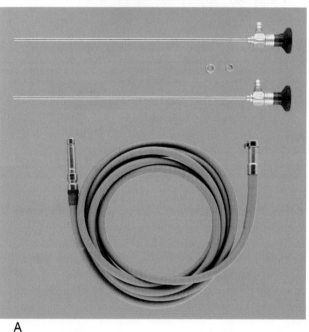

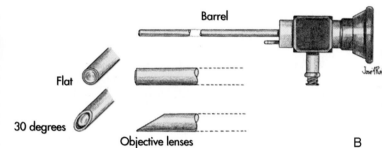

FIGURE 22-19
A, *Top to bottom,* hysteroscopic operative set: hysteroscopy lens, 4 mm, 0 degree; two sealing caps; hysteroscopic lens, 4 mm, 30 degree; fiberoptic cord. **B**, Common viewing angles are 0 degrees (flat) and 30 degrees. (**A** from Tighe SM: *Instrumentation for the operating room,* ed 6, St Louis, 1999, Mosby; **B** from Baggish MS, Barbot J, and Valle RF: *Diagnostic and operative hysteroscopy, a text and atlas,* ed 2, St Louis, 1999, Mosby.)

Sorbitol, glycine, and dextrose are fluids used for continuous irrigation of the uterus. However, because of their low viscosity, they may mix with blood and cause some obscurity of the telescopic field.

Lactated Ringer's solution is an **electrolytic media** (conducts electricity). Electrolytic solutions are *not* used during electrosurgical resection! Dispersal of electricity and burns can occur.

HYSTEROSCOPY INSTRUMENTS
A basic hysteroscopic set-up includes the following:

▶ 30-degree telescope
▶ 0-degree telescope
▶ Accessory equipment
▶ Auvard or Sims speculum
▶ Uterine sound
▶ Single-toothed straight tenaculum
▶ Solution bowl
▶ Four 50-ml syringes
▶ Pratt dilators
▶ 1-inch silicone tubing with Luer-Lok and fittings
▶ Stopcocks
▶ Short bridge
▶ Catheterization bridge
▶ Aspirating cannula
▶ Scissors
▶ Biopsy forceps

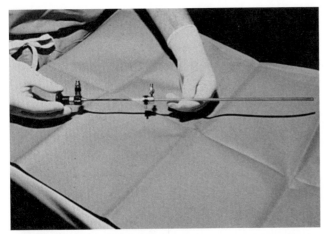

FIGURE 22-20
The hysteroscope being inserted into the sheath. (From Baggish MS, Barbot J, and Valle RF: *Diagnostic and operative hysteroscopy, a text and atlas,* ed 2, St Louis, 1999, Mosby.)

▶ Grasping forceps
▶ Fulgurating tip with high-frequency cord

Hysteroscope

The hysteroscope brings the image to the surgeon's eye and illuminates the target area (Figure 22-19, *A*). Traditional lens systems as well as fiberoptic imaging are now available. Fiberoptic systems produce extremely bright, cool light without distortion.

A common hysteroscope has an outer diameter of 4 mm. The most common viewing angles are 0 degrees (straight scope) and 30 degrees (offset). The scope is 30 to 35 cm long (Figure 22-19, *B*).

Sheath

The hysteroscope is inserted into the sheath before insertion into the uterine cavity (Figure 22-20). The main operating channel receives the telescope, while side channels, controlled by stopcocks, accept the accessory instruments. The main channel is fitted with rubber gaskets that prevent the backflow of distension media. Both double-channel and single-channel sheaths are available. Some models contain separate channels for the telescope and liquid media. This type of system allows the surgeon to flush fluid and debris from the uterus while operating at the same time.

Operating Instruments

Most hysteroscopic procedures employ 3-mm instruments; 2-mm accessories are available for very fine tissue dissection. Accessory instruments include biopsy forceps, scissors, and grasping forceps (Figure 22-21, *A*). Flexible instruments can be fitted easily into the deflector bridge. Suction cannulas and a flexible catheter are used to remove blood clots, debris, blood, and mucus, and to inject liquid media (Figure 22-21, *B*). Rigid and semi-rigid instruments are inserted directly into the sheath (Figure 22-21, *C*).

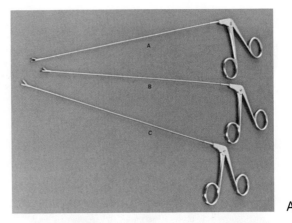

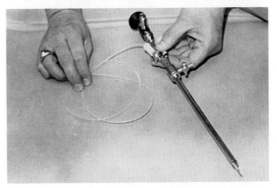

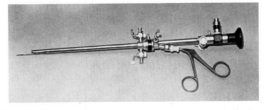

FIGURE 22-21
A, *Top to bottom,* grasping forceps; biopsy forceps; scissors. **B**, Suction cannulae and a flexible catheter. **C**, Semirigid instrument. (From Baggish MS, Barbot J, and Valle RF: *Diagnostic and operative hysteroscopy, a text and atlas,* ed 2, St Louis, 1999, Mosby.)

Light

The light source for the surgical hysteroscope is delivered through a xenon generator, halide generator, or tungsten generator. The xenon light is used most often. A fiberoptic light cable connects the light source to the hysteroscope. The scrub should remember that all fiberoptic light cables are easily damaged. These cables should be handled gently and never allowed to strike a hard surface. Review Chapter 18 for safe handling of fiberoptic cables.

Electrodes are inserted into the operating sheath for tissue coagulation and cutting. A variety of tips are available for bipolar and monopolar instruments. These include the ball tip, spring tip, needle, and hook active electrodes.

Snares and corkscrew instruments are available for removing polyps and dense tumors.

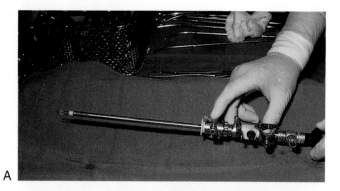

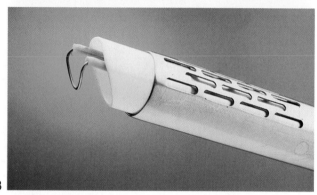

FIGURE 22-22
A, A small resectoscope for gynecological surgery. **B**, Tip of a cutting-loop resectoscope. (From Baggish MS, Barbot J, and Valle RF: *Diagnostic and operative hysteroscopy, a text and atlas,* ed 2, St Louis, 1999, Mosby.)

Video Camera
Similar to the laparoscope, the hysteroscope is capable of video-assisted surgery and documentation. Many procedures are observed and surgery is performed by indirect viewing on the video monitor. Refer to Chapter 18 for a discussion on videoscopic surgery.

Resectoscope
The intrauterine resectoscope is a modification of the cystoscopic resectoscope usually used in transurethral procedures. It is used to remove polyps, subcutaneous leiomyomas, and uterine adhesions, and to **ablate** (remove by heat and coagulation) the endometrium to treat abnormal uterine bleeding.

The resectoscope contains a 0-degree or 12-degree telescope that is inserted into a separate sheath. A spring-loaded mechanism in the handle retracts and exposes the electrode tip (Figure 22-22, *A* and *B*). The loop-shaped electrode on the tip shaves and coagulates tissue when activated. As tissue is removed by pieces from the uterine wall, it remains free floating in the media until flushed from the uterine cavity. The advantage of the loop resectoscope is that it can both shave and coagulate tissue bit by bit so that bleeding can be controlled.

Continuous irrigation permits clear visualization during procedures. The resectoscope is constructed with an outer sheath that allows fluid outflow and an inner sheath that provides continuous irrigation.

During resection it is essential that a nonelectrolytic solution be used for uterine irrigation. This prevents current

from the loop electrode from dispersing and causing injury to the uterine walls.

LASER AND ELECTROSURGERY DURING HYSTEROSCOPY
Lasers
Lasers and laser safety are discussed in Chapter 17. The technologist should review this chapter before learning to assist in laser hysteroscopy.

The Nd:YAG and argon lasers usually are used during hysteroscopic surgery. KTP-532 and tunable dye lasers also are effective. Safety considerations must be a primary focus when these technologies are in use. Backscatter of the laser beam (laser beam reflected back to the operator) is a risk. Special filters therefore must be fitted onto the hysteroscope.

The argon laser is capable of transmission through aqueous solution and therefore is useful during continuous irrigation hysteroscopy. The Nd:YAG laser has a variety of uses, including the severing of endometrial and myometrial structures.

Coagulation with the laser is achieved on lower power settings.

Electrosurgery
Safety principles for electrosurgery are discussed in Chapter 17. Techniques used in electrosurgery apply to hysteroscopy as in other types of surgery. These include pure cutting, blended cutting, coagulation, and **fulguration** (spray coagulation).

Hysteroscopic Endometrial Ablation
SURGICAL GOAL
Endometrial **ablation** is coagulation of the endometrium of the uterus to treat uterine bleeding that cannot be controlled by hormonal means.

PATHOLOGY
Abnormal uterine bleeding can be related to hormonal abnormalities or pathological changes in the endometrium.

Technique

1. After prepping and draping, the surgeon inserts a vaginal speculum and grasps the anterior cervix with a tenaculum.
2. The cervix is dilated with Pratt, Hank, or Hegar dilators.
3. The operating hysteroscope sheath (or resectoscope) is inserted into the os cervix.
4. The uterine cavity is irrigated to remove any blood and tissue debris.
5. Continuous irrigation with a nonelectrolytic solution is initiated.
6. A 3-mm ball electrode is inserted into the operating channel. If the laser is used, a 1-mm laser fiber is positioned on the fundus.
7. The surgeon ablates the myometrium, using a systematic approach to cover all interior segments of the uterus.
8. The suction cannula is used to remove debris and bubbles throughout the procedure.

DISCUSSION

Before beginning the procedure, the scrub should ensure that all equipment is in good working order and that sufficient irrigation fluid is immediately available *in the OR suite* to complete the procedure. Electrical cables, light cords, fiberoptic systems, and suction systems must be checked to make sure that they do not malfunction during surgery.

The patient is placed in lithotomy position and prepped for a vaginal procedure. Routine draping for a perineal procedure is performed, with the addition of a urological pocket, which is positioned under the patient's buttocks. If a pocket drape is not available, a sterile Mayo stand cover can be used to collect fluid.

The scrub secures all connections, cords, suction tubing, and irrigation tubing. All cables and cords must be secured with nonpenetrating towel clamps. The scrub should measure the amount of slack needed to allow the instruments to be used correctly. Once cords are placed, they cannot be readjusted without breaking aseptic technique.

Do not loop the electrosurgical cables through or around a stainless-steel clamp. A nonvisible weak or thinned area in the cord can cause sparking and patient fire.

The surgeon begins the procedure by inserting a weighted or bivalve speculum into the vagina. The surgeon then grasps the cervix with a single-toothed tenaculum and inserts the hysteroscope sheath into the os. The resectoscope may be used in place of the sheath.

The entire uterine cavity is irrigated with the irrigation fluid selected for the type of ablation to be performed (nonelectrolytic for electrosurgical ablation). All clots and tissue debris are cleared from the intrauterine cavity. If electrosurgical ablation is performed, a 3-mm ball electrode is selected. The surgeon then proceeds with the ablation.

Resectoscope Myomectomy
SURGICAL GOAL

Myomectomy is the removal of a benign tumor (fibroid) of the myometrium to control bleeding and prevent pressure on other structures in the pelvis. Submucous myomas can be removed with the hysteroscopic resectoscope or laser.

PATHOLOGY

Refer to Uterine Leiomyoma in the earlier section, Abdominal Hysterectomy (Open).

Technique

1. The patient is prepared for hysteroscopy as described above.
2. After cervical dilation, a double-sheath resectoscope is inserted.
3. All cords and tubing are connected.
4. The uterine cavity is irrigated and infused with nonelectrolytic solution or Hyspak.
5. The resectoscope is activated to shave off bands of the tumor.
6. The outer sheath is removed to flush out the sectioned tumor pieces. Alternatively, the cervix may be further dilated and sponge forceps used to remove pieces of tumor.

7. The myoma is reduced until it is level with the endometrium.

DISCUSSION

Before beginning the procedure, the scrub must test the resectoscope to make sure that all working parts move smoothly and that the cutting electrodes are intact. All cords must be checked for signs of impairment or weakness.

A continuous irrigation system is set up and tested before surgery.

The patient is placed in lithotomy position, prepped, and draped as described previously in Hysteroscopic Endometrial Ablation.

The procedure begins as the surgeon dilates the cervix and inserts the resectoscope sheath with or without an **obturator.** This is a blunt-tipped rod that is advanced ahead of the sheath to protect the tissue from injury. If used, the obturator is removed after the sheath is inserted.

A resectoscope with a 0-degree or fore-oblique telescope is inserted into the cervix. The resectoscope is surrounded by an 8-mm or 9-mm sheath, which has an insulated tip to prevent contact between the active electrode and the outer sheath. The outer sheath provides inflow of intrauterine fluid. A bridge allows entry of the electrodes.

Power settings for coagulation and cutting are set according to the surgeon's directions.

The scrub should never change the power settings unless the surgeon requests a change. When beginning the procedure, the scrub always should ask for the correct settings and never start the procedure without checking the settings.

As described above, the resectoscope is operated via a spring-loaded handle, which pushes and retracts an active electrode loop. The surgeon removes sections or slices of tissue by repeatedly looping the tissue and drawing it into the resectoscope. This cuts and coagulates the tissue and releases it into the uterine cavity where it is flushed out through the resectoscope sheath or by manual removal.

The cutting and coagulation action of the resectoscope may cause bleeding, which is controlled by the ball electrode. The surgeon flushes out the irrigation fluid and bits of tissue by removing the outer sheath and allowing the fluid to drop into the perineal drape.

The procedure is complete when the tumor is level with the endometrium. All specimen pieces must be retrieved and collected for pathological examination.

Refer to Figure 22-23 for photos of this procedure.

Dilation and Curettage
SURGICAL GOAL

In this procedure, the surface of the endometrium is removed to obtain tissue for biopsy and to control uterine bleeding.

PATHOLOGY

The procedure also may be performed to remove tissue after an incomplete abortion or missed abortion (the fetus is no

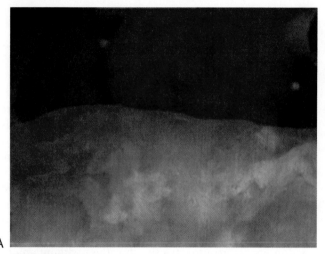

FIGURE 22-23
Resectoscope myomectomy. **A**, The loop electrode is placed on the fundus superior to the myoma. **B**, Passes are made with the loop to remove fragments of tissue to debulk the myoma. **C**, The stalk of the myoma is transected. (From Goldberg JM and Falcone T: *Atlas of endoscopic techniques in gynecology*, Philadelphia, 2001, Saunders.)

longer viable but is retained in the uterus), or in cases of retained placenta after normal vaginal delivery. An incomplete abortion (an abortion in progress that has occurred spontaneously) also may be treated with a D & C and uterine evacuation with suction. The tissue is removed for diagnostic purposes in cases of unexplained persistent uterine bleeding.

Technique

1. The uterine depth is measured with a uterine sound.
2. The cervix is dilated with graduated dilators.
3. Curettes are used to remove endometrial tissue.

DISCUSSION
Dilation and curettage is performed for therapeutic treatment and diagnosis. Products of conception (fetus or embryo) are removed with a suction apparatus.

The patient is placed in lithotomy position. The bladder may be emptied with a straight catheter. The patient is then prepped and draped for a vaginal procedure.

The surgeon stands or sits at the foot of the operating table. The scrub should stand next to the surgeon to assist. To begin the procedure the surgeon places a weighted specu-

lum in the vagina. The surgeon then grasps the anterior lip of the cervix and retracts it slightly forward and downward.

A uterine sound is inserted into the cervix to measure its depth and position. This prevents accidental perforation during the procedure. Using Hegar, Pratt, or Hank uterine dilators, the surgeon slowly dilates the cervix.

As soon as the cervix is sufficiently dilated to accept the curettes, the surgeon places a strip of Telfa-coated cotton over the right angle of the speculum or on the posterior edge of the vagina. The uterus is then gently curetted, allowing the specimen to collect on the Telfa. The technologist should have several types and sizes of curettes available, including smooth, sharp, and serrated. When curettage is complete, the Telfa is removed and passed to the scrub. Both the Telfa and specimen are placed in a container for pathological examination. The perineum is dressed with a perineal pad.

Therapeutic Abortion
SURGICAL GOAL
In this procedure, pregnancy is terminated by removal of the fetus from the uterus through the vagina.

Technique

1. The uterus is sounded, and the cervix is dilated.
2. Curettage is performed.
3. The uterine contents are aspirated mechanically via a special suction apparatus.

DESCRIPTION

This procedure employs a special vacuum device to evacuate the contents of the uterus. A routine dilation and curettage is performed, as previously described. Sterile suction tubing and a suction tip are given to the scrub or surgeon. One end of the suction tubing is passed to the circulator, who then attaches it to the vacuum device. The circulator activates the vacuum, and the surgeon suctions the uterus clean. The scrub must retrieve the specimen from the suction bottle at the close of the procedure. The vagina is dressed with a perineal pad.

A suction dilation and curettage also may be performed on patients who have had a miscarriage (also called missed abortion). These patients may have retained products of conception (POC), which may be lodged in the uterus and can cause the patient to continue to bleed or have uncomfortable labor symptoms until the contents of the uterus have been evacuated. These patients need special emotional support, as they are dealing with the loss of life, in addition to the anxiety of the surgical procedure.

A scrub may refuse to participate in elective abortions if the procedure violates his or her religious, ethical, or moral beliefs.

Loop Electrode Excision Procedure (LEEP)
SURGICAL GOAL

A core of tissue is removed from the cervix when pathological examinations show precancerous or cancerous cells on the cervix or endocervix. The tissue is removed to prevent the progression of disease.

PATHOLOGY

The squamous cell intraepithelial lesion (SIL) is the most common type of cervical cancer. It is diagnosed by any of three tests:

▶ The *Pap* test uses a thin layer of cells retrieved from the endocervix for microscopic examination.
▶ During *colposcopy* (an office or clinic procedure), the cervix is painted with acetic acid or iodine solution (called the Schiller test), which stains abnormal cells. The culposcope produces high magnification to allow examination of the cervix.
▶ Cervicography is used less often. This is a photographic technique that uses pictures of both normal and abnormal cervical patterns.

Technique

1. The surgeon grasps the cervix with a single-toothed tenaculum.

2. A local anesthetic is injected into the cervical canal.
3. A loop electrode is used to remove tissue from the cervix.
4. A ball electrode is used to control bleeding.

DISCUSSION

The decision to perform a LEEP excision is made after one or more abnormal Pap smears.

The patient is placed in lithotomy position, prepped, and draped for a vaginal procedure. The surgeon infuses the cervix with local anesthetic using a 1½-inch 22-gauge needle. The surgeon then grasps the anterior lip of the cervix and uses a disposable loop electrode to make a circumferential incision around the os. The specimen is removed, and the scrub passes it to the circulator for pathological examination. The loop electrode is then replaced with a ball coagulator, which is used to coagulate the area of the excision.

Uterine Balloon Therapy
SURGICAL GOAL

Balloon therapy is a form of endometrial ablation. Endometrial ablation is performed to treat abnormal uterine bleeding, to create amenorrhea, or to reduce bleeding to a normal, tolerable flow for the patient.

PATHOLOGY

The patient demonstrates a history of:

▶ Excessive bleeding as evidenced by either profuse bleeding lasting more than 7 days or anemia caused by acute or chronic blood loss
▶ Failure of hormonal treatment or contraindications to hormonal therapy
▶ No current medication use that may cause bleeding
▶ Nonmalignant cervical cytology
▶ Negative preoperative pregnancy test
▶ No abnormal coagulation studies

Technique

1. The patient is placed in the lithotomy position.
2. A standard vaginal prep is performed.
3. After draping, the patient's bladder is drained.
4. The surgeon may perform a pelvic exam before the procedure.
5. A dilation and curettage is performed.
6. The uterine balloon is introduced until the tip touches the fundus.
7. The balloon is inflated, and the ablation begins.
8. After the procedure, the balloon is removed.
9. A perineal pad is placed.

DISCUSSION

Balloon therapy employs direct heat, as opposed to the laser, which uses light to create heat, and electrocautery devices, which use electricity to create heat. A uterine balloon catheter actually conforms to the internal contours of the uterus and contains a thermal heating element.

A dilation and curettage with suction curettage is necessary before the therapy; this ensures that the balloon will have maximal contact with the uterine lining.

The cervix is dilated to 5 mm to accommodate the balloon.

Many companies offer uterine balloon devices. Each has its own parameters for inflation amount, inflation medium, temperature, and duration of therapy. Please follow the manufacturer's guidelines for the device used in your institution.

Uterine balloon therapy may be performed as an ambulatory surgical procedure, and the patient may be discharged the same day.

Laser Ablation of Condylomata
SURGICAL GOAL
Laser ablation of condylomata or cancers is the eradication of diseased tissue through the use of a laser beam.

PATHOLOGY
Laser therapy has proven through clinical trials to be an effective treatment for this type of diseased tissue when other treatments have been less successful.

Technique
1. The patient is positioned supine with legs placed in stirrups for adequate exposure.
2. Appropriate laser safety precautions should be used, and the laser should be tested before the patient is brought into the room.
3. After positioning and draping of the patient, the surgeon will tell the staff the desired laser settings.
4. The laser is used to treat all lesions.
5. An antibiotic ointment may be used to dress the area.

DISCUSSION
Laser safety precautions include:

▶ Correct laser safety goggles for the laser in use
▶ Covering of the windows in the room to protect the outside environment
▶ A basin of wet towels for draping and for emergencies
▶ Signs on the doors to the room warning of a laser in use
▶ Use of only laser-safe instruments in the procedure
▶ Pre-firing and testing the laser to ensure that it is in proper working order

Wet towels are used to drape the patient for protection. *No* paper products at all should be used in the procedure area. The wet or damp towels will absorb the laser beam to prevent the possible burning of tissue that is not being treated.

In treating the lesions, the surgeon moves the beam across the tissue transversely, then in a criss-cross matrix to treat all perimeters of the lesion. Acetic acid in a 3% to 5% concentration can be used to wipe the area; this makes the diseased tissue stand out and allows treatment to deeper layers.

Laser ablation causes less edema and necrosis to the tissue, and healing is fairly rapid.

Removal of Cystic Bartholin's Gland
SURGICAL GOAL
This procedure is used to remove a cyst and Bartholin's gland to prevent recurrence of the cyst and infection.

PATHOLOGY
Bartholin's gland, which secretes mucus, is a common site of cyst formation. The cyst may become infected, and in such cases, surgical removal is indicated.

Technique
1. The labia minora are retracted and secured to the skin.
2. The surgeon incises the mucosa overlying the cyst.
3. The cyst and sometimes the gland are removed.
4. The wound edges are secured open with small sutures.

DISCUSSION
The patient is placed in lithotomy position, prepped, and draped for a perineal incision.

The surgeon may begin the procedure by securing the labia minora laterally with sutures or small skin staples. The surgeon then makes a curved incision in the mucosa over the cystic gland. The incision is lengthened with Metzenbaum scissors. Small bleeders are coagulated with a needle or flat-blade ESU tip.

Both the gland and the cyst may be removed together, or the cyst may be dissected away from the gland with dissecting scissors. The wound edges are secured open with sutures to allow secondary closure, as in marsupialization. The surgery is illustrated in Figure 22-24.

Repair of Vesicovaginal Fistula
SURGICAL GOAL
A vesicovaginal fistula is a small, hollow tract connecting the bladder to the vagina. Fistula tracts can result from infection or trauma. Chronic fistula tracts are lined with epithelial tissue, which prevents the tract from closing. The surgical goal is to incise the length of the tract and remove this tissue. The fascia layer separating the bladder from the vagina is approximated. Healing then can occur normally, and urine is prevented from draining into the bladder.

PATHOLOGY
Vesicovaginal fistula may result from traumatic penetrating injury, infection, radiation therapy that thins and weakens the pelvic structures, vaginal birth, or chronic inflammation. Urine drains into the vagina, causing irritation and incontinence. The fistula may extend into the ureter. The repair may be approached through pelvic laparotomy or vaginally. A pelvic approach is required when the tract occurs in the proximal vaginal vault. A vaginal exposure is described here.

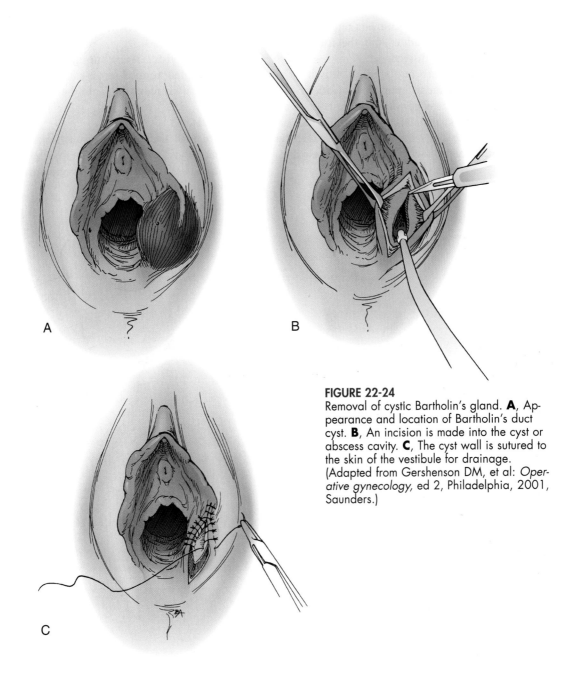

FIGURE 22-24
Removal of cystic Bartholin's gland. **A**, Appearance and location of Bartholin's duct cyst. **B**, An incision is made into the cyst or abscess cavity. **C**, The cyst wall is sutured to the skin of the vestibule for drainage. (Adapted from Gershenson DM, et al: *Operative gynecology*, ed 2, Philadelphia, 2001, Saunders.)

Technique

1. The surgeon grasps the edge of the tract with two or more Allis clamps.
2. A metal probe may be placed in the fistula to identify its course. Diagnostic procedures, including instillation of contrast media, may have preceded the surgery. Films obtained from the procedure describe the route of the fistula.
3. The tissue around the fistula is sharply dissected.
4. The surgeon creates a tissue plane between the bladder and the fistula with sharp and blunt dissection.
5. The mucosa is inverted, and sutures are placed through smooth muscular layer and mucosa.

6. An internal layer of sutures is placed in the bladder.
7. The edges of the vaginal wall are repaired.
8. An indwelling Foley catheter is placed.

DISCUSSION

The patient is placed in lithotomy position, prepped, and draped for a perineal incision. The surgeon places an Auvard or Sims retractor in the vagina to expose the fistula. A malleable probe is inserted into the fistula. The surgeon then uses dissecting scissors to make a circular incision around the probe and fistula. The surgeon carries this incision the full length of the fistula with dissecting scissors until the anterior bladder wall is exposed. Two lateral retractors may be placed in the vagina for better exposure. The surgeon creates a tissue plane between the bladder and the fistula with sponge dissectors or by sharp dissection.

When the bladder mucosa and smooth muscle layer have been exposed, the surgeon inverts the bladder tissue layers and approximates the edges with double-layer interrupted sutures of absorbable material, size 3-0. The vaginal wall is repaired with size 0 or 2-0 sutures. A Foley catheter may be inserted into the bladder at the close of the procedure.

This procedure is illustrated in Figure 22-25.

Repair of Rectovaginal Fistula
SURGICAL GOAL

Rectovaginal fistula is an abnormal tract between the rectum and the vagina. Surgical repair closes the defect to prevent fecal material from draining into the vagina.

PATHOLOGY

Rectovaginal fistula may result from vaginal or rectal trauma, childbirth, radiation therapy, chronic inflammation, or infection. A fistula tract causes fecal material to drain into the vagina, causing infection.

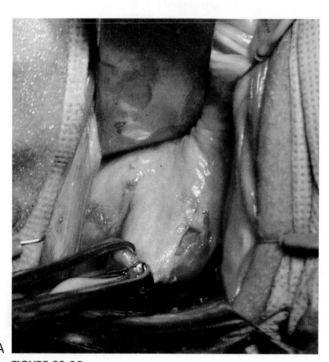

A

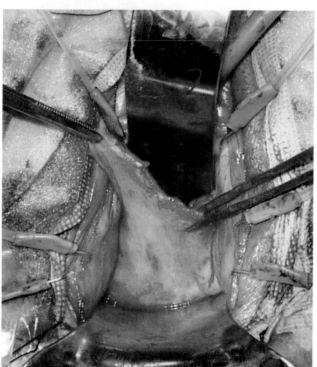

B

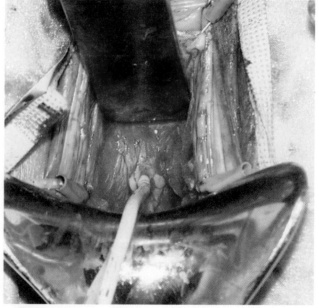

C

FIGURE 22-25
Repair of vesicovaginal fistula. **A**, Two flaps are created at the anterior and posterior sides of the fistula. The anterior flap is prepared, starting in a healthy area of tissue of the vaginal wall. **B**, The surgeon prepares the posterior flap by dissecting around the fistula for 2 to 4 cm. **C**, The fistula tract is isolated by further lateral dissection. (From Raz S: *Atlas of transvaginal surgery*, ed 2, Philadelphia, 2002, Saunders.)

1. The fistula is exposed.
2. The surgeon creates a tissue plane around the defect.
3. The surgeon incises the vaginal wall, exposing the deep layers of the rectum.
4. The plane is carried to the rectal outlet.
5. The fistula is completely excised and removed.
6. The levator muscle, mucosa defect, and vaginal wall are repaired.
7. A Foley catheter is inserted.

DISCUSSION

The patient is placed in high lithotomy position, prepped, and draped for perineal exposure. To begin the procedure, the surgeon places a weighted retractor in the vagina. He or she then inserts a malleable probe into the fistula. The assistant grasps the posterior wall of the vagina with Allis clamps to produce traction across the fistula. The surgeon then makes a circular incision around the fistula with the scalpel or dissecting scissors. Toothed tissue forceps are used to pick up the edge of the tissue as it is incised. Metzenbaum scissors are used to follow the tract and create a tissue plane between the tract and the deep tissue.

The vaginal wall is then grasped and incised with scissors, exposing the wall of the rectum. The surgeon circumscribes the fistula in the mucosa and removes the specimen. For a small fistula, a simple repair is made using a purse-string suture around the circular rectal opening. The surgeon reconstructs the perineal floor to restore strength to the muscles, using interrupted sutures of synthetic absorbable material or chromic gut. Sutures are placed until the defect is closed and the repair is secure. A Foley catheter is placed at the close of the procedure.

Episiotomy and Repair
SURGICAL GOAL

This is the surgical incision and repair of the wound (episiotomy) made between the vagina and anus to enlarge the vaginal opening during delivery.

PATHOLOGY

This procedure is intended to prevent vaginal tearing during delivery.

1. An incision is made from the vagina approximately 2 to 3 cm toward the anus.
2. Delivery occurs through the enlarged vaginal opening.
3. The incision is closed after delivery of the baby and placenta.

DISCUSSION

The obstetrician uses a local anesthetic, numbing the immediate area of the incision.

Just before the baby is delivered, the surgeon makes the incision to enlarge the vaginal opening, most often using curved Mayo scissors.

The episiotomy is closed with an absorbable suture, such as chromic gut.

Episiotomies usually heal without complications, and normal activities can be resumed shortly after birth.

Any pain and discomfort can be relieved with warm baths and medication.

Cervical Cerclage (Shirodkar's Procedure)
SURGICAL GOAL

In some obstetrical patients, spontaneous abortion occurs when the cervical musculature is unable to support the growing weight and pressure of the fetus. To prevent this outcome, a strip of synthetic material is embedded and sutured around the cervix just below the mucosa tissue. This prevents abortion.

PATHOLOGY

Stretching, loss of muscle tone, trauma, and radiation therapy to the cervix can result in an **incompetent cervix** (one that cannot bear the weight of the fetus).

1. The cervix is grasped with tissue forceps or a single-toothed tenaculum.
2. The surgeon incises the anterior cervix with the knife or Mayo scissors.
3. A mucosa flap is raised circumferentially around the cervix.
4. A synthetic tape is passed around the internal os.
5. The mucosa is closed.

DISCUSSION

The patient is prepped and draped for a vaginal procedure. The surgeon places a weighted speculum in the vagina. The surgeon then grasps the anterior lip of the cervix with a single-toothed tenaculum.

An incision is made with a #10 or #15 scalpel around the circumference of the cervix. This creates a plane between the mucosa and the underlying musculofascial layer of the cervix. A number 5-mm synthetic cerclage tape is passed around the internal os. The tape is not sutured to the tissue. The mucosa incision is closed with absorbable sutures, size 0 or 2-0.

Repair of Cystocele and Rectocele (Anterior-Posterior Repair)
SURGICAL GOAL

Vaginal hernia results when the support structures of the bladder and rectum allow these structures to bulge into the vagina, causing discomfort, stress incontinence, and cystitis. The patient also experiences difficulty voiding and defecating. The surgical goal is to strengthen the supportive tissues through vaginal exposure. If the defect is very severe, hysterectomy may be performed when the patient no longer plans childbearing. A more conservative treatment, trans-vaginal repair of the cystocele and rectocele, is presented here.

PATHOLOGY

Cystocele (herniation of the bladder) and **rectocele** (hernia-tion of the rectum) occur because musculature and connec-tive tissues that support the uterus are relaxed. This relax-ation occurs after multiple childbirths or after menopause. The pelvic floor or diaphragm provides support to the intes-tinal and genitourinary structures, especially during preg-nancy when gravity pulls the fetus downward and stretches the ligaments and muscles. As the pelvic floor becomes weakened, the bladder and rectum bulge into the vaginal canal. Actual herniation of the intestine into the vagina (called an enterocele) can be congenital or caused by birth trauma. Repair and reconstruction of the supportive struc-ture restores normal function and relieves discomfort and pain.

Technique

1. The anterior vaginal mucosa is incised.
2. The surgeon grasps the incision edges with Allis clamps.
3. A surgeon creates a tissue plane by blunt and sharp dissec-tion between the vaginal mucosa and the supportive con-nective tissue lying just underneath.
4. The dissection is continued to the bladder neck.
5. The vaginal wall is reconstructed with sutures.
6. The posterior vaginal wall is incised, and steps 2 and 3 are repeated.
7. The tissue plane is continued to the rectum.
8. Sutures are placed across the rectal musculature to recon-struct the pelvic floor.
9. The vaginal mucosa is sutured closed.

DISCUSSION

Anterior Repair

The patient is placed in lithotomy position, prepped, and draped for a vaginal procedure. Before the procedure begins, the circulator inserts a straight catheter into the bladder to drain it. The surgeon inserts a weighted speculum into the vaginal outlet. The surgeon then grasps the cervix with a tenaculum and places forward traction on it. Using the scalpel or curved Mayo scissors, the surgeon makes an inci-sion in the anterior vaginal wall. The edges of the incision are grasped with several Allis clamps, and the assistant fans out the clamps to spread the tissue edges (Figure 22-26).

The tissue plane between the vaginal mucosa and con-nective tissue beneath is now spread. Most surgeons wrap a Raytec sponge over their index finger and push the connec-tive tissue off the mucosa. This technique of blunt dissection effectively separates the tissue and creates a flap (the vaginal mucosa) with a minimum of bleeding and trauma to the tis-sue. The technologist should have ample sponges available. As the sponge becomes moist, its surface becomes smooth, and the sponge is less effective for dissection. The curved

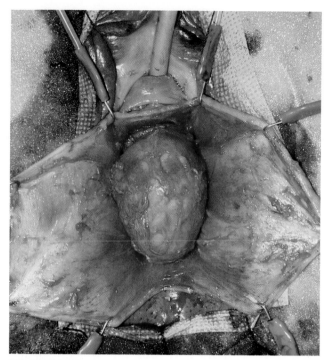

FIGURE 22-26
Anterior repair of cystocele: the vaginal wall is dissected free to expose the bladder and urethra. (From Raz S: *Atlas of transvaginal surgery*, ed 2, Philadelphia, 2002, Saunders.)

Mayo scissors are used alternately with sponges to continue the dissection to the level of the bladder.

During this portion of the procedure, the assistant or scrub may be required to retract the superior vaginal vault upward with a lateral (Heaney) right-angle retractor. This el-evates the roof of the vagina and effectively exposes the dis-section plane.

When retracting the superior vaginal wall, one must *not* toe the retractor upward. This can puncture the vaginal wall or cause bruising and formation of hematoma. Instead, one should lift up the blade of the retractor evenly to exert even pressure.

When the dissection has reached the bladder neck, several sutures of size 0 chromic gut or synthetic absorbable sutures are placed through the fascia and pulled laterally. This tight-ens the tissue and prevents the bladder from bulging. The edge of the vaginal mucosa is measured over the repair, and the edges are trimmed. The mucosa is then approximated with running or interrupted sutures of absorbable material, usually of the same size as that used on the bladder repair.

Posterior Repair

To begin the posterior repair, the surgeon places two Allis clamps in the posterior vaginal wall and makes a small transverse incision between them. The assistant provides traction on the clamp as described in the anterior repair. The techniques used in anterior repair are repeated to the level of the rectum. The levator muscles and fascia then are brought together and tightened with absorbable interrupted sutures, and the vaginal mucosa is repaired. A self-retaining catheter may be inserted after the procedure.

Vulvectomy
SURGICAL GOAL
Surgical excision of the labia, clitoris, and inguinal and pelvic lymph nodes is performed to treat cancer of the vulva.

PATHOLOGY
Cancer of the vulva represents about 5% of all genitourinary carcinomas. It is more common among women over the age of 60. Most invasive carcinoma that involves the lymph nodes is seen in this age group. Local vulvar cancer (vulvar intraepithelial neoplasm) appears to be associated with some strains of human papilloma virus (HPV), which is sexually transmitted.

Technique   INVASIVE CARCINOMA

1. The surgeon makes a wide incision around the vulva, extending laterally to include the labia majora.
2. A second incision is made on the interior edge of the first.
3. The incision is carried to subcutaneous and connective tissue.
4. The tissue specimen is retracted with Kocher and Allis clamps.
5. Hemorrhage is controlled with the ESU and suture ties.
6. The specimen is removed in one piece (**en bloc**).
7. An incision is made in the posterior vaginal wall.
8. The levator muscles are sutured.
9. Bilateral groin incisions are made.
10. Lymph nodes are removed.
11. Suction drains are placed.
12. All incisions are closed. A skin graft is placed as needed.
13. A Foley catheter is inserted into the urethra.

DISCUSSION
Vulvectomy may be performed as a simple or radical procedure. During simple vulvectomy, only the lesion itself and a small margin surrounding it are removed. The specimen is examined for clear margins, and no further surgery is indicated unless there is extensive involvement. Radical vulvectomy (described below) is a complex procedure involving groin exploration, lymph-node removal, and wide resection of the lesion and adjacent tissue.

The patient is placed in lithotomy position, prepped, and draped for lower abdominal and perineal incisions. Instruments and equipment used in the perineal portion of the procedure are kept separate from those of the groin procedure. Two set-ups may be created to isolate the perineal equipment. Gloves and gowns are changed for the groin procedure, according to the surgeon's directions.

The surgeon begins the procedure by making a large elliptical incision around the vulva (Figure 22-27, *A*). The incision encompasses the labia minora, labia majora, and clitoris. A second incision is made superior to the urethral orifice and encompasses the vagina. The surgeon grasps the skin edges of the incision with Allis clamps and carries dissection through the subcutaneous and connective tissues of the vulva. The assistant provides traction on the tissue edges while the surgeon incises and coagulates the tissue, creating a block of tissue that will be removed.

Large bleeding vessels are clamped with small hemostats and ligated with fine absorbable sutures or coagulated with the ESU. The vulva is removed en bloc when the dissection and mobilization are complete. The specimen is isolated from the set-up that will be used on the groin dissection.

The assistant next inserts a right-angle retractor into the superior portion of the vagina. A Heaney lateral retractor is

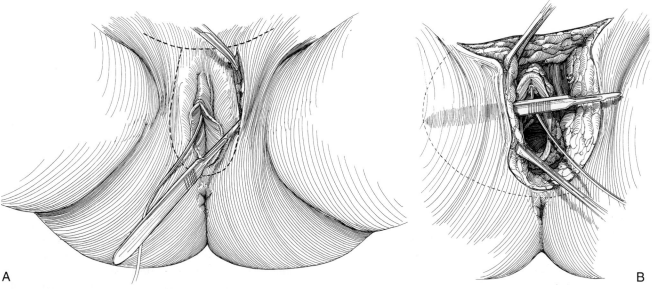

FIGURE 22-27
Vulvectomy. **A**, Incision is made in the vulvular organs. **B**, The suprapubic incision is lengthened for the groin dissection, and skin flaps are mobilized. (From Economou SG and Economou TS: *Atlas of surgical technique,* ed 2, Philadelphia, 1996, Saunders.)

typically used. The surgeon then incises the posterior vaginal mucosa and uses interrupted sutures of absorbable material, size 0 or 2-0, to strengthen the connective tissues of the posterior pelvic floor. The mucosal incisions are closed with size 2-0 or 0 absorbable sutures. If the excision is narrow, the skin edges may be directly closed. Several subcutaneous sutures may be needed to prevent an open pocket between the tissue layers. The skin is closed with interrupted monofilament synthetic sutures.

The groin excision is carried out through bilateral inguinal incisions (Figure 22-27, *B*). After incising the skin, the surgeon extends the incision to the inguinal chain. Exposure to these lymph nodes follows a dissection similar to that of inguinal hernia. Lymph nodes are located within the connective tissue. The surgeon removes the nodes individually using sharp dissection and controls bleeding with the ESU and suture ties of absorbable material. The wounds are closed in layers as in inguinal surgery.

Vaginoplasty
SURGICAL GOAL
This surgical technique repairs a surgical or congenital defect of the vagina.

PATHOLOGY
The procedure is performed to repair a congenital or surgical defect.

Technique
1. The patient is placed supine with legs in stirrups for exposure. An abdominal and vaginal prep is required.
2. The surgeon selects the type of reconstruction to be performed.
3. A skin graft is obtained and applied to a mold.
4. A simple incision and mold are used.
5. The bladder is catheterized.
6. A peripad is applied for dressing.

DISCUSSION
The abdomen is prepped if a skin graft will be used to form the new vaginal space. After the graft is taken, the site is dressed with nonadherent gauze and a pressure dressing. The skin graft itself is placed in a moist gauze and set aside.

A vaginal orifice is made with sharp dissection. Extreme care is taken to avoid damaging the bladder or rectum.

A mold is then used to form the cavity, either with the donor skin placed over the mold and sutured into place, or with just the mold in place, holding the dissected area open and allowing for spontaneous epithelialization.

Vaginal Hysterectomy
SURGICAL GOAL
In this procedure, the uterus is removed through a vaginal incision.

PATHOLOGY
Refer to the section, Abdominal Hysterectomy (Open).

Technique
1. The surgeon makes a circumferential incision at the base of the cervix.
2. The surgeon partially mobilizes the uterus by sequentially incising and ligating the uterine ligaments.
3. The peritoneal reflection of the bladder (bladder flap) is dissected from the uterus.
4. The uterus is completely mobilized and removed.
5. The bladder flap is reconstructed.
6. The peritoneum is closed.
7. The deep vaginal incision is closed.

DISCUSSION
A major portion of the vaginal hysterectomy procedure is the serial clamping, division, and ligation of ligaments and vessels of the uterus. The surgeon may use Heaney, Heaney-Ballentine, or Masterson forceps to secure the uterine segments before dividing them from the uterus. The uterine arteries are contained in many of these segments. Each segment therefore is ligated with heavy suture material or a suture ligature is used to ensure that the ligatures do not slip off postoperatively.

The open procedure begins with the patient placed in lithotomy position, prepped, and draped for a vaginal procedure. The bladder is drained with a straight catheter during the prep. A pocket drape should be attached to the perineal drape.

The surgeon grasps the cervix with a heavy uterine tenaculum (Figure 22-28, *A*). Using the scalpel or curved Mayo scissors, the surgeon makes a circumferential incision around the cervix, separating the vaginal mucosa and fascia from the body of the cervix (Figure 22-28, *B*). This incision exposes the first set of ligaments, which are double-clamped, divided, and ligated with suture ligatures of size 0 synthetic absorbable material on a tapered needle (Figure 22-28, *C*).

The surgeon picks up the posterior peritoneum with toothed tissue forceps and incises it with the scalpel or scissors. With the peritoneal cavity open, the surgeon detaches the peritoneal attachment to the bladder from the uterus with Metzenbaum scissors. The assistant retracts the bladder upward with a Sims or Heaney retractor. The scrub must have long tissue forceps and long dissecting scissors available as the mobilization is carried deep into the pelvis.

Mobilization of the uterus continues until the uterus is completely free. The uterus then is removed and delivered to the scrub as a specimen. The specimen must be retained in a basin.

Before closing the peritoneum, the surgeon reperitonealizes the bladder (closes the bladder flap) with a running suture of size 2-0 synthetic material on a small curved needle. The peritoneum is then closed with a running absorbable suture. The wound is dressed with a perineal pad.

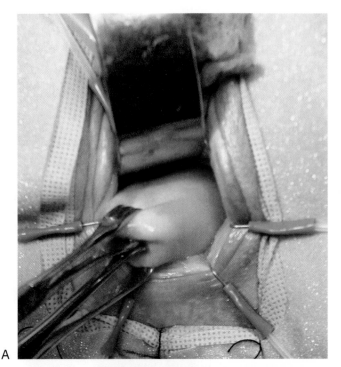

A

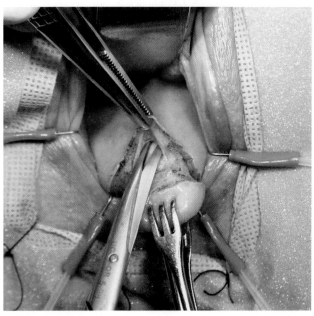

B

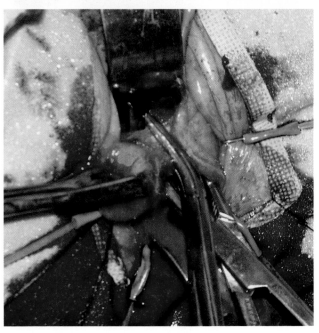

C

FIGURE 22-28
Vaginal hysterectomy. **A**, The cervix is grasped with a tenaculum, and mobility of the uterus is assessed. **B**, Dissection creates a plane between the anterior cervix and posterior bladder wall. **C**, The cardinal and sacrouterine ligaments are clamped and tied. (From Raz S: *Atlas of transvaginal surgery*, ed 2, Philadelphia, 2002, Saunders.)

Laparoscopic Assisted Vaginal Hysterectomy (LAVH)

SURGICAL GOAL

This procedure is the surgical removal of the uterus via a laparoscopic approach rather than a full abdominal approach.

PATHOLOGY

The scope is used to determine whether any disease is present. LAVH can be used for such conditions as postmeno-

pausal bleeding, pelvic pain, absence of genital prolapse, salpingitis or endometriosis, and endometrial cancer.

Technique

1. The patient is placed in a low lithotomy position.
2. The patient's abdomen is opened and explored as in a diagnostic laparoscopy.
3. Other trocars and sheaths are used for accessory instrumentation, such as laparoscopic scissors.

4. During the laparoscopic portion of the procedure, the following steps may be performed:
   ▶ Hydrodissection of the broad ligament
   ▶ Use of the bipolar ESU to desiccate the round and infundibulopelvic ligaments
   ▶ Dissection of the broad ligaments
   ▶ Mobilization of the bladder from the lower uterine segment
   ▶ Use of either endoscopic scissors or a monopolar electrode to open the vaginal vault
5. The surgeon next moves to the vaginal approach.
6. The remainder of a vaginal hysterectomy is performed and the uterus is delivered.
7. The vaginal vault is closed.
8. A final visual inspection is performed in the abdomen through the scope, and the sheaths are removed.
9. The abdominal wounds are either stapled or closed subcuticularly.
10. A perineal pad is placed, and Band-Aids are placed on abdominal wounds.

DISCUSSION

A vaginal hysterectomy set-up and laparoscopic gear are required for this procedure. The patient does not undergo the long abdominal incision with this procedure. The hospital stay and recovery time also are shorter when LAVH is performed.

REFERENCES

Baggish MS, Barbot J, and Valle RF: *Diagnostic and operative hysteroscopy, a text and atlas,* ed 2, St Louis, 1999, Mosby.

Economou SG and Economou TS: *Atlas of surgical technique,* ed 2, Philadelphia, 1996, Saunders.

Gershenson DM, et al: *Operative gynecology,* ed 2, Philadelphia, 2001, Saunders.

Goldberg JM and Falcone T: *Atlas of endoscopic techniques in gynecology,* Philadelphia, 2001, Saunders.

Hunt RB: *Text and atlas of female infertility surgery,* ed 3, St Louis, 1999, Mosby.

Moody FG: *Atlas of ambulatory surgery,* St Louis, 1999, Mosby.

Murray SS, McKinney ES, and Gorrie TM: *Foundations of maternal-newborn nursing,* ed 3, Philadelphia, 2002, Saunders.

Raz S: *Atlas of transvaginal surgery,* ed 2, Philadelphia, 2002, Saunders.

Chapter 23

Genitourinary Surgery

Terminology

BPH—Benign prostatic hypertrophy; a condition in which the prostate gland enlarges and impinges on the urethra.

Calculi—Abnormal stones in body tissues resulting from the precipitation of minerals, such as calcium, and other substances.

Circumcision—Removal of all or part of the prepuce (foreskin) of the penis.

Epispadias—Congenital abnormality in which the opening of the urethra is on the dorsum of the penis.

ESWL—Extracorporeal shockwave lithotripsy; a procedure in which ultrasonic sound waves are used to pulverize kidney or gall bladder stones.

Hematuria—Condition of blood in the urine.

Hypospadias—Abnormal congenital condition in which the urethra opens infe-

rior to its normal location. Normally seen in males, where the urethra opens on the undersurface of the penis.

Hypothermia—Condition of abnormally low body temperature.

Lithotripsy—A procedure in which stones are crushed within a body cavity such as the bladder.

Nonelectrolytic—Nonconductive; nonelectrolytic solutions must be used for bladder distension or continuous irrigation whenever the electrosurgical unit (ESU) is used.

Resectoscope—An instrument that removes tissue by cutting and coagulating small slices.

Retrograde pyelography—X-ray or fluoroscopic studies of the renal pelvis using contrast media; "pyel" refers to renal pelvis.

Stent—A supportive catheter placed in a duct or tube.

Tamponade—An instrument or other means of placing pressure on tissue.

Torsion—Twisting of an organ or structure that may cause local ischemia and necrosis.

Transurethral—Describes a procedure in which access is gained through the urethral opening. The term also may describe an instrument that enters the bladder through the urethral meatus.

TURBT—Transurethral resection of a bladder tumor.

TURP—Transurethral resection of the prostate.

UTI—Urinary tract infection.

INTRODUCTION TO GENITOURINARY SURGERY

Genitourinary (GU) surgery encompasses surgery of the internal GU system, including the kidney, adrenal gland, bladder, prostate, urethra, and accessory structures of these organs. The external system includes the male genitalia—the testicles, their internal structures, and penis. Procedures of the female external genitalia are described in the previous chapter.

There are three basic approaches to the GU system:

▶ **Transurethral** (instruments are passed through the urethra)
▶ **Laparoscopic** (through the surgical laparoscope, as discussed in Chapter 17)
▶ **Open** transabdominal (through an abdominal, flank, or combination thoracoabdominal incision)

Urinary procedures are classified as *open* or *closed*. In an open procedure, the focal point of the surgery is exposed through an incision, while closed procedures are performed through cystoscopy (direct visualization of structures by means of the fiberoptic cystoscope inserted into the urethra and bladder). The patient is placed in the lateral position for operations involving the kidney and ureter. The supine position is preferred for procedures of the bladder and reproductive structures. Closed procedures are performed with the patient in the lithotomy position. Procedures of the urinary system are performed via closed technique more often than open technique.

ANATOMY OF THE GENITOURINARY SYSTEM

Kidney

The kidneys are paired organs that lie behind the parietal peritoneum at the level of the twelfth thoracic vertebra and third lumbar vertebra. Each kidney weighs approximately 150 grams and is about 11 cm long in the adult. Each kidney is covered by three separate tissue layers that protect it from injury and help hold it in place. The outer layer, the *renal fascia,* anchors the kidney. The next layer, called the *perirenal fat,* is an adipose layer that surrounds the kidney and helps to protect it from injury. The innermost layer, or true *capsule* (sometimes called *Gerota's capsule*), is a smooth, fibrous tissue that adheres closely to the body of the kidney.

The *hilum* is the notched area of the kidney located on the medial side. The renal artery, vein, and ureter emerge from the hilum. An enlarged portion of the ureter called the *renal pelvis* joins the kidney in this location. It branches into sections called renal *calyces.*

The inner structure of the kidney consists of several tissue layers within which lies the complex filtering system that rids the blood of impurities (Figure 23-1). The outer layer is called the *cortex.*

The medulla is composed of 8 to 12 large collecting areas called the *renal pyramids.* Each pyramidal apex faces the renal pelvis. The wide part of the wedge interfaces with the cortex. The pyramids extend out away from the renal pelvis

FIGURE 23-1
Inner structure of the kidney. (Modified from Herlihy B and Maebius NK: *The human body in health and illness,* ed 2, Philadelphia, 2003, Saunders.)

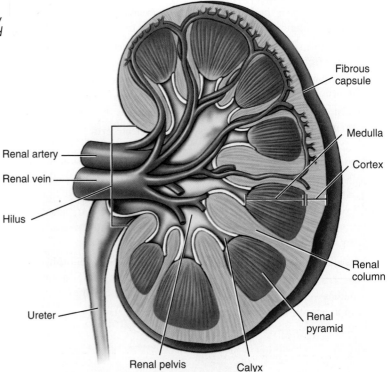

and the area where the ureter joins the kidney. The cavities of the kidney into which the pyramids converge are called the *calyces* (singular, *calyx*). The microscopic filtering system of the kidney lies within the cortex and the medulla. This system is composed of many single units called *nephrons* (Figure 23-2). Urine drains from the renal calyces into the renal pelvis.

Adrenal Glands

The adrenal glands are paired organs that lie on the medial side of the upper kidney, posterior to the stomach and pancreas. The gland has two layers: the outer cortex and the inner medulla. The adrenal glands secrete both steroids and hormones necessary for body function. The blood supply of each gland is supplied by the aorta and branches of the renal and inferior phrenic arteries. The adrenal gland is important in the production of norepinephrine and epinephrine, which act to stimulate or slow the heart rate, the activities of the gastrointestinal system, and certain portions of the respiratory system.

Ureter

The *ureter* emerges from the renal pelvis, where filtered urine is shunted away from the kidney and out of the body. The ureter is continuous with the renal pelvis. The *renal pelvis* is the proximal collection area for filtered urine from the kidney. The ureters lead directly to the urinary bladder, which lies below. Each ureter is about 30 cm long and about 5 mm in diameter. Because of its small diameter, the ureter is often a site of lodged kidney stones. The ureter is a three-layered tubular structure, including an outer fibrous layer, a middle muscular layer, and an inner epithelial mucosa layer.

From the renal pelvis, the ureter extends past the sacroiliac joint (called the ureteropelvic junction) and curves to the base of the bladder. It enters the bladder at the trigone muscle at the ureterovesical junction. Dense connective tissue is found at the ureterovesical junction. The ureterovesical valve lies at the distal end of the ureter, where the lumen of the ureter opens into the bladder. Urine is moved down the ureter by the peristaltic action of the muscular layer. Distension of the renal pelvis with urine causes a muscle contraction, which causes a peristaltic response by the middle muscular layer.

Urinary Bladder

The urinary bladder lies behind the symphysis pubis in the pelvic cavity (Figure 23-3). In the female, this hollow organ is separated from the rectum by the vagina and uterus. In the male, the seminal vesicles separate the bladder from the rectum. The prostate gland in the male surrounds the bladder neck and urethra.

The wall of the bladder is composed of four tissue layers: the outer serosa, the muscular layer, the submucosa, and the inner mucosa. The bladder is attached loosely to the peritoneal wall by the *urachus*. The base or neck of the bladder (the lowest portion) is called the *trigone*. This triangular region has both superficial and deep muscle layers. The superficial layer extends into the bladder neck of the female and into the proximal portion of the urethra in the male. The trigone has three corners that correspond with the two *ureteral* openings and one *urethral* opening. The detrusor muscles of the bladder wall extend into the neck of the bladder and form the internal sphincter, which communicates with the urethra.

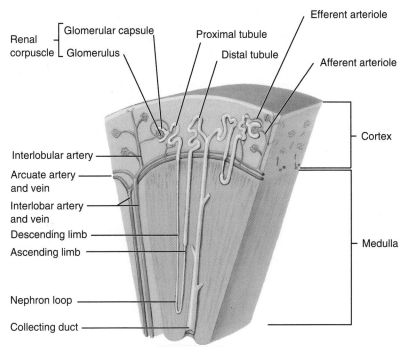

FIGURE 23-2
Nephron. (Modified from Applegate EJ: *The anatomy and physiology learning system,* ed 2, Philadelphia, 2000, Saunders.)

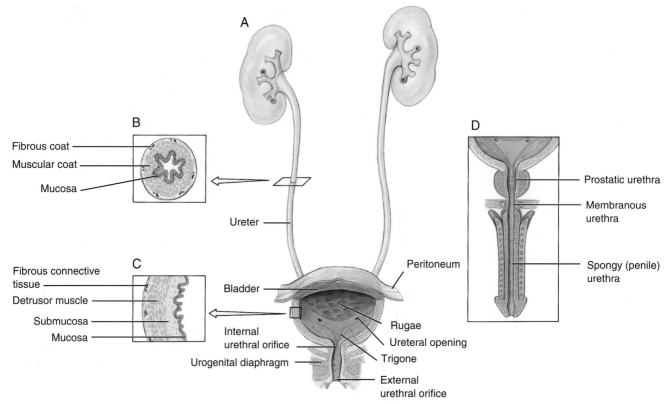

A

B

Fibrous coat

Muscular coat

Mucosa

Ureter

C

Fibrous connective
tissue

Detrusor muscle

Submucosa

Mucosa

Bladder

Internal
urethral orifice

Urogenital diaphragm

D

Prostatic urethra

Membranous
urethra

Spongy (penile)
urethra

Peritoneum

Rugae

Ureteral opening

Trigone

External
urethral orifice

FIGURE 23-3
Ureter, urinary bladder, and urethra. **A,** Urinary tract. **B,** Cross-section through the ureter. **C,** Cross-section of the bladder wall.
D, Regions of the male urethra. (Modified from Applegate EJ: *The anatomy and physiology learning system,* ed 2, Philadelphia,
2000, Saunders.)

The urinary bladder functions as a reservoir for urine. Urination empties the bladder. This process is controlled by the muscular fibers and sphincters, under the influence of the autonomic nervous system. Urination is accomplished by a complex series of nervous impulses that are finally transmitted to the trigonal area, where a sphincter contracts or relaxes to allow the retention or release of urine.

Urethra

As previously mentioned, the urethra emerges from the bladder at the trigone. The female urethra is quite short, while the male homologue is considerably longer. Its function is to convey urine from the urinary bladder to the outside of the body.

FEMALE

In the female, the urethra is 3 to 5 mm long and 6 to 8 mm in diameter and follows a direct course from the bladder to the external meatus, or urethral opening. It is located on the posterior side of the symphysis pubis and passes in front of the vagina. The proximal urethra is composed primarily of smooth muscle tissue. The middle third contains skeletal muscle. The distal portion attaches to the vagina.

The distal urethra contains the Skene's glands, which produce mucus. These are located on each side of the urethra just inside the opening or *meatus.* The periurethral muscles

on the pelvic floor support the distal urethra and aid in sphincter control.

MALE

The male urethra is approximately 25 to 30 cm long. The diameter varies from 7 to 10 mm. It exits the bladder at the proximal end of the bladder and extends to the end of the penis at the meatus. The male urethra is divided into several distinct parts. The *prostatic* urethra is the most proximal (uppermost) portion and is approximately 3 cm long. The *prostatic* urethra begins at the bladder neck and is followed by the *membranous* urethra, which is the shortest portion and is approximately 2 cm long. The *cavernous* urethra, or penile portion, is approximately 15 cm long and lies within the spongiosum layer of the penis.

External Reproductive Organs of the Male
TESTES AND SCROTUM

The *scrotum* is a pouch that lies at the base of the penis. It is an extension of the abdominal wall that houses and protects the testicles—the male reproductive organs. The scrotum is divided into two subpouches by a septum, with one testicle resting in each pouch. The wall of the scrotum contains a subcutaneous tissue of smooth muscle fibers called the *dartos layer.* When the ambient temperature is unsuitable for maximum sperm protection, the dartos layer causes the scrotum to tighten and pull upward (in the case of a cold ambient temperature) or to relax and hang farther away from the body (in the case of a warm ambient temperature).

Each testicle is suspended in the scrotum by the *epididymis*. The epididymis is a convoluted duct that secretes seminal fluid and is the medium that gives sperm the mobility to travel along the reproductive tract of the male. The testicle also serves as the housing for the production of sperm. Each testicle manufactures testosterone, the male hormone, and contains the *seminiferous tubules*, which are the site of sperm production.

PENIS

The penis, or male copulatory organ, is a highly vascular structure that is flaccid except during sexual stimulation, when it becomes engorged with blood and becomes rigid. It lies just in front of the scrotum and is suspended at the pubic arch by fascial tissue. The penis is composed of several columns of tissue. Two dorsal columns, called the *corpora cavernosa*, are composed of spongy vascular tissue that makes up the greatest portion of the organ. The two columns are separated by a septum but are bound together by a fibrous sheath. A third tissue column that runs ventrally is the *corpus spongiosum*. Within this section lies the penile portion of the urethra. A slightly enlarged distal end of the corpus spongiosum forms the *glans penis*, which is normally covered by a skin fold called the *prepuce*, or *foreskin*. At the tip of the glans penis lies the *urethral orifice*.

Figure 23-4 illustrates the external and internal reproductive organs of the male.

Internal Reproductive Glands of the Male

The internal reproductive organs of the male (see Figure 23-4) include the prostate, bulbourethral glands, vas deferens, seminal vesicles, and ejaculatory duct.

PROSTATE GLAND

The prostate gland is a musculoglandular structure approximately the size of a chestnut. It is conical and lies with its base in close proximity to the bladder. The prostate surrounds the prostatic portion of the urethra and secretes an alkaline fluid needed to nourish and give mobility to the sperm. The gland is divided into six main lobes: anterior, posterior, middle, subcervical, right lateral, and left lateral. The gland is covered by a fibrous tissue called the *capsule*. Behind the prostatic capsule lies a sheath called the *true prostatic capsule*, which separates the gland and seminal vesicles from the rectum.

BULBOURETHRAL GLANDS

The bulbourethral glands (also called Cowper's glands) are paired structures that lie just below the prostate. They are about the size of a pea and rest on each side of the urethra. These glands secrete mucus, a portion of the fluid that makes up semen.

VAS DEFERENS

The vas deferens, also called the ductus deferens or seminal duct, is a portion of the path that the seminal fluid travels. It is a continuation of the epididymis and begins along the back or posterior edge of a testicle, traverses the inguinal canal, and enters the abdomen. As the vas deferens enters the abdomen through the *inguinal canal* and *internal ring*, it is encompassed by the *spermatic cord*. This cord contains not only the vas deferens but also blood vessels and lymphatics. The vas deferens continues across the bladder and ureter, where it meets the opening of the *seminal vesicle* and forms the *ejaculatory duct*.

EJACULATORY DUCT

As previously discussed, the ejaculatory duct is formed by the joining of the vas deferens and the seminal vesicle's duct or lower end. The ejaculatory duct travels through the base of the prostate gland, then enters the prostatic urethra.

EQUIPMENT

Genitourinary surgery is often daunting to the learner because of the many types and large amounts of equipment used. As with any specialty, a systematic study of the equipment (one step at a time) and thorough knowledge of the anatomy greatly improves the learning process.

Electrosurgical Unit

The ESU is used in both open and transurethral procedures. Review Chapter 17, which describes safety considerations for both the patient and team members.

Transurethral procedures that require an ESU during continuous irrigation are discussed below. This is a *critical discussion*. Extreme hazards are associated with the use of electrosurgical equipment in the presence of fluids. The scrub must understand these principles before assisting in any procedure.

Microscope

An operative microscope is used during fine reconstructive surgery, laser ablation, and vaporization of lesions. Sterile procedures require that the microscope be draped. Laser ablation of the external genitalia does not require a microscope drape. Use and care of the microscope are described in Chapter 24.

Laser

The Nd:YAG, CO_2, tunable dye, and argon lasers are typically used in GU surgery. Review surgical and safety precautions, including the use of a smoke-evacuation system (during surgery that does not require continuous irrigation), in Chapter 17. Certain aspects of laser use will be discussed in particular procedures in this chapter, but the reader should review all safety precautions.

Radiography

Radiography is an important component of GU surgery. Both x-ray and C-arm fluoroscopy are often used. The cys-

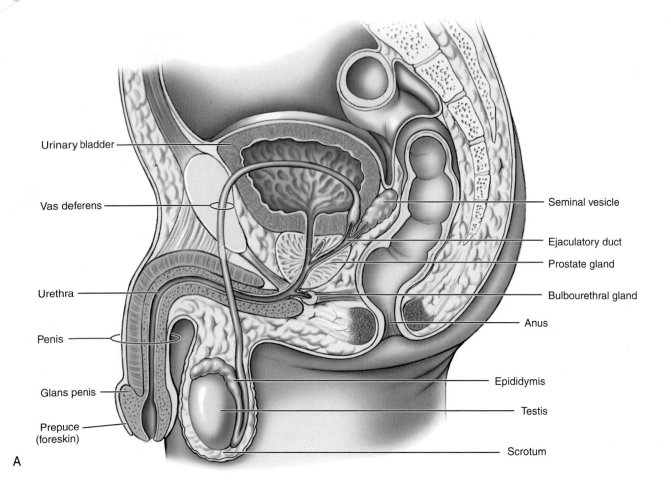

Urinary bladder

Vas deferens

Urethra

Penis

Glans penis

Prepuce
(foreskin)

Seminal vesicle

Ejaculatory duct

Prostate gland

Bulbourethral gland

Anus

Epididymis

Testis

Scrotum

A

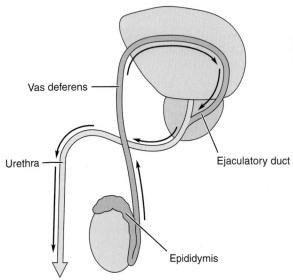

Vas deferens

Urethra

Ejaculatory duct

Epididymis

B

FIGURE 23-4
A, Male reproductive organs. **B,** The pathway for semen. (From Herlihy B and Maebius NK: *The human body in health and illness,* ed 2, Philadelphia, 2003, Saunders.)

toscopy table is specially constructed to accommodate the C-arm, and many operating rooms now have permanent x-ray capability in their GU cystoscopy room. Images taken before and during the procedure are included in the patient's medical record.

Video Camera

Digital video technology is available for all types of endoscopic GU surgery. Video assistance is typically used during laparoscopic, nephroscopic, and ureteroscopic surgery. Refer to Chapter 17 for a discussion of the video camera.

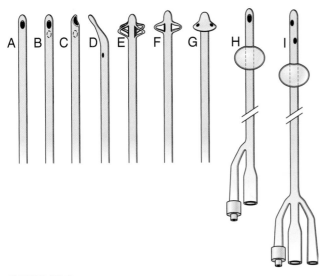

FIGURE 23-5
Urinary catheters. **A,** Conical-tip urethral catheter. **B,** Robinson urethral catheter. **C,** Whistle-tip urethral catheter. **D,** Coudé hollow olive-tip catheter. **E,** Malecot self-retaining, four-wing urethral catheter. **F,** Malecot self-retaining, two-wing catheter. **G,** Pezzer self-retaining drain, open-end head, used for cystotomy drainage. **H,** Foley-type balloon catheter. **I,** Foley-type, three-way balloon catheter. (Modified from Walsh PC, Retik AB, Vaughan ED, et al: *Campbell's urology,* ed 8, Philadelphia, 2002, Saunders.)

Suction Unit

Suction is available for all procedures. The scrub is responsible for checking suction pressure before each case.

Catheters

Urinary catheters are used for a variety of purposes, both in and out of surgery (Figure 23-5). These purposes include (1) short-term urinary drainage, (2) long-term urinary drainage, (3) hemostasis, (4) evacuation of blood clots or blood, (5) diagnosis, and (6) maintenance of continuity of the urethra. Most hospitals maintain a supply of sterile catheters packaged by the manufacturer and designed for one-time use only. A catheter is a hollow tube made of flexible synthetic material, such as latex rubber, Teflon-coated rubber, or plastic. A variety of ureteral and urethral catheters may be used during GU procedures.

The lumen or bore of the catheter is measured in "French" (abbreviated Fr) sizes ranging from 10 to 26 Fr. As the number of the catheter decreases, the diameter also decreases. The most common catheters are those that range in size from 16 to 18. Retention catheters also have a retention balloon size that is measured in cubic centimeters.

URETERAL CATHETERS

Assorted ureteral catheters are used for both open and closed procedures. General uses are:

▶ To provide a method of instilling contrast media into the ureter and kidney for retrograde pyelography x-ray studies.

▶ To provide immediate drainage of a ureter.
▶ To provide temporary drainage of the ureter after a procedure. In this case, the catheter may be left in place during healing. This type is called an indwelling catheter or **stent.** The catheter can be attached to a collection bag.
▶ To keep the ureter open to allow a stone to pass.
▶ To bypass a stone or tumor.
▶ To block the ureteral opening during x-ray studies.
▶ To identify a structure during open procedures.
▶ To obtain urine specimens or renal washings from a specific kidney.

Ureteral catheters have graduated marks so the surgeon can see how deeply the catheter is inserted.

The *indwelling pigtail* catheter is a stent, specifically a J-stent. This means that it maintains the form of the ureter and keeps it open to allow a stone or urine to pass through the ureter. It contains a wire, which aids in passing it through the narrow urethra (Figure 23-6, *A*). When the wire is removed, the distal end forms a J or slight spiral, which holds it in place. The distal end may be sutured to the patient's skin to allow for a noninvasive removal. This type of catheter is also used during ESWL (extracorporeal shockwave lithotripsy). After the stone has been pulverized, the stent allows it to drain from the ureter.

The *Braasch bulb* or *cone-tipped* catheter is used to occlude the ureteral orifice during dye studies, when contrast media is inserted during retrograde pyelography.

Other commonly used catheters are the whistle tip, round tip, spiral tip, and olive tip (Figure 23-6, *B*).

URETHRAL CATHETERS

The urethral catheter is a flexible latex or rubber tube. Two major types are the indwelling catheter, which contains a balloon or flange at the proximal tip, and the straight catheter, which is used for temporary bladder drainage.

The Foley catheter is available in a variety of types and balloon sizes. The three-way balloon catheter is used for intermittent or continuous bladder irrigation. Those with large, 30-ml balloons are used postoperatively as a **tamponade** (used to apply pressure against a tissue or orifice). This type is used after transurethral resection of the prostate (Figure 23-7).

The Foley catheter is the retention catheter used most often and has a variety of uses. The catheter is held in place in the bladder by means of an inflatable balloon located at the end of the catheter, which prevents it from sliding back out of the bladder. This type of catheter is available in sizes 8 through 30 Fr, and the retention balloon may be from 5 to 30 cc, depending on the specific use of the catheter. The smaller balloon is used for simple retention, while the larger retention balloon is used postoperatively to maintain hemostasis. The balloon should be tested before it is inserted to ensure its integrity. It is inflated with air or sterile water. The larger balloons may be inflated up to as much as 120 cc for greater hemostatic efficiency.

The Phillips catheter is straight but differs from the utility catheter in that one end has a screw tip designed to accept

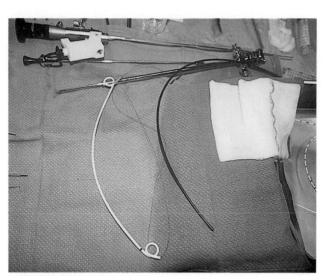

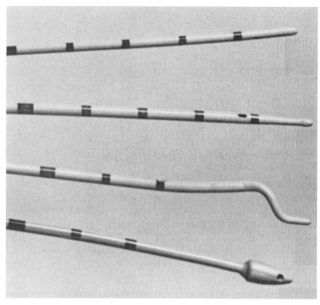

FIGURE 23-6
A, Ureteral stent with tether. **B,** Ureteral catheters, *from top to bottom:* round-tip, olive-tip, spiral-tip, and conical- or "bulb-" tip. (**A** from Nagle GM: *Genitourinary surgery: perioperative nursing series,* St Louis, 1997, Mosby; **B** from Walsh PC, Retik AB, Vaughan ED, et al: *Campbell's urology,* ed 8, Philadelphia, 2002, Saunders.)

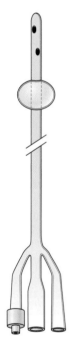

FIGURE 23-7
Foley three-way balloon catheter. (Modified from Walsh PC, Retik AB, Vaughan ED, et al: *Campbell's urology,* ed 8, Philadelphia, 2002, Saunders.)

a filiform (a small catheter used to locate a true passage through the urethra in case of stricture or the presence of a small passage). The filiform is of a much smaller diameter than the catheter and is easily manipulated in the urethra.

The Coudé catheter can be straight or may be a Foley retention type. This type of catheter has a firm rubber tip or beak usually used to facilitate its passage through a false urethral passage or past anatomic prominences in the urethra or in an enlarged prostate.

The Gibbon catheter is a long, thin catheter used mainly for long-term drainage of the bladder. A major disadvantage of the Gibbon catheter is that it has no device for self-retention and must be taped to the patient's thigh.

INSTRUMENTS

Instruments for open GU procedures are similar to those used for general surgery. Right-angled, Allis, and Babcock clamps are needed for most procedures. Special prostatic retractors, stone-grasping forceps, and kidney pedicle clamps also may be required.

Stainless-steel surgical instruments needed for GU procedures also may include plastic, general, thoracic, and special GU instruments. GU-specific instruments are shown in Figures 23-8 through Figure 23-11.

Because the approach to most urinary structures often crosses muscle tissue, which is highly vascular, the scrub should have an ample supply of lap sponges and hemostatic clamps available. Sponge dissectors and stick sponges are needed for nearly all of these procedures. Chromic gut and synthetic absorbable sutures (Dexon or Vicryl) are used when the surgeon is suturing in and around the tissues of the urinary tract, because nonabsorbable sutures can cause the formation of stones (calculi).

CYSTOSCOPIC PROCEDURES

Psychological Considerations

The lithotomy position, necessary for cystoscopic procedures, is embarrassing for most patients. However, operating room personnel help the patient by making the position as comfortable as possible. The patient's dignity should be protected, and the patient must not be exposed unless necessary.

Text continued on p. 564

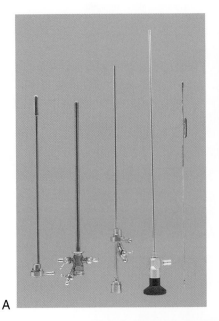

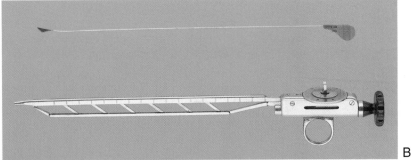

FIGURE 23-8
Urethroscope. **A,** *Left to right,* obturator; urethroscope sheath; telescope adapting bridge; telescope, 0 degree; urethrotome blade. **B,** *Top to bottom,* Otis urethrotome: blade, urethrotome. (From Tighe SM: *Instrumentation for the operating room,* ed 6, St Louis, 2003, Mosby.)

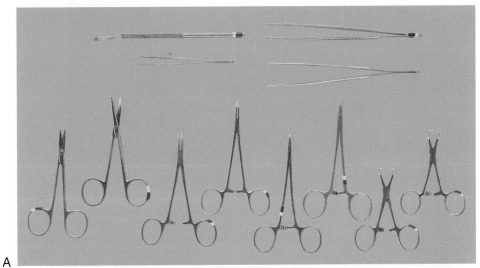

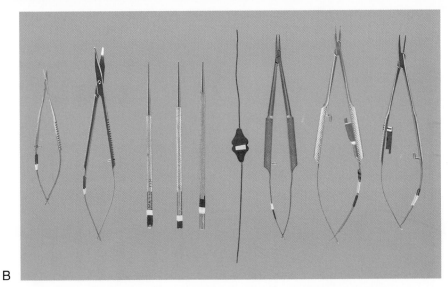

FIGURE 23-9
Vasectomy and vasovasotomy instruments. **A,** *Top to bottom, left to right,* Beaver knife handle, knurled, with tip; jeweler's forceps; two DeBakey vascular Atraugrip tissue forceps, short. *Bottom, left to right,* iris scissors, straight, sharp; Stevens tenotomy scissors; four Providence hemostatic forceps; two Backhaus towel forceps. **B,** *Left to right,* Vannas capsulotomy scissors; Westcott tenotomy scissors; two Henle probes, assorted sizes; lacrimal probe, 0-00; titanium microneedle holder, nonlocking; Barraquer needle holder, extra delicate, tapered, curved, with lock; Troutman tier needle holder with lock. (From Tighe SM: *Instrumentation for the operating room,* ed 6, St Louis, 2003, Mosby.)

Continued

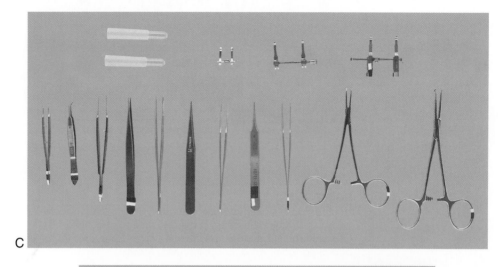

C

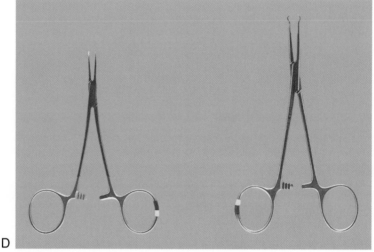

D

FIGURE 23-9, cont'd

Vasectomy and vasovasotomy instruments. **C,** *Top, left to right,* two chamber maintainers; Silber vasovasostomy clamp; two Strauch vasovasostomy approximators, hinged, small; vasovasostomy approximator, hinged, large. *Bottom, left to right,* two McPherson tying forceps, angled, front view and side view; Castroviejo suturing forceps, 0.12 mm, front view; three jeweler's forceps, no. 3, side view, front view, and side view; two jeweler's forceps, no. 4, front view and side view; jeweler's forceps, no. 5, front view; Snowden Pencer dissecting forceps; Snowden Pencer fixation forceps. **D,** *Left to right,* Snowden Pencer dissecting forceps; Snowden Pencer fixation forceps.

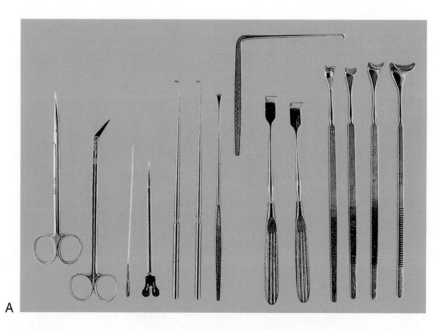

A

FIGURE 23-10

Nephrectomy and ureteroplasty instruments. **A,** *Left to right,* Lincoln Metzenbaum scissors, narrow dissecting tip; Potts-Smith cardiovascular scissors, 45-degree angle; probe dilator; grooved director; two Hoen nerve hooks; two Love nerve retractors, straight, front view, and 90-degree angle, side view; two Little retractors, medium; four Gil-Vernet retractors, assorted sizes.

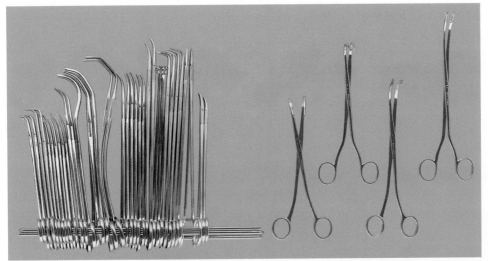

B

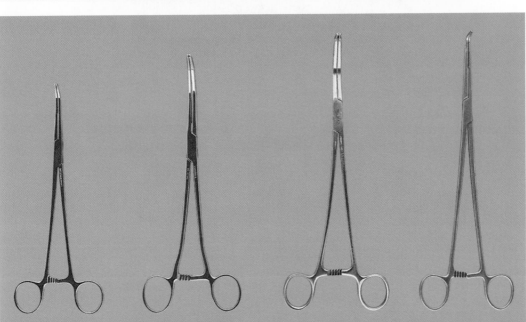

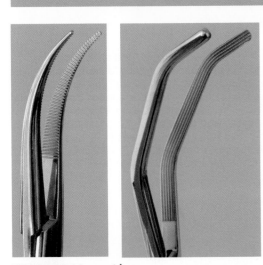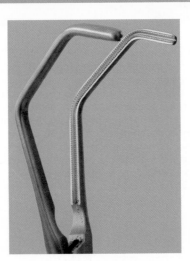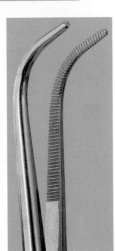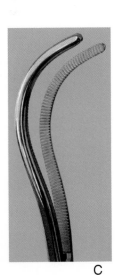

C

FIGURE 23-10, cont'd

Nephrectomy and ureteroplasty instruments. **B,** *Left to right,* four Westphal hemostatic forceps; six hemostatic tonsil forceps; two Adson hemostatic forceps, fine curved; Mayo (Guyon) kidney clamp; two Herrick kidney clamps; two Satinsky (vena cava) clamps; six hemostatic tonsil forceps, 9½ inch; two hemostatic tonsil forceps, 10½ inch; two Babcock tissue forceps, extra long; four Mixter hemostatic forceps, 10½ inch, fine tip; two Ayer needle holders, extra long; two Heaney needle holders, long; four Randall stone forceps: full curve, ¾ curve, ½ curve, and ¼ curve. **C,** *Top, left to right,* Adson hemostatic forceps, fine curve; Herrick kidney clamp; Satinsky (vena cava) clamp, medium, 4 cm, 9½ inch; Mixter hemostatic forceps, fine tip, 10½ inch. *Bottom,* tips of Adson hemostatic forceps, fine curve; Herrick kidney clamp; Satinsky (vena cava) clamp, medium, 4 cm, 9½ inch; Mixter hemostatic forceps, fine tip, 10½ inch; and Mayo (Guyon) vessel clamp, ½ inch. (From Tighe SM: *Instrumentation for the operating room,* ed 6, St Louis, 2003, Mosby.)

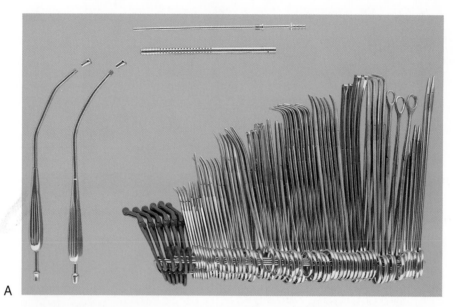

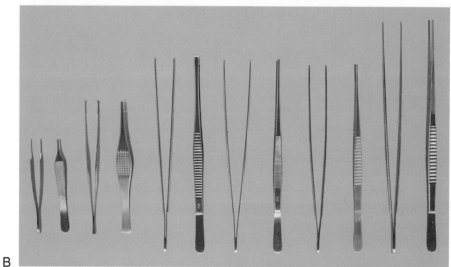

FIGURE 23-11
Radical prostatectomy set. **A,** *Top,* Poole abdominal suction tube and shield. *Left to right,* two Yankauer suction tubes and tips; six paper drape clips; four Halsted mosquito hemostatic forceps, curved; four Halsted mosquito hemostatic forceps, straight; Halsted hemostatic forceps; six Crile hemostatic forceps, 6½ inch; four hemostatic tonsil forceps; two Mayo-Péan hemostatic forceps, curved; two Allis tissue forceps, medium; Babcock tissue forceps, medium; four Ochsner hemostatic forceps, straight, long jaw; six Mixter hemostatic forceps, 9 inch; six hemostatic tonsil forceps, long; four Allis tissue forceps, extra long, curved; four Mixter hemostatic forceps, extra long; three Foerster sponge forceps; two Crile-Wood needle holders, 7 inch; two Crile-Wood needle holders, 8 inch; two Mayo-Hegar needle holders, 12 inch. **B,** *Left to right,* two Adson tissue forceps (1 × 2), front, side view; two Ferris-Smith tissue forceps (1 × 2), front, side view; two Russian tissue forceps, front, side view; two thumb tissue forceps with teeth (1 x 2), long, front, side view; two DeBakey vascular Atraugrip tissue forceps, long, front, side view; two DeBakey vascular Atraugrip tissue forceps, extra long, front, side view.

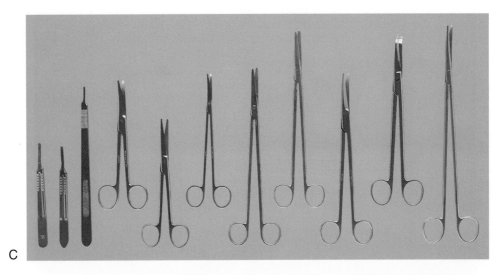

C

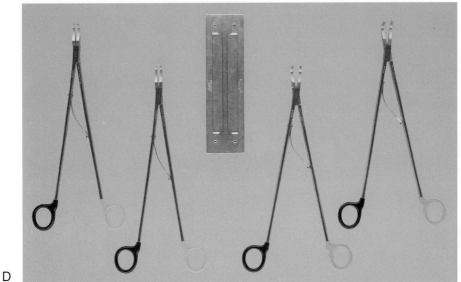

D

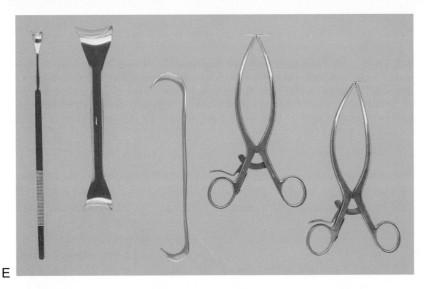

E

FIGURE 23-11, cont'd
Radical prostatectomy set. **C,** *Left to right,* two Bard-Parker knife handles, no. 4; Bard-Parker knife handle, no. 3, long; two Mayo dissecting scissors, curved and straight; two Metzenbaum dissecting scissors, 7 inch and extra long; two Snowden Pencer scissors, straight and curved; Jorgenson dissecting scissors; Mayo dissecting scissors, long, curved. **D,** *Left to right,* two Samuels hemoclip-applying forceps, medium; hemoclip cartridge base for hemoclips; two Samuels hemoclip-applying forceps, large. **E,** *Left to right,* Gil-Vernet retractor; two Goelet retractors, front view and side view; two Gelpi retractors.

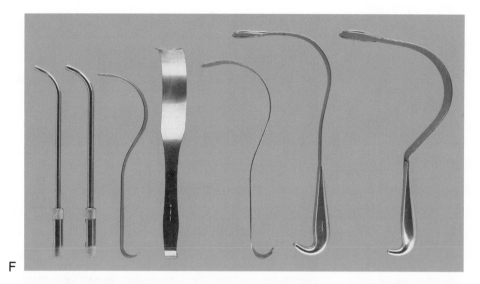

F

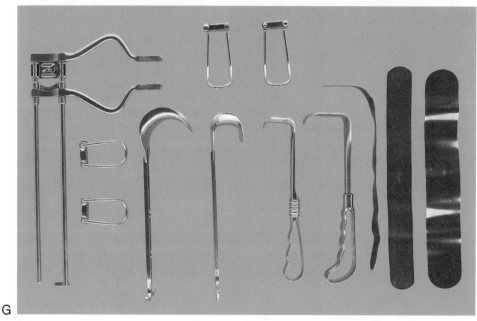

G

FIGURE 23-11, cont'd
Radical prostatectomy set. **F,** *Left to right,* two Greenwald suture guides, 24 Fr and 28 Fr; three Deaver retractors: narrow, side view; medium, front view; and wide, side view; two Harrington splanchnic retractors, small and large. **G,** *Top,* two Balfour abdominal retractor fenestrated blades, large. *Left to right,* Balfour abdominal retractor frame; two Balfour abdominal retractor fenestrated blades, small; two Balfour abdominal retractor center blades, large and small; two Richardson retractors, medium and large; three Ochsner malleable retractors: narrow, side view; medium; and large. (From Tighe SM: *Instrumentation for the operating room,* ed 6, St Louis, 2003, Mosby.)

Talking to the patient often eases apprehension, and one should explain preparatory steps for the procedure to the patient. Warm blankets should be available because the room temperature is low.

Cystoscopy ("Cysto") Room

Cystoscopic procedures take place in a specialized cystoscopy ("cysto") room. This dedicated surgical suite contains all the equipment needed to perform diagnostic or therapeutic procedures. GU instruments and equipment are very specialized. The cystoscopy table has accommodations for continuous drainage, intraoperative fluoroscopy, and x-ray. The cystoscopy table differs from the standard operating table in that it is designed to maintain the patient in the lithotomy position, receive x-ray cassettes, and allow for drainage of irrigation fluid. The stirrups of the table are removable and differ in design according to the manufacturer. X-ray cassettes are placed in a hollow space built into the table. Irrigation fluid is directed into a drainage tray located at the foot of the table. The tray is covered with a wire mesh plate that can be sterilized for resection procedures when tissue specimens are collected piece by piece and evacuated with the irrigation solution. Proper positioning of the patient is discussed later.

More extensive and modern cystoscopic rooms include digital data recording and equipment for video-assisted transurethral and ureteroscopic surgery.

Positioning

It is the scrub's duty to assist in positioning the patient on the cystoscopy table. The lithotomy position is used for rigid cystoscopic procedures and procedures that require bladder distension. The male patient may be placed in supine position for procedures of the urethra. The female is placed in the lithotomy position. All safety precautions regarding positioning are discussed in detail in Chapter 10. The cystoscopy or urology table is constructed with a "break" in the middle (Figure 23-12). The patient's buttocks must be in line with this break with the legs supported by lithotomy crutches. All patients are moved gently and with consideration for their individual physical ability. The cystoscopy stirrups are a modified (lower) version of those used commonly in open procedures involving the lower genital and perianal area. However, many patients who arrive for cystoscopic procedures suffer from hip deformities, including ankylosis or total hip fusion. In these cases, the cystoscopy stirrups are replaced with standard right-angled stirrups, such as those used in gynecological procedures.

One must take extreme care when positioning the patient. The scrub must be particularly careful not to overextend the fixed joints in the patient with a hip deformity. The hip usually can be flexed but not necessarily abducted. One should check the patient's chart before positioning the patient, and, if a hip deformity is present, the surgeon may assist and direct the safe positioning. The patient with arthritis or other musculoskeletal problems must be assisted so that the range of motion does not produce pain. Particular attention is given to leg abduction. Great care must be exercised to prevent overabduction. The sedated patient may be more flexible but unable to report pain. The patient's legs must *never* be forced into position. All bony prominences must be padded properly.

Electrosurgical Grounding and Settings

During cystoscopic procedures, the ESU may be in frequent use, particularly during resection procedures. The grounding plate may be placed on the patient's thigh or waist. It must be placed over a fleshy area and never over a bony prominence. The ESU should be placed on the lowest setting, which is increased gradually as directed by the urologist.

Duties of the Cystoscopic Assistant

The circulator who assists in cystoscopic and transurethral resection procedures may be responsible for setting up the instrument table and all other equipment. The circulator may serve in a dual capacity as the scrub and the circulator.

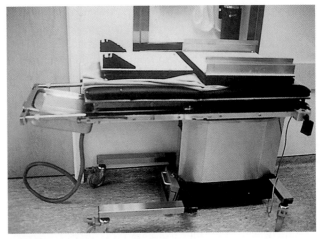

FIGURE 23-12
The cystoscopy or urology table. (From Nagle GM: *Genitourinary surgery: perioperative nursing series*, St Louis, 1997, Mosby.)

The circulator dons sterile gloves to set up the instruments and other sterile supplies. The urologist usually does not require a scrubbed assistant, so after setting up the supplies, the assistant removes his or her gloves and functions as a circulator during the case.

DURING A PROCEDURE
During a cystoscopic procedure, the circulator has the following responsibilities:

1. Remain in the room at all times, unless otherwise directed by the urologist.
2. Connect the nonsterile ends of the power cables or suction tubing.
3. Open sterile supplies for the urologist, as needed.
4. Replace irrigation bottles as they empty. Note the number of bottles used.
5. Receive any specimens from the urologist and label them properly.
6. Monitor the patient's vital signs every 15 minutes if the procedure is performed with the use of a local anesthetic.

AFTER A PROCEDURE
After a cystoscopic procedure, the circulator has the following responsibilities:

1. Assist in transferring the patient from the cystoscopy table to the stretcher and accompany the urologist or anesthesiologist to the postanesthesia care unit.
2. Transfer any tissue or fluid specimens to the designated area and record them in the specimen log.
3. Put away nonsterile supplies used during the procedure.
4. Transfer soiled equipment to the workroom and carry out proper terminal sterilization or decontamination on the equipment (see Chapter 8).

5. In some operating rooms, the cystoscopic equipment is washed and decontaminated in the cystoscopy room itself. If the instruments are to be decontaminated in a liquid chemical, remove them from the liquid promptly after the amount of time specified by the manufacturer. Oversoaking can damage delicate instruments.

Anesthesia

Most patients receive a local or topical anesthetic for diagnostic cystoscopy. In the male patient, local anesthetic in solution may be instilled in the bladder. For the female patient, cotton-tipped applicators dipped in anesthetic are inserted into the urethral meatus. Lidocaine gel, 1% or 2%, is typically used for this purpose. Monitored sedation or general anesthetic is used for more complex procedures.

Patient Skin Prep

The patient is prepped and draped for a perineal procedure. Aseptic technique is maintained throughout the procedure.

Irrigation

During most closed procedures, the bladder is distended with solution. Whenever electrosurgical instruments are used, the irrigation fluid must be **nonelectrolytic,** that is, unable to disperse and transmit electricity from the active electrode tip during use of the ESU. Sterile distilled water may be used during observation of the bladder and retrograde pyelography. The nonelectrolytic solutions used most often during resection are 3% sorbitol and glycine. These are nonelectrolytic, hypotonic (do not cause lysis of blood cells) solutions.

Continuous irrigation is achieved by an irrigation unit that holds the fluid and regulates the amount of inflow. Fluid packs that contain 1000 or 3000 ml should be hung 2½ to 3 feet above the cystoscopic table to maintain the correct pressure. Pressure also may be regulated by a pressure device. The technologist is responsible for ensuring that there is a continuous flow of fluid during the procedure. The technologist should take care to accurately measure the intake and output of bladder irrigation. Certain bladder irrigation fluids are absorbed and can cause systemic hypertension.

Fluid warmers prevent hypothermia during long procedures. The warmer must be carefully maintained and checked intraoperatively to ensure that the temperature is safe. All solutions should be stored at a temperature no higher than 65° C. Temperatures greater than this tend to damage the solutions. Solutions should not be used except at body temperature. Fluid warmers may contribute to increased hemorrhage as the warm water suppresses or delays the body's natural clotting mechanism. Bladder spasm or hypothermia may occur when cold irrigation solutions are used. The surgeon should be asked whether he or she prefers that the irrigation solution be warmed in a fluid warmer.

The Rigid Cystourethroscope

Diagnostic rigid cystourethroscopy (commonly called *cystoscope*) requires a minimum of equipment. Basic equipment common to all closed procedures is discussed in this section.

The cystourethroscope is a rigid, straight endoscope that is passed through the urethral meatus to perform diagnostic or operative procedures (Figure 23-13). The *cystoscope* is the precursor to the modern cystourethroscope. In this text we will use *cystoscope* to describe the modern transurethral scope to maintain continuity of understanding. However, the technologist should understand that the current scopes have more advanced technological and surgical capabilities than the cystoscope used in the past.

The cystoscope is a delicate and complex tool that allows the surgeon to examine, make diagnoses, and perform surgery on the urinary system. Different types of cystoscopes are available and vary according to the manufacturer. Because of these variations and because every technologist and nurse working in the cystoscopy room must become familiar with the equipment used in that particular operating room, a long discussion of various cystoscopes will not be given. However, some basic guidelines help one become familiar with the handling and care of any cystoscope:

1. Read and study the manufacturer's guidelines and instructions for the assembly of the cystoscope and its accessories *before* attempting to work with the equipment.
2. Handle the equipment gently. Remember that these instruments are delicate and costly. Never use force on the various components of the instrument when assembling or dismantling the instrument.
3. Seek help from other surgical personnel if you do not understand how to assemble or disassemble the equipment. It is better to learn from someone who is familiar with the equipment than to risk damaging it.
4. Attend in-service lectures given by the manufacturer or the operating room's in-service educator and, if possible, take written notes. Many operating rooms employ a cystoscopy technologist or nurse whose main duty is to work in the cystoscopy room. Consequently, other technologists or nurses in the department may either forget or never have the opportunity to learn about the equipment. The system is efficient as long as the cystoscopy technologist is available at all times. If, however, this person is ill or otherwise unable to assist the urologist in the cys-

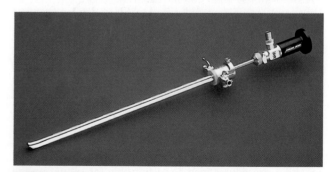

FIGURE 23-13
Rigid cystourethroscope. (From Nagle GM: *Genitourinary surgery: perioperative nursing series*, St Louis, 1997, Mosby.)

toscopy room, other staff members must take his or her place. Having some written notes to use as guidelines in these circumstances can be very helpful.

The cystoscope has many components for performing diagnostic and surgical procedures. Basic equipment is described as follows.

CYSTOSCOPE

The cystoscope is the optical portion of the scope (Figure 23-14). It contains the lenses, which magnify and offer an unimpaired view of structures within the bladder and urethra. The cystoscope is a delicate instrument and must be

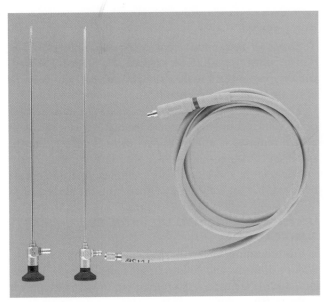

FIGURE 23-14
Left to right: cystoscope, 30 degree; cystoscope, 70 degree; fiberoptic cable. (From Tighe SM: *Instrumentation for the operating room,* ed 6, St Louis, 2003, Mosby.)

handled gently at all times. The shaft of the telescope is subject to bending and always must be picked up in the *middle*; if the shaft of the scope becomes bent, it cannot be used. One should take additional care to avoid scratching the lens, which will distort the view.

FIBEROPTIC LIGHT CABLE AND SOURCE

The fiberoptic light cable connects the cystoscope to the fiberoptic light source (see Figure 23-14). Light sources are the same as those used in other endoscopic procedures and include xenon and halide. Tungsten rarely is used as a light source because it lacks the brightness of other sources. Cables may be fiberoptic or liquid light (refer to Chapter 18). One should handle the light cables very carefully and should not coil them tightly. Coiling them too tightly will cause the fiberoptics inside the cables to break, and they will not transmit light properly.

SHEATH

The sheath is a hollow tube that serves as a passageway for the instruments used during cystoscopy and resection. The telescope is inserted into the sheath before it is passed into the urethra. The sheath allows the use of operative accessories, instruments, suction, and irrigation. The sheath has attachments that accept the instruments and irrigation tubing. The tip may be beveled or oblique. The main operating channel receives the telescope, while side channels, controlled by stopcocks, accept the accessory instruments. A *bridge* attaches to the head of the scope and permits the entry of accessory tools (Figure 23-15).

OBTURATOR

The insertion of the sheath into the urethra may be aided by the obturator (see Figure 23-12), a metal rod with a blunt, rounded tip. It is inserted into the sheath and advanced so that it precedes the sheath during urethral entry. This prevents the end of the sheath from abrading the mucosal lin-

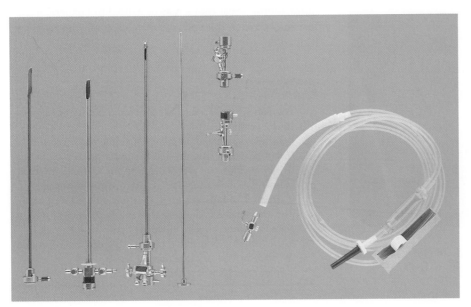

FIGURE 23-15
Left to right, obturator; cystoscope sheath; catheter deflecting mechanism with two instrument channels; obturator for cystoscope; two Storz short telescope bridges. (From Tighe SM: *Instrumentation for the operating room,* ed 6, St Louis, 1999, Mosby.)

ing of the urethra as it is inserted. The obturator may be straight or deflecting (able to be turned to the side).

CYSTOSCOPIC OPERATIVE PROCEDURES

The cystourethroscope is capable of a variety of operative procedures. These include:

▶ Use of stone-crushing forceps
▶ Biopsy and stone grasping
▶ Fulguration of lesions via Bugbee electrodes
▶ Release of urethral strictures through the use of dilators and urethrotomes

The Flexible Cystourethroscope

The flexible cystourethroscope is used most often in outpatient and clinic settings (Figure 23-16). The disadvantage of this scope is that it is capable of primarily diagnostic rather than therapeutic use. NOTE: Do not confuse the *cystourethroscope with the flexible operating ureteroscope or nephroscope.*

CYSTOSCOPIC SURGICAL PROCEDURES

Diagnostic Cystoscopy

SURGICAL GOAL

The goal of cystourethroscopy (cystoscopy) is to examine the inside of the urinary bladder and urethra for evidence of disease.

PATHOLOGY

Cystoscopy is performed in the male to evaluate blood in the urine (**hematuria**), difficulty voiding, and strictures, and to evaluate the patient for prostatic surgery. In the female, hematuria, painful urination, incontinence, and frequent voiding are indications for this procedure. Hematuria may be caused by chronic infection or tumor.

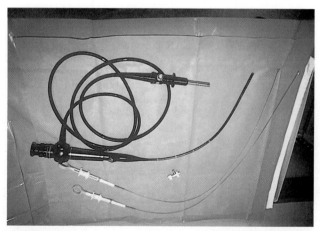

FIGURE 23-16
The flexible cystourethroscope. (From Nagle GM: *Genitourinary surgery: perioperative nursing series,* St Louis, 1997, Mosby.)

Technique

1. The patient is placed in the supine position on the urology table. Low lithotomy attachments are used to abduct and externally rotate the patient's legs. The patient's hips are flexed as the patient's musculoskeletal capabilities allow.
2. The patient is prepped and draped for a perineal procedure.
3. A topical anesthetic or water-soluble anesthetic solution is instilled into the urethra.
4. Urethral dilation is performed as needed.
5. The sheath and telescope or obturator are lubricated and inserted into the urethra.
6. The obturator is removed.
7. The bladder is filled with distension media.
8. The surgeon examines the urethra and bladder from all angles.

DISCUSSION

The basic set-up for cystoscopy is described in Box 23-1.

The patient is positioned, prepped, and draped. The bladder may be emptied with a straight catheter, and a sterile urine specimen may be obtained.

The rigid cystoscope is well lubricated with water-soluble or lidocaine gel and inserted into the urethra. The obturator is then removed, and any residual urine is collected in the specimen container.

The urethra and bladder are examined. Instruments are removed, and the solution is drained from the bladder.

Ureteral Dilation and Urethrotomy

SURGICAL GOAL

In this procedure, the urethra is dilated to relieve a stricture. Phillips filiforms and followers, graduated sounds, or balloon dilators are used. Urethrotomy is a small incision made in the internal urethra to release scar tissue.

PATHOLOGY

Urethral stricture is usually caused by an enlarged prostate that impinges on the urethra, previous trauma, or infection of the urethra. Scar tissue may be caused by congenital malformation. When dilation is ineffective, urethrotomy is performed.

Technique

1. The patient is placed in the lithotomy (female) or supine (male) position.
2. Routine draping and prepping are performed.
3. A routine examination cystoscopy is performed.
4. If Phillips filiforms are passed into the urethral stricture, followers of increasing size are attached and advanced.
5. If urethral sounds are used, they are inserted, beginning with the smallest. The largest sound is allowed to stay in place for a short time to dilate the tissue.
6. A urethrotome is inserted through the urethroscope, and the blade is used to incise the scar tissue.
7. A Foley catheter is inserted.

Box 23-1   Basic Set-Up for Cystoscopy

- ▶ Cystoscopy pack (gowns, towels, drapes)
- ▶ Sterile gloves
- ▶ Cystourethroscope
- ▶ Cystoscopy irrigation tubing
- ▶ Albarran bridge
- ▶ Catheter adapters
- ▶ Lateral and foroblique telescope
- ▶ ESU
- ▶ Bugbee electrodes
- ▶ Rubber nipples for catheterization
- ▶ Penile clamp
- ▶ Luer-Lok stopcock
- ▶ Water-soluble lubrication gel
- ▶ Irrigation solution
- ▶ Fiberoptic light source
- ▶ Small prep basin with sponges
- ▶ Specimen containers
- ▶ X-ray protective aprons
- ▶ Laser units if required
- ▶ Syringes
- ▶ Assorted catheters

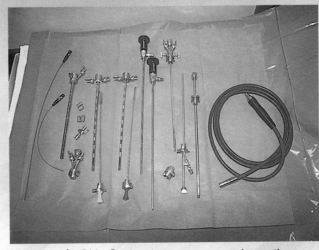

(From Nagle GM: *Genitourinary surgery: perioperative nursing series*, St Louis, 1997, Mosby.)

DISCUSSION

The patient is positioned and draped in routine manner. A routine diagnostic cystoscopy precedes the dilation and urethrotomy.

Urethral dilation often is necessary to allow the passage of instruments through the urethra. Stricture of the urethra is a common condition in GU disease, and dilation of the urethral stricture may be performed as an isolated procedure.

To gain entry to the bladder and ureter, the surgeon may need to perform dilation. Many different types of dilators are available. Filiforms are very small rods with a threaded distal end. The threaded portion accepts all sizes of followers, which are larger dilators in graduated sizes. The van Buren sounds are graduated metal rods that are inserted and removed. The largest sound is left in place for a short time to stretch the tissue.

All sounds are first lubricated, then introduced slowly to avoid tearing the delicate tissue of the urethra.

Management of Bladder Calculi Using the Cystourethroscope
SURGICAL GOAL

In this procedure, bladder **calculi** or stones are removed because they cause pain or urinary blockage.

Extracorporeal shockwave lithotripsy (**ESWL**) is commonly used to dissolve bladder, kidney, and other calculi. In this procedure, the patient is exposed to ultrasonic waves, which pulverize the calculi. Not all stones can be removed by ESWL. Surgical intervention may be required.

PATHOLOGY

Bladder calculi (stones) are much less common than kidney stones. Approximately 95% of cases occur in men. They may be caused by urinary tract infection, bladder diverticula, or an enlarged prostate gland. Bladder stones can form when urine is concentrated and minerals crystallize and precipitate.

Technique

1. A cystoscopy is performed.
2. A 17- to 23-Fr panendoscope is inserted after urethral dilation as needed.
3. Sterile water is infused into the urinary bladder.
4. The lithotrite instrument is inserted and the stone is crushed.
5. Stone fragments are removed with a stone basket or forceps.
6. Bleeding is controlled with the Bugbee electrode.

DISCUSSION

Bladder calculi may be managed in several ways. Small stones may be grasped with stone-grasping forceps. The lithotrite is a specialized instrument that grasps and crushes the stone. During the set-up, the technologist must be certain that the lithotrite is in good working order and that all working parts glide smoothly.

To begin the procedure, the surgeon performs a routine cystoscopy. The urethra may require dilation to accommodate the 24-Fr cystourethroscope. The surgeon distends the bladder with sterile water. After locating one or more stones, the surgeon introduces the lithotrite into the scope. Under direct vision, the stone is crushed. Small pieces are flushed out of the bladder with an Ellik evacuator. Bleeders are coagulated with the Bugbee active electrode.

FLEXIBLE URETEROSCOPY PROCEDURES

The flexible ureteroscope is used to perform diagnostic and surgical procedures of the ureter and renal pelvis (Figure 23-17). The ureteroscope is a fiberoptic instrument with a deflecting tip. The flexibility allows the scope to be positioned in the renal pelvis and advanced into the calyces. Like other fiberoptic instruments, the ureteroscope has working channels for insertion of instruments, suction, and irrigation.

Equipment

Equipment required for flexible ureteroscopy is listed in Box 23-2.

Irrigation

Irrigation fluid can be delivered through a special pumping device or manually through the same channel used by the working instruments (e.g., biopsy forceps). Sterile saline is used for most procedures that do not require the ESU. Sorbitol or glycine is used when electrosurgery is required. Contrast media may be added to the irrigation fluid for fluoroscopic examination.

Use of the Ureteroscope

A guide wire is used to provide support in passing the flexible ureteroscope. The guide wire is made of Teflon-coated stainless steel. It is passed into the ureter with the cystoscope and advanced into the renal pelvis through the ureter. This is performed with the aid of fluoroscopy. The ureteroscope is capable of passing through the urethra and ureter, and into the renal pelvis. The deflecting tip can reach into the calyces of the kidney, where endoscopic surgery can be performed through the working channels of the scope. The distal end of the scope enters the lower calyces of the renal pelvis by deflection.

Working instruments are passed through the channel of the scope. The technologist guides the instruments into the channel so the surgeon can maintain control of the scope head.

Procedures

TISSUE BIOPSY

Tissue biopsy is performed to remove a tissue specimen and to determine whether the tissue is benign or malignant. Tissue biopsy is performed with cup forceps or with a flat wire basket.

Cell biopsy can be taken with the cytology brush. After the specimen is retrieved on the brush, the technologist agitates the brush gently in a prepared specimen container holding normal saline to release the cells from the brush. The specimen container must be labeled.

TUMOR REMOVAL

Neoplasm can be removed through fulguration or the holmium:YAG laser. Laser precautions must be observed. Refer to Chapter 17 for a complete discussion of laser use and safety considerations.

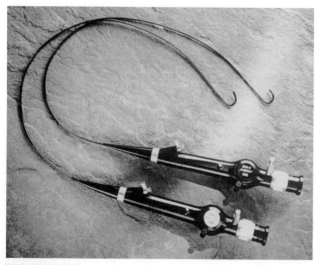

FIGURE 23-17
Flexible ureteroscopes.

Box 23-2 Ureteroscopy Instruments

▸ Ureteroscope
▸ Guide wires
▸ Cystoscope
▸ Saline for irrigation
▸ Connectors and tubing
▸ Three-way stopcock
▸ Syringes, sizes 20 ml and 50 ml
▸ Contrast media
▸ Lithotriptor (as needed)
▸ Grasper
▸ Stone basket
▸ Double-lumen catheter
▸ Ureteral dilators
▸ Active fulgurating electrode
▸ Luer-Lok connectors
▸ Specimen containers

STONE RETRIEVAL

The ureteroscope is used to remove stones that occur in the renal pelvis or ureter.

PYELOPLASTY

Strictures in the ureter are relieved by fine electrosurgical or laser devices introduced through the endoscope. This approach avoids the traditional method of percutaneous pyeloplasty (discussed below) and offers the patient a much quicker recovery period with less trauma.

URETHROTOMY

If urethrotomy (release of stricture) is planned, an optical urethrotome is inserted into the stricture, and the blade incises the scar tissue.

FLEXIBLE URETEROSCOPY SURGICAL PROCEDURES

Transurethral Resection of the Prostate

SURGICAL GOAL

In transurethral resection of the prostate (TURP), the prostate is removed with a resectoscope.

PATHOLOGY

Benign **hypertrophy** (tissue enlargement) of the prostate, or **BPH,** usually occurs in men over the age of 30 years. The cause may be related to increased release of androgens such as testosterone. As the prostate enlarges, nodules in the gland develop. These nodules put pressure on the urethra, causing urinary blockage and difficulty voiding. The bladder becomes distended and causes diverticuli in the bladder wall. Urinary retention results in infection, stones, and hematuria.

Technique
1. The surgeon may perform routine cystoscopy.
2. The urethra is dilated with van Buren sounds.
3. A resectoscope sheath is inserted into the urethra.
4. The surgeon resects the middle and lateral lobes of the prostate.
5. Pieces of resected tissue are evacuated from the bladder with the Toomey syringe or Ellik evacuator.
6. During continuous irrigation, the outflow is produced by suction or gravity.
7. After resection, the surgeon controls bleeders with the ESU.
8. A three-way Foley catheter with 30-ml balloon is inserted into the urethra.

DISCUSSION

Transurethral resection is carried out with the resectoscope and ESU or laser energy. The resectoscope has a 0-degree or 12-degree telescope that is inserted into the separate sheath (Figure 23-18, *A*). Two common types of working elements are the Iglesias and the McCarthy elements. The electrode tip shaves and coagulates tissue when the working element

is activated. Assorted tips are illustrated in Figure 23-18, *B*. Resectoscope accessories are shown in Figure 23-18, *C* through *E*.

During resection, continuous irrigation or bladder distension with nonelectrolytic solution such as sorbitol or glycine is used to maintain a clear surgical field and to evacuate small pieces of tissue. Continuous irrigation permits clear visualization during resection. The resectoscope is constructed with an outer sheath that allows fluid to flow out of the instrument.

Irrigation fluid must be maintained. A solution warmer is used to prevent hypothermia, as described at the beginning of this chapter.

Before beginning the procedure, the surgeon may perform a routine cystoscopy . The urethra is then dilated with van Buren sounds. The resectoscope is inserted, and surgical removal is initiated at the middle and lateral lobes. The small pieces of tissue that are released into the irrigation fluid may be evacuated with the Ellik evacuator or Toomey syringe. The technologist must retain all pieces of specimen for pathological examination. These should be maintained in a small basin.

NOTE: Transurethral resection of a bladder tumor (**TURBT**) is performed in the same manner as the TURP.

OPEN PROCEDURES OF THE EXTERNAL GENITALIA

Urethral Meatotomy

SURGICAL GOAL

Urethral meatotomy is a procedure in which the external urethral meatus is enlarged with an incision.

PATHOLOGY

Strictures of the ureteral meatus result from infection or trauma related to previous surgery or traumatic pelvic injury. Congenital stricture of the meatus is relatively rare.

Technique
1. The patient is positioned, prepped, and draped for a urethral procedure.
2. The surgeon grasps the ventral frenulum with a straight mosquito hemostat.
3. The surgeon makes a small incision in the frenulum.
4. Small bleeders are coagulated with the ESU.
5. The mucosal layer of the meatus is sutured to the skin.

DISCUSSION

After positioning and draping of the patient, the surgeon grasps the ventral portion of the frenulum with a straight mosquito hemostat. He or she then makes a small incision at the frenulum to enlarge the meatus. Small bleeders are coagulated with the ESU. In the infant, the wound heals by secondary intention. In the adult, several absorbable sutures attach the mucosal layer to the skin. The wound is covered with petrolatum gauze dressing.

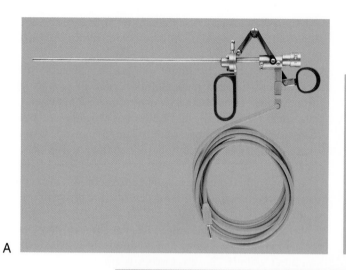
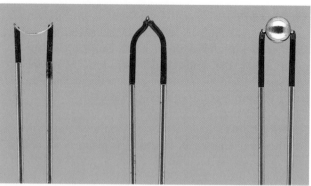
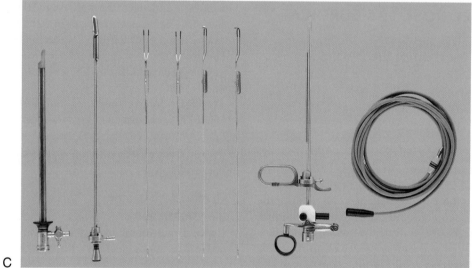
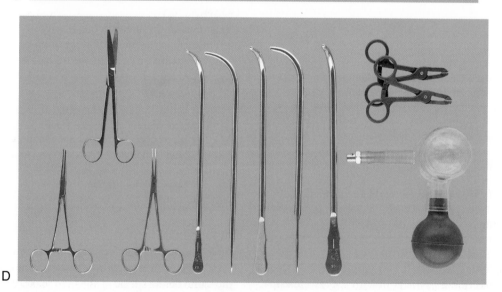

FIGURE 23-18

A, Resectoscope and connecting cord. **B,** *Left to right,* enlarged tips: cutting electrode with round wire; cutting electrode with pointed end; coagulating electrode with ball end. **C,** *Left to right,* resecting sheath, 27 Fr; deflecting obturator; two resecting loops; roller ball electrode; coagulating electrode with pointed end; resectoscope working element; high-frequency cautery. **D,** *Top, left,* Mayo dissecting scissors, curved. *Bottom, left to right,* Crile hemostatic forceps, straight; Crile hemostatic forceps, curved; five van Buren urethral sounds, male, sizes 8 to 16. *Right, top to bottom,* two nonperforating towel forceps; Ellik evacuator.

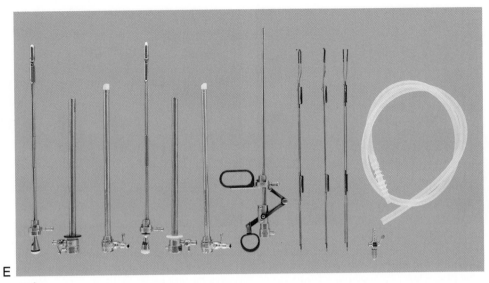

FIGURE 23-18, cont'd
E, *Left to right,* low-pressure resecting set: deflecting obturator; resecting sheath, 28 Fr; resecting sheath, 28 Fr, insulated; deflecting obturator; resecting sheath, 26 Fr; resecting sheath, 26 Fr, insulated; working element; three electrodes: sharp, ball, and loop; stopcock; tubing. (From Tighe SM: *Instrumentation for the operating room,* ed 6, St Louis, 2003, Mosby.)

Circumcision in the Adult
SURGICAL GOAL
Circumcision is the removal of the prepuce (foreskin).

PATHOLOGY
Phimosis is the inability to retract the foreskin in the uncircumcised male. It is caused by irritation of the foreskin or the inability of the foreskin to be retracted. This is usually related to accumulation of smegma under the prepuce. Circumcision is performed to prevent infection.

Technique
1. The surgeon grasps the prepuce with straight hemostats or straight mosquito hemostats.
2. A dorsal slit incision is made.
3. A circumferential incision is made with dissecting scissors.
4. The skin edges are approximated.

DISCUSSION
The patient is placed in the supine position, prepped, and draped with a small fenestration sheet. The surgeon places several Kelly, Crile, or mosquito hemostats on the edge of the prepuce. Using fine dissecting scissors, the surgeon makes a longitudinal incision on the dorsal side of the skin. The incision is carried circumferentially around the prepuce. Small bleeders are controlled with the ESU. The surgeon then approximates the wound edges with interrupted absorbable sutures, size 4-0 or 5-0. The wound is dressed with petrolatum gauze. Circumcision is illustrated in Figure 23-19.

The skin is not approximated on the very young infant. A nonadherent dressing is applied.

Urethral Meatoplasty
SURGICAL GOAL
This procedure is the incisional enlargement and repair of the external meatus of the urethra.

PATHOLOGY
Urethral meatoplasty is performed to relieve a congenital or acquired stenosis or stricture at the external meatus.

Technique
1. Males are placed in the supine position; females are placed in a lithotomy position.
2. Local anesthesia generally is used.
3. A straight hemostat is placed on the ventral surface of the meatus.
4. An incision is made to relieve the stricture or stenosis.
5. The wound is closed.

DISCUSSION
The straight hemostat is placed to tamponade the tissue to reduce bleeding at the incision. The surgeon makes the incision along the frenulum to enlarge the opening and overcome the stricture or stenosis.

Any bleeding sites are controlled with clamp and ties or electrocautery.

At closure, the mucosal layer is sutured to the skin with fine 3-0 or 4-0 absorbable sutures.

A dressing of petrolatum gauze may be used.

Repair of Hypospadias
SURGICAL GOAL
Hypospadias is a birth defect in which the urethral meatus is located on the underside of the penis. The goal of repair is to

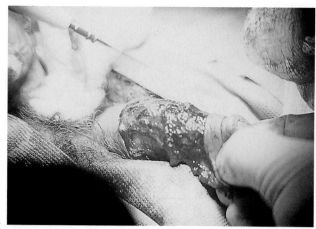
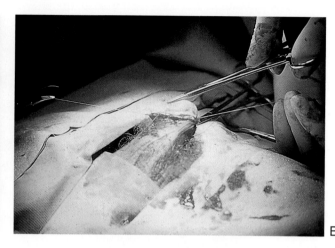

A   B

FIGURE 23-19
Circumcision. **A,** Dorsal skin is elevated and freed from the dartos fascia. Bleeders are fulgurated with an ESU or tied with 4-0 absorbable sutures. **B,** The raw edges of skin are approximated to a coronal cuff of mucosal prepuce with a 3-0 or 4-0 absorbable suture. (From Nagle GM: *Genitourinary surgery: perioperative nursing series,* St Louis, 1997, Mosby.)

correct the defect and position the meatus at the tip of the penis. Repair is performed when the patient is 12 months to school age.

PATHOLOGY

Hypospadias is a common birth defect in males. It is associated with a condition called **chordee** in which the urethra is shortened, causing the penis to bow inward toward the body. In mild chordee, the meatus is near the tip of the penis. In moderate to severe cases, the meatus is located along the shaft of the penis or at the base near the scrotum.

Technique

1. The surgeon releases the chordee by sharp dissection.
2. The prepuce is used to create an autograft and extend the urethra.
3. The defect left by the chordee repair is covered with the prepuce.
4. A portion of the prepuce is wrapped around a catheter.
5. The remaining prepuce is pulled over the glans and sutured into place.

DISCUSSION

Many different procedures are used to correct chordee and hypospadias. The severity of the condition determines the best approach. Many repairs are performed as multi-stage procedures. Figure 23-20 illustrates a simple correction.

Repair of Epispadias
SURGICAL GOAL

This is the surgical correction of an opening in the dorsum of the penis to restore anatomical correctness and to relieve possible incontinence associated with the deformity (Figure 23-21).

PATHOLOGY

An epispadias is a congenital anomaly. The corrective surgical procedures employed depend on the severity of the deformity.

Technique

1. Mild deformities can be repaired using the hypospadius repair technique.
2. *Stage 1 Repair:* The surgeon makes a vertical incision distal to the epispadial meatus and carries it circumferentially to the dorsal coronal margin. The foreshortened dorsal urethral strip is lifted from the corpora cavernosa, and the ventral foreskin is rotated to cover the dorsal skin defect created by penile straightening.
3. *Stage 2 Repair:* The surgeon makes a vertical suprapubic incision, exposing the anterior bladder wall and the widened vesical neck. A wedge of prostatic urethra is removed on each side so that the reconstruction produces a prostatic urethra of more normal caliber.
4. The surgeon excises the roof of the membranous urethra.
5. The surgeon closes the prostatic urethra, also suturing together muscle at the midline. An indwelling suprapubic catheter is placed, and the bladder is closed. The abdomen is closed in layers.
6. The anterior urethra is closed after an appropriate section of dorsal penile skin is identified.
7. The creation of the urethra and its coverage with lateral penile skin make up the remainder of the repair.

DISCUSSION

The least severe forms of epispadias are:

▶ Balanic epispadias: the urethra opens in the dorsum of the glans
▶ Penile epispadias: the urethra opens on the penile shaft

Complete epispadias deformity is the most severe form of epispadias and is always associated with urinary incontinence because the patient has little to no development of the bladder neck. In a more severe form, the urethra opens onto the proximal end of the shaft or in the penopubic position.

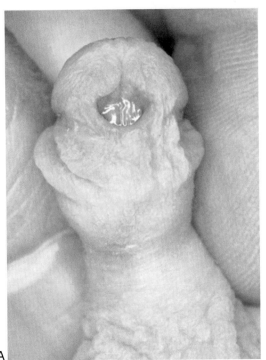

A

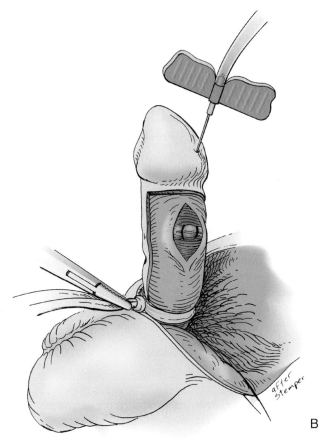

B

FIGURE 23-20
Simple repair of hypospadias. **A,** Photo of hypospadias. **B,** Incisions are approximated, and the intervening strip of tunica albuginea and suture knots are buried. (From Walsh PC, Retik AB, Vaughan ED, et al: *Campbell's urology,* ed 8, Philadelphia, 2002, Saunders.)

Orchidopexy
SURGICAL GOAL
Orchidopexy is the surgical correction of an undescended testicle. The goal of surgery is to bring the testicle into the scrotum and attach it to the scrotal wall. The procedure is performed before the child reaches school age.

PATHOLOGY
During normal fetal life, the testicles are retained within the abdomen. Just before birth, the testicles normally descend into the scrotum. Occasionally one or both testicles fail to descend into the scrotum. An undescended testicle can become sterile as a result of the increased temperature in the abdominal cavity.

Technique

1. The surgeon enters and explores the inguinal region.
2. The surgeon identifies the undescended testicle.
3. The spermatic cord is dissected free.
4. The testicle is mobilized by sharp and blunt dissection.
5. A tunnel is made through the inguinal canal into the scrotum.
6. The testicle is brought through the tunnel and secured with sutures.
7. The inguinal layers are closed.

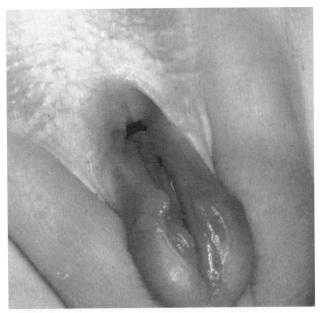

FIGURE 23-21
Three-month-old male with complete epispadias. (From Walsh PC, Retik AB, Vaughan ED, et al: *Campbell's urology,* ed 8, Philadelphia, 2002, Saunders.)

DISCUSSION

The patient is placed in the supine position, prepped, and draped with the inguinal and groin area on the affected side exposed. The surgeon makes an incision over the external ring as for a hernia repair. The incision is carried into the deep inguinal tissues with sharp dissection.

Small bleeders are coagulated with the ESU or clamped with mosquito hemostats and ligated with fine absorbable sutures. The spermatic cord is then identified and dissected with blunt and sharp dissection. The cord is dissected high in the internal ring to create sufficient slack to bring the testicle into the scrotum.

To create a tunnel for the testicle, the surgeon uses his or her finger or a blunt clamp such as a Mayo or sponge forceps. The surgeon advances the clamp through the external oblique fascia and separates the tissue manually, forming a pocket in the scrotum.

The testicle is then brought through the tunnel, and the scrotum is incised to expose the scrotal septum. Several sutures of size 3-0 or 4-0 absorbable material are placed through the septum and testicle, securing it into place.

Vasectomy
SURGICAL GOAL

Vasectomy is an elective procedure in which a portion of the vas deferens is removed to produce male sterilization.

Technique

1. The surgeon incises the scrotum.
2. The vas deferens is identified and isolated.
3. Two hemostats are placed across the duct, and a small section of the duct is removed.
4. The cut ends of the duct are coagulated.
5. The incision is closed.
6. The severed vas may be sent as specimen.

DISCUSSION

The patient is placed in the supine position, prepped, and draped for a scrotal incision. Local anesthetic is used. The surgeon makes a small incision in the proximal scrotum over the vas deferens (Figure 23-22). Small bleeders are coagulated with the needle-point ESU. The surgeon then isolates the duct with small hemostats and fine dissecting scissors.

The duct is cross-clamped, leaving a short section between the clamps. This surgeon transects and removes this section. The two severed ends of the vas deferens are coagulated with the ESU. The scrotum is closed with fine nonabsorbable sutures.

Vasovasostomy
SURGICAL GOAL

Vasovasostomy is the surgical reanastomosis of the vas deferens, using the operative microscope.

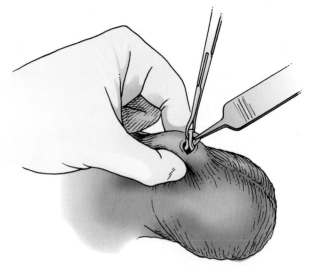

FIGURE 23-22
Vasectomy: incision to access the vas. (From Walsh PC, Retik AB, Vaughan ED, et al: *Campbell's urology*, ed 8, Philadelphia, 2002, Saunders.)

PATHOLOGY

Reanastomosis is performed to alleviate chronic testicular pain (a common side effect of vasectomy). In addition, many men who have undergone vasectomy wish to regain their fertility.

Technique

1. The patient is placed in the supine position, and the groin, including the scrotum, is prepped.
2. The vas deferens is identified by external manipulation, and a vertical incision is made in the scrotum.
3. The testicle, epididymis, and vas are displaced. The scarred vas is excised.
4. The operative microscope is brought into the field.
5. The vas ends are prepared, and the anastomosis is performed.
6. The wound is closed in layers, and a supportive pressure dressing is applied.

DISCUSSION

The proximal end of the vas deferens is cut back until fluid is expelled. The fluid is collected, placed on a glass slide, and sent to the lab for examination to determine whether live sperm are present. The surgery continues even if the results are negative. The distal end of the vas is resected until a normal lumen is visible. Both distal and proximal ends are dilated.

The two ends are placed in close proximity to each other and held in place with an approximator clip. A microbackground material is placed under the vas to isolate it during the anastomosis.

A two-layer anastomosis is used; this technique has a 40% to 70% success rate. The inner layer is identified and sutured with 10-0 nonabsorbable interrupted stitch, approximately six stitches. The second layer is anastomosed with 9-0 nonabsorbable interrupted stitches, with the surgeon taking care *not* to enter the lumen of the vas.

The wound is closed in two layers with absorbable 3-0 and 4-0 suture.

To help ensure the success of the anastomosis, the patient is cautioned not to do any lifting or have any ejaculations for at least 2 weeks. Sperm counts and viability are checked at 3-month and 6-month intervals.

Varicocelectomy
SURGICAL GOAL
Varicocelectomy is a high ligation of the gonadal veins of the testes to reduce venous backflow of blood into the venous plexus of the testes and to improve spermatogenesis.

PATHOLOGY
Varicoceles occur mainly on the patient's left side because of the backpressure built up from the anatomical junction of the gonadal vein and the renal vein.

Technique

1. The patient is supine and prepped as for an inguinal hernia; the scrotum also is prepared.
2. The incision may be either suprainguinal or oblique inguinal over the external inguinal ring.
3. The surgeon identifies the spermatic cord and structures, and mobilizes the vessels from the vas deferens.
4. The surgeon clamps and ligates any abnormal veins; redundant portions are excised.
5. A drain may be placed, and the wound is closed in layers.

DISCUSSION
Because of the backpressure, the pampiniform plexus of the spermatic cord becomes tortuous and engorged, resembling a bag of worms.

Varicocelectomies now can be performed laparoscopically and are performed as for laparoscopic hernia repairs.

Hydrocelectomy
SURGICAL GOAL
A hydrocele is a fluid-filled sac that develops over the testicle. It is drained and removed to prevent rupture and hemorrhage.

PATHOLOGY
A hydrocele is caused by trauma, infection, or tumor within the scrotum. It is often seen in association with inguinal hernia.

Technique

1. The surgeon incises the scrotum.
2. The intact hydrocele sac is delivered out of the scrotum and drained.
3. The sac is completely mobilized and removed from the scrotum.
4. The scrotal incision is closed.

DISCUSSION
The patient is placed in the supine position, prepped, and draped for a scrotal incision. The surgeon makes a small incision of the sac. The ESU is used to coagulate bleeders. The surgeon delivers the hydrocele out of the scrotum without rupturing it. The surgeon then makes a small incision in the sac membrane. The scrub should have suction immediately available to drain the sac, which is excised and removed. The surgeon may insert a small Penrose drain in the wound, which then is closed in two layers with fine absorbable sutures.

Orchiectomy
SURGICAL GOAL
Orchiectomy is surgical removal of one or both testicles.

PATHOLOGY
Removal of one testicle is most commonly performed to treat testicular carcinoma, **torsion** (twisting of the testis resulting in ischemia and necrosis), trauma, or infection. Bilateral orchiectomy is performed to control metastatic carcinoma of the prostate.

Technique

1. The surgeon makes a transverse skin incision in the anterior testicle.
2. Blunt dissection is used to remove the fascia and subcutaneous layers away from the testicle.
3. The surgeon delivers the testicle from the scrotum.
4. The spermatic artery and veins are cross-clamped.
5. A suture ligature is placed in the spermatic artery and veins.
6. The stalk of the testicle is incised.
7. The wound is closed with subcuticular suture.

DISCUSSION
Orchiectomy may be performed under local anesthesia with sedation. The patient is placed in the supine position, prepped, and draped for a scrotal incision. A towel should be placed under the scrotum to elevate it on the surgical field.

If a local anesthetic is used, the agent is injected into the skin and spermatic cord.

The surgeon makes a transverse anterolateral incision in the scrotal skin. Using sponge dissectors and manual dissection, the surgeon separates the testicle from the fascia and subcutaneous tissue. This technique exposes the tunica vaginalis and testicle. The surgeon then delivers the testicle out of the scrotal sac. Bleeders are controlled with the ESU.

The spermatic cord is identified, and the artery and veins are cross-clamped with Kelly or Mayo clamps. The surgeon divides the tissue with the ESU or scissors. The technologist should have a suture ligature of size 0 absorbable material available. This suture ligature is placed through the vessels. Two such ligatures may be placed.

The wound is closed with a subcuticular suture of absorbable material on a fine cutting needle. Antibiotic ointment may be applied to the wound. Dressing consists of

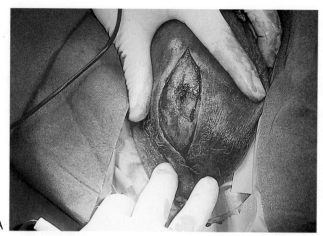
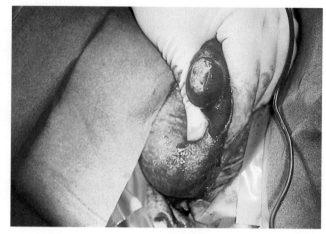

FIGURE 23-23
Orchiectomy. **A,** A transverse incision is made to expose both testes. **B,** The testis and tunica vaginalis are displaced from the scrotum. (From Nagle GM: *Genitourinary surgery: perioperative nursing series,* St Louis, 1997, Mosby.)

gauze fluffs and a scrotal support. Orchiectomy is illustrated in Figure 23-23.

Insertion of Penile Implant
SURGICAL GOAL

In this procedure, a penile implant is surgically placed to treat impotence caused by organic disease. Two types of implants are available: the semi-rigid implant and the inflatable reservoir type.

PATHOLOGY

A malfunction in the erectile system of the penis is most often caused by neurological disease, diabetes mellitus, vascular disease with atherosclerosis, or hypertension. Patients for whom no organic cause can be found are carefully screened for this procedure.

Technique

1. The surgeon inserts a Foley catheter.
2. A small incision is made at the base of the scrotum.
3. The tunica albuginea is incised longitudinally to expose the corpus cavernosum.
4. The length of the corpus cavernosum is measured with a sizing instrument.
5. The inserter is pushed into the corporal tunnel, and the cylinders are inserted.
6. A small pocket is made in the scrotum for the pump, which is then placed.
7. The surgeon uses blunt dissection to make a passageway through the external inguinal ring.
8. The transversalis fascia is incised, and the reservoir is positioned in the perivesical space.
9. The surgeon closes the scrotum.
10. The cylinder and reservoir are connected to the pump and tested.

DISCUSSION

Many types of inflatable penile implants are available. Each manufacturer provides detailed instructions on the tools and techniques used to place the implant. The technique described here uses an inflatable pump manufactured by American Medical Systems. This surgery has three parts, and the system has three components. The cylinders are placed in the corpora cavernosa of the penis and can be inflated by the patient. The pump is placed surgically in the scrotum, and the reservoir, which contains the cylinder media, is placed in the inguinal area.

See photos of this procedure in Figure 23-24.

TRANSABDOMINAL SURGICAL PROCEDURES

Transabdominal procedures of the GU tract are performed as open or laparoscopic surgery. Techniques and instruments used for laparoscopic procedures follow those of the abdominal laparotomy.

Pyelolithotomy
SURGICAL GOAL

Pyelolithotomy is surgical entry to the hilum of the kidney.

PATHOLOGY

Pyelolithotomy is performed most often to remove large impacted calculi in the renal pelvis. When a stone is lodged in the ureteropelvic junction, a **pyeloplasty** may be necessary. This is a remodeling of the renal pelvis to repair tissue damage. Stones in the renal pelvis are extremely painful and cause tissue trauma with their sharp surfaces. **Nephrolithotomy** is the removal of calculi from the kidney parenchyma.

Technique

1. The kidney is approached from a flank incision.
2. The surgeon identifies and mobilizes the ureter.
3. Traction sutures are placed on either side of the incision site in the renal pelvis.
4. The surgeon makes an incision into the renal pelvis and removes the stone.

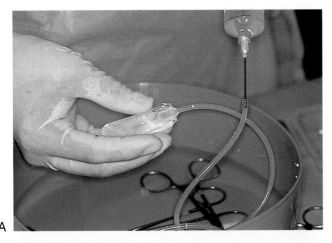
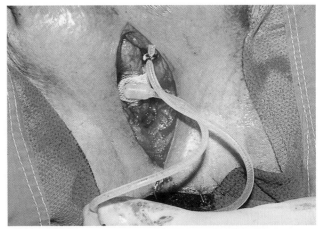
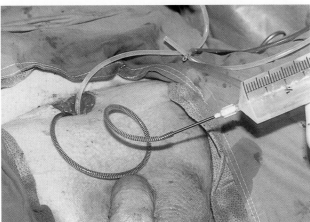
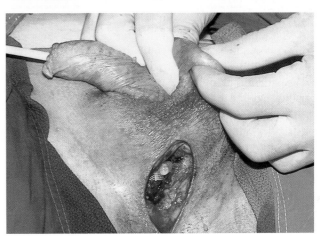

FIGURE 23-24
Insertion of penile implant. **A,** Preparation of the reservoir. **B,** Placement of reservoir and cuff in perineal incision. **C,** The reservoir and pump are filled with 12.5% Hypaque to the appropriate volume. **D,** The pump is activated and deactivated to determine integrity. (Courtesy American Medical Systems, Minnetonka, Minn.)

5. The renal pelvis and all collecting tubes are irrigated with warm saline.
6. Nephrolithotomy is performed as necessary. The kidney parenchyma is incised, and stones are removed.
7. The collecting system is closed, and the renal pelvis is sutured.
8. A nephrostomy tube is placed in the wound for drainage.
9. The wound is closed in layers.

DISCUSSION

Before open procedures, **retrograde pyelography** and cystoscopy (cystoscopic examination with contrast media injected into the renal collection system) are performed to locate the stone and assess for operability.

Before prepping of the patient, a Foley catheter is inserted. A flank incision is made, and a self-retaining retractor is placed in the wound. The renal pelvis is identified, and an incision is made over the area of the stone. Before making the incision, the surgeon may place two or more traction sutures on either side of the incision site. These are used to hold the renal tissue back while the stone is removed.

The surgeon grasps the stone with a stone forceps. The scrub should preserve the stone in a small, dry basin. If stones are located within the renal tissue, the incision may be extended to locate them. These stones usually are visible on x-ray. The surgeon carefully divides the parenchyma with dissecting scissors. All stones are removed with forceps. Before closing the wound, the surgeon irrigates the entire system with warm saline to flush out any remaining small fragments.

The surgeon closes the parenchyma with absorbable sutures, size 2-0 or 3-0. The renal pelvis is closed with similar sutures. A nephrostomy tube may be placed in the renal pelvis before closure. A Malecot or similar tube is typically used.

If postoperative bleeding or excessive drainage is expected, a Jackson-Pratt drain also may be placed in the wound.

Simple Nephrectomy (Flank Incision)
SURGICAL GOAL
Simple nephrectomy is surgical removal of one kidney.

PATHOLOGY
Nephrectomy is indicated for many renal diseases. The procedure is performed most often for severe hydronephrosis,

localized tumor, calculus disease with infection, and trauma to the kidney. A kidney also may be removed from a live donor for transplant.

Technique

1. The surgeon enters the flank through a transcostal incision.
2. The incision is carried through the skin, fat, and fascial layers.
3. The oblique and transverse muscles are incised.
4. A rib resection may be performed if needed.
5. The ureter is identified, clamped, severed, and ligated.
6. The kidney pedicle is dissected and clamped.
7. Suture ligatures are placed in the pedicle.
8. The kidney is removed.
9. The wound is closed.

DISCUSSION

The transcostal incision gives good exposure of the kidney; the scrub must be familiar with this incision.

The patient is placed in the lateral position with the flank over the table break or kidney lift (Figure 23-25, *A*). He or she is prepped and draped for a flank incision. Before the prep, a Foley catheter is inserted.

The surgeon makes the flank incision along the twelfth rib extending to the border of the rectus muscle. If a rib must be resected, the eleventh or twelfth rib is first stripped of periosteum with a Doyen rib raspatory or with osteotomes. This is necessary for the rib cutter to cut through the bone effectively. The surgeon grasps the rib with a heavy Oschner or Kocher clamp. The surgeon then uses a Bethune shears or rib cutter to cut the rib. The scrub should have bone wax available to be placed over the cut portions. These also may require some trimming to remove sharp edges.

The incision is carried through the subcutaneous and oblique muscles with the ESU. A self-retaining retractor is placed in the wound after the surgeon protects the edges of the wound with laparotomy sponges.

Gerota's capsule (perirenal fascia) is identified, and perirenal fat is removed. The scrub must preserve all perirenal fat in a small basin because it may be used to help control bleeding later in the surgery.

The ureter is identified, double-clamped with Mayo clamps, divided, and ligated with absorbable 0 or 2-0 sutures (Figure 23-25, *B*).

The surgeon mobilizes the kidney pedicle, including the renal vessels, by sharp and blunt dissection (Figure 23-25, *C*). To ensure that the renal artery is occluded securely, the vessels are triple-clamped and suture ligatures are placed through each vessel. These vessels are then divided. The ligatures are not cut but are left long and tagged with a small hemostat to make sure that they are secure.

The surgeon then removes the kidney from the wound. All bleeding is controlled with the ESU. The pedicle ligatures are cut, and the wound is irrigated with warm saline.

Before closure the table break may be closed for easier tissue approximation.

A Penrose drain is placed in the kidney fossa and brought out through a separate stab wound. If a rib was removed, the periosteum may be closed separately. The incision is then closed in layers. The fascial and muscle layers are closed with interrupted absorbable sutures. The skin is closed with staples.

Kidney Transplant
SURGICAL GOAL

Kidney transplant is the removal of a kidney from a living donor or cadaver and implantation into the patient. Laparoscopic transplant allows more rapid recovery for both the recipient and the live donor.

PATHOLOGY

Kidney transplant is performed for acute or chronic end-stage renal failure. Ideally the donor is a close family member. Donors and recipients are matched as closely as possible via cross-matching and histocompatibility.

Technique   LIVING DONOR

1. A nephrectomy is performed as described above, except the renal pedicle (vascular supply) is isolated and ligated before the kidney is removed. Gerota's fascia is left intact on the donor kidney.
2. The ureter is divided to achieve maximum length.
3. The renal vessels are carefully dissected to preserve their length and viability.
4. After removal, the donor kidney is placed in cold saline solution. It is then flushed with electrolyte solution through a needle catheter.
5. The kidney and cold slush are covered with a sterile drape and transported by the surgeon to the recipient room.
6. The donor wound is closed.

Technique   RECIPIENT

1. The surgeon carries a right lower-quadrant incision through the abdominal wall.
2. The retroperitoneum is dissected.
3. The hypogastric artery is dissected to the internal iliac artery.
4. If necessary, the donor kidney is remodeled to accommodate the anastomosis.
5. The donor renal vein and artery are anastomosed to the recipient iliac vein.
6. An incision is made in the bladder wall.
7. The donor ureter is implanted in the bladder, and a catheter stent is placed from the implant site to the renal pelvis. The stent is brought through the urethra.
8. The bladder is closed.
9. The bladder is irrigated and observed for any leakage.
10. The wound is closed.

DISCUSSION

Performing kidney transplant requires skills in vascular, GU, and abdominal surgery. The procedure usually is performed by a transplant team, and routines are well estab-

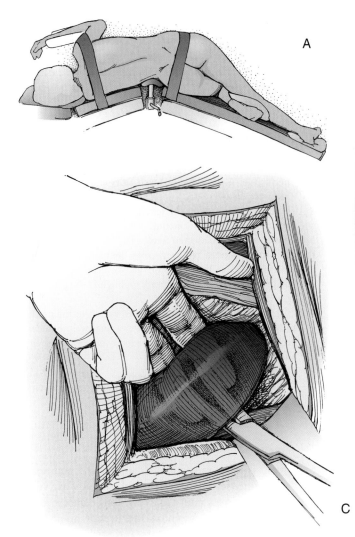

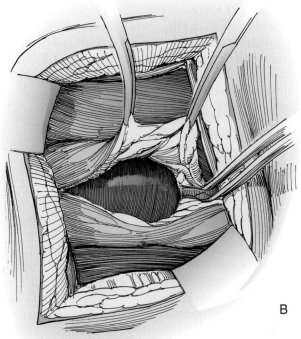

FIGURE 23-25
Simple nephrectomy. **A,** Patient is placed in kidney position. **B,** The ureter is identified on the peritoneal side of the wound. **C,** The pedicle is isolated by blunt dissection. (Adapted from Hinman F Jr: *Atlas of urologic surgery,* ed 2, Philadelphia, 1998, Saunders.)

lished. This discussion is limited to essential points in the procedure.

In this procedure, surgeons operate on the living donor and recipient simultaneously. However, the kidney can be perfused to preserve the organ.

The donor kidney is removed as described under the section on nephrectomy, with several major differences. The renal pedicle, which contains the vascular supply, is isolated and ligated before the kidney is removed. The other variation is that Gerota's fascia is left intact on the donor kidney.

After removal, the donor kidney is preserved in cold solution and perfused with the surgeon's choice of electrolyte solution. When the recipient team is ready to receive the kidney, the surgeon transports it in a covered container, maintaining the correct temperature. The donor wound is closed as previously described.

The recipient patient is prepped and draped for a right iliac incision. An incision is made in the right lower quadrant and carried to the retroperitoneum. A self-retaining retractor is placed in the wound. Vascular forceps and fine dissect-

ing scissors are used to mobilize the hypogastric artery to the level of the bifurcation of the aorta.

The internal iliac artery is divided after cross-clamping with a curved or angled vascular clamp. The proximal side of the artery remains clamped. The donor kidney then is brought to the field, and the vessels are trimmed as needed to accommodate the recipient structures. The kidney then is returned to cold solution until the surgeon is ready for implantation.

The internal iliac vein is cross-clamped, and a small incision is made between the clamps. Heparin solution is used to irrigate the vein. The incision is extended as needed to fit the donor renal vein, which is anastomosed via an end-to-side technique. Vascular sutures, size 6-0 or 5-0, are used. The renal artery then is anastomosed to the proximal arm of the iliac artery. The iliac artery clamps are removed, and the anastomosis is observed.

To begin ureteral implantation, the surgeon incises the anterior bladder. The donor ureter is then placed through the bladder wall, and the edges are anastomosed to the inner bladder lining with fine absorbable sutures.

A catheter stent is placed into the ureter through the anastomosis. It is advanced into the renal pelvis superiorly and brought out through the urethra inferiorly. The surgeon then closes the bladder incision in two layers, using 4-0 or 5-0 absorbable sutures for the bladder lining and 2-0 for the muscular layer. The bladder is irrigated to check for leakage. One or more suction drains are placed in the wound, which is closed in layers.

Adrenalectomy

SURGICAL GOAL

Adrenalectomy is removal of one or both adrenal glands.

PATHOLOGY

Excision of the adrenal gland is indicated for diseases such as pheochromocytoma, Cushing's syndrome, and hypersecretion of ACTH (adrenocorticotropic hormone). Hypersecretion of ACTH may cause neuroblastoma and affect other tumors whose growth depends on adrenal secretions. Adrenal diseases are often life threatening, and the procedure has many potential postoperative metabolic complications.

Technique

1. The surgeon enters the retroperitoneal space through a flank incision.
2. The transverse fascia is incised, and Gerota's fascia is identified.
3. The upper pole of the kidney is mobilized.
4. The blood supply to the adrenal gland is identified, clamped, ligated, and divided.
5. The gland is removed, and the wound is closed in layers.

DISCUSSION

The patient is placed in the lateral position, prepped, and draped for a flank incision as previously discussed. The adrenal glands also may be approached from an abdominal posterior incision or through laparoscopy, which is typically used for adrenalectomy.

The surgeon enters the flank and places a self-retaining retractor in the wound. Gerota's fascia and the perirenal fat are identified. Babcock clamps are used to grasp the adrenal gland and upper pole of the kidney to prevent tearing of the tissue. Using dissecting scissors and the ESU, the surgeon isolates the blood vessels supplying the gland. These are individually clamped, divided, and ligated with suture ties or with hemostatic clamps.

The adrenal gland lies in contact with the vena cava. The circulator should have vascular suture available in the room to repair the vena cava in case it is inadvertently nicked during dissection.

When the vascular supply has been occluded, the gland is removed. The wound is irrigated and closed as previously described for a flank incision.

Cystectomy

SURGICAL GOAL

Cystectomy is total or partial removal of the bladder. This procedure is performed most often to treat bladder cancer.

PATHOLOGY

Total cystectomy is indicated for small invasive tumors that penetrate the bladder wall. A more conservative partial cystectomy may be performed when there is no involvement of the lymph nodes.

Technique

1. The surgeon performs a laparotomy through a lower midline incision.
2. The urachus is divided.
3. The bladder is dissected on each side, and major blood vessels are ligated.
4. The bladder (uterus in the female) is elevated to expose the cul-de-sac and peritoneum.
5. The rectal wall is dissected free.
6. The rectum is retracted away from the bladder and male accessory organs. The lateral bladder pedicles are divided.
7. The prostate is dissected from the pubis, and the prostatic ligaments are divided.
8. In the female, the broad ligament is incised to the ovary and fallopian tubes. The posterior vaginal wall, bladder neck, and proximal urethra will be removed with the specimen.
9. The vagina is closed.
10. The urethra is isolated and clamped, and the specimen is removed.
11. A urinary diversion procedure is performed.

DISCUSSION

If the patient is male, prostatic instruments are required. A major laparotomy set is used. The scrub should have vessel loops, umbilical tapes, and a narrow, long Penrose drain available to retract and mobilize the ureters, urethra, or other structures. Sponge dissectors and stick sponges are typically used.

The patient is placed in the supine or lithotomy position. The abdomen and perineum are prepped, depending on the position and the surgeon's technique.

To begin the surgery, the surgeon makes a midline or lower midline incision. The urachus (fibromuscular attachment at the umbilicus) is clamped and divided. A self-retaining retractor is placed in the wound, and the bowel is packed away from the bladder. If a lateral approach to the bladder is used, the duodenum and colon are packed to one side. The bladder is elevated to begin dissection. Each side (lateral pedicle) of the bladder is dissected separately. The internal iliac artery is identified, ligated, and divided. Branches also are ligated. Right-angle clamps often are used to pass suture ties under vessels during the dissection. The scrub should have a variety of sizes available. Heavy silk sutures or vascular clips are typically used to occlude the vessels. In the male, the vas deferens is divided with the urethra.

The bladder is retracted upward, and the peritoneum is incised. The anterior rectal wall is dissected free from the bladder. This exposes the seminal vesicles and prostate in the male, or the posterior vaginal wall in the female. The lateral pedicles of the bladder are mobilized, divided, and ligated with silk sutures or surgical clips. In the female patient, the broad ligament is excised to the level of the ovary and fallopian tubes. The surgeon separates the posterior vaginal wall from the bladder using blunt dissection. The vaginal vault is closed after the excision.

The anterior dissection continues with dissection of the prostate away from the pubis. The ESU is used frequently to control small vessels that communicate with the prostate. The ESU tip must be kept clean. During the later stages of the dissection, the ESU is used often.

The urethra is isolated with vessel loop or umbilical tape, clamped, and divided. The remaining fascia attachments are released, and the specimen is removed. A urinary diversion surgery is initiated. Major steps of the procedure are illustrated in Figure 23-26.

Ileal Conduit
SURGICAL GOAL
Ileal conduit is a procedure in which a functional bladder is constructed with a loop of bowel that is brought out of the abdominal wall. A stoma is created for urine drainage.

PATHOLOGY
Urinary diversion away from the bladder is performed most often after radical cystectomy in which the bladder and surrounding tissue have been removed as treatment for cancer. Other reasons include neurogenic bladder and severe stricture of the distal ureters.

Technique
1. The surgeon mobilizes a portion of the colon and ileum.
2. The surgeon resects and anastomoses the ileum using traditional bowel technique or stapling instruments.
3. The surgeon closes the proximal ileal segment using a two-layer technique.

4. The mesentery is closed.
5. The distal and proximal sections of the functional ileum are anastomosed.
6. The ureters are divided from the bladder.
7. Each ureter is implanted into the ileal pouch.
8. The surgeon creates the stoma by incising a circular disk of abdominal wall. The stoma is created at a predetermined location below the patient's belt line.
9. The distal arm of the ileal segment is brought through the circular incision.
10. The exteriorized ileum is modeled into a stoma.
11. A suction wound drain is placed in the abdominal cavity, and the wound is closed in layers.

DISCUSSION
Many of the techniques used in this procedure are discussed in Chapter 21. In preparation for the procedure, the scrub should have gastrointestinal and long instruments available.

The patient is placed in supine position, and a Foley catheter is inserted. The patient then is prepped and draped for an abdominal incision. To begin the procedure, the surgeon enters the abdomen and retroperitoneal cavity. A Balfour retractor is placed in the wound. A portion of the large intestine and adjoining ileum are mobilized, as for a bowel resection.

Four intestinal clamps are placed across a segment of the ileum, two at each end. The surgeon then divides the ileum in both locations, cutting between the sets of clamps with the ESU or knife. The proximal end of the ileum is closed with a double layer of chromic gut or absorbable synthetic suture. A linear stapling instrument also may be used to resect the proximal limb of the ileum. The two severed ileal limbs are then reanastomosed.

The surgeon identifies the ureters and may place a small Penrose drain around them for retraction. The ureters are

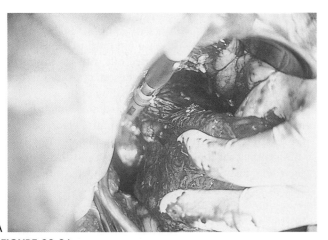 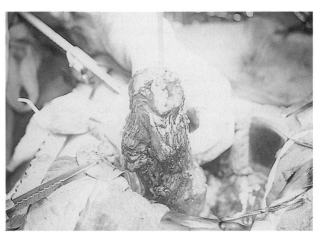

FIGURE 23-26
Cystectomy. **A,** The vesical arteries are clip ligated. **B,** Surgical specimen consisting of the bladder, distal ureters, prostate, seminal vesicles, and distal vas deferens is removed en bloc. (From Nagle GM: *Genitourinary surgery: perioperative nursing series,* St Louis, 1997, Mosby.)

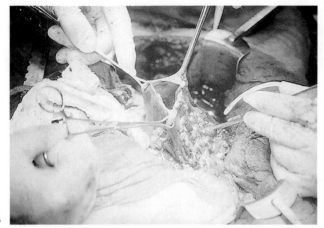 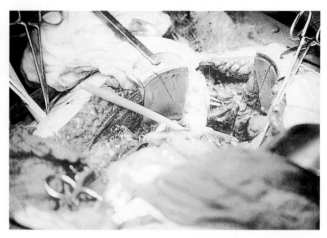

FIGURE 23-27
Ileal conduit. **A,** The ileal segment is opened. **B,** Ureteral stents are left in the stoma. (From Nagle GM: *Genitourinary surgery: perioperative nursing series,* St Louis, 1997, Mosby.)

divided from the bladder, and an end-to-side anastomosis is made between the ureters and the isolated segment of the ileum. The anastomosis is performed with interrupted sutures of 4-0 absorbable material.

To perform the ileostomy, the surgeon first incises the skin over the area of the proposed stoma, taking a small disk of tissue from the abdominal wall. The open end of the ileal segment is then brought through the hole and everted. The edge of the stoma is sutured to the abdominal wall with interrupted absorbable sutures, size 3-0. The wound is then irrigated, and a suction drain is placed in the abdomen. Closure is routine as described for a laparotomy. This procedure is illustrated in Figure 23-27.

Ureteral Reimplantation
SURGICAL GOAL
Reconstructive operations of the ureter are performed to repair forms of renal obstruction and thus avoid subsequent renal failure.

PATHOLOGY
Renal obstructions can have various causes, including congenital malformations, stasis, and metabolic imbalances. The type of obstruction dictates the type of procedure required:

▶ Ureterostomy: Procedure that opens the ureter for continued drainage into another part of the body.
▶ Cutaneous ureterostomy: Procedure that routes the flow of urine from the kidney, through the ureter, away from the bladder, and out the skin of the abdomen through a stoma.
▶ Ureterectomy: Complete removal of the ureter, the kidney, and a portion of the bladder cuff.
▶ Ureteroureterostomy: Segmented resection of a diseased portion of the ureter with reconstruction of the continuity of the ureter.
▶ Ureteroenterostomy: Diversion of the ureter into a segment of the ileum or sigmoid colon

Conditions that require reconstruction of the urinary tract include malignancy, stricture, trauma, and cystitis.

Technique

1. Patient positioning and the site of the incision depend on the proposed surgery.
2. The surgeon exposes the ureter through the desired incision site.
3. The ureter is mobilized and severed at the desired level.
4. The distal end is ligated, and the proximal stoma is anastomosed to the appropriate site dictated by the procedure. Fine nonabsorbable sutures are used.
5. A soft splinting stent may be placed until free drainage is ensured.
6. The wound is closed in layers and dressed as per routine.

DISCUSSION
Depending on the procedure to be performed, the patient may be placed in a supine position for abdominal access to the ureter, modified Trendelenburg position for low abdominal or pelvic procedures, or lateral position for high or mid-ureteral procedures.

Hypothermia is sometimes useful during prolonged renal surgeries to extend the safe period of renal ischemia during manipulation. This can be carried out with ice slush, cold saline, surface cooling coils, perfusion of cold solutions through the renal atery, or a combination of these.

When the ureter has been identified and mobilized, the surgeon secures it with fine traction sutures before severing it so as not to lose it in the surrounding anatomy.

Depending on the size of the patient and the approach taken, long instrumentation is recommended for these procedures.

Suprapubic Prostatectomy
SURGICAL GOAL
In this procedure, the prostate gland is removed through a suprapubic incision.

PATHOLOGY

Prostatectomy is performed to treat benign prostatic hypertrophy and for cancer of the prostate. Inguinal nodes may be removed for diagnosis of metastasis.

Technique

1. The surgeon incises the bladder.
2. The prostatic mucosa is incised.
3. The prostate is removed.
4. A suprapubic catheter is inserted.
5. The bladder is closed.

DISCUSSION

The patient is placed in the supine position. Shoulder braces may be required if the patient will be tipped into Trendelenburg position. A Foley catheter is inserted before the prep. The patient is prepped and draped for a suprapubic incision.

The surgeon makes a transverse or longitudinal suprapubic incision into the space of Retzius. A self-retaining retractor is placed in the wound. Two traction sutures or Allis clamps are placed in the bladder wall, and an incision is made between them. The bladder edges are then grasped with Allis clamps and retracted upward. The scrub should have suction available to drain the bladder. A Judd or Deaver retractor is placed in the bladder, and the prostatic mucosa is incised with the ESU. The bladder retractors are then removed.

Using his or her fingers, the surgeon **enucleates** the prostate. In this technique, the tissue is removed en bloc without trauma to the fossa or bed of the tissue. The bladder retractors are replaced, and the wound is checked for bleeding. The fossa may be packed with sponges to secure hemostasis. Large bleeding vessels are ligated with suture ligatures of 2-0 or 0 absorbable material. Capillary bleeding is controlled with hemostatic agents such as Surgicel, Avitene, or Gelfoam. A Malecot or Pezzer catheter is placed in the wound and brought out through a small stab incision near the wound edge. The bladder is then closed in two layers with absorbable sutures. The wound is irrigated, and a wound drain is placed in the cavity. The incision then is closed in layers. Figure 23-28 illustrates the procedure.

Retropubic Prostatectomy
SURGICAL GOAL

Refer to the section on suprapubic prostatectomy.

PATHOLOGY

Refer to the section on suprapubic prostatectomy.

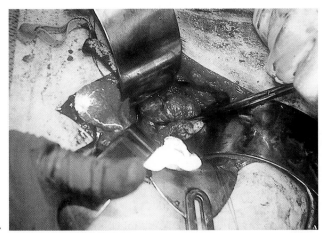

A

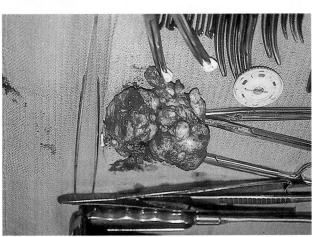

C

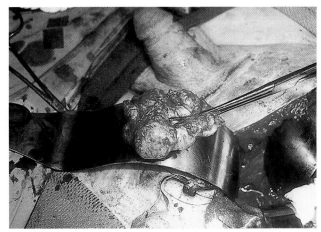

B

FIGURE 23-28
Suprapubic prostatectomy. **A,** The mucosa of the adenoma is incised. **B,** The adenoma is excised. **C,** The prostatic adenoma is removed. (From Nagle GM: *Genitourinary surgery: perioperative nursing series*, St Louis, 1997, Mosby.)

1. The surgeon makes a transverse abdominal incision.
2. The surgeon enters the space of Retzius.
3. The anterior surface of the prostate is exposed.
4. The prostatic capsule is incised.
5. The prostate is dissected free.
6. The wound is closed.

DISCUSSION

The patient is placed in the supine position, prepped, and draped as for a suprapubic prostatectomy. In the retropubic approach, however, the bladder is not entered for access to the prostate.

A low transverse pelvic incision is made and carried to the space of Retzius as previously described. A Balfour retractor is placed in the wound. Before incising the prostatic capsule, the surgeon may place two traction sutures through the capsule. The capsule is then excised between the sutures with the ESU, and the incision is extended with Metzenbaum scissors. The gland is then removed from the capsule with sharp and blunt dissection. Bleeding is controlled with the ESU and hemostatic agents. Before closing the wound, the surgeon inserts a Foley catheter with a 30-ml balloon. A large Penrose drain is placed in the space of Retzius, and the wound is then closed in layers.

Perineal Prostatectomy
SURGICAL GOAL

Perineal prostatectomy is the removal of prostatic adenoma through a perineal approach.

PATHOLOGY

The perineal approach is appropriate for open prostatic biopsy for diagnosis. Radical excision then can be performed if a confirmation of cancer returns from pathology.

1. The patient is placed in an exaggerated lithotomy position with the legs well above the pelvis and the buttocks extended several inches over the edge of the bed. A large bump or bolster is placed under the sacrum to bring the perineum as parallel as possible with the operating room bed.
2. A Lowsley traction device is passed through the urethra and into the bladder, and held by the assistant. This pushes the prostate down toward the perineum.
3. The incision is an inverted-**U** from one ischial tuberosity to the other.
4. Three to four Allis clamps are placed on the edge of the incision and retracted downward over the anal drape.
5. The surgeon carries the incision through subcutaneous tissue using electrocautery. The central tendon is isolated, clamped, and cut distal to the external anal sphincter.
6. The rectourethral muscle is cut from the central tendon and pushed downward.
7. The levator ani muscle is exposed and retracted laterally.

8. The prostate gland then is exposed.
9. Biopsies are taken and sent to pathology for frozen section confirmation. If negative, the adenoma is removed. If the specimen shows signs of malignancy, a radical prostatectomy may be performed.
10. If a simple adenoma enucleation is all that is required, the capsule to the prostate is incised. The Lowsley retractor is removed, the urethra is divided, and a Young prostatic retractor is inserted.
11. The Young retractor blades are opened, drawing the prostate down, and the adenoma is manually enucleated from the surgical capsule.
12. A 22-Fr Foley catheter with a 30-ml balloon is inserted through the urethra into the bladder.
13. Bleeding is controlled with suture or electrocautery.
14. The capsulotomy incision is repaired with a continuous 2-0 absorbable suture.
15. A drain is left in place at the level of the capsulotomy incision.
16. The subcutaneous tissue is closed with 3-0 absorbable suture, and the skin is closed with 4-0 absorbable suture. The wound is dressed according to the surgeon's preference.

DISCUSSION

Advantages of this procedure include preservation of the bladder neck, improved urethrovesical anastomosis, and easier control of bleeding.

Positioning for this procedure requires special draping to cover the legs and allow access to the anus. A TURP pack with extra three-quarter sheets to wrap the legs works well.

The bladder is drained before the Lowsley retractor is inserted into the bladder.

The technologist should have plenty of Surgilube or K-Y lubricant on the field for the catheters, along with Lowsley and Young prostatic retractors.

The urethra is reapproximated with 2-0 interrupted sutures.

A perineal Bookwalter retractor designed specifically for this procedure is available, and it gives very adequate exposure for such a small wound.

See Figure 23-29, *A-C*, for photos of this procedure.

Suprapubic Cystostomy
SURGICAL GOAL

Suprapubic cystostomy is the placement of a suprapubic catheter into the bladder for drainage. A suprapubic catheter is used when a urethral catheter is undesirable, as in the event of a urethral stricture. A suprapubic catheter is more comfortable for the patient than a urethral catheter and may be used when urinary diversion is required for a long period of time.

1. The surgeon enters the space of Retzius.
2. The bladder is incised.

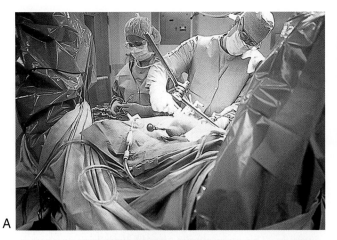

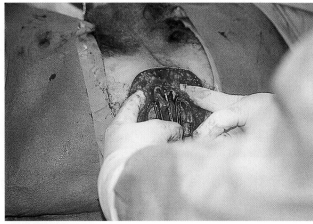

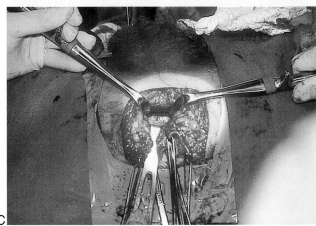

FIGURE 23-29
Perineal prostatectomy. **A,** A Lowsley retractor is placed in the male urethra. **B,** The superficial perineal fascia is exposed. **C,** The central tendon is exposed. (From Nagle GM: *Genitourinary surgery: perioperative nursing series,* St Louis, 1997, Mosby.)

3. The catheter is positioned in the bladder.
4. The bladder is closed.
5. The wound is closed.

DISCUSSION

The patient is placed in the supine position, prepped, and draped for a suprapubic incision. This area lies just above the pubic symphysis. The incision passes through the skin, fatty subcutaneous layer, fascia, and muscle fibers. The peritoneal cavity is *not* entered, because the area lying between the bladder and the symphysis pubis (the space of Retzius, which is the operative site) is bounded superiorly (at the top) by the abdominal peritoneum. Because the muscle fibers are quite vascular and contain many large veins, the technologist should have an ample supply of lap sponges available. The surgeon makes the incision with the scalpel and carries it through to the bladder with the cautery pencil or dissecting scissors.

The surgeon places two Allis clamps on the bladder wall and makes a small incision between the clamps. A purse-string suture then is placed around the bladder incision, and the catheter is threaded into the bladder. Malecot or Pezzer catheters are usually used. The purse-string suture is tied snugly around the catheter, and the bladder incision is closed with in-

terrupted sutures of size 0 or 2-0 chromic gut swaged to a tapered needle. The suprapubic incision then is closed in layers.

An alternative method of suprapubic colostomy uses a Silastic catheter that is placed in the bladder through a stab wound made in the skin over and through the bladder wall. A Cystocath catheter (made by Dow Corning Wright, Arlington, TN) is usually used. To insert the catheter, the surgeon makes a small stab incision using a #11 knife blade. The Cystocath kit comes complete with a trocar and cannula, which are thrust through the stab incision. The trocar then is removed, and the catheter is inserted through the cannula. The surgeon removes the cannula and places a special Silastic disk over the catheter and glues it to the patient's skin with surgical adhesive. The wound is neither sutured nor dressed.

Vesicourethral Suspension of the Bladder
SURGICAL GOAL
Suspension of the bladder is performed to treat urinary stress incontinence in the female caused by reduction in the angle at the urethrovesical junction. This procedure is commonly performed with the laparoscope.

PATHOLOGY
In the female, the bladder and the posterior urethra (urethrovesical junction) normally form a 90-degree to 100-

degree angle. During voiding, the angle is reduced as the bladder empties. Loss of muscle tone associated with childbirth, age, and surgery can cause the angle to become increasingly reduced, resulting in displacement of the neck of the bladder. This causes intermittent loss of urine, especially during straining activity.

Technique

1. The surgeon enters the space of Retzius through a low transverse abdominal incision.
2. The bladder is retracted downward and the bladder neck grasped with long Allis clamps.
3. Interrupted sutures are placed through the bladder neck and attached to the cartilage of the symphysis.
4. The wound is closed.

DISCUSSION

The patient is placed in the supine position, and a Foley catheter is inserted. She is prepped and draped for a suprapubic incision. The scrub should have long general surgical instruments available, including long needle holders and Allis clamps.

After entering the space of Retzius, the surgeon begins the procedure by manually retracting the bladder upward. This exposes the urethra. The surgeon then grasps the bladder neck with several long Allis clamps. Several interrupted heavy absorbable sutures are then placed through the tissue surrounding the urethra. The needle is passed through the cartilage attached to the symphysis. Several of these sutures are placed in succession. The wound is then closed in layers.

Vesicourethral Suspension (Marshall-Marchetti-Krantz Procedure)
SURGICAL GOAL

Vesicourethral suspension (Marshall-Marchetti-Krantz procedure) is a suspension of the bladder neck and urethra to the cartilage of the pubic symphysis to treat urinary stress incontinence in the female. The patient with urinary stress incontinence experiences urine leakage while straining in such activities as coughing, laughing, or bending.

Technique

1. The surgeon enters the space of Retzius.
2. The bladder neck and urethra are sutured to the symphysis.
3. The wound is closed.

DISCUSSION

Before the procedure begins, the circulator places a Foley catheter in the patient's bladder. The patient is placed in the supine position, prepped, and draped for a suprapubic incision. The technologist should have long instruments available, including long needle holders and long Allis clamps.

After entering the space of Retzius, the surgeon begins the procedure by placing his or her hand over the bladder to retract it upward. This exposes the urethra. The surgeon may grasp the bladder neck with several long Allis clamps. Several interrupted sutures of Dexon or Dacron, size 2-0, mounted on a small, stout, tapered needle, are then placed through the tissue surrounding the urethra. The needle is passed through the cartilage attached to the symphysis. Several of these sutures are placed in succession. The sutures are left long. The assistant is then required to place a finger in the vagina to release the pressure on the sutures while the surgeon ties them in place. After this maneuver, the scrub must, of course, reglove the assistant. This completes the procedure. A large Penrose drain is placed in the space of Retzius, and the wound is closed in routine fashion.

This procedure is illustrated in Figure 23-30.

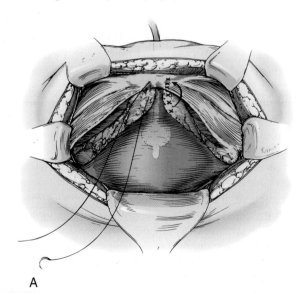

A

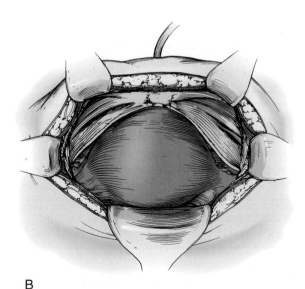

B

FIGURE 23-30
Vesicourethral suspension. **A,** Suture is placed for Marshall-Marchetti-Krantz procedure. **B,** The vaginal wall is approximated to retrosymphysis. (Adapted from Walsh PC, Retik AB, Vaughan ED, et al: *Campbell's urology*, ed 8, Philadelphia, 2002, Saunders.)

Suburethral Sling

SURGICAL GOAL

In the suburethral sling (pubovaginal sling), a graft strip of fascia lata or synthetic material is placed between the urethra and the anterior vaginal wall to treat women with severe urinary stress incontinence.

PATHOLOGY

This procedure is indicated for women who may have been unsuccessfully treated for incontinence by traditional elevation and stabilization procedures. Candidates for this procedure often are diagnosed upon examination with a partial or total opening of the urethral sphincter at rest. This causes the patient to have severe urinary incontinence. Candidates for this procedure often are patients who have prior conditions such as pelvic trauma, corrective bladder suspension surgery, injury from radiological treatment, neurological injury, congenital tissue weakness, obesity, and chronic pulmonary disease.

Technique

1. The surgeon uses a lower transverse incision and blunt dissection to expose lateral rectus muscle.
2. The surgeon makes a bilateral excision of the anterior vaginal mucosa lateral to the urethra.
3. An anterior vaginal-wall flap is raised.
4. The dissection continues to the pubic bone bilaterally.
5. The pubic bone is drilled bilaterally to create a defect for anchoring of suture.
6. The graft is measured and positioned.
7. A cystoscopy is performed to assess proper tension of the graft for urinary continence.
8. The graft is sutured into place.
9. A suprapubic catheter is inserted.
10. The abdominal and vaginal incisions are closed.

NOTE

The suburethral (pubovaginal) sling procedure (Figure 23-31) requires a graft strip of fascia lata or a synthetic material such as Gore-Tex to be placed in the patient. The graft of fascia lata may be an allograft or an autograft. An autograft is fascia lata removed from the patient's own fascia by either of two different ways. In the abdominal approach, the rectus fascia is removed laterally from one iliac crest to the other through a Pfannenstiel incision. The fascia also may be removed in the lateral thigh through two vertical incisions mid-thigh and above the knee. The graft is dissected out through a tunnel created between the two incision sites.

The allograft may be freeze dried or fresh frozen fascia lata obtained from a cadaver. Fresh frozen fascia lata is the preferred material for repairbecause it produces a stronger repair with minimal dissection and a faster recovery time than an autograft or synthetic material. If an allograft is used, the patient may have the procedure performed on an outpatient basis, but if an autograft is used, the patient may need to be hospitalized for up to 3 days for postoperative pain management.

This procedure requires the graft to be attached to the pubic bone, so in addition to the normal instrumentation required for cystoscopic and bladder-suspension procedures, the scrub will need to have a power drill and anchoring system such as Mitek available on the back table for the surgeon's use.

DISCUSSION

The patient is anesthetized and placed in the lithotomy position with Allen stirrups. A lower abdominal and vaginal prep is performed. If a fascia lata autograft is to be obtained from the thigh, a separate set-up for prepping, draping, and instrumentation will be needed for the operative leg. The patient is draped with lithotomy drapes. A cystoscopy is performed, and a Foley catheter is inserted.

The labia majora are sutured laterally for retraction purposes with a silk suture. An Auvard weighted vaginal speculum is inserted, and localanesthetic with epinephrine is injected into the lower abdominal incision site and the vaginal mucosa to maintain hemostasis.

A lower transverse incision is made just above the symphysis pubis. The tissue is spread by blunt dissection to expose the anterior rectus muscle. The incision is then packed with sponges moistened with an antibiotic solution.

The surgeon then performs the vaginal portion of the procedure. The surgeon inserts a Foley catheter into the urethra and measures the length of the urethral meatus by placing the Foley catheter and inflating the balloon at the internal vesical neck. The surgeon marks, deflates, and removes the catheter. The balloon on the catheter is then reinflated, and a measurement is taken from the meatal mark to the balloon. After the measurement is taken, the balloon is again deflated, and the catheter is reinserted in the patient.

To create space for the sling, the surgeon bilaterally incises the anterior vaginal mucosa lateral to the urethra, raises the vaginal mucosa flap, and continues dissection to expose the pubic bone bilaterally. The surgeon perforates the endopelvic fascia and enters the retropubic space. The power drill is used to create defects (small holes) in the pubic bone bilaterally to assist in the anchoring of the Mitek suture. After the drill has created the defects, the sutures are anchored to the site; this anchoring technique causes the sutures to be embedded in the pubic bone.

A Stamey needle is passed through one of the vaginal incisions to the pubic bone. The free end of the Mitek suture is threaded, and the needle is passed parallel to the posterior symphysis pubis. The needle is guided through the fascia and periurethral tissues along the bladder neck. The Foley catheter is again removed, and a cystoscope is used to check the position of the needle. The same process is followed at the other vaginal incision site. The free end of the Mitek suture then is sutured to one end of the graft. The Stamey needle then is used to pass the graft to the pubic site. The graft

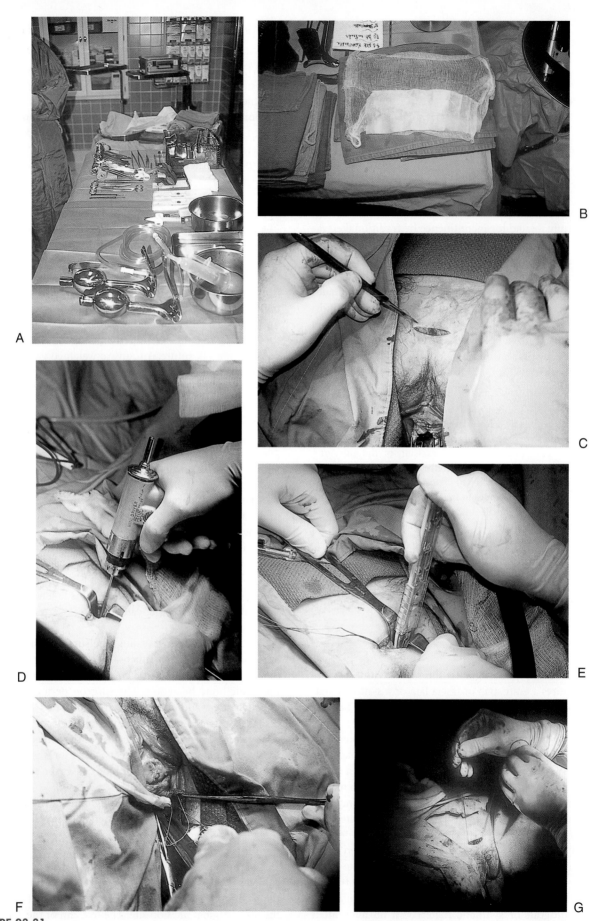

FIGURE 23-31
Suburethral sling. **A,** Back table set-up for suburethral sling. **B,** Fresh frozen fascia lata graft. **C,** Transverse midline abdominal incision at the upper border of the symphysis pubis. **D,** Power drill used to create defects in the pubic bone to assist in the anchoring of the Mitek suture. **E,** The Mitek suture is anchored into the pubic bone. **F,** The free end of the graft is passed between the urethra and the vaginal mucosa. **G,** The tension of the graft is tested for the ability to stop the urinary stream from above.
(From Nagle GM: *Genitourinary surgery: perioperative nursing series,* St Louis, 1997, Mosby.)

is then sutured to the pubic tubercle or paraurethral fascia. The free end of the graft is passed between the urethra and vaginal mucosa (Figure 23-31, *F*). The surgeon then determines the length of the graft while the assistant secures the abdominal end of the graft. The surgeon places the free end of the graft into the opposite vaginal wound. The excess graft is excised, and the process is repeated for the other side. The tension of the graft (ability to stop the urinary flow) is checked before the sling is sutured in place (Figure 23-31, *G*). The surgeon performs this step with the cystoscope and by inflating the bladder with fluid. The surgeon may directly visualize the flow of urine, and as the assistant applies tension and pulls the suture upward, the flow of urine should stop. The surgeon then sutures the graft in place on one side through the suprapubic incision, uses the cystoscope again, fills the bladder with fluid, and repeats the tension testing of urine flow before the opposite side of the graft is sutured in place. A suprapubic catheter is inserted while the bladder is still full of fluid. The abdominal incision is closed with an absorbable suture. The vaginal mucosa is closed with an absorbable suture, and a packing coated with sulfa cream is inserted into the vagina.

REFERENCES

Hinman F Jr: *Atlas of urologic surgery,* ed 2, Philadelphia, 1998, Saunders.

Nagle GM: *Genitourinary surgery: perioperative nursing series,* St Louis, 1997, Mosby.

Walsh PC, Retik AB, Vaughan ED, et al: *Campbell's urology,* ed 8, Philadelphia, 2002, Saunders.

Chapter 24

Ophthalmic Surgery

By Mary Grace Hensel

Learning Objectives

After studying this chapter the reader will be able to:

- Analyze and explain the psychological effects and considerations of having eye surgery
- Practice safe procedures and techniques in eye surgery
- Describe the anatomy of the eye
- Explain how to prepare the microscope for use and care for it properly
- Name and recognize commonly used eye instruments
- Differentiate the types of ophthalmic drugs and their uses

Terminology

Aqueous humor—Clear, watery fluid that fills the anterior and posterior chambers in the front of the eye.

Bridle suture—A traction suture placed in tissue and used to retract or maintain tension on the tissue.

Buckling component—Silicone bolster that encircles the eye.

Capsulorrhexis—Derived from the Greek word "rhexis," meaning a bursting, a rupture, or a tearing. This is a surgical technique used in cataract extraction when the capsule of the cataract is torn, and a complete capsulotomy is performed.

Cataract—A condition in which the crystalline lens of the eye, its capsule, or both become opaque, with consequent loss of vision.

Choroid—The vascular, intermediate tissue layer that provides nourishment to the other parts of the interior eye.

Conformer—A device placed in the socket after enucleation or evisceration to preserve the shape of the fornices.

Conjunctiva—The mucous membrane that lines the eyelids and covers the front of the eyeball.

Cryotherapy—A technique whereby an instrument or cryoprobe is used to freeze tissue such as the sclera, ciliary body (for glaucoma), or retinal layers after detachment. The cryoprobe also can be used to remove an opaque lens during intracapsular cataract removal.

Diathermy—Low-power cautery used to mark the sclera over the area of the retinal detachment.

Enucleation—Surgical removal of the eyeball after the eye muscles and optic nerve have been severed.

Evisceration—Surgical removal of the contents of the eyeball, with the sclera left intact.

Exenteration—Removal of the entire contents of the orbit.

Glaucoma—A localized eye disease characterized by increased sustained intraocular pressure that causes damage to the eye.

Globe—The eyeball.

Hydroxyapatite implant—A porous implant made of calcium phosphate and a naturally occurring body substance that is coupled to an artificial eye with a peg.

Keratoplasty—Corneal transplant surgery.

Phacoemulsification—A process whereby high-frequency waves are used to emulsify tissue, such as a cataract. The dissolved tissue then can be removed by aspiration.

Posterior chamber—The fluid-filled space between the back of the iris and the front of the lens.

Pterygium—A triangular membrane that arises from the medial canthus and that can extend over the cornea, causing blindness.

Trabeculectomy—Surgical removal of a portion of the trabeculum to improve outflow of aqueous in glaucoma patients.

Vitreous humor—A transparent, colorless gel that normally fills the eyeball in front of the retina.

INTRODUCTION TO OPHTHALMIC SURGERY

The goal of ophthalmic surgery is to restore vision lost from disease, injury, or congenital defect and to produce good cosmetic effect. Eye procedures are delicate and precise. In most cases, surgeons prefer that talking and movement be kept to an absolute minimum during surgery. The patient about to undergo eye surgery may need extra comfort and emotional support if he or she is partially blind. Because most eye procedures are performed under a local anesthetic, the patient's physical comfort is of utmost importance. The technologist and nurse should pay strict attention to the position of the patient on the operating table to ensure that he or she does not become restless because of discomfort during the procedure.

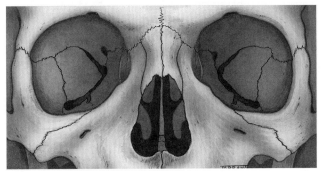

FIGURE 24-1
Anterior view of the bony orbit. (From Tyers AG and Collin JRO: *Colour atlas of ophthalmic plastic surgery*, ed 2, Oxford, 2001, Butterworth-Heinemann.)

ANATOMY OF THE EYE

External Structures of the Eye

The external structures of the eye include the bony orbit, the ocular muscles, the eyelids, the **conjunctiva,** and the lacrimal apparatus.

THE BONY ORBIT

The bony orbit (also called the orbital cavity) houses the eye. It is situated in the front of the skull within the frontal bone (Figure 24-1). The cavity is lined with fatty tissue to cushion the eye. Although most of the orbit is composed of thin bone tissue, the rim is particularly thick and therefore more protective.

THE OCULAR MUSCLES

Six muscles attached to the sclera and the bony orbit move the eyeball around various axes and allow both eyes to focus on a single point. Each eye contains four *rectus* muscles. These are the superior, inferior, lateral, and medial rectus muscles. There are also two *oblique* muscles, the superior and inferior. These are illustrated in Figure 24-2.

THE EYELIDS

The eyelids are two plates of fibrous connective tissue that are covered with skin (Figure 24-3). The lids open and close over the eye to protect it from injury and light. The space or interval between the upper and lower lids is called the *palpebral fissure*. Each juncture of the eyelids is called the *canthus*. The medial canthus is closest to the nasal bridge. The lateral canthus is opposite. At the medial canthus lies a small pink mass of tissue called the *lacrimal caruncle*. This tissue contains glands that secrete sebaceous material that causes the lids to become airtight when closed. The *tarsal plate* extends

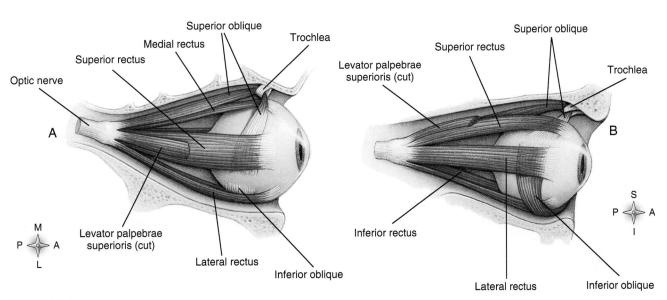

FIGURE 24-2
Muscles of the right eye. **A,** Superior view. **B,** Lateral view. (From Thibodeau GA and Patton KT: *Anatomy and physiology*, ed 5, St Louis, 2003, Mosby.)

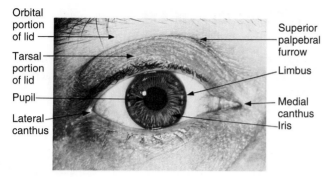

FIGURE 24-3
The eyelid. (From Stein HA, Slatt BJ, and Stein RM: *The ophthalmic assistant: a guide for ophthalmic medical personnel,* ed 7, St Louis, 2000, Mosby.)

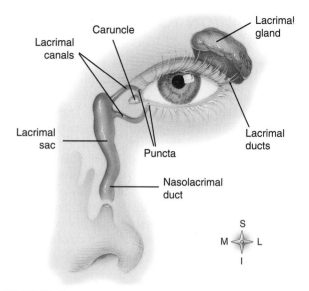

FIGURE 24-4
Lacrimal apparatus. (From Thibodeau GA and Patton KT: *Anatomy and physiology,* ed 5, St Louis, 2003, Mosby.)

along the free edge of the eyelid. This consists of dense fibrous tissue that gives the eyelids their characteristic shape. The *eyelashes,* which extend along the tarsus, protect the eye from dust and other pollutants.

CONJUNCTIVA

The conjunctiva is a thin transparent mucous membrane that lines each eyelid and covers the sclera. The conjunctiva is divided into palpebral and bulbar parts. The portion of the conjunctiva that lines the inside surfaces of the lids is called the *palpebral conjunctiva.* The palpebral conjunctiva appears red in color because of the vascularity of the eyelids. The bulbar conjunctiva covers the anterior portion of the optic globe up to the junction of the sclera and cornea. The bulbar conjunctiva appears white because the sclera is located behind it. An additional layer of mucous membrane covers the eyeball itself.

THE LACRIMAL APPARATUS

The lacrimal apparatus is the eye's tear system (Figure 24-4). It is composed of several parts. The lacrimal gland, located within the frontal bone at each angle of the orbit, secretes tears. The gland contains about 12 separate ducts, which supply tears to the conjunctiva. The lacrimal ducts extend from the inner canthus to the lacrimal sac. The opening of each duct is called the lacrimal punctum. The lacrimal sac is a large opening at the upper end of the nasolacrimal duct, which is a passageway between the lacrimal sac and the inferior meatus of the nose.

Internal Structures of the Eye
EXTERNAL LAYERS OF THE EYEBALL

The eyeball contains several outer protective layers (Figure 24-5). These layers are the sclera, cornea, ciliary body, **choroid,** and iris. The *sclera* is a thick, white fibrous tissue that encompasses about three fourths of the eyeball. It is the external supportive structure of the eyeball and is continuous with the cornea, which covers the front of the eye.

The *cornea* is a fine, transparent membrane that covers the front of the eyeball. This layer contains no blood vessels and is the tissue that refracts light rays as they enter the eye.

The choroid layer is situated beneath the sclera and is a vascular, darkly pigmented tissue. The primary function of the choroid is to prevent the reflection of light within the eyeball. An extension of the choroid layer, the *ciliary body,* is located at the periphery of the anterior portion of the choroid. It consists of smooth muscle tissue to which suspensory ligaments are attached. These ligaments hold the lens in place. In addition, the ciliary processes, which are folds of tissue that attach to the internal portion of the ciliary body on the anterior side, produce **aqueous humor.** This fluid fills the anterior chamber of the eye.

The *iris* or colored part of the eye is a pigmented contractile membrane composed mainly of muscle tissue. The iris is circular and contains a flat bar of muscular fibers surrounding the pupil. The actions of these muscular fibers can cause the pupil to close or open, to exclude light or admit light into the inner eye. The *pupil* lies at the center of the iris and may appear dilated or constricted according to the action of the iris.

RETINA

The inner layer of the eye is called the *retina* (see Figure 24-5). This is the so-called photoreceptive layer of the eye. It lies on the inside posterior wall of the eyeball. The retina receives images and transmits them to the brain for interpretation. Light is projected onto the retina through the front of the eye; the retina then converts the light into nervous impulses and transmits them to the brain, creating sight.

THE ANTERIOR AND POSTERIOR CHAMBERS

The anterior cavity of the eye is divided into two chambers by the iris. The *anterior chamber* lies directly in front of the iris, while the **posterior chamber** is directly posterior to the iris but anterior to (in front of) the lens (see Figure 24-5). The space between the cornea and the lens is filled with

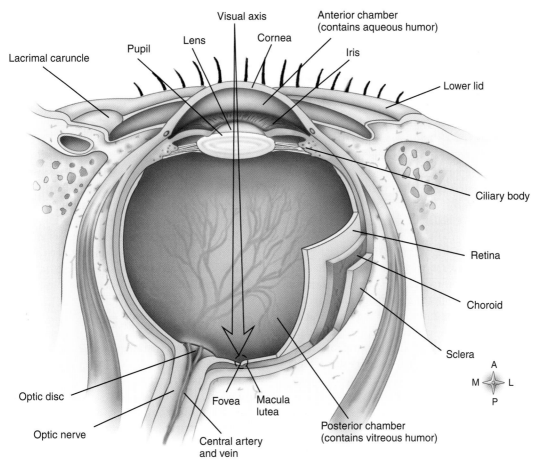

FIGURE 24-5
Horizontal section through the left eyeball. (From Thibodeau GA and Patton KT: *Anatomy and physiology,* ed 5, St Louis, 2003, Mosby.)

aqueous humor, which is produced by the ciliary processes. Because this fluid is continually produced, it must have a route of exit from the internal eye. The fluid drains through a small space between the lens and iris. It enters the canal of Schlemm within the sclera and is shunted directly into the venous system.

The large posterior cavity of the eyeball, located behind the lens, is filled with a gel substance called **vitreous humor**. This substance is vital to maintaining the shape of the eye.

THE LENS

The lens lies directly behind the iris and is a biconcave, clear structure encompassed by a transparent capsule (see Figure 24-5). It is held in place by suspensory ligaments attached to the capsule. In this area, the ciliary body and the choroid meet. The suspensory ligaments change the shape of the lens to bend light that passes through the lens. This focuses the images that are projected onto the retina.

CARE OF THE OPHTHALMIC PATIENT

Psychological Considerations

Ophthalmic surgery is extremely frightening for the patient. Creating a relaxing environment is important to the patient's

psychological and physical well-being. This is particularly important in ophthalmic surgery because anxiety can result in increased hemorrhage, a serious complication. All patients know that blindness is a possible complication of their surgery. This risk is always present during surgery and contributes to their anxiety.

Most ophthalmic surgeries are performed under conscious sedation and regional anesthetic. The patient therefore is awake and can hear everything in the surgical environment. In addition, the patient can *see* the objects and instruments that are placed in the eye (before regional block). Patients are asked to remain very still. The patient must concentrate on remaining still, knowing that objects and medications are near or in the eye. The body's normal reflex is to pull away from stimulation, but the patient must consciously override this reflex until anesthesia is secured.

The scrub can help the patient by creating a calm and supportive atmosphere. The surgeon will explain each step and always warn the patient of sensations he or she might feel, such as the initial sting of anesthetic or numbness. One must never disregard the patient's own reports of sensations because the sensations might be related to an adverse reaction to drugs used during the surgery.

Patient Safety

Ophthalmic surgery is performed in the operating room, surgery center, or other outpatient setting. Regardless of the setting, the patient's safety is the most important concern during the perioperative period.

MEDICATION REACTION

Reactions to medications are a serious consideration during eye surgery. The scrub should notify the circulator and surgeon of any symptoms reported by the patient. Although the technologist does not assess the patient medically, the technologist should immediately report any observed changes in the patient's appearance or behavior.

VERIFICATION OF THE OPERATIVE SITE

The entire surgical team is responsible for verifying that surgery is performed on the correct eye. The Joint Commission on the Accreditation of Healthcare Organizations recommends that the surgeon write on or mark the skin near the operative site to identify the correct side. The circulator should again verify the correct eye with the surgeon, scrub, and operating room team; through the chart documents; and with the patient. If there is any discrepancy, surgery must not proceed until the correct site is confirmed.

POSITIONING THE PATIENT

Surgery of the eye is performed with the patient in the supine position with the head resting on a foam headrest called a *doughnut*. This headrest helps to stabilize the head. The operating microscope magnifies the surgical field up to 100 times. Even the slightest movement can cause disruption and possible injury to the eye.

Positioning must be safe and comfortable. An uncomfortable patient may become restless and move during surgery, and this can result in injury to the eye. Many patients require soft support under the knees to relieve pressure on the lower back. When tucking the arms at the patient's sides, remember to consider pressure points and contact with the table frame. This not only causes pain but also can result in nerve and tissue injury. Refer to Chapter 10 for a complete discussion of surgical positioning.

The surgical team must transfer the eye patient from the stretcher to the operating table and return the patient to the stretcher after surgery. The patient should not exert any effort because this can increase intraocular pressure.

Prepping and Draping the Patient

A complete discussion of the eye prep is found in Chapter 11. Recall that the prep is performed so that sponges do not return to an area previously prepped. In particular, the medial (inner) canthus is considered a contaminated area, and any sponge that touches this point must not be returned to a previously prepped area.

Hospital policy and surgeon preference determine the choice of prepping solution. If Betadine is used, it must be diluted to 10%.

Many different techniques are used to drape the eye. It is important to isolate the hairline and nonoperative side of the face. Some surgeons may use a head drape, which is discussed in Chapter 11. This usually followed by a fenestrated drape to expose the operative eye. A body sheet is used to maintain a wide sterile field, or the procedure drape may be large enough to extend over the sides of the operating table.

Anesthesia

Many eye procedures are performed with regional anesthetic with monitored sedation. Administration methods for ophthalmic anesthesia include topical, infiltration, peribulbar, and retrobulbar methods.

Pediatric patients are given a general anesthetic.

A retrobulbar block is typically used for eye surgery in adults. The surgeon administers the block with a 10-ml syringe fitted with a long 25-gauge needle.

OPHTHALMIC DRUGS

Medications are instilled or injected into the eye before, during, and after surgery. These medications are available as solutions (drops) or ointments. A variety of medications are used during eye surgery. These include anesthetics, antibiotics, anti-inflammatory agents, diagnostic agents, enzymatics, irrigants, mitotics (agents that constrict the pupil), and mydriatics (agents that dilate the pupil). Uses of medications vary according to the type of surgery performed. Refer to Table 13-8 in Chapter 13 for a complete description of ophthalmic drugs and their uses.

INSTRUMENTS

Ophthalmic instruments are delicate and expensive. All surgical personnel must take special care to ensure that the edges and tips of microsurgical eye instruments are not dulled or damaged by careless handling. Before the procedure begins, the scrub should check all instruments. Sharp items must be smooth, and scissor blades must align properly. Needle holders are particularly susceptible to injury. Ensure that catches and spring mechanisms are working properly. Suction tips should be checked for patency. All instruments must be kept in order on the Mayo stand. Surgery often is performed in the dark. A neat instrument table is essential. Ophthalmic instruments are illustrated in Figure 24-6.

EQUIPMENT AND SUPPLIES

Electrosurgical Unit

A single-use, hand-held cautery unit or bipolar electrosurgical unit (ESU) is used in ophthalmic procedures. During vitrectomy, the unit is equipped with an electrocautery probe.

Eye Sponges

Eye sponges are spear-shaped and made of lint-free nonwoven material such as cellulose. These are available mounted

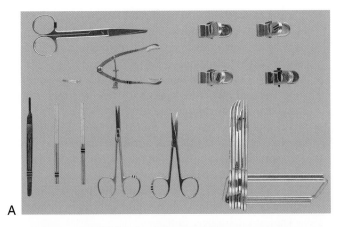

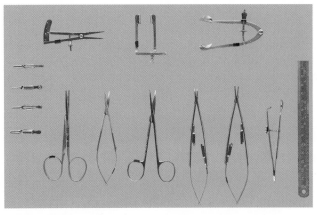

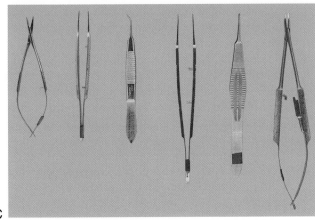

FIGURE 24-6
A, *Top, left to right,* 1 plastic scissors, straight, sharp, 5½ inch; 1 Lancaster speculum; 4 Edwards holding clips. *Bottom, left to right,* 1 Bard-Parker knife handle, No. 9; 2 Beaver knife handles, knurled, one insert above; 1 Stevens tenotomy scissors, curved, blunt; 1 iris scissors, straight, 4½ inch; 4 Halsted mosquito hemostatic forceps, curved; 2 Halsted mosquito hemostatic forceps, straight. **B,** *Top, left to right,* 1 Castroviejo caliper; 1 Cook eye speculum, child sized; 1 Lancaster speculum. *Bottom, left to right,* 4 serrefines; 1 strabismus scissors, straight; 1 Westcott tenotomy scissors, curved; 1 Stevens tenotomy scissors, curved; 1 Castroviejo needle holder with lock, curved; 1 Castroviejo needle holder with lock, straight; 1 Erhardt chalazion clamp; 1 metal ruler, small. **C,** *Left to right,* 1 Vannas scissors, curved; 1 McPherson forceps without teeth, straight; 1 McPherson forceps without teeth, angled; 2 Castroviejo suturing forceps, 0.12 mm teeth (1 × 2), front view and side view; 1 Barraquer needle holder, extra delicate, tapered, curved, with lock. (From Tighe SM; *Instrumentation for the operating room,* ed 6, St Louis, 1999, Mosby.)

on a plastic rod, or the technologist may be required to mount them on a mosquito hemostat for use. During surgery they are used to wipe away excess fluids or blood.

Sutures
Eye sutures are available in a wide range of materials in sizes from 4-0 to 12-0. These delicate sutures must be handled gently and carefully. Sutures should be handled as little as possible, and the points should be protected from damage. Both single-arm and double-arm sutures are used. Double-arm sutures are used to close circumferential incisions.

Syringes and Irrigation Tips
The technologist should have several sizes of syringes and irrigation tips available for instillation of medications and for irrigation. Syringes commonly used are 3-ml, 5-ml, and 10-ml sizes. Irrigation tips must be kept clean and free of debris.

MICROSURGERY

Microsurgery presents challenges to the scrub because:

1. The surgeon's field of vision is magnified, but the scope—the area of vision—is very limited. Special technique is required when passing instruments because the surgeon must not look away from the field to receive them.

2. When the surgeon is required to look away from the field, the surgeon loses concentration and the rhythm of the surgery. To avoid such interruptions, the scrub should prepare for each step of the procedure. Using the proper method while passing instruments reduces the risk of patient injury.

3. The patient and surgical field must be completely still. The scrub must prevent even slight movement of the microscope. When passing instruments or preparing items near the field, the scrub must have a steady hand and create as little movement as possible. Remember that if the patient raises his or her head, or if any instruments are jarred while touching the eye, the patient can lose his or her eyesight.

The Operating Microscope
The operating microscope is a heavy piece of equipment, but it is also very delicate (Figure 24-7). The technologist should become familiar with all components of the microscope to prevent injury to the patient and protect the microscope from damage. See Box 24-1 for common microscope terminology.

HANDLING THE MICROSCOPE
Follow these guidelines when handling the microscope:

▶ Before moving the microscope, secure the arms. This prevents them from swinging out and striking the wall or other equipment.

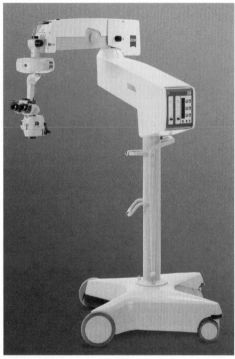

FIGURE 24-7
Microscope used in ophthalmic procedures. (From Rothrock JC: *Alexander's care of the patient in surgery,* ed 12, St Louis, 2003, Mosby; courtesy of Carl Zeiss.)

▶ The microscope must be balanced before use. This is necessary to ensure that the head of the microscope does not drift up or down. Always consult the manufacturer's instructions for balancing.

▶ The microscope must be adjusted to accommodate the surgeon's and assistant's eyesight. Always test the microscope before moving it to the surgical field.

▶ Check the brake and other controls to ensure that they are tight before using the microscope.

▶ Take special care to ensure that the microscope head control knob is secure before surgery.

▶ Check all cords for fraying or loose wires. Light bulbs also should be tested before surgery, and an extra bulb should be kept in the surgical suite.

▶ Some microscopes are equipped with an X-Y axis carrier. This carrier must be centered before the microscope is positioned at the field.

▶ When moving the microscope, the technologist should handle it only by the vertical column. Moving the microscope by the head can cause it to tip over and fall. A fall can result in serious injury to the patient or team members. To move the microscope, one should grasp the vertical column in the center with both hands.

▶ Use two hands to apply observer hands or cameras.

▶ Before surgery, the scrubbed technologist should adjust the height of the oculars to a comfortable level.

▶ Remember: "right is tight, left is loose."

CARE OF THE MICROSCOPE

Follow these guidelines when caring for the microscope:

▶ The microscope should be damp dusted before use. Follow the manufacturer's recommendations for use of dis-

---

Box 24-1   Microscope Terminology

Assistant binoculars

A separate optical body with nonmotorized hand-controlled zoom.

Beam splitter

A device that transmits an image from the primary ocular to an observer tube, producing an identical picture.

Broadfield viewing lens

A low-powered magnifying glass attached to the front of the oculars, producing an overview of the field.

Coaxial illuminator

A light source (usually fiberoptic) transmitted through the lens or body of the microscope. It illuminates the area within the field of view of the objective lens.

Compound microscope

A microscope that uses two or more lenses within a single unit.

Illumination system

The lighting system of the microscope.

Magnifying power

The ability to enlarge an image.

Objective lens

Lens that establishes the working distance and produces the greatest magnification.

Ocular or eyepiece

The component of the microscope that magnifies the field of view.

Paraxial illuminators

One or more light tubes that contain incandescent bulbs and focusing lenses. Light is focused to coincide with the working distance of the scope.

X-Y attachment

A mechanism that allows the scope to move precisely along a horizontal plane.

Zoom lens

A lens that increases or decreases magnification and is operated by the foot pedal.

infectant. Never use detergent or disinfectant on the lenses. They should be cleaned with a lens cleaner or water and wiped with lens paper. Do not use cloth because this leaves lint on the lens.
▶ Do not place fingers on the lenses.

The scope and all its openings and attachments should be covered at the end of the day to prevent dust accumulation.

Special Techniques
Scrubs should follow certain techniques when performing microsurgery:

▶ When preparing microsurgical instruments, the technologist should check for burrs (rough or jagged spots on sharp instruments). The technologist can do this by inspecting the instruments visually under microscope magnification or by running a lint-free microsurgical wipe gently along the edges of the instrument to feel for any sharp edges.
▶ The scrub or circulator should never place heavy objects on top of microinstruments because this damages the instruments.
▶ Instruments are kept clean during each procedure. One should use a special lint-free microsurgical wipe. A surgical sponge can damage very delicate instruments.
▶ Learning to properly handle and load sutures requires practice. When a locking needle holder is used, one should apply *gentle pressure on the shaft.* Excessive pressure on the shaft prevents the needle holder from locking. A needle that is too large for the needle holder also may prevent locking.
▶ The scrub passes the needle holder to the surgeon as if it were a pencil.
▶ When loading a needle onto a curved needle holder, one should point the curve away from the tip of the needle.
▶ Cutting suture under a microscope requires particular skill. The scrub first should place the scissors within the scope's field of vision. Only then should the scissors tip be positioned at the suture. One should gently lower the scissors until it is time to cut the suture.
▶ The scrub is responsible for maintaining irrigation over the eye during surgery. This requires constant attention to the condition of the eye. If the eye has a shiny appearance under the scope, the cornea is probably becoming too dry. The scrub must irrigate the eye frequently with balanced salt solution (BSS) to prevent drying.
▶ The scrub must keep all instruments in a specific order on the Mayo stand. When returning instruments to the Mayo stand, the scrub should place them in their original position and not rearrange them.
▶ Microsurgery requires dexterity and a steady hand. Caffeine can cause small tremors in the hand, which are magnified under the microscope lens. What appears as a small tremor to the naked eye can be severe under magnification.
▶ The experienced scrub does not remove his or her eyes from the microscope to orient the instrument to the surgeon's hand.

▶ The eye normally produces lubricating fluid that nourishes and protects the eye from infection and drying. The scrub is required to irrigate the eye periodically during surgery to prevent drying. BSS is used for this purpose. During irrigation, one should never touch the eye with the irrigator.
▶ *Meticulous* aseptic technique is essential in eye surgery. A postoperative infection may result in permanent blindness.

SURGICAL PROCEDURES
Orbital Decompression
SURGICAL GOAL
In this procedure, one, two, or three bony sections of the orbital cavity are removed to reduce pressure on the optic nerve and allow the eyelids to approximate normally.

PATHOLOGY
Orbital decompression is performed most often to treat hypothyroidism or *Graves' disease.* In this disease, the **globe** is displaced and protrudes anteriorly. This condition prevents the eyelids from closing. Other indications for orbital decompression are pressure on the optic nerve caused by tumor or swelling. The bony orbit does not yield to pressure. To prevent damage to the optic nerve and other structures, one, two, or three sections of the bone may be removed to decompress the globe.

Technique
1. The surgeon incises the lower lid.
2. The orbital rim is exposed, and the periosteum is incised.
3. The orbital floor is exposed.
4. The infraorbital nerve is located, and bone is removed with rongeurs or chisels.
5. The incision is closed.

DISCUSSION
The patient is placed in the supine position, prepped, and draped. A general anesthetic is used. The lower lid and anterior orbit are injected with Xylocaine with epinephrine to maintain hemostasis. The most common approach to orbital decompression is through the lower lid. A horizontal incision is made approximately 2 mm under the eyelashes, extending from the punctum to the medial canthus.

The orbital rim is exposed, and the incision path is drawn with a marker. The surgeon incises the lower lid with a tenotomy or Westcott scissors to the bony rim. A malleable retractor is used to displace the globe. This exposes the orbital floor and nerve bundle.

An osteotome or power drill is used to cut through the orbital floor. When the drill is in use, the technologist must provide irrigation over the drilling site. The bone then is removed in small pieces with a Kerrison or other small tipped rongeur. This exposes the nerve and vessels across the antrum. Incisions are made on each side of the inferior rectus muscle with a blunt scissors, such as a Stevens tenotomy scissors. The periosteum is closed with 4-0 chromic gut. The wound is closed in two layers. The muscle is approximated with 5-0 chromic gut, and the skin is closed with 6-0 nylon. The procedure is illustrated in Figure 24-8.

Excision of Chalazion

SURGICAL GOAL

In the excision of a chalazion, inflamed tissue is incised to preserve the tarsal plate.

PATHOLOGY

A chalazion is a chronic inflammatory granuloma of the tarsal or meibomian (sebaceous) glands. The meibomian gland becomes occluded as a result of inflammation. Sebum accumulates and ruptures the meibomian gland. The rupture into the tarsal plate creates a granuloma. The lid becomes swollen and painful, and a cyst forms. The conservative treatment for a chalazion in its early stages consists of compresses and steroid injections. When the cyst is large and a thick wall develops, surgery is indicated.

Technique
1. Topical anesthesia is applied.
2. The lid is injected with a local anesthetic.
3. A chalazion clamp is applied to the lid.
4. A vertical incision is made into the tarsal plate.
5. The contents of the chalazion are removed with a curette.

DISCUSSION

The patient is placed in a supine position, prepped, and draped for an eye procedure. Regional anesthetic is used. The surgeon clamps the lid with a chalazion clamp. The lid is everted, and a vertical incision is made through the tarsal plate with a #11 blade. A curette is used to remove the contents. The tarsal plate may be removed for recurring chalazion. Bleeding on the edges of the tarsal plate is controlled

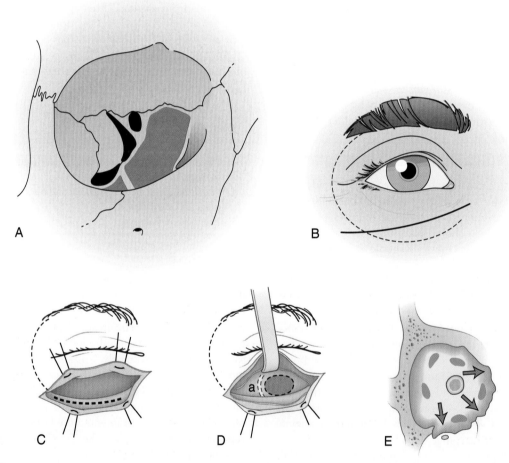

FIGURE 24-8
Orbital decompression. **A,** Orbital decompression, floor and medial wall, the bone to be removed is marked. **B,** Skin incision location for floor and medial wall decompression. **C,** The orbital rim is exposed and the periosteal incision is marked. **D,** The orbital floor is exposed for removal of the bone medial to the infraorbital nerve (a) **E,** Coronal section with the floor and medial wall removed. The orbital contents prolapse into the created space. (Modified from McNab AA: *Manual of orbital and lacrimal surgery,* ed 2, Oxford, 1998, Butterworth-Heinemann.)

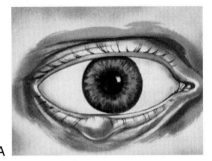

FIGURE 24-9
A, Chalazion of the lower eyelid.
B, Removal of the chalazion. (From Stein HA, Slatt BJ, and Stein RM: *The ophthalmic assistant: a guide for ophthalmic medical personnel,* ed 7, St Louis, 2000, Mosby.)

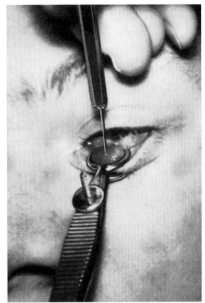

with the ESU. A pressure dressing is applied, as suturing is not necessary.

See Figure 24-9 for highlights of this procedure.

Excision of Pterygium
SURGICAL GOAL
In this procedure, the **pterygium** membrane is surgically removed to *prevent* loss of vision.

PATHOLOGY
A pterygium is a patch of degenerative elastic tissue that proliferates from the conjunctiva (Figure 24-10). It originates from a pinguecula (inherited benign elastic nodule) in response to irritation. The lesion begins at the medial canthus and moves laterally. It appears as a white or yellowish vascular mass. Pterygiums usually are bilateral and often are found in individuals who are exposed to high levels of ultraviolet light and dust. If a person is asymptomatic and vision is not impaired, treatment consists of artificial tears and vasoconstrictors. Because a pterygium usually is progressive, surgery is indicated when there is documented growth, the lesion is close to the visual axis, or vision is impaired.

Technique

1. A topical or regional anesthetic is administered.
2. The surgeon completely excises the pterygium from the cornea.
3. The surgeon dissects and excises the lesion from adjacent structures.
4. Mitomycin or the excimer laser may be used to prevent recurrence.
5. The conjunctiva is closed.

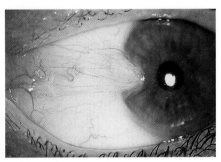

FIGURE 24-10
Pterygium. (From Stein HA, Slatt BJ, and Stein RM: *The ophthalmic assistant: a guide for ophthalmic medical personnel,* ed 7, St Louis, 2000, Mosby.)

DISCUSSION
The patient is placed in the supine position, prepped, and draped for bilateral surgery.

The surgeon places an eye speculum and instills local anesthetic into the conjunctival tissue around the pterygium. The technologist should have a ½-inch 27-gauge needle available for injection. A Superblade or #15 surgical blade is used to incise the neck of the pterygium. Using Westcott scissors and toothed forceps, the surgeon incises the conjunctiva on both sides of the pterygium, including any scar tissue. The incision is extended from the limbus. The tissue is then removed and retained as a specimen.

If the pterygium is expected to recur, mitomycin or the excimer laser may be used at this time.

The conjunctiva is approximated with a 5-0 or 6-0 nonabsorbable suture. The speculum is removed, and antibiotic ointment is instilled into the eye.

This procedure is illustrated in Figure 24-11.

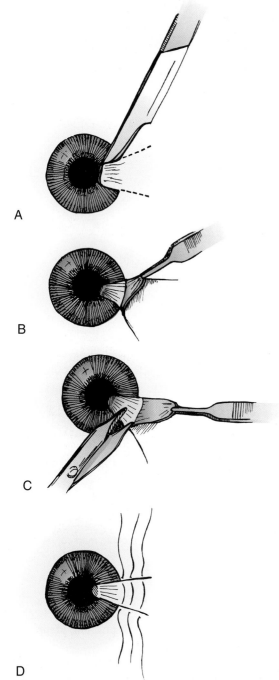

FIGURE 24-11
McReynolds technique for pterygium excision. **A,** Cornea around head of pterygium is incised. **B,** Pterygium flap is dissected upward, leaving clear cornea. **C,** Lower margin of pterygium is dissected, and whole pterygium is freed from sclera. **D,** Sutures are placed for closer closing of conjunctiva. (Modified from Rothrock JC: *Alexander's care of the patient in surgery*, ed 12, St Louis, 2003, Mosby.)

Repair of Entropion
SURGICAL GOAL
Entropion is an abnormal inversion of the lower eyelid. This condition causes the eyelashes to rub on the cornea, resulting in irritation and pain. The condition is caused by injury or the aging process.

DISCUSSION
In preparation for this procedure, the scrub should have chalazion clamps, dye marking pen, calipers, and a metal ruler available. A large package of sterile cotton-tipped applicators is necessary, along with a basic eye soft-tissue set. The procedure is usually performed under local anesthesia. A solution of 1% lidocaine with epinephrine usually is injected with a 5-ml syringe and a $\frac{1}{2}$-inch 27-gauge needle.

The patient is placed in the supine position with the head stabilized on a doughnut-type headrest. Before the procedure begins, the circulator instills tetracaine ophthalmic drops into the operative eye. The eye is then prepped and draped, as discussed previously (see Chapter 11).

The surgeon usually sits on the side of the operative eye. If surgery is planned for both eyes, the surgeon switches sides when the first side has been completed.

The most common and successful surgical procedure for the treatment of entropion is the excision of a base-down tarsoconjunctival triangle. The surgeon retracts the lid with a chalazion clamp. The surgeon may wish to outline the triangle with a dye marking pen before making the incision. The incision is made with a #15 Bard-Parker blade mounted on a #3 handle. Straight iris scissors may be used to free the tissue excised by the scalpel. Small bleeders are controlled with the electrocautery pencil.

During the procedure, the scrub usually is asked to dry the site when necessary with a cotton-tipped applicator. He or she also may be required to irrigate the cornea to prevent it from drying out. Because the surgeon is busy with the surgery, the scrub should watch for the need for irrigation, and irrigate when necessary.

After the triangle has been excised, the scrub should pass three or four interrupted absorbable sutures of size 5-0 or 6-0 swaged to spatula-type needles to the surgeon. The surgeon places the sutures one at a time with the aid of smooth tissue forceps and leaves the suture ends untied. When the last suture has been placed, the scrub should pass tying forceps so that the surgeon can tie the sutures in place. The scrub may be required to cut the knots very short to prevent further irritation to the cornea.

When hemostasis has been maintained, the surgeon releases the chalazion clamp and instills an antibiotic ointment into the eye. The eye is dressed with a cotton eye patch, which is then taped into place.

This procedure is illustrated in Figure 24-12.

Repair of Ectropion
SURGICAL GOAL
Ectropion is the abnormal sagging of the lower eyelid away from the eye. A major concern for the patient with ectropion is the overflow of tears down the patient's face. In addition,

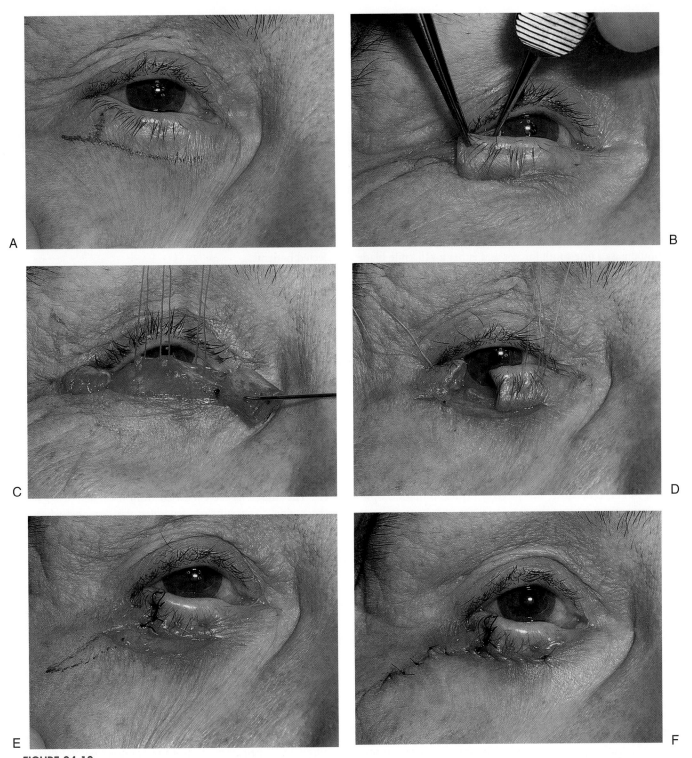

FIGURE 24-12
Repair of entropion. **A,** The incision is marked. **B,** A marginal strip of lid is overlapped to estimate the amount of lid shortening. **C,** Double-armed 4-0 sutures are placed in the conjunctiva and lower lid as retractors. **D,** The double-armed sutures are passed anterior to the tarsal plate and through the skin inferior to the lashes. **E,** The lid margin is closed. A small lateral "dog-ear" is marked for excision. **F,** The wound is closed. (From Tyers AG and Collin JRO: *Colour atlas of ophthalmic plastic surgery,* ed 2, Oxford, 2001, Butterworth-Heinemann.)

the exposed conjunctiva may become irritated. The goal of surgical treatment is to produce proper tear drainage and good cosmetic appearance.

Technique

1. A triangular tissue specimen is removed from the lower lid.
2. The lid is closed.

DISCUSSION

As for repair of entropion, the scrub should have a basic soft-tissue eye set, cotton-tipped applicators, a metal ruler, a caliper, and a marking pen available. The eye prep, draping, and anesthetic are the same as for entropion repair.

To begin the procedure, the surgeon usually marks the area of incision in the lid with a marking pen. The scrub should pass a fine-tooth forceps and either a #15 knife blade or straight tenotomy scissors. The surgeon then excises the tissue and cauterizes any small bleeding vessels with the hand-held cautery unit. The scrub is required to irrigate the cornea and blot any excess blood or irrigation fluid as necessary.

To begin the closure, the surgeon places one or more sutures of size 4-0 absorbable suture swaged to a spatula-type needle through the tarsal plate and canthal ligament. This prevents the ectropion from recurring. The surgeon then closes the deep tissue layers with several size 4-0 or 5-0 absorbable sutures. After the deeper layers are closed, the technologist should pass several interrupted sutures of size 5-0 or 6-0 silk swaged to cutting needles for skin closure. Fine-tooth tissue forceps are used in skin closure. At the completion of the procedure, the surgeon instills antibiotic ophthalmic ointment into the eye. The surgeon may or may not wish to patch the eye.

Repair of ectropion is illustrated in Figure 24-13.

NOTE: Many procedures and techniques are used in ectropion surgery, and the scrub should study the particular techniques used by his or her surgeons.

External Levator Resection for Ptosis
SURGICAL GOAL

The goal of ptosis surgery is to resect the levator tissues to correct the patient's vision and to produce good cosmetic effect.

PATHOLOGY

Ptosis is a condition of abnormal drooping of the upper eyelid. This condition may be caused by deficient nerve stimulation, lack of muscle strength, or paralysis of the levator palpebrae muscle.

Technique

1. The surgeon makes a skin incision just below the upper tarsal border.
2. The levator muscle is exposed and clamped.
3. The muscle is incised.
4. The conjunctiva is separated from the muscle and sutured to the tarsus.
5. The levator muscle is sutured to the tarsus.
6. The skin incision is closed.

DISCUSSION

In preparation for this procedure, the scrub should have available a basic eye-muscle tray, skin hooks, selected muscle clamps, a caliper, a metal ruler, cotton-tipped applicators, and surgical loupes for the surgeon (if requested).

The patient is placed in the supine position with the head stabilized on a headrest. The operative eye is prepped and draped in routine fashion. A general anesthetic may be administered, although local anesthesia may be used with selected patients.

To begin the procedure, the surgeon places two skin hooks just above the eyelashes. The assistant uses these to retract the lid. When an assistant is not available, the scrub is required to retract during the procedure. If this is the case, the Mayo tray should be neatly organized with all instruments readily available so that the surgeon may locate them. The surgeon then incises the upper eyelid from canthus to canthus. Straight tenotomy scissors and fine-tooth forceps are used to separate the pretarsal levator fibers from the fascia. The technologist is required to irrigate the surgical site frequently so that the anatomy is clearly visible to the surgeon. The cautery unit and cotton-tipped applicators are used to control excess bleeding.

The dissection is continued to expose the orbital fat. The surgeon then places a muscle clamp across the levator muscle. The muscle is then released from its attachments with the scalpel. The surgeon separates the conjunctiva from Müller's muscle using tenotomy scissors. Using a continuous suture of Dexon, size 5-0 or 6-0, the surgeon sutures Müller's muscle to the upper portion of the tarsus.

The scrub then passes a double-arm silk suture, size 5-0 or 6-0, which the surgeon uses to suture the levator to the tarsus. Additional sutures of the same material then are placed in the levator to secure it to the tarsus, and the excess levator is resected. The muscle specimen is retained by the scrub as a specimen.

The skin incision is closed with silk or nylon sutures, size 5-0 to 8-0, according to the surgeon's preference. The surgeon may place two temporary fine silk sutures through the lid margin and tape the ends to the patient's forehead to prevent stress on the lid for a short time after surgery. An antibiotic ointment is then instilled, and the eye is closed and dressed with a cotton eye pad and metal Fox shield. A Telfa dressing may be placed over the skin incision and taped in place.

Highlights of this procedure are illustrated in Figure 24-14.

Muscle Surgery: Lateral Rectus Resection and Medial Rectus Recession
SURGICAL GOAL

Muscle surgery is performed to correct deviation of the eye caused by *strabismus*—a condition in which the eye (or

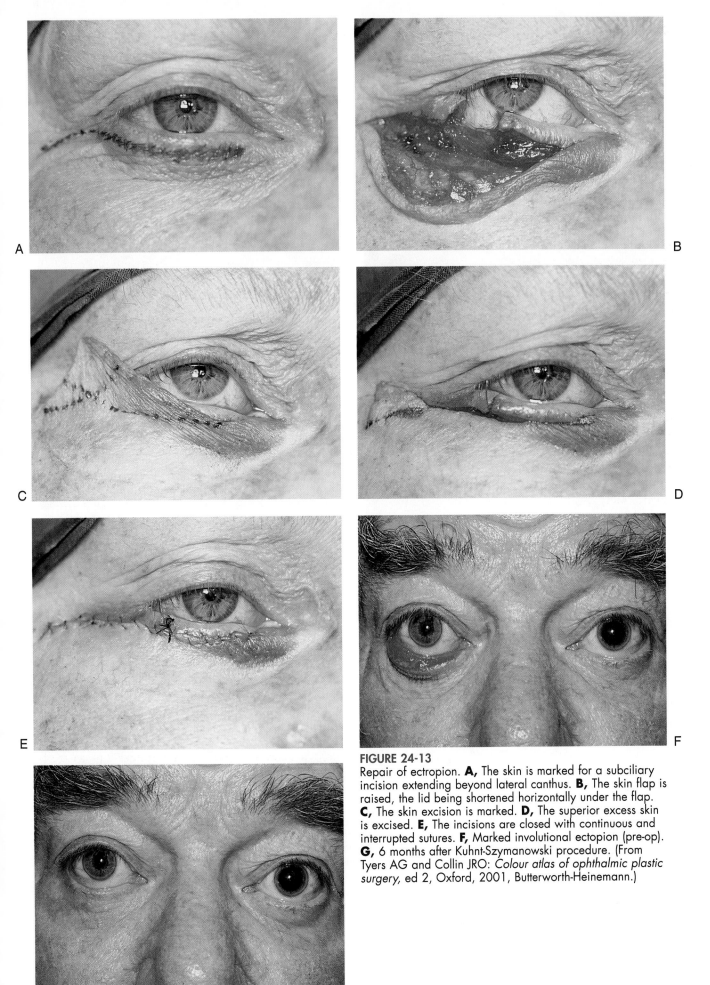

FIGURE 24-13
Repair of ectropion. **A,** The skin is marked for a subciliary incision extending beyond lateral canthus. **B,** The skin flap is raised, the lid being shortened horizontally under the flap. **C,** The skin excision is marked. **D,** The superior excess skin is excised. **E,** The incisions are closed with continuous and interrupted sutures. **F,** Marked involutional ectropion (pre-op). **G,** 6 months after Kuhnt-Szymanowski procedure. (From Tyers AG and Collin JRO: *Colour atlas of ophthalmic plastic surgery,* ed 2, Oxford, 2001, Butterworth-Heinemann.)

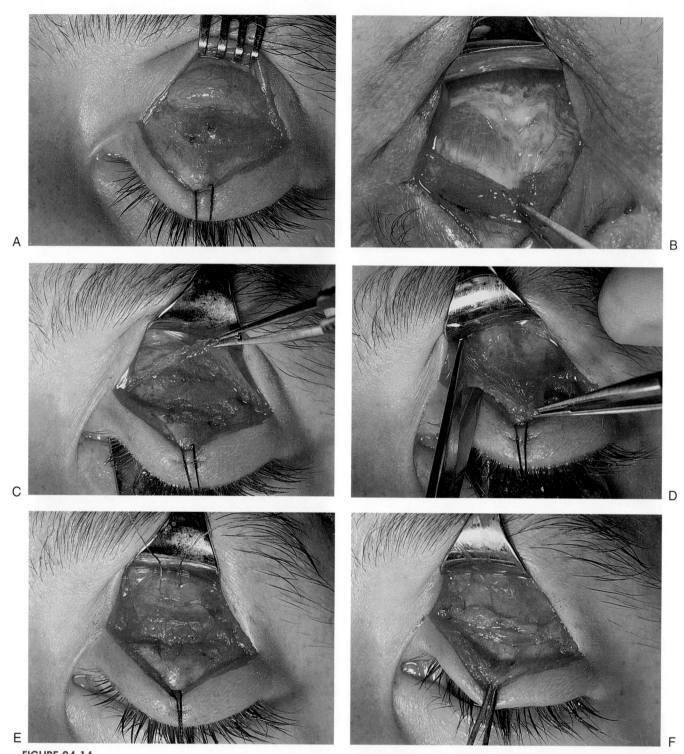

FIGURE 24-14
External levator resection for ptosis. **A,** The preaponeurotic fat pad is exposed by opening the septum. **B,** Whitnall's ligament and levator muscle are exposed by retraction of the preaponeurotic fat pad. **C,** The aponeurosis and Müller's muscle are separated from the conjunctiva; horns identified. **D,** Division of the medial horn of the levator aponeurosis. **E,** A central fixation suture is inserted. **F,** The levator is reattached to the tarsal plate with three sutures. (From Tyers AG and Collin JRO: *Colour atlas of ophthalmic plastic surgery,* ed 2, Oxford, 2001, Butterworth-Heinemann.)

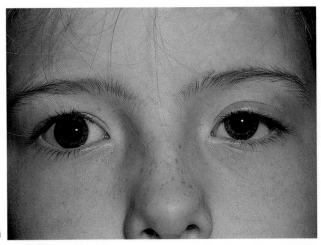
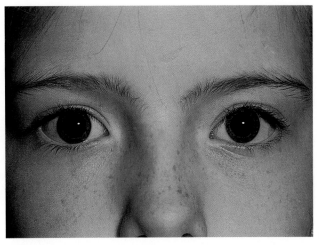

G   H

FIGURE 24-14, cont'd
G, Left congenital ptosis. **H,** Three months after left anterior levator resection. (From Tyers AG and Collin JRO: *Colour atlas of ophthalmic plastic surgery,* ed 2, Oxford, 2001, Butterworth-Heinemann.)

eyes) cannot focus on an object because the muscles lack coordination. The affected muscles are removed and reattached to the proper location.

PATHOLOGY

Strabismus is a condition in which the eyes fail to spontaneously focus on an object because the muscles lack coordination. One eye (the fixing eye) looks directly at the object of attention; the other eye (the deviating eye) does not.

There are two surgical procedures typically used to treat strabismus. In lateral rectus *resection,* a portion of the muscle is excised and the severed end is reattached at the original site of insertion. This shortens the drift of the eye. In medial rectus *recession,* the muscle is detached from its insertion, moved posteriorly, and reattached. This releases the eye and allows it to move further back laterally.

In preparation for either type of muscle surgery, the scrub should have some special instruments available. These include calipers, a metal ruler to check the accuracy of the caliper, at least four muscle hooks of the surgeon's choice, a marking pen, two straight mosquito hemostats, two curved mosquito hemostats, assorted muscle clamps, and a large pack of cotton-tipped applicators.

Technique

1. The surgeon incises the conjunctiva.
2. The muscle is measured with calipers.
3. A portion of the lateral rectus muscle is excised.
4. The medial rectus muscle is detached.
5. The muscle is moved posteriorly and reattached.
6. The conjunctiva is closed.

DISCUSSION

The patient is placed in the supine position, and the head is stabilized on a headrest. Before the prep, the circulator instills tetracaine ophthalmic drops into the operative eye. Af-

ter the administration of a general anesthetic, the eye is prepped and draped in routine fashion. The surgeon may wish to use a retrobulbar injection (see the discussion of enucleation) in addition to the general anesthetic. The surgeon usually sits on the operative side, facing the assistant.

During the procedure, traction on the muscles can cause a vagal response, which can affect the patient's cardiac status. If this occurs, the surgeon will release traction on the muscles.

Resection of the Lateral Muscle

To begin the *lateral rectus resection,* the surgeon inserts an open-ended eyelid retractor and grasps the limbus with Castroviejo forceps. He or she then makes a "buttonhole" incision in the conjunctiva at the limbus using the scissors. Bleeding is controlled with cautery. A muscle hook is used to separate the attachments between Tenon's capsule and the muscle sheath. The surgeon makes an incision with scissors to expose the tip of the muscle hook. Two Stevens hooks are guided down the lateral rectus muscle, exposing the sclera. A caliper then is used to measure and mark the muscle.

The muscle is clamped with a hemostat and then is cut with tenotomy scissors. A piece of the muscle may be retained for a specimen. The muscle is then reattached to its original site with a 6-0 S-24 double-armed nonabsorbable synthetic suture. The conjunctiva can be closed with an absorbable suture or left open, depending on the physician's preference.

Resection of the lateral muscle is illustrated in Figure 24-15.

Recession of the Medial Muscle

The procedure for medial rectus recession is identical to that for lateral rectus resection to the point of the conjunctival incision. The surgeon uses tenotomy scissors to undermine the conjunctiva. Using a previously adjusted caliper, the surgeon measures the distance from the original insertion point to its new one. The surgeon may wish to mark the new insertion point with a marking pen.

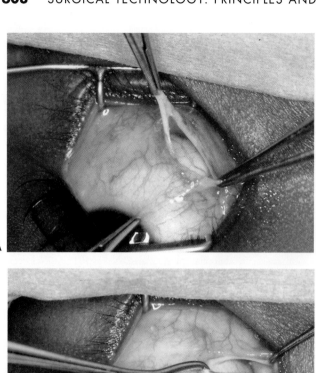

A

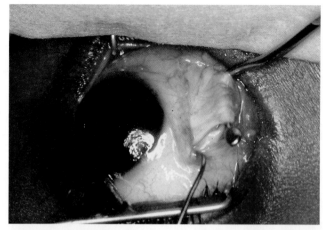

B

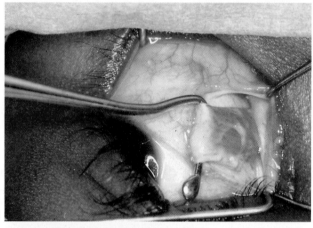

C

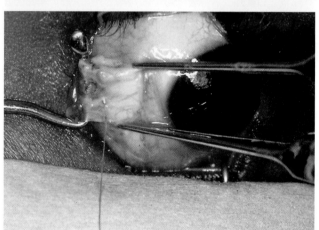

D

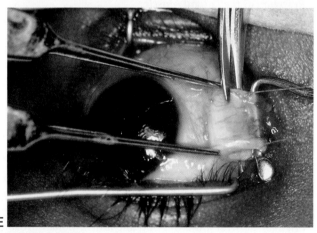

E

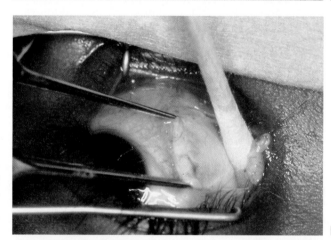

F

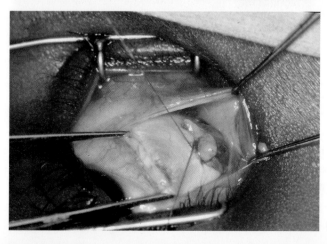

G

FIGURE 24-15
Resection of the lateral muscle. **A,** Visualization of the bare
sclera is maintained with forceps to prevent dragging fascia
into the insertion. **B,** The small hook exposes the anterior fascia at the insertion for anterior dissection and exposure of
the insertion. **C,** Two small tenotomy hooks are passed posteriorly along the tendon, against bare sclera, and elevated to
expose the intermuscular fascia. **D,** The surgeon places a suture at the insertion. **E,** Westcott scissors are used to remove
the tendon. **F,** Visualization, support, and hemostasis of the
tendon may be preserved by passing a dry cotton pledget,
or sponge, between the tendon and the globe. **G,** The sutures are then drawn in the direction they were passed to
avoid pulling them up and through their scleral tunnels and
tied. (From Jaffe N: *Atlas of ophthalmic surgery,* ed 2, St
Louis, 1995, Mosby.)

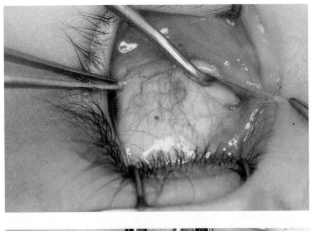
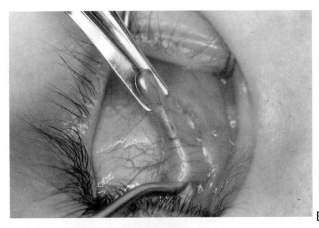
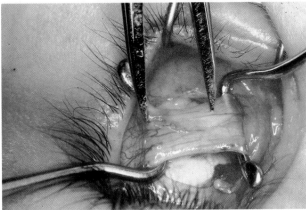
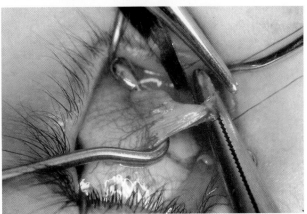

A

B

C

D

FIGURE 24-16
Recession of the medial muscle. **A,** A large muscle hook is passed beneath the tendon, going no further posteriorly than the insertion itself. **B,** Tenon's capsule beneath the olive tip of the large muscle hook is incised. **C,** A second large muscle hook is passed beneath the tendon, and traction is applied between the two. The anterior arm of the caliper is placed in the midportion of the anterior hook, and the posterior arm delineates the site for needle passage. **D,** The tendon is cut ahead of the clamp, and the resection of the tendon is completed at the original insertion. (From Jaffe N: *Atlas of ophthalmic surgery,* ed 2, St Louis, 1995, Mosby.)

The surgeon now places two sutures of size 5-0 or 6-0 absorbable material at the end of the muscle but does not tie them. A straight mosquito hemostat may be placed across the muscle between the sutures and the insertion point. The clamp is allowed to remain on the muscle for up to 3 minutes. This crushes tiny vessels that would otherwise bleed profusely when the muscle is severed. The clamp is removed and the technologist passes a muscle hook, which the surgeon places under the muscle to elevate it away from the globe. The surgeon then incises the muscle with a straight iris scissor. At this point the cautery pencil may be necessary to ensure hemostasis.

The technologist now passes an empty needle holder and smooth tissue forceps to the surgeon, who moves the muscle back to the dye marks and sutures it at its new location with the previously placed muscle sutures. The conjunctival incision is closed with size 5-0 or 6-0 absorbable sutures swaged to a spatula needle. An antibiotic ophthalmic ointment is instilled, and the eye is dressed with a cotton eye pad and metal Fox shield.

Recession of the medial muscle is illustrated in Figure 24-16.

Dacryocystorhinostomy
SURGICAL GOAL
Dacryocystorhinostomy is performed to create a permanent opening in the tear duct for the drainage of tears.

PATHOLOGY
Dacryocystitis is an inflammation of the lacrimal sac, causing pain, redness, and swelling at the site of the medial canthus of the eye. This condition appears as a red mass in the septal-orbital area. Pus or a mucoid material sometimes is present at the punctum. This condition arises from an obstruction or stricture of the nasolacrimal duct, a part of the lacrimal system that is prone to infection.

Lacrimal-sac inflammation and infection are usually seen in two groups of patients: adults over the age of 40 and infants. Dacryocystorhinostomy surgery reestablishes drainage into the lacrimal duct system by enlarging the opening into the nasal sinus. A tube may be inserted to eliminate the obstruction. In infants, the lacrimal duct is usually probed and the duct irrigated.

Technique
1. The surgeon incises the skin over the lacrimal sac.
2. The muscle is dissected to the level of the periosteum.
3. The periosteum is incised.
4. A probe is inserted through the punctum.
5. The anterior lacrimal crest is perforated with a drill.
6. The lacrimal sac and nasal mucosa are incised.
7. The anterior flaps are closed.
8. The incision is closed.

DISCUSSION

The patient is positioned supine, and the head is placed on a head ring or rest for stability. A local anesthetic (usually 2% Xylocaine with epinephrine) may be infiltrated into the operative site to promote hemostasis. Most surgeons pack the nasal sinus with gauze impregnated with topical anesthetic. The skin prep starts at the medial canthus and includes the nose, orbital rim, and cheek.

To begin the procedure, the surgeon makes an incision along the medial canthus of the nose with a #15 blade. Small bleeding vessels are cauterized. A 4-0 suture is placed in the flap for traction. A Stevens tenotomy scissors is then used to dissect the muscle down to the bone. A self-retaining retractor is placed into the wound if a traction suture was not placed. The surgeon incises the periosteum and uses a Freer or periosteal elevator to elevate the periosteum, which can be retracted back with a small malleable retractor. This exposes the lacrimal sac.

Nasal packing is removed at this time for better visualization of the nasal mucosa. The sac is then separated from the fossa. A Bowman probe is inserted into the punctum of the sac to identify the location and to retract the sac laterally.

The technologist should pass the power drill with a 4-mm to 5-mm ball burr to the surgeon and should pass a bulb syringe filled with normal saline to the assistant. The surgeon uses the drill to excise the lacrimal crest. The drill site is irrigated and suctioned simultaneously to remove bits of bone. A small Kerrison rongeur is used to enlarge the nasolacrimal crest.

A vertical incision perpendicular to the previous incision is made into the lacrimal sac, forming an "H." The surgeon then approximates the lacrimal sac flaps to the nasal mucosa using 4-0 or 6-0 chromic sutures. The anterior limb of the medial canthal tendon is attached to the edge of the periosteum with 6-0 chromic gut, and the incision is closed with 6-0 nylon.

This procedure is illustrated in Figure 24-17.

Alternative Techniques

The lacrimal duct may be stented with silicone tubing, which is passed into the nose, similar to a probe and irrigation procedure. The probe and irrigation procedure is indicated for congenital lacrimal obstruction. A small number of infants are born with a dacryocele and have an obstruction causing dacryocystitis. In these cases, the punctum is dilated with a probe and fluorescein dye is used to ascertain patency. The probe and tube are passed down the nasolacrimal duct and retrieved under the inferior turbinate in the nose (Figure 24-18).

Lacrimal Duct Probing
SURGICAL GOAL

The lacrimal duct is opened, and the obstruction is removed.

PATHOLOGY

During development of the lacrimal system, three anomalies may occur. First, the passage may not develop. Second, the

punctum of the lower eyelid is absent. Finally, a congenital dacryocystocele or mucocele may occur, causing an obstruction. The most common sign of abnormality of the lacrimal system is a constant tearing. Infection will soon follow with this obstruction.

Technique

1. A chalazion clamp is applied over the punctum.
2. A 2-ml syringe filled with saline is inserted into the canthus.
3. Pressure is exerted. (This is probing.)
4. A Bowman probe is passed through the punctum.
5. Silicone tubing is placed on the probes.

DISCUSSION

This procedure is common with infants because of the underdevelopment of the lacrimal system while in utero. Adults also may have this condition and usually are treated in the office. Local or IV sedation is used with adult patients and general anesthesia with infants.

Pressure is applied over the upper canthus, or a chalazion clamp is applied over the punctum. A 2-ml syringe with a lacrimal cannula tip filled with air or saline is inserted. Pressure is cautiously applied; this is called probing. The superior punctum is dilated with a dilator. A 0 or 00 Bowman probe usually is used with an infant. The probe is at an angle and rotated vertically. The probe is inserted vertically until the obstruction is met, and then gentle pressure is exerted. The surgeon will feel a slight pop, and the probe is advanced to the nares. The probe is removed, and a fluorescein solution is used to gently irrigate the system. A yellow–green solution should be suctioned through the nares via a suction cannula, indicating patency.

Silicone intubation is indicated for patients who have inadequate probing. After the Bowman probe is threaded with silicone tubing, it is inserted the same way as previously described. The probe is advanced through the nares, and a Crawford hook is attached to the olive tip and advanced further through the nares. The tubing is cut from the probe, and the suture within the stent is tied into a secure square knot. After intubation, the patient is placed on a steroid antibiotic solution to prevent infection.

Enucleation
SURGICAL GOAL

Enucleation is complete removal of the eyeball (globe).

PATHOLOGY

Enucleation is performed to treat intraocular malignancy, such as retinoblastoma and melanoma, penetrating ocular wound, painful blind eye, or an eye that is blind and painless but disfigured. An artificial prosthesis may be inserted to replace the globe.

A similar procedure is used for a severely traumatized eye. **Evisceration** is the removal of the contents of the eye, leaving the outer shell of the sclera with its muscle attachments intact.

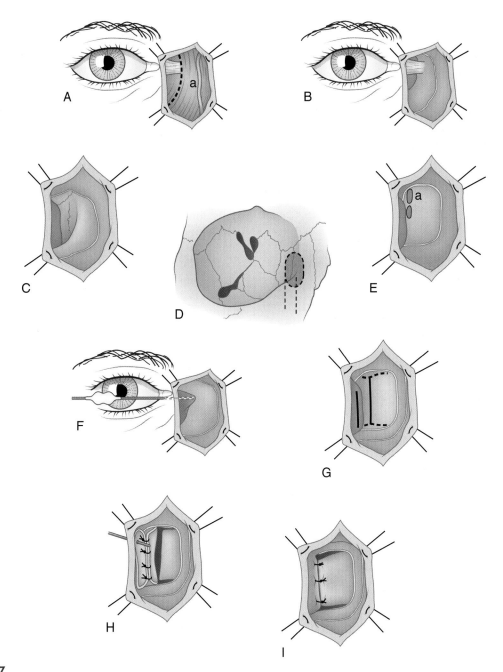

FIGURE 24-17

Dacryocystorhinostomy. **A,** The medial canthal tendon is exposed. The angular vein (a) lies anteriorly on the orbicularis muscle. The orbicularis muscle is separated at the point of insertion of the canthal tendon (dotted line). **B,** The periosteum is incised and reflected anteriorly. **C,** The canthal tendon and periosteum are reflected laterally with the lacrimal sac to expose the lacrimal fossa. **D,** The area of bone removed for dacryocystorhinostomy. **E,** The bony osteum is formed. **F,** A probe is passed into the lacrimal sac. **G,** The vertical lacrimal sac and nasal mucosal incisions are marked. **H,** The posterior mucosal flaps are sutured with a probe in place. **I,** The anterior mucosal flaps are sutured. (Modified from McNab AA: *Manual of orbital and lacrimal surgery,* ed 2, Oxford, 1998, Butterworth-Heinemann.)

Technique

1. The surgeon incises the conjunctiva.
2. The four rectus muscles are identified, clamped, and severed.
3. The rectus and inferior oblique muscles are anastomosed.
4. The optic nerve is severed.
5. A sphere is introduced into the socket.
6. The conjunctiva and Tenon's capsule are sutured over the sphere.
7. A tarsorrhaphy is performed (the eyelids are sutured together).

DISCUSSION

Enucleation is usually a psychologically traumatic experience for the patient. Many hospitals now perform the sur-

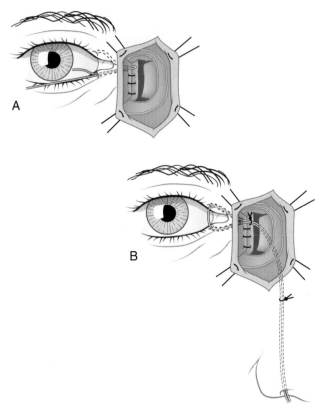

FIGURE 24-18
Alternative technique for dacryocystorhinostomy. **A,** The lacrimal tubing is passed through the canaliculi on the end of a fine probe. **B,** The lacrimal tubing is passed through both canaliculi and into the nose and sutured together to prevent proplapse onto the eye. (Modified from McNab AA: *Manual of orbital and lacrimal surgery,* ed 2, Oxford, 1998, Butterworth-Heinemann.)

gery in an outpatient setting. This increases the anxiety and grief experienced by the patient and family because there is no professional support after surgery. Great care is taken to provide a comforting environment in the operating room. All team members must be sensitive to the psychosocial and emotional effect of losing the eye. A general anesthetic is preferred for obvious psychological reasons. However, hospital protocol may require regional anesthetic with monitored sedation.

The patient is placed in supine position and prepared for routine eye surgery as previously discussed. A closed eye retractor is placed in the eye. The surgeon makes a circular incision as close to the limbus as possible. This conserves as much conjunctiva as possible for closure later in the procedure. The incision is made with a #15 blade or iris scissors. The surgeon undermines the conjunctiva and Tenon's capsule and prepares to sever the rectus and oblique muscles from the globe.

Because the rectus muscles will be sutured to the inferior oblique muscles, both muscles are tagged with sutures of silk or absorbable synthetic material, size 4-0 or 5-0. The superior oblique muscle is severed and allowed to retract. The

surgeon then severs the previously tagged inferior oblique muscle, secures it to the lateral rectus muscle with size 4-0 sutures, and pulls the globe anteriorly (forward).

The technologist should have a muscle hook available at this time. The surgeon passes the hook around the globe to ensure that all connections except the optic nerve have been severed. The surgeon places a Mayo clamp across the optic nerve for 30 to 60 seconds to effect hemostasis. The clamps are then removed, and curved enucleation scissors are used to sever the optic nerve across the area crushed by the Mayo clamp. This frees the globe, which is passed to the technologist as a specimen. If any intraocular contents have been extruded into the socket, they must be cleaned out with irrigation solution and a 4 × 4 gauze sponge. Hemostasis is secured with pressure and the ESU.

After the globe has been removed, an implant must be placed and sutured to the socket to shape the socket. This implant is called a **sphere.** A **conformer** is placed over the sphere. The conformer covers the surface of the sphere. The sphere will be replaced by an artificial eye at a later date. The technologist should have several sizes of implant spheres available from which the surgeon can choose the correct size. The sizes for an adult usually range from 14 to 18 mm.

The surgeon selects the implant and conformer, and the sphere is introduced into the orbit. Some surgeons use a *sphere introducer* to insert the implant. The rectus muscles are sutured to the appropriate positions on the sphere with size 4-0 or 5-0 absorbable sutures. Next, Tenon's capsule is pulled over the sphere and sutured into place with scleral biting forceps and absorbable synthetic suture, size 4-0. A purse-string suture may be used here. The conjunctiva is closed with size 5-0 sutures. A conformer sometimes is placed over the sphere. The silk retraction sutures are removed, and the surgeon instills an antibiotic ointment into the eye. The eyelids are then sutured together (**tarsorrhaphy**). The eye is patched with a cotton eye pad secured with tape.

Highlights of this procedure are shown in Figure 24-19.

Evisceration
SURGICAL GOAL
In evisceration, the contents of an eye are removed while the sclera shell and muscles are left intact.

PATHOLOGY
Indications for evisceration are endophthalmitis, or infection in the eye. Cosmetic reasons for an evisceration are the replacement of a blind eye with a **hydroxyapatite implant,** which is a porous coralline structure. This gives the eye a more normal appearance to the layperson. Evisceration is contraindicated in malignancies and blind painful eyes. The ciliary nerves are left intact with an evisceration, so it is contraindicated for a painful eye because the patient would still experience pain.

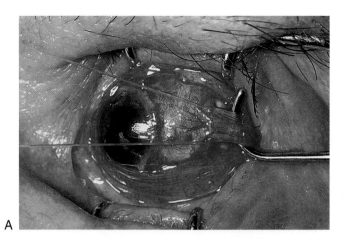

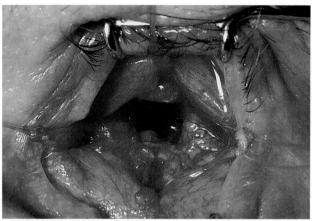

A   B

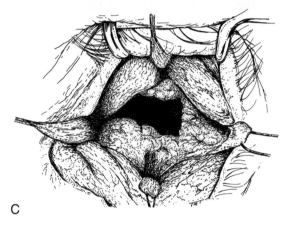

C

FIGURE 24-19
Enucleation. **A,** Suture placed through a rectus muscle tendon. **B,** Enucleation completed. **C,** An implant of the surgeon's choice is inserted. If no implant is used, the rectus muscles are left free within the orbit, and the conjunctiva is closed with interrupted absorbable sutures. (From Tyers AG and Collin JRO: *Colour atlas of ophthalmic plastic surgery,* ed 2, Oxford, 2001, Butterworth-Heinemann.)

1. The surgeon excises the cornea and makes a 360-degree conjunctival incision.
2. The evisceration spoon is used to separate and scoop out the contents of the eye.
3. The sclera is pulled through and closed.
4. The conjunctiva is closed.

DISCUSSION

The cornea is excised and a 360-degree conjunctival incision is made. The surgeon dissects to Tenon's capsule. The surgeon uses a blade to extend the limbus to make removal of the eye contents easier. A spatula is used to separate the iris from the sclera. An evisceration spoon is used to scoop out the intraocular contents of the eye; suction also may be used to remove any remaining contents of the eye. The sclera shell is irrigated with saline. Bleeding is controlled with cauterization. The sclera is pulled through and closed, and then the conjunctiva is closed with a 6-0 absorbable suture. A conformer and light bandage are applied.

Orbital Exenteration
SURGICAL GOAL

Orbital **exenteration** is the removal of the entire eye and orbital contents, including eyelids, ocular muscles, and orbital fat in the treatment of life-threatening cancers.

PATHOLOGY

An orbital exenteration is generally performed to treat life-threatening cancers and infections, or to treat severe orbital pain and deformities. Because this is a radical procedure and because of the relatively poor reconstruction alternatives, an orbital exenteration is performed only after all other therapies have failed.

The number of orbital exenteration procedures has decreased over the years. In the past, squamous cell cancers and melanomas were treated with an exenteration, but recently the preferred treatment for these cancers has become local resection without exenteration, as long as the tumor remains superficial.

Another reason for an orbital exenteration is fungus invading the paranasal sinuses and extending into the orbit. A typical patient with this diagnosis is one who is diabetic or immunosuppressed. Benign tumors such as meningioma and lymphangioma may warrant an exenteration because of the extreme pain they cause the patient.

1. The surgeon uses a knife or cautery to remove the skin, orbital fat, and periosteum down to the bony orbit.
2. A periosteal elevator separates tissue from the circumference of the bony orbit.

3. The surgeon completes dissection at the superior orbit.
4. Scissors are used to separate the orbital contents from the orbit. The specimen is removed.
5. The orbital cavity is packed, and reconstruction is performed.

DISCUSSION

The patient is under general anesthesia, the eyelids are sewn closed, and often the sutures are left long and in place so as to move the eye. The bony orbit is marked. The surgeon uses a knife or cautery to remove the skin, orbital fat, and periosteum down to the bony orbit. Depending on the extent of the tumor, some skin and muscle sometimes may be saved for reconstruction. Otherwise, dissection of the tumor is continued until the frozen sections are negative for cancer.

A ribbon retractor and periosteal elevator separate tissue from the circumference of the bony orbit. Careful dissection at the superior area of the orbit is completed. A possible complication of the use of excessive force is a puncture of the bony orbit and a resulting leak of cerebrospinal fluid. In ad-

dition, a fistula may develop after reconstruction. Thus this procedure is a very tense part of the operation.

The nasolacrimal duct should be removed. The lacrimal drainage system and part of the nose sometimes need to be removed as well.

The enucleation scissors are used to separate the orbital contents from the bony orbital rim. The surgeon removes the specimen and packs the orbital cavity with moist gauze to achieve hemostasis. After 5 to 10 minutes, the packs are removed, and any bleeding vessels are cauterized.

If additional excision is needed for tumor removal, this is performed at this time, until the margins are free of tumor. The area is inspected for cerebrospinal leaks, and the surgeon obtains hemostasis.

At this time, the surgery turns to the reconstructive phase. Possible closures are as follows:

▶ The orbit may be packed and dressed with antibiotics, and the patient returns later for more reconstructive surgery.
▶ A split-thickness skin graft may be used for closure.
▶ A dermal graft can be substituted for skin grafts.

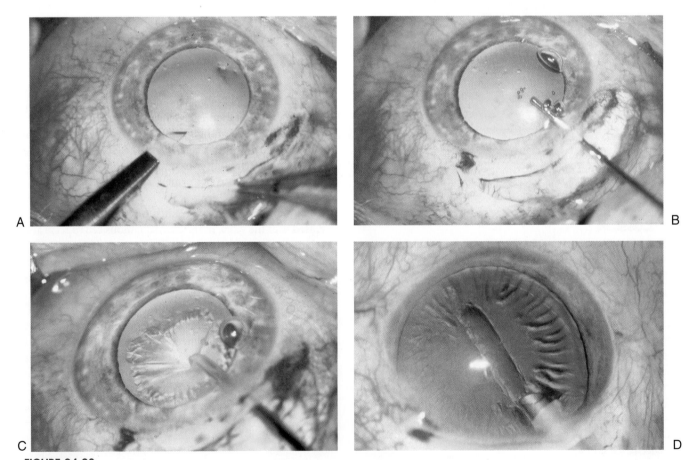

FIGURE 24-20
Intracapsular cataract extraction. **A,** An ab externo incision is made at the anterior limbal border at 1:30 o'clock. **B,** Viscoelastic material is injected into the anterior chamber. **C,** The oval portion of the incised anterior capsule is freed with the capsulectomy needle. **D,** The ultrasonic hand-piece is passed into the anterior chamber, and sculpting of the anterior surface of the nucleus begins. (From Jaffe N: *Atlas of ophthalmic surgery,* ed 2, St Louis, 1995, Mosby.)

► Regional flaps and composite grafts may be used as well for reconstruction. Refer to Chapter 26 for reconstruction.

Cataract Extraction

Two methods are used for **cataract** removal. *Intracapsular cataract extraction* requires a large incision through which the entire lens is removed, usually with suction and a cryosurgical probe (Figure 24-20). This method is used under limited circumstances because it requires a large incision and many sutures.

The second method of cataract removal is *extracapsular cataract extraction* (Figure 24-21). Extracapsular cataract extraction is often performed with a phacoemulsifier.

Phacoemulsification is the fragmentation of tissue through ultrasonic vibration. Current technology allows the phacoemulsifier to be tuned to the frequency that destroys only the target tissue. After the tissue is fragmented and emulsified (liquefied), it is aspirated (suctioned) with an aspirating system. Extracapsular cataract extraction often reduces operative, postoperative, and recovery times. This procedure is performed in 95% of cataract extractions.

Extracapsular Cataract Extraction
SURGICAL GOAL

The goal of cataract extraction is to remove an opaque lens (cataract) and replace it with an intraocular lens implant to restore vision.

PATHOLOGY

A cataract is an opaque lens that leads to progressive loss of vision. It is a result of the aging process, trauma, **glaucoma**, or certain medications. Cataracts also may occur as a congenital anomaly.

Technique

1. The surgeon places a traction suture in the superior rectus.
2. A conjunctival incision is made at the limbus.
3. The anterior chamber is inflated with Healon.
4. A capsulorrhexis is performed.
5. BSS is used to irrigate the eye to free the lens.
6. The phacoemulsification probe is introduced, and the lens is emulsified.
7. Residual fragments of lens are removed.

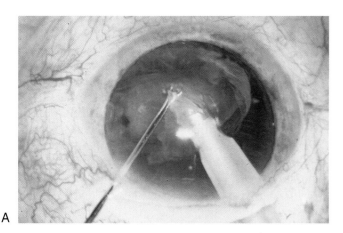
A

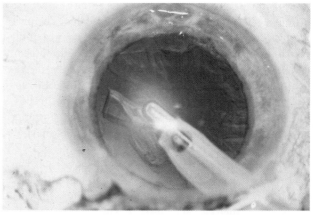
B

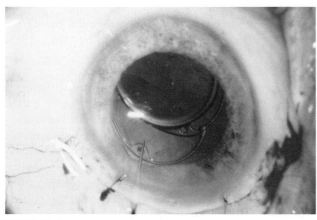
C

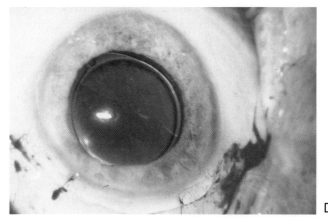
D

FIGURE 24-21
Extracapsular cataract extraction. **A,** The nucleus is displaced toward 6 o'clock with the bent-tipped needle, performed inside the capsular bag. **B,** Irrigation-aspiration of the residual cortex is performed inside the capsular bag, and the posterior capsule is polished. **C,** The loop is passed under the superior capsular flap. **D,** The lens is now completely within the capsular bag. The opening in the anterior capsule is shown. (From Jaffe N: *Atlas of ophthalmic surgery*, ed 2, St Louis, 1995, Mosby.)

8. A viscoelastic (Healon) is used to reinflate the chamber.
9. An intraocular lens is put in place.
10. The incision may be sutured or left open to heal.

DISCUSSION

The patient is placed in the supine position with a headrest (*phaco vacuum* pillow) to immobilize the head. During the prep, several drops of Betadine 10% are instilled into the eye for antibacterial effect. The patient is draped for an eye procedure with a head drape and adhesive eye drape. The patient receives conscious sedation or a combination of topical and regional anesthetic.

To begin the procedure, the surgeon places a **bridle suture** of size 3-0 or 4-0 silk in the superior rectus and creates a conjunctival flap with Westcott scissors and toothed forceps. The surgeon then makes a stab incision into the cornea with a diamond knife. This creates a triangular cut. A second incision is made into the anterior chamber, and a viscoelastic (Healon) is injected. The surgeon performs a **capsulotomy** (incision into the capsule) or **capsulorrhexis** (procedure in which the capsule is torn and a capsulotomy performed). The surgeon mobilizes the lens by instilling BSS into the eye with a 27-gauge needle.

The surgeon then introduces the phacoemulsification probe. Many surgeons groove the nucleus of the cataract and separate it into four quadrants before proceeding. The phacoemulsification probe fragments and emulsifies most of the lens. However, some small pieces may remain. The surgeon manipulates the probe toward the edges to aspirate the remaining pieces. This is called "polishing the posterior capsule." If the surgeon places the probe in the center, it is possible to bring the vitreous forward from the posterior capsule. This is a complication of the surgery and may necessitate an anterior vitrectomy.

The scleral incision is enlarged, and an intraocular lens (IOL) is manipulated into the posterior chamber of the capsule. Healon is injected into the chamber and onto the lens. The incision is then closed with size 6-0 or 7-0 suture, or the incision may be left open to heal. If the lens becomes dislocated (the lens falls into the pars plana), a posterior vitrectomy is performed at this time.

Intracapsular Cataract Extraction
SURGICAL GOAL

During intracapsular cataract extraction, an opaque lens is removed with a cryoextractor—a hand-held freezing probe or cryosurgical unit. The **cryotherapy** probe is touched to the lens, which adheres to the probe so the lens can be removed.

PATHOLOGY

Refer to the section on extracapsular cataract extraction.

Technique

1. The surgeon incises the conjunctiva
2. The cornea is incised at the limbus.

3. Closing sutures are placed but not tied.
4. An iridotomy is performed, and the lens is removed.
5. The anterior chamber is filled.
6. The corneal incision is closed.
7. The conjunctiva is closed.

DISCUSSION

After routine prep and draping of the patient, the surgeon places a lid speculum in the eye. The surgeon dissects the conjunctiva with Wescott scissors. The cornea is then incised with the knife. The incision is lengthened with right and left corneal scissors. Small bleeders are managed with the cautery unit.

The surgeon may place closing sutures at this time. Size 9-0 or 10-0 sutures with a spatula needle are used. Approximately six sutures are placed.

After the corneal sutures have been placed, the surgeon performs an iridotomy (incision into the iris) using Colibri forceps and Vannas scissors. The assisting surgeon retracts the cornea with smooth forceps by holding the central corneal suture. The surgeon irrigates the anterior chamber of the eye with alpha-chymotrypsin, which is used to dissolve the zonules that hold the lens in place.

The scrub should prepare Miochol, which is used to constrict the pupil and prevent loss of vitreous. A 27-gauge cannulated irrigation needle is used for instillation. This fluid will be injected as soon as the corneal flap has been approximated.

The cryoextractor and smooth forceps are used to remove the lens. Using two tying forceps, the surgeon closes the corneal incision. The anterior chamber is filled with saline or intravitreous gas. The conjunctiva is pulled over the corneal incision and sutured with interrupted or running sutures. The bridle suture is cut, and the speculum is removed. The eye is dressed with an eye pad and shield.

Anterior Vitrectomy
SURGICAL GOAL

Anterior vitrectomy is performed to remove the vitreous from the anterior chamber.

PATHOLOGY

Anterior vitrectomy may be performed for a variety of conditions such as opacity of the anterior segment of the vitreous and loss of vitreous during cataract extraction. For example, during a cataract extraction with phacoemulsification, a physician may unintentionally place the phacoemulsification probe in the center of the posterior capsule and overhydrate the vitreous through irrigation or a tear through the capsule. The vitreous then would move forward from the posterior chamber into the anterior chamber. Vitreous is very viscous, has strands, and causes tension within the anterior chamber and surrounding structures. In such cases, an anterior vitrectomy would be indicated, which is considered a complication of cataract surgery.

1. A vitrector, infusion line, and suction line are attached to the phacoemulsification machine.
2. The vitrectomy is performed.
3. A spatula is placed in the anterior chamber to check for vitreous strands.
4. An anterior chamber lens is placed in the eye (extracapsular cataract extraction [ECCE]).
5. The conjunctiva is closed.

DISCUSSION

A vitrectomy probe, infusion line, and vacuum line are attached to the phacoemulsification machine. After the vitrectomy has been completed, a spatula is placed in the incision to sweep for any vitreous strands. The pupil is constricted with acetylcholine (Miochol or Miostat). The surgeon rechecks the pupil for elevation, and the anterior chamber will be re-formed with BSS. If the anterior chamber is intact, a posterior intraocular lens is placed in the eye. If there is not enough capsular support for a posterior chamber lens, then an intraocular anterior chamber lens is inserted. The anterior chamber then is filled with air drawn through a filter. Viscoelastic (Healon) is applied around the pupil, and a lens glide (small plastic sheet 1 mm in size) is inserted into the eye, and the anterior chamber lens is placed into the eye. The lens guide is removed, and sometimes an iridectomy is performed if the lens is large. In an iridectomy, the iris is grasped with forceps, care is taken to avoid damaging the ciliary body, and part of the iris is cut by Vannas scissors. The conjunctiva is closed with a 10-0 nylon suture.

Scleral Buckling Procedure for Detached Retina

SURGICAL GOAL

Scleral buckling surgery is performed when the sensory layer of the retina and the pigment epithelial layer become separated from each other. The surgical goal is to restore the layers to their normal positions and prevent blindness.

PATHOLOGY

The vitreous normally adheres to the retina in several locations. However, the layers of the retina may become separated. This causes sudden, painless loss of vision, or "shadowing," which appears as a curtain that descends over the patient's field of vision. Light flashes and "floaters" often accompany the vision loss.

A tear in the retina (called a rhegmatogenous detachment) creates a passage for the vitreous to seep between the pigment epithelium and the neural layer of the retina. This seepage wedges the layers apart and increases the area of detachment. Vitreous traction, which pulls the layers apart, is caused by the aging process (the vitreous begins to shrink, causing traction on the retina). Detachment also may be caused by trauma, diabetes mellitus, hemorrhage, or inflammation.

1. The surgeon separates Tenon's capsule from the sclera using blunt dissection.
2. Diathermy is applied to the area of detachment or tear.
3. Sutures are placed in the sclera.
4. The **buckling components** are placed.
5. The site is examined under the indirect headlight for the position of the retinal detachment and break.
6. Intravitreous gas may be injected.
7. Tenon's capsule and the conjunctiva are closed.

DISCUSSION

A retinal detachment requires immediate repair. Several techniques are used to repair detached tissue. A common technique is to produce adhesions (scar tissue) between the layers using cryotherapy (freezing of the tissue) or **diathermy** (mild heat created by a diathermy unit or laser). Neither treatment damages the eye but creates points of scar tissue. This is followed by immediate **scleral buckling.** This Silastic or foam band is attached to sclera. Several synthetic "buckles" are placed over the band, causing it to indent. This technique puts the tissue in close contact with the retina during healing.

Another common technique used to treat retinal detachment is to perform a **vitrectomy** in conjunction with scleral buckling. In this procedure, the vitreous gel is replaced with saline solution or gas through a small puncture wound. This method is used to eliminate traction and tearing on the retina. Two puncture sites are made in the sclera to accommodate microinstruments used to perform cryotherapy or diathermy. The eye remains pressurized throughout the microsurgical procedure. The procedure described here is for scleral buckling and cryotherapy.

The patient is placed in the supine position, prepped, and draped for an eye procedure. Conscious sedation is usually used for the surgery unless the procedure is expected to last longer than 2 hours. A retrobulbar block also may be used.

An open-ended retractor is placed in the eye. Using toothed forceps and Wescott scissors, the surgeon makes two incisions in Tenon's capsules, one under each rectus muscle. Some surgeons place two 4-0 bridle sutures under the rectus muscles so the eye can be rotated as needed.

Using the diathermy unit, the surgeon makes many small burn marks or "spot welds" over the area of detachment. The diathermy electrode produces a high-frequency electrical current that produces mild burning. If the cryosurgical probe is used, the detached area is treated in the same manner.

The assistant steadies the eye by holding the bridle sutures while the surgeon compresses the globe with cotton-tip applicators.

The sclera then is approximated with fine suture of 4-0 Prolene. A double-armed suture of Dacron or other synthetic material is placed into the sclera and secured over

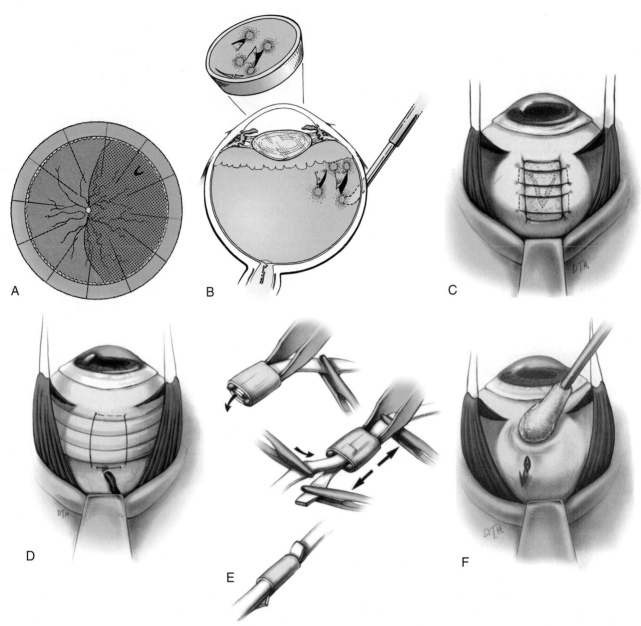

FIGURE 24-22
Scleral buckling operation for treatment of retinal detachment. **A,** Diagram of retina showing detachment of retina of temporal half of left eye, with retinal tear at equator of glove at 1:30 o'clock position. **B,** Surgeon visualizes field and places electrode beneath retinal tear; burn mark is made on sclera at the site of the retinal tear with the diathermy electrode. **C,** Sponge sutured in place over the treated site of the retinal tear. **D,** Band and tire used to encircle the eye. **E,** Placement of Watzke silicone sleeve to secure the encircling band. **F,** Incision made in sclera and fine incision made in choroids to allow subretinal fluid to drain. (From Ryan S et al: *Retina,* ed 2, St Louis, 1994, Mosby.)

Silastic sponges. This causes the eye to be compressed inward at the area of detachment. A Silastic band may be placed 360 degrees around the eye and a scleral buckle sutured into place under the muscles. A Watzke sleeve or sutures are secured to the buckle so that it remains in place.

Intravitreous Gas Injection
This is the injection of intraocular gas to create pressure on the retina while subretinal fluid is reabsorbed and scars form. The gases include SF6 (sulfur hexafluoride) and C3F8 (perfluoropropane). The gas is obtained through a hand-held syringe with a filter, and then the surgeon injects it into the eye.

This completes the buckling procedure. The eye is dressed with a patch. This procedure is illustrated in Figure 24-22.

Pars Plana Vitrectomy
SURGICAL GOAL
In pars plana vitrectomy, opaque vitreous humor is removed to restore vision.

PATHOLOGY
The most common cause of vitreous opacity is hemorrhage. The hemorrhage may result from diabetic retinopa-

thy, retinal vein occlusion, amyloidosis, Eales's disease, and sickle cell anemia. Other indications for vitrectomy include penetrating trauma with retained foreign objects, dislocated lens as a result of cataract extraction, HIV, and detached retina. The vitreous normally is transparent, and its consistency is gel-like. When the vitreous becomes opaque, the patient's vision becomes severely compromised.

Technique

1. The surgeon marks the sclera from the limbus with a suture for securing the port.
2. The surgeon makes the incision with a microvitrector knife.
3. An infusion port is inserted and secured with the preplaced suture.
4. The incision for the vitrector and light source is completed.
5. Upon entering the eye, the surgeon verifies that the tip is cutting well by removing vitreous well away from the vitreous base. This step is performed to prevent accidental tears in the retina.
6. Picks, forceps, and MPC scissors are used to complete the membrane dissection.
7. Scleral incisions are closed.
8. The conjunctiva is approximated and closed.

DISCUSSION

The vitrectomy equipment has many functions during vitrectomy (Figure 24-23). These include:

▶ Excision
▶ Illumination
▶ Irrigation
▶ Hemostasis

The vitrectomy system contains a hand-held probe connected to a larger unit. During surgery the machine is placed to the side of the patient or on an overhead table above the patient. The *vitrector* is connected to the vitrectomy machine by a set of silicone tubes. Other instruments used during the vitrectomy are the microvitrector knife and the micro scissors. These are delicate instruments; the micovitrector knife is extremely thin and sharp. The MPC scissors are used intraocularly. These are attached to the vitrectomy machine and deliver up to 300 cuts a minute. The endoilluminator is attached to the vitrectomy machine and is the light source for the interior of the eye or posterior chamber.

During vitrectomy, the technologist is required to hold a lens on the patient's eye.

Absolute steadiness is imperative. A comfortable hand position therefore is important. The scrub places the lens over the patient's eye with just enough pressure to create a bubble on the eye. Excessive pressure on the lens displaces the vitreous and distorts the surgeon's view. The technologist must follow the instruments with the lens as the surgeon moves them.

The vitrectomy can be performed under a local or general anesthetic. The advantage of using a general anesthetic is that it allows for a longer operating time.

A metal horseshoe-shaped hand rest may be attached to the operating table near the patient's head. A plastic drape covers the patient's face and the head to create a trough for fluid.

The surgeon makes an incision in the conjunctiva. Three incisions then are made in the sclera with a special microvitrectomy blade. The infusion cannula is inserted and sutured into place with 4-0 silk. The endoilluminator and vitrector are inserted into the superior incisions.

When the retina has been identified, the vitrectomy can start. The cutting rate is set at 200 to 400 cuts per minute. A low suction is maintained, allowing the vitreous debris to be aspirated in very small pieces. This prevents retinal tears and is safer for the patient. Bleeding occasionally may occur, and diathermy may be used for hemostasis.

After completion of the vitrectomy, the surgeon may perform an air–fluid exchange. The sclerotomies are closed with 8-0 or 9-0 nylon. The conjunctiva is closed with absorbable suture. A subconjuctival steroid injection is given, and antibiotic ointment is instilled into the eye. An eye patch and shield are applied. During the immediate postoperative period, the head should be elevated to avoid increased pressures in retinal vascularity.

This procedure is illustrated in Figure 24-24.

Filtering Procedures and Trabeculectomy
SURGICAL GOAL

The goal of this procedure is to create an adequate channel from which the aqueous humor may drain from the anterior chamber.

PATHOLOGY

Glaucoma is a local eye disease characterized by increased intraocular fluid, optic nerve cupping, and visual field loss. Increased pressure resulting from the fluid in the eye leads to pressure on the optic nerve and atrophy, causing loss of vision.

Types of Glaucoma

▶ *Primary angle closure glaucoma:* This condition accounts for 30% of all glaucoma cases. The incidence is higher in women. A sudden rise in intraocular pressure is caused by total blockage or obstruction of aqueous humor at the root of the iris (the limbal drainage system). This is considered a medical emergency, as blindness may result.

▶ *Open angle or chronic glaucoma:* Primary open angle glaucoma is an insidious bilateral disease that usually develops in the middle years or later. In this condition, outflow of aqueous humor is obstructed in the trabecular meshwork. This causes intraocular tension and a gradual loss of vision.

▶ *Secondary glaucoma:* This condition results from injury, infection (such as iritis), tumors, drugs, or inflammation that causes scarring and blockage of the drainage system. A gradual loss of vision occurs.

▶ *Congenital glaucoma:* In this condition, the fluid-drainage system is abnormal at birth. The infant's eye distends, and corneal haziness occurs. The classic sign is called an "ox

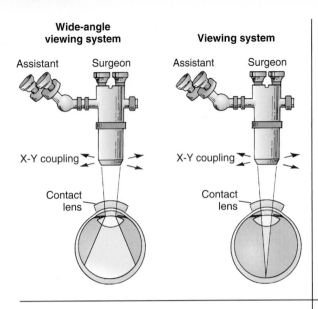

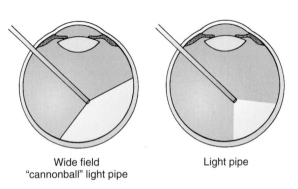

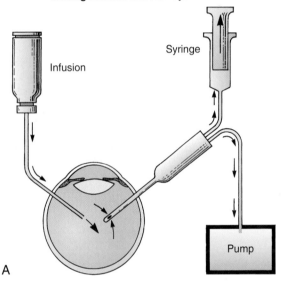

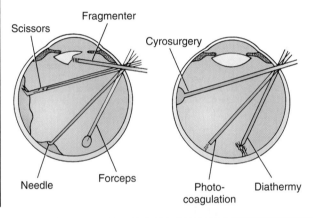

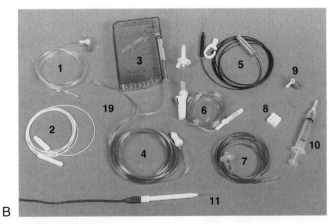

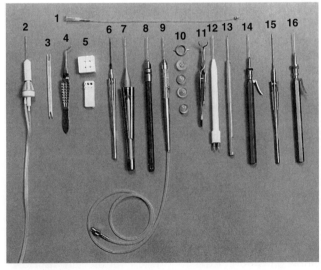

FIGURE 24-23

A, Vitrectomy equipment and accessories. **B,** Disposable vitrectomy accessories: (1) tubing with three-way stopcock for fragmentor extrusion; (2) fiberoptic light pipe; (3) collection cassette; (4) vitrectomy tubing and probe; (5) endolaser probe; (6) infusion tubing; (7) air pump tubing; (8) scleral plugs; (9) three-way stopcock; (10) syringe; (11) wet-field cord with hemostatic eraser. **C,** Accessory instruments for vitrectomy: (1) 4-mm infusion cannula; (2) variable port vitrector; (3) 3.5- and 4-mm premeasured calipers; (4) scleral plug holder; (5) scleral plugs in tablets; (6) Lambert subretinal forceps; (7) Thomas subretinal handle; (8) Charles vacuum cannula; (9) Flynn needle; (10) lens set with sew-on ring; (11) Landers lens holder; (12) wet-field endocautery; (13) MVR blade; (14) Grieshaber side-gripping forceps; (15) DORC end-gripping forceps; (16) Grieshaber vertical cutting scissors. (**A** Modified from Rothrock JC: *Alexander's care of the patient in surgery,* ed 12, St Louis, 2003, Mosby; **B** and **C** courtesy of Visual Communications, The Methodist Hospital, Houston, Tx.)

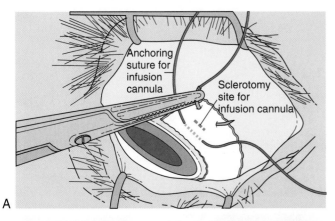

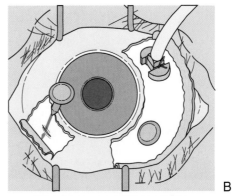

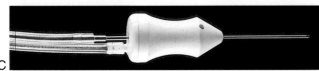

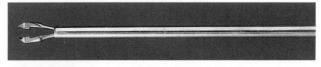

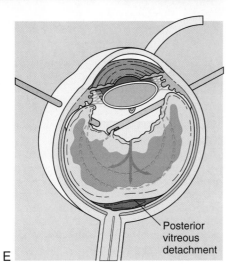

FIGURE 24-24
Pars plana vitrectomy. **A,** A preplaced suture, such as a 4-0 silk, is prepared so that the infusion cannula can be placed through the first sclerotomy. **B,** Scleral plugs may be used to temporarily close the sclerotomies while other extraocular procedures, such as scleral buckling or indirect ophthalmoscopy, are performed. **C,** Vitrectomy probe. **D,** Intraocular accessory instrument for membrane dissection and other intraocular manipulations. **E,** Two additional sclerotomies are made—one in the superonasal quadrant and one in the superotemporal quadrant—with one dedicated to illumination and the other dedicated to the cutting or dissection instrument. (From Jaffe N: *Atlas of ophthalmic surgery,* ed 2, St Louis, 1995, Mosby.)

eye." Symptoms include light sensitivity and excessive tearing. Surgery is indicated to prevent blindness.

Technique

1. The surgeon makes an incision through the cornea or conjunctiva at the limbus.
2. The limbus is incised.
3. A scleral flap is created.
4. A small portion of the trabecular meshwork is excised and removed.
5. An iridectomy may be performed.
6. The conjunctiva is closed.
7. The anterior chamber is reinflated as needed.

DISCUSSION

Before the start of the procedure, the patient's intraocular pressure is measured with a tonometer, and if the pressure is high, medications are administered to reduce the pressure.

The patient is prepped and draped in routine manner. To begin the procedure, the surgeon inserts a lid speculum. Size

4-0 traction sutures may be placed in the superior rectus muscle. The surgeon incises the conjunctiva using toothed forceps and the knife. The surgeon then dissects Tenon's capsule from the sclera with Westcott scissors in the direction of the limbus. This creates a conjunctival flap.

The limbal area is then gently scraped with a Beaver blade to remove any blood clots. This technique prevents accidental puncture of the conjunctiva. The sclera is then cauterized in the shape of the flap. The surgeon uses the Beaver blade to make an incision in the sclera, following the outlines of the cautery. Dissection of the scleral flap starts at the apex and extends upward toward the iris.

A stab wound is made through the cornea to drain the aqueous humor. This incision is self-sealing and can be used later to reinflate the anterior chamber if necessary. The scleral flap is retracted, and Vannas scissors are used to excise a portion of the trabecular meshwork.

A complication of the procedure may occur at this point, in which the iris spontaneously prolapses into the wound. In this case an iridectomy would be performed. The surgeon

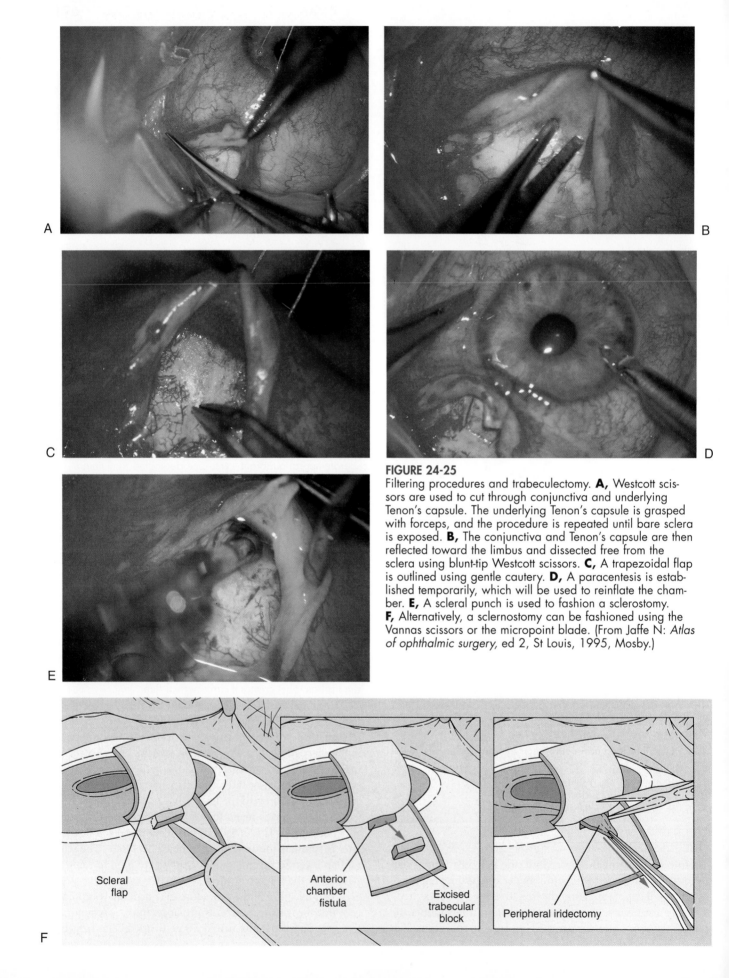

FIGURE 24-25

Filtering procedures and trabeculectomy. **A,** Westcott scissors are used to cut through conjunctiva and underlying Tenon's capsule. The underlying Tenon's capsule is grasped with forceps, and the procedure is repeated until bare sclera is exposed. **B,** The conjunctiva and Tenon's capsule are then reflected toward the limbus and dissected free from the sclera using blunt-tip Westcott scissors. **C,** A trapezoidal flap is outlined using gentle cautery. **D,** A paracentesis is established temporarily, which will be used to reinflate the chamber. **E,** A scleral punch is used to fashion a sclerostomy. **F,** Alternatively, a sclernostomy can be fashioned using the Vannas scissors or the micropoint blade. (From Jaffe N: *Atlas of ophthalmic surgery,* ed 2, St Louis, 1995, Mosby.)

Scleral flap

Anterior chamber fistula

Excised trabecular block

Peripheral iridectomy

grasps the iris with forceps and removes a portion, taking care not to damage the ciliary body.

At this point in an uncomplicated procedure, BSS is instilled into the anterior chamber to reinflate it. The scleral flap is closed with 10-0 nylon sutures. The conjunctiva and Tenon's capsule are approximated with 8-0 absorbable suture. BSS then is instilled into the anterior chamber. An eye sponge is placed over the incision site to check for leakage. Subconjunctival antibiotics and steroids are injected, and antibacterial ointments are instilled into the eye. Figure 24-25 illustrates this procedure.

Adjunctive Chemotherapy

If the filtering procedure is at risk of failure or if a low IOP (intraocular pressure) is indicated, the surgeon may use a chemotherapeutic agent such as 5-fluorouracil (5-FU) and mitomycin. If this is the case, a sponge soaked with the agent is placed at the surgical site for approximately 1 minute. After the sponge has been removed, the entire field is irrigated with BSS and the instruments that have been exposed to the mitomycin are removed from the field. Because of the potential toxicity of the drugs, protocols for their disposal and instrument decontamination procedures are required in most hospitals.

Argon Laser Trabeculoplasty

SURGICAL GOAL

In this procedure, the argon laser is used to shrink collagen and stretch the canal of Schlemm, thereby expanding the canal, increasing drainage, and reducing intraocular pressure.

PATHOLOGY

Glaucoma is classified as open angle or closed angle and then further classified as primary or secondary. The argon laser trabeculoplasty is indicated for primary and secondary open angle glaucoma. Primary open angle glaucoma has a genetic component and is more common in diabetics and blacks. Secondary open angle glaucoma is differentiated by the obstruction of the outflow of aqueous humor, thus causing an increase in intraocular pressure. Refer to Filtering Procedures and Trabeculectomy above.

Technique

1. The surgeon makes a conjunctival incision and another incision into the anterior chamber.
2. The trabecular meshwork is exposed.
3. An indirect gonioscopy lens with antireflective laser coating is used for the procedure.
4. Laser burns are placed at 180 to 360 degrees on the trabecular meshwork.
5. The surgeon places 20 to 25 laser burns in each quadrant.

DISCUSSION

The surgeon makes a superior conjunctival incision and dissects the conjunctiva up to the level of the limbus. The sclera is incised, and a flap is dissected. An incision is made into the anterior chamber; the trabecular meshwork is exposed.

Laser burns are placed at 180 to 360 degrees on the trabecular meshwork. An indirect gonioscopy lens with antireflective laser coating is used for the procedure. Laser burns are evenly spaced and applied to the anterior portion of the trabecular meshwork. The surgeon places 20 to 25 laser burns in each quadrant.

A laser spot is a burn of 50-mm spot (size) applied for 0.1 second. Laser energy of 800 to 1200 mV is recommended, with an argon blue-green laser. After the procedure, a drop of alpha-adrenergic agonist (epinephrine) is instilled into the eye. Steroid therapy is started postoperatively.

Penetrating Keratoplasty (Corneal Transplant)

SURGICAL GOAL

Penetrating **keratoplasty** is transplantation of a donor cornea to restore vision.

PATHOLOGY

The cornea is the clear, convex portion of the eye, similar to a window. Injury, infection, or degenerative diseases can cause the cornea to become cloudy. A corneal transplant is performed when the patient's other visual structures are intact, but the cornea has become opaque and thickened, causing loss of vision. The cornea is an excellent recipient of donor tissue, and this procedure has extremely high success rates. The reason is that the cornea is devoid of blood vessels, and this reduces the risk of rejection.

Two types of corneal transplants are performed. These are the *lamellar,* or partial penetrating keratoplasty, and the *penetrating,* or full-thickness transplant. In the partial penetrating technique, the anterior chamber is not entered and one half to two thirds of the cornea is transplanted. In penetrating keratoplasy, a full-thickness corneal graft is transplanted. The anterior chamber is entered, and many sutures are required to prevent escape of aqueous humor.

Technique

1. The donor cornea is prepared.
2. A scleral support ring may be sutured for additional support of the trephine (circular cutting instrument).
3. The trephine is placed on the recipient's eye, and partial penetration is completed with the sharp trephine.
4. The anterior chamber is entered, and the diseased cornea is excised.
5. The patient cornea is lifted off, and the donor cornea replaces the patient cornea.
6. The corneal graft is secured with a running or interrupted suture.
7. The surgeon re-forms the anterior chamber by injecting BSS.
8. Antibiotics and steroids are instilled into the eye topically after the corneal transplant has been completed.

DISCUSSION

In this procedure, a separate instrument table and Mayo set-up are required for preparing and transplanting the donor tissue. Each set-up is isolated from the other, and instruments are not shared between the two set-ups. These precautions are followed to prevent cross-contamination.

The patient is placed in supine position with the head stabilized on a foam ring. Before beginning the patient prep, the circulator or scrub positions the microscope above the patient and the surgeon adjusts it to his or her needs. The microscope is then locked into position and rotated out of the field.

The circulator instills tetracaine ophthalmic drops into the operative eye. The eye is then prepped in routine manner. If a regional block anesthetic is to be used, the postauricular area also is prepped. The patient is then draped for an eye procedure. Adhesive towel drapes may be used to isolate the operative eye.

The donor cornea is prepared for transplant. After determining the size of cornea required, the surgeon places donor tissue on a silicone block and uses a disposable circular trephine to cut the cornea. The donor trephine is larger than the recipient's cornea. After preparation, the donor tissue is placed in a container moistened with BSS.

The patient's cornea then is excised. After the surgeon inserts a lid speculum, the microscope is placed in position. A sclera support ring is sutured to the cornea with 6-0 silk sutures. A calibrated marker then can be used to indicate the location of suture sites for closure. The surgeon excises the superficial corneal layer using a trephine. The surgeon then makes a small stab incision into the anterior chamber with the diamond knife and extends the incision with corneal scissors. The surgeon gently lifts off the full-thickness cornea and passes it to the technologist as a specimen.

At this point in the procedure, the eye is extremely vulnerable to environmental contamination. This part of the procedure is often called "open sky." Viscoelastic material is placed over the iris and lens. The donor tissue is lifted out of its container with a size .12 forceps and manipulated onto the recipient's eye. The surgeon uses 10-0 nylon interrupted or running suture to close the cornea. If needed, BSS can be injected into the anterior chamber to replace lost fluid. The sclera ring support is removed. Antibiotic and steroid injections are given. Antibiotic ointment is applied, and an eye patch with shield is secured with tape.

This procedure is illustrated in Figure 24-26.

Lasik or Laser in Situ Keratomileusis
SURGICAL GOAL
Lasik surgery is performed to reduce the curvature of the cornea and correct a refractory problem.

PATHOLOGY
Lasik is the removal of corneal tissue to correct a refractory problem, such as myopia, hyperopia, and astigmatism (nearsightedness and farsightedness). This procedure is performed with an excimer laser. The excimer laser beam is a product of the reaction of argon and halogen gases with strong electrical discharge. This reaction creates a short-lived molecule that emits strong impulses of light. When the excimer laser is focused on the cornea, it can remove tissue more cleanly and precisely than a diamond knife.

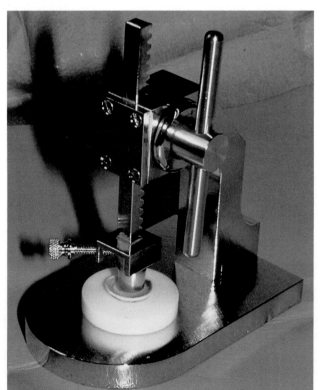

A

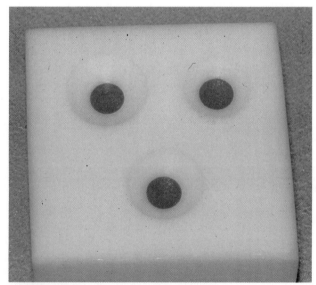

B

FIGURE 24-26
Penetrating keratoplasty (corneal transplant): **A,** Bourne punch, a mechanical punch that utilizes disposable trephines on the donor tissue. **B,** Cutting block with wells of various radii reduces distortion of the donor button. (From Jaffe N: *Atlas of ophthalmic surgery,* ed 2, St Louis, 1995, Mosby.)

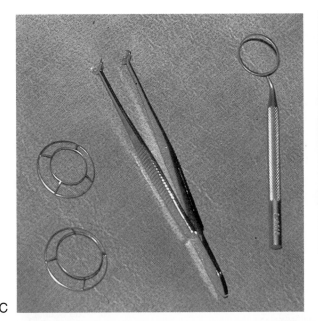

C

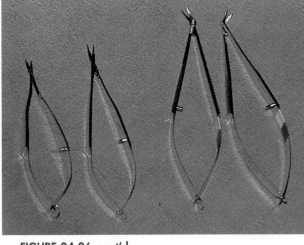

D

FIGURE 24-26, cont'd
C, Stabilization instruments. *Left to right,* Flieringa rings, Flieringa-LeGrand fixation forceps, and a Thornton fixation ring. **D,** Vannas scissors and mini-Westcott scissors minimize trauma to the iris and lens. **E,** Excision of the host button by suction trephine. **F,** A running suture is placed. (From Jaffe N: *Atlas of ophthalmic surgery,* ed 2, St Louis, 1995, Mosby.)

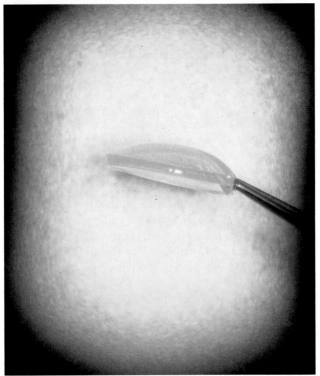

E

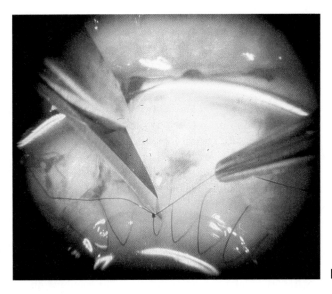

F

Lasik surgery is becoming increasingly common because of its advantages and the convenience of office surgery. Lasik surgery produces less postoperative discomfort and faster results than other conventional methods.

Lasik is a corrective procedure in which microkeratomes are used to lift a flap of corneal tissue. The excimer laser then is used to ablate part of the stromal bed to change the curvature of the cornea. The corneal flap then is repositioned. This procedure thus eliminates the original condition (e.g., myopia) and the patient's need for glasses or contacts also is eliminated.

Technique

1. The surgeon tests the microkeratome before use.
2. Eyelids, eyelashes, and canthic areas should be prepped and the eyelashes draped to hold back the lashes. An eyelid speculum then is inserted.
3. Corneal alignment is marked.
4. The microkeratome is inserted, and the corneal flap is created.
5. The excimer laser is used to ablate the stromal bed.
6. The corneal flap is refloated into the correct position.

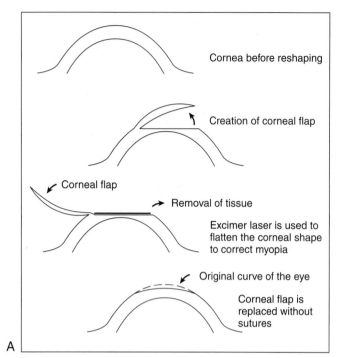

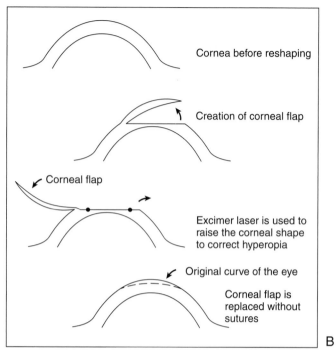

FIGURE 24-27
Lasik or laser in situ keratomileusis. **A,** Diagram of lasik correction for nearsightedness. **B,** Diagram of lasik correction for farsightedness. (From Wilson TS: LASIK surgery, *AORN Journal,* 1(5):977, 2000.)

7. The flap is sealed after 2 to 3 minutes.
8. Antibiotic-steroid ointment is instilled, and the flap alignment is rechecked in 20 to 30 minutes.

DISCUSSION

The patient is positioned under the laser and prepped with a Betadine solution similar to the preparation followed in ocular surgeries described previously (refer to Chapter 11, Surgical Preparation and Draping). The head is realigned on a head ring under the laser, and additional topical anesthetic is instilled into the eye. The unoperative eye is patched for protection from the laser. All the instrumentation is tested, with particular attention paid to the microkeratome, to prevent errors. The surgeon inserts the speculum into the eye, making sure the eyelashes are out of the operative view. Corneal alignment marks are placed on the cornea. A tonometer verifies the intraocular pressure of the eye. The suction ring is placed on the eye and displaced nasally but in the visual field. The eye is irrigated with BSS. Insertion of the microkeratome shaper head into the suction ring has been completed.

The patient is reminded that he or she will hear a buzzing noise before activation. The microkeratome then is activated. The corneal flap is incised. The corneal flap is retracted nasally with a spatula, and the patient is instructed to gaze ahead at the light. The physician verifies the laser alignment for the last time and then proceeds to ablate the stroma. The stroma is dried at completion, and the flap is folded back over the stroma with an irrigation cannula. The flap is irrigated to remove debris and realigned back in place for the last time. The flap is redried with a spear, and the flap is left to seal for 2 to 3 minutes. The final flap and adhesion check is performed in another 20 to 30 minutes.

This procedure is illustrated in Figure 24-27.

REFERENCES

Jaffe N: *Atlas of ophthalmic surgery,* ed 2, St Louis, 1995, Mosby.

McNab AA: *Manual of orbital and lacrimal surgery,* ed 2, Oxford, 1998, Butterworth-Heinemann.

Rothrock JC: *Alexander's care of the patient in surgery,* ed 12, St Louis, 2003, Mosby.

Stein HA, Slatt BJ, and Stein RM: *The ophthalmic assistant: a guide for ophthalmic medical personnel,* ed 7, St Louis, 2000, Mosby.

Tyers AG and Collin JRO: *Colour atlas of ophthalmic plastic surgery,* ed 2, Oxford, 2001, Butterworth-Heinemann.

Chapter 25

Otorhinolaryngologic, Oral, and Maxillofacial Surgery

By Rebecca Carr Ferguson

Behavioral Objectives

After studying this chapter the reader will be able to:

- Define the common terminology used in surgery involving the ear, nose, throat, and mouth
- Identify the key anatomical structures of the ear, nose, throat, and mouth
- Describe the primary procedures of the ear, nose, throat, and mouth
- Discuss equipment and instrumentation used in procedures of the ear, nose, throat, and mouth
- Identify the purpose and procedure for a cochlear implant
- Identify the principles of endoscopic sinus surgery
- Describe the process of a radical neck dissection
- Identify the purpose and procedure for performing a tracheostomy
- Identify surgical techniques to repair maxillofacial fractures

Terminology

Bicortical screw—A screw that goes through both the inner and outer layers of a bone.

Canalplasty—A procedure in which the external auditory canal is reconstructed.

Cerumen—Substance produced by the cerumen glands of the ear (i.e., ear wax).

Cholesteatoma—An ectopic growth of squamous epithelium (skin) in the ear.

Chondroradionecrosis—Necrosis of cartilage resulting from radiation.

Cricoid cartilage—A ring of cartilage between the trachea and the larynx. This is the only true complete circle of cartilage of the entire airway.

Dentition—Teeth.

Effusion—Fluid in the middle ear.

Epistaxis—Bleeding arising from the nasal cavity.

Eustachian tube—A tube lined with mucous membrane that joins the nasopharynx and the middle ear cavity. It allows for equalization of the air pressure in the middle ear.

Evert—To turn outward or inside out.

Glottis—Area of the larynx from the superior surface of the true vocal cords to about 1 cm below the medial extent of the true vocal cords.

Hyperkeratotic—A condition of thickening of squamous epithelium (i.e., callus).

Hypertrophy—An enlargement.

Hypopharynx—The digestive tract between the oropharynx and the esophagus. This is where the airway departs from the aerodigestive tract to form the larynx.

Terminology—cont'd

Innervation—State in which a body part or organ is supplied with nerves or nervous stimuli.

Keratin—A substance created by squamous epithelium.

Leukoplakia—A white plaque on mucosa.

Ligation—The procedure of tying off blood vessels or ducts with suture or wire ligatures. This procedure may be used to stop or prevent bleeding or block the passage.

Mastoidectomy—A procedure in which the air cells of the mastoid bone are removed.

Maxillomandibular fixation—Fixation of the upper and lower dentition.

Medialize—To move to the midline.

Microlaryngoscopy—Procedure in which a rigid laryngoscope is placed and suspended from the patient and an operating microscope is used to produce better visualization of the larynx. Also called microsuspension laryngoscopy and microdirect laryngoscopy.

Monocortical screw—A screw that goes through only the outer layer of bone.

Mucocele—A cyst that is filled with mucus and lined with mucosa.

Myringoplasty—Closure of a myringotomy.

Myringotomy—An incision or hole in the tympanic membrane created to allow aspiration or aeration of the middle ear.

Nasal polyp—A polyp of the nasal cavity or paranasal sinuses.

Nasolaryngoscope—A flexible scope that is passed through the nose to visualize the larynx.

Nasopharynx—The portion of the pharynx above the palate.

Neoplasm—An abnormal growth of cells.

Oropharynx—Portion of the pharynx between the palate and base of the tongue, separated from the oral cavity by the tonsillar pillars.

Osteotomy—Surgical breaking of bone.

Otitis media—Inflammation of the middle ear.

Otorrhea—Drainage from the external auditory canal.

Otosclerosis—Abnormal thickening of the bone in the otic capsule (middle and inner ear).

Ototoxic—A substance that is noxious to the sensory organs of the inner ear.

Papilloma—A benign epithelial neoplasm characterized by a branching or lobular tumor. Also called papillary tumor.

Paranasal sinus—Air cells surrounding or on the periphery of the nasal cavities. These are maxillary, ethmoid, sphenoid, and frontal sinuses.

Perforation—A defect in the tympanic membrane caused by trauma or infection.

Perichondrium—Tissue overlying the cartilage that provides its vascular and nervous supply.

Periosteum—Tissue overlying the bone that provides its vascular and nervous supply.

Peritonsillar abscess—A collection of purulent fluid that arises from the blockage of a pit (or crypt) of the tonsil.

Pharyngitis—Inflammation of the pharynx.

Phonation—Vibration of the vocal cords; speaking.

Rhinorrhea—Drainage from the nose.

Sensorineural hearing loss—Hearing impairment arising from the cochlea, auditory nerve, or central nervous system.

Septoplasty—A procedure in which the septum is manipulated to improve airflow through the nasal cavity.

Stapedectomy—A procedure in which the ear is replaced with a prosthesis. This procedure is used as treatment for otosclerosis.

Stenosis—Narrowing.

Supraglottic—Portion of the larynx above the surface of the true vocal cords.

Tracheostomy—An opening through the neck into the trachea through which an indwelling tube may be inserted.

Tracheotomy—An incision made into the trachea through the neck below the larynx to gain access to the airway.

Turbinectomy—A procedure in which a portion of the inferior nasal turbinates is removed.

Tympanoplasty—A procedure in which a perforated tympanic membrane is repaired.

Tympanostomy tube—A tube that is placed into a myringotomy to produce aeration of the middle ear.

Uvulopalatopharyngoplasty—A procedure in which the tonsils, uvula, and a portion of the soft palate are removed to reduce and stiffen the excess oropharyngeal and oral-cavity tissue in patients with obstructive sleep apnea or snoring.

SECTION I
Surgery of the Ear

INTRODUCTION TO SURGERY OF THE EAR

Surgical procedures involving the middle and inner ear are performed with the goal of restoring hearing. Hearing loss may be conductive or sensorineural in nature. Conductive hearing loss is caused most often by infection, **otosclerosis**, trauma, or occlusion of the external auditory canal. **Sensorineural hearing loss** may be caused by damage to the cochlea, eighth cranial nerve, or central nervous system. A surgeon specializing in otology or otorhinolaryngology may perform surgery of the ear.

ANATOMY OF THE EAR

The anatomy of the ear may be divided into three regions. These are the external ear, the middle ear, and the internal ear.

External Ear

The structures of the external ear include the outer surface of the tympanic membrane and all structures lateral to it (Figure 25-1). This includes the auricle or pinna, the external auditory meatus, and the external auditory canal. The auricle is a cartilaginous structure that is covered by skin. Its function is to gather sound waves. The center of the auricle contains the entrance to the external auditory meatus, which leads to the external auditory canal. The external auditory canal is lined with glands that secret a waxy substance called **cerumen.** The external auditory canal measures approximately 2.5 cm and terminates at the tympanic membrane.

Middle Ear

The middle ear extends from the tympanic membrane (TM) to the middle ear cleft (see Figure 25-1). It includes the TM, the ossicles (malleus, stapes, and incus), the opening to the eustachian tube, the opening of the mastoid cavity, and the intratympanic portion of the facial nerve. The TM is elliptical and conical in shape. The malleus (hammer bone), the most lateral of the ossicles, is partially embedded in the TM. The incus (anvil) is attached to the malleus. The stapes (stirrup) transmits the vibrations of the TM and the other ossicles to the inner ear via the oval window.

Inner Ear

The inner ear or otic capsule is composed of a series of tunnels called *labyrinths* (Figure 25-2). These labyrinths are re-sponsible for the body's equilibrium and for the final reception of sound waves. The *bony labyrinth* is a series of canals hollowed out of the temporal bone. It consists of the *cochlea*, a snail-shaped structure that contains the *organ of Corti*, the organ of hearing. Within the bony labyrinth lies the membranous labyrinth. The bony labyrinth contains a fluid called *perilymph*, and the membranous labyrinth contains *endolymph*. In addition to the cochlea, the bony labyrinth also contains a structure called the *vestibule*. This in turn contains two other structures, the *utriculus* and the *sacculus*, which function along with the *semicircular canals* to control equilibrium and the body's ability to sense its position.

EQUIPMENT AND INSTRUMENTS

The equipment and instruments required for ear surgery are very specialized. The equipment includes an operating microscope and several types of drills, as well as other specialty equipment. The instrumentation is a combination of micro and macro instruments.

Power Drills

Power drills are needed in virtually every ear surgery that involves bone. They are used to remove the large mastoid bone or to drill through the small stapes footplate. Several power drills are available for use during ear surgery, and the choice depends on the procedure to be performed. The most frequently used drills are the Stryker (shown in Figure 25-3), the Anspach, and the Skeeter drills. All of the drills are used

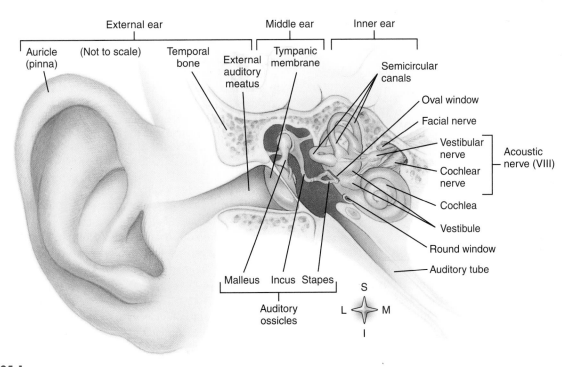

FIGURE 25-1
Structures of the external, middle, and internal ear. (From Thibodeau GA and Patton KT: *Anthony's textbook of anatomy and physiology,* ed 17, St Louis, 2003, Mosby.)

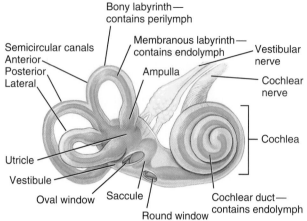

FIGURE 25-2
Labyrinths of the inner ear. (From Applegate EJ: *The anatomy and physiology learning system*, ed 2, Philadelphia, 2000, Saunders.)

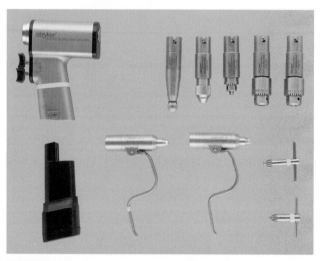

FIGURE 25-3
Left, top to bottom, one Stryker drill; one power pack. *Right top, left to right,* one sagittal saw attachment; one Synthes chuck; one Jacob 5/32 chuck; two Jacob 1/4 chucks; *right bottom, left to right,* one pin collet, 3 mm (1.2); one pin collet, 7 mm (1.8); two chuck keys. (From Tighe SM: *Instrumentation for the operating room*, ed 6, St Louis, 2003, Mosby.)

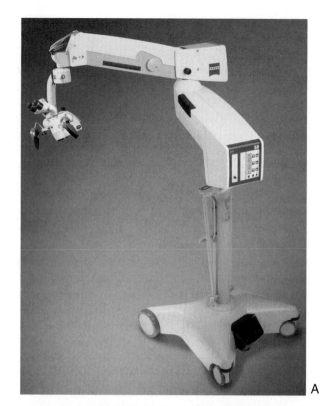

A

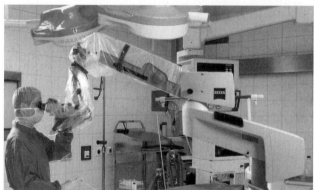

B

FIGURE 25-4
A, Operating microscope used during various otologic procedures. **B,** Draped microscope for otologic surgery. (From Rothrock JC: *Alexander's care of the patient in surgery*, ed 12, St Louis, 2003, Mosby; courtesy of Carl Zeiss.)

with small burs, either cutting or diamond, that vary in size from .5 mm to 7 mm. The surgical technologist should lightly irrigate the bone while drilling is being performed unless a suction irrigator is being used.

Microscopes

Microscopes are a vital piece of equipment in ear surgery. They are used in every procedure involving the middle or inner ear. The standard operating lens for ear surgery is 250 mm in focal length; however, some surgeons may prefer either 200-mm or 300-mm lenses. For procedures such as **myringotomy,** a small operating microscope on a floor stand may be used, but for more involved procedures such as **tympanoplasty** or **mastoidectomy,** a larger, more mobile operating microscope on a floor stand or ceiling mount will be preferred (Figure 25-4, *A*). The microscope is draped with a sterile microscope drape (Figure 25-4, *B*). The drapes usually are clear in color, so it is important to remind others in the room that the microscope has been draped and is sterile.

Speculum Holder

The speculum holder is used to stabilize a speculum in the ear to allow the surgeon to use both hands while operating. Several styles of speculum holders may be used. They usually include a bed bracket, a blade, a flexible arm, and a speculum holder (Figure 25-5). These are used frequently in stapedectomy, which is a transcanal procedure.

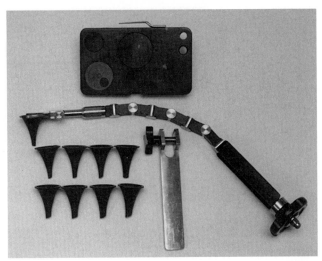

FIGURE 25-5
Universal ear speculum holder and assorted specula. (From Rothrock JC: *Alexander's care of the patient in surgery*, ed 12, St Louis, 2003, Mosby.)

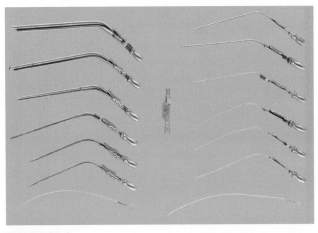

FIGURE 25-6
Suction irrigators. *Left to right,* six House suction/irrigators with finger valve control and one stylet; one metal suction connector; six Baron ear suction tubes with finger valve control and one stylet. (From Tighe SM: *Instrumentation for the operating room*, ed 6, St Louis, 1999, Mosby.)

Suction Irrigators

Suction irrigators are used during drilling (Figure 25-6). They are composed of a Frazier suction device and a smaller irrigator. They allow the surgeon to irrigate the wound through the smaller lumen and suction the irrigation and wound fluids or debris at the same time. Lactated Ringer's solution or normal saline generally is used as the irrigation fluid.

Microinstruments

The primary set of instruments is the basic ear instruments (Figure 25-7); however, several other instruments, including microinstruments, also are required for ear surgery (Figure 25-8). Microinstruments include various picks, knives, forceps, probes, and curettes.

Otologic Endoscopes

Otologic endoscopes occasionally are used in conjunction with other procedures of the ear. They allow the surgeon to visualize parts of the ear anatomy that may otherwise be very difficult to see. The scopes can be of size 4.0 mm or 2.7 mm, depending on the area of the ear that is being examined, and measure 11 cm in length. The endoscopes are connected to a light source via a fiber optic cable. A video tower and camera may or may not be used to assist visualization.

PREPPING AND DRAPING

The surgeon typically shaves a portion of the patient's hair before prepping. (Shaving is never performed for myringotomy and rarely performed for **stapedectomy**) The surgeon also places the facial nerve wires if the facial nerve is to be monitored during the procedure. The circulator preps the surgical site, extending to the cheek medially, the occiput laterally, the temporal bone superiorly, and the upper neck inferiorly. Betadine or Hibiclens solution generally is used to prep the patient.

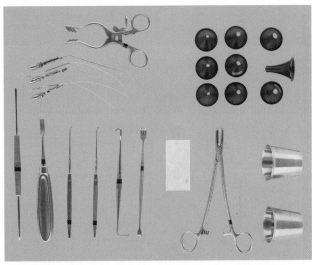

FIGURE 25-7
Left, top to bottom, 1 Weitlaner retractor, dull prongs, angled; 3 Baron ear suction tubes with finger valve control; 3, 5, and 7 Fr; 1 stylet. *Right, top to bottom,* 9 Richard ear spculums, assorted sizes, 4 to 8 mm, one side view. *Bottom, left to right,* 1 Cottle elevator, double ended; 1 Lempert elevetor (converse periosteal); 2 Johnson skin hooks; 2 Senn-Kanavel retractors, side view and front view; 1 House Teflon block; 1 House Gelfoam press or Sheehy fascia press; 2 metal medicine cups, 2 oz. (From Tighe SM: *Instrumentation for the operating room*, ed 6, St Louis, 2003, Mosby.)

The scrub always should ask the surgeon whether he or she wants any prep solution in the ear before prepping. The scrub must take care not to allow prep solution to pool in the ear; prolonged exposure to the solutions can be **ototoxic.** The ear is draped with four towels (usually left unsecured) covered by a transparent drape with a hole. The transparent drape is positioned so that the auricle is exposed through the hole. The drape may be stapled into place. Next, a split sheet is draped over the patient and around the ear (Figure 25-9).

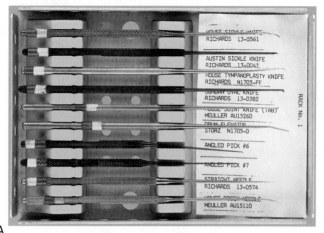

A

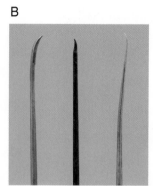

B

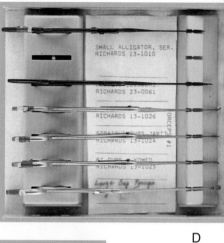

D

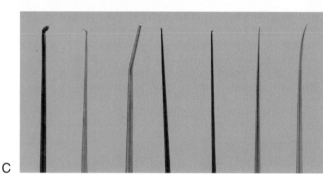

C

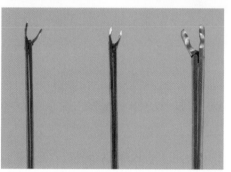

F

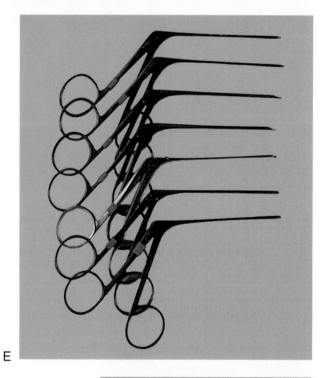

E

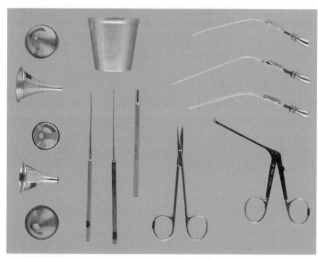

G

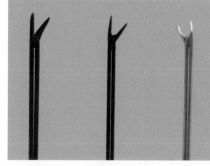

H

FIGURE 25-8

A, Rack no. 1 of delicate ear instruments with labels. **B,** *Left to right,* tips of delicate ear instruments: House sickle knife; Austin sickle knife; House tympanoplasty knife. **C,** *Left to right,* tips of delicate ear instruments; Jordan oval knife; House joint knife; drum elevator; angled pick, no. 6; angled pick, no. 7; straight needle; House Rosen needle. **D,** Tray no. 1 of delicate ear forceps with labels. **E,** Delicate ear forceps out of tray. **F,** *Left to right,* tips of delicate ear forceps: straight-cup forceps; right-cup forceps; large-cup forceps. **G,** *Left, top to bottom,* 5 Boucheron ear speculums, assorted sizes. *Top, left to right,* 1 metal medicine cup, 8 oz; 3 Frazier suction tubes. *Bottom, left to right,* 1 ear curette, small; 1 ear curette, large; 1 myringotomy knife in folding handle with straight Royce blade; 1 iris scissors, straight; 1 alligator forceps, straight. **H,** *Left to right,* tips of delicate ear forceps: small alligator, serrated; Bellucci scissors; left-cup forceps. (From Tighe SM: *Instrumentation for the operating room,* ed 6, St Louis, 2003, Mosby.)

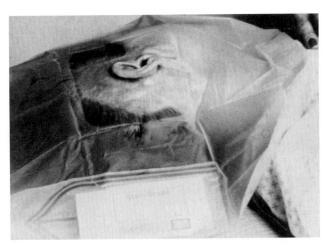

FIGURE 25-9
An ear draped for surgery. (From Brackmann D, Shelton C, and Arriaga MA: *Otologic surgery*, ed 2, Philadelphia, 2001, Saunders.)

MEDICATIONS, SPONGES, AND DRESSINGS

Medications

The primary medications used during ear surgery are anesthetics, hemostatic agents, antibiotic solutions, and irrigation solutions. A local anesthetic with epinephrine is used in most ear surgeries. This practice not only anesthetizes the incision site, but the epinephrine also produces vasoconstriction, which reduces the blood flow to the area.

The hemostatic agents are used to reduce active bleeding. The primary hemostatic agents used are Gelfoam and Helistat. In addition, pledgets may be soaked in epinephrine and applied to the wound to control bleeding. Antibiotic solutions often are instilled into the ear; these may contain steroids as well. Pledgets may be soaked in the antibiotic solution if the solution includes steroids to reduce inflammation.

Sponges

In addition to 4 × 4 Raytec sponges and lap sponges, cotton pledgets and cottonoids may be used during ear surgery. All sponges, needles, and other sharps are counted at the beginning of the case, during the case, and at the end of the case.

Dressings

Two types of dressings are used after ear procedures: the mastoid dressing and the Glasscock dressing. The mastoid dressing is used after complex procedures of the ear, especially those that involve drilling of the mastoid. It consists of several fluffed gauze sponges placed over the ear and incision, and rolled gauze (Kling or Kerlix), which is wrapped around the patient's head to hold the dressing in place. The Glasscock dressing is used after minor procedures of the ear, such as stapedectomy. This dressing comes packaged with a plastic bowl filled with gauze sponges with Velcro straps to secure the dressing in place.

SURGICAL PROCEDURES

Myringotomy

SURGICAL GOAL

Myringotomy is performed to alleviate **effusion.**

PATHOLOGY

A myringotomy is a small incision made in the tympanic membrane to allow the drainage of fluid from the middle ear. This accumulation of fluid is called an effusion. The effusion may be caused by inflammation of the middle ear mucosa or **eustachian tube** dysfunction caused by congenital anomalies, inflammation of nasal mucosa (allergies), or, most often, enlarged adenoids. If left untreated, the effusion may lead to infection (including mastoiditis), hearing loss, or **perforation.** Effusions are seen in patients of all ages; however, most adults are treated in the office. A **tympanostomy tube** often is inserted to maintain the patency of the myringotomy, to allow the fluid to drain freely, and to equalize pressure within the middle ear. Tubes usually are not removed, but rather are left in place until they fall out.

Technique
1. The surgeon places speculums in the ear canal and uses the microscope to visualize the TM.
2. Excess cerumen is removed from the ear canal.
3. A small incision is made in the TM.
4. A tympanostomy tube is placed if necessary.

DISCUSSION

The patient is placed in the supine position with a doughnut headrest. Skin prep and draping usually, but not always, are omitted. General anesthesia is administered via mask, as the procedure is brief. The surgeon sits while operating and uses a microscope with a 250-mm lens. The microscope is brought into position as soon as the surgeon is seated.

To begin the procedure, the surgeon inserts a speculum (usually a Farrior speculum) into the external ear canal. The speculum size is determined by the diameter and depth of the ear canal. With the speculum in place, the surgeon visualizes the TM and removes any wax or debris from the external auditory canal with a cerumen curette. The surgeon makes a 2-mm to 3-mm incision in the TM with a myringotomy blade (Figure 25-10, *A*.) Any fluid behind the TM is suctioned out with a small Frasier micro-suction device of size #3 or #5. If a tympanostomy tube is to be used, the scrub uses an alligator forceps to grasp the tube. The method to be used to load the tube onto the alligator forceps depends on the surgeon's preference. The surgeon then inserts the tube into the myringotomy incision (Figure 25-10, *B*). Next, a fine Rosen needle is used to refine the position of the tube. The instruments needed for myringotomy are shown in Figure 25-11. Antibiotic drops or a combination of antibiotic and steroid drops are then instilled into the external canal, the speculum is removed, and the external canal is packed with cotton.

Circumferential
incision

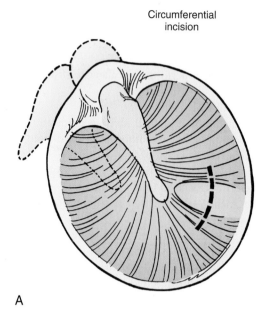

A

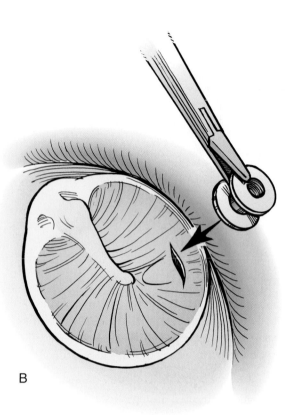

B

FIGURE 25-10
Myringotomy. **A,** Circumferential incision is made in the tympanic membrane. **B,** A tympanostomy tube is inserted into the myringotomy incision. (Modified from Coker NJ and Jenkins HA: *Atlas of otologic surgery,* Philadelphia, 2001, Saunders.)

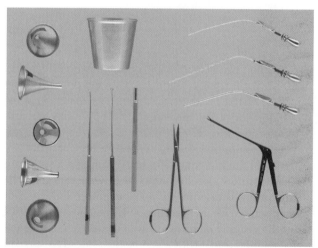

FIGURE 25-11
Myringotomy instrument set. *Left, top to bottom,* five Boucheron ear speculums, assorted sizes. *Top, left to right,* one metal medicine cup, 8 oz; three Frazier suction tubes. *Bottom, left to right,* one ear curette, small; one ear curette, large; one myringotomy knife in folding handle with straight Royce blade; one iris scissors, straight; one alligator forceps, straight. (From Tighe SM: *Instrumentation for the operating room,* ed 6, St Louis, 2003, Mosby.)

Myringoplasty
SURGICAL GOAL
Myringoplasty is performed to close a **perforated** TM.

PATHOLOGY

A myringoplasty is performed to repair a hole, or perforation, of the TM. This perforation may be caused by the removal of a tympanostomy tube or trauma (water skiing fall, cotton swab injuries, blast trauma, or penetrating injuries). Perforations often heal spontaneously. If a perforation is large or not healing properly, a myringoplasty is performed.

Technique

1. The surgeon places a speculum in the external canal to allow visualization of the TM through the microscope.
2. Debris is removed from the ear canal.
3. The TM edges are **everted** and roughened.
4. Fat graft is removed if necessary.
5. A small patch is placed over the perforation.

DISCUSSION

The patient is placed in the supine position with a doughnut headrest. The patient is prepped and draped for an ear procedure. The scrub must avoid allowing prep solution to collect in the ear canal by packing a small piece of cotton into the external auditory canal when prepping, because many prep solutions are ototoxic. General anesthesia via mask is used. Endotracheal intubation seldom is required because the anesthesia time is short.

The surgeon operates while sitting. The operating microscope is fitted with a 250-mm lens; draping of the micro-

Table 25-1   TYMPANOPLASTY

Type	Condition of Middle Ear	Repair/Graft Placement
I	Ossicular chain intact/perforated membrane.	Graft covers the defect and is placed against the malleus.
II	Malleus is damaged.	Graft contacts the body of the incus.
III	Malleus and incus are missing; stapes is intact and mobile.	Graft is placed against the mobile stapes.
IV	Ossicular chain is missing, except for a mobile stapes footplate.	Graft is placed tightly into the oval window.
V	Ossicular chain is intact; the stapes footplate is not mobile.	Graft is placed tightly into the oval window.

scope generally is not necessary. To begin the procedure, the surgeon places a Farrior speculum into the external auditory canal. The surgeon cleans the external canal using a cerumen curette and Frasier suction. The edges of the perforated TM are then everted and scratched with either a fine Rosen needle or a fine right-angle pick. When the edges have been everted, a small patch is placed over the tympanic perforation. Several different types of patches are used (Gelfoam, Gelfilm, Steri-Strip, or a fat graft). The fat generally is removed from the posterior lobe of the affected ear. With the patch or graft in place, the external auditory canal is packed with gelatin sponges soaked in steroid-antibiotic solution, and a Glasscock-style dressing is applied.

Fat Graft

The surgeon makes a small incision (approximately 5 to 8 mm) on the posterior portion of the ear lobe using a #15 blade. Using single skin hooks to expose the wound, the surgeon excises a small portion of adipose tissue with a #15 blade, a hemostat, or toothed Adson forceps. With hemostasis accomplished, the graft site is then closed with a 4-0 Vicryl stitch. When the graft is removed it is placed in normal saline to keep it moist until the surgeon is ready to place it over the wound. The fat is then placed over the perforation in the tympanic membrane.

Tympanoplasty

SURGICAL GOAL

Tympanoplasty is performed to eradicate disease, close a tympanic defect, and improve hearing.

PATHOLOGY

Tympanoplasty is performed to correct several disorders affecting the TM. These conditions include non-healing perforation of the TM, dysfunction of the eustachian tube causing retraction of the TM, and **cholesteatoma.** In dysfunction of the eustachian tube, inadequate airflow between the nasopharynx and the middle ear causes a negative pressure in the middle ear and the retraction of the TM. The retraction causes the TM to vibrate improperly, possibly leading to a perforation or cholesteatoma.

A cholesteatoma is a mass of skin growing in the wrong place. The accumulation of **keratin** causes infection, **otorrhea,** bone destruction, hearing loss, and paralysis of the facial nerve.

Technique

1. The surgeon makes an incision posterior to the ear.
2. A fascia graft is taken.
3. The native TM is removed or prepared for grafting.
4. The ear canal is enlarged with a drill (for **canalplasty**).
5. The tympanic membrane is reconstructed.
6. The incision is closed, and the ear canal is packed.

DISCUSSION

Several methods of performing a tympanoplasty are used, depending on the condition of the TM and its underlying structures (Table 25-1). Following is an overview of the procedure.

The patient is placed in the supine position, with a doughnut headrest, with the operative-side arm tucked at the patient's side. General anesthesia is used. If a skin graft is to be taken from the arm or abdomen, it may be taken before prepping and draping. The arm is prepped and draped with towels. The surgeon then takes the graft, using a sharp double-edged razor blade, such as a Gillette, a Watson, or a Cobbett or Weck skin-graft knife.

After the graft is taken, it is placed on the sterile field and kept moist with either normal saline or antibiotic ointment, depending on surgeon preference. The arm is then dressed. The patient is then prepped and draped for an ear procedure.

The surgeon makes an incision behind the ear and extends it through the temporalis fascia to the level of the mastoid tip, using a #15 blade (Figure 25-12, *A*). The surgeon takes a temporalis fascia graft, using brown Adson forceps and a #15 blade. The graft must be large enough to cover the tympanic defect. A fascia press may used to flatten and shape the graft. The fascia press with the graft on it should be left in the open position, unless the surgeon requests otherwise. This allows the graft to dry so that it may be trimmed and placed in the ear at a later time (Figure 25-12, *B*). An operative microscope with a 250-mm lens is used to visualize the middle ear. The microscope is draped with a sterile microscope drape.

The surgeon then exposes the native TM using a gimmick or weapon and then removes it using Bellucci scissors, the weapon, and/or a lancet knife. If a canalplasty is to be per-

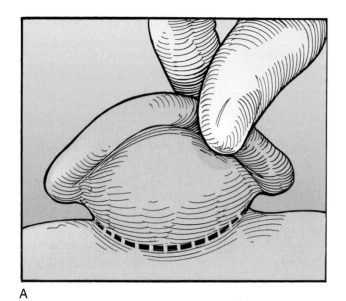

A

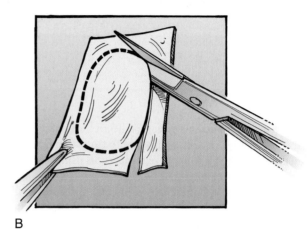

B

FIGURE 25-12
Tympanoplasty. **A,** The incision is made behind the ear and extends through the temporalis fascia. **B,** The temporalis fascia graft is trimmed. (Modified from Coker NJ and Jenkins HA: *Atlas of otologic surgery,* Philadelphia, 2001, Saunders.)

formed, the ear canal is enlarged with a small cutting drill and a small, 4 × 5 suction irrigator. This allows the surgeon better visualization of the middle ear and a greater space in which to work.

Next, the surgeon prepares the middle ear to receive the graft. The surgeon trims the fascia graft to the appropriate size using the fascia press and a #15 blade. The graft is then grasped with a smooth alligator forceps and removed from the fascia press. The surgeon then reconstructs the middle ear by placing the graft into position using the alligator forceps and a fine Rosen needle. The skin grafts are then laid over the fascia graft with alligator forceps and a fine Rosen needle. The ear is then packed with small pledgets of gel foam or Helistat to hold the graft in position. The surgeon does this using alligator forceps and a gimmick. The wound is then closed in layers with 3-0 absorbable sutures, and the skin is closed with 4-0 absorbable sutures. The wound is then dressed with a mastoid dressing.

Mastoidectomy/Tympanomastoidectomy
SURGICAL GOAL
Mastoidectomy, or tympanomastoidectomy, is performed to remove the mastoid process and eradicate disease.

PATHOLOGY
Mastoidectomy is indicated in cholesteatoma, unreconstructable posterior canal wall, contracted mastoid, **neoplasms,** and nonfunctioning eustachian tube. The most common reason for performing mastoidectomy is cholesteatoma. This procedure may be performed in adults or children. Mastoidectomy is often performed in conjunction with tympanoplasty.

Technique
1. The ear is injected with lidocaine with epinephrine.
2. The surgeon makes the postauricular incision.
3. The flaps are elevated.
4. Temporalis fascia is harvested.
5. Diseased mastoid is removed with a drill.
6. The ossicles are removed if diseased.
7. The cholesteatoma is removed.
8. The mastoid cavity and middle ear are packed.
9. Incisions are closed.
10. Dressings are applied.

DISCUSSION
The patient is placed in the supine position with a doughnut headrest, and the operative-side arm is tucked at the patient's side. The ear is injected with lidocaine with epinephrine via a small, 27-gauge needle. General anesthetic is used. The skin grafts are taken before the patient is prepped. The patient is prepped and draped for an ear procedure.

The surgeon makes a postauricular incision. As with tympanoplasty, the temporalis fascia is harvested, smoothed onto the fascia press, and left to dry. The diseased mastoid then is drilled out with a power drill with a large cutting bur and with a large, 7 × 10 or 12 × 14 suction irrigator. As the surgeon drills the disease away, he or she may want to change to smaller burs or diamond burs. The surgeon will use Rosen needles, gimmicks, or picks to assess patency of the mastoid antrum and to assess the facial recess if this has been resected as the drilling progresses. At this time the surgeon takes the ossicles, if necessary, using a joint knife. A malleus nipper, Bellucci scissors, weapon, or other microsurgical instruments also may be used. The surgeon removes all evidence of cholesteatoma using a gimmick or Rosen needle to remove it from the tissue.

With the cholesteatoma removed, the surgeon places the fascia graft over the remaining ossicles. This is done in the same fashion as with tympanoplasty. The skin graft then is laid over the fascia. The surgeon then uses a serrated alligator and a gimmick to pack the mastoid cavity and middle ear with gelatin sponges that have been soaked in saline solution or steroid-antibiotic drops. The incisions are then closed in layers with 3-0 absorbable sutures. The skin is closed with 4-0 absorbable sutures. The surgeon then uses a serrated alligator and a gimmick to pack the external auditory canal with gelatin sponges that have been soaked in saline solution or steroid-antibiotic solution. A mastoid dressing then is applied.

Stapedectomy/Ossicular Reconstruction
SURGICAL GOAL
Stapedectomy, or ossicular reconstruction, is performed to restore mobilization of the ossicular chain.

PATHOLOGY
Stapedectomy or ossicular reconstruction may be performed in patients who have hearing loss that can progress to deafness. This hearing loss may be caused by otosclerosis, which causes the formation of abnormal bone growth that locks the stapes into place and prevents it from vibrating and carrying the stimulus. Otosclerosis generally begins when the patient is in his or her thirties and progresses with age. After surgery, 90% of surgically treated ears have permanent hearing gain, while 1% have permanent hearing loss.

Technique
1. The auditory canal is injected with lidocaine with epinephrine.
2. The external auditory canal is cleaned.
3. The surgeon places the speculum in the external auditory canal.
4. The TM is elevated.
5. The affected ossicles are freed or removed.
6. A small drill is used to drill a hole in the stapes footplate.
7. The prosthesis is placed and secured.
8. The TM is replaced.
9. The external canal is packed, and the dressing is applied.

DISCUSSION
The patient is placed in the supine position with a doughnut headrest, and the operative-side arm is tucked. General anesthesia is used. The patient is prepped and draped for an ear procedure. The external ear canal is injected with local anesthetic. The operative microscope with a 250-mm lens is used to visualize the middle ear. The external ear canal is cleaned with irrigation and 7-Fr Frazier suction.

The surgeon places a speculum in the external canal; the surgeon usually starts with a small speculum and progresses to a larger speculum. When the correct speculum is in place, the surgeon applies the universal speculum holder to stabilize the speculum. This allows the surgeon to operate with both hands while the speculum is maintained in the external canal. The surgeon then changes to 5-Fr Frazier suction to clear any fluid from the ear.

The surgeon elevates the TM and removes the posterior bony ledge using a House knife (weapon). With the TM elevated, the surgeon now has visualization of the ossicular chain. The surgeon cuts the incostapedial joint using a joint knife and severs the stapedial tendon with Bellucci scissors. The stapes superstructure is then the fractured with a fine Rosen needle and microcupped forceps.

Next, the surgeon drills a hole into the stapes footplate using a Skeeter drill or similar drill with a 1-mm cutting bur. The surgeon has loaded the prosthesis onto a serrated alligator or hook, and the surgeon now places the prosthesis by connecting it to the hole that has been drilled into the footplate. The surgeon then secures the prosthesis into place by using a serrated alligator and gimmick or Rosen needle to pack the ear with gelatin sponges soaked in normal saline or steroid-antibiotic ointment. The surgeon replaces the TM using the gimmick and a fine Rosen needle. The external auditory canal then is packed with gelatin sponges that have been soaked in saline or antibiotic-steroid solution. A Glasscock or mastoid dressing then is applied.

Cochlear Implant
SURGICAL GOAL
A cochlear implant is used to restore sound perception.

PATHOLOGY
A cochlear implant is performed to treat profound deafness. Deafness can be either congenital or acquired (profound **sensorineural deafness**). Sensorineural deafness is characterized by the inability of hair cells to stimulate the cochlear nerve. Cochlear implants in children are contraindicated until age 2. The primary reason for placing a cochlear implant in a child is to treat congenital deafness.

Technique
1. The surgeon makes a postauricular incision, extending superiorly over the temporal squama.
2. The cranium is exposed.
3. The site of the internal receiver is drilled out.
4. The mastoid is drilled.
5. The facial nerve is identified.
6. The medial wall of the middle ear is identified.
7. The internal electrodes of the implant are placed into the cochlea via the round window.
8. The internal receiver is placed and secured.
9. Hemostasis is achieved.
10. The incision is closed.

DISCUSSION
The patient is positioned supine with a doughnut headrest and with the operative-side arm tucked at the side. The head

is positioned so that the operative ear is exposed. General anesthesia is used. The surgeon shaves the hair in the temporal region. The intended site of the surgical incision is marked with a surgical marker. The surgical site is injected with 1% lidocaine with epinephrine 1:100,000. The facial nerve monitor is used to monitor stimulation of the facial nerve during the procedure. The surgeon places the electrodes for facial-nerve monitoring and connects them to the monitor. The patient is prepped and draped for an ear procedure.

The surgeon makes a postauricular incision and extends it superiorly to the temporal region using a #15 blade. The flap is elevated using needle-tip electrocautery with retraction provided by double-prong skin hooks or three-prong wire rakes.

With the flaps elevated, the surgeon places a Beckman-Adson retractor or similar self-retaining retractor under the flaps to expose the cranium. The internal receiver template is placed and marked with either a sterile surgical marking pen or the electrocautery. The surgeon then drills the temporal bone using a medium-size cutting bur and a 4 × 5 or 5 × 7 suction irrigator. The template is placed periodically in the drilled portion of the temporal bone to ensure that the proper depth and width have been drilled. A medium-size diamond bur is used to finish the edges of the temporal bone. Suture tunnel holes are placed, two on each side of the internal processor recess, to allow for the securing of the processor.

Next, the mastoidectomy is performed. The surgeon drills the mastoid with a large cutting bur and a 5 × 7 or 7 × 10 suction irrigator, preserving the bony ear canal and the opening of the facial recess. With the medial wall of the middle ear identified, the implant is opened. The implant is opened onto the sterile field very slowly, to limit the amount of static electricity created. The sterile implant package is then submerged in normal saline and opened slowly under water; this further reduces the amount of static charge. (Static charge could interfere with the function of the implant electrodes.)

The surgeon then places the internal processor into the recessed temporal bone and places the active electrode through the facial recess and through the round window into the cochlea using the electrode positioner included in the cochlear implant instrument set (provided by the manufacturer of the implant). The surgeon then secures the active electrode into place by placing temporalis fascia into the round window using a gimmick or fine Rosen needle.

The surgeon next secures the internal processor by placing a 2-0 or larger Prolene suture through the suture tunnel holes, tying the knots diagonally across the holes (Figure 25-13). Hemostasis is achieved with a bipolar cautery (monopolar cautery could cause current to be passed through the receiver). With the implant secured, the fascia overlying the cranium is closed with 2-0 absorbable suture. A 3-0 absorbable suture is used to close the subcutaneous tissue. The skin then is closed with a nonabsorbable suture. A mastoid dressing is placed over the wound.

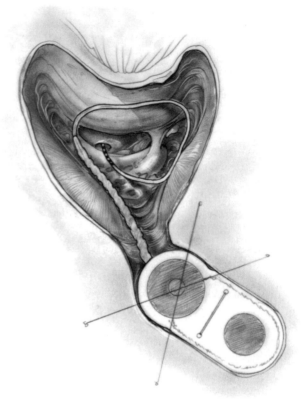

FIGURE 25-13
The cochlear implant is secured with suture, and knots are tied diagonally. (From Brackmann D, Shelton C, and Arriaga MA: *Otologic surgery*, ed 2, Philadelphia, 2001, Saunders.)

SECTION II
Surgery of the Nose, Throat, and Mouth

INTRODUCTION TO SURGERY OF THE NOSE, THROAT, AND MOUTH

Procedures of the nose, throat, and mouth involve the external and internal nasal cavities, sinuses, tonsils, and adenoids. These procedures are performed primarily by otorhinolaryngologists. Procedures involving facial reconstruction are performed primarily by maxillofacial or plastic surgeons. Procedures involving the teeth are performed primarily by oral surgeons.

ANATOMY OF THE NOSE

External Nose

The external nose is formed by two U-shaped cartilaginous structures called the *nares*. Within each naris is the *nostril*, the actual opening through the naris. The nares are formed by the *alar cartilage*. Another cartilaginous structure, the *septum*, separates the two nostrils (Figure 25-14, *A*). The roof of the nose is formed by the *nasal bone*, which consists

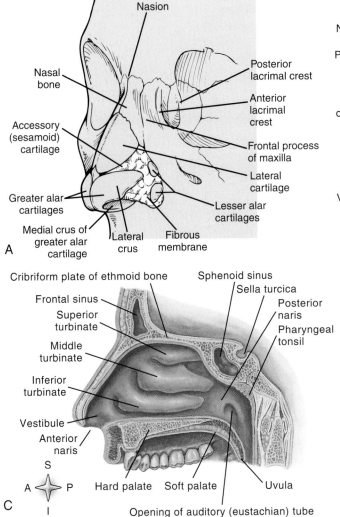

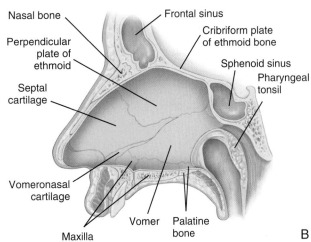

FIGURE 25-14
A, External anatomy of the nose. **B,** Nasal cavity. **C,** Nasal septum. (**A** from Fortunato N and McCullough SM: *Plastic and reconstructive surgery: perioperative nursing series,* St Louis, 1998, Mosby; **B** and **C** from Thibodeau GA and Patton KT: *Anthony's textbook of anatomy and physiology,* ed 17, St Louis, 2003, Mosby.)

of portions of the ethmoid, sphenoid, and palatine bones. The floor of the nose is formed by the maxilla and palatine bones, and the lateral walls are formed by the *nasal conchae,* which divide the two nasal cavities into passageways called *meatuses.* The nasal cavity is lined with mucous membrane, which aids in the warming and humidifying process. Small hairs or *vibrissae* are also present, and these filter out large foreign material as the air passes over them. The *posterior nares,* the back portion of the passageways, open directly into the *pharynx* (discussed subsequently).

Nasal Cavity/Septum

The nasal cavity extends from the piriform aperture to the choanae posteriorly and is separated in the midline by the septum, which is composed of quadrangular cartilage anteriorly and bone posteriorly. The floor of the nose is the palate, which separates the nose from the mouth. The roof of the nose separates it from the anterior cranial fossa.

Extending from the roof of the nose and the lateral nasal walls are the conch shell–shaped turbinates. The inferior, middle, and superior (and occasionally the supreme)

turbinates form spaces lateral to the inferior, middle, and superior meatuses, respectively. The nasolacrimal duct (tear duct) drains into the inferior meatus. The frontal sinus, maxillary sinus, and anterior and middle ethmoid sinuses drain into the middle meatus. The posterior ethmoid sinuses and sphenoid sinus drain into the superior meatus. The nasal cavity and septum are shown in Figure 25-14, B and C.

Paranasal Sinuses

The paired maxillary sinuses are the large sinuses below the orbits. The apices of the tooth roots are found in the floor of these sinuses. The paired frontal sinuses lie behind the lower forehead. The ethmoid sinuses consist of many small air cells in the roof of the nasal cavity between the lateral nasal wall and turbinates. The sphenoids lie at the posterosuperior extent of the nasal cavity. The optic nerves are within the lateral wall of these sinuses, and the pituitary gland lies behind and above them. The sphenoids are often traversed to allow surgical access to these structures. The anatomy of the sinuses is shown in Figure 25-15.

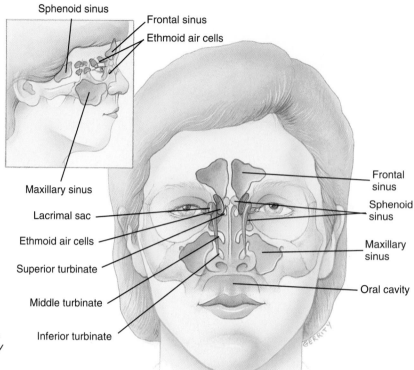

FIGURE 25-15
Anatomy of the sinuses. (From Thibodeau GA and Patton KT: *Anthony's textbook of anatomy and physiology*, ed 17, St Louis, 2003, Mosby.)

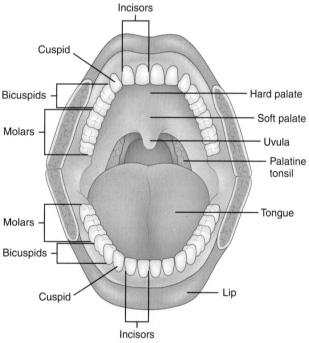

FIGURE 25-16
Oral cavity. (Modified from Herlihy B and Maebius NK: *The human body in health and illness*, ed 2, Philadelphia, 2003, Saunders.)

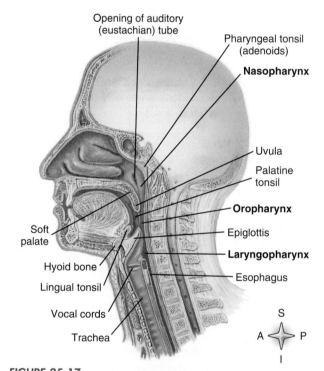

FIGURE 25-17
Anatomy of the pharynx. (From Thibodeau GA and Patton KT: *Anthony's textbook of anatomy and physiology*, ed 17, St Louis, 2003, Mosby.)

ANATOMY OF THE MOUTH

The mouth consists of all structures between the lips and the mucosal folds posterior to the tonsils, and is divided into two sections: (1) the vestibule, which lies between the inner sur-

face of the lips and buccal mucosa (cheeks) and the lateral aspects of the mandible (jaw bone) and maxilla, and (2) the oral cavity proper, which lies within the medial surface of the maxillary and mandibular teeth. The roof of the oral cavity proper consists of the hard and soft palates and separates it

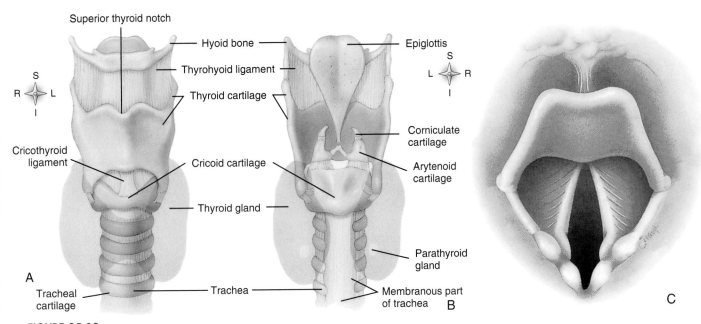

FIGURE 25-18
A, Anterior view of the pharynx. **B,** Posterior view of the pharynx. **C,** The vocal cords. (From Thibodeau GA and Patton KT: *Anthony's textbook of anatomy and physiology,* ed 17, St Louis, 2003, Mosby.)

from the nasal cavity (Figure 25-16). The soft palate meets in the middle to form the uvula.

The floor of the mouth contains the ducts for the paired submandibular and lingual glands. The tongue lies within the floor of the mouth and is a muscular structure capable of fluid movement. The tongue is divided into the anterior two thirds and the posterior third, or base of tongue, by the circumvillate papilla, a V-shaped row of large taste buds. The anterior two thirds of the tongue lies within the oral cavity proper and is attached in the midline to the floor of the mouth by a membranous structure called the frenulum.

ANATOMY OF THE PHARYNX

The pharynx is a tubular structure extending from the nose to the esophagus and is separated into three areas: the **nasopharynx,** the **oropharynx,** and the **hypopharynx** (Figure 25-17). The nasopharynx extends from the posterior chonae of the nose to the palate. The adenoids lie in the posterosuperior aspect of the nasopharynx, and the eustachian tubes open on each side of the adenoids. The oropharynx extends from the palate to the hyoid bone. The soft palate, tonsils, and posterior third of the tongue (base of tongue) lie in the anterior portion of the oropharynx. The hypopharynx extends from the hyoid bone to the esophagus. The paired piriform sinuses are mucosal patches that are found in the lateral aspects of the hypopharynx. The larynx is anterior to the hypopharynx.

ANATOMY OF THE LARYNX

The larynx is composed of nine segments of cartilage, three paired sets and three unpaired segments (Figure 25-18, *A* and *B*). The unpaired cartilages are the cricoid, thyroid, and

epiglottis segments, and the paired are the arytenoids, corniculate, and cuneiform segments. The larynx is separated into three spaces.

The supraglottis lies above the true vocal cords and contains the vestibule, the false vocal cords, and the epiglottis, consisting of spoon-shaped cartilage. The **glottis** extends from the true vocal cords to 1 cm below the free edge of the true vocal cords. The subglottis extends below this position to the inferior edge of the **cricoid cartilage.** The arytenoid cartilages lie in the posterior larynx and have processes that extend anteriorly (the vocal processes) and that lie within the true vocal cords (Figure 25-18, *C*). The area between the arytenoids is called the posterior commissure. The true vocal cords meet anteriorly at the anterior commissure and connect to the thyroid cartilage. The free edge of the true vocal cords has a loosely covered membrane that vibrates to produce **phonation.**

EQUIPMENT AND INSTRUMENTS

Microdebrider

Microdebriders are used in nasal and laryngeal surgeries to excise tissue. They consist of a small powered handpiece that is loaded with a debriding blade. This is a small blade that rotates within a larger blade. The microdebrider suctions as it cuts away the tissue, removing blood and debris from the surgical field. Most microdebriders also irrigate through the blade. This helps the surgeon maintain visualization. Different blades are used, depending on the operation being performed. The nasal blades are relatively short and are straight or have a 15-degree bend, while the laryngeal blades are long and usually have a 15-degree or 30-degree bend.

Suction Cautery

Suction cautery is used primarily in tonsillectomies and adenoidectomies. This particular cautery device is connected to suction, allowing the surgeon to suction blood and debris from the field while cauterizing tissue. It is generally used with the foot pedal.

Microscope

An operative microscope fitted with a lens of 400-mm focal length is used for microlaryngeal surgery. The microscope gives the surgeon better visualization of the small structures of the larynx. The microscope typically is not draped sterilely. When the surgeon is under the microscope, the surgical technologist must guide the instruments into the laryngoscope, because the surgeon will not be focused on the end of the laryngoscope.

Sinus Scopes

Sinus scopes are used in endoscopic sinus surgery to give the surgeon visualization of the various sinuses. They come in 0-degree, 30-degree, and 70-degree angles (Figure 25-19). The 0-degree scope is used initially for all procedures. The 30-degree scope is used for maxillary, sphenoid, and ethmoid sinus procedures; and the 70-degree scope is used for procedures of the frontal sinus.

Nasal Instruments

Nasal instruments are used for all procedures involving the nose. They include various nasal speculums, scissors, cupped forceps, probes, chisels, and elevators. Basic nasal instruments are depicted in Figure 25-20.

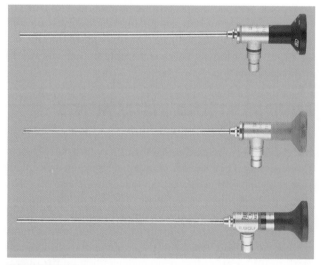

FIGURE 25-19
Sinus scopes, *bottom to top*, 0 degree; 30 degree; and 70 degree. (From Tighe SM: *Instrumentation for the operating room*, ed 6, St Louis, 2003, Mosby.)

Tonsil and Adenoid Instruments

Tonsil and adenoid instruments include the Crowe-Davis mouth gag, tonsil snares, adenoid curettes, elevators, clamps, and scissors. The Crowe-Davis mouth gag is suspended from the Mayo stand during the procedure to hold the mouth open and allow the surgeon the use of both hands. Tonsil snares are loaded with wire and are used to transect the tonsils. Basic tonsil and adenoid instruments are shown in Figure 25-21.

PREPPING AND DRAPING

The prepping and draping varies depending on the procedure being performed. Patients undergoing nasal procedures generally are prepped with Betadine or Hibiclens from the level of the forehead to the upper neck, including the entire face. Intranasal (endoscopic) procedures may not be prepped, according to the preference of the surgeon. The patient may be draped with a head drape. The head drape consists of towels folded into a triangular shape, wrapped around the patient's head like a turban, and secured with a towel clip (that goes through only the towel). A three-quarter sheet is placed under the patient's head. The face then is draped with four towels secured with towel clips, and a split sheet is placed over the patient and around the face. Generally there is no prep for tonsillectomy, adenoidectomy, **laryngoscopy, bronchoscopy,** and **esophagoscopy.** These procedures may not be draped at all or may be draped with a "down" sheet (a three-quarter sheet draped over the patient's chest).

MEDICATIONS, SPONGES, AND DRESSINGS

Medications

Medications used for procedures of the nose, mouth, and throat include anesthetic agents, vasoconstrictive agents, decongestants, and bismuth. Local anesthetic with epinephrine is injected into the nasal mucosa and turbinates for most nasal procedures. This step is performed to anesthetize the area and to produce some vasoconstriction. Cocaine in a solution may be used as a vasoconstrictive agent in the nose or larynx. For use with the nose, the solution is placed on cottonoid sponges and packed into the nose; for the larynx, it is place on strung cotton pledgets and placed into the larynx. One may use decongestants such as Afrin to decongest the nose by soaking cottonoids in the solution and then packing them into the nose. Bismuth is used in tonsillectomies as a hemostatic agent. It is applied to strung cotton sponges that are packed into the tonsillar fossa after removal of the tonsil.

Sponges

In addition to Raytec sponges, the surgeon uses cottonoids, cotton pledgets, and strung cotton sponges in procedures of the nose, mouth, and throat. These sponges are counted

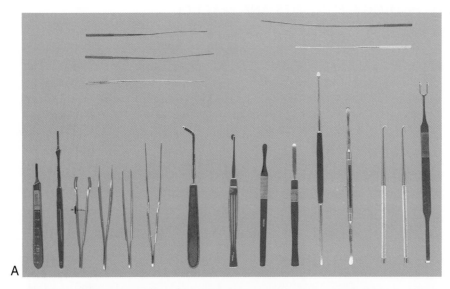

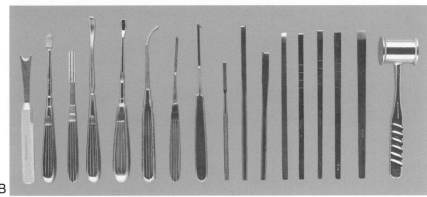

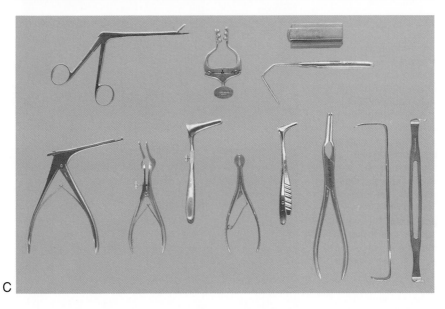

FIGURE 25-20

Basic nasal instruments. **A,** *Top,* five Ludwig wire applicators. *Bottom, left to right,* one Bard-Parker knife handle, no. 3; one Bard Parker knife handle, no. 7; one Cottle columella forceps; one Brown-Adson tissue forceps with teeth (7 × 7); one Beasley-Babcock tissue forceps; one Jansen thumb forceps, bayonet shaft, serrated tips; one Joseph button-end knife, curved; one Freer septum knife; one Cottle nasal knife; one McKenty elevator; one Cottle septum elevator; one Freer elevator; two Joseph skin hooks; one Cottle knife guide and retractor. **B,** *Left to right,* one Bauer rocking chisel; one Lewis rasp; one Maltz rasp; one Aufricht rasp, large; one Aufricht rasp, small; one Wiener antrum rasp; two Ballenger swivel knives; one Ballenger chisel, 4 mm; two Converse guarded osteotomes; one Cottle osteotome, round corners, curved, 6 mm; four Cottle osteotomes, straight: 4, 7, 9, and 12 mm; one mallet, lead-filled head. **C,** *Top, left to right,* one Ferris-Smith fragment forceps; one mastoid articulated retractor; one Cottle bone crusher, closed; one Aufricht retractor. *Bottom, left to right,* one Kerrison rongeur, upbite; one Killian nasal speculum, 2 inch, front view; one Killian nasal speculum, 3 inch, side view; one Vienna nasal speculum, 1⅜ inch, front view; one Vienna nasal speculum, 1⅛ inch, side view; one Asch septum forceps; two Army-Navy retractors, side view and front view. (From Tighe SM: *Instrumentation for the operating room,* ed 6, St Louis, 2003, Mosby.)

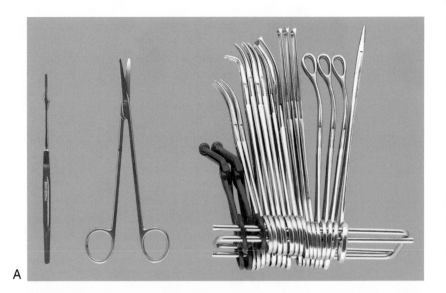

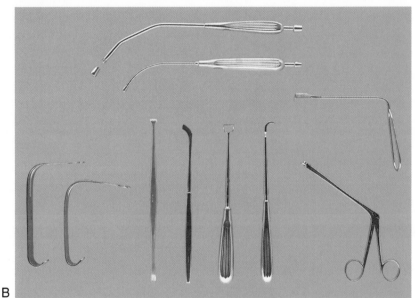

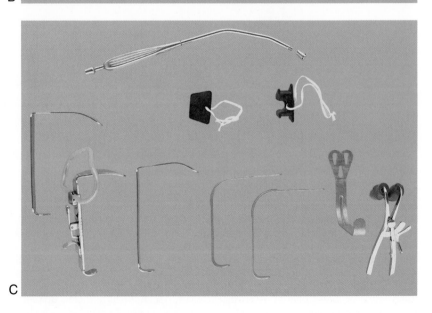

FIGURE 25-21
Basic tonsil and adenoid instruments. **A,** *Left to right,* one Bard-Parker knife handle, no. 7; one Metzenbaum scissors, 7 inch; two paper drape clips; two Crile hemostatic forceps, 6½ inch; one Westphal hemostatic forceps; four tonsil hemostatic forceps; one Allis tissue forceps, long, curved; one Allis tissue forceps, long; three Ballenger sponge forceps, curved; one Crile-Wood needle holder, 8 inch. **B,** *Top to bottom,* one Andrews-Pynchon suction tube with tip; one adenoid suction tube, tip connected. *Bottom, left to right,* two Weider tongue depressors; one Hurd tonsil dissector and pillar retractor; one Fisher tonsil knife and dissector; one LaForce adenotome, small, front view; one LaForce adenotome, large, side view. *Right, top to bottom,* one Lothrop uvula retractor; one Meltzer adenoid punch, round, with basket. **C,** *Top to bottom,* one Andrews-Pynchon suction tube with tip; two bite blocks: child and adult. *Left to right,* one McIvor mouth gag frame with blade and two additional blades; three Weider tongue depressors, two side views and one front view; one side mouth gag. (From Tighe SM: *Instrumentation for the operating room,* ed 6, St Louis, 2003, Mosby.)

along with needles and other sharps at the beginning of the procedure, during the procedure, and at the conclusion of the case.

Dressings

Typically, no dressings are applied to the mouth and throat after the procedure. A variety of nasal dressings may be used, depending on the procedure that has been performed. Internal splint packs may be placed to hold the nasal passages open or to aid in the control of bleeding or drainage after **septoplasty** or **rhinoplasty**. These include bivalve splints, Doyle splints, and nasal packing. Packing may be soaked in antibiotic ointment before it is placed in the nose. External splints generally are placed after a rhinoplasty. Several types of external splints are available. These include metal splints, fiberglass splints, and tape. These splints help support the nose and protect it from damage, much like a cast supports and protects a long bone.

SURGICAL PROCEDURES

Endoscopic Sinus Surgery
SURGICAL GOAL
Endoscopic sinus surgery is performed to treat disease of the **paranasal sinuses,** nasal cavity, and skull base, and to improve nasal airflow.

PATHOLOGY
Most endoscopic procedures of the nose are performed to treat inflammatory or infectious diseases. These conditions can include polyps, as these arise from inflammation of the nasal mucosa. Rarely, intranasal neoplasms, **epistaxis,** and CSF (cerebrospinal fluid) leaks may be treated endoscopically.

Technique
1. The nasal mucosa is injected with local anesthetic.
2. The nasal cavities are packed with decongestant.
3. The surgeon inserts the endoscope into the nasal cavity.
4. Diseased tissue is removed.
5. Hemostasis is achieved.

DISCUSSION
The patient is placed in the supine position with a doughnut headrest, and the arms are tucked at the sides. General anesthesia is used. Local anesthesia, usually 1% lidocaine with epinephrine 1:100,000, is injected into the nasal mucosa. The surgeon then uses a nasal speculum and bayonet forceps to pack the nose with cottonoids, $\frac{1}{2}$-inch- by 6-inch, soaked in a nasal decongestant (cocaine, topical adrenaline 1:1000, or Afrin). The patient is prepped and draped for a nasal procedure. The 0-degree sinus endoscope is inserted into the nasal cavity to allow visualization.
Polypectomy
Under direct visualization, the surgeon removes the **nasal polyps** using either a Wilde forceps or a powered irrigating microdebrider. A 12-Fr Frazier tip suction device is used to suction nasal contents.
Maxillary Antrostomy
Under direct visualization with the 0-degree endoscope, the surgeon displaces the middle turbinate using a Freer elevator. The surgeon then removes the uncinate process either sharply, using the sickle knife and Cottle elevator, or by using the microdebrider after disruption of the mucosa with a Lusk osteum-seeking probe. A ball-tip suction probe then is used to identify the maxillary antrum. The surgeon may wish to change to a 30-degree endoscope to view the maxillary sinus. The antrum is then enlarged with either a microdebrider or a back biter. Inflammatory disease and polyps may be removed from within the maxillary sinus with a microdebrider, Wilde forceps, or Takahashi forceps.
Ethmoidectomy
Under direct visualization with a 0-degree endoscope, the surgeon **medializes** the middle turbinate and removes the uncinate, as in the maxillary antrostomy. This allows the surgeon to visualize the middle meatus. The ethmoids then are removed with either the microdebrider or Wilde forceps.
Frontal Sinus
Under direct visualization with a 0-degree endoscope, the surgeon medializes the middle turbinate and removes the uncinate, as in the maxillary antrostomy. This allows the surgeon to visualize the middle meatus. The surgeon then changes to a 30-degree or 70-degree endoscope. Any bony obstruction at the frontal sinus osteum is excised if necessary, with a microdebrider with a curved blade or with Wilde forceps.
Sphenoidectomy
Under direct visualization with a 0-degree endoscope, the surgeon medializes the middle turbinate and removes the uncinate, as in the maxillary antrostomy. This allows the surgeon to visualize the middle meatus. The posterior ethmoids then are removed with either the microdebrider or Wilde forceps. The surgeon may change to a 30-degree endoscope to better visualize the sphenoid sinus. The osteum is then opened with the microdebrider or Wilde forceps. Any disease then is removed with the Wilde forceps or Takahashi forceps.

Hemostasis is achieved with nasal packs soaked in decongestant. These are removed after several minutes, and, if necessary, the surgeon packs the nose by filling the nasal cavity with antibiotic ointment or by packing the nose with $\frac{1}{2}$-inch gauze packing saturated in antibiotic ointment.

Caldwell-Luc
SURGICAL GOAL
A Caldwell-Luc procedure is performed to produce access to the maxillary sinus.

PATHOLOGY
The Caldwell-Luc procedure is performed for several reasons. These include intractable infection, failure of a chronic

infection to resolve after intranasal antrostomy, polypoid tissue that fills the antrum, cystic disease of the antrum, osteonecrosis, and suspicion of maxillary sinus neoplasm. This procedure typically is not performed in children. This procedure produces access to the maxillary sinus and pterygomaxillary fissure.

Technique

1. The surgeon makes the incision in the gingivo-buccal sulcus.
2. The periosteum over the canine fossa is elevated.
3. The infraorbital nerve is identified.
4. The anterior wall of the antrum is opened.
5. Cysts and tumors are removed.
6. The gingivo-buccal incision is closed.

DISCUSSION

The patient is positioned supine with a doughnut headrest and arms tucked at the side. General anesthetic is used. Usually no prep is performed because the incision is through the mouth. The patient is draped for a nasal procedure. The lip is retracted with a gauze sponge, and the surgeon makes a horizontal incision in the gingivo-buccal sulcus using electrocautery, being sure to be superior to the roots of the teeth. The incision extends from the lateral incisor to the second molar through to the **periosteum.** The mucous membranes are retracted superiorly with an Army-Navy retractor to expose the periosteum overlying the canine fossa. The periosteum is elevated with a Freer periosteal elevator to the level of the infraorbital nerve. The nerve then is identified and preserved. The anterior wall of the maxillary sinus is fenestrated with a drill fitted with a small cutting bur. With the anterior wall opened, the surgeon enlarges the opening using a Kerrison bone-cutting forceps. Cysts and tumors then are removed with Wilde-Blakesley and Takahashi forceps. The gingivo-buccal incision is then closed with 3-0 absorbable sutures.

This procedure is illustrated in Figure 25-22.

Turbinectomy/Turbinate Reduction
SURGICAL GOAL
Turbinectomy is performed to improve nasal airflow.

PATHOLOGY
Nasal airflow may be impaired by the chronic engorgement of the middle and/or inferior turbinate, which causes nasal congestion and **rhinorrhea.**

Technique

1. The nose is packed with a vasoconstrictive agent, and a local anesthetic (1% lidocaine with epinephrine 1:100,000) is instilled into the turbinate.
2. A nasal speculum is inserted into the nose to expose the affected turbinate.
3. The surgeon removes or reduces the affected turbinate.
4. The nose is packed if necessary.

DISCUSSION

The patient is positioned supine with a doughnut headrest and the arms tucked at the sides. General or local anesthesia may be used. The patient is prepped and draped for a nasal procedure. The surgeon begins by instilling the turbinate with local anesthetic, usually 1% lidocaine with epinephrine 1:100,000, and the nose may be packed with vasoconstrictive agents. The surgeon then places a nasal speculum into the nose to retract the nostril and expose the turbinates. If a turbinectomy is to be performed, a #15 blade is used to make an incision into the mucosa at the anterior border of the inferior turbinate. The mucosa is elevated off the underlying bone with a Freer or Cottle elevator. A portion of the bone then is removed with a Wilde forceps. The mucosa may be closed with a 3-0 chromic suture.

If a turbinate reduction is to be performed, a sharp two-prong electrocautery, sometimes called a turbinate bipolar, may be inserted into the turbinate and used for several seconds, causing desiccation of the tissue. The surgeon also may use Coblation or Somnus cauterization to desiccate the turbinate by placing the probe onto the turbinate for a few seconds. The nasal speculum is removed, and the nasal cavity is packed if necessary.

Septoplasty
SURGICAL GOAL
Septoplasty is performed to produce a patent nasal airway.

PATHOLOGY
Septoplasty, the removal of a portion of the bony nasal septum, and submucosal resection, the removal of a large portion of the bony nasal septum, may be performed for several reasons. These may include nasal obstruction caused by deviated or obstructing nasal septal cartilage or bone, obstructive sleep apnea, cosmetic correction of a deviated or twisted septum, chronic sinusitis with deviated septum, and in very rare instances, neoplasms. The most common of these reasons is nasal obstruction with or without sleep apnea. Septoplasty may be performed with other procedures such as rhinoplasty or sinus surgery.

Septoplasty is very rarely performed in children because the septum is the major growth center of the midface; disrupting it may lead to maxillary hyperplasia.

Technique

1. The nose is anesthetized with 1% lidocaine with epinephrine 1:100,000 and then is packed with 1/2-inch × 6-inch cotton strips soaked in a vasoconstrictive agent.
2. A nasal speculum is inserted into the nose.
3. The surgeon makes an incision ahead of the obstruction on one side.
4. The nasal septum is freed.
5. The deviated bone is removed.
6. The incision is closed.
7. Internal nasal splints are placed.

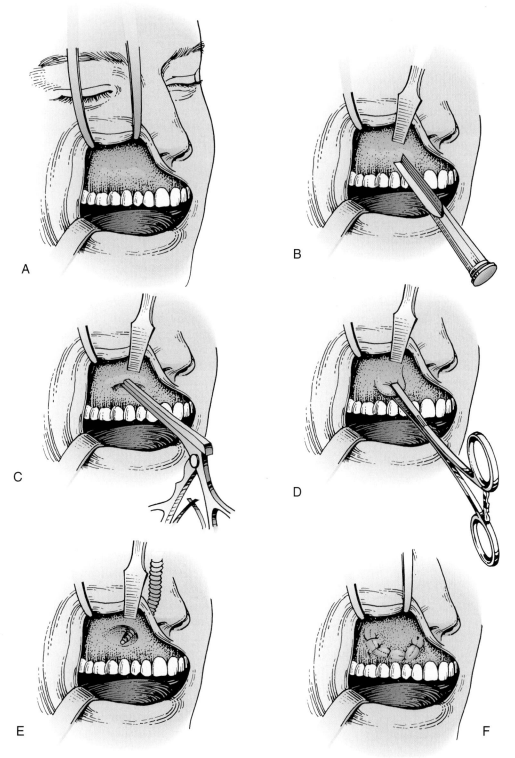

FIGURE 25-22
Caldwell-Luc. **A,** Incision is made under upper lip, creating a flap. **B,** Flap is retracted, and a perforation is made in the canine fossa. **C,** Enlargement of the perforation with a Kerrison rongeur. **D,** The diseased antral membrane is removed. **E,** An antral window is created with a rasp. **F,** The incision is closed. (Modified from Rothrock JC: *Alexander's care of the patient in surgery,* ed 12, St Louis, 2003, Mosby.)

DISCUSSION

The patient is positioned supine with a doughnut headrest, and the arms are tucked. General anesthesia typically is used, but local anesthetic with IV sedation also may be used. Before prepping and draping, the surgeon instills the nose and turbinates with local anesthetic, 1% lidocaine with epinephrine 1:100,000, and then packs the nose with ½-inch × 6-inch cotton strips soaked in a vasoconstrictive solution, such as adrenaline 1:1000, cocaine, Afrin, or local anesthetic with epinephrine. The patient is then prepped and draped for a nasal procedure. The surgeon then removes the nasal packs and places a nasal speculum into the nose; usually the side with the least obstruction is preferred. The surgeon then makes an incision into the nasal septum below the level of the obstruction using a #15 blade. Next, the surgeon uses small tenotomy scissors to gently dissect the membranous nasal septum and expose the cartilaginous end of the septum. A Freer or Cottle elevator then is used to elevate the septum off the underlying tissue (Figure 25-23). With the nasal septum free, the surgeon removes the deviated bone using a chisel, usually 4 mm, and a small mallet. The fractured portions of the septum are then grasped with a Takahashi forceps and removed. The incision then is closed with 4-0 chromic suture, and internal nasal splints are placed bilaterally to stabilize the septum and are stitched to the membranous septum with a 3-0 nonabsorbable suture.

Rhinoplasty
SURGICAL GOAL

Rhinoplasty is performed to cosmetically correct the nose.

PATHOLOGY

Rhinoplasty is typically used for cosmetic reasons. It is performed for patients who want elevation of the nasal tip, hump removal, or a smaller, straighter, or narrower nose.

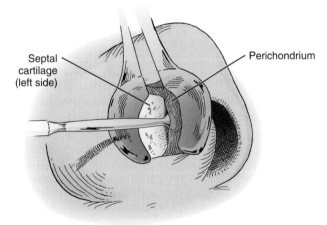

Septal cartilage (left side)

Perichondrium

FIGURE 25-23
Septoplasty: A Cottle elevator elevates the septum off of the underlying tissue. (Modified from Marks SC: *Nasal and sinus surgery*, Philadelphia, 2000, Saunders.)

This procedure may be performed with a septoplasty, if nasal obstruction is present.

Technique

1. The nose is anesthetized with 1% lidocaine with epinephrine 1:100,000 and then packed with a vasoconstrictive using ½-inch × 6-inch cotton strips.
2. The surgeon makes the incision through the skin and cartilage, using a #11 or #15 blade.
3. The periosteum and perichondrium are elevated.
4. The hump is removed if necessary.
5. Septoplasty is performed if necessary.
6. Soft-tissue correction and grafting are performed if necessary.
7. The incisions are closed.
8. An external nasal splint is applied.

DISCUSSION

Because each rhinoplasty is approached differently, depending on the patient, this section gives a generic overview of the steps in the procedure.

The patient is positioned in the supine or beach-chair position with a doughnut headrest and with arms tucked. General anesthesia is used. Before prepping and draping, the surgeon instills local anesthetic, 1% lidocaine with epinephrine 1:100,000, into the nose and turbinates, and then packs the nose with ½-inch × 6-inch cotton strips soaked in a vasoconstrictive solution, such as adrenaline 1:1000, cocaine, Afrin, or local anesthetic with epinephrine. The patient then is prepped and draped for a nasal procedure, including head drape.

The surgeon begins by removing the nasal packs. The surgeon makes the incision in the naso-labial angle using a #11 or #15 blade and then retracts using double-prong skin hooks. The nasal cavity is suctioned with Frazier-tip suction. The **perichondrium** and periosteum then are elevated with a Freer elevator, tenotomy scissors, and chisels. If a hump is present, it is removed with either a rasp or chisel and a small mallet. Next, the surgeon performs a septoplasty if necessary. Any cartilage or bone removed from the septum should be preserved on the back table in normal saline because it may be used for grafts later in the procedure. The surgeon then reconstructs the nasal tip if necessary by placing cartilage or bone grafts to provide support and projection.

Finally, lateral **osteotomies** may be performed using a 3-mm or 4-mm chisel and small mallet; this further straightens a curved nose and prevents widening of the nose. The nose is then closed with 3-0 and 4-0 chromic sutures. After the wounds have been closed, an external nasal splint is placed. This splint may be of metal, fiberglass, or tape.

Tonsillectomy
SURGICAL GOAL

Tonsillectomy is performed to eradicate infection, improve the airway, or remove a cancer.

PATHOLOGY

There are three pathological indications for removing the tonsils: infection, **hypertrophy,** and cancer. The patient may suffer from recurrent episodes of tonsillitis, chronic tonsillitis, or **peritonsillar abscess.** Individuals who suffer from recurrent episodes of streptococcal **pharyngitis,** "strep throat," may have tonsils that are colonized with the bacteria and thus may benefit from tonsillectomy. Enlarged tonsils may lead to disturbed sleep patterns, including sleep apnea. Hypertrophy also may interfere with oral intake, causing difficulty in swallowing a food bolus. Finally, the tonsil is a frequent site of cancer in adults, especially those who smoke.

Technique

1. The Crow-Davis mouth gag, including tongue blade, is inserted into the mouth and suspended from the Mayo stand.
2. The surgeon retracts the tonsil medially with an Allis clamp.
3. The tonsil is separated from the underlying musculature.
4. Hemostasis is established.

DISCUSSION

The patient is positioned supine with a doughnut headrest and with a shoulder roll, and the arms are tucked at the side. General anesthesia is used to protect the airway. The patient then is rotated 90 degrees to give the surgeon access to the head. The patient is draped with a head drape and a down sheet (usually a three-quarter sheet); prepping is not necessary. The surgeon stands at the head of the bed and uses a headlight to light the field.

The Crow-Davis retractor is inserted into the oral cavity and secured onto the edge of the Mayo stand, over the patient's chest. One should not elevate the Mayo stand until the surgeon states that the retractor is ready to be secured. When the retractor has been secured, the Mayo stand cannot be moved. The oral cavity then is suctioned with Yankauer suction.

The surgeon then grasps the tonsil with a straight or curved Allis clamp, and retracts it toward the midline. The surgeon makes the incision anterior to the tonsil to expose the tonsillar capsule. This incision can be made with electrocautery with an insulated tip, a #12 blade, a laser, or a Coblation wand. The surgeon then separates the capsule from the underlying musculature. This step may be performed with electrocautery, a laser, a Coblation wand, a Fisher knife, a Hurd elevator, or a tonsil snare.

Throughout the procedure, the assistant uses suction to remove smoke from the oral cavity and to maintain a "dry" field. The tonsillar fossa then is packed with a strung gauze sponge or tonsil sponge. Bismuth, mixed with saline to the consistency of a thick paste, may be applied to the tonsil sponges before packing. The surgeon then removes the other tonsil, if indicated, in an identical fashion. The tonsil sponges then are removed and hemostasis is achieved. The surgeon may achieve hemostasis using electrocautery or suction cautery.

It is important to protect the lip from burn when using the suction cautery. This may be achieved by draping a moistened Raytec sponge over the lip. Some surgeons may use 2-0 Vicryl sutures on a tapered needle with a Heaney needle holder to ligate any large vessels. The oral cavity then is copiously irrigated, and any residual bleeding is addressed. The tension of the retractor then is released. The tonsils then are passed off the field and sent to pathology. The field must not be broken down until the patient has been extubated and is out of the room.

Adenoidectomy
SURGICAL GOAL

Adenoidectomy is performed to eradicate infection and remove adenoid tissue.

PATHOLOGY

The primary reasons for performing an adenoidectomy are infection and obstruction caused by hypertrophy. The adenoid tissue may harbor bacteria, causing infection, or the adenoids may be hypertrophied to the point of obstructing the orifice of the eustachian tube, which can lead to **otitis media.** Adenoid hypertrophy also can cause upper-airway obstruction, resulting in snoring and sleep apnea. Children are affected more often than adults by adenoiditis and hypertrophy because the tissue usually atrophies during adolescence. However, some adults do retain their adenoid tissue. An adenoidectomy may be performed alone or in conjunction with placement of tympanostomy tubes or tonsillectomy.

Technique

1. The Crow-Davis mouth gag, including tongue blade, is inserted into the mouth and suspended from the Mayo stand.
2. The surgeon applies retraction to the soft palate, usually using a red rubber catheter passed through the nose and out the mouth and secured with a tonsil clamp.
3. The surgeon uses a mirror to visualize the adenoids in the nasopharynx.
4. The adenoid tissue is removed.
5. Hemostasis is established.

DISCUSSION

The patient is positioned supine with a doughnut headrest and a shoulder roll, and the arms are tucked at the sides. General anesthesia is used to protect the airway. The patient then is rotated 90 degrees to give the surgeon access to the head. The patient is prepped and draped in the same fashion used for tonsillectomy. The surgeon stands at the head of the bed and uses a headlight to light the field. The Crow-Davis retractor is inserted into the oral cavity and secured on the edge of the Mayo stand, over the patient's chest.

One should not elevate the Mayo stand until the surgeon says that the retractor is ready to be secured; after the retractor has been secured, the Mayo stand cannot be moved. The oral cavity is suctioned with Yankauer suction to remove any secretions.

The surgeon then retracts the palate using a red rubber catheter (12 or 14 Fr) inserted through the nose and brought out of the mouth. The ends of the red rubber catheter are secured with a tonsil clamp. Next, the surgeon uses a dental mirror to manually and visually inspect the adenoids. Dipping the mirror in anti-fog or Hibiclens solution helps to prevent fogging.

If the adenoid tissue is substantial, the surgeon uses an adenoid curette to remove the tissue. The size of the curette depends on the size of the nasopharynx. For minimal amounts of adenoid tissue, suction cautery may be used to remove the tissue. After the tissue has been removed, the oral cavity and nasopharynx are profusely irrigated. The surgeon then uses the mirror to ensure that hemostasis has been achieved and that all of the target tissue has been removed. Tension is released from the Crow-Davis mouth gag, and the red rubber catheter and mouth gag are removed.

Uvulopalatopharyngoplasty
SURGICAL GOAL

Uvulopalatopharyngoplasty (UPPP) is performed to improve the upper airway.

PATHOLOGY

UPPP is performed to correct upper-airway obstruction, most often in the form of obstructive sleep apnea, caused by the obstruction of anatomical structures of the soft palate and oropharynx. Obstructive sleep apnea can cause a variety of sleep disorders, ranging from sleep deprivation to fatal pulmonary and cardiovascular complications, including hypertension, cardiac arrhythmias, and neurological dysfunction.

Technique

1. The Crow-Davis mouth gag, including tongue blade, is inserted into the mouth and suspended from the Mayo stand.
2. The surgeon retracts the tonsil medially using an Allis clamp.
3. The tonsil is separated from the underlying musculature.
4. Hemostasis is established.
5. The procedure is repeated for the other side.
6. The uvula and soft palate are retracted posteriorly with an Allis clamp.
7. The uvula and a portion of the soft palate are excised.
8. Hemostasis is established.
9. The soft palate is closed.

DISCUSSION

The patient is positioned supine with a doughnut headrest and a shoulder roll, and the arms are tucked at the sides. General anesthesia is used to protect the airway. A tracheotomy set-up should be available in case of difficulty with the intubation. The patient then is draped; prepping is unnecessary. The surgeon stands at the head of the bed and uses a headlight to light the field.

The surgeon inserts the Crow-Davis retractor into the oral cavity and secures it onto the edge of the Mayo stand, over the patient's chest. The oral cavity then is suctioned with Yankauer suction. The tonsils are removed in the same fashion as described for a tonsillectomy.

When the tonsils have been removed, the surgeon turns his or her attention to the uvula and soft palate. The surgeon grasps the uvula with an Allis clamp and retracts it posteriorly. Using electrocautery, the surgeon excises the soft palate and uvula; the amount of tissue to be excised depends on the width and depth of the patient's oropharyngeal space.

The surgeon closes the soft palate with 2-0 Vicryl sutures, using the Heaney needle holder and a tonsil clamp. The oral cavity then is copiously irrigated, and any residual bleeding is addressed. The tension on the retractor then is released. The tonsils and uvula then are passed off the field and sent to pathology. The field must not be broken down until the patient has been extubated and removed from the room.

Laryngoscopy
SURGICAL GOAL

Laryngoscopy is performed to visualize the laryngeal mucosa and to treat or remove lesions.

PATHOLOGY

Laryngoscopy is performed for the diagnosis, biopsy, and treatment of laryngeal lesions. These lesions can include foreign bodies, **papilloma** of the vocal cords, laryngeal polyps, **leukoplakia,** and laryngeal web. Papilloma is a benign proliferative overgrowth of epithelium. Leukoplakia is a benign growth of **hyperkeratotic** epithelium of the laryngeal mucosa. It is seen more often in patients who smoke. If an area of leukoplakia is surrounded by erythema, there is a strong suspicion of malignancy. Laryngeal web is the adherence of the anterior aspects of the vocal cords as a result of removal of mucous membrane or after inflammation. Laryngoscopy almost always is performed when a neck dissection is performed.

Technique — INDIRECT LARYNGOSCOPY

1. A mirror is placed into the oral cavity.
2. The tongue is grasped and gently held with a gauze sponge.
3. The patient is asked to phonate.
4. The vocal cords are visualized.

DISCUSSION

The patient is placed either in the sitting position or supine with a doughnut headrest. If the patient can cooperate throughout the procedure, no anesthetic is necessary. However, if the patient cannot cooperate, sedation or general anesthesia may be needed. The surgeon opens the patient's mouth and uses a tongue blade to retract the tongue. The mirror is placed in the mouth. The tongue blades then are removed, and the surgeon gently grasps the patient's tongue with a moist gauze sponge. The surgeon then positions the mirror against the uvula, allowing him or her to visualize and inspect the larynx, base of tongue, and pharyngeal wall. The patient may be asked to speak if possible, so that the surgeon can see the larynx in motion. The mirror then is removed from the mouth.

Technique DIRECT LARYNGOSCOPY

1. The tooth guard is placed.
2. The surgeon introduces the laryngoscope into the right side of the patient's mouth.
3. The laryngoscope is advanced through the vocal cords.
4. Biopsies are taken if needed.
5. The laryngoscope is removed.

DISCUSSION

The patient is positioned supine with a shoulder roll and a doughnut headrest. General anesthesia is used. Generally no prepping or draping is used, but some surgeons do prefer a head drape and a down sheet. The surgeon places the tooth guard over the patient's upper teeth; this prevents injury to the teeth as the scope is introduced. The surgeon introduces the rigid laryngoscope into the mouth via the right side. The laryngoscope is advanced into the throat. With the laryngoscope in the throat, the surgeon visualizes the hypopharynx, epiglottis, **supraglottic** larynx, and glottis.

Oral secretions are suctioned with open-tip or velvet-tip laryngeal suction. The assistant aids in the placement of the suction into the end of the laryngoscope. The surgeon then continues to advance the scope to the level of the larynx, allowing visualization of the vocal cords. The surgeon also examines the subglottic region and the upper portion of the trachea. If the surgeon finds any areas of suspicion, the surgeon biopsies them using a long cupped biopsy forceps. Any bleeding is controlled with the placement of cotton patties that have been soaked in a vasoconstrictor (adrenaline, Afrin, or cocaine) over the affected area. With hemostasis established, the scope and tooth guard are removed.

Suspension Microlaryngoscopy

For suspension **microlaryngoscopy,** the same procedure is followed as with direct laryngoscopy. The only difference is that the laryngoscope becomes self-retaining through suspension in a special device that rests on the patient's chest. This allows the surgeon to have both hands free to use both instruments and an operative microscope fitted with a 400-mm lens. Use of the microscope allows the surgeon to have increased magnification of areas that are otherwise difficult to visualize.

Bronchoscopy
SURGICAL GOAL

Bronchoscopy is performed to visualize the bronchus.

PATHOLOGY

Bronchoscopy may be used for diagnostic or treatment purposes. Diagnostic bronchoscopy primarily involves the tak-

ing of a biopsy of a suspicious lesion. Bronchoscopy as treatment involves the removal of a foreign body, excision of a small tumor, or application of medications.

Technique

1. The tooth guard is inserted into the mouth.
2. The surgeon introduces the bronchoscope into the mouth and advances it.
3. Secretions are aspirated.
4. Procedures are performed as necessary.
5. The scope is removed.

DISCUSSION

The patient is positioned supine with a doughnut headrest. General anesthesia is used to allow the patient to tolerate manipulation. Prep and drape generally are not needed. The surgeon places the tooth guard over the patient's upper teeth to protect them throughout the procedure.

The bronchoscope then is introduced through the mouth, usually from the right side. The scope is advanced while angled backward. With the scope in place, the surgeon suctions secretions from the bronchus using velvet-eye suction. The assistant aids the surgeon in placing the suction into the bronchoscope. The surgeon visualizes the bronchus, searching for lesions and foreign bodies. If lesions are seen, a biopsy is taken using a long cupped biopsy forceps. If regions of **stenosis** are encountered, the surgeon attempts to insert a larger bronchoscope to open the bronchus. The CO_2 laser also may be used to treat stenotic regions. Foreign bodies are removed with a long alligator forceps or cupped forceps. The scope then is carefully removed, and the tooth guard also is removed.

Esophagoscopy
SURGICAL GOAL

Esophagoscopy is performed to visualize the esophagus.

PATHOLOGY

Esophagoscopy, or direct visualization of the esophagus and cardia of the stomach, is indicated for removal of a foreign body, injection of esophageal varices, dilation of esophageal stenosis, and examination of lesions. In children the primary reason for esophagoscopy is removal of a foreign body.

Technique

1. A tooth guard is placed in the patient's mouth.
2. The esophagoscope is introduced into the mouth and advanced with the patient's head extended.
3. The secretions of the esophagus are suctioned.
4. The surgeon visualizes the esophagus.
5. If any other procedure is planned, it is performed at this time.
6. The esophagoscope is removed.

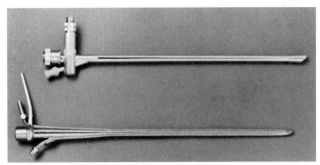

FIGURE 25-24
Esophagoscopes. (Modified from Rothrock JC: *Alexander's care of the patient in surgery,* ed 12, St Louis, 2003, Mosby.)

DISCUSSION

The patient is positioned supine with a doughnut headrest, with the head at the top of the table. General anesthesia is used because the patient must be paralyzed to allow for manipulation. Generally no prep or drape is needed because this is a clean procedure.

The surgeon first places a tooth guard on the upper teeth to protect them from injury during the procedure. The esophagoscope is then introduced into the mouth, usually from the right side, and is advanced through the cricoid cartilage to the beginning of the esophagus with a gentle pressure and a slight turning motion (Figure 25-24). The surgeon continues to advance the scope to the cardia. The head of the patient is maximally extended to allow the passage of the scope.

With the scope in place, the surgeon suctions the secretions using open-ended suction. The assistant must aid the surgeon in placing the suction into the esophagoscope by guiding the tip of the suction into the scope. The surgeon next visualizes the esophagus, inspecting for foreign bodies, varices, lesions, and stenosis. If any of these are seen, they are treated. The surgeon grasps a foreign body with a long alligator forceps or cupped forceps and removes it. Any lesions that are encountered may be biopsied with a long cupped biopsy forceps. The surgeon achieves esophageal dilation by inserting various sizes of esophageal dilators (e.g., bougie dilators) or a larger esophagoscope into the esophagus. The esophagoscope then is carefully removed, as is the tooth guard.

SECTION III
Surgery of the Head and Neck

INTRODUCTION TO SURGERY OF THE HEAD AND NECK

Procedures of the head and neck include procedures involving the trachea, salivary glands, and neck. These procedures may be performed by otorhinolaryngologists and general surgeons.

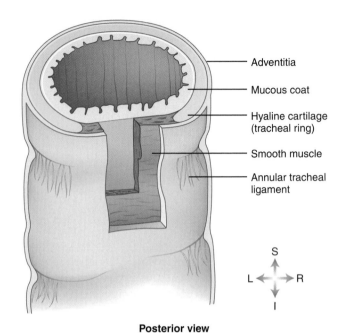

FIGURE 25-25
Posterior view of the trachea. (From Thibodeau GA and Patton KT: *Anthony's textbook of anatomy and physiology,* ed 17, St Louis, 2003, Mosby.)

ANATOMY OF THE TRACHEA

The trachea extends from the cricoid to the mediastinum. It is composed of approximately 20 incomplete cartilaginous rings. The posterior aspect of the trachea is membranous and contains no cartilaginous structure (Figure 25-25).

ANATOMY OF THE SALIVARY GLANDS

There are three pairs of salivary glands: parotid, submandibular, and sublingual (Figure 25-26). Hundreds of minor salivary glands are found throughout the oral cavity and pharynx. The largest of the glands, the parotid gland, overlies the mandible anterior to the ear. It extends anteriorly to the masseter muscle. The tail of the parotid extends below the mandible into the upper neck. The parotid duct, Stensen's duct, arises from the anterior border of the gland 1.5 cm below the zygoma and drains into the mouth and the cheek opposite the upper second molar. The facial nerve enters into the posterior aspect of the gland, branches, and exits from the anterior aspect of the gland. The nerve separates the parotid gland into a superficial, or lateral, lobe and a deep lobe.

The submandibular gland is the second largest salivary gland. It is C-shaped and wraps around the inferior border of the mandible. The submandibular, or Wharton's, duct emerges from the deep anterior portion of the gland and drains into the anterior floor of the mouth. The marginal mandibular nerve, a branch of the facial nerve, lies within the superficial fascia of the gland. The hypoglossal nerve (cranial nerve XII) and the lingual nerve lie deep to the gland.

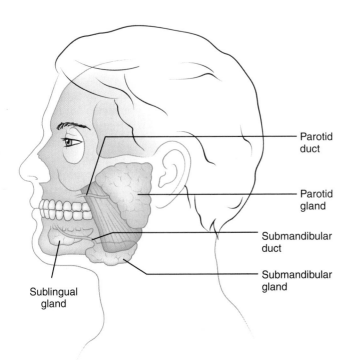

FIGURE 25-26
Location of the salivary glands. (Modified from Herlihy B and Maebius NK: *The human body in health and illness,* ed 2, Philadelphia, 2003, Saunders.)

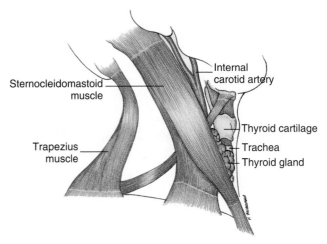

FIGURE 25-27
Anatomy of the neck. (From Potter PA and Perry AG: *Fundamentals of nursing,* ed 5, St Louis, 2001, Mosby.)

The smallest pair of salivary glands, the sublingual glands, lies just beneath the mucosa of the anterior floor of the mouth and empties into the oral cavity via multiple small ducts (ducts of Rivinus).

ANATOMY OF THE NECK

The anatomy of the neck is shown in Figure 25-27. The neck is traditionally organized into triangles. Each side of the neck is divided into two large triangles separated by the sternocleidomastoid muscle, which runs from the mastoid process below the ear to the sternum and medial clavicle. Below the sternocleidomastoid muscle is the carotid sheath, which contains the carotid artery and its bifurcation to the internal and external carotid arteries, the internal jugular vein and its tributaries, and the vagus nerve. The vagus nerve extends into the thorax. On the right side it passes behind the subclavian artery and a branch, the recurrent laryngeal nerve, arises below and passes anterior to the subclavian artery en route superiorly to the larynx.

On the left, the vagus nerve passes behind the arch of the aorta, and a branch, the left laryngeal nerve, passes anterior to the aortic arch en route superiorly to the larynx. Deep to the carotid sheath, the phrenic nerve travels inferiorly en route to the diaphragm. Posterior to the sternocleidomastoid muscle, the posterior triangle of the neck is traversed diagonally by the spinal accessory nerve, cranial nerve XI. Anterior to the sternocleidomastoid, the anterior cervical triangle is found. This triangle is traversed by the digastric muscle. Above this is the submandibular triangle, which contains the

submandibular gland and the hypoglossal nerve (cranial nerve XII). The space below the digastric muscle contains the carotid sheath and the structures medial to it, including the larynx, the pharynx, the thyroid gland, the parathyroid glands, the ansa cervicalis (a nerve that loops down into the neck and provides **innervation** to the strap muscles and a small branch to the hypoglossal nerve), and the sympathetic chain (which provides sympathetic innervation of the head and neck).

Throughout the anterior neck are groups of lymph nodes, which provide lymphatic drainage of the head and neck. The thoracic duct connects the body's entire lymphatic system to the vascular system and is found predominantly in the left lower neck posterior to the carotid sheath, where it inserts at the junction of the left internal jugular vein and subclavian vein.

EQUIPMENT AND INSTRUMENTS

No special equipment and very little special instrumentation is required for procedures of the head and neck. Only the tracheal instruments differ from the basic major and minor instrumentation. These tracheal instruments include cricoid hooks and a tracheal spreader (Figure 25-28).

PREPPING AND DRAPING

The surgeon shaves the patient's chest if necessary before the prep. The prep is usually Betadine paint and scrub. The circulator preps from the level of the nose to the level of the umbilicus, including the area behind the shoulders and ears and to the level of the bed laterally. If the endotracheal tube (ET) is in the field, it is also prepped. The prep is wide so that, in the event a flap is needed, the donor area has been prepped. The surgical site then is draped with towels (generally more than four are needed to surround the area that has been prepped), which are secured with towel clips or skin staples.

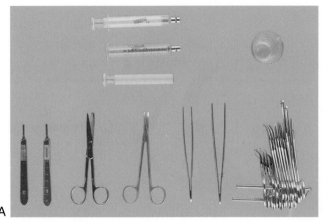
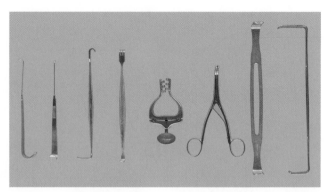
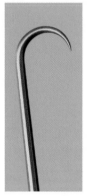
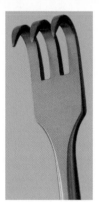
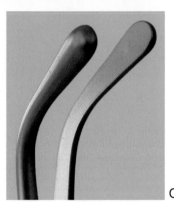

FIGURE 25-28
Tracheotomy set. **A,** *Top, left to right,* 2 glass 10-ml syringes, together and separate; 1 glass medicine cup. *Bottom, left to right,* 2 Bard-Parker knife handles, no. 3; 1 plastic suture scissors, 5½ inch; 1 Metzenbaum dissecting scissors, 5 inch; 2 thumb tissue forceps, without teeth and with teeth (1 × 2); 4 Backhaus towel clips; 3 Halsted mosquito hemostatic forceps, curved; 3 Halsted mosquito hemostatic forceps, straight; 2 Allis tissue forceps; 1 Johnson needle holder, 5 inch. **B,** *Left to right,* 2 News tracheal hooks, side view and front view; 2 Senn retractors, double-ended, sharp, side view and front view; 1 articulated mastoid retractor; 1 Trousseau tracheal dilator, adult; 2 Army-Navy retractos, front view and side view. **C,** *Left to right,* tips: tracheal hook; sharp tip of Senn retractor, double-ended; Trousseau tracheal dilator, adult. (From Tighe SM: *Instrumentation for the operating room,* ed 6, St Louis, 2003, Mosby.)

The patient then is draped with a split sheet that surrounds the head. It may be helpful to cover the patient's chest with a towel and place a magnetic drape on top of the towel to capture instruments that the surgeon places on the chest.

MEDICATIONS, SPONGES, AND DRESSINGS

Medications
The primary medications used in procedures of the head and neck are local anesthetics and hemostatic agents. Particularly during awake tracheotomies, local anesthetics are injected into the incision and possibly into the trachea. Hemostatic agents such as Gelfoam and thrombin should be available for major procedures of the head and neck, as many great vessels pass through the neck.

Sponges
The sponges needed for head and neck cases include Raytec sponges, lap sponges, and cottonoids. All sponges and sharps are counted before, during, and at the end of the procedure. Some facilities require that instruments also be counted with these procedures.

Dressings
The dressings used after procedures of the head and neck vary according to the procedure. Tracheotomy incisions generally are dressed with drain sponges (4 × 4 gauze that has been slit to allow the tracheotomy tube to be surrounded) and tracheal ties. Other procedures of the head and neck may be dressed with Telfa and Tegaderm or 4 × 4 sponges and tape. If staples are used to close the skin, no dressings may be applied, and the wound is coated with antibiotic ointment.

SURGICAL PROCEDURES

Tracheotomy/Tracheostomy
SURGICAL GOAL
Tracheotomy, or **tracheostomy,** is performed to provide a patent airway for the patient.

PATHOLOGY
Tracheostomy is indicated for patients who require emergent or elective airway management of prolonged ventilator dependence or acute or chronic upper-airway obstruction. Upper-airway obstruction may be due to mechanical obstruction by a tumor, foreign body, infection, or secretions. Obstruction also may be due to congenital, neurological, or traumatic conditions. These obstructions can include a foreign body in the larynx or hypopharynx, acute laryngotracheal bronchitis in children, laryngeal edema, or any other condition that obstructs normal respiration.

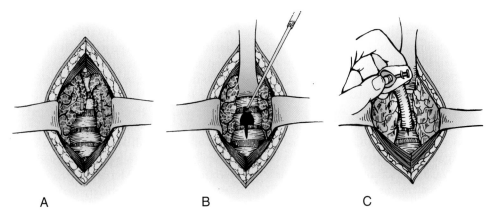

FIGURE 25-29
Tracheotomy/tracheostomy. **A,** Isthmus of thyroid is divided to expose the trachea. **B,** Two tracheal rings are cut, and the upper ring is partially resected. Tracheal hook pulls the trachea from the depth of the wound toward the surface. **C,** Tube is inserted. (Modified from DeWeese DD: *Textbook of otolaryngology,* ed 6, St Louis, 1982, Mosby.)

Technique

1. An incision is made over the anterior tracheal wall.
2. The surgeon visualizes the tracheal wall.
3. The tracheal incision is made, usually between the third and fourth tracheal rings.
4. The ET is partially removed to the point superior to the tracheal incision.
5. The tracheotomy tube is inserted.
6. Hemostasis is achieved.
7. The tracheotomy tube is secured.
8. Dressings are applied.
9. The obturator from the ET is sent with the patient.

DISCUSSION

The patient is positioned supine with the head on a doughnut headrest, and the arms are tucked at the sides. General anesthesia is used. The patient is prepped and draped for a head and neck procedure. Using a #15 blade, the surgeon makes the incision to the midline of the neck; the incision may be vertical or horizontal. The skin flaps are elevated with double-prong skin hooks and a #15 blade. With the flaps elevated, the strap muscles are separated in the vertical midline, at the median raphe, with a hemostat or electrocautery. The isthmus of the thyroid also may be divided to allow visualization of the anterior tracheal wall (Figure 25-29, *A*). A tracheal hook then is placed into the cricoid cartilage to elevate the trachea.

The incision then is made into the trachea between the second and third or third and fourth tracheal rings with a #15 blade (Figure 25-29, *B*). In adults, the tracheal incision is vertical and may include the removal of an anterior square of tracheal cartilage. In infants, the tracheal incision is made vertically and no tracheal cartilage is removed. The anesthesia provider withdraws the ET to the level just above the tracheal incision. A tracheotomy tube then is placed into the tracheal incision with the obturator in place (Figure 25-29, *C*). If a cuffed tracheotomy tube is used, one must ensure

that the balloon has no leaks before placing the tube. One can do this by instilling 5 cc of air into the balloon, applying pressure, and then removing the air.

The obturator then is removed, and the internal cannula is placed. The obturator is saved and sent with the patient. The tracheotomy tube then is connected to the anesthesia circuitry to ensure that the patient is properly and adequately ventilated. When ventilation through the tracheotomy tube has been established, the ET is fully removed. Hemostasis then is established with electrocautery. The tracheotomy tube then may be sutured to the skin with a 2-0 nonabsorbable suture, such as Prolene or silk. Drain sponges and tracheotomy ties are then applied.

Submandibular Gland Excision
SURGICAL GOAL
The submandibular gland is excised.

PATHOLOGY
The submandibular gland may be excised for several reasons, including chronic infection (bacterial or viral), stone formation, or neoplasm (benign or malignant). These conditions are much more common in adults than in children. In children, however, about 60% of salivary-gland masses are malignant.

Technique

1. A skin incision is made 2 cm below the mandible.
2. The submandibular gland is exposed.
3. The facial artery and vein are ligated.
4. The gland is separated from the mandible.
5. The duct and nerve to the gland are ligated.
6. The gland is removed.
7. Hemostasis is achieved.
8. The incision is closed.

DISCUSSION

The patient is positioned supine on a doughnut headrest with the arms tucked at the sides. General anesthesia is used. The patient is prepped and draped for a head and neck procedure. The surgeon makes the incision with a #15 or #10 blade 2 cm below the inferior border of the mandible in a skin crease. The incision is sharply carried down through the platysma. The surgeon elevates the skin-muscle flaps using the knife with retraction employing double-prong skin hooks. The surgeon does this carefully to avoid injuring the marginal mandibular branch of the facial nerve.

A knife or small Metzenbaum scissors are used to make an incision in the tissue overlying the inferior border of the gland. The facial artery and vein are then identified and ligated with 2-0 or 3-0 silk ties. The tissue and the vessels overlying the gland then are retracted superiorly with a dull Senn retractor or three-prong dull rake. The gland then is retracted inferiorly with an Allis clamp or a Raytec sponge. Metzenbaum scissors and bipolar cautery are used to separate the gland from the inferior border of the mandible. The submandibular branch of the lingual nerve is identified and ligated with 2-0 or 3-0 silk ties. Next, an Army-Navy retractor is inserted to retract the myohyoid muscle anteriorly; the submandibular duct then is identified and ligated. The remaining soft-tissue attachments of the submandibular gland then are excised with monopolar cautery. Hemostasis is achieved with electrocautery. The wound then is copiously irrigated, and a drain is placed if necessary. The incision then is closed in layers with absorbable sutures. The skin may be closed with absorbable or nonabsorbable sutures.

Parotidectomy
SURGICAL GOAL
Parotidectomy is performed to excise the parotid gland.

PATHOLOGY
Parotidectomy is performed to remove a parotid mass, most often a neoplasm (usually benign) or a lymph node. The facial nerve splits the parotid gland into superficial and deep lobes. Most pathology occurs in the superficial lobe; rarely does pathology involve the deep lobe. When the deep lobe is involved, it is usually indicative of malignancy.

Technique

1. The surgeon makes a skin incision anterior to the ear and extending down the neck.
2. The parotid gland is exposed.
3. The gland is mobilized, and the sternocleidomastoid muscle is retracted.
4. The gland is separated from the cartilaginous portion of the external auditory canal.
5. The facial nerve is identified.
6. The superficial portion of the parotid gland is removed.
7. The deep portion of the parotid gland is excised if necessary.
8. Hemostasis is achieved.
9. The wound is closed over a drain.

DISCUSSION

The patient is positioned supine on a doughnut headrest or a Mayfield headrest, with arms tucked at the sides. General anesthesia is used. The patient is prepped and draped for a head and neck procedure. The surgeon uses a #15 blade to make the incision anterior to the ear, extending down into the neck.

The surgeon elevates the skin flaps using the knife with retraction employing double-prong skin hooks. The flaps then are retracted with four-prong dull rakes. The gland then is separated from the sternocleidomastoid muscle with electrocautery and Metzenbaum scissors. The gland is then separated from the cartilaginous portion of the external auditory canal with Metzenbaum scissors. The facial nerve then is identified.

Dissection is continued along the facial nerve branches, either superiorly or inferiorly, with a mosquito clamp or hemostat with bipolar cautery until the superficial portion of the gland is removed. If the deep lobe of the parotid must be excised, the facial nerve is elevated and retracted with vessel loops. With the facial nerve retracted, the facial nerve branches are elevated off the underlying deep lobe of the parotid gland with a mosquito clamp or hemostat with bipolar cautery.

The gland then is elevated off the underlying masseter muscle with Metzenbaum scissors and bipolar cautery. Allis clamps are used to grasp the gland and provide counter traction as it is elevated. When the gland has been removed, the wound is irrigated and a drain is placed. The wound then is closed in layers with absorbable sutures. The skin may be closed with either absorbable or nonabsorbable sutures.

This procedure is illustrated in Figure 25-30.

Thyroidectomy
SURGICAL GOAL
Thyroidectomy is the surgical removal of one or more lobes of the thyroid gland.

PATHOLOGY
This procedure is performed to treat various diseases of the thyroid, such as hyperthyroidism and cancer that cannot be treated by chemotherapy.

Technique

1. The surgeon incises the neck.
2. The thyroid is mobilized and removed.
3. The wound is closed.

DISCUSSION

The patient is placed in the supine position with the neck hyperextended. To achieve this position, a rolled bath blanket is placed under the patient's neck and shoulders.

Before beginning the procedure, the surgeon marks the proposed incision line by grasping a length of suture and pressing it against the patient's neck. The resulting indentation will serve as a guideline for an incision that produces a nearly unnoticeable scar.

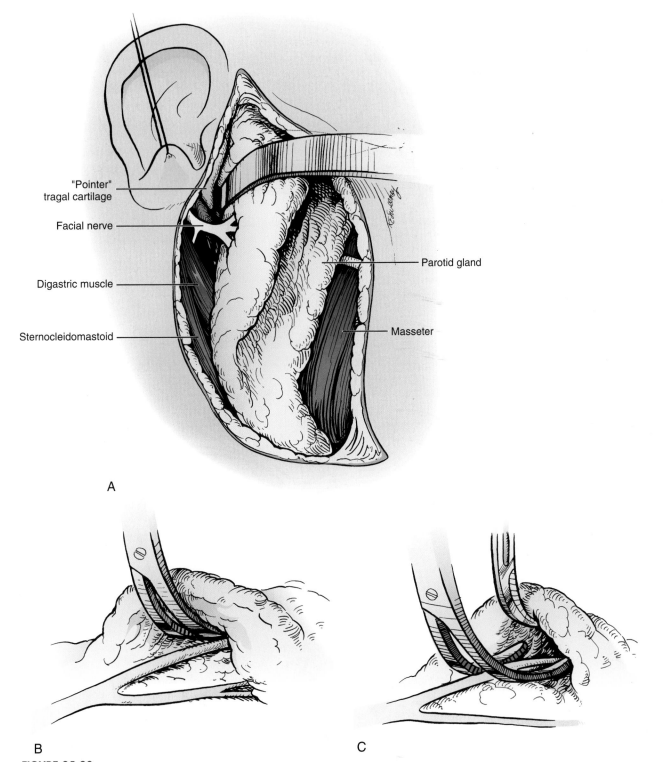

"Pointer"
tragal cartilage

Facial nerve

Digastric muscle

Sternocleidomastoid

Parotid gland

Masseter

A

B

C

FIGURE 25-30
Parotidectomy. **A,** Blunt dissection of the parotid gland exposing the facial nerve. **B,** Technique for following each branch of the facial nerve. **C,** Parotid tissue overlying the facial nerve is cut with a #12 blade.

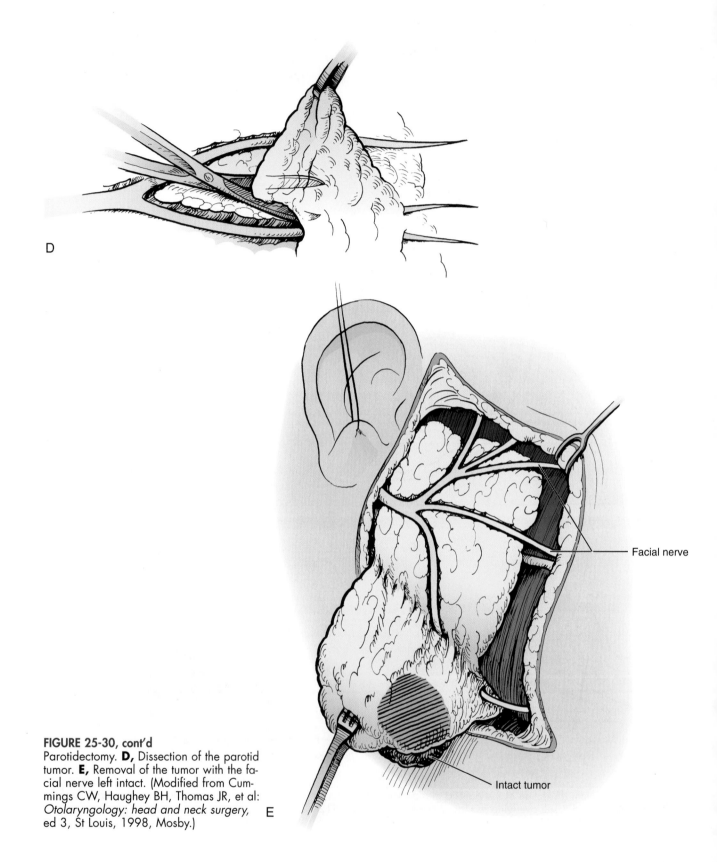

D

E

FIGURE 25-30, cont'd
Parotidectomy. **D,** Dissection of the parotid
tumor. **E,** Removal of the tumor with the facial nerve left intact. (Modified from Cummings CW, Haughey BH, Thomas JR, et al:
Otolaryngology: head and neck surgery,
ed 3, St Louis, 1998, Mosby.)

Facial nerve

Intact tumor

The surgeon incises the neck with a #10 blade. The subcutaneous tissue is incised with the cautery pencil, exposing the platysma muscle. The assistant retracts the tissue layers with rake retractors. The surgeon then divides the muscle layer with the deep knife. Using both sharp and blunt dissection, the surgeon deepens the flaps of the incision above and below the platysma muscle. The cautery pencil is used often to coagulate bleeders in the vascular tissue.

As the dissection continues, deeper retractors are used. A special thyroid (Green) retractor may be used if the wound is very deep. The scrub should have U.S. retractors available.

When the thyroid gland is finally exposed, two Lahey spring (self-retaining) retractors are placed in the wound. The surgeon then grasps the gland with one or two Lahey tenaculi that are designed for thyroid procedures.

The thyroid gland is an extremely vascular structure, and its attachments to the trachea consist of a bed of tissue that is rich with blood vessels. Therefore, to mobilize the gland, the surgeon successively double-clamps small sections of tissue, divides between the clamps, and ligates the stump. Most surgeons prefer to use *straight* Kelly clamps or mosquito clamps for mobilization. The scrub should have at least 12 clamps available and may need as many as 24 if the surgeon prefers to clamp and divide many sections before ligating the stumps and returning the clamps to the scrub. Mobilization is performed as described above. A #15 scalpel blade is used to divide the tissue **ligation.** Because the scalpel is used so often during mobilization, the surgeon may request that it remain on the field where he or she can pick it up rather than having the scrub hand it to him or her repeatedly. If left on the field, the scalpel should be placed on a folded towel to prevent accidental injury to the patient.

Large arteries of the thyroid are occluded with suture ligatures of 2-0 or 3-0 silk mounted on a fine needle. When mobilization is complete, the gland is passed to the scrub. If the tissue looks suspicious, the surgeon may order a frozen section to identify the type of disease.

The wound is irrigated, a small Penrose drain is inserted, and the layers of the neck tissue are closed individually. The surgeon uses interrupted silk sutures on a fine needle for muscle and fascial layers. Subcutaneous tissue is closed with fine interrupted absorbable sutures. The skin is closed with the surgeon's preferred material, or wound clips may be used.

The incision is dressed, and the dressings are secured by a gauze strip passed around the patient's neck. Because of the danger of tracheal swelling and consequent obstructed airway, a tracheostomy tray is sent to the recovery room with the patient.

A thyroidectomy is illustrated in Figure 25-31.

Parathyroidectomy
SURGICAL GOAL

Parathyroidectomy is performed to remove one or more diseased or malfunctioning parathyroid glands.

PATHOLOGY
Parathyroidectomy is performed most often to treat hyperparathyroidism and adenoma of the parathyroid.

Technique
1. The surgeon incises the skin and raises skin flaps using sharp dissection.
2. The platysma muscle is divided.
3. The thyroid sheath is dissected.
4. Bleeders are serially ligated and sutured.
5. The upper and lower poles of the thyroid are explored bilaterally for parathyroid glands.
6. Affected glands are dissected and removed.
7. The wound is closed.

DISCUSSION
The patient is placed on the operating room table in the supine position with the neck hyperextended and the arms tucked. The patient then is prepped and draped for a neck procedure. The surgeon begins by palpating the thyroid gland and determining the incision line based on the exposure needed and the natural skin creases of the neck. The incision is made with a #15 blade, and the skin flaps are elevated with the knife and double-prong skin hooks for retraction. This incision is extended through the platysma muscle. The skin is retracted with either a Mayhorn thyroid retractor or rakes. The muscle is then divided with the ESU. Dissection is taken down to the thyroid capsule; the surgeon controls any bleeding by either using the ESU or tying off the vessel. When the surgeon has entered the thyroid capsule, Army-Navy retractors are used to retract the thyroid and the strap muscles.

The surgeon then uses blunt dissection to explore the superior and inferior poles of the thyroid for the affected parathyroid. This is done bilaterally. The surgeon also explores the region for the superior laryngeal nerves and the recurrent laryngeal nerve. These nerves must be identified because their injury can lead to difficulty with swallowing and speaking.

When the affected parathyroid has been identified, the blood vessels supplying it are clamped, tied off, and transected. When all affected parathyroids have been identified and removed, the wound is irrigated, hemostasis is achieved with the bipolar cautery, and the wound is closed. If the wound bed is not dry, a small drain or a Penrose drain may be placed. The wound is closed in a layered closure with absorbable suture. The skin then is closed with a suture of the surgeon's choice. A small dressing may be placed.

Thyroplasty
SURGICAL GOAL

Thyroplasty is performed to **medialize** a paralyzed vocal cord.

PATHOLOGY
Unilateral vocal cord paralysis or paresis is the primary reason for performing a thyroplasty. The paralysis/paresis may

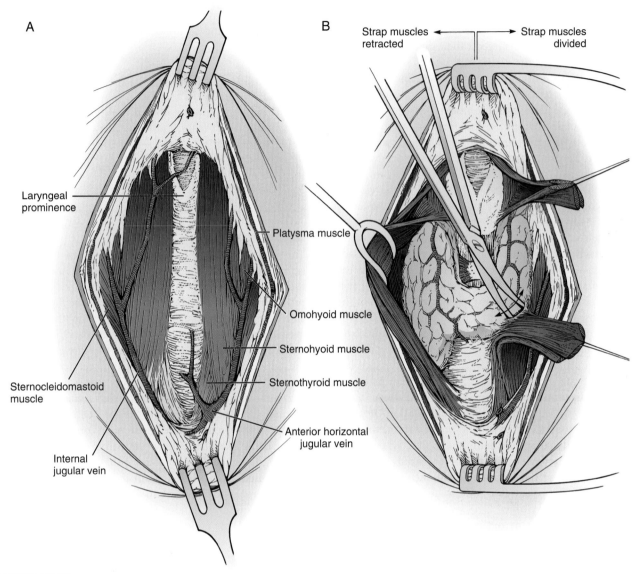

FIGURE 25-31
Thyroidectomy. **A,** Division of the midline muscles with creation of superior and interior flaps. **B,** The strap muscles retracted on the right *(left side of illustration)* and divided on the left *(right side of illustration)*.

be caused by a variety of conditions, including surgical trauma to the laryngeal nerves or prolonged intubation. Cord paralysis or paresis prevents the vocal cords from meeting at the midline on phonation. Open, closed, or unilateral paralysis can cause difficulty with speech (hoarseness) and aspiration.

Technique

1. The surgeon makes an incision in the midline neck.
2. Exposure is made to the level of the thyroid cartilage.
3. A "window" is cut into the thyroid cartilage to expose the paraglottic space.
4. The surgeon inserts a **nasolaryngoscope** to view the vocal cords.
5. The true vocal cord is medialized.

6. The patient is asked to speak to verify medialization.
7. The implant is positioned in the paraglottic space.
8. The incision is closed.

DISCUSSION

The patient is positioned supine with a doughnut headrest and arms tucked at the sides. The patient is awake for most of the procedure, so it is important that the patient be comfortable. IV sedation is given, and local anesthetic (1% lidocaine with epinephrine 1:100,000) is infiltrated into the surgical site. When adequate sedation has been achieved, the surgeon makes a 2-cm to 3-cm incision in the neck at the midline, using a #15 blade. The skin edges are retracted with double-prong skin hooks to allow the creation of the skin flaps. With the skin flaps elevated, the surgeon exposes and

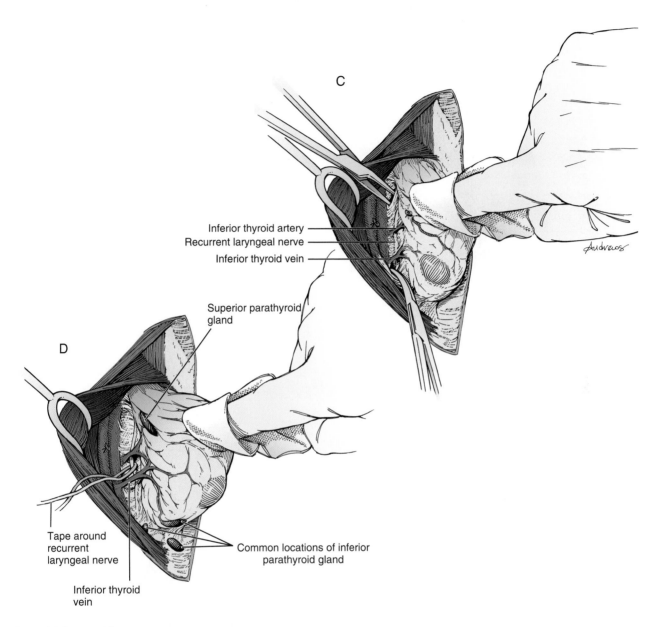

Inferior thyroid artery
Recurrent laryngeal nerve
Inferior thyroid vein

Superior parathyroid
gland

Tape around
recurrent
laryngeal nerve

Common locations of inferior
parathyroid gland

Inferior thyroid
vein

FIGURE 25-31, cont'd
Thyroidectomy. **C,** Blunt dissection of the thyroid; the right recurrent laryngeal nerve is identified. **D,** Blunt dissection continues, exposing the relationship of the laryngeal nerve to the inferior thyroid vein.

splits the platysma using a #15 blade and toothed Adson forceps. A small Weitlaner retractor is placed to expose the strap muscles, which are retracted laterally to expose the thyroid muscle.

Using a Freer elevator, the surgeon releases the thyroid muscle from the thyroid cartilage. With the thyroid cartilage exposed, the surgeon marks the cartilage for the window (Figure 25-32, A-E). The surgeon can do this with a caliper or free hand. When the window has been marked, the surgeon uses a small sagittal saw to cut the window, measuring 5 by 10 mm.

The assistant should keep the cartilage moist with sterile normal saline to prevent burning of the cartilage during the cutting of the window. The surgeon then elevates the window using a single prong skin hook and a Freer elevator (Figure 25-32, F-H). With the window removed, the surgeon attempts to medialize the paralyzed cord by pushing the thyro-arytenoid cartilage to the midline. The anesthesiologist passes a flexible nasolaryngoscope to visualize the medialization.

The surgeon asks the patient to speak while the nasolaryngoscope is in place. This step is taken to confirm that the paralyzed cord has been medialized. Upon confirmation of medialization, the surgeon places an implant. The method of medialization varies; some surgeons carve a Silastic block and others place a folded Gore-Tex patch into the paraglottic space; several prefabricated systems include pre-cut implants.

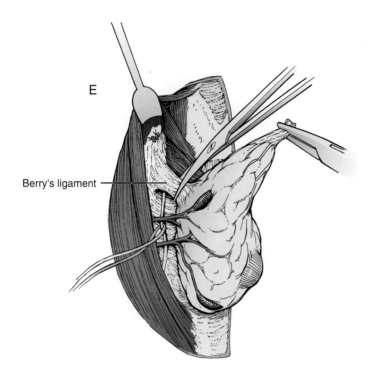

E

Berry's ligament

FIGURE 25-31, cont'd
Thyroidectomy. **E,** The division of Berry's ligament. **F,** The isthmus is divided. **G,** The strap muscles are closed. (Modified from Moody FG: *Atlas of ambulatory surgery*, St Louis, 1999, Mosby.)

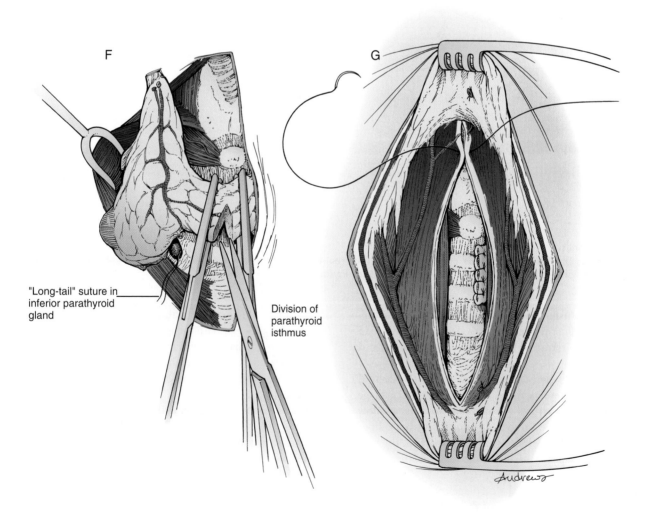

F

"Long-tail" suture in inferior parathyroid gland

Division of parathyroid isthmus

G

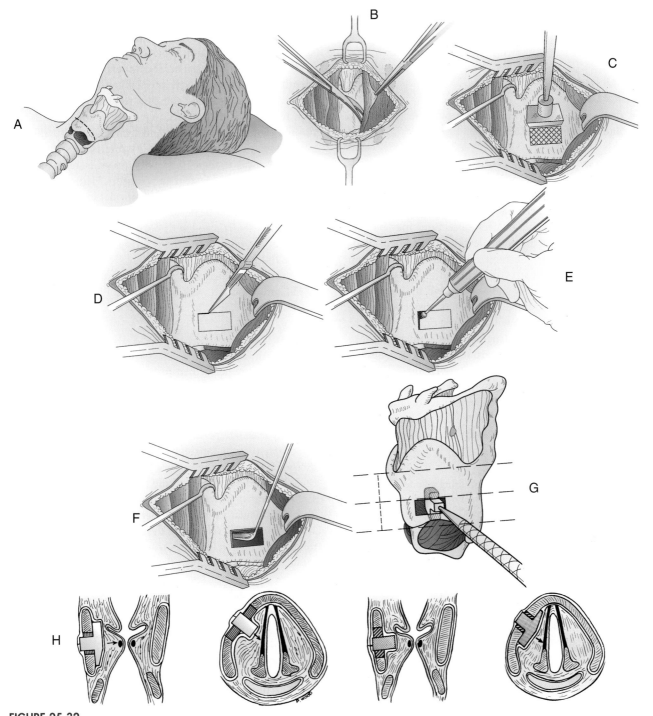

FIGURE 25-32
Thyroplasty. **A,** Location of incision site midline in the neck. **B,** Creation of skin flaps to expose the platysma. **C,** A template for window is positioned. **D,** The cartilage is marked. **E,** The window is removed. **F,** The window is elevated. **G,** The vocal cord is shifted medially, and the implant is placed. **H,** Methods for placement of implants for medialization. (Modified from Cummings CW, Haughey BH, Thomas JR, et al: *Otolaryngology: head and neck surgery,* ed 3, St Louis, 1998, Mosby.)

The surgeon reapproximates the strap muscles using a 3-0 or 4-0 absorbable suture. A small drain may be placed below the platysmal layer. The platysma is closed with absorbable suture. The skin then is closed and dressed.

Neck Dissection

SURGICAL GOAL

Neck dissection is performed to remove affected lymph nodes and halt the spread of disease.

PATHOLOGY

Many head and neck cancers, including malignant tumors of the oral and pharyngeal cavities, cutaneous malignant melanoma, and skin cancer, metastasize to the cervical lymph nodes. Three types of neck dissections may be performed, depending on the nodes' level of involvement. Radical neck dissection is the removal of all cervical lymph nodes and surrounding structures, including the spinal accessory nerve, the internal jugular vein, and the sternocleidomastoid muscle. Modified radical neck dissection is the excision of all lymph nodes with the preservation of one or more of the nonlymphatic structures (i.e., spinal accessory nerve, internal jugular vein, or sternocleidomastoid muscle). In selective neck dissection, one or more chains of cervical lymph nodes are preserved and all nonlymphatic structures are preserved. The removal of the primary lesion and any affected cervical lymph nodes on one or both sides of the neck can offer a chance of cure and stop the spread of the disease.

> **Technique**
>
> 1. The surgeon makes a skin incision using a knife. The incision may be a curved incision, an apron incision, a Y incision, or an **H** incision.
> 2. The structures of the neck are exposed.
> 3. The affected structures are removed.
> 4. A tracheotomy is performed, if necessary.
> 5. A drain is placed, and the wound is closed.

DISCUSSION

The patient is placed in the supine position on a doughnut or Mayfield headrest, with the affected side of the neck facing upward. The arms are tucked at the patient's sides, and a shoulder roll is placed to hyperextend the neck slightly. General anesthesia is used. The patient is prepped, including the face, neck, and chest, and draped for a head and neck procedure.

The surgeon begins the procedure by outlining the proposed incisions with a surgical marker. The surgeon makes the skin incision using a #15 blade (Figure 25-33). The surgeon extends the incision through the platysma using electrocautery with double-prong skin hooks for retraction. Bleeding vessels are ligated with hemostats and 2-0 or 3-0 silk ties or electrocautery.

The surgeon mobilizes the sternocleidomastoid muscle (SCM) using blunt dissection and then retracts it laterally using an Army-Navy retractor. If the SCM is to be sacrificed, it is cut with electrocautery. This allows the surgeon visuali-zation of the neurovascular sheath enclosed in a delicate layer of connective tissue. Dissection continues along the neurovascular sheath to expose the anterior portion of the specimen. This dissection is performed with hemostats.

With the neurovascular sheath exposed, the surgeon identifies the carotid artery, internal jugular vein, and vagus nerve. The neurovascular sheath is retracted with a Cushing vein retractor. If the internal jugular is to be sacrificed, it is double clamped, transected, and ligated with 2-0 silk ties. The surgeon then retracts the SCM anteriorly, exposing the lateral cervical triangle. The fatty tissue is removed with blunt dissection or Metzenbaum scissors. Hemostasis is then achieved with hemostats and 2-0 silk ties or electrocautery. A tracheotomy may be performed if necessary. The wound is then copiously irrigated with normal saline. A drain then is placed in the wound, and the wound is closed in layers with absorbable suture.

A modified radical neck dissection is illustrated in Figure 25-34, and a radical neck dissection is illustrated in Figure 25-35.

Glossectomy

SURGICAL GOAL

Glossectomy is performed to remove the cancer and produce a watertight seal.

PATHOLOGY

The only reason to perform a glossectomy is to treat cancer of the oropharynx or tongue base. A partial glossectomy is the excision of tissue in the anterior two thirds of the tongue. Because of the development of the tongue, this is almost exclusively unilateral. However, if the base of the tongue is involved, both the vascular supply and innervation of the hemi-tongue are compromised. Therefore the affected side or the entire tongue (for bilateral involvement) must be removed. A pectoralis myocutaneous (PM) flap or free flap is constructed to produce a watertight seal. A total glossectomy may be combined with a total laryngectomy to treat laryngeal involvement with the cancer or problems with aspiration.

> **Technique**   **PARTIAL GLOSSECTOMY**
>
> 1. The tongue is grasped with a towel clip or heavy silk in the midline.
> 2. The affected portion of the tongue is excised with electrocautery.
> 3. The defect is closed.

DISCUSSION

The patient is positioned supine on a doughnut or Mayfield headrest with arms tucked at the sides. General anesthesia is used. The patient is prepped and draped for a head and neck procedure.

The surgeon grasps the tongue either by using a large towel clip at the midline or by suturing the midline with a size-0 silk suture and grasping the ends of the suture with a hemostat. The tongue is then pulled anteriorly to expose the

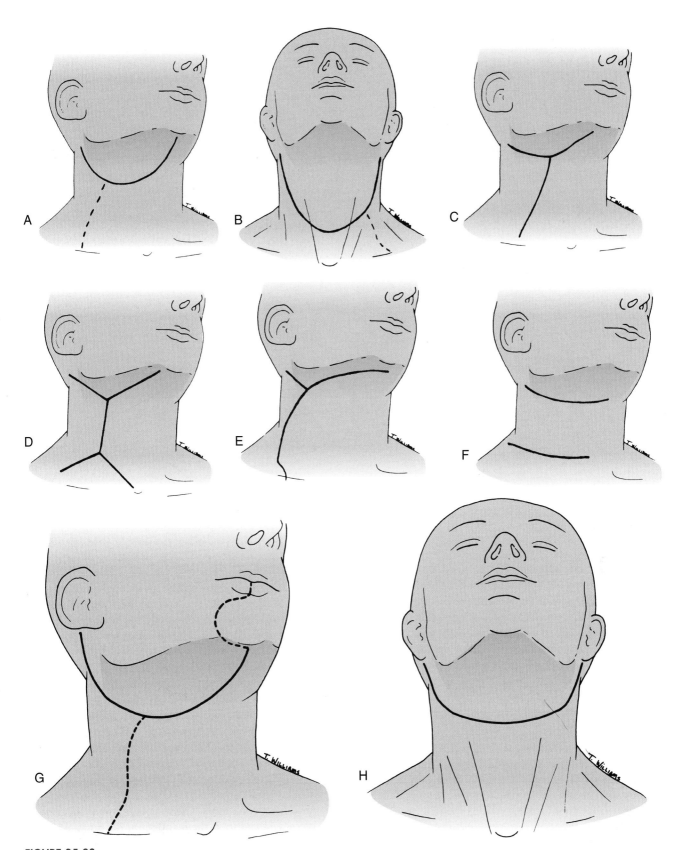

FIGURE 25-33
Neck dissection incisions. **A,** Latyschevsky and Freund incision. **B,** Freund incision. **C,** Crile incision. **D,** Martin incision. **E,** Babcock and Conley incision. **F,** MacFee incision. **G,** Incision used for unilateral supraomohyoid neck dissection. **H,** Incision used for bilateral supraomohyoid neck dissection. (Modified from Cummings CW, Haughey BH, Thomas JR, et al: *Otolaryngology: head and neck surgery,* ed 3, St Louis, 1998, Mosby.)

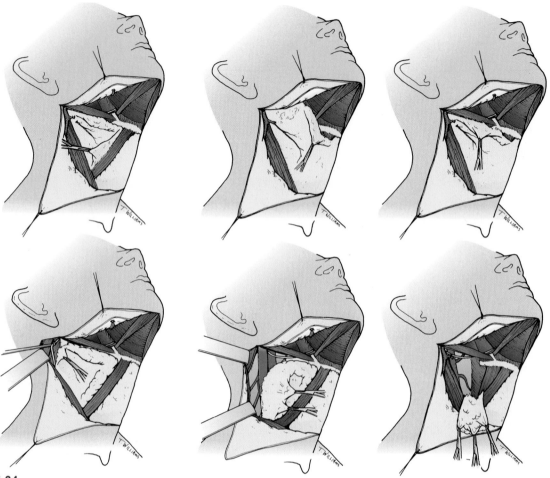

FIGURE 25-34
Modified radical neck dissection. (Modified from Cummings CW, Haughey BH, Thomas JR, et al: *Otolaryngology: head and neck surgery,* ed 3, St Louis, 1998, Mosby.)

affected region. The surgeon then excises the affected area using electrocautery with either an insulated blade tip or an insulated needle tip. Hemostasis is achieved with the electrocautery. The tongue is then closed. If primary closure is possible, the tongue is closed with 3-0 absorbable sutures. If primary closure is not possible, the defect is closed with a split-thickness skin graft. The graft is sutured into place with 3-0 absorbable suture.

Technique	HEMI/TOTAL GLOSSECTOMY

1. The incision is made at the midline of the lip and is extended to the submental region.
2. The surgeon retracts the soft tissue to expose the anterior surface of the mandible.
3. A titanium plate is placed over the proposed site of division and then removed.
4. The mandible is divided at the midline with a saw.
5. The tongue is divided at the midline for hemiglossectomy.
6. An incision is made in the floor of mouth between the tongue and mandible.
7. The tumor is excised.
8. The mandible is reapproximated and internally fixated.
9. The incision is closed.

DISCUSSION

The patient is positioned supine on a doughnut headrest or Mayfield headrest with arms tucked at the sides. General anesthesia is used. Often a tracheotomy has been performed or will be performed before the glossectomy. The patient is prepped and draped for a head and neck procedure, including the chest in case a PM flap is included.

The surgeon makes an incision in the midline lip (through and through [i.e., completely]), extending it to the submental border using a #15 blade. Electrocautery is used to produce hemostasis. The surgeon elevates the skin flaps using electrocautery and with retraction using dull Senn retractors.

With the mandibular surface exposed, a titanium plate is placed in the region of the planned division. The screw holes are drilled with a small power drill. The plate is secured to the mandible with screws. The surgeon removes the plate after placement and splits the mandible at the midline, using a small power saw with medium-sized saw blade.

The surgeon then grasps the mandible with four-prong dull rakes or a self-retaining retractor such as a Wheatlander retractor. For a hemiglossectomy, the anterior part of the oral floor and the body of the tongue are divided at the midline with electrocautery. The incision is extended to the

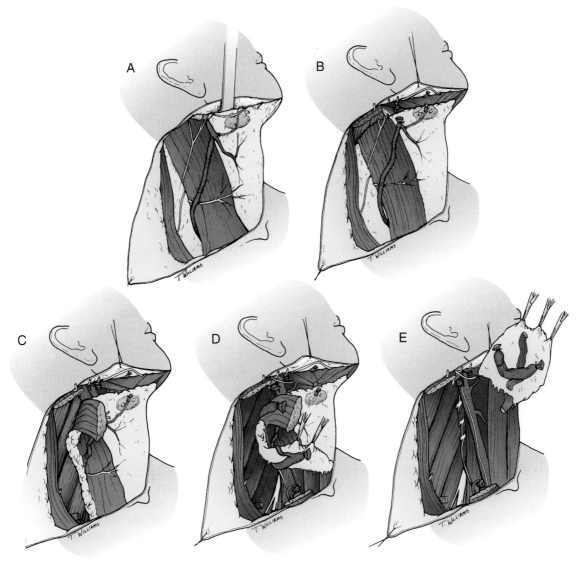

FIGURE 25-35
Radical neck dissection. **A,** Elevation of the skin flaps. **B,** Dissection and ligation of the facial vessels and dissection of the sub-mandibular fascia. **C,** Sacrifice of the sternocleidomastoid muscle (SCM) superiorly. **D,** Sacrifice of the SCM inferiorly and ligation of the internal jugular. **E,** The specimen is removed. (Modified from Cummings CW, Haughey BH, Thomas JR, et al: *Otolaryngology: head and neck surgery,* ed 3, St Louis, 1998, Mosby.)

tongue base. The affected side of the tongue is then excised with electrocautery.

The incision usually is closed primarily or with a skin graft. The mandible is reapproximated and internally fixed with the plate. The incision is closed in layers with absorbable suture. For a total glossectomy, the incision is made between the floor of the mouth and the mandible and extended to the base of tongue with electrocautery. The tongue is excised from the epiglottis with electrocautery. A neck dissection then is performed on one or both sides of the neck (see neck dissection). A PM flap is harvested (see the section Pectoralis Myocutaneous/Deltopectoral Flap on the following page). The flap is sutured into the defect with the skin taking the place of the tongue. The skin is sutured to the remaining mucosa of the floor of the mouth, and also to the epiglottic mucosa or pharyngeal mucosa if total laryngectomy was performed concomitantly, with 3-0 absorbable su-

ture. The mandible is reapproximated and internally fixed with the titanium plate.

The lip incision, oral mucosa, and deep portions of the skin incisions are closed with 3-0 absorbable sutures. The skin is closed with fine nonabsorbable suture. A nasal feeding tube is placed and secured with a 2-0 silk suture through the nasal septum. The skin incisions are then coated in antibiotic ointment.

Laryngectomy
SURGICAL GOAL

Laryngectomy is performed to remove the larynx and to produce a watertight pharynx.

PATHOLOGY

There are three reasons to perform a laryngectomy. These are cancerous lesions of the larynx, diversion for total separation of the respiratory and digestive tracts, and **chondro-radionecrosis** of the laryngeal framework, usually caused by radiation treatments,.

Technique

1. The surgeon makes the skin incision.
2. The larynx and neck contents are exposed.
3. A neck dissection is performed if necessary.
4. A tracheotomy is performed.
5. The larynx is removed.
6. The pharynx is closed
7. Hemostasis is achieved.
8. Drains are placed.
9. The wound is closed.

DISCUSSION

The patient is placed in the supine position on a doughnut headrest or Mayfield headrest with the arms tucked at the sides. A shoulder roll may be placed to hyperextend the neck. General anesthesia is used. The patient is prepped from the level of the nose to the level of the umbilicus and draped for a head and neck procedure, including the face, neck, and chest.

The surgeon begins by making an apron incision, either from mastoid to mastoid (for laryngectomy with neck dissection) or from mid sternocleidomastoid muscle to mid sternocleidomastoid muscle (for laryngectomy alone), with a #15 blade. The surgeon then elevates the flaps, using either a knife or electrocautery, to 1 to 2 cm above the sternal notch from below and 1 to 2 cm below the hyoid bone from above. The flaps generally are secured back with fish hook retractors or suture to allow for easier visualization of the underlying anatomy.

The surgeon then detaches the strap muscles from the sternum using the electrocautery or Mayo scissors and retracts them laterally with Army-Navy retractors. This exposes the carotid sheath, thyroid, and a portion of the trachea. The carotid sheath is lateralized with blunt dissection and retracted with a Cushing vein retractor. The thyroid veins may be ligated with hemostat clamps and 2-0 silk ties. The surgeon removes the thyroid lobe on the affected side by dividing the isthmus of the thyroid down the middle with electrocautery or scissors. Hemostasis is achieved with the electrocautery.

The thyroid lobe is then dissected out from medial to lateral beginning at the tracheoesophageal groove. Scissors are used to remove the fat and lymph tissue from the gland. The inferior thyroid artery is ligated and transected, and the recurrent laryngeal nerve is transected. The dissection of the thyroid continues with blunt dissection to the level of the trachea. The remaining portion of the gland is grasped with a Kocher clamp and dissected off the trachea with electrocautery.

A cricoid hook then is placed into the right-side larynx to allow rotation of the larynx and exposure of the constrictor muscles on the thyroid cartilage. The muscle is removed from the cartilage with the electrocautery. A periosteal elevator then is used to remove the soft tissue from the underside of the thy-

roid cartilage. The larynx then is rotated to the left with a cricoid hook to allow the freeing of the larynx from the remaining muscle and soft tissue of the thyroid. The surgeon then uses Metzenbaum scissors or a hemostat clamp to dissect between the thyroid cartilage and the hyoid bone. Any vessels and nerves that are exposed at this portion of the dissection are ligated. With electrocautery, the surgeon removes all of the muscular attachments of the tongue base from the hyoid bone, which is grasped with a tenaculum clamp.

With the hyoid bone exposed and free, the surgeon uses heavy Mayo scissors to cut the attachments of the hyoid bone. The tracheotomy is performed at this point because the surgeon is ready to enter the airway. The surgeon sews the anterior tracheal wall to the posterior skin flap to secure it in place. The ET then is removed, and the anesthesia circuit is switched to the tracheotomy tube.

The surgeon next uses scissors or electrocautery to make an incision into the hypopharynx in the midline over the hyoid bone. The hypopharynx then is opened with a hemostat clap, and the epiglottis is grasped with an Allis clamp and rotated out of the larynx. The lateral pharyngeal walls then are incised with heavy Mayo scissors, sparing as much mucosa as possible. The larynx then is opened like a book. The tracheal tube is removed, and the posterior membranous trachea is incised with a #15 blade. The trachea then is dissected from the anterior esophageal wall with Metzenbaum scissors. The surgeon also transects any fibrous attachments to the larynx at this point. The larynx then is removed, and the tracheal tube is replaced.

With the larynx removed, the pharyngeal mucosa is closed with or without a PM flap (discussed below) in two layers. The first layer is closed with a long 3-0 absorbable suture on a tapered needle, and the second layer is closed with a horizontal mattress with a 3-0 absorbable suture. With the pharynx closed, the surgeon creates a stoma by closing the anterior tracheal wall to the inferior skin flap and the posterior tracheal wall to the superior skin flap, using either absorbable or nonabsorbable sutures, depending on the surgeon's preference. The wound then is irrigated with normal saline. Drains then are placed, and the skin is closed in layers with absorbable suture.

A laryngectomy is illustrated in Figure 25-36.

Pectoralis Myocutaneous/Deltopectoral Flap
SURGICAL GOAL

PM and deltopectoral (DP) flaps create coverage for a soft-tissue defect.

PATHOLOGY

PM and DM flaps replace soft tissue, usually after surgical excision of cancer in the head and neck region. A DP flap usually is used to close post-irradiation fistulas and to resurface large cutaneous defects in the neck. A PM flap may be used in the reconstruction of the pharynx, tongue, face, or neck. It is especially useful in covering the carotid artery when it may be at risk because of prior irradiation.

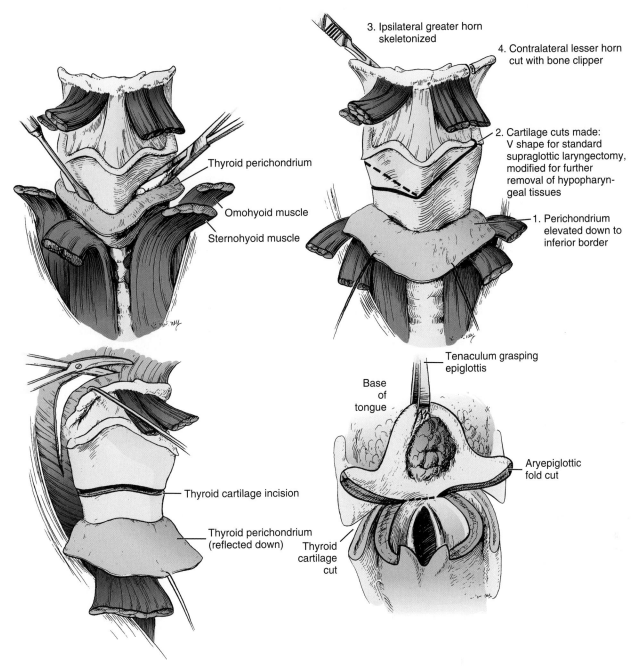

3. Ipsilateral greater horn
skeletonized

4. Contralateral lesser horn
cut with bone clipper

2. Cartilage cuts made:
V shape for standard
supraglottic laryngectomy,
modified for further
removal of hypopharyn-
geal tissues

1. Perichondrium
elevated down to
inferior border

Thyroid perichondrium

Omohyoid muscle

Sternohyoid muscle

Tenaculum grasping
epiglottis

Base
of
tongue

Aryepiglottic
fold cut

Thyroid cartilage incision

Thyroid perichondrium
(reflected down)

Thyroid
cartilage
cut

FIGURE 25-36
Laryngectomy. (Modified from Cummings CW, Haughey BH, Thomas JR, et al: *Otolaryngology: head and neck surgery*, ed 3, St Louis, 1998, Mosby.)

Technique	DELTOPECTORAL FLAP

1. The surgeon makes an incision.
2. The flap is elevated.
3. The flap is rotated.
4. The flap is inset.
5. The donor site is closed with a skin graft.

DISCUSSION

The patient is positioned, prepped, and draped as with a neck dissection or laryngectomy, because the DP flap often is performed in conjunction with either of these procedures.

The surgeon begins by outlining the proposed incision with a surgical marker. The incision typically goes from the acromion process to the sternum, extending to the space between the third and fourth ribs.

The incision is made with a #10 blade, and the flap (skin, vascular supply, subcutaneous tissue, and fascia) is elevated from the underlying pectoralis major muscle in a lateral to medial fashion. This is done with either electrocautery or a scalpel. Hemostasis is achieved with electrocautery. The flap is left attached at the medial border, because this is where its vascular supply enters, and is rotated to cover the defect of the

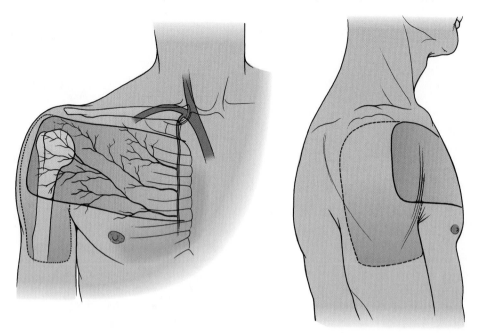

FIGURE 25-37
Deltopectoral (DP) flap. (Modified from Silver CE and Rubin JS: *Atlas of head and neck surgery,* ed 2, Philadelphia, 1999, Churchill Livingstone.)

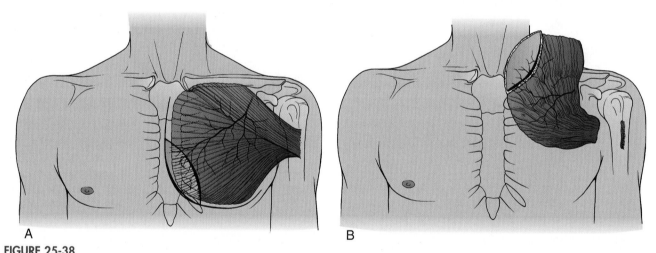

A

B

FIGURE 25-38
Pectoralis myocutaneous (PM) flap. **A,** Location of skin flap outlined and incised down to the underlying fascia. **B,** The skin flap is elevated, and the lower border of the pectoralis is identified. (Modified from Silver CE and Rubin JS: *Atlas of head and neck surgery,* ed 2, Philadelphia, 1999, Churchill Livingstone.)

neck. The flap then is sutured into place with 3-0 absorbable sutures. The donor site then is covered with a skin graft, which is secured with 3-0 absorbable sutures or skin staples.

The DP flap is illustrated in Figure 25-37.

Technique	PECTORALIS MYOCUTANEOUS FLAP

1. The surgeon makes the incision.
2. The flap is elevated.
3. The flap is "tunneled."
4. The flap is inset into the defect.
5. The donor site closed.

DISCUSSION

The patient is positioned, prepped, and draped as with a neck dissection or laryngectomy, because the PM flap often is performed with one of these procedures. The surgeon begins by measuring from the inferior border of the defect to the mid-clavicle with a lap sponge. This distance marks the superior portion of the skin paddle, which is drawn as a rectangle with rounded edges between the nipple and the sternum inferiorly to the inferior border of the pectoralis major muscle. A line is then drawn from the superolateral portion of the rectangle to the axilla.

The incision is made with a #10 blade. The skin, subcutaneous tissue, and fascia superior to the incision are elevated off the underlying muscle over the clavicle, making a tunnel into the neck. The flap (skin, vascular supply, subcutaneous tissue, fascia, and pectoralis muscle) is elevated from the underlying chest wall in an inferior to superior fashion. This may be performed with either a scalpel or electrocautery. The surgeon uses electrocautery to separate the muscle from the sternum and the humerus. The muscular portion of the flap should be slightly larger than the skin paddle. Hemostasis is achieved with electrocautery. Care is taken to preserve the skin of the deltopectoral region in case it may be needed at another time.

When the flap has been elevated to the level of the clavicle, it is rotated 180 degrees and tunneled under the skin and over the clavicle to reach the defect. The flap then is sutured into place with 3-0 absorbable sutures. Two drains are placed into the donor site, and it is usually closed with 3-0 absorbable suture.

The PM flap is illustrated in Figure 25-38.

SECTION IV
Maxillofacial Trauma and Oral Surgery

INTRODUCTION TO MAXILLOFACIAL TRAUMA AND ORAL SURGERY

Cases of facial trauma may involve the many bones of the face and frontal sinus. These injuries are repaired with wires, plates, and screws.

ANATOMY OF THE MIDFACE

The anatomy of the midface and mandible is shown in Figure 25-39, *A*. The facial skeleton includes the frontal bone of the forehead, all of the bones of the midface, and the mandible. The frontal bone forms the upper part of the orbits. It is divided by sutures that join the sphenoid and ethmoid bones, and by the paired nasal, lacrimal, maxillary, and zygomatic bones.

The posterior orbits are formed by the sphenoid bone (a butterfly-shaped bone) and the palatal bones. The medial walls of the orbit are formed by the ethmoid, lacrimal, and nasal bones, and by the maxilla. The lateral orbital rim is formed by the zygoma. The ethmoid bone also forms the roof and posterior lateral wall of the nasal cavities. The nasal bones form the bridge of the nose, which is between the orbits. The maxilla, the upper jawbone, holds the palate and extends laterally to the zygoma and temporal bone. The two maxillary bones join to form the palate. The teeth are embedded in the alveolus of the maxillary bones.

The design of the midface not only protects the orbits and cranium, but also serves to resist vertical forces. A series of buttresses must be restored in midface fractures to accommodate the primary force of the face, mastication. These buttresses are paired and consist of the lateral zygomaticomaxillary buttress, the medial nasomaxillary buttress, and the posterior pterygomaxillary buttress. The latter is difficult to access surgically and therefore is rarely repaired. These buttresses are suspended from the frontal bar, which consists of the superior orbital rims and the thick bone between the rims. In addition to being an important part of the lateral buttress, the malar complex (cheek) provides for the width and projection of the face.

Malar-complex fractures often are called tripod and tetrapod fractures. These are misnomers, because the complex actually is composed of five fractures. For this "cheek" complex to be mobile, fractures must occur through the zygomatic arch, lateral orbital rim, inferior orbital rim and orbital floor, lateral orbital wall, and anterior wall of the maxillary sinus.

ANATOMY OF THE MANDIBLE

The mandible is a U-shaped bone that is suspended from the temporal bone (Figure 25-39, *B*). The condyles insert into the glenoid fossa of the temporal bones to form the temporomandibular joints. The ramus extends inferiorly from the condyle to the angle, where it joins the body of the mandible and extends anteriorly and medially to join the other half of the mandible at the symphysis. This region is called the parasymphysis. The teeth are embedded in the alveolus of the body and parasymphysis.

There is a small projection from the ramus anterior to the condyle called the coronoid process, which is where the temporalis muscle inserts. The inferior alveolar nerve enters the mandible on the deep surface of the ramus. This nerve travels through the body of the mandible and provides sensation to the teeth. It exits the mandible on the superficial surface

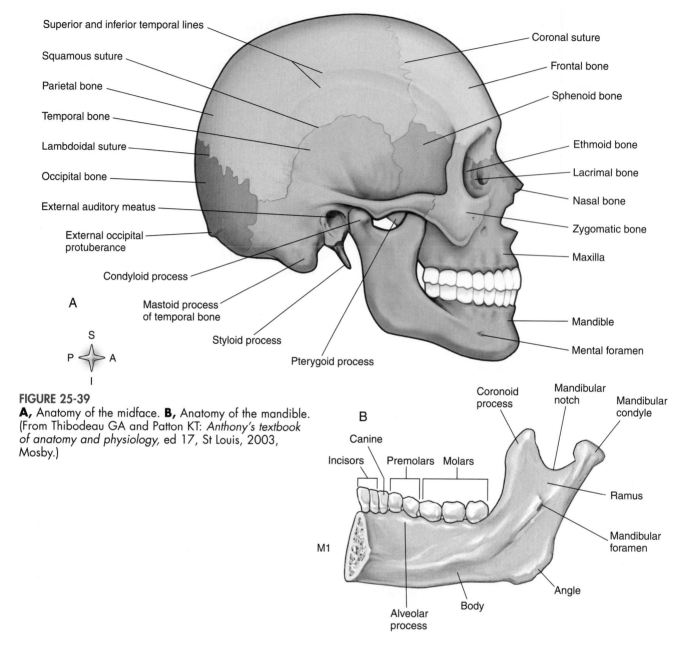

FIGURE 25-39
A, Anatomy of the midface. **B,** Anatomy of the mandible. (From Thibodeau GA and Patton KT: *Anthony's textbook of anatomy and physiology,* ed 17, St Louis, 2003, Mosby.)

of the parasymphysis, forming the mental nerve, which provides sensation to the chin. Patients with mandibular fractures often have chin numbness.

EQUIPMENT AND INSTRUMENTS

Power Drills

For procedures involving facial fractures, some sort of power drill is needed to drill the holes for the screws. Usually the choice is a Stryker microdrill (or TPS). The drill bits for the screws are included in the modules of the plate system being used.

Plates and Screws

Plates and screws are vital parts of the repair of facial fractures; very few fractures can be reduced and fixed without them. Many systems are available for fixation. These include Synthes, Leibinger, W Lorenz, Osteomed, and KLS

brands. Each of these systems includes the instrumentation required for placement of the plates and screws, such as plate benders and cutters, plate-holding forceps, screwdriver handles, screwdriver blades, and depth gauges.. The modules also include plates and screws of various sizes (Figure 25-40).

For mandibular fractures, the plates and screws are most often at least 2.0 mm in size. For midface, orbital, and frontal-sinus fractures, the plates and screws range from 1.0 mm to 2.0 mm. The scrub must keep track of all plates and screws that are used with the patient for the purposes of charging and recording of implants. Any screw that enters the bone must be charged to the patient because it cannot be used again on another patient, even though it has been removed and will be discarded. Screws and plates are very costly and are charged to the patient even though they are not included on the implant record.

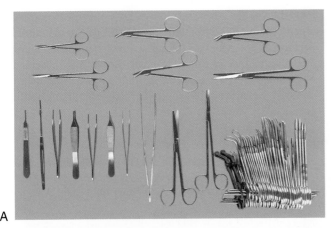

A

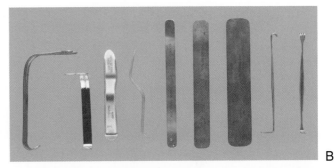

B

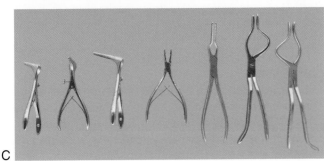

C

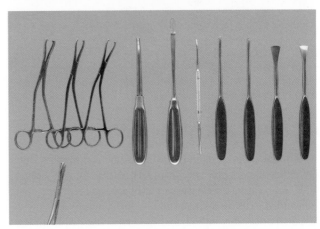

D

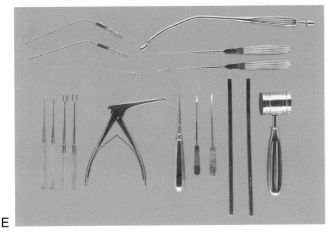

E

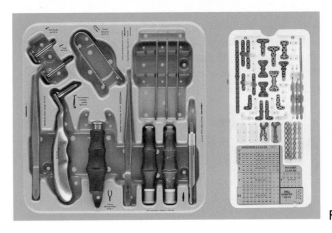

F

FIGURE 25-40

Facial fracture set. **A,** *Top, left to right,* 1 Stevens tenotomy scissors, curved; 1 plastic scissors, straight, sharp; 3 wire-cutting scissors; 1 Mayo dissecting scissors, straight. *Bottom, left to right,* 1 Bard-Parker knife handle, no. 3; 1 Bard-Parker knife handle, no. 7; 2 Adson tissue forceps with teeth (1 × 2), front view and side view; 2 Adson tissue forceps without teeth, front view and side view; 1 Brown-Adson tissue forceps with teeth (9 × 9), front view; 1 bayonet dressing forceps, 7½ inch; 1 Mayo dissecting scissors, curved; 1 Metzenbaum scissors; 2 paper drape clips; 2 Backhaus towel forceps, small; 2 Backhaus towel forcps; 6 Halsted mosquito hemostatic forceps, curved; 2 Halsted mosquito hemostatic forceps, straight; 2 Providence hemostatic forceps, curved; 2 Halsted hemostatic forceps, straight; 4 Crile hemostatic forceps, curved; 2 Allis tissue forceps; 2 Webster needle holders, 4 inch; 2 Crile-Wood needle holders, 6 inch; 2 Johnson needle holders, 6 inch. **B,** *Left to right,* 1 Weider tongue retractor, large, side view; 1 Weider tongue retractor, small, front view; 2 University of Minnesota cheek retractors, front view and side view; 3 ribbon retractors, assorted sizes; 2 Senn-Kanavel retractors, side view and front view. **C,** *Left to right,* 1 Cottle nasal speculum, no. 1, side view; 1 Cottle nasal speculum, no. 2, front view; 1 Cottle nasal speculum, no. 3, side view; 1 Friedman rongeur, single action; 1 Asch forceps; 2 Rowe disimpaction forceps, left and right. **D,** *Top, left to right,* 3 Dingman bone-holding forceps; 1 Dingman zygoma elevator; 1 Gilles malar elevator; 1 Freer elevator; 2 Langenbeck elevators; 1 Langenbeck periosteal elevator, straight; 1 Langenbeck periosteal elevator, angled. *Bottom left,* tip of Dingman bone-holding forceps. **E,** *Top, left to right,* 2 Frazier suction tubes with stylets; 1 Yankauer suction tube with tip; 2 zygomatic arch awls. *Bottom, left to right,* 2 Joseph skin hooks, single; 2 Joseph skin hooks, double; 1 Kerrison rongeur, 90-degree upbite; 1 Lucas curette, no. 0, short; 2 mandibular awls; 1 Cottle osteotome, curved; 1 Cottle osteotome, straight; 1 metal mallet. **F,** Titanium 2.0-mm micro-fixation system instrumentation, trays 1 and 2 of 3 (labeled). *Continued*

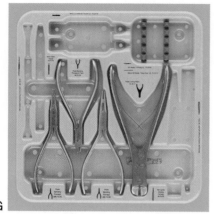

G

FIGURE 25-40, cont'd
Facial fracture set. **G,** Titanium 2.0-mm micro-fixation system instrumentation, tray 3 of 3 (labeled). (From Tighe SM: *Instrumentation of the operating room,* ed 6, St Louis, 2003, Mosby.)

PREPPING AND DRAPING

Facial fractures are prepped with Betadine scrub and paint. The entire face is prepped, from the hairline to the sternal notch. An ET usually is in the surgical field and therefore must be included in the prep. If a bicoronal incision is planned, first the patient's head is shaved, and the prep is carried from the occiput to the sternal notch. The mouth may be rinsed with diluted Betadine paint, and the teeth may be brushed after the patient has been draped. The patient is draped with four towels secured with towel clips to mark the surgical field. A split sheet then is draped over the patient and around the face, with the mouth, nose, and eyes in the surgical field.

MEDICATIONS, SPONGES, AND DRESSINGS

Medications

Generally no medications are used for facial fractures. However, some surgeons may use antibiotic ophthalmic ointment if the eye is involved, and local anesthetic with epinephrine in the incision sites.

Sponges

In addition to 4 × 4 Raytec sponges, cottonoids may be used. All sponges and sharps are counted before, during, and at the end of the procedure.

Dressings

Typically no dressings are used for facial fracture procedures. External incisions are coated with antibiotic ointment.

SURGICAL PROCEDURES

Open Reduction Internal Fixation: Mandibular Fractures
SURGICAL GOAL

In this procedure, a mandibular fracture is repaired and **dentition** is restored.

PATHOLOGY

Open reduction internal fixation (ORIF) of the mandible is performed to treat facial trauma involving the mandible. This trauma may be caused by a fall, motor vehicle accident, or assault. These events occur in adults more often than to children, because adults tend to be exposed to the causative agents more often than children.

Technique
1. The patient is placed in **maxillomandibular fixation** (MMF) if necessary.
2. The surgeon makes an incision either transorally or externally.
3. The fracture is exposed and reduced.
4. The fracture is internal fixated with mini plates and screws.
5. The incisions are closed.
6. The patient may be taken out of MMF.

DISCUSSION

The patient is placed in the supine position with a doughnut headrest; arms are tucked at the patient's sides. General anesthesia with a nasal Rae tube is used. The surgeon needs full access to the mouth, and if the patient is to be placed in MMF, an oral tube is contraindicated. The patient is prepped and draped for a facial procedure.

Maxillomandibular Fixation (Arch Bars)

The surgeon cleans the mouth with irrigation using an Asepto syringe and suction with a Yankauer suction tip. He or she then bends an arch bar wire to the shape of the patient's upper teeth and gums. With the cheek and tongue retracted by a cheek retractor and a sweetheart retractor, the bar is wired into place with 24-gauge or 26-gauge wires, which are stretched and then cut into thirds with wire cutters. The wires then are loaded onto a Rubio needle holder, threaded between the teeth, wrapped around the bar, and twisted to tighten; the excess wire is cut with a wire cutter. If the patient's dentition allows, three wires are placed on each side of the mouth. The procedure is repeated for the lower teeth and gums.

When the arch bars have been applied to both the upper and lower teeth, the two are "wired" together (Figure 25-41). This is accomplished with 24-gauge or 26-gauge wire, twisted into a clockwise loop, which is wrapped around the upper and lower bars with a Rubio needle holder. The wire is twisted clockwise until tight against the arch bars. The wire is then cut with a wire cutter, leaving a small amount to twist onto itself. One makes this "rosebud" by grasping the wire with a hemostat and crimping it inward; it may be buried in the patient's gingiva.

ORIF of the Mandible

The surgeon makes an incision either in the gingival-buccal mucosa using electrocautery, or in the external surface using a #15 or #10 blade. The incision varies depending on the type of fracture and the exposure needed to repair it. With the incision made, the surgeon exposes the mandible and elevates the periosteum using a Freer or periosteal elevator. The surgeon then mobilizes the fracture using a bone hook

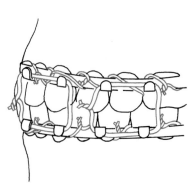
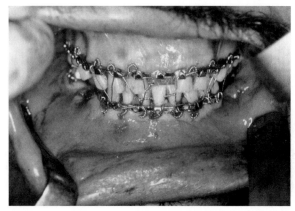

FIGURE 25-41
Arch bar intermaxillary fixation. (From Peterson LJ, Ellis E, Hupp JR, et al: *Contemporary oral and maxillofacial surgery*, ed 4, St Louis, 2003, Mosby.)

or a Hohmann retractor and approximates the fracture with a bone clamp.

When the fracture has been approximated, the surgeon chooses the plates necessary for fixation, usually 2.0 mm, 2.4 mm, or 2.7 mm. Most mandibular fractures require two plates per fracture: a larger plate inferiorly using **bicortical screws,** which go through the entire bone, and a smaller superior plate, or tension-band plate, using **monocortical screws,** which go through only the outer layer of the bone.

Depending on the size of plate chosen, the appropriate drill bit is fitted to a small power drill. The plate is stabilized against the mandible with a plate-holding forceps, and the screw holes are drilled. A drill guide may be used to stabilize the drill bit. If a drill guide is used, a depth gauge then is used to measure the screw length needed. The appropriate screw then is loaded onto a screwdriver, which is included in the module. The surgeon then screws it into position. This sequence (drill, measure, screw) is repeated until the plate has been secured.

When all of the fractures have been reduced and fixed, the incisions are closed. Transbuccal incisions are closed with a 3-0 absorbable suture; external incisions are closed in layers with 3-0 absorbable suture, and the skin is closed with 4-0 absorbable suture. The patient may be taken out of MMF if the fractures are stable enough and the patient is not at risk for noncompliance. If the patient is left in MMF, it is imperative that a wire cutter be sent with him or her to the recovery room and then home in case of an airway emergency.

Open Reduction Internal Fixation: Midface Fractures
SURGICAL GOAL

In this procedure, a fracture is reduced and the facial buttresses (the weight-bearing structures of the face) and facial width and projection are restored.

PATHOLOGY

ORIF of midface fractures is performed to treat fractures of the maxilla, zygoma, and malar complex, and LeFort fractures. Trauma to the midface primarily is due to motor vehicle accidents, falls, and assault. LeFort fractures are classified based on the fractures that are present. LeFort I is a fracture involving the lower maxilla. LeFort II is a fracture through the inferior orbital floor. LeFort III is a fracture of the lateral rim of the orbit. These fractures may occur unilaterally or bilaterally, and more than one type of LeFort fracture may be present.

Technique
1. The patient is placed in MMF if necessary.
2. The surgeon makes an incision transorally or externally.
3. The fracture is exposed and reduced.
4. The fracture is internally fixated with mini plates and screws.
5. The incisions are closed.
6. The patient may be taken out of MMF.

DISCUSSION

The patient is positioned supine on a doughnut or Mayfield headrest, with arms tucked at the sides. General anesthesia with a nasal Rae tube is used. The patient is prepped and draped for a facial procedure. If other fractures are present, the patient may be placed in MMF. The surgeon makes the incision in the upper gingival mucosa on the affected side using a #15 blade. The incision is extended through the mucosa to the level of the maxilla. The surgeon then elevates the periosteum using a Freer or periosteal elevator. The zygoma then is reduced with Hohmann retractors and/or a bone hook.

The surgeon then chooses the size and type of plate to be used. The plates typically are size 1.5 mm, 1.7 mm, or 2.0 mm. Monocortical screws are used to secure the plate to the bone. The plate is secured into place with a plate-holding forceps or hemostat. The appropriate drill bit is loaded onto a small power drill, and the screw holes are drilled. The surgeon then chooses the screw length; a depth gauge may be used. The screw is loaded onto the screwdriver, and it is screwed into place. This process is repeated until all of the screws have been placed and the plate has been secured to the bone. The incision then is closed with 3-0 absorbable suture. If the patient is to remain in MMF, a wire cutter must follow the patient to the recovery room.

Frontal Sinus Fracture

SURGICAL GOAL

This procedure is performed to reduce one or more fractures, repair a cerebrospinal fluid (CSF) leak, and prevent future **mucocele.**

PATHOLOGY

Fractures of the frontal sinus result from a traumatic event. As with other facial fractures, the cause can be motor vehicle accidents, falls, or assaults. These fractures involve the anterior and/or posterior wall of the frontal sinus. They must be repaired to prevent the formation of a mucocele or brain herniation and to repair leaks of CSF.

Technique

1. The surgeon makes a bicoronal incision.
2. The periosteum is elevated off the skull.
3. The fractures are exposed.
4. The fractures are repaired.
5. The incision is closed.

DISCUSSION

The patient is positioned supine with a Mayfield headrest, and with arms tucked at the sides. General anesthesia is used. Either the patient's head is shaved in a coronal strip going ear to ear, or the entire head is shaved. The hair is collected, saved in a plastic bag, and placed on the patient's chart. The patient is then prepped and draped for a cranial procedure.

The surgeon makes the incision from the root of the helix of one ear to the root of the helix of the other ear, using a #10 blade or electrocautery with a Colorado needle tip. If a blade is used, Raney clips are applied to the scalp with a Raney clip applier to aid in hemostasis. The incision extends to the level of the periosteum. The periosteum is elevated to the level of the superior orbital rims and anterior wall of the frontal sinus with a periosteal elevator.

The surgeon then examines the anterior and posterior walls of the frontal sinus for fractures. If the posterior wall of the frontal sinus is fractured, the frontal sinus will need to be obliterated. The surgeon does this by removing the posterior wall of the sinus and then obliterating the mucosal lining of the frontal sinus. The surgeon removes the posterior wall by using hemostats to remove the fractured portions. The mucosa is obliterated with a medium cutting or diamond bur loaded onto a small powered drill. The mucosa of the frontal osteum is removed with a small acorn bur. The frontal osteum then is packed with muscle or fascia. This cuts off the frontal sinus cavity from the rest of the sinuses. The cavity then is packed with fat, which is taken from the abdomen.

The anterior wall of the frontal wall then is repaired with micro mesh plates; usually size 1.0 mm or 1.3 mm is used. The free portions of the bone are secured to the mesh before it is secured to the stable portions of the bone. The appropriate drill bit is loaded onto a small power drill, and holes are drilled into the bone. The surgeon selects the screw size.

The screws are loaded onto a screwdriver, which is included in the plating module. These steps are repeated until the mesh has been secured into place and the fracture has been reduced.

The incision then is closed in layers. The periosteum is replaced over the cranium, and the subcutaneous tissue is closed with 3-0 absorbable suture. The skin then is closed with skin staples or a locking silk stitch. The wound then is covered with antibiotic ointment; generally no dressing is applied.

Fat Graft

The surgeon makes a small incision in the abdomen (approximately 2 to 3 mm) using a #15 blade. Using double-prong skin hooks to expose the wound, the surgeon excises a small portion of adipose tissue with a #15 blade, a hemostat, or a toothed Adson forceps. When hemostasis has been accomplished by electrocautery, the graft site is closed with a 4-0 Vicryl stitch. When the graft is removed, it is placed in normal saline to keep it moist until the surgeon is ready to place it into the frontal sinus.

Orbital Fractures

SURGICAL GOAL

This procedure is performed to reduce a fracture, prevent entrapment of the extraoccular muscles, and support the orbital contents.

PATHOLOGY

Orbital fractures can involve the orbital floor, inferior orbital rim, or lateral orbital rim, and can include naso-orbital-ethmoidal (NOE) fractures. As with other facial fractures, these fractures usually are associated with traumatic events, including motor vehicle accidents, falls, and assaults.

Technique

1. The surgeon makes either a subciliary or a transconjunctival incision.
2. The surgeon exposes the orbit.
3. The fractures are reduced and repaired.
4. The incision is closed.

DISCUSSION

The patient is positioned supine on a doughnut or Mayfield headrest with arms tucked at the sides. General anesthesia is used. The patient is prepped and draped for a facial procedure. Care is taken not to get prep solution in the eye because it can cause burning. If possible, lubrication should be placed into the eyes before prepping. The surgeon begins by placing corneal protectors in the operative eye. The surgeon does this by grasping the protector with a hemostat, opening the eye using the fingers, and placing the protector over the cornea. Balanced salt solution then is instilled into the eye to provide moisture; this may be done several times throughout the case.

With the cornea protected, the surgeon makes the incision. Two incisions are possible: subciliary and transconjunctival. A subciliary incision is made 2 mm under the eyelashes with #15 blade; a transconjunctival incision is made at the conjunctiva of the inferior eyelid with a #15 blade. The surgeon exposes the orbit by placing small malleable retractors, brain spatula retractors, into the wound and retracting superiorly and inferiorly. The wound is exposed to the level of the orbital rim, and the periosteum is elevated with a Freer elevator. The surgeon then elevates and retracts the orbital contents superiorly using a small malleable retractor.

The surgeon then examines the orbital floor (Figure 25-42). The floor of the orbit is recreated with nylon sheeting, mesh, Gelfilm, Silastic sheeting, or an orbital floor plate. Typically a 1.0 mm, 1.3 mm, or 1.5 mm plate or mesh is selected for orbital fractures. The surgeon cuts the selected material to size using plate cutters or scissors, depending on the material, and then positions it into place between the orbital floor and the orbital contents. Only orbital floor plates are secured into place, with screws placed into the infraorbital rim. This is carried out in the same fashion as described previously for the other types of facial fractures.

With the orbital contents supported, the retractors are removed, and the wound is closed. Subciliary incisions are closed with a 5-0 absorbable suture. Transconjunctival incisions are not closed. The surgeon removes the corneal protector after the incisions have been closed. Antibiotic ophthalmic ointment may be placed in the eye and on the incision.

Dental Implants

SURGICAL GOAL

Dental implants are used to replace lost dentition.

PATHOLOGY

Dental implants are used to replace injured or lost dentition. An implant may replace a single tooth or multiple teeth.

DISCUSSION

Three types of dental implants are commonly used. They are endosteal implants, subperiosteal implants, and transosteal implants.

Endosteal implants are a threaded screw, cylinder, or flat blade that is implanted in the alveolus of the maxilla or mandible and then covered with soft tissue. After several months (3 months for the mandible and 6 months for the maxilla) a post is connected to the implanted fixture. This post extends slightly above the gingiva, allowing the artificial tooth to be attached.

Subperiosteal implants are placed beneath the periosteum directly on the alveolar bone. This type of implant is used primarily when bone is insufficient to support an endosteal implant.

Transosteal implants are bone plates with retaining posts and resemble a staple. This type of implant is used only when the patient has severe mandibular alveolar-ridge atrophy.

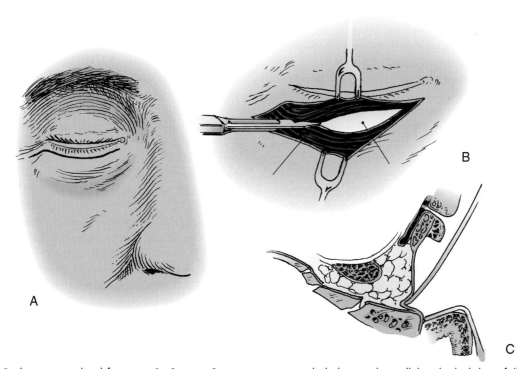

FIGURE 25-42 Reducing an orbital fracture. **A,** 2-cm to 3-cm incision is made below and parallel to the lash line, following a natural crease. **B,** The incision is deepened through the orbicularis muscle to the orbital septum to the level of the orbital rim. **C,** The orbit is retracted, and the periosteum is pulled tightly against the underlying muscle. (Modified from Marks SC: *Nasal and sinus surgery*, Philadelphia, 2000, Saunders.)

Odontectomy

SURGICAL GOAL

Odontectomy is performed to remove affected teeth.

PATHOLOGY

Odontectomy, or tooth extraction, may be performed for a variety of reasons. These can include damage or decay in teeth, or impaction, which often affects the third molars (wisdom teeth).

Technique

1. The surgeon makes an incision in the gingiva of the affected tooth.
2. The tissue surrounding the tooth is elevated to the level of the bone.
3. The tooth is elevated out of the alveola, making it mobile.
4. The tooth is extracted with a dental extractor of the appropriate size.
5. The incision is closed if necessary.

DISCUSSION

The patient is placed in the supine position with the arms tucked at the sides. Generally no prep is performed because the procedure is performed in the mouth. Betadine may be available on the field for irrigation. The patient is draped to allow adequate access to the mouth. The surgeon reviews x-rays to ensure that the correct teeth will be extracted. The surgeon uses a #15 blade to make a gingival incision to the level of the bone. A Molt elevator is used to elevate the tissue, including the periosteum, surrounding the tooth.

The surgeon then elevates the tooth out of the alveolus using an elevator; this breaks the attachment of the ligament holding the tooth in place, allowing the tooth to become mobile. The tooth then is extracted with a dental extractor of the appropriate size. The size varies with the tooth being extracted and the age of the patient. If necessary, the incision is closed with an absorbable 3-0 suture; this is usually required with impactions. Dental packs may be placed to prevent bleeding postoperatively.

ORTHOGNATHIC SURGICAL PROCEDURES

Mandibular Advancement

SURGICAL GOAL

Mandibular advancement is performed to correct a bony deformity of the mandible.

PATHOLOGY

Mandibular defects may be either acquired or congenital and usually are represented by a recessed mandible. Surgical correction of the defects may help the patient for medical and psychological reasons. Surgery generally is delayed until the patient has developed sufficiently and has most of his or her permanent teeth.

Technique

1. Arch bars are placed.
2. The surgeon makes intraoral incisions.
3. The mandible is cut at the predetermined location.
4. The bone is advanced.
5. Grafts are placed if necessary, and the bones are wired in place.
6. The intraoral incisions are closed.

DISCUSSION

The patient is placed on the operating room table in the supine position with arms tucked at the sides. The patient is prepped and draped to allow full exposure of the lower third of the face. Preoperative x-rays must be available in the room for the surgeon's use.

The surgeon begins by placing the patient in MMF (with arch bars). This allows the patient's dentition to be aligned and stabilized and provides postoperative immobilization.

After stabilization has been achieved, the surgeon makes intraoral incisions to produce exposure of the mandible. This may be performed with the scalpel or electrocautery. The incisions extend to the level of the periosteum. The periosteum then is elevated with a periosteal elevator to allow exposure of the mandible itself. The surgeon then uses an oscillating saw to make cuts through the mandible at predetermined locations. With the mandible split, it can then be advanced to the proper position. Bone graft is placed to fill any space between the advanced mandible and the fixed mandible.

The grafts and mandible then are fixed into place with either wire or a mandibular plating system. The incisions then are closed with a 3-0 absorbable suture. The patient remains in MMF for several weeks. Therefore it is extremely important that wire cutters be sent with the patient to allow release in case of an airway emergency.

Midface (Maxillary) Advancement

SURGICAL GOAL

Midface advancement is performed to correct a bony deformity of the maxilla.

PATHOLOGY

Maxillary defects may be either acquired or congenital and usually are represented by a recessed mandible. Surgical correction of the defects may help the patient for medical and psychological reasons. Surgery generally is delayed until the patient has developed sufficiently and has most of his or her permanent teeth.

Technique

1. Arch bars are placed.
2. The surgeon makes intraoral incisions.
3. The maxilla is cut at a predetermined location.
4. The bone is advanced.

5. Grafts are placed if necessary, and the bones are wired in place.
6. The intraoral incisions are closed.

DISCUSSION

The patient is placed on the operating room table in the supine position with arms tucked at the sides. The patient is prepped and draped to allow full exposure of the lower third of the face. Preoperative x-rays must be available in the room for the surgeon's use.

The surgeon begins by placing the patient in MMF (with arch bars). This allows the patient's dentition to be aligned and stabilized and provides postoperative immobilization. After stabilization has been achieved, the surgeon makes intraoral incisions to allow exposure of the maxilla. This may be done with the scalpel or electrocautery. The incisions extend to the level of the periosteum. The surgeon then elevates the periosteum using a periosteal elevator to allow exposure of the maxilla itself. The surgeon then uses an oscillating saw to make cuts through the maxilla at predetermined locations. With the maxilla split, it can then be advanced to the proper position. Bone graft is placed to fill any space between the advanced maxilla and the fixed maxilla.

The grafts and maxilla then are fixed into place with either wire or a mandibular plating system. The incisions then are closed with a 3-0 absorbable suture. The patient remains in maxillomandibular fixation for several weeks. Therefore it is extremely important that wire cutters be sent with the patient to allow release in case of an airway emergency.

Temporomandibular Joint Arthroplasty

SURGICAL GOAL

Temporomandibular joint (TMJ) arthroplasty is performed to reduce pain and increase mobility.

PATHOLOGY

TMJ disease is characterized by persistent pain and dysfunction of the joint. It is usually associated with stress-related muscle tension and grinding of the teeth (bruxism), malocclusion, trauma, or arthritis and other degenerative changes in the joint.

Technique

1. The surgeon makes a preauricular or postauricular incision.
2. The temporalis fascia is exposed.
3. The joint capsule is incised and opened.
4. The disk is replaced or repositioned.
5. Drains are placed.
6. The wound is closed.

DISCUSSION

The patient is placed on the operating room table in the supine position with arms tucked at the sides. The patient is placed under general anesthesia. The patient then is pepped and draped to allow adequate exposure of the affected joint, including a head drape.

The surgeon begins by making a preauricular or postauricular incision using a #15 blade. The surgeon elevates the skin flaps using either the electrocautery or scissors to expose the temporalis fascia. Retractors are placed to allow visualization of the wound. A #9 Molt elevator is used to dissect the underlying periosteum to the level of the arch. Blunt dissection next is performed with a hemostat.

The surgeon makes a horizontal incision into the joint capsule and creates a flap to expose the condyle. The condyle is distracted inferiorly. Any adhesions then are lysed with the electrocautery or freed with a scalpel. If any perforations are noted in the disk of the joint, the joint usually is removed and an artificial joint placed. If the disk has rotated, it is repositioned and sutured into place with a 2-0 nonabsorbable suture. A drain then is placed if necessary, and the wound is closed.

REFERENCES

Bailey BJ et al: *Head and neck surgery: otolaryngology,* ed 2, vol 1 and 2, Philadelphia, 1998, Lippincott–Raven.

Boston Medical Products: *Montgomery thyroplasty system: surgeon's implant guide,* ; Westborough, Mass, 1998, Boston Medical Products.

Brackmann D, Shelton C, and Arriaga MA: *Otologic surgery,* ed 2, Philadelphia, 2001, Saunders.

Coker NJ and Jenkins HA: *Atlas of otologic surgery,* Philadelphia, 2001, Saunders.

Cummings CW, Haughey BH, Thomas JR, et al: *Otolaryngology: head and neck surgery,* ed 3, St Louis, 1998, Mosby.

Fortunato N and McCullough SM: *Plastic and reconstructive surgery: perioperative nursing series,* St Louis, 1998, Mosby.

Gruendemann BJ and Fernsebner B: *Comprehensive perioperative nursing,* vol 2, Boston, 1995, Jones and Bartlett.

Herman C: Medialization thyroplasty for unilateral vocal cord paralysis, *AORN J* Mar, 75(3): 511-522, 2002.

Marks SC: *Nasal and sinus surgery,* Philadelphia, 2000, Saunders.

Montgomery WW: *Surgery of the upper respiratory system,* ed 3, Baltimore, 1996, Williams & Wilkins.

Moody FG: *Atlas of ambulatory surgery,* St Louis, 1999, Mosby.

Phillips N: *Berry & Kohn's operating room technique,* ed 10, St Louis, 2004, Mosby.

Robbins KT et al : Standardizing neck dissection terminology: official report of the Academy's committee for head and neck surgery and oncology, *Arch Head Neck Surg* June, 117:601-605, 1991.

Rothrock JC: *Alexander's care of the patient in surgery,* ed 12, St Louis, 2003, Mosby.

Seiden AM et al: *Otolaryngology: the essentials,* New York, 2002, Thieme.

Silver CE and Rubin JS: *Atlas of head and neck surgery,* ed 2, Philadelphia, 1999, Churchill Livingstone.

Staffel JF: *Basic principles of rhinoplasty,* San Antonio, 1996, University of Texas Health Science Center.

Thumfart WF et al: *Surgical approaches in otorhinolaryngology,* New York, 1999, Thieme.

Weerda H: *Reconstructive facial plastic surgery: a problem-solving manual,* New York, 2001, Thieme.

Wigand ME et al: *Endoscopic surgery of the paranasal sinuses and anterior skull base,* New York, 1990, Thieme.

Chapter 26

Plastic and Reconstructive Surgery

By Rebecca Carr Ferguson

Learning Objectives

After studying this chapter the reader will be able to:

- Define the terminology of plastic surgery
- Identify the anatomical structures of the skin
- Discuss the procedures involving the skin
- Differentiate the types of skin-grafting techniques
- Identify various cosmetic procedures of the face
- Identify equipment and instruments used in plastic surgery
- Identify procedures for breast augmentation and reduction
- Identify procedures for reconstruction of the breast after mastectomy

Terminology

Aesthetic—Having a pleasing shape and form.

Allograft—Transfer of tissue between two genetically dissimilar individuals of the same species.

Augmentation—An addition or increase in size.

Autograft—Surgical transplantation of any tissue from one part of the body to another location in the same individual.

Bicoronal—An incision made between the frontal bone and the parietal bone on one side of the head and extending to the same location on the other side.

Bilobate—Having two lobes.

Blepharoplasty—Surgery to restore or repair the eyelid or eyebrow.

Conjunctival sulcus—Depression at the level of the conjunctiva.

Debridement—Process of removing dead skin, debris, or foreign bodies from a wound.

Deepithelialized—State in which epithelial tissue has been removed.

Eschar—A scab or dry crust caused by a thermal or chemical burn, infection, or excoriating skin disease.

First-degree burn—Burn that involves only the outer layer of the epidermis.

Full-thickness skin graft—Skin graft that consists of the entire epidermis and dermis.

Gynecomastia—An abnormal enlargement of the mammary gland in males, resulting in enlargement of one or both breasts.

Hydrodressing—Dressings that have been impregnated with water-based gel.

Imbricate—To build a surface with overlapping layers of material.

Philtrum—The vertical groove in the center of the upper lip.

Photodamage—Damage to the skin caused by the sun.

Terminology—cont'd

Plicate—To fold, shorten, or reduce the size of a muscle or hollow organ by taking it in tucks.

Pretrichial—The region anterior to the hairline.

Ptosis—An abnormal condition involving one or both upper eyelids in which the eyelid droops because of a congenital or acquired weakness of the levator muscle or paralysis of the third cranial nerve.

Second-degree burn—Burn that involves the entire epidermis and part of the dermis.

Split-thickness skin graft—Skin graft that consists of the epidermis and a portion of the papillary dermis.

Subcuticular—Beneath the skin.

Supratarsal crease—A horizontal crease above the lash line of the upper eyelid.

Third-degree burn—Burn that causes the destruction of the entire thickness of the skin.

Turgid—Swollen, hard, and/or congested.

INTRODUCTION TO PLASTIC AND RECONSTRUCTIVE SURGERY

Plastic and reconstructive surgical procedures include operations to correct congenital defects or deformities caused by disease or injury and operations to alter the patient's appearance for simple cosmetic purposes. Whether the patient arrives in surgery for an elective or nonelective procedure, special psychological needs must be met. The technologist or nurse should treat the patient in an honest and straightforward manner and should offer as much emotional support as possible. Recently, many plastic surgeries (e.g., rhytidectomy, blepharoplasty, dermabrasion) have been increasingly performed on an outpatient basis or in the plastic surgeon's office. Consequently, in some geographical areas these procedures are seen in the operating room only occasionally.

ANATOMY OF SKIN OR THE INTEGUMENTARY SYSTEM

The skin, or integumentary system, serves several functions. It protects underlying tissues and organs; excretes salts, water, and organic waste; stores nutrients; and detects touch, pressure, pain, and temperature. The skin is composed of two layers: the epidermis and the dermis.

Epidermis

The epidermis is the outer layer of the skin (Figure 26-1). It comprises five sublayers. These layers are the stratum corneum, stratum lucidum, stratum granulosum, stratum spinosum, and stratum germinativum.

The stratum corneum is a relatively transparent layer and is the body's primary protective barrier against water. It is composed of dead cells that are filled with a protein called keratin. The stratum corneum is thicker on areas of the body that are weight-bearing or that undergo a lot of friction, such as the hands and feet.

The stratum lucidum is composed of dead or dying cells that are flattened, densely packed, and filled with eleidin. This layer is extremely thin, approximately five cells thick. This layer may not be found on regions of the body that have thin skin.

The stratum granulosum is the layer of the skin in which keratinization takes place. This is the production of keratin.

The stratum spinosum is composed of a layer that is several cells thick. These cells resemble miniature pincushions. This layer is the middle layer of the epidermis.

The stratum germinativum, or stratum basale, is the deepest layer of the epidermis. It lies directly above the dermis. This is the regenerative layer of the epidermis and gives rise to all other layers of the epidermis. As the cells undergo mitosis and their subsequent changes, the cells of the stratum germinativum move to the upper layers of the epidermis. The melanocytes also are found in this layer. These are the cells responsible for the production of melanin, which gives the skin its pigment.

Dermis

The dermis lies directly beneath the epidermis (see Figure 26-1). This layer contains the nervous and blood supply of the skin. It is also the layer of the skin that consists of all of the accessory structures. It contains the hair follicles and the sebaceous and sweat glands. The hair follicles extend deep into the dermis and sometimes into the subcutaneous layer.

The hair follicles consist of the root, which encloses the matrix and is surrounded by the follicle; and the shaft, which is the visible portion of the hair and may vary in size, shape, and color. The sebaceous glands discharge a waxy, oily secretion called sebum into the hair follicles. Sebum acts as a lubricant for the skin. Sweat glands are found virtually throughout the body; however, they are most numerous on the hands and soles of the feet. The sweat glands excrete sweat to the surface of the skin. Sweating is an important part of the body's cooling system; when the body is hot, the sweat glands secrete sweat to the skin's surface in an effort to cool the skin. Sweat glands also are active during extreme emotional periods, such as when one is nervous.

ANATOMY OF THE HAND

The hand and wrist comprise many bones, nerves, tendons, ligaments, and muscles (Figure 26-2). The wrist comprises the eight carpal bones in two rows of four; the distal row of carpal bones from the radial to the ulnar side is the trape-

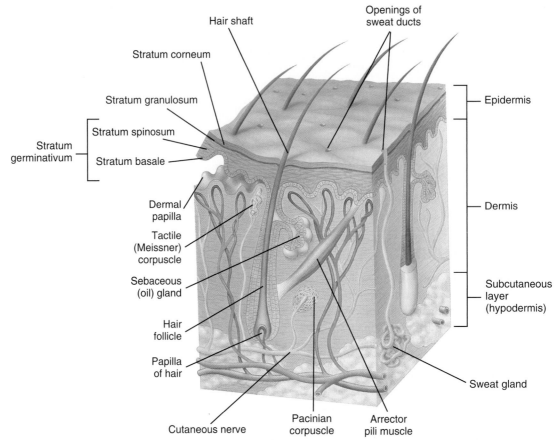

FIGURE 26-1
The epidermis. (From Thibodeau GA and Patton KT: *Anthony's textbook of anatomy and physiology,* ed 17, St Louis, 2003, Mosby.)

zium, trapezoid, capitate, and hamate; the proximal row consists of the scaphoid (or navicular), lunate, triquetrum, and pisiform. The scaphoid bone is the bone that is responsible for stabilization and coordination of movement of the two rows of carpal bones. Each of these carpal bones has several smooth articular surfaces that allow movement against the adjacent bones and rough surfaces that allow for the attachment of the ligaments.

The metacarpals are the bones of the palm and are the only long bones of the wrist and hand. There are five metacarpal bones. Their proximal ends articulate with the distal row of the carpal bones, and their distal end articulates with the phalanx (or finger). The heads of the metacarpals form the knuckles.

The phalanges, or fingers, consist of 14 bones in each hand. The thumb consists of two bones, and the four fingers each have three bones.

EQUIPMENT AND INSTRUMENTS

Dermabrader

The dermabrader may be a larger powered dermabrader such as the Osada or a small powered dermabrader such as

the Xomed Xps (Figure 26-3). The Osada dermabrader consists of a handpiece with several sizes of burs, a motor, and a foot pedal. The bur size depends on the area to be treated. The burs resemble sanders; they contain diamonds and are cylindrical in shape. For smaller areas, the small powered dermabrader may be used. The small dermabraders follow the same principles as the large dermabraders but have only have one size of bur (usually a barrel bur).

Liposuction Instruments

The liposuction instruments consist of rigid cannulas that are connected to a large-bore suction tube (at least $\frac{3}{8}$ inch in diameter) (Figure 26-4). This suction tube is connected to a high-vacuum suction. Large-bore tubing and high-vacuum suction are required because adipose tissue is dense and would clog normal suction tubing, and the vacuum power of wall suction is not sufficient to pull the tissue through the tubing.

CO_2 Laser

CO_2 lasers are used for facial resurfacing procedures. The principles of laser safety must be followed during the procedure. Laser safety is discussed in Chapter 17.

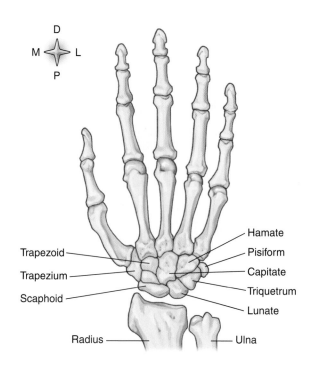

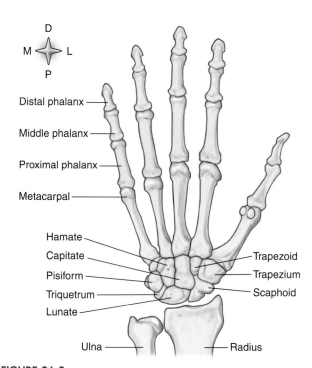

FIGURE 26-2
Bones of the hand and wrist. (From Thibodeau GA and Patton KT: *Anthony's textbook of anatomy and physiology*, ed 17, St Louis, 2003, Mosby.)

Facial Implants

Several different materials can be used as facial implants. These include silicone, acrylic, Medpore, Gore-Tex, allografts, and hemografts.

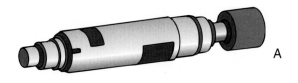

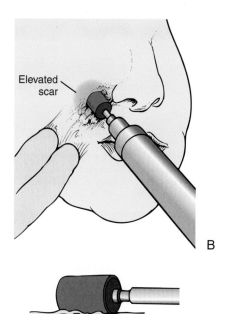

FIGURE 26-3
A through **C,** Dermabrasion. (From Fortunato N and McCullough SM: *Plastic and reconstructive surgery: perioperative nursing series*, St Louis, 1998, Mosby.)

SILICONE

Silicone has been used as an implant material since the 1950s. It has proven to be both safe and effective. The harder the silicone is, the more stable it is. Soft silicone has gel-like qualities and may leak into surrounding areas. The silicone implant must have sufficient soft-tissue coverage to prevent chronic inflammation. These implants are easily sculpted. Silicone can be used for a variety of purposes, including chin and cheek implants.

ACRYLIC

Acrylic is a powder that is mixed with a liquid catalyst to produce a pliable paste that hardens quickly on standing. Acrylic is not often used as a facial implant because its rigidity makes it difficult to insert into small areas. The rigidity of acrylic also makes it difficult to mold directly to the bone.

POLYETHYLENE

Polyethylene or Medpore implants are porous and are proven to be very stable and cause little inflammatory reaction. These characteristics make it a desirable implant; however, it is difficult to sculpt, and when it is removed it can cause damage to surrounding soft tissue.

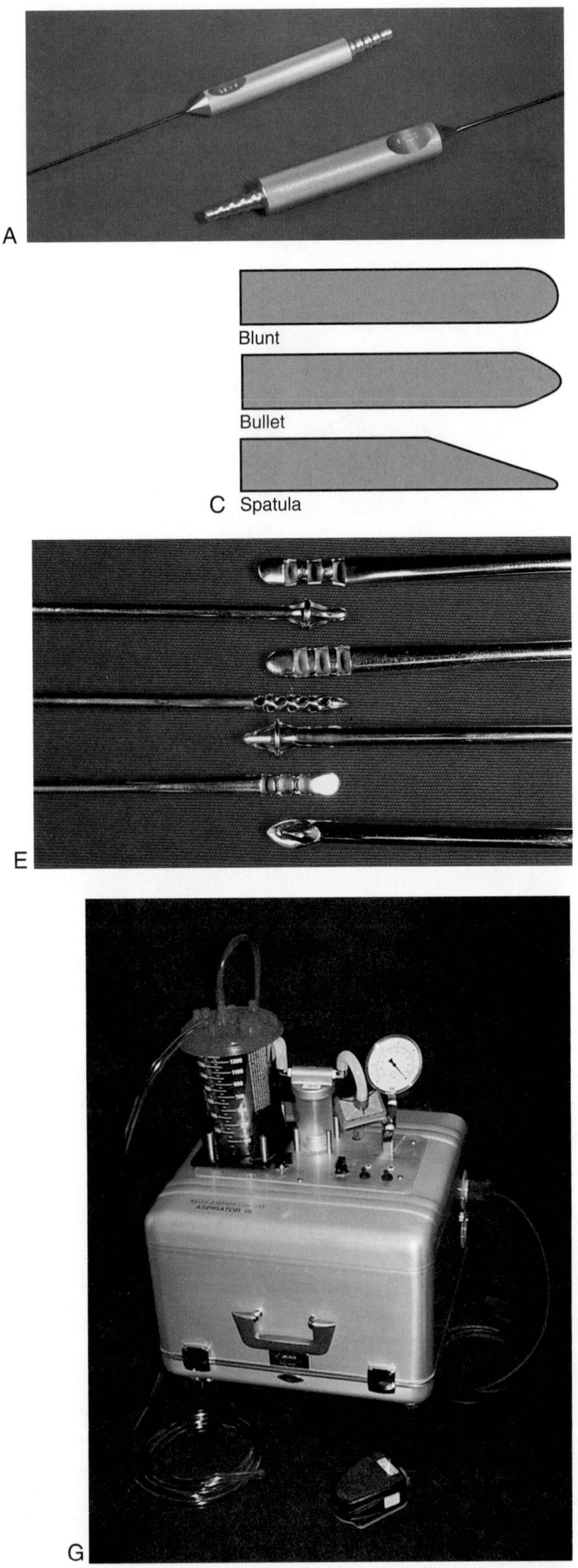

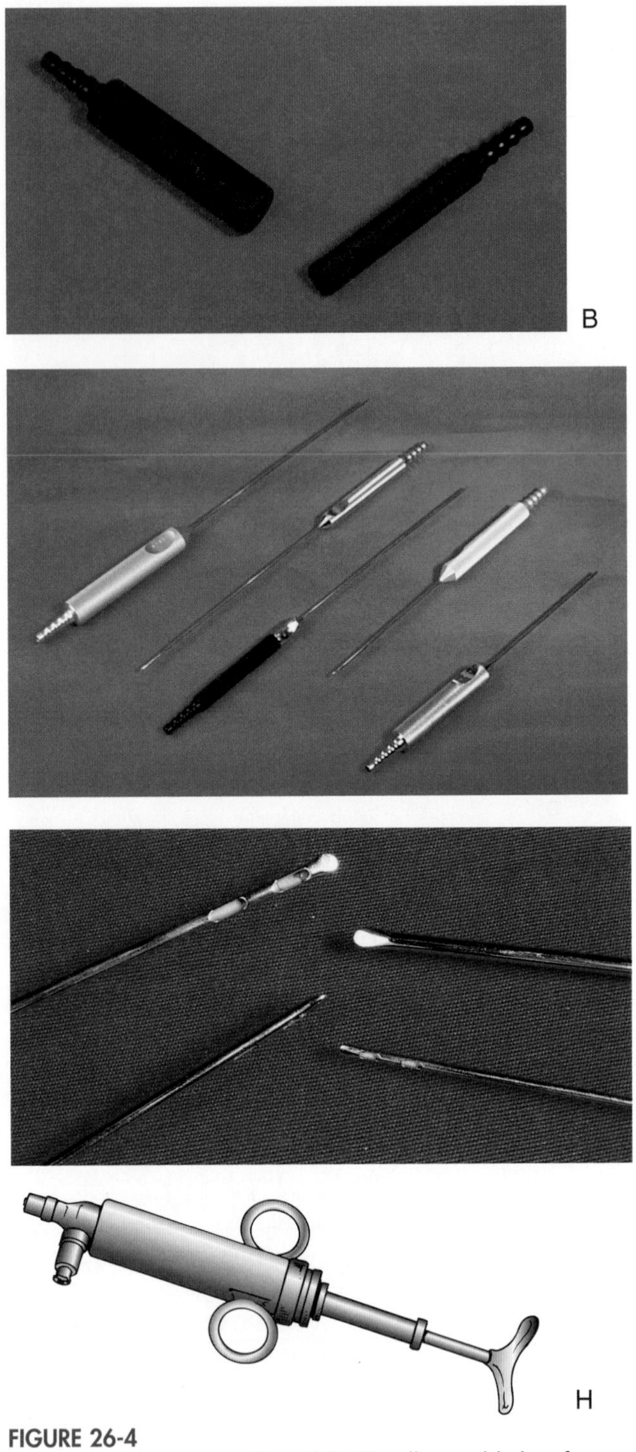

FIGURE 26-4
Liposuction instruments. **A** and **B,** Handles and hubs of suction hand pieces. **C,** Three styles of blunt cannulae tips. **D,** Custom-designed cannulae. **E** and **F,** Custom-designed cannulae tips. **G,** Mechanical suction machine. **H,** Manual syringe. (From Fortunato N, McCullough SM: *Plastic and reconstructive surgery,* St Louis, 1998, Mosby; courtesy Wells Johnson, Tucson, Ariz.)

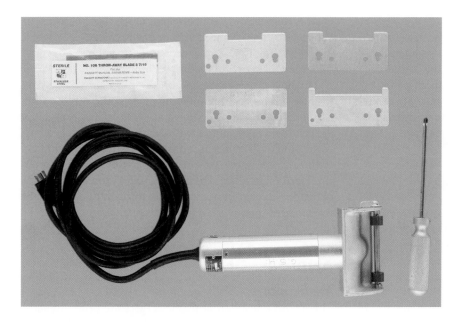

FIGURE 26-5
Padgett electric dermatome with disposable blade. (From Tighe SM: *Instrumentation for the operating room*, ed 6, St Louis, 2003, Mosby.)

GORE-TEX

Gore-Tex implants initially were used in cardiovascular procedures. However, Gore-Tex now is used often as an implant for facial augmentation. Gore-Tex causes little tissue inflammation, and there is little tissue growth into the implant. The lack of growth into the implant makes it easy to remove at a later date if necessary.

AUTOGRAFTS AND HOMOGRAFTS

Autografts include autogenous bone, cartilage, and fat. These grafts are taken from one area of the body and transplanted to another area to fill a defect. Homografts include injectable collagen and AlloDerm. Allografts and homografts are subject to partial reabsorption over time. The timing and amount of absorption vary from patient to patient.

Dermatome

The dermatome is used to take autograft skin. The set should include the dermatome itself, the power box, blade guards, a screwdriver, and a disposable blade (Figure 26-5). The blade is positioned onto the dermatome and is then fitted with the blade guard of appropriate width. The guards are chosen based on the width of the defect to be covered. The guards usually are available in 1-inch, 2-inch, and 3-inch sizes. The guard is screwed into place with the screwdriver. The dermatome is then plugged into the power source and tested to ensure that the blade moves freely. When the dermatome is handed to the surgeon, the depth gauge should be set to zero to prevent the graft from being too deep. The surgeon sets the depth gauge to the desired depth.

Mesher

The mesher is used to increase the surface area of grafted skin by placing holes into the skin graft (Figure 26-6). One does this by feeding the skin through the mesher; some meshers use a plastic plate to feed the skin through, while

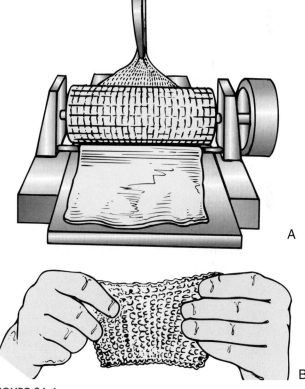

FIGURE 26-6
A and **B,** Manual skin mesher. (From Fortunato N and McCullough SM: *Plastic and reconstructive surgery: perioperative nursing series*, St Louis, 1998, Mosby.)

others take only the skin. As the skin is fed through the mesher, holes are placed into the skin by combs on the mesher itself. The skin must be fed into the mesher in a uniform fashion. If the skin bunches up or gets caught in the mesher, the holes will not be placed evenly, and the skin graft could be ruined.

Endobrow Instruments

The endobrow instruments include a variety of periosteal elevators and instruments for blunt and sharp dissection. These instruments usually are included in an all-inclusive set. Many of the instruments are adapted to cautery to aid in hemostasis. In addition to the instruments, the set includes a cannula through which the endoscope may be passed. The endoscope may or may not be included in the set of instruments. A 4-mm or 5-mm endoscope in 0-degree and 30-degree angles is the endoscope of choice.

Other Instruments Used for Plastic Surgery

Other instruments used for plastic surgery are shown in Figure 26-7.

PREPPING AND DRAPING

Betadine, pHisoHex, and Hibiclens are the prep solutions of choice for plastic surgery procedures. Betadine often is used in prepping of the body in cases such as liposuction or debridement of burns. However, in prepping of the face, pHisoHex or Hibiclens is typically the prep solution of choice. Regardless of the prep solution used, one must take care not to let the prep solution pool in or around the eyes or in the ear.

Draping varies depending on the procedure to be performed. For procedures involving the face, the surgeon usually prefers a head drape (see Figure 11-15). This drape keeps the hair from falling into the field and allows the surgeon visualization of the entire face during the procedure regardless of the area being treated. For other procedures, the draping is performed in a way that allows visualization of the surgical field. This may be accomplished through the use of split sheets, three-quarter sheets, or extremity sheets.

MEDICATIONS, SPONGES, AND DRESSINGS

Medications

The medications used in plastic surgery are primarily local anesthetic, epinephrine, and mineral oil. The anesthetics are used to produce anesthesia at the surgical site. Epinephrine

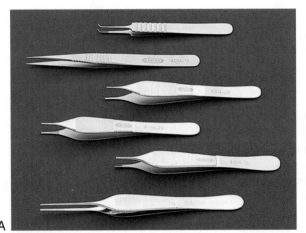

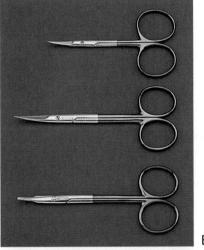

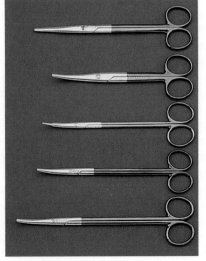

FIGURE 26-7
Other instruments used for plastic surgery. **A,** Forceps. *Top to bottom,* 45 angled jeweler's foceps; straight jeweler's forceps; Adson forceps with 1:1 teeth; Adson foceps with 1:1 teeth 1.2 mm; Adson-Brown tissue forceps with side teeth; Broli-Adson foceps with diamond dust tips. **B,** Jabaley scissors, 4¾-inch, curved, Jabaley scissors, 5-inch, curved; Jabaley scissors, 5-inch, straight. **C,** Comparison of common scissors used in plastic surgery: Mayo scissors, 6¾-inch, straight; Mayo scissors, 6¾-inch, curved; Stevens tenotomy scissors, 7-inch, curved; Metzenbaum scissors, 7-inch, curved; Metzenbaum scissors, 8-inch, curved. (From Fortunato N, McCullough SM: *Plastic and reconstructive surgery,* St Louis, 1998, Mosby; courtesy Scanlon, International, St Paul, Minn.)

is used for its hemostatic effects. Mineral oil is often used in skin grafting. It provides lubrication, which allows the dermatome to glide easily over the graft site.

Sponges

In addition to Raytec sponges and lap sponges, cotton pledgets and cottonoids may be used. All sharps and sponges are counted on each case.

Dressings

Dressings vary depending on the procedure that has been performed. Dressings often used in plastic surgery procedures are Steri-Strips, Telfa, Tegaderm, fluffs, Kerlix rolls, and Ace wraps.

SURGICAL PROCEDURES

Dermabrasion
SURGICAL GOAL
Dermabrasion is performed to reduce the appearance of scars and **photodamage** on the skin.

PATHOLOGY
Dermabrasion is performed to treat superficial lesions of the skin. These lesions are caused most often by photodamage, scarring, and in some cases, both. Dermabrasion is performed primarily on the face. Because of the mechanisms of injury, this procedure is performed most often on adults.

Technique
1. Local anesthetic may be injected, or "freezing" may be performed.
2. The affected regions are demarcated.
3. The dermabrasion is performed.
4. The wound is then dressed.

DISCUSSION
The patient is placed in the lounge-chair position with the arms at the sides. The patient receives IV sedation for the procedure. The patient's face is prepped with pHisoHex or Hibiclens prep to remove all debris and oil. The patient may be draped with only a down sheet, or a head drape and split sheet may be used.

The areas to be dermabraded are either frozen; with chemicals that cause the skin to become cold and taut, or injected with local anesthetic, usually 1% lidocaine with epinephrine 1:100,000. This surgeon does this by anesthetizing one area at a time. The surgeon then uses the powered micro dermabrader loaded with the appropriate bur to dermabrade the skin.

The assistant retracts the area being treated, using either gauze sponges or towels. The assistant must be careful to maintain even tension over the entire area being treated and not allow the gauze or towel to get tangled in the bur. This procedure is repeated over each area to be treated.

When all of the areas have been treated, the face is covered in gauzes that have been soaked in epinephrine with or without local anesthetic. These gauzes are left in place for several minutes to allow for hemostasis. The wound is then dressed with either ointment (possibly containing antioxidants, antibiotics, and/or steroids) or a **hydrodressing** and then covered with gauze and tape.

Laser Skin Resurfacing
SURGICAL GOAL
Laser skin resurfacing is performed to reduce the effects of aging on the skin.

PATHOLOGY
The aging process of the skin is due to inherent changes within the skin itself and photodamage. This ultimately leads to pigmentary changes, thinning and laxity of the skin, and fine lines and wrinkles. Laser resurfacing is a treatment option for these changes because it removes the epidermis and possibly a portion of the dermis.

Technique
1. The patient is anesthetized.
2. The patient is draped with wet towels.
3. The skin is resurfaced with either the CO_2 or erbium-YAG laser.
4. The wounds are dressed.

DISCUSSION
The patient is placed in either the supine or lounge-chair position with arms at the sides. The anesthetics used for the procedure vary depending on the extent of the resurfacing planned and whether any other procedures are to be performed at the same time. Some cases are performed with only local anesthetic, while others are performed with general anesthesia. If general anesthesia is used, a laser endotracheal tube may be used, or a regular endotracheal tube may be wrapped in moist gauze to reduce the risk of airway fire in the event of laser malfunction.

The face is prepped with pHisoHex to remove debris and oil. Prep solutions that contain large amounts of alcohol should be avoided because they can be a fire hazard. The patient then is draped with a head drape and a split sheet. Wet towels are placed around the area to be resurfaced to reduce the risk of thermal damage to other tissue and to reduce the risk of fire. The patient's eyes also are covered with either wet towels or laser safety goggles. This is done to protect the patient's eyes from the possible retinal damage that may be caused by the laser. All of the staff in the room also must wear safety goggles.

The laser then is used to resurface the skin. The surgeon does this by setting the laser on a particular pattern and wattage and then making multiple passes over the patient's skin using a handpiece with a computer-generated imaging system. Each pass removes a layer of the epidermis, reducing the appearance of wrinkles. When the entire face has been resurfaced, the face is dressed with either a hydrodressing or ointment.

Blepharoplasty

SURGICAL GOAL

Blepharoplasty is performed to rejuvenate the eye and improve vision.

PATHOLOGY

Blepharoplasty is performed to rejuvenate the eye and to improve vision in patients who have visual disturbances caused by sagging upper lids. This procedure is performed primarily on the aging adult.

> ### Technique
> 1. The lids are injected with local anesthetic.
> 2. The surgeon makes the incision.
> 3. The surgeon removes the excess tissue.
> 4. The incision is closed.
> 5. The procedure is repeated on the other eye and lid if necessary.

DISCUSSION

The patient is placed in the supine position on a doughnut headrest with arms tucked at the sides. General or local anesthesia may be used. The choice depends on whether blepharoplasty is to be performed alone or in conjunction with other procedures. Local anesthetic is instilled into the lids to be treated. The patient is prepped with pHisoHex. Care must be taken to prevent pooling of prep solution in the canthi because the eye mucosa may be burned by these solutions. The patient is draped with a head drape and a split sheet.

Upper-Lid Blepharoplasty

The surgeon determines how much tissue is to be removed by grasping the excess lid skin between forceps. Based on the amount of excess skin, the surgeon marks the skin to be removed using a surgical marker. The surgeon then makes the incision in the **supratarsal crease,** 10 mm above the lash line in men and 8 mm above the lash line in women, using a #15 blade. The excess skin is excised with the #15 blade. If there is also excess muscle, it may be excised with Adson toothed forceps and curved iris scissors. The incision then is closed with a nonabsorbable **subcuticular** stitch with placement of a few interrupted sutures to reinforce the subcuticular suture line. The ends of this stitch are not tied to allow easy removal at a later date.

Upper-lid blepharoplasty is illustrated in Figure 26-8.

Lower-Lid Blepharoplasty: Subciliary Approach

The surgeon makes the incision in the subciliary region, 2 to 3 mm below the lower lash line, using a #15 blade. The surgeon elevates the lower lid skin upward and outward to determine the amount to be removed. The lower lid skin is then excised with a #15 blade. To gain access to the infraorbital fat pads, the surgeon makes an incision into the orbicularis oculi muscle. Retraction is provided via double-prong skin hooks placed into the incision. The excess fat is removed with toothed Adson forceps and iris scissors. The orbicularis oculi muscle then is reattached to the periosteum at the lateral orbital rim with a clear, nonabsorbable stitch. This prevents the lower lid from drooping after blepharoplasty. The incisions then are closed with a nonabsorbable subcutaneous stitch with placement of a few interrupted sutures to enforce the subcuticular suture line.

The subciliary approach to lower-lid blepharoplasty is illustrated in Figure 26-9.

Lower-Lid Blepharoplasty: Transconjunctival Approach

This approach is used in patients who do not require removal of excess skin, but rather of fat pad. The surgeon retracts the lower lid with a double-prong skin hook and makes the incision in the **conjunctival sulcus.** This is done with electrocautery with a needle tip. A nonabsorbable suture is placed in the lower flap, and the end of the suture is tagged and placed over the patient's head. This allows retraction of the lower flap over the eye. The fat is then teased from the wound with a mosquito forceps and Adson toothed forceps. The excess fat then is grasped with the mosquito for-

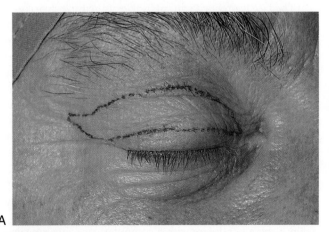
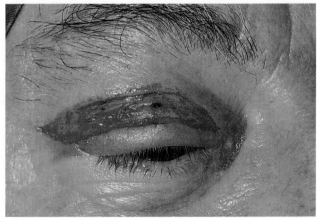

A   B

FIGURE 26-8
Upper-lid blepharoplasty. **A,** Blepharoplasty incision marked. **B,** The skin is removed, exposing the orbicularis muscle. (From Tyers AG and Collin JRO: *Colour atlas of ophthalmic plastic surgery,* ed 2, Oxford, 2001, Butterworth-Heinemann.)

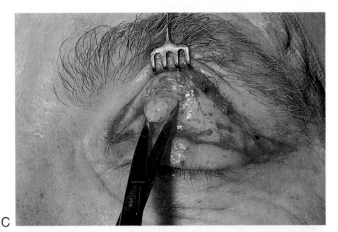

C

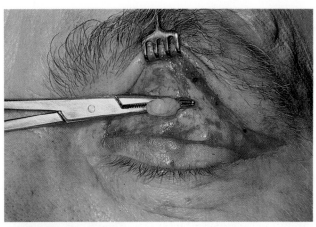

D

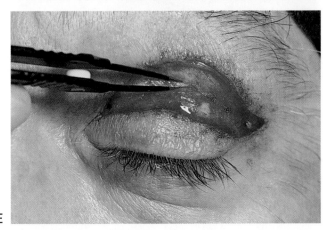

E

FIGURE 26-8, cont'd
C, The preaponeurotic fat is prolapsed through a small incision in the septum. **D,** The prolapsed rag is clipped.
E, Cautery is applied through the unopened septum to reduce fat prolapse and tighten the septum. (From Tyers AG and Collin JRO: *Colour atlas of ophthalmic plastic surgery,* ed 2, Oxford, 2001, Butterworth-Heinemann.)

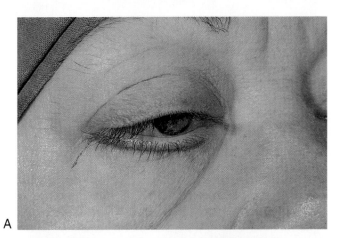

A

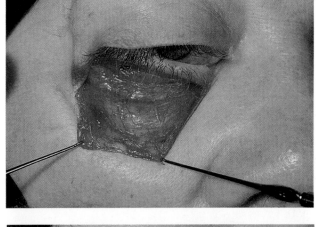

B

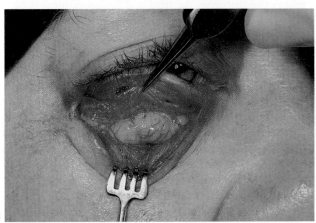

C

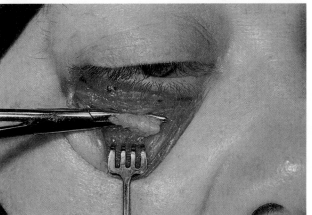

D

FIGURE 26-9
The subciliary approach to lower-lid blepharoplasty. **A,** The subciliary incision is marked and extended laterally. **B,** The skin-muscle flap is raised, exposing the tarsal plate and spectum. **C,** The septum is opened over the prolapsed fat. **D,** The prolapsed fat is excised without traction. (From Tyers AG and Collin JRO: *Colour atlas of ophthalmic plastic surgery,* ed 2, Oxford, 2001, Butterworth-Heinemann.)

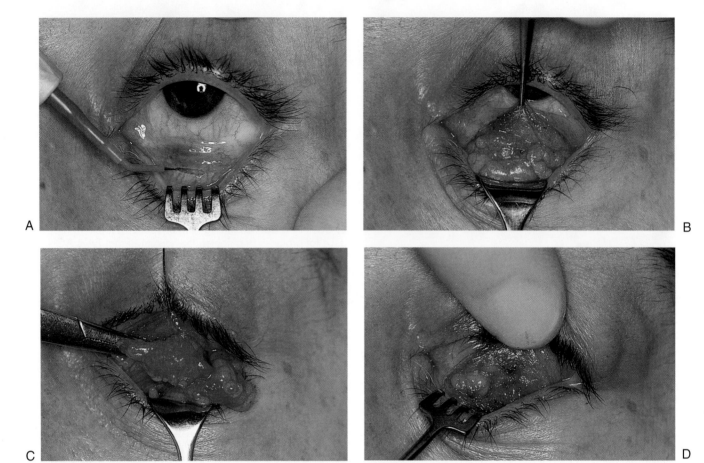

FIGURE 26-10
The transconjunctival approach to lower-lid blepharoplasty. **A,** An incision is made into the lower fornix with a cutting cautery needle tip. **B,** The orbital fat prolapsing though the incision in the conjunctiva and lower-lid retractors. **C,** Artery forceps are applied to the central fat pad. **D,** The medial fat pad is prolapsed by application of pressure on the globe. (From Tyers AG and Collin RO: *Colour atlas of ophthalmic plastic surgery*, ed 2, Oxford, 2001, Butterworth-Heinemann.)

ceps and cut with iris scissors. Before removing the clamp, the surgeon uses the electrocautery to produce hemostasis. The clamp then is removed. The stay suture is removed, and the wound is left to close by primary intention.

The transconjunctival approach to lower-lid blepharoplasty is illustrated in Figure 26-10.

Brow Lift (Open and Endoscopic)
SURGICAL GOAL
Brow lift is performed to rejuvenate the upper third of the face.

PATHOLOGY
Over time, gravity pulls the brows down. This not only ages a patient, but also often gives a scowl-like appearance. This procedure often is performed before a blepharoplasty because it reduces the excess skin of the upper eyelid.

Technique
1. The surgeon makes the incisions.
2. The skin, muscle, and periosteum are elevated to the level of the orbital rims.
3. The brows are suspended.
4. The incisions are closed.

DESCRIPTION
Open Brow Lift
The patient is placed in the lounge-chair position with arms tucked at the sides. General or local anesthesia may be used, depending on the procedures to be performed. The surgeon pulls the hair back and ties it with rubber bands. This removes the hair from the field and produces surgical exposure. The patient is prepped with pHisoHex, with care taken to prevent the solution from pooling in the eyes. The patient is draped with a head drape and a split sheet.

The surgeon chooses from one of four incisions: **bicoronal**, **pretrichial** (at the hair line), mid brow (usually in men), and direct (at the level of the brow itself). Incisions are made with a #15 blade. A periosteal elevator is used to elevate the periosteum off the cranium to the level of the superior orbital rims. The periosteum is then incised at the level of the orbital rim with the elevator. This allows for mobility of the brows. The muscles at the bridge of the nose are incised with scissors, electrocautery, or the elevator. Excess skin of the inferior flaps is excised with the #15 blade. The inferior flap then is suspended to the superior periosteum with a nonabsorbable suture. The wound is then closed to layers. Absorbable sutures are used for the deep layers. Absorbable or

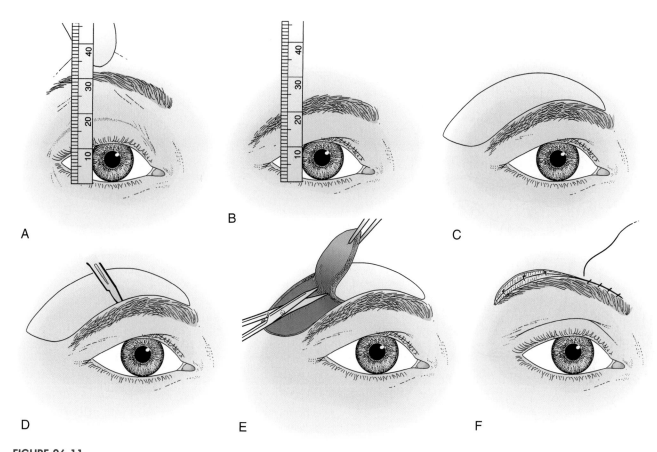

FIGURE 26-11
Open brow lift. **A,** The brow is elevated with some overcorrection to the desired position. **B,** The brow is relaxed, and a measurement is taken. **C,** The ellipse of tissue to be removed is marked. **D,** The skin incision is made and extended to the frontalis and orbicularis muscles. **E,** The skin and muscle are excised to the periosteum, with careful attention paid to avoid damage to the frontal nerve. **F,** The incision is closed. (Modified from Nerad JA: *Oculoplastic surgery: ophthalmology requisites series,* St Louis, 2001, Mosby.)

nonabsorbable sutures are used for the skin, or staples may be used in a bicoronal approach.

See Figure 26-11 for illustrations of an open brow lift.

Endoscopic Brow Lift
The patient is placed in the lounge-chair position with arms tucked at the sides. General or local anesthesia is used, depending on the extent of the planned procedures. The hair is tied back with rubber bands. The patient is prepped with pHisoHex and is draped with a head drape and a split sheet.

The surgeon makes three central scalp incisions behind the anterior headline, one in the midline and two just medial to the superior temporal line, with a #10 blade (Figure 26-12, *A*). Using the periosteal elevator included in the set, the surgeon extends the incisions to the level of the vertex. The surgeon also elevates the forehead flap with a curved periosteal elevator from the endoscopic brow set. The surgeon performs this step with the endoscope, usually a 30-degree, 4 mm or 5 mm scope that has been placed in a sheath and passed through the rim of one of the incisions (Figure 26-12, *B*). This elevation is continued to a point approximately 2 cm above the supraorbital rim.

The surgeon next uses a straight periosteal elevator to elevate the temporal fascia with the endoscope in place to assist with visualization. The surgeon then connects the two temporal dissections, using a straight periosteal elevator and the 30-degree endoscope. Using the 30-degree endoscope and an orbital periosteal elevator, the surgeon elevates the frontal fascia to the level of the supraorbital rim. When the periosteum has been freed and the brow is mobile, the surgeon elevates and fixes the lateral brow. (The medial brow usually is not fixed because if it is elevated too much, the brow will look unnatural). The surgeon performs the fixation by creating a bony bridge through which to pass the suture by drilling suture pass holes into the bone and then passing a long-lasting absorbable suture through the soft tissue and the holes to create the suspension. The surgeon can create the same effect by placing a screw behind the incision line, pulling the soft tissue up to the level of the screw, and stapling the tissue behind the screw (the screw is removed a week later). The incision lines then are closed with staples. A head dressing consisting of Kerlix fluffs and rolls is then applied.

Incisions

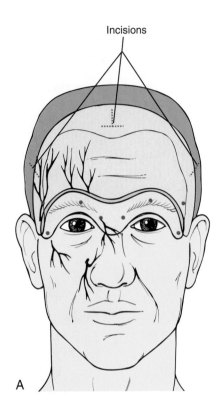

A

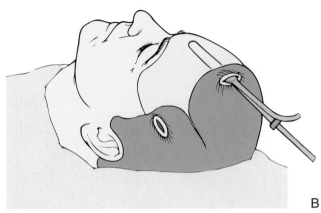

B

FIGURE 26-12
Endoscopic brow lift. **A,** Locations of scalp incisions. **B,** The endoscope is inserted into the brow. (From Fortunato N and McCullough SM: *Plastic and reconstructive surgery: perioperative nursing series,* St Louis, 1998, Mosby.)

Rhytidectomy (Face Lift)

SURGICAL GOAL

A rhytidectomy, or a face lift, is performed to rejuvenate the lower third of the aging face.

PATHOLOGY

A face lift is performed to rejuvenate an aging face. The aging process and gravity affect the skin and the structures that lie beneath it. This results in brow **ptosis,** hollow infraorbital regions, nasolabial folds, jowls, and submental skin excess. Fine wrinkles and irregular pigmentation also may be present.

Technique
1. The surgeon marks the skin with a surgical marker before the prepping.
2. The skin is injected with local anesthetic containing epinephrine.
3. The surgeon makes the incision.
4. The surgeon elevates the skin.
5. The superficial musculoaponeurotic system (SMAS) is imbricated; incised, and plicated; or incised, elevated, and then plicated.
6. The skin is closed.
7. Dressings are applied.

DISCUSSION

The patient is placed in the lounge-chair position on a doughnut headrest or Mayfield horseshoe headrest with arms tucked at the sides. General anesthesia is used. The surgeon marks the skin using a surgical marker before the prep

is performed. The patient is prepped with pHisoHex or Hibiclens solution. The patient is draped with a head drape and a split sheet.

The surgeon then injects the area of the face to be elevated from the cheek to the submentum and posteriorly over the mastoid and into the neck. This is done with local anesthetic with added epinephrine (usually 1% lidocaine with epinephrine 1:100,000) in a 10-ml syringe with a 22-gauge or 25-gauge spinal needle. The surgeon makes the incision with a #15 blade, following the marked incision line. Initially the skin flap is elevated with double-prong skin hooks and the #15 blade. The surgeon may staple a sponge to the posterior aspect of the incision to reduce the amount of blood that collects in the hair.

When the surgeon has reached the desired depth, the dissection continues with face lift scissors. Hemostasis is achieved with a bipolar cautery. The surgeon may use the face-lift retractor, which may be lighted, to aid in the exposure of the field during the dissection. At this point the surgeon may imbricate the underlying SMAS with a 2-0 or 3-0 absorbable suture. The surgeon may choose to excise a strip of SMAS in the preauricular and infraauricular regions using Metzenbaum scissors. This tissue should be saved on the back table in saline in case it is needed for further augmentation procedures.

If the surgeon is performing a deep-plane face lift, he or she elevates the SMAS off the parotid gland and into the neck using either the face-lift or Metzenbaum scissors. The assistant should observe the face for twitching. The two ends of the SMAS are then plicated with a 2-0 or 3-0 absorbable suture. The skin flaps are then redraped over the incision lines, and the excess skin is marked for incision. This skin is then excised with Metzenbaum scissors. The skin is then closed with 3-0, 4-0, and 5-0 absorbable sutures in the dermal layer. A drain may be placed in the postauricular portion of the incision. The skin is then closed with a combination of staples and 5-0 absorbable or nonabsorbable sutures. A head dressing is placed to support the incisions. This dressing may be gauze sponges with an Ace wrap or a fascioplasty splint.

Some steps of a face lift are illustrated in Figure 26-13.

Facial Augmentation (Lips, Chin, and Cheek)
SURGICAL GOAL
A facial augmentation is performed to produce adequate projection of the lips, chin, or cheek.

PATHOLOGY
Facial augmentation is performed to correct underprojection of either the chin (mandible) or cheek (malar). The surgeon achieves this projection by placing an implant in the region. Many different materials are used as implants. These include silicone, acrylic polymers, polyethylene, Gore-Tex, mesh, and autografts (fat, bone, or cartilage). There are also several subdermal and subcutaneous injectable filler materials, such as Dermalogen, Alloderm, Restylane, collagen, and liquid silicone. The type of implant used is based on physician preference and the type of defect to be filled.

Technique

1. The surgeon marks the incision site.
2. The surgical site is injected with local anesthetic.
3. The surgeon makes the incision.
4. The periosteum is elevated.
5. The implant is inserted.
6. The wound is closed.
7. The dressings are applied.

DESCRIPTION
Mentoplasty (Chin Augmentation)
The patient is placed on the operating table in the lounge-chair position with arms tucked at the sides. Before induction of anesthesia, the surgeon marks the anatomical landmarks by having the patient flex the neck. General anesthesia may be used. Local anesthetic is instilled into the region of the mental nerve, the incision line, and surrounding soft tissue. The skin is then prepped with Betadine scrub and paint or pHisoHex, including the entire face. The face is exposed during the procedure to allow the surgeon to assess the projection given by the implant.

The patient then is draped with a head drape and a split sheet. The incision, measuring 10 to 15 mm, is made vertically in the midline on the chin using a #15 blade. The incision extends through the subcutaneous fat and muscle to the layer of the periosteum. The skin flaps are retracted by the assistant, using double-prong skin hooks. The periosteum then is incised with a #15 blade.

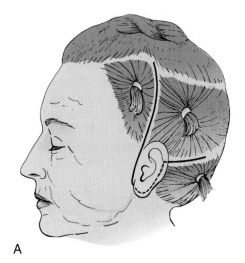

A

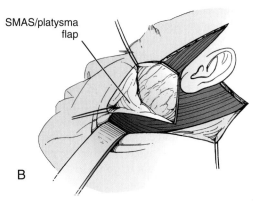

SMAS/platysma flap

B

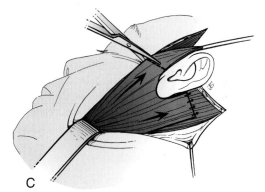

C

FIGURE 26-13
Face lift. **A,** Incision location from above the ear and in front of and behind the pinna. **B,** Dissection beneath and elevation of the platysma flap. **C,** The platysma muscle is sutured back to the mastoid. (From Phillips N: *Berry & Kohn's operating room technique*, ed 10, St Louis, 2004, Mosby.)

With the incision made, the surgeon elevates the periosteum off the bone using a periosteal elevator such as a Joseph elevator. The surgeon elevates the periosteum superiorly to the midportion of the mandible. The inferior portion of the periosteum is elevated with a periosteal elevator and Senn retractors to allow visualization. The surgeon should take care to avoid damaging the mental nerve because the mental nerve foramen is in this region. Hemostasis is achieved with the bipolar cautery.

The surgeon then inserts the implant by retracting the periosteum with a Senn retractor, placing one end of the implant into the subperiosteal pocket slightly more than half way, and then bending the implant so that the other end of the implant may be inserted into the superior portion of the periosteal envelope. When the implant is under the periosteum, the surgeon moves it back and forth until it is centered into the midline. A long-lasting absorbable stitch may be placed in the distal end of the implant through the periosteum to prevent the implant from rising. The wound is then closed in two layers. The periosteum is closed with interrupted 3-0 absorbable sutures, and the skin is closed with 6-0 nonabsorbable suture or a 5-0 fast absorbing suture. The dressings are then applied.

Cheek Augmentation

As with chin augmentation, the patient is placed in the lounge-chair position, marked, injected with local anesthetic, and then prepped and draped. The intraoral incision is made with a #15 blade just inferior and slightly anterior to the parotid duct. It measures 3 cm and is carried through the mucosa and muscle to the periosteum. The periosteum then is cut with the #15 blade and elevated with a periosteal elevator such as a Joseph elevator. This elevation is continued superiorly and laterally over the malar and zygoma. The surgeon must keep in mind the location of the orbital rim and the infraorbital nerve to avoid injuring the nerve. The surgeon also must take care not to go under the periosteum or close to the zygomatic arch when elevating the periosteum to avoid injuring the seventh cranial nerve, the facial nerve.

The implant then is placed into position with an Army-Navy retractor to retract the periosteum and allow for placement of the implant. The implant is then positioned so that the prominence of the implant corresponds with the prominent area of the cheek, which was drawn before the beginning of the procedure. The Army-Navy retractor then is removed, and the wound is closed in layers with 3-0 absorbable sutures. No dressing is applied because the incision is intraoral.

Cheiloplasty (Lip Augmentation)
SURGICAL GOAL
Cheiloplasty is performed to improve the shape and fullness of the lips.

PATHOLOGY
Cheiloplasty, or lip augmentation, typically is performed for cosmetic reasons, to improve the fullness and the shape of the lip. It can aid in reducing the appearance of fine lines and rhytids, or wrinkles, in the perioral region. Several different products, temporary and permanent, can be used. These include liquid fillers such as Cymetra, collagen, fat, and sheets or strips of implant materials such as Alloderm and Gore-Tex.

Technique

1. The lips are numbed with 1% lidocaine with epinephrine 1:100,000. This can be done by direct infiltration or nerve block.

2. If the augmentation is to use fillers, the filler is injected with a 23-gauge needle. If sheets are to be used, small incisions are made at the corners of the mouth, and the product is threaded through the incisions.
3. The material is molded into place.
4. Any incisions are closed.

DISCUSSION
This procedure typically is performed in the office. The patient is placed in the sitting position in the exam chair with the head all the way back on the head rest. The surgeon numbs the lips with 1% lidocaine with epinephrine 1:100,000 and waits approximately 5 minutes to begin the augmentation. If fillers are to be used, they are mixed according to the manufacturer's directions (included in packaging) and then injected with a 23-gauge needle. The upper and lower lips usually are injected. When the injections are complete, the surgeon molds the material to give it a natural shape. The patient then lightly places an ice pack to the lips for swelling. No dressing is used, and the patient is instructed to apply only light pressure to the lips as the material may shift if heavy pressure is applied.

When strips of implant materials are to be used, the surgeon makes small incisions at each of the four corners of the lips (upper and lower), using a #15 or #11 blade. The lips then are tunneled with a curved tendon passer. When the passer has been tunneled to the other side, the sheet, which has been rolled tightly, is placed into the tendon passer and pulled through the lip. This is repeated for the other lip. The incisions then are closed with an absorbable 4-0 stitch. No dressing is applied, and the patient is given an ice pack to help control swelling.

Excision of Superficial Lesions
SURGICAL GOAL
In this procedure, a lesion is removed in its entirety to prevent recurrence.

PATHOLOGY
Lesions of the integumentary system may be classified as either benign or malignant. Malignant lesions usually result from sun damage to the skin and include basal cell carcinoma, squamous cell carcinoma, and malignant melanomas. Many benign pathologies may require excision for cosmetic purposes, to prevent recurrent infections, and for diagnostic purposes.

Technique

1. The lines of excision are planned and marked.
2. The site is injected.
3. The surgeon makes the incision.
4. The surgeon excises the lesion.
5. The wound is closed.
6. Dressings are applied.

DISCUSSION

The patient is positioned to allow the surgeon access to the surgical site. This may include prone positioning for lesions on the back and buttocks, lateral positioning for lesions of the hip and shoulder, and supine positioning for most other lesions. Local anesthetic is used if the surgical wound can be closed by primary intention. If the procedure is to be more extensive, general anesthesia may be warranted.

The surgeon may choose to mark the incision and possible flaps before the prepping. The planning considers the possibility of total excision of the lesion with adequate margins, and the resultant defect and how it will be closed. The patient is prepped with Betadine scrub and paint, and the surgical site is draped to allow access to the lesion. The surgeon makes the incision, using a #15 blade or electrocautery, through the epidermis and dermis to the subcutaneous layer. The surgeon dissects out any subcutaneous extension of the lesion using tenotomy scissors, hemostat clamps, or the scalpel. The assistant may use double-prong or single-prong skin hooks to aid in the retraction of the skin flaps. Electrocautery is used to produce hemostasis.

When the lesion has been removed in its entirety and delivered from the wound, it may be marked for pathology with a silk stitch to denote margins. The lesion then is sent to pathology for review. The wound then is irrigated and closed. For primary closure and local flaps, any skin incisions are made with a #15 blade, and the epidermis and dermis are undermined around the wound with the #15 blade or Metzenbaum scissors. The wound then is closed with subcutaneous and dermal absorbable sutures. The skin then is closed with fine absorbable or nonabsorbable sutures at the surgeon's discretion. Dressings are applied if the surgeon deems them necessary; however, some wounds simply are covered with antibiotic ointment.

Scar Revision
SURGICAL GOAL
Scar revision is performed to improve the appearance of a scar.

PATHOLOGY
Scar revision is performed on scars that have not healed properly after injury. This includes keloids and hyperpigmented scars.

Technique

1. The scar revision plan is marked.
2. The surgeon excises the original scar.
3. Surrounding tissue is undermined.
4. The edges of the skin are brought together and closed.

DISCUSSION

The patient is brought to the operating room and positioned in a manner that will allow exposure of the affected area. The patient is then prepped, including the area of the original scar and the surrounding tissue to be included in the revi-

sion. The patient is then draped to allow exposure of the affected area and the areas of proposed revision.

The surgeon begins by marking the planned revision. Next, he or she excises the scar using a #15 blade and Adson toothed forceps. The surgeon then undermines the surrounding tissue using Metzenbaum scissors. The wound edges are then approximated, ensuring that the wound is covered, and the wound is closed. The incision then is closed with 3-0 or 4-0 absorbable suture. The skin then is closed with 4-0 or 5-0 sutures that may be absorbable or nonabsorbable, depending on the surgeon's preference.

Pedicle Grafts: Advancement, Rotation, and Transposition
SURGICAL GOAL
Pedicle grafts provide coverage of a soft-tissue defect.

PATHOLOGY
Pedicle grafts (also called flap grafts) are those that are raised from the donor site but not immediately severed free. This type of graft is used when the recipient site requires tissue other than just skin (e.g., subcutaneous fat). Pedicle grafts are classified as either near or distant. A near graft is created in adjacent tissue (e.g., from the palm for use on the finger). Distant grafts are created from the trunk or other areas for use on a limb.

Flap grafts are used to provide coverage of soft-tissue defects. The soft-tissue defects may be the result of surgical resection or trauma. Various types of flap grafts may be used to cover a defect. Advancement flaps are flaps that are raised from the tissues in the immediate area of the defect. They are especially effective in the coverage of circular defects resulting from Mohs' surgery. Rotation flaps are semicircular skin flaps that are rotated into the soft-tissue defect on a pivot. Rotation flaps are a type of pedicle flap.

Pedicle flaps are flaps that have large vessels directly supplying the skin paddle. They include rotation, transposition, **bilobate,** rhomboid, and tubed bipedicle flaps. Composite flaps are flaps that are a mixture of tissues. The mixture could include skin, muscle, cartilage, and bone in any combination. Composite flaps usually are free flaps.

Technique

1. The defect is measured.
2. The proposed incision lines of the flap are measured and marked.
3. The surgeon makes the incision.
4. The surgeon elevates the flap.
5. The flap is positioned over the defect.
6. The flap is sutured into place.
7. The donor site is closed.

DISCUSSION
Advancement Flap

The patient is placed in a position that allows access to both the defect and the donor site. Depending on the size of the

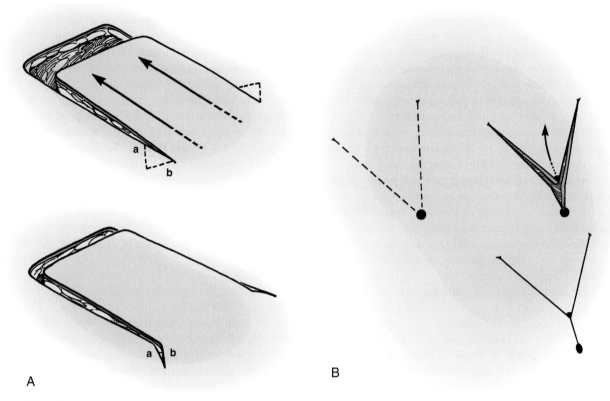

FIGURE 26-14
A, The single-pedicle advancement flap. **B,** A V-to-Y advancement flap. (Modified from Marks MW and Marks C: *Fundamentals of plastic surgery*, Philadelphia, 1997, Saunders.)

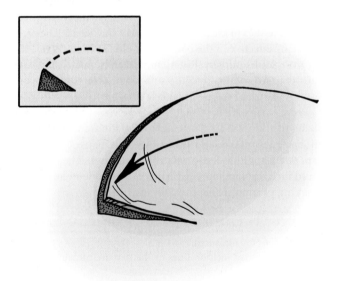

FIGURE 26-15
A rotation flap. (Modified from Marks MW and Marks C: *Fundamentals of plastic surgery*, Philadelphia, 1997, Saunders.)

defect, general or local anesthesia may be used. The surgeon begins by measuring the size of the defect and then measures the proposed flap, to ensure that the flap will create proper coverage. The proposed flap then is marked with a surgical marker (Figure 26-14). Both surgical sites are then prepped with Betadine scrub and paint. The patient then is draped.

The surgeon cleans any rough uneven edges of the defect using a #15 blade and an Adson toothed forceps.

Next, the surgeon makes the incisions of the donor site. The surgeon follows the marks with a #15 blade. The flap is elevated with either the #15 blade or tenotomy scissors, and retraction is applied with double-prong skin hooks. When the flap has been freed, it is advanced into position. The surgeon does this by simply approximating the two edges of the skin flap to cover the defect. The defect is then closed in layers with 3-0 or 4-0 absorbable sutures at the deep layers and 5-0 or 6-0 nonabsorbable sutures on the skin.

Rotation Flap
Rotation flaps follow the same procedure as advancement flaps, except that the flap is rotated into position from a pivot point (Figure 26-15).

Transposition Flap
Transposition flaps are very similar to rotation flaps except the flap rotates over normal tissue to the defect (Figure 26-16).

Debridement for Burns
SURGICAL GOAL
Debridement is performed to excise burned and damaged tissue.

PATHOLOGY
Burns are caused by the transfer of heat from an external source to the body. This heat transfer may be caused by flame, scalding (liquid), electric current, radiation, or chem-

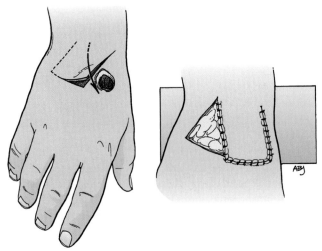

FIGURE 26-16
A transposition flap. (Modified from Marks MW and Marks C: *Fundamentals of plastic surgery*, Philadelphia, 1997, Saunders.)

icals. Burns are classified by the depth of the tissue affected. **First-degree burns** involve only the outer layer of the epidermis, as in sunburn. These burns are characterized by reddened skin and pain; they usually heal primarily in a few days.

Second-degree burns involve the entire epidermis and part of the dermis. This type of burn is defined by pain, blister formation, and reddish-pink, mottled skin. These burns usually heal in a few weeks. First-degree and second-degree burns are called partial-thickness burns.

Third-degree burns cause the destruction of the entire thickness of the skin. These burns are characterized by dry, white skin; generally there is little pain associated with these burns. In a few days an **eschar**—a thick, black, leathery crust—forms. These burns do not lend themselves to spontaneous regeneration of the epithelium, and **debridement** generally is performed. Third-degree burns are called full-thickness burns. Debridement also may be performed on second-degree and third-degree burns. The damaged tissue is removed to a layer of healthy, viable tissue. This is generally performed in stages. When the tissue bed is viable, grafts may be applied to create skin coverage.

Technique
1. Nonviable tissue is debrided down to a viable layer.
2. Hemostasis is achieved.
3. The debrided regions may be covered with allograft or autograft skin.
4. Dressings are applied.

DISCUSSION
The patient is positioned to allow for adequate exposure of the burns. The position may be supine, prone, or lateral. General anesthesia is used for these patients. Often the patient has already been intubated before coming to the oper-

ating room, as the airway of a burn patient must be secure. The patient is prepped with Betadine paint; usually this solution is sprayed on, rather than painted on. The wounds are considered contaminated and usually become infected within a few days. The patient is draped with towels and three-quarter sheets. Sterile tourniquets may be applied to the extremities.

The surgeon begins the procedure by removing all of the nonviable skin. This is done with a Braithwaite blade or a USF debrider, which is a hemostat forceps with wings. The tissue is taken down to a viable layer. To control bleeding as the debridement proceeds, lap sponges that have been soaked in a solution of sterile saline and topical epinephrine 1:1000 are applied. The concentration used most often is 1000 ml of normal saline, with 4 ml of topical epinephrine 1:1000 added. The scrub must check with the surgeon to ensure that the proper concentration is being used.

When hemostasis has been achieved, an allograft may be applied. This is cadaver skin that has been banked. The allograft is stapled over the debrided burns to create a layer of protection until autografting can be performed (usually several days after the initial debridement). Nonadherent dressings, such as Xeroform, and fluffs are applied. The extremities then are wrapped with Ace bandages.

Skin Grafts
SURGICAL GOAL
Skin grafting is performed to create epithelial coverage.

PATHOLOGY
Skin grafting is performed to create coverage of **deepithelialized** areas. These areas can become deepithelialized through thermal injury, from trauma that causes a soft-tissue defect, or through a surgical defect. Skin grafts may be either split thickness or full thickness. **Split-thickness skin grafts** (STSG) consist of the epidermis and a portion of the papillary dermis. **Full-thickness skin grafts** (FTSG) consist of the entire epidermis and dermis.

Technique
1. The donor site is pulled taut.
2. The donor site is covered with mineral oil or a similar solution.
3. The surgeon takes the graft using a dermatome.
4. The graft is placed in moist gauze sponges to keep it moist.
5. The donor site is dressed.

DISCUSSION
The patient is positioned to allow for exposure of the donor site. The position may be supine for the lower extremities and trunk or prone for the buttock and back. General anesthesia is used because the procedure is performed in conjunction with some other type of procedure. The patient is prepped with either Betadine paint or alcohol to cleanse the donor site. If alcohol is used, it must be completely dry before draping is performed. The donor site is then draped

with towels and three-quarter sheets or split sheets, depending on the surgical sites.

The surgeon then takes the skin graft with either a free-hand skin-graft knife or an automatic dermatome (Figure 26-17). The choice of instrument depends on the size of the graft needed. If only a small area is to be covered, a free-hand knife likely will be used; if the area to be covered is large, a dermatome will be used. To assist the surgeon in taking the graft, the assistant pulls the donor skin taut using either 4 × 4 gauze sponges or tongue blades, and the skin is moistened with mineral oil or a solution such as Shur-Clens. This is done to reduce the resistance of the skin to the blade and to allow the blade to glide over the skin.

The surgeon then uses the blade to take the graft. If the surgeon plans to use a dermatome, the scrub always should hand it to the surgeon with the depth gauge set at 0, and allow the surgeon to select the depth setting for the blade, usually .012 to .015. This prevents the inadvertent taking of a deeper graft than was intended. The dermatome should be held at a 45-degree angle to the skin when one is taking the graft. This also prevents the graft from being too deep. When the appropriate length of graft has been taken, the dermatome is brought parallel with the skin, and the graft is truncated from the body. If this cannot be done, the graft is removed from the dermatome, and iris scissors are used to free it. The donor site then is covered with a lap sponge soaked in saline. The saline may have epinephrine 1:1000 topical solution added to assist in hemostasis. The graft is placed on the back table and covered with moist gauze.

When the surgeon is ready to place the graft, he or she spreads the graft over the defect and trims any excess using curved iris scissors. The graft then is attached to the skin surrounding the defect with either staples or absorbable suture. The surgeon chooses the method based on the location of the graft. If the graft is placed on a visible area of the body, such as the hands or face, it is sutured into place; if it is to be

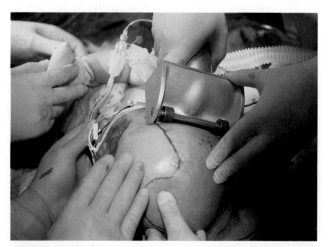

FIGURE 26-17
A dermatome taking a skin graft. (From Barret JP and Herndon DN: *Color atlas of burn care,* Philadelphia, 2001, Saunders.)

placed on a nonvisible area, such as the abdomen or back, it is stapled. The donor site is dressed with an Opsite dressing or a nonadherent dressing covered with Kerlix gauze roll. No dressing is applied to the recipient site.

Liposuction
SURGICAL GOAL
Liposuction is performed to remove excess deep fat.

PATHOLOGY
Liposuction is the removal of excess fat through suction cannulas to improve the appearance of any area of the body. Liposuction is particularly successful in patients who have taut skin; additional procedures may be needed to achieve the desired results in those who have lax skin. Liposuction was first performed in the 1970s and has since become the most common aesthetic surgery in the United States.

Technique

1. The surgeon marks the patient preoperatively with a surgical marker.
2. The areas that will be liposuctioned are injected with local anesthetic mixed with lactated Ringer's solution.
3. The surgeon makes the incisions.
4. The fat is aspirated.
5. The incisions are closed.
6. Dressings are applied if needed.

DISCUSSION
The patient is placed in the supine position with arms out at 90-degree angles to the body. Depending on the extent of the procedure, general anesthesia or IV sedation is used. The patient is prepped with Betadine paint. The patient is then draped with towels and three-quarter sheets to allow exposure of all the sites to be treated. If multiple sites are to be treated, the patient may have to be repositioned, reprepped, and redraped during the procedure.

The surgeon begins by injecting anesthetic into the soft tissue. The surgeon injects large volumes of lidocaine and epinephrine that has been diluted in lactated Ringer's solution. The solution is injected into the targeted tissue until the tissue is **turgid** . This injection into the tissue gives the surgeon several advantages: it provides local anesthesia and hemostasis, and it expands the target area, making the passing of liposuction cannulas easier. Hemostatic effects appear within 10 minutes of injection, but one should allow 20 minutes for maximum effectiveness.

When the surgeon believes that adequate hemostasis has been achieved, he or she makes the incisions using a #15 blade. Multiple incisions are made into each target area. This is done to allow the surgeon easier access to the target area and to prevent depressions around the access sites. The surgeon then begins aspirating the targeted area. The surgeon does this by connecting a liposuction cannula to large-bore suction tubing that has been connected to high-vacuum suction. High-vacuum suction is used because the adipose tissue is thick and cannot be pulled from the body with regular suction. For deeper areas, the surgeon chooses cannulas that are 4 mm to 5 mm in diameter, and for shallower, superficial areas the surgeon chooses cannulas that are 2 mm to 3 mm.

The surgeon continues to aspirate until the desired volume of fat has been removed or the desired shape of the target area has been achieved (Figure 26-18). When the surgeon has finished aspirating, the cannula is removed and the incisions are closed with 3-0 absorbable suture. If the extremities have been treated, a compression stocking then is applied to provide support and reduce swelling postoperatively.

Panniculectomy (Abdominoplasty)
SURGICAL GOAL
Panniculectomy is performed to remove excess skin and adipose tissue from the abdominal wall and tighten the muscles of the abdominal wall.

PATHOLOGY
Abdominoplasty is usually performed as a cosmetic procedure, sometimes called a tummy tuck, but also can be performed for medical reasons. After significant weight loss, the skin of the abdomen hangs flaccid and can interfere with movement by forming an "apron" that in some cases can hang to the level of the knees. This "apron" makes movement and activities of daily living very difficult.

Technique
1. With the patient in the standing position, the surgeon marks the incision line in the natural skin fold of the lower abdomen.
2. The patient is placed in a semi-flexed position before the surgeon makes the incision.
3. The surgeon makes a low transverse incision in the lower abdomen, across both inguinal areas laterally.
4. The skin or subcutaneous tissue flap is elevated away from the anterior abdominal wall.

5. The umbilicus is left in position.
6. Plication of the rectus abdominis may be performed from the level of the xyphoid process to the mons pubis if there is diastasis.
7. The skin and subcutaneous tissue flaps are pulled inferiorly, and the excess tissue is excised.
8. The surgeon makes a small midline incision through which the umbilicus may be delivered.
9. The umbilicus is then sutured in place.
10. If drains are to be used, they are placed.
11. The abdominal incision is closed in two layers.
12. Postoperatively the patient is placed in high Fowler's position to reduce tension on the abdomen.

DISCUSSION
The surgeon marks the preoperative area while the patient is in a standing position. This allows the surgeon to adequately assess the pannus or "apron" created by the excess tissue.

In the operating room, the patient is placed under general anesthesia. The patient is then prepped from nipples to groin to ensure that the entire affected area is included. An additional person may be needed to hold the "apron" to allow a proper prep. The patient is then draped for an abdominal procedure. The patient is positioned in a semi-Fowler's position to reduce tension of the abdomen.

There are two acceptable incisions for an abdominoplasty. The first incision extends laterally to the inguinal areas bilaterally. This is a U-shaped incision from inguinal areas with a dip in the lateral incision at the mons pubis. This type of incision is for the patient who desires to wear a French cut bikini. The second acceptable incision is along the natural abdominal skin creases below the iliac crest, with a dip in the incision at the mons pubis. This incision is performed for those desiring to wear a bikini. The depth of the incision is extended to the fascia. The surgeon then elevates the large skin flap using the electrocautery unit or Metzenbaum scissors. The umbilicus is excised and left in its natural position with a #15 blade. The skin flap is fur-

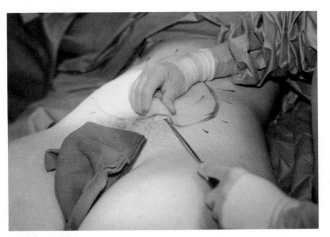
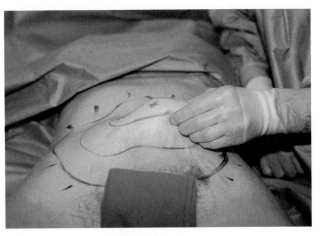

FIGURE 26-18
Touch-up at the conclusion of a liposuction procedure. (From Fortunato N and McCullough SM: *Plastic and reconstructive surgery: perioperative nursing series*, St Louis, 1998, Mosby; courtesy of Brian W. Davies.)

ther elevated to the level of the xyphoid process and the inferior sternal borders.

If the abdominal wall is loose or spreading, it may be plicated from the xyphoid process to the mons pubis. The surgeon does this using a 2-0 nonabsorbable suture such as Prolene. The skin flap then is pulled inferiorly, and the excess skin is excised with electrocautery. A small midline incision is made in the skin flap with a #15 blade to allow for delivery of the umbilicus into its natural position. The umbilicus then is sutured into place with 3-0 absorbable suture.

If the surgeon chooses to use drains, they are placed at this time. Hemostasis is achieved with the electrocautery. The abdominal wound is then closed in two layers with absorbable suture. Dressings then are applied. Postoperatively, the patient is to maintain a high Fowler's position for 24 hours; this includes the transfer from the operating-room table to the patient's hospital bed. This prevents any undue stress on the abdomen.

Mastopexy
SURGICAL GOAL
Mastopexy is performed to lift the breast and remove excess skin.

PATHOLOGY
Mastopexy is performed to correct breast ptosis. This procedure can play a significant role in improving the patient's body image.

Technique
1. The surgeon marks the incision site to include the nipple, using an anchor-shaped incision extending inferiorly from the inferior midline edge of the nipple.
2. Excess skin is deepithelialized, and the nipple is brought superiorly.
3. The incisions are closed.

DISCUSSION
The surgeon usually marks the incision lines in the holding area before the patient comes into the operating room. This step is performed at this time so that the patient can stand with the arms at the sides to allow the breasts to fall into their natural position.

In the operating room, the patient is placed in the supine position and prepped from chin to navel. The patient is then draped for a breast incision, ensuring that the sternal notch and the xyphoid process are included in the field. The field also must be draped as wide as possible. The surgeon begins by making an anchor-shaped incision that begins at or above the level of the nipple, with the curve of the anchor in the inframammary fold. The surgeon does this with a #15 blade or an ESU.

The surgeon deepithelializes and excises the excess skin using Metzenbaum scissors. The nipple is then brought superiorly, and the incisions are closed. The periareolar incisions are closed with 3-0 and 4-0 absorbable suture, as are

the vertical and inframammary-fold incisions. The skin may be closed with a 3-0 or 4-0 polydioxanone (PDS) or Monocryl suture. Dressings then are applied, usually Steri-Strips, Raytec sponges, and an Ace wrap or mammary support.

Augmentation Mammoplasty
SURGICAL GOAL
Augmentation mammoplasty is performed to increase the size and improve the shape of the breast.

PATHOLOGY
Mammoplasty (breast augmentation) may be performed either for cosmetic reasons (the patient desires larger breasts) or to reconstruct the breast after a mastectomy. When used after mastectomy, this procedure can give the patient's self-esteem and body image a boost. Postmastectomy augmentation may be immediate or delayed.

The implants used for augmentation may be saline filled, silicone filled, or a combination of the two that uses a silicone outer layer and a saline balloon in the center. The choice of implant depends on the doctor's preference and the desires of the patient. In addition, the implants may be round or anatomical (tear drop) in shape. Round implants are used when the augmentation is elective, and anatomical implants are used after mastectomy.

Technique
Postmastectomy
1. The mastectomy scar is excised.
2. The surgeon creates a pocket under the pectoralis major muscle.
3. A tissue expander is implanted in the pocket with the saline port in the subcutaneous tissue of the midaxillary line (allowing easy access for expansion over the following weeks).
4. The saline reservoir is filled; the initial amount is 150 to 300 ml of saline solution.
5. The wound is closed.

Cosmetic
1. The incision is made (axillary or hemiareolar, or in the inframammary fold).
2. The surgeon creates a pocket under the pectoralis major muscle.
3. A temporary sizer is placed and filled with the appropriate amount of saline.
4. The sizer is removed, and the permanent implant is placed.
5. The wound is closed.

DISCUSSION
Postmastectomy Augmentation
The patient is placed in the supine position, prepped, and draped for a breast procedure. One must ensure that the sternal notch and the xyphoid process are included in the field. This allows the surgeon to have midline anatomical marks that have not been altered by previous surgeries.

The surgeon makes the incision by excising the mastectomy scar. The surgeon grips it with either Allis clamps or Adson toothed forceps and excises it using a #15 blade. The scar generally is sent for pathological evaluation to ensure that no abnormal cells are presents. Hemostasis is achieved with the ESU.

The surgeon then creates a pocket in the submusculofascia of the pectoralis major. The surgeon performs this step bluntly by using either the finger or a hemostat. The tissue expander then is inserted into the pocket that has been created. The saline reservoir then is filled with 150 to 300 ml of saline. The injection port is placed in the subcutaneous tissue at the midaxillary line of the affected side. The incision then is closed with 3-0 and 4-0 absorbable suture, such as Vicryl. The skin usually is closed with a running subcuticular closure.

The surgeon uses the saline-filled tissue expander to produce gradual stretching of the skin and underlying tissue by gradually filling the saline reservoir and allowing the tissue to stretch. When the tissue has stretched sufficiently, the tissue expander is removed and replaced with a permanent implant. This procedure follows the same steps as the procedure for placing the tissue expander.

Cosmetic Augmentation

The patient is placed in the supine position, prepped, and draped for a breast procedure. One must ensure that the sternal notch and the xyphoid process are included in the field. This allows the surgeon to have midline anatomical marks to ensure that the breasts are in the midline. The surgeon makes the incision either in the axillary region, around the lower half of the areola and nipple, or in the inframammary fold. This is performed with a #15 blade. Hemostasis is achieved with the ESU. The surgeon then creates a pocket under the pectoralis major. The surgeon does this bluntly by using either the finger or a hemostat.

The tissue expander then is inserted into the pocket that has been created. The temporary tissue expander then is placed with the "tail" through the incision. The expander then is filled with saline in 60 ml increments. The scrub must record the amount of fluid placed in the expander, because this amount of saline will be used in the saline implant.

The surgeon may sit the patient up in full Fowler's position to assess the symmetry and position of the breast. If this is done, the arms must be properly supported, and the anesthesia provider must support the patient's head. The surgeon then inserts the permanent implant and fills it with the same amount of saline as the temporary sizer. The circulator and scrub should verify the size of the implant before opening. The incision then is closed with 3-0 and 4-0 absorbable suture. The skin is closed with a running subcuticular stitch.

The procedure is repeated for the other breast. At the conclusion of the procedure, the scrub must communicate to the circulator the amount of saline instilled into each breast.

Reduction Mammoplasty
SURGICAL GOAL
The size of the breast is reduced.

PATHOLOGY

Reduction mammaplasty is performed to remove excess breast fat and skin to reduce the size of the breast. This procedure may be performed for cosmetic or medical reasons. The condition macromastia (enlarged breasts) is a result of an excess of fatty tissue and breast parenchyma. The "normal" breast size varies among cultures and fashion trends, making macromastia difficult to define.

Symptoms of macromastia are related to the weight and size of the breast. The increased forward weight can cause cervical and thoracic pain. These patients also may suffer socially and psychologically. Clothes may not fit properly; participating in sports may be difficult or impossible. These factors can cause patients to suffer from a negative body image. Although women have macromastia more often than men, it is not uncommon for men to develop this disorder.

Technique

1. The surgeon marks the incision lines with a surgical marker. This may be done in the preoperative holding area or in the operating room.
2. The surgeon makes an incision around the areola and a second incision in the shape of a triangle with a wide base at the inframammary line.
3. The triangle is deepithelialized.
4. The surgeon removes breast tissue by sharp dissection through the inframammary incision.
5. The inframammary incision and triangular incision are closed.
6. The surgeon makes a circular incision at the apex of the breast, brings the nipple up, and sutures it into place.
7. The wound is closed and dressed with a bulky dressing or pressure dressing.

DISCUSSION

Many different techniques are used to perform reduction mammoplasty. The surgeon may infiltrate the incision areas with lidocaine with epinephrine to produce additional hemostasis. The concentrations of lidocaine and epinephrine vary based on surgeon preference. Before the start of surgery, the surgeon marks the incisions on the patient's breasts. This step may require calculations, templates, or measuring devices. When prepping, one must take care not to remove the marks. The patient is positioned in the supine or semi-Fowler's position, prepped, and draped for a breast procedure. The field must include the sternal notch and the xyphoid process and extend laterally as far as possible.

The surgeon begins by making a circular incision around the areola with the breast held in extension. Next, the surgeon makes the triangle incision and deepithelializes the skin. This step is performed with a #15 blade, Adson toothed forceps, or Metzenbaum scissors. The breast then is manually retracted superiorly, and the glandular and fatty tissue is excised through the incision in the inframammary fold (the base of the triangle). This step is performed with sharp dissection. Any tissue that is removed is passed off the field to be weighed. This is done to ensure that approximately the same amount of tissue is removed from each breast.

The surgeon then approximates the breast tissue at the midline by bringing the sides of the triangle together and suturing them with absorbable 3-0 suture on a curved needle. Any excess skin at the inframammary incision is trimmed with Metzenbaum scissors or a #15 blade. The surgeon then closes the incision using a 3-0 absorbable suture. Both skin incisions then are closed with a 4-0 subcuticular stitch.

The surgeon then creates a circular incision at the apex of the triangular incision by using a nipple marker (sometimes called a cookie cutter) to mark the incision site and then excising the tissue using a #15 blade. This creates a new position for the areola and nipple, which are pulled through the incision line and sutured into place with a nonabsorbable subcuticular suture. Dressings of the surgeon's preference then are applied.

Transverse Rectus Abdominis Myocutaneous Flap
SURGICAL GOAL
A transverse rectus abdominis myocutaneous (TRAM) flap is performed to reconstruct the breast without the use of implants.

PATHOLOGY
The TRAM flap can be used in a variety of plastic and reconstructive procedures; it is used most often in breast reconstruction after mastectomy. In this procedure, a tissue flap containing skin and subcutaneous tissue, including muscle, is taken from the lower abdomen and transferred to the mastectomy site. The flap continues to receive its blood supply from its pedicle (the portion of the flap that remains attached to its point of origin). This allows the reconstruction of the breast without the use of implants.

Technique

1. The mastectomy scar is excised.
2. The surgeon makes an elliptical incision in the transverse plane in the lower abdomen, at the level of the umbilicus, to include the umbilicus and the area above the symphysis pubis.
3. The surgeon extends the incision along the border with attention to avoiding the large vessels of the rectus muscle.
4. The skin superior to the incision site is undermined at the level of the fascia.
5. The surgeon incises the rectus sheath.
6. The inferior epigastric artery and vein are ligated.
7. The flap is dissected up the costal margin, leaving the central edge of the rectus sheath attached to the rectus muscle.
8. The flap is delivered through the subcutaneous tunnel that has been created.
9. The TRAM flap is inserted into the area created by the elevated skin flaps of the mastectomy site.
10. The surgeon trims the flap to fit the defect, and a new breast is reconstructed.
11. Excess portions of the flap may be defatted and used to create a breast mound.
12. The flap is sutured into place.
13. The abdominal wound is closed, and a new umbilicus is created.

DISCUSSION
The patient is placed in the supine position and prepped from the neck to the pubis. Draping is done so as to allow exposure of the abdomen and the breasts.

The surgeon first excises the mastectomy scar by grasping it with Adson toothed forceps or Allis clamps and excises it using the scalpel, usually with a #15 blade. The surgeon makes the abdominal incision by making a linear curved incision from one iliac crest to the other, with the upper margin including the umbilicus and the lower margin above the symphysis pubis. The surgeon then creates a subcutaneous tunnel that connects the mastectomy site with the abdominal incision, usually along the costal margin. This surgeon performs this step bluntly using hemostats and occasionally Metzenbaum scissors. The surgeon next elevates the flap. The upper border of the elliptical incision is carried into the abdominal wall. A small amount of subcutaneous tissue is left intact over the rectus sheath to preserve vascular supply to the area.

The lower incision is carried to the level of the anterior fascia. Lateral elevation then is performed bilaterally so that the lateral margins or "tails" are freed. The rectus sheath and muscle then are incised. The inferior epigastric artery, which is found on the posterior surface of the rectus muscle, is ligated with a 2-0 silk tie. The surgeon uses sharp dissection to mobilize the rectus muscle, including the sheath, to the level of the costal margin.

The surgeon then delivers the flap through the subcutaneous tunnel. The surgeon usually does this with the hands by passing the flap superiorly in the direction of the mastectomy site. When the flap is in place over the mastectomy incision site, it is trimmed. Excess skin from the flap is excised with scissors or a knife, and the flap edges are brought into position with the skin flaps of the mastectomy incision. The surgeon then molds and shapes the breast, trimming excess skin and subcutaneous tissue as needed, using Metzenbaum scissors or the scalpel. The scrub must save all trimmed portions of the flap because the subcutaneous tissue can be used to fill in the axillary region and to add more tissue to the breast mound itself.

A suction drain is placed before closure of the wound. The drain is placed in the wound with the distal end brought out laterally through a stab wound. Absorbable synthetic sutures, such as Vicryl, are used to secure the flap to the chest wall. Next, the skin flaps are closed with a 4-0 nonabsorbable suture, such as Monocryl. Nipple reconstruction may be performed at a later date, if the patient desires. Additional surgeries also may be needed to contour the breast mound. The surgeon then closes the abdomen primarily by suturing the anterior rectus sheath with a 2-0 absorbable synthetic suture. The skin then is closed with staples or an absorbable subcuticular suture. A mesh may be used to reinforce the closure.

Nipple Reconstruction

After mastectomy with TRAM flap reconstruction, some women may wish to have the nipple and areola reconstructed to create a more natural appearance to the breast. To do this, a full-thickness skin graft is taken from the medial thigh crease or postauricular region and is used to create an areola. The nipple is created with a full-thickness skin graft taken from the labia.

The nipples also may be tattooed either in conjunction with a reconstruction or alone. This tattooing may be performed in the operating room, outside the hospital in the office, or even at a tattoo parlor. The nipple is tinted a deeper color than the areola to create a contrast between the two.

Repair of Cleft Lip
SURGICAL GOAL
In this procedure, a cleft defect in the lip is closed.

PATHOLOGY
The **philtrum** of the upper lip is formed during embryologic development by the joining of the median nasal processes. The lateral portions of the upper lip are formed by the maxillary processes. These formations occur during the first 8 weeks of development. Interruption of the normal development of the lip may result in a cleft lip. The cleft may be complete or incomplete, and unilateral or bilateral. The cleft also may include the alveolus. Bilateral cleft lip is often associated with clefts of the soft palate. The infant with a cleft lip is referred to a surgeon immediately after birth. The cleft is repaired in stages, and the initial repair is performed at 10 to 12 weeks of age.

Technique
1. The incision and anatomical landmarks are marked.
2. The surgeon makes incisions along the marked incision lines.
3. The surgeon performs the dissection.
4. The defect is closed.
5. The splints or dressings are applied.

DISCUSSION
The patient is placed in the supine position with the head on a doughnut headrest and the arms at the sides. General anesthesia is used. Before the prep, the surgeon marks the anatomical landmarks and the planned incisions using a surgical marker. If local anesthetic is to be used, it is injected at this time. The amount of the injection is minimal because the surgeon does not want to cause the lips and surrounding soft tissue to be deformed by the infiltration. The patient is prepped with Betadine solution and then draped for a head and neck procedure.

The incision is made with a #11 blade along the vermilion border toward the cleft-side midline. Retraction is performed with double-prong or single-prong skin hooks, and the mucosa is separated off the orbicularis oris muscle with either the #11 knife or tenotomy scissors. The surgeon then detaches the medial lip from the maxilla by making an incision from the cleft to at least the midline at the top of the labial sulcus; this releases the medial lip. The Z-plasty incision then is made through the skin, muscle, and mucosa with a #11 or #15 blade. Hemostasis is achieved with an electrocautery. The procedure is repeated on the lateral portion of the cleft. When the dissection has been completed and the Z-plasty flaps have been created, the wound is ready to be closed. The mucosa is closed with interrupted absorbable sutures. The muscle then is closed with subcuticular absorbable sutures in the tips of the Z-plasty flaps. The vermilion border also is closed with a subcuticular suture. The skin then is closed with a fast-absorbing suture.

Two methods of cleft lip repair are illustrated in Figure 26-19.

Repair of Cleft Palate
SURGICAL GOAL
In this procedure, the palate is closed and the development of normal speech is restored.

PATHOLOGY
In the development of the midface, the palate arises from the joining of the medial nasal prominences on each side of the oral cavity to the maxillary prominence. Failure of these prominences to meet results in a cleft palate. The degree of clefting can be complete or incomplete, depending on the level of fusion that occurred during embryologic development. Although cleft palate sometimes is seen in conjunction with cleft lip, they are separate malformations and are rarely related to one another. Infants with this condition are referred to a surgeon shortly after birth if not before birth. However, the defects usually are not repaired until the infant is 11 to 12 months old. This delay in repair results in a low risk of interference with facial growth. Before the surgical repair of the palate, the infant may require myringotomy with tube placement, because these infants often have problems with ear infections and sometimes hearing. The infant also may be fitted with a palatal prosthesis to allow for easier feeding until the time of repair.

Technique
1. The incision is injected with local anesthetic.
2. The surgeon makes incisions in the palate and the muscle.
3. The flaps are prepared.
4. The palatal incisions are closed.
5. The flaps are closed.
6. The dressings are applied.

DISCUSSION
The patient is placed in the supine position with the head on a doughnut headrest and with a shoulder roll to allow for

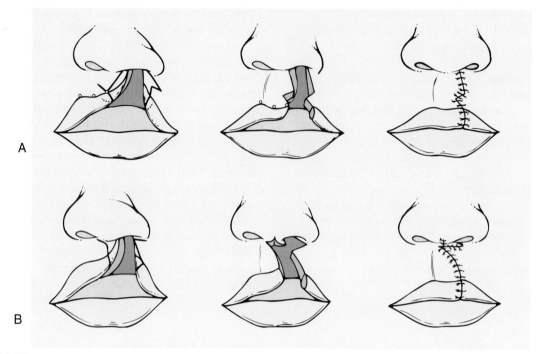

FIGURE 26-19
Cleft lip repair. **A,** Randall-Tennison triangular flap method. **B,** Millard rotation-advancement method. (From Fortunato N and McCullough SM: *Plastic and reconstructive surgery: perioperative nursing series,* St Louis, 1998, Mosby.)

hyperextension of the head, which gives the surgeon better visualization of the palate. General anesthesia is used. The surgeon may insert the cleft-palate mouth gag, or Dingman mouth gag, before the prep. The palate is injected with local anesthetic with added epinephrine. This injection is given before the prep so that the hemostatic effects of the epinephrine will have time to begin working before the initial incision. The patient is then prepped with Betadine scrub and paint. If the mouth gag is already in place, it also must be prepped.

The surgeon first suspends the mouth gag from the Mayo stand. The surgeon then makes the initial incisions along the borders of the mucosa using a #15 blade. The incisions are extended through the oral mucosa, the muscle, and the nasal mucosa with a cleft-palate blade (#6910 Beaver blade). After the incisions have been made, the surgeon elevates the nasal mucosa off the underlying muscle with the cleft-palate blade and the Freer or Cottle elevator. This step is performed on both sides of the cleft.

Next, the surgeon separates the oral mucosa from the overlying muscle. This step is performed in the same fashion as in the nasal mucosa. This creates three layers for closure. When all of the mucosa has been elevated to the most lateral edges, the incisions are closed. The nasal mucosa is closed first with a 4-0 absorbable suture on a 6-inch Crile-Wood needle holder and a pair of 6-inch DeBakey forceps. It is important that there not be too much tension on the incision line during closing. Tension will cause the wound to break down. Next, the muscle is closed with a 4-0 absorbable suture. When the

muscle has been closed, the oral mucosa is closed over the other two layers with a 4-0 or 5-0 absorbable suture. When the palate has been closed, the surgeon examines the wound for tension and releases any areas that are under tension. The wound is then irrigated, and the mouth gag is removed. The anesthesiologist must be careful when extubating the patient to avoid damaging the newly repaired palate.

Closure of a cleft palate is shown in Figure 26-20.

Repair of Microtia
SURGICAL GOAL
Microtia is a congenital defect that results in the absence of all or part of the ear. The deformity also affects the inner ear, resulting in deafness. Reconstructive surgery is performed before the child reaches school age.

DISCUSSION
Reconstruction of the ear is usually performed in multiple stages with several operations. The technique varies, depending on the type and severity of the defect. A common method of reconstruction is to elevate the skin where the ear normally would lie and insert either an artificial implant or a graft taken from the patient's costal cartilage.

When an autograft is to be taken, the patient is placed in the supine position. The surgeon creates a template (pattern) for the graft by placing a sheet of transparent material over the *unaffected* ear and tracing its outline on the material. The template is then placed over the affected ear, and the ear remnants are traced on the template.

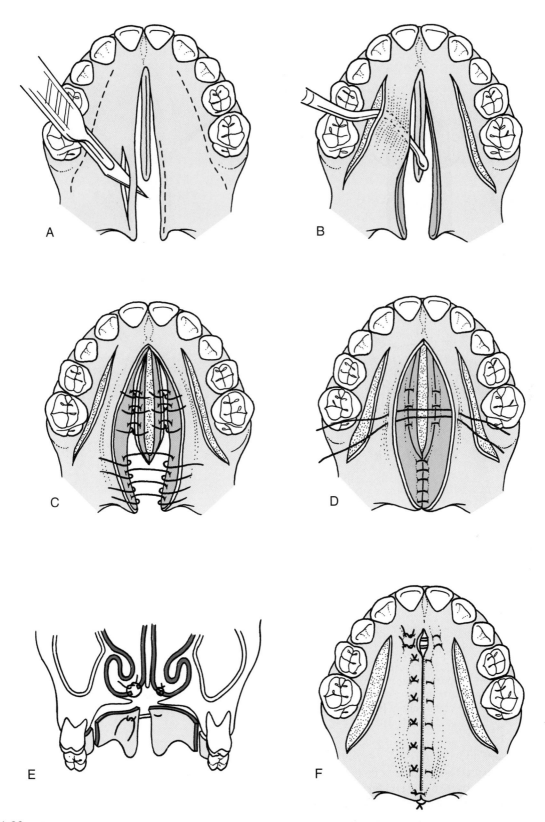

FIGURE 26-20
Closure of a cleft palate. **A,** Mucosa is removed from the margin of the cleft. **B,** Lateral releasing incisions are made and mucoperiosteal flaps are developed on the hard palate. **C,** Nasal flaps are created from the vomer and nasal floor; sutures are placed into the nasal mucosa. **D,** Closure of the nasal mucosa. **E,** Frontal view of repair of nasal mucosa. **F,** The oral mucoperiosteum is closed. (From Peterson LJ, Ellis E, Hupp JR, et al: *Contemporary oral and maxillofacial surgery,* ed 4, St Louis, 2003, Mosby.)

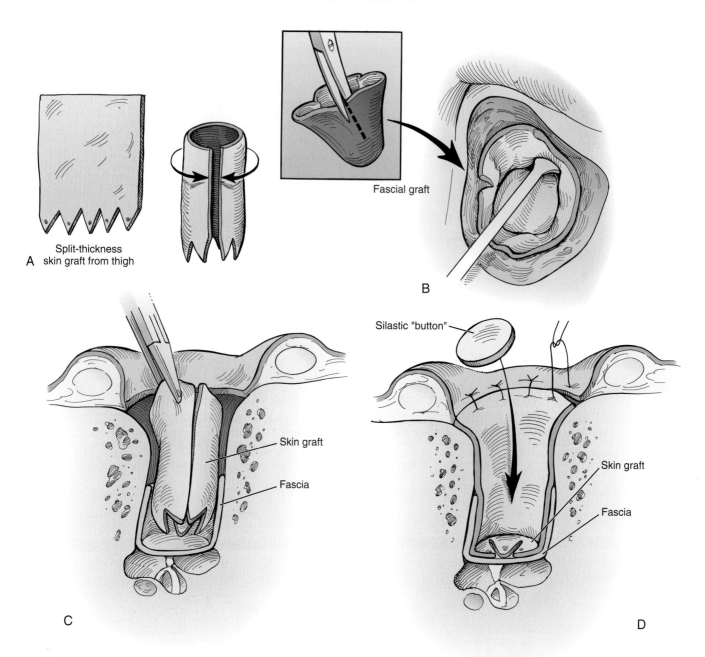

Split-thickness skin graft from thigh

A

Fascial graft

B

Skin graft

Fascia

C

Silastic "button"

Skin graft

Fascia

D

FIGURE 26-21
Aural atresia. **A,** Split-thickness skin graft. **B,** The graft is tailored to line the newly created external auditory canal using an ear speculum as a template; the graft is inserted into the auditory canal. **C,** The graft is positioned over the fascia and walls of the canal, and is adjusted and trimmed as needed to fit the canal. **D,** The graft is secured, and a Silastic button is cut to fit the eardrum and placed on top of the repair. (Modified from Coker NJ and Jenkins HA: *Atlas of otologic surgery,* Philadelphia, 2001, Saunders.)

The surgeon makes an incision over the seventh, eighth, or ninth intercostal space. The template is then placed over the costal cartilage, and the tissue is excised, following the outline of the template. The incision is closed in layers in routine fashion.

The surgeon may wish to carve the graft so that it resembles the shape of the ear more closely. This is done with a power drill and small bur attachments. The surgeon outlines the postauricular (behind the ear) area where the graft will be inserted. The technique of undermining the skin and inserting the newly constructed graft is illustrated in Figure 26-21. The surgeon pulls the skin over the graft and sutures it in place. This completes the first stage of the reconstruction.

When the first stage has healed, subsequent operations are performed to raise the frame of the ear and to construct the folds and recesses of the outer ear. The surgeon accomplishes this by incising flaps of adjacent skin and shifting them into position. Fine sutures of nylon, Prolene, or other synthetic material are used to suture the flaps in place. Bulky dressings are employed after ear repair to protect it from injury during healing.

REFERENCES

Aston SJ, Beasely RW, and Thorne CHM: *Grabb and Smith's plastic surgery,* ed 5, Philadelphia, 1997, Lippincott-Raven.

Phillips N: *Berry & Kohn's operating room technique,* ed 10, St Louis, 2004, Mosby.

Bailey BJ, et al: *Head and neck surgery – otolaryngology,* ed 2, vol 1 and 2, Philadelphia, 1998, Lippincott-Raven.

Fortunato N and McCullough SM: *Plastic and reconstructive surgery: perioperative nursing series,* St Louis, 1998, Mosby.

Gruendemann BJ and Fernsebner B: *Comprehensive perioperative nursing,* vol 2, Boston, 1995, Jones and Bartlett.

Jobe R: *Davies repair of cleft lip,* September 12, 2002, www.teachsurgery.org/public/interplastcd/interplast/surgical/.

Marks MW and Marks C: *Fundamentals of plastic surgery,* Philadelphia, 1997, Saunders.

Rothrock JC: *Alexander's care of the patient in surgery,* ed 12, St Louis, 2003, Mosby.

Papel ID et al: *Facial plastic and reconstructive surgery,* ed 2, New York, 2002, Thieme.

Sandberg DJ, McGee WP, and Denk MJ: Neonatal cleft lip and cleft palate repair, *AORN Journal* March 75 (3):490-499, 2002.

Sykes JM: The endoscopic brow and forehead lift surgical technique, September 10, 2002, Medtronic, www.xomed.com/SurgicalTechniques/surgtech_plastic1.asp.

Tyers AG and Collin JRO: *Colour atlas of ophthalmic plastic surgery,* ed 2, Oxford, 2001, Butterworth-Heinemann.

Weerda H: *Reconstructive facial plastic surgery: a problem-solving manual,* New York, 2001, Thieme.

Chapter 27

Orthopedic Surgery

By Robert Doheny and Janet Anne Milligan

Learning Objectives

After studying this chapter the reader will:

- Discuss orthopedic terminology
- Identify the muscle groups, the bones, and their functions
- Identify the names and uses of orthopedic instruments, hardware, and supplies
- Describe the proper sequence of events in orthopedic procedures
- Describe the types of diagnostic tests and laboratory tests used preoperatively in the orthopedic patient

Terminology

Abduction—To take away from; away from midline.

Acetabulum—A hollow, cuplike portion of the hip joint; the hip socket.

Adduction—To move toward the midline.

Allograft—Transplant tissue obtained from the same species.

Amputation—The surgical removal of a limb or portion of a limb.

Ankylosis—The immobility or fusion of a joint caused by injury, disease, or surgical procedure.

Arthritis—Inflammation of a joint.

Arthrocentesis—Puncture of a joint space through use of a needle.

Arthrodesis—The surgical immobilization of a joint.

Arthrogram—Visualization of a joint by radiographic study after injection of a contrast medium into the joint space.

Arthroplasty—The operative procedure of reshaping or reconstructing a diseased joint.

Arthroscopy—An examination of the interior of a joint for therapeutic and di-agnostic purposes with a specially designed endoscope.

Arthrotomy—A surgical incision into a joint.

Articular cartilage—Hyaline cartilage covering the articular surfaces of bones.

Articulation—The place of union between two or more bones; a joint.

Baker's cyst—Synovial cyst (pouch) arising from the synovial lining of the knee.

Bursa—A padlike sac or cavity found in connective tissue near the joint.

Cancellous bone—A latticework structure of spongy or soft bone.

Cardiac muscle—The muscles of the heart.

C-arm—A type of radiograph that produces "real time" fluoroscopic images for the surgeon or radiographer.

Condyle—A rounded protuberance at the end of a bone forming an articulation.

Contracture—Fibrosis of muscle, fascia, skin, or joint capsule that cannot be mobilized if flexed or extended.

Delayed union—A fracture that has not healed within an average amount of time.

Diaphysis—The shaft of a long bone.

Electromyogram—A graphic record of the contraction of a muscle as a result of electrical stimulation.

Endosteum—A fine membrane that lines the medullary cavity of bone.

Epiphysiodesis—Fusion of the growth plates in bones.

Epiphysis—The center for ossification at each extremity of long bone. The growth plate.

Eversion—A turning outward.

Exostosis—A benign bony growth that arises from the surface of a bone.

Exsanguination—The process of expressing blood from a part.

Fascia—Fibrous membrane covering, supporting, and separating muscles.

Fasciotomy—A surgical incision and division of the fascia.

Fracture—A break in a bone.

Terminology—cont'd

Gout—Hereditary metabolic disease that is a form of acute arthritis. Marked by inflammation of the joints, usually starting in the foot or the knee.

Hematopoiesis—The production and development of blood cells, normally in the bone marrow.

Inversion—To turn inward.

Joint cavity—The saclike structure that encloses the ends of bones in diarthrodial joints, consisting of an outer fibrous layer, an inner synovial layer, and synovial fluid.

Joint mouse—Free bits of cartilage or bone present in the joint space, especially the knee. Also called loose bodies.

Ligament—Strong band of fibrous connective tissue connecting the articular ends of bones and serving to bind the bones together and to facilitate or limit motion.

Malunion fracture—An imperfect union in which the fragments of a fractured bone grow in a faulty position.

Marrow—The soft tissue occupying the medullary cavities of long bones

Neuropathy—Any disease of the nerves.

Nonunion fracture—Failure of fragments of a fractured bone to knit together.

Osteoarthritis—Inflammation of a joint.

Osteoarthrotomy—Excision of a joint end of a bone.

Osteoblast—A cell of mesodermal origin that is concerned with the formation of bone.

Osteogenesis—Formation and development of bone.

Osteomalacia—A disease marked by increasing softness of the bones; the adult form of rickets.

Osteomyelitis—Inflammation of bone, especially the marrow.

Osteonecrosis—Death of generalized bone tissue rather than of isolated areas.

Osteophyte—A bony outgrowth, usually found around a joint; a "joint mouse" if loose in the joint.

Osteosclerosis—The abnormal thickening of bone (*skleros,* hardening).

Osteotomy—Surgical incision into bone.

Patella—A lens-shaped sesamoid bone situated in front of the knee in the tendon of the quadriceps femoris muscle. Also called kneecap.

Periosteum—Fibrous membrane that covers bones except at the articular surfaces.

Sesamoid—Resembling a grain of sesame in size or shape.

Smooth muscle—Muscle activated involuntarily, such as the muscle of the digestive tract.

Striated muscle—Muscle that is under voluntary control, such as those used to move an arm or leg.

Suture—A joint that connects bones of the skull.

Symphysis—A joint whose bones are connected by a disk of cartilage.

Synchondrosis—A type of cartilaginous joint in which the cartilage is usually converted into bone before adulthood.

Syndesmosis—A fibrous articulation in which two bones are joined by ligaments.

Tendon—Fibrous portion of muscle, serving to attach muscles to bones and other parts.

Traction—The process of drawing or pulling.

SURGICAL ANATOMY

The Skeleton

The human skeleton is the bony support of the body (Figure 27-1). It consists of 206 bones. These bones are divided into groups (classifications) according to their location in the body.

CLASSIFICATION OF BONES

Bones are classified according to their shape, including long bones, short bones, sesamoid bones, flat bones, and irregularly shaped bones.

Long bones include bones whose length is greater than their width or circumference. This group includes the clavicle, humerus, radius, ulna, femur, tibia, and fibula. Also included are the bones of the fingers and toes: the metacarpals, metatarsals, and phalanges. Each long bone has geographic landmarks. The *shaft* of the long bone is called the *diaphysis.* The end of the bone is called the *epiphysis.* Figure 27-2 illustrates the anatomy of the long bone.

Short bones include bones whose dimensions are approximately equal. Included in this group are the many small

bones of the hands and feet. Figure 27-3 illustrates the anatomy of the forearm and the hand.

Sesamoid bones sometimes are called "floating" bones and are an oval-shaped nodule of bone or fibrocartilage in a tendon playing over a bone surface. The patella is an example of a sesamoid bone and is the largest one in the human body.

Flat bones are usually curved, thin, and flat. These bones serve to protect soft body parts or to attach wide muscles. Included in this group are the ribs, pelvic bones, scapula, and many skull bones.

Irregular bones are bones that do not actually fit into any of the other groups. These bones are uncommon in shape. Included in this group are the vertebrae, the ossicles of the ear, and some of the skull bones. The anatomy of vertebrae and the bones of the skull are illustrated in Chapter 31. The ossicles of the ear are illustrated in Chapter 25.

BONE TISSUE AND MEMBRANES

There are two types of bone tissue, *cancellous bone* and *compact bone.* Cancellous bone (also called soft bone) is not soft but contains many small open spaces. These open spaces

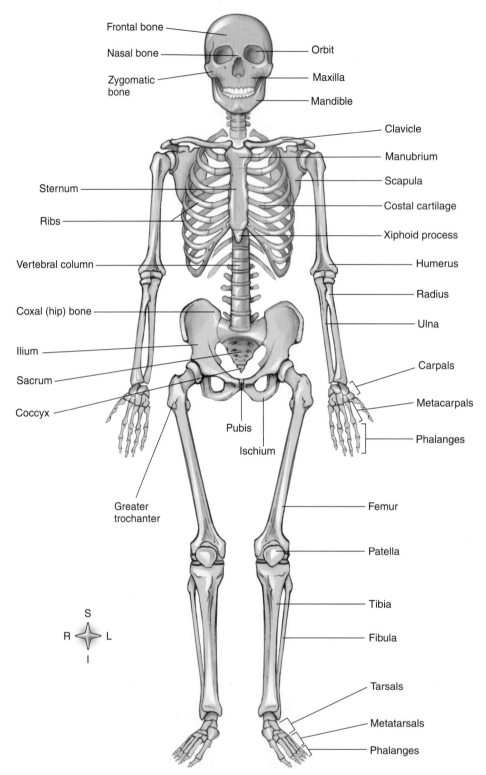

FIGURE 27-1
Anterior and posterior views of a skeleton. (From Thibodeau GA and Patton KT: *Anthony's textbook of anatomy and physiology,* ed 17, St Louis, 2003, Mosby.)

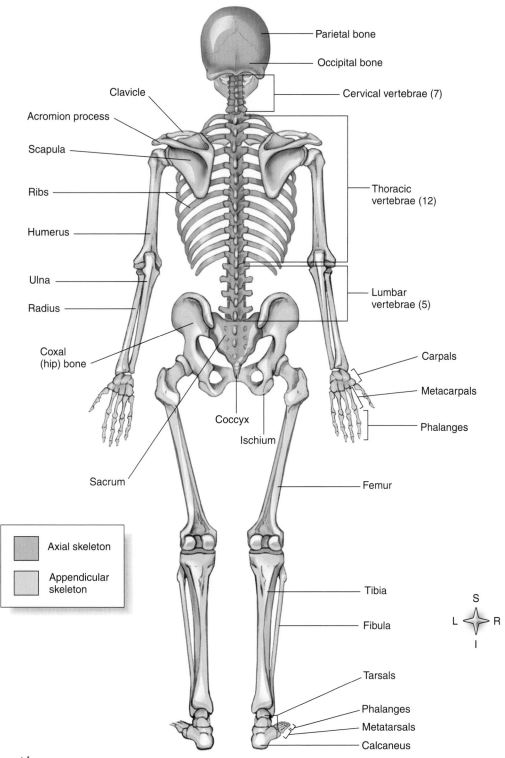

Parietal bone
Occipital bone
Cervical vertebrae (7)
Clavicle
Acromion process
Scapula
Thoracic vertebrae (12)
Ribs
Humerus
Ulna
Lumbar vertebrae (5)
Radius
Coxal (hip) bone
Carpals
Metacarpals
Phalanges
Coccyx
Ischium
Sacrum
Femur

Axial skeleton
Appendicular skeleton

Tibia
Fibula

S
L   R
I

Tarsals
Phalanges
Metatarsals
Calcaneus

FIGURE 27-1, cont'd

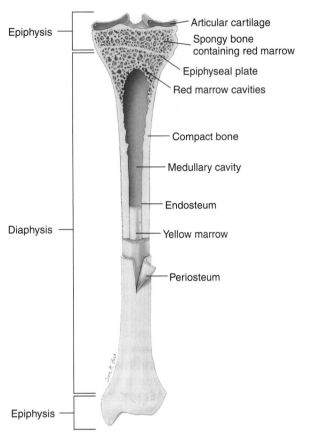

FIGURE 27-2
Anatomy of a long bone. (From Fortunato N: *Berry & Kohn's operating room technique*, ed 9, St Louis, 2000, Mosby.)

make the bone appear soft. Bone grafts typically use cancellous bone.

Compact bone is very dense with few open spaces. The shaft of a long bone is compact bone. Within the shaft of the bone and surrounded by compact bone is the *medullary canal*. Figure 27-4 illustrates compact and cancellous bone in the hip joint.

The medullary canal contains red or yellow marrow. *Red marrow* is found mostly in the small spaces of the spongy or cancellous bone. It is highly vascular and functions as the site of production of blood cells and hemoglobin. The production of these cells is called hematopoiesis. *Yellow marrow* consists mainly of fat cells and connective tissue. It is found primarily in the medullary cavity of long bones.

The periosteum consists of a dense external layer containing blood vessels and an inner layer of connective tissue cells that function as *osteoblasts* when bone is injured and participate in the formation of new bone. Periosteum serves as a supporting structure for blood vessels that nourish bone and serves to attach muscles, tendons, and ligaments. The location of the periosteum is illustrated in Figure 27-2.

BONE LANDMARKS
Bones have certain landmarks, which are irregularities or markings that serve many functions and are named separately according to their shape and function. Some of these markings may serve as attachments for muscle or tendon, while others are passageways for nerves or blood vessels.

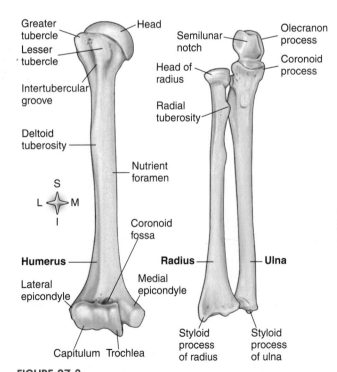

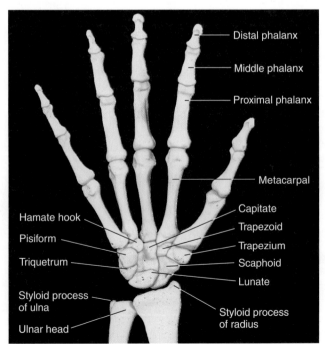

FIGURE 27-3
Anatomy of the hand and forearm. (From Thibodeau GA and Patton KT: *Anthony's textbook of anatomy and physiology*, ed 17, St Louis, 2003, Mosby; photo from Vidic B, Suarez FR: *Photographic atlas of the human body*, St Louis, 1984, Mosby.)

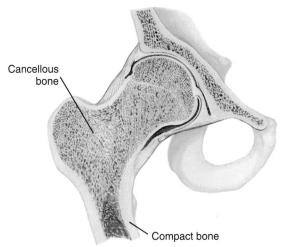

FIGURE 27-4
Compact and cancellous bone in the hip joint. (From Thibodeau GA and Patton KT: *Anthony's textbook of anatomy and physiology,* ed 17, St Louis, 2003, Mosby.)

Whenever skeletal anatomy is discussed, these landmarks are used for clarity.

- **Crest:** a ridge of bone (e.g., iliac crest)
- **Spine:** a sharp, narrow projection (e.g., spinous process)
- **Condyle:** a knuckle-shaped portion of bone, generally found in association with a joint
- **Process:** a projection of bone (e.g., coracoid process)
- **Tubercle:** a small, rounded projection (e.g., deltoid tubercle)
- **Tuberosity:** a large, rounded projection (e.g., ischial tuberosity)
- **Foramen:** a rounded orifice in bone (e.g., olfactory foramen); a passageway for blood vessels or nerves.
- **Sinus:** a cavity within a bone (e.g., nasal sinus)
- **Sulcus:** a groove in a bone

The Muscular System

Muscles are responsible for most movement in the human body (Figure 27-5). Some muscles may move an entire limb, while others are responsible for the movement of fluid or to maintain a heartbeat.

There are three major muscle types in the human body: striated, smooth, and cardiac. Each is described as follows.

STRIATED MUSCLE

Striated muscle, also commonly called *skeletal muscle,* is composed of fibers that are bound together by sheaths of protective tissue. Each group of fibers and its associated sheath are bound together to form one muscle.

SMOOTH MUSCLE

Smooth muscle tissue is also called *involuntary muscle* because it is not under conscious control. These muscles are found principally in the internal organs, especially the digestive tract, respiratory passages, urinary and genital ducts,

urinary bladder, and gallbladder, and in the walls of blood vessels. When found in structures such as the bladder and intestine, smooth muscle contains two layers—one outside, longitudinal layer and another inner, circular layer. When the muscles contract, they actually reduce the diameter and length of the structure of which they are a part, thus moving contents through the structure.

CARDIAC MUSCLE

As the name implies, cardiac muscle is the muscle of the heart. Like voluntary muscle, cardiac muscle is striated, but these muscles are involuntary. Cardiac muscle is responsible for the sustained contractions of the heart and for the movement of blood in and out of the heart. This mechanism, and also the rate of contraction, is driven by a complex series of impulses from the autonomic nervous system.

Joints

The articular system or joint system includes those areas of the body where two bones meet and where movement occurs. The degree of movement may be small, such as in the ossicles of the ear, or large, such as in the hip joint.

CLASSIFICATION OF JOINTS

Joints are classified according to the degree of movement they allow and also by the shape of the articulating surfaces (Figure 27-6). Following are joint classifications:

- **Synarthrosis:** a joint that is immovable, such as the union of the major skull bones
- **Amphiarthrosis:** a joint that is slightly movable, such as a vertebral joint
- **Diarthrosis:** a joint that is freely movable, such as the hip or the shoulder

The diarthroses include most joints of the body. These joints also are called *synovial joints,* because the joint capsule contains a fluid called *synovia,* or *synovial fluid.*

SYNOVIAL JOINT

The synovial joint consists of the articulating bone ends and the connective tissues that surround and bind them. Surrounding the joint is a tough fibrous tissue called the *joint capsule.* The joint capsule is lined with a membrane called the *synovial membrane.* This membrane produces a thick, clear fluid, *synovial fluid,* which lubricates and nourishes the joint. Each bone surface within the joint is covered with *cartilage,* a strong, smooth tissue that, combined with the lubricating effect of the synovial fluid, aids in the smooth gliding of one bone surface over the other. Joints are grouped according to their motion, including ball and socket, hinge, condyloid, pivot, gliding, and saddle joints. Joints can move in four ways: *gliding, angular motion, circumduction,* and *rotation.* Angular movement that moves forward or backward is called *flexion* or *extension.* The terminology of joint movement is used extensively in orthopedic joint surgery, and all operating room personnel should know these terms well.

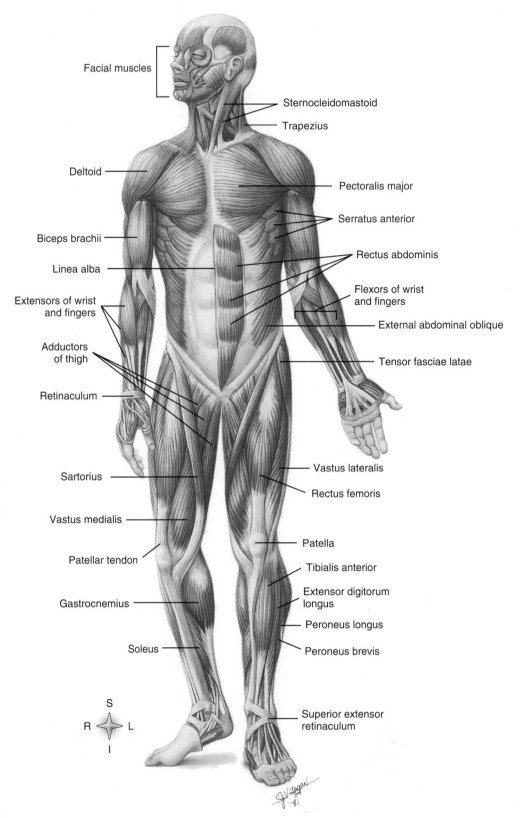

Facial muscles

Sternocleidomastoid

Trapezius

Deltoid

Pectoralis major

Serratus anterior

Biceps brachii

Rectus abdominis

Linea alba

Flexors of wrist
and fingers

Extensors of wrist
and fingers

External abdominal oblique

Adductors
of thigh

Tensor fasciae latae

Retinaculum

Sartorius

Vastus lateralis

Rectus femoris

Vastus medialis

Patella

Patellar tendon

Tibialis anterior

Extensor digitorum
longus

Gastrocnemius

Peroneus longus

Peroneus brevis

Soleus

Superior extensor
retinaculum

S
R ✦ L
I

FIGURE 27-5
Muscles of the human body in anterior and posterior positions. (From Thibodeau GA and Patton KT: *Anthony's textbook of anatomy and physiology*, ed 17, St Louis, 2003, Mosby.)

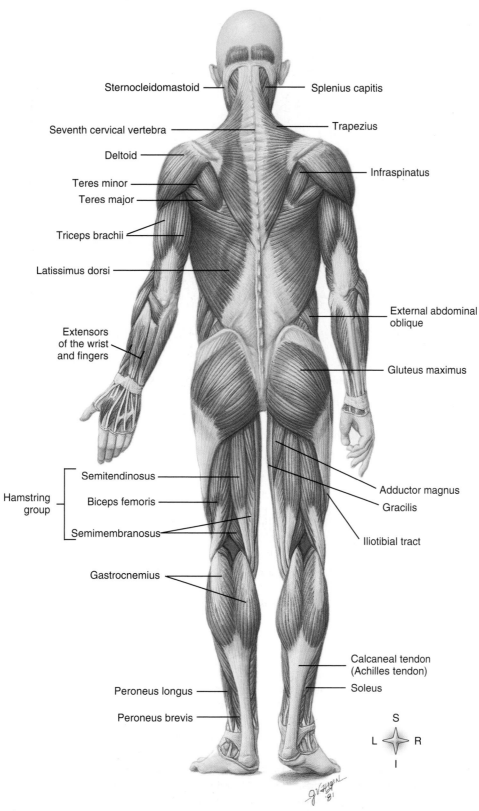

FIGURE 27-5, cont'd

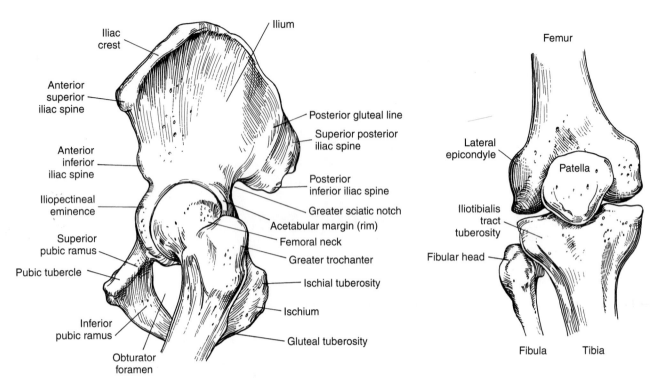

FIGURE 27-6
A ball-and-socket hip joint and a hinged knee joint. (From Fortunato N: *Berry & Kohn's operating room technique*, ed 9, St. Louis, 2000, Mosby.)

Following are common terms referring to the movement of a joint:

▶ **Flexion:** forward movement
▶ **Extension:** backward movement
▶ **Abduction:** movement away from the body
▶ **Adduction:** movement toward the median plane of the body
▶ **Valgus:** an abnormal position in which a part of a limb is bent outward or twisted, away from the midline of the body
▶ **Varus:** a position in which a part of a limb is turned inward
▶ **Volar:** pertaining to the palm of the hand or the sole of the foot. Also called palmar, palmaris, or volaris

The synovial joints are further classified according to the shape of their articular surfaces, which in turn governs their type of movement.

Because of their location and constant use, joints are prone to stress, injuries, and inflammation. The main diseases affecting the joints are rheumatic fever, rheumatoid arthritis, osteoarthritis, and gout. Common injuries to joints are contusions, sprains, dislocations, and penetrating wounds.

NONSYNOVIAL JOINTS

Nonsynovial joints (also called synarthrodia) are a type of immovable cartilaginous joint in which bones are separated by only connective tissue membrane. In nonsynovial joints, a continuous intervening substance such as cartilage, fibrous tissue, or bone unites the skeletal elements. Movement is absent or limited, and a joint cavity is lacking. These joints are said to have a fixed articulation. Nonsynovial joints include the *sutures, synchondroses, symphyses,* and *syndesmoses.* The nonsynovial joints are illustrated in Chapter 31.

Ligaments are the strong fibrous bands of tissue that join bones together and limit or help facilitate the motion of the joints. In addition, where a muscle joins a bone, an intermediary tissue—the *tendon*—forms the actual attachment. An example of a ligament and a tendon attachment of the knee is illustrated in Figure 27-7.

DIAGNOSTIC TESTS

Orthopedic surgeons use a variety of tests to diagnose a musculoskeletal injury or condition. Following are the tests used most often.

Arthrography

Arthrography (arthrogram) often is used to determine the cause of unexplained joint pain. A needle is placed through the skin and into the joint space. An x-ray then is used to identify the placement. Contrast dye then is injected into the joint space to highlight the joint structures, such as the ligaments, cartilage, tendons, and joint capsule. During this test, several x-rays are taken with the joint in various positions.

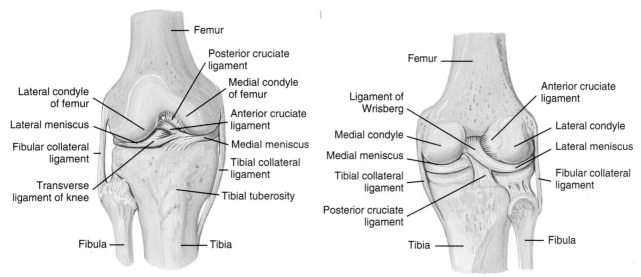

FIGURE 27-7
Tendon and ligament attachments of the knee. (From Thibodeau GA and Patton KT: *Anthony's textbook of anatomy and physiology*, ed 17, St Louis, 2003, Mosby.)

Blood Tests

As part of most exams, blood tests may be taken. Some conditions, such as rheumatoid arthritis, infection, diabetes mellitus, and gout, may be detected and treatment may be started after a simple blood test.

Electromyography

Electromyography (EMG) records and analyzes the electrical activity in muscles. It is used to learn more about the functioning of the nerves in the arms and legs. EMG can be used to identify damage to nerves caused by blunt trauma or any other kind of trauma to the extremities.

During an EMG, small, thin needles are placed into the muscle to record activity. Some pain or discomfort may occur but will subside. The EMG technologist may ask the patient to tense and relax the muscle being tested. The signals are recorded, and the electrical activity is projected onto a monitor. Results usually are available immediately after the testing is completed.

Magnetic Resonance Imaging

Magnetic resonance imaging (MRI) uses magnetic fields and a sophisticated computer to take high-resolution pictures of bones and soft tissues, resulting in a cross-sectional image of the body. MRI helps diagnose torn muscles, ligaments, and cartilage; herniated disks; hip or pelvic problems; and many other conditions. An MRI creates a picture of the body using a combination of magnetic fields and radio waves. A non-iodine–based contrast injection may be given before the study to highlight tumors and infectious processes within the body. There is no pain associated with this diagnostic examination, and this examination usually takes about 30 to 90 minutes.

Computed Topography

A computed topography (CT) scan combines x-rays with computer technology to produce a more detailed, cross-sectional image of the body. CT scanners are better at detecting fresh bleeding than other diagnostic exams. A CT scan may be ordered if the physician suspects a tumor or a fracture that will not appear on x-ray. The scan is painless. As with an MRI, the patient lies motionless on a table, and the patient is positioned into the center of the scanner. The x-ray tube slowly rotates around the patient, taking pictures from all directions. The pictures are viewed on a television screen, and the test produces a clear two-dimensional photograph of the area in question. Iodine-based contrast may be injected before the scan to improve the images produced by the scan.

Radiographs (X-Rays)

X-rays are the most widely used of available diagnostic imaging techniques. X-rays are always used for fractures and joint dislocations, and also may be used if the physician suspects damage to a bone or joint from other conditions such as arthritis or *osteonecrosis*. The part of the body that is being x-rayed is placed between the machine and the film. Radiation then is sent through the body and to the film. The radiation exposes the film, creating a radiograph of the structure. On the x-ray image, the bones, tumors, and other dense matter appear white because they absorb the radiation. Soft tissue and breaks in the bone appear darker.

FRACTURES

Classification of Fractures

Fractures are classified by the extent and type of injury to the bone and surrounding tissues (Figure 27-8). These classifi-

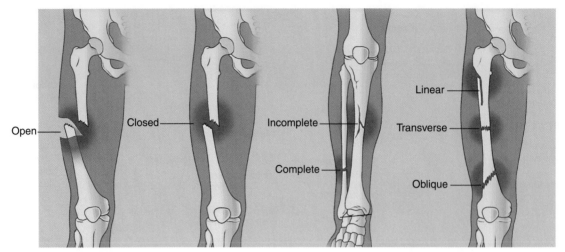

FIGURE 27-8
Types of bone fractures. (From Thibodeau GA and Patton KT: *Anthony's textbook of anatomy and physiology,* ed 17, St Louis, 2003, Mosby.)

cations are clinically significant because some fracture sites are contaminated and present the risk of infection. Compound or open fractures are always an emergency and will *bump* into the surgery schedule as an emergency case.

Classifications of fractures are listed in Table 27-1.

Fracture Management

The biology of fracture healing is not particularly complex and parallels that of any non-ossified tissue. Fracture healing occurs in three basic phases: the vascular phase, the metabolic phase, and the mechanical phase.

The vascular phase begins at the time of injury and proceeds through the development of a hematoma. The formed hematoma becomes organized, and collagen is formed. The end result of the vascular phase is the development of a soft callus.

The metabolic phase begins about 4 to 6 weeks after injury. In this period, the soft callus is reworked and a hard callus is formed.

The mechanical phase begins after the hard callus has formed. During this phase, a solid, mechanically strong bone is formed.

Bone healing is related to the age and physical condition of the patient. In addition, some medication may hinder or inhibit bone healing. Healing bone is classified by degree as delayed union, malunion, or nonunion, and is confirmed by radiological examination.

Complications of fractures and fracture management include:

▶ Problems of union (delayed union, malunion, or nonunion)
▶ Stiffness and loss of motion
▶ Infection
▶ Myositis ossificans
▶ Avascular necrosis

▶ Implant failure
▶ Reflex sympathetic dystrophy
▶ Compartment syndrome

MANAGEMENT OF COMPARTMENT SYNDROME

Compartment syndrome is a condition of increased resting pressure in a contained compartment, such as the leg or the forearm. This increase in pressure results in decreased lymphatic drainage, decreased venous drainage, loss of arterial inflow, and death to the muscle contained in the compartment, in that order. Compartment syndrome is an emergent injury to the vascular system. When the diagnosis of compartment syndrome has been confirmed, immediate fasciotomy of the compartment in question is required. Figure 27-9, *A,* illustrates a double-incision technique for performing fasciotomies of all four compartments of the lower leg.

Figure 27-9, *B,* illustrates a patient who had a closed fracture of the tibia that required a fasciotomy; the fracture had to be treated in traction. It is fundamental to the objectives of the procedure to leave the wounds open. The patient returns to surgery for a delayed skin closure and possible skin grafting after the compartment syndrome has resolved.

While preparing for the procedure, the surgical technologist should make sure that there are plenty of dressings in the room to accommodate these large open wounds. The wounds are left open, but sterile surgical dressings are used to cover the wounds.

REDUCTION AND FIXATION

Reduction is the physical approximation of the fracture ends so that bone healing, called *osteogenesis,* can begin. Reduction is the process of returning fractured bones to their correct anatomical position, using internal or external means to stabilize them. Reduction can be performed *externally,* through manipulation of the bone from outside the body, a technique called closed reduction (CR); or *internally,* in

Table 27-1 CLASSIFICATION AND SURGICAL OPTIONS OF FRACTURES

Classification of Fracture	Description of Fracture	Surgical Option	Surgical Repair
Simple fracture	A fracture in which there is a single fracture line	▶ Closed reduction (CR); application of a plaster splint or cast	▶ Treatment may include only a plaster splint or cast. ▶ In pediatric cases, the patient will require a general anesthetic for the CR and cast application.
Comminuted fracture	This type of fracture consists of multiple bone fragments and fracture lines.	▶ ORIF ▶ OR external fixation	▶ The force needed to produce this type of injury usually results in soft-tissue damage and may require extensive repair of both soft tissue and bone. ▶ Soft-tissue repair may require the reattachment of ligaments with sutures, staples, or screws.
Open or compound fracture	A fracture in which the bone fragments protrude through the skin	▶ ORIF ▶ Debridement ▶ Skin grafts ▶ Delayed closure	▶ This is an emergency case. This type of fracture is considered an emergency because of the immediate risk of infection. ▶ Orthopedic hardware is needed. The hardware depends on the type of fracture and the bone involved.
Greenstick fracture	Primarily pediatric fractures, where the bones are resilient and covered with a durable, tough periosteum. Because of this resiliency, children's bones may "bend" rather than break. When this occurs, the concave side of the fracture surface is compressed and the convex side is pulled apart. Thus, the bone appears angled but is not broken.	▶ ORIF ▶ CR and application of a plaster cast or splint	▶ Treatment may include only CR with a plaster splint or cast. ▶ In pediatric cases, the patient will require a general anesthetic for the CR and cast application. ▶ ORIF is indicated if the fracture is across the growth plate.
Pathologic fracture	A fracture caused by disease such as metastatic disease. The fracture occurs most often at the tumor site, where the bone is weak.	▶ ORIF ▶ IM rodding	▶ These fractures are painful, and the ORIF procedure may include a potential for extreme blood loss. ▶ With IM rodding, the rod must go across the cancerous tumor. Often it is impossible to put a plate and screws across the tumor site because of the soft bone involved, and the IM rod is the only option.
Impacted fracture	This is a fracture caused by violent impact along the longitudinal axis of a bone. This occurs at the junction of the metaphysis and the diaphysis, where the cortex is quite thin. The diaphysis usually is forced into the metaphysis, tightly wedging the two fragments together.	▶ ORIF	▶ This is a more extensive repair than a typical ORIF because the surgeon must repair the impacted area. ▶ This procedure is like "un-breaking an eggshell" and putting a plate and screws across the fracture site. ▶ This type of fracture has the potential for a long operation.
Spiral fracture	Results from the twisting or torquing of a bone. In this type of fracture, the bone is twisted apart into two fragments.	▶ ORIF	▶ This type of fracture must be opened and internally fixed with plates and screws. ▶ IM rodding will *not* work on this type of fracture if the spiral is long.

IM, intramedullary; *ORIF,* open reduction internal fixation.

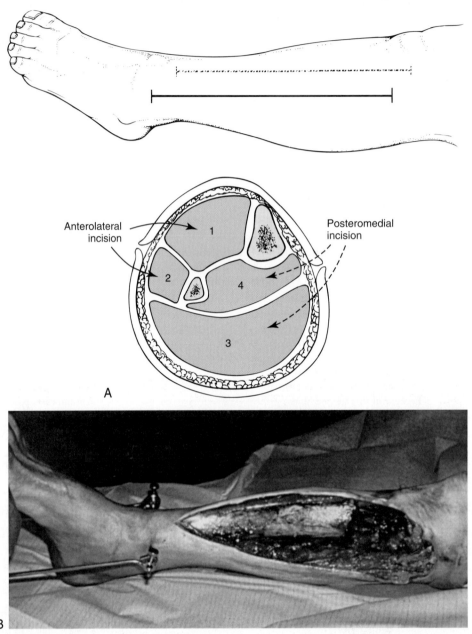

FIGURE 27-9
A, *Top,* the double-incision technique for performing fasciotomies. *Bottom,* cross-section of lower extremity showing all four compartments involved. **B,** Compartment syndrome of the lower leg. (From Browner BD, Jupiter JB, Levine AM, et al: *Skeletal trauma: basic science, management, and reconstruction,* ed 3, Philadelphia, 2003, Saunders.)

which the bone ends themselves are manipulated and approximated during surgical intervention, a technique called open reduction internal fixation (ORIF).

External manipulation is possible only when the orthopedist can overcome the force of the spasms that occur in the muscles that bridge the fracture site. When the fracture occurs in areas such as the proximal humerus or femur, these spasms often are too strong for manual reduction.

In these cases, prolonged pull on the fractured bones is necessary. This can be achieved through *traction* (Figure 27-10). In skeletal traction, a transverse pin or rod is placed through the limb, and continuous weight is applied to the end. This draws the fractured bones apart. In some cases (as in pediatric patients), the muscles will not relax or the patient is unable to cooperate, and a general anesthetic and a muscle relaxant are given. After these drugs are administered, the fracture may be more easily reduced without the use of an incision (Figure 27-11, *A*).

Many types of traction are used in the preoperative and intraoperative phases. For example, a patient who has been in

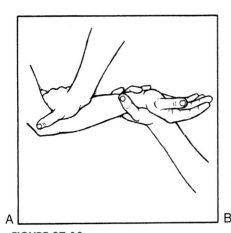
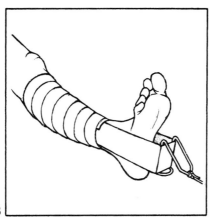
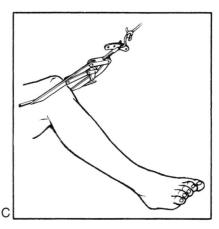

FIGURE 27-10
Traction techniques. **A,** Manual. **B,** Skin. **C,** Skeletal. (From Rothrock J: *Alexander's care of the patient in surgery,* ed 12, St Louis, 2003, Mosby; courtesy *Zimmer Traction Handbook,* 1989, Zimmer, Inc., Warsaw, Ind.)

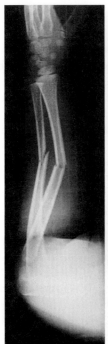
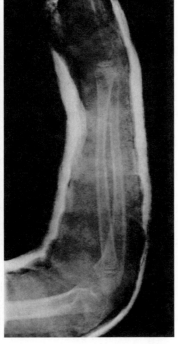
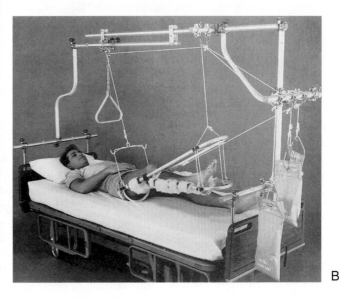

FIGURE 27-11
A, *Left,* a greenstick fracture of the radius and ulna of a 6-year-old. *Right,* closed reduction of the fracture with the patient under general anesthesia and a long arm cast applied. **B,** A patient in skeletal traction, in a balanced suspension traction bed. (**A** from Green NE and Swiontkowski MF: *Skeletal trauma in children,* ed 3, Philadelphia, 2003, Saunders; **B** from Rothrock J: *Alexander's care of the patient in surgery,* ed 12, St Louis, 2003, Mosby; courtesy *Zimmer Traction Handbook,* 1989, Zimmer, Inc., Warsaw, Ind.)

a motor vehicle accident often is unable to withstand a surgical or medical fixation of a fracture. The surgeon might choose to place the patient in skeletal traction until he or she is more stable. This option is used only if the fracture is a closed wound. In this scenario, the patient later comes to surgery and is anesthetized in his or her own bed with the traction in place. The traction is removed only after the patient is under a general or a spinal anesthetic (Figure 27-11, *B*).

The traction methods that are used with surgical patients during the preoperative phase, such as the previous example, are listed in Table 27-2.

IMMOBILIZATION
Bone fragments must be stabilized while the patient's bone heals. In surgery, immobilization is called *fixation.* Reduction and fixation are discussed below.

Type of Traction	Equipment Needed	Description and Uses
Skeletal traction	▶ Traction bow ▶ Manual or power drill ▶ Steinmann pin ▶ Rope ▶ Pulley ▶ Weights	▶ Pulling force applied directly to the bone through surgically applied pins and tongs ▶ Typically seen in patients with a fractured femur
Manual traction		▶ The hands apply the forces pulling on the bone being realigned ▶ Used primarily on forearm fractures and pediatric patients
Skin traction	▶ External traction boot ▶ Tape, digital straps, moleskin, or Ace wrap ▶ Rope ▶ Pulley ▶ Weights	▶ The pulling force is applied externally and applied directly on the skin ▶ Typically seen in elderly patients with nondisplaced hip fractures

Table 27-2 TRACTION TYPES AND EQUIPMENT NEEDED

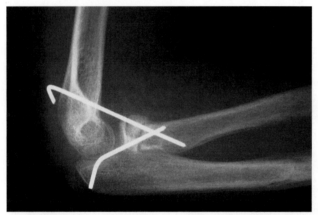

FIGURE 27-12
Lateral radiograph of the elbow of a 9-year-old after reduction of a displaced fracture of the radial head. Reduction was performed with K-wires. (From Green NE and Swiontkowski MF: *Skeletal trauma in children,* ed 3, Philadelphia, 2003, Saunders.)

CLOSED REDUCTION

In this type of procedure, the bone ends are reduced externally (without surgery), by manipulation. The reduction is painful, and the patient may require a general anesthetic for the procedure; however the reduction often can be achieved in the ER with IV conscious sedation.

When the fracture has been reduced, the bone is then immobilized or *fixated* by external means, such as a plaster cast, plaster splint, or traction.

CLOSED REDUCTION EXTERNAL FIXATION

In this procedure, the bone ends are approximated (reduced) externally and then held in place by an internally placed device, such as a rod or pin. This type of procedure requires surgical intervention because the stabilizing (fixation) appliance must be inserted. However, instead of making an incision to insert the fixating device, the pins are

pushed or drilled through the skin (*percutaneous puncture*) and then into the bone fragments, holding the bone pieces together. This is an excellent way to achieve fixation of a fractured finger. The pins or K-wires are either bent just outside the skin or buried into the bone, depending on whether the surgeon wants to remove the pins after x-ray has confirmed that the fracture has healed (Figure 27-12). Postoperative dressing includes an immobilizing splint.

EXTERNAL FIXATION DEVICE

In closed reduction external fixation, a special system is applied. Many operating room staff members have nicknamed this system "Tinker-toys" because the system uses the same principles as the children's toy set.

The procedure requires a percutaneous stick and the insertion of a series of small Steinmann pins through the bone. (One pin is placed at each end of the fracture.) Distraction rods are then placed lengthwise across the fracture to distract or hold traction on the bone as it heals. The patient must learn to take care of the puncture sites. This external fixation device typically is used in fractures that are close to a wrist or an ankle joint. The external fixation device is being used successfully in pelvic fractures as well. An external fixation placement is illustrated in Figure 27-13, *A.* This procedure reduces and stabilizes the fracture with the same equipment, and although a sterile dressing is required to cover the small wounds, no splint or plaster cast is needed for the postoperative healing phase. An x-ray of a healing tibial fracture with an external fixation device is illustrated in Figure 27-13, *B.*

OPEN REDUCTION INTERNAL FIXATION

This procedure requires both the internal manipulation of the bone fragments and the application of a stabilizing or fixating device called an *orthopedic implant.* This type of reduction is performed most often in the operating room and requires the most complex surgical intervention.

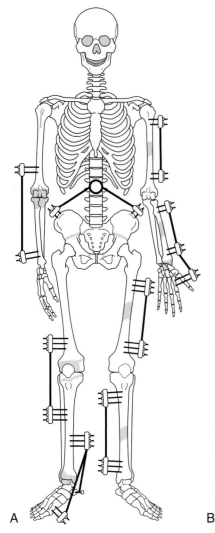

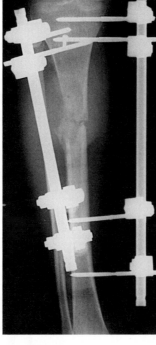

FIGURE 27-13
A, Simple unilateral external fixation can be applied rapidly to most upper and lower extremity fractures.
B, External fixation device on a tibial fracture. (From Browner BD, Jupiter JB, Levine AM, et al: *Skeletal trauma: basic science, management, and reconstruction*, ed 3, Philadelphia, 2003, Saunders.)

Orthopedic implants are applied across, over, or through a fracture during surgery to hold the bone fragments together while the bone heals. These implants may be left in the body or removed at a later date. Examples include plates, pins, screws, rods, wire, nails, or staples. Many types of implants are available, and new ones are constantly being developed.

Internal fixation devices are surgical steel, titanium, or steel alloy appliances used to stabilize the fracture during bone healing. ORIF procedures are discussed later in this chapter.

Important research is exploring *bio-absorbable orthopedic implants.* These implants are placed with the same surgical technique as surgical steel or titanium implants but are ultimately absorbed by the patient. This type of implant is discussed in Chapter 31.

Some fractures require removal of bone fragments or complete replacement of the bone with a prosthesis. Fractures of the radial or femoral head, which result in painful irregular surfaces between the two joint components, often require this type of surgery. Although this procedure is considered an open fixation, the surgical technologist must realize that the surgical set-up is just like that of a total hip, total shoulder, or total elbow replacement. Typically the "ball" part of the joint and not the "socket" part is involved in this type of open reduction. Care must be taken to avoid scarring of the "socket" part of the joint in this procedure (Figure 27-14).

IMMOBILIZATION METHODS
Casts
The application of a plaster or fiberglass cast or splint is a procedure of its own. The procedure is treated as part of the surgical dressing, but the proper placement of a cast or a splint brings many patient safety issues. Surgical technologists are involved in the procedure by directly applying the cast or splint, by holding the limb, or by handing up the supplies.

When a cast is applied, it must immobilize the joint above and the joint below the fracture site. This often is a difficult task, as in fractures of the proximal humerus. Casting materials available in the operating room include plaster of Paris

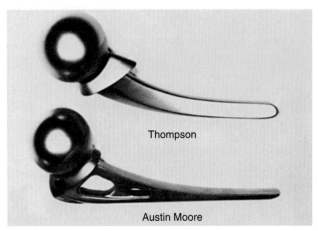

FIGURE 27-14
Thompson and Austin Moore femoral endoprostheses. (From Rothrock J: *Alexander's care of the patient in surgery,* ed 12, St Louis, 2003, Mosby; courtesy Zimmer Inc., Warsaw, Ind.)

and fiberglass. Both come in 2-inch to 6-inch rolls as well as strips of material called splints. Splints are used as a postoperative dressing in open reduction procedures and many soft-tissue procedures. If a splint is used as a postoperative dressing, it is used to immobilize the surgical site until postoperative swelling is decreased and to limit the motion of the limb for a few days as the wound heals. The different types of casts are illustrated in Figure 27-15.

Plaster casting is the most popular material because of its manipulability and strength. Fiberglass also has excellent properties. Fiberglass is very strong and waterproof, which makes it excellent for pediatric patients.

Traditional cast construction, using plaster of Paris or fiberglass, often results in cutaneous complications, including macerations, ulceration, infections, burns, blisters, rashes, and allergic contact dermatitis. Patients report that plaster casts itch, smell, and are difficult to keep dry. Plaster of Paris casts break down if they get wet. Although fiberglass casts with stockinet and cast padding can withstand mois-

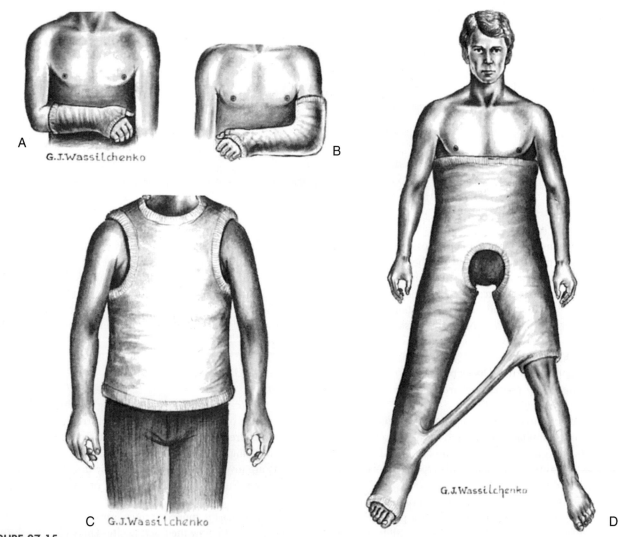

FIGURE 27-15
Types of casts. **A,** Short arm cast. **B,** Long arm cast. **C,** Plaster body jacket cast. **D,** One and one-half hip hip spica cast. (From Mourad LA: *Orthopedic disorders,* St Louis, 1991, Mosby.)

ture, they must be dried, perhaps with a hair dryer, to minimize cutaneous complications. A fiberglass cast with a waterproof liner that "breathes" is a treatment option for patients who have nondisplaced or stable fractures or severe sprains. The liner is used with fiberglass casting material and is made of Gore-Tex by W.L. Gore and Associates. The surgeon will determine the type of casting to be used on an individual basis.

PROCEDURE AND PATIENT SAFETY IN APPLICATION OF A CAST

1. The limb should be elevated during this process.
2. If a surgical dressing is needed (for open reductions), it is applied through aseptic technique before the cast is applied.
3. The limb is wrapped with expandable webbing (such as stockinet)
4. *Webril* rolls are applied
   a. Webril is a soft cotton roll. When it is applied, care must be taken to avoid folds or wrinkles in the wrap. If the cast is applied over folds in the Webril, the patient can develop a pressure sore or blisters under the cast.
5. The casting splints (or plaster rolls) are then dipped in *cold* water and applied as directed by the surgeon.
   a. Cold water must be used when dipping the plaster. When the plaster begins to dry, it gives off heat. Additional heat caused by hot water could cause a burn under the cast.
6. The casting material is placed along the long axis of the bone (as in a posterior splint) or around the limb (as in a short arm cast).
   a. During the process of "wrapping" a limb with casting material, the limb must be elevated. The surgical technologist who is holding the limb must not put direct pressure on the material as it dries. The pressure placed on the cast may cause a pressure sore or blister to develop under the cast.
   b. The technologist then must hold the cast lightly with the palm of the hand and not with the fingers.
7. The limb remains elevated and held securely in a position of comfort for the patient.
   a. The limb should be elevated as the patient wakes up from the anesthetic or IV sedation.
   b. Pillows or towels are used to elevate a limb after the casting material has dried.
      i. Reflective materials (such as a pillow with a plastic coating or plastic pillow case) should not be used as they will reflect the heat given off by the casting material back into the patient's limb and cause a burn.
   c. Postoperative swelling may occur at the fracture site, causing prominent blood vessels to become compressed and compromise the limb's circulatory function.
      i. The tip of the limb must be cleaned of all prepping solutions and casting materials so that the patient can be monitored for signs of circulatory disruption.

   b. The surgeon often will place a cast such as a short arm cast and then bifurcate the cast (cut the cast lengthwise across the sides) to allow for postoperative swelling. The cast is changed in 5 to 7 days during a postoperative visit.
      i. Signs of circulatory disruption are: increasing pain in the limb, pain that progresses into numbness, and cyanotic or cold skin (especially fingers and toes).

COMPLICATIONS

Complications that arise from fractured bones include hemorrhage, edema, and soft-tissue injury. The displaced bone ends often cause tendon and muscle tissue to be pulled, twisted, or bruised. Nerves, blood vessels, or organs that lie adjacent to the fracture site may be injured during the trauma, or the displaced bones themselves can cause further injury.

During clinical evaluation of the orthopedic patient, extensive examination may be necessary to discover these additional injuries. Orthopedic repair often is performed on an emergency basis to prevent further injury.

ORTHOPEDIC EQUIPMENT AND INSTRUMENTS

Orthopedic Table

The orthopedic or fracture table allows the patient to be positioned for placement of hip nails, IM rods, and other orthopedic appliances.

A common hip nailing position is illustrated in Figure 27-16. The patient rests with the injured leg restrained in a boot-like device. The leg may be rotated, pulled into traction, or released, as the surgery requires.

Fracture tables vary widely from manufacturer to manufacturer, and the scrub and the circulator should become well acquainted with the use of the tables with which they work.

The process of positioning a patient on the fracture table brings many safety issues. Some general safety guidelines are:

▶ The patient's affected leg is held by a traction device that is well padded to protect the foot.

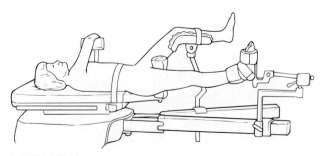

FIGURE 27-16
The orthopedic fracture table. The unaffected leg is raised. (From Rothrock J: *Alexander's care of the patient in surgery,* ed 12, St Louis, 2003, Mosby.)

▶ The unaffected leg rests comfortably on the leg support and is well cushioned. If the existing cushion on the leg rest puts pressure on the heel, a pillow must be placed under the lower leg to lift it from the leg rest.

▶ A restraint strap secures the unaffected leg.

▶ A center post is placed at the perineum and is well padded for protection with soft towels and abdominal pads.

▶ The arm rests lightly over the abdomen or may rest on an armboard in the manner previously described.

▶ Radiographs may be taken during the procedure because the unaffected leg is well out of the field of the radiograph.

Pneumatic Tourniquet

The pneumatic tourniquet is used during most orthopedic extremity procedures. The tourniquet allows a bloodless surgical site, which helps with proper visualization. A pneumatic tourniquet can be used in either an unsterile application (most common) or a sterile application, which requires that a sterile tourniquet be placed after the skin prep.

The surgeon wraps the limb with a sterile Ace wrap or Esmarch bandage to exsanguinate the limb. The limb then is wrapped tightly, beginning at the distal end and working in a proximal direction. The Ace or Esmarch bandage compresses the blood vessels of the limb and pushes most or all the blood out of and away from the limb. The tourniquet is inflated, and the time started is noted.

An average, healthy 50-year-old patient can tolerate continuous tourniquet pressure less than 1 hour on the upper extremity and 2 hours on the thigh. The surgeon must be told how long the tourniquet has been inflated beginning every 30 minutes. The tourniquet may be periodically deflated. If this is the case, the interval between deflation and reinflation should be 5 minutes for every 30 minutes of tourniquet time to minimize adverse effects on the muscles, nerves, and circulatory system of the limb.

The total time that the tourniquet is inflated must be documented in the patient's operative report. Pneumatic tourniquets are illustrated in Figure 27-17.

Power Equipment

Power equipment is used often in orthopedic surgery. Power tools may be powered by electricity, batteries, or nitrogen, depending on the manufacturer and the type of procedure being performed.

Power sources should be checked for problems regularly, and a program of thorough maintenance following the manufacturer's instructions should be performed by the hospital or surgical staff.

Improper usage or maintenance can lead to outages or serious damage to the equipment and can lead to situations in the operating room that are unsafe for the patient or the staff. Whenever power-driven cutting instruments are in use, the scrub should lightly irrigate the cutting blade with saline solution (with the surgeon's approval). Irrigation reduces friction and prevents the tissue and bone from burning and drying.

The surgical technologist must understand and be familiar with the proper assembly and function of all power equipment. Figure 27-18 illustrates many of the different types of Stryker drills that are available.

Arthroscopic Equipment and Instrumentation

The arthroscope is a lensed, fiberoptic telescope that is inserted into a joint space for diagnostic purposes. The surgeon must have well-functioning equipment that gives him or her the best possible view. The types of equipment needed for these cases include:

▶ Video monitor
▶ Light source
▶ Arthroscopy pump
▶ Pump tubing
▶ Water or saline (surgeon's preference)
▶ Patella shaver
▶ Camera
▶ Printer and print paper for pictures
▶ Electrocautery

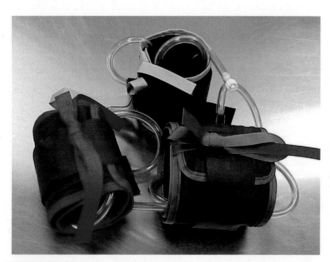
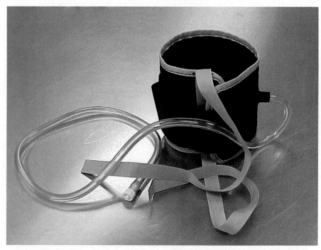

FIGURE 27-17
Disposable pneumatic tourniquets. Note the Velcro attachment to allow snug placement of the tourniquet and the Luer-Lok attachment on the tubing that attaches to the air source. (Picture courtesy of the College of Southern Idaho, Twin Falls, Idaho.)

There are many manufacturers of arthroscopy instruments, but all instruments have similar components (Figure 27-19). The following instrumentation is needed for a simple arthroscopy:

▶ Inflow cannula: for irrigation, to enter and expand the joint space
▶ Scope cannula: used as an insertion port through which the arthroscope may enter the joint
▶ Probe/hook: used as a feeler to move and manipulate structures within the joint
▶ Arthroscope: used to view the joint, comes in different degrees (e.g., 30-degree and 70-degree)
▶ Camera: a lens that attaches to the arthroscope and allows the image being viewed to be transmitted to a video screen.

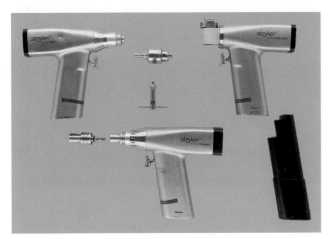

FIGURE 27-18
Types of Stryker drills. *Top, left to right,* Stryker battery-powered drills: drill, adapter, chuck key, sagittal saw. *Bottom, left to right,* Stryker battery-powered drill: adapter, reamer, battery pack. (From Tighe S: *Instrumentation for the operating room,* ed 6, St Louis, 2003, Mosby.)

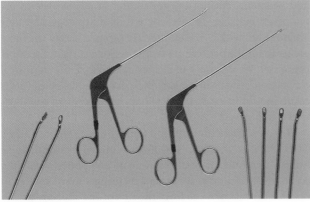

FIGURE 27-19
Arthroscopy instruments and arthroscopes. *Left to right,* tips: 1 Acufex Duckbill biter, right; 1 Acufex Duckbill biter, left. 1 Acufex Duckbill biter, upbite; 1 Acufex Duckbill biter, straight bite. Tips: 4 Acufex Ducklings bill biters: right, upbite, straight, left. (From Tighe S: *Instrumentation for the operating room,* ed 6, St Louis, 2003, Mosby.)

Orthopedic Instrumentation

Orthopedic instruments vary according to the type of orthopedic operation. Each type of procedure has a special set-up of instruments; large bone trays are used with large procedures, and small bone trays are used with delicate bones and soft-tissue procedures. Some complex procedures require multiple trays of instrument sets.

The surgical technologist must be familiar with the procedure as well as the instruments to be used so that careful planning and preparation for the procedure will ensure efficient use of time and instrumentation. However, an entry-level surgical technologist could not yet be familiar with all the specialized instrumentation that is used in orthopedic procedures. This knowledge comes with time and experience in the operating room. After the technologist understands the "flow" of the operation, the instrumentation and techniques become simple, even though the procedures can be complex.

A large bone set is illustrated in Figure 27-20. A small bone set is illustrated in Figure 27-21. The sets differ in the size of their instruments, but note that both sets have the same basic instrumentation, such as Kelly clamps, Kocher clamps, Metzenbaum scissors, and forceps for working on soft tissue; and specialty orthopedic instruments designed to cut, rasp, and measure bone, as well as similar types of retractors and rongeurs.

IMPACTORS, EXTRACTORS, AND SCREWDRIVERS

Impactors (or drivers), extractors, and screwdrivers are instruments used to place or remove orthopedic implants.

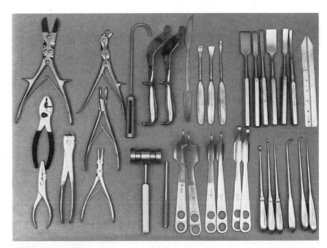

FIGURE 27-20
Large bone set, *left to right. Top,* Stille-Liston bone-cutting forceps; Stille-Luer rongeur; bone hook; Bennett retractors; rasp; Langenbeck periosteal elevators (wide and narrow); Cushing periosteal elevators, osteotomes (straight, curved); ruler. *Middle,* pliers; Adson cranial rongeur. *Bottom,* needle-nosed pliers; pin cutter; Zaufal-Jansen rongeur; mallet; bone tamp; Hohmann retractors (wide sharp, narrow sharp, blunt); curettes (straight, curved). (From Rothrock J: *Alexander's care of the patient in surgery,* ed 12, St Louis, 2003, Mosby.)

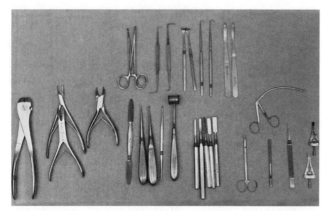

FIGURE 27-21
Extremity or small bone set, *left to right. Top,* baby Mixters; Ragnell retractors; Alm retractors; Volkman hooks; mini-Hohmann retractors. *Bottom,* pin cutter; Lempert and Carroll rongeurs; Liston bone cutter; bone rasp; small curettes; fine double-ended curette; small mallet; Hoke osteotomes; Littler scissors; tendon passer; Beaver blade handle; Carroll elevator; Miltex self-retaining retractors. (From Rothrock J: *Alexander's care of the patient in surgery,* ed 12, St Louis, 2003, Mosby.)

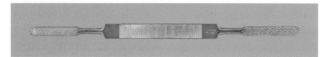

FIGURE 27-22
Double-ended Cottle bone rasp. (From Tighe S: *Instrumentation for the operating room,* ed 6, St Louis, 2003, Mosby.)

Impactors and drivers are placed over the head or fixed to the end of the implant, which may then be driven into or onto the bone with a mallet. This prevents the mallet from contacting the fixation device and scratching, nicking, or denting it. Extractors are designed to fit over the head of the fixation device for its removal.

There are many types of implantable screws. These screws may or may not be used with plates or rods, but they always require the use of a screwdriver. Screwdrivers have different heads (cross hatches or a hole on the head of the screw) that must fit the type of screw being removed. It is helpful if the surgeon notes in the preoperative history and physical the type of screw being removed so that the surgical technologist can prepare for the operation.

CUTTING AND DISSECTING INSTRUMENTS

These types of instruments all have sharp edges. They are used to separate, incise, dissect, and excise tissue. For safety and to prevent injury, they always should be kept in a secluded area.

Rasps are used to smooth the surface of bone. They are hand held and often double ended. A surgeon often will opt to use a high-speed bur to smooth bone instead of a hand-held rasp. The effect is the same. Irrigation is needed to cool the bur and keep the heat produced by the bur from burning the bone (Figure 27-22).

Reamers are used to form a hollow area in the bone. Reamers may be bell shaped, such as those used in creating a space in the acetabulum for a prosthesis, or they may be long

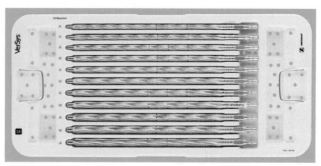

FIGURE 27-23
Reamers. (From Tighe S: *Instrumentation for the operating room,* ed 6, St Louis, 2003, Mosby.)

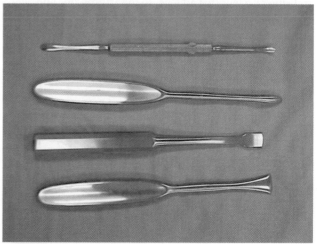

FIGURE 27-24
Periosteal elevators, *top to bottom:* Freer, Langenbeck, Key, and Cushing elevators. (Picture courtesy of the College of Southern Idaho, Twin Falls, Idaho.)

and narrow, such as those used to create a hole to accommodate a large intramedullary nail. A reamer is illustrated in Figure 27-23.

Elevators are used to lift the periosteum from the surface of the bone and to perform fine dissection during tendon and ligament repair. They are similar in appearance to osteotomes, but they do not have a fine, sharp edge, and they are not used with a mallet; they are scraped across the bone gently to lift the periosteum from the bone surface. Elevators come in a wide variety of shapes and sizes. Freer periosteal elevators are small to $\frac{1}{8}$ inch and curved, and Key elevators come in widths of $\frac{1}{4}$ inch to 2 inches. Elevators are illustrated in Figure 27-24.

Rongeurs are used to cut and remove bone (Figure 27-25). These are *double action* (two hinges) or *single action* (single hinge). The rongeur removes bone in small bites, which the scrub must retrieve as specimens by using a moist sponge to remove the bits of bone from the tips of the rongeur.

Saws are used to cut through fine bone. These are power driven and are available in two types. The *reciprocating* saw blade vibrates in and out. The *oscillating* saw blade vibrates back and forth. These saws are used to remove small spurs or to smooth the surface of a bone. Both types of orthopedic saws are shown in Figure 27-26.

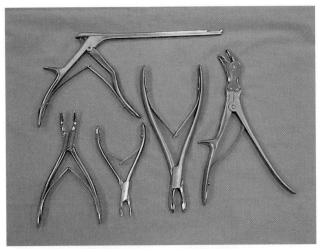

FIGURE 27-25
Rongeurs. (Picture courtesy of the College of Southern Idaho, Twin Falls, Idaho.)

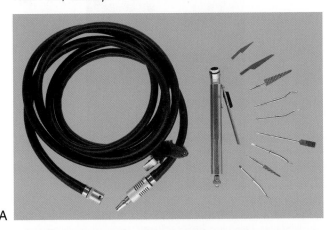

A

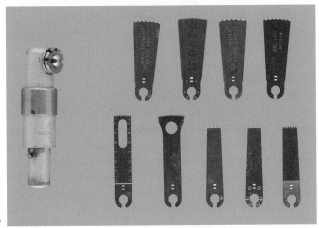

B

FIGURE 27-26
A, Reciprocating micro saw, power cord, saw handle, and assorted blades. **B,** Oscillating saw and blades. (From Tighe S: *Instrumentation for the operating room,* ed 6, St Louis, 2003, Mosby.)

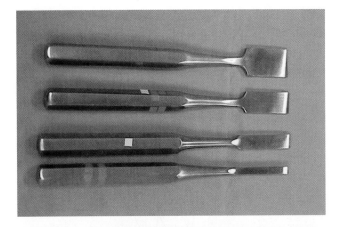

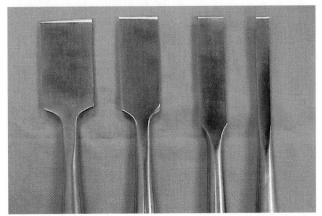

FIGURE 27-27
Top, top to bottom, 3 osteotomes and a gouge. *Bottom,* Tips of the instruments in the top photograph. (Courtesy the College of Southern Idaho, Twin Falls, Idaho.)

Osteotomes, curettes, and *gouges* are used to trim and sculpt bone or to remove bone to be used as an autologous graft (Figure 27-27). While they are all classified as cutting instruments, they all have very distinctly different uses. The osteotome creates a sliver of bone that can be used as a graft and leaves a flattened surface. The curette is used to spoon out bits of bone from a curved area. The gouge creates a grooved surface on the bone. These instruments are heavy and sharp, and should be handled carefully. Their cutting edges should be protected. Osteotomes and gouges usually are handed to the surgeon with a mallet.

Drills may be hand operated or power operated, and are used in conjunction with a *drill bit.* These are small, graduated pins that have a spiral cutting edge. A drill bit is used to drill a hole in which a screw or pin may be inserted. Drill bits are kept in a rack that protects their sharp edges and allows the surgical team easy access to them. Drills may have a drill chuck and key for tightening the drill bit into the chuck. The anatomy of a drill bit is illustrated in Figure 27-28.

Measuring devices are used during implant procedures. Two commonly used measuring devices are the *caliper* and the *depth gauge.* The caliper is used to measure the width of a ball joint head, such as the femoral or humeral head, in preparation for a prosthetic implant. The depth gauge is used to measure the depth of the hole made by a drill bit to determine the length of screw that is needed.

Retractors are used to retract soft tissue away from the wound site or to hold the wound edges open. Many types of retractors are available for orthopedic procedures and are very specific to the type of patient and the type of operation

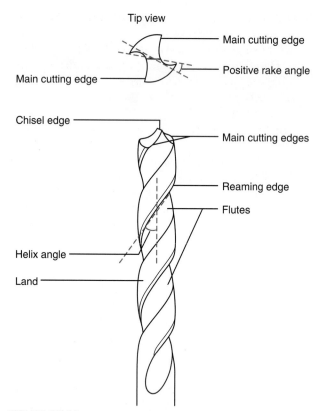

FIGURE 27-28
The anatomy of a drill bit. (From Browner BD, Jupiter JB, Levine AM, et al: *Skeletal trauma: basic science, management, and reconstruction,* ed 3, Philadelphia, 2003, Saunders.)

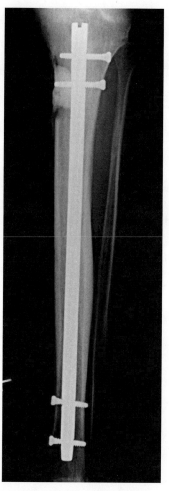

FIGURE 27-29
IM rod of a femur. (From Browner BD, Jupiter JB, Levine AM, et al: *Skeletal trauma: basic science, management, and reconstruction,* ed 3, Philadelphia, 2003, Saunders.)

being performed. For example, a Charnley hip retractor is used specifically during a total hip joint replacement, and a Blount knee retractor is used only for knee procedures.

Bone clamps are used to hold a bone in place during ORIF or while the bone is being cut (as in a bunionectomy). Bone clamps are available in large, heavy sizes, such as the Lane clamp, and in delicate sizes, such as the Lewin clamp. Many operating rooms ask that bone clamps be packaged together so that the surgeon has a choice of bone clamps during the procedure. It is not uncommon to use something as familiar as a baby towel clip or a Kocher clamp to hold a small bone, and these instruments are found in the bone set.

INTERNAL FIXATION DEVICES (IMPLANTS)

Pins and bolts are inserted across two small bone fragments, such as those of the hand, ankle, elbow, or wrist. They also may serve as an attachment point for traction. They are inserted with a drill or pin driver. See the illustration of pins used in the reduction of a fracture of the radial head in Figure 27-12.

Nails and *rods* are used to span the longitudinal axis of the humerus, femur, or tibial shaft. They also may be driven into the medullary canal to span two fracture ends. Nails and rods are driven with a *driver* or *impactor* and have a set of specialized instruments for insertion. IM rod replacement for femoral fracture is illustrated in Figure 27-29.

Staples are used to reconnect soft tissue to bone, such as during ligament repair of the knee. Staples are available in various sizes and weights. They are driven with a *staple driver* and a mallet. They typically are packaged with a specialty extractor as well.

Plates and *screw fixation* are used to span the surface of two large bone fragments. This technique might be used in a fracture of the femur. The plates are held in place with *screws.* In Figure 27-30, *A,* a forearm fracture is successfully reduced via a dynamic compression plate and screws.

Any discussion about different screws and their applications should be based on an understanding of basic screw types and their anatomy. There are two basic types of screws, cancellous and cortical. Figure 27-30, *B* illustrates the two types of screws.

The ability of a screw to achieve interfragmentary fixation or stable attachment of a plate depends on its ability to hold firmly in bone and resist pullout. The *pullout strength* of a screw is proportional to the surface area of thread that is in contact with the bone. Surgeons describe the surface area of thread in contact with bone as "bite" during ORIF.

Screws are placed across the fracture ends of small bones such as those of the ankle. They also are used to attach a plate to bone or to attach soft tissues to bone. Screws are implanted with a surgical *screwdriver.*

Figure 27-30, *C* shows the steps of inserting a cortical lag screw after reduction of a fracture.

Although the procedure may look complex to the beginner, the steps actually are quite simple. As in other surgical specialties, the placement of implantable orthopedic screws (or plates and screws) is a sequential procedure. If the surgical team understands the principles of placement of screws for compression, the procedure becomes less laborious and actually quite satisfying. The simplified, sequential steps are listed below.

The sequence for instrumentation has been highlighted.

1. Reduce the fracture.
2. Determine the *diameter of screw* that will be used.

3. **Drill a hole** with a drill bit smaller than the diameter of the screw that will be used.
   a. The surgical technologist always should announce the size of drill bit and tap being handed to the surgeon in case the technique has changed from the norm.
4. **Use the depth gauge** to determine *the length of screw* that will be used.
5. **Use the tap** to "score" the bone and make "ridges" for the screw to follow.
   a. Under most circumstances, the same diameter of tap will be used as is used for the screw.
   b. While the surgeon is tapping the bone, the surgical technologist should check the length of the screw by measuring it and then placing it on the self-retaining screwdriver.

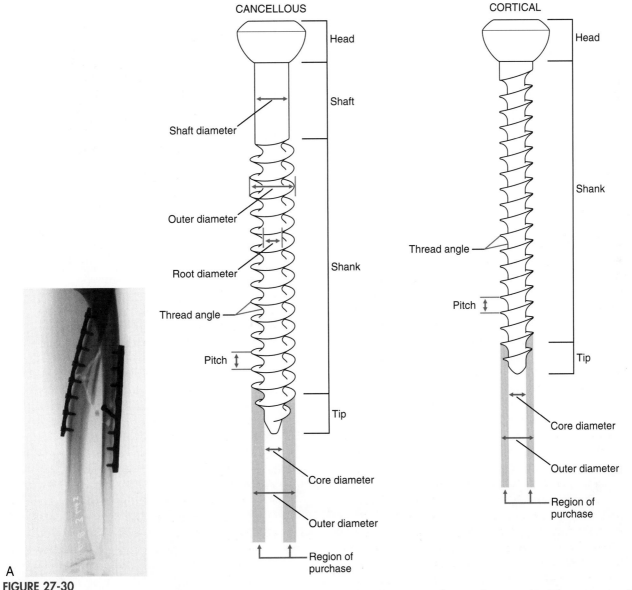

FIGURE 27-30
A, Plate and screw placement in a forearm fracture. **B,** Anatomy of the cancellous and cortical screws. (**A-C** from Browner BD, Jupiter JB, Levine AM, et al: *Skeletal trauma: basic science, management, and reconstruction,* ed 3, Philadelphia, 2003, Saunders)

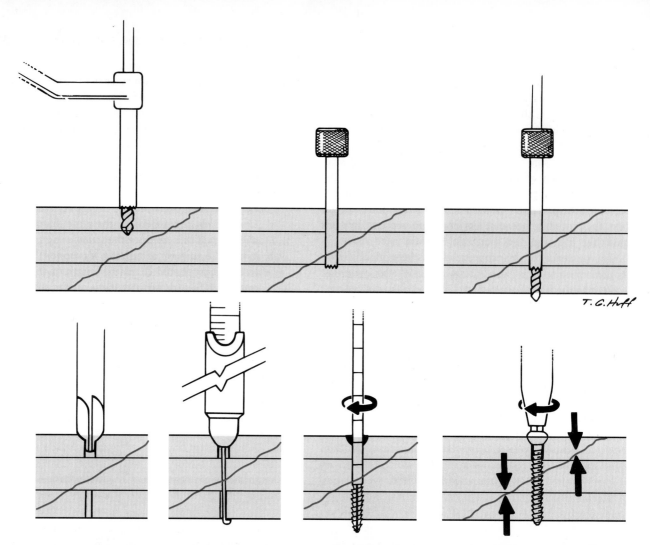

C

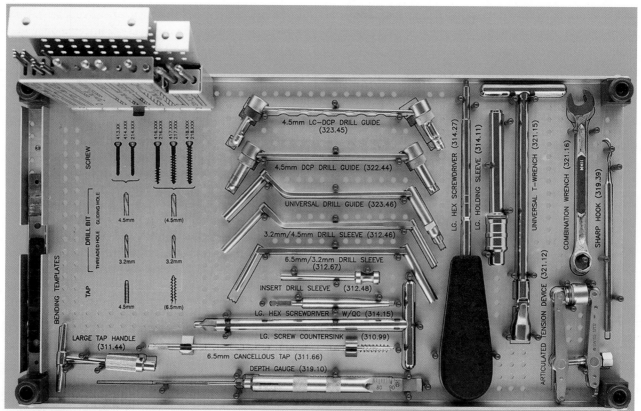

D

FIGURE 27-30, cont'd

C, Technique for screw placement. **D,** Association for the Study of Internal Fixation (ASIF) basic low contact–dynamic compression plate (LD-DCP) and DCP instrument set. (**D** from Tighe S: *Instrumentation for the operating room,* ed 6, St Louis, 2003, Mosby.)

6. **Using the screwdriver,** place the screw into the plate or across the fracture.

Screw placement can be performed in multiple ways, just as there are multiple types of fractures, but the basics listed above remain the same. The instrumentation needed for the procedure described above is an ASIF basic instrumentation set (Figure 27-30, *D*).

Care of Orthopedic Implants

The Food and Drug Administration (FDA) requires strict documentation and tracking of implant devices. Documentation should include:

▶ The patient's permanent record
▶ The operative report
▶ The implant registry
▶ The manufacturer

Information to be recorded includes the lot and serial number of the implants used; the manufacturer; and the size, type, and anatomical position of the implant.

Many different types of alloys are used in the manufacture of orthopedic implants. It is in each patient's best interest, however, that only one particular type of alloy be used in the patient. This will prevent galvanic corrosion. For example, a surgical steel plate should never be used with titanium screws.

Orthopedic implants are extremely expensive. For that reason, all surgical personnel should follow these basic guidelines to prevent implant damage:

1. *Internal fixation devices should never be reused.* Any imperfections created while placing or removing the device will increase the potential for corrosion and weaken the implant.
2. *Bending of the implants to make them conform to the contour of the bone should be avoided.* When bending is necessary, the proper bending press should be used. When an implant has been bent, it should not be reshaped. This may weaken the implant.
3. *Special care should be used in storage, processing, and handling of implants.* Implants should be individually wrapped and processed. During processing, the implants should be protected. They should be put in appropriate sterilization trays and padded to avoid moving around in the tray.
4. *Any internal fixation device that has become damaged in processing or storage should be discarded.*

Bone Cement

Bone cement, also known polymethyl methacrylate (PMMA), is used to secure and cement some orthopedic implants. Implants that would need cement include:

▶ Total knee arthroplasty
▶ Total hip arthroplasty

The acrylic cement is composed of a liquid monomer and a copolymer, methylmethacrylate-styrene (a powder). The bone cement polymer does not present a fire hazard, but the liquid monomer is highly flammable. The electrosurgical unit (ESU) should never be brought near the liquid or the surface of the uncured cement, as it could present a fire hazard.

When the two compounds are mixed, the liquid will exhibit a strong vapor. While the cement is not toxic to the patient, excessive exposure to the fumes is potentially dangerous for the OR staff.

Excessive exposure to the vapors can produce:

▶ Eye irritation
▶ Skin irritation
▶ Respiratory tract irritation
▶ Depression of the central nervous system
    ▶ Drowsiness
    ▶ Fatigue
    ▶ Sleep disturbance
    ▶ Irritability
    ▶ Headaches
▶ Possible effects on the liver or kidneys

Pregnant women should not be present in the OR during the mixing of the bone cement. Most hospitals have a standing policy or procedure in place regarding employees working with the bone glue. Students should follow the same policy. There are many special hoods and evacuators that will disperse the fumes and reduce the potential for harm.

Adverse patient reactions have been associated with the use of PMMA. These include hypotension, cardiac arrest, cardiovascular accident (CVA), pulmonary emboli, thrombophlebitis, and hypersensitivity. These reactions, and especially cardiac arrest and death, have resulted after insertion of the bone cement. The reactions are uncommon, and the exact cause of the reactions is unknown.

Technique   **MIXING THE BONE CEMENT**

1. The scrub begins by emptying the entire package of powder into the sterile mixing bowl.
2. The vial of monomer is opened and added to the powder.
3. The top of the mixing bowl is closed.
4. The cement is then stirred in the mixing bowl for about 2 minutes.
5. When the cement has reached the proper consistency, it is ready to be loaded into an injector (sometimes called a cement gun) or placed in the patient or on the prosthesis by hand.
6. After the cement has been applied and the prosthesis has been impacted (hammered into place with a surgical mallet and a specialized impactor that is made to properly place the prosthesis), the total setting time for the prosthesis in the cement is 8 to 16 minutes.
7. As the bone hardens and chemically changes, it becomes quite hot. The scrub should retain a piece of the glue to check for heat and subsequently to see if the glue is hardening and report the progress to the surgeon

According to the Environmental Protection Agency (EPA), bone cement is classified as a hazardous substance and requires proper disposal and special handling. Principal safety practices when working with bone cement include always wearing safety glasses and surgical gloves that are suitable for working with bone cement. Non-latex gloves are not recommended, as liquid may be absorbed through them.

POSITIONING

Positioning is a very important aspect of orthopedic surgery and can be quite involved. The position of the patient should allow proper exposure of the operative site and should prevent pressure on the muscles, nerves, and blood vessels. If necessary, extra padding and support can be used. The type of position selected depends on the type of procedure, location of surgery, and surgeon's preference.

Lateral Position

The lateral position is regularly used for operations on the hip, shoulder, and sometimes ankle. The patient usually is placed on a bean bag or a positioning board, or is held in position with rolled towels. The bean bag takes the shape of the patient's body structure. The bean bag inflates in the opposite manner that a beach ball inflates: the bag is attached to a suction device, and as the air is sucked out of the bag, the bag hardens and keeps the patient in position. If repositioning of the patient is required, one would simply let air back into the bag to soften it up.

Prone Position

Procedures on the back, shoulder, ankle, and Achilles tendon can be performed while the patient is in the prone position. See Chapter 10 for information on and illustrations of these positions.

SURGICAL PROCEDURES

Arthroscopic procedures
KNEE ARTHROSCOPY
Surgical Goal
Knee arthroscopy is a diagnostic visual exam of the joint through the use of a camera.

Pathology
An arthroscopy is used for diagnosing and repairing injury to the knee joint. Some procedures that are typically performed through the arthroscope are:

▶ Possible meniscal tears (lateral or medial)
▶ Anterior cruciate ligament (ACL) repair
▶ Posterior cruciate ligament (PCL) repair
▶ Medial collateral ligament (MCL) repair
▶ Synovitis
▶ Chondroplasty (lateral, medial condylar, tibial, or patellar)
▶ Excessive osteophytes
▶ Lateral release
▶ Removal of foreign body

Technique

1. An incision is made lateral to the patella with a #11 or a #15 blade.
2. An inflow cannula is inserted into the knee joint.
3. An incision is made medially, and the scope sheath is inserted into the knee joint.
4. The 30-degree scope is passed through the sheath.
5. An 18-gauge spinal needle is inserted into the knee joint, marking the third incision.
6. A probe is used to check stability of the meniscus and ACL.
7. Any repair work that is needed (e.g., arthroscopic meniscectomy) is performed after this endoscopic exam.
8. The knee is irrigated and closed.
9. At the surgeon's preference, Marcaine may be injected into the knee joint and infiltrated at the incision sites.
10. With many older patients, a steroid such as Depo-Medrol is instilled into the knee joint at this time.
11. A pressure dressing and knee immobilizer are applied.

Discussion
The patient is placed in the supine position on the table. Spinal or general anesthesia is administered. Before the patient is prepped and after the patient is relaxed, the surgeon may choose to perform a knee examination under anesthesia (EUA), checking for problems with flexion, extension, and manipulation.

A tourniquet is applied to the operative leg. The tourniquet setting depends on the patient's blood pressure. The foot of the bed is flexed 90 degrees. The nonoperative leg is placed in a padded leg holder, and the operative leg is placed in a holding device. There are several types of knee holders. They are designed to secure the leg and allow counter traction, which "opens" the knee joint for better visualization during the procedure.

When the patient has been positioned, the prep is performed from mid thigh to the ankle circumferentially, the patient is draped, and the extremity is exsanguinated. The tourniquet then is inflated. The incision is made lateral to the patella and just above the joint line, allowing an inflow cannula to be inserted into the knee joint without damaging the cartilage.

When the knee has been infiltrated with fluid, a second incision is made medially, and a sharp trocar and sheath are inserted into the knee joint. The trocar then is removed and replaced with a blunt trocar. The knee is irrigated and any effusion is removed, and then the blunt trocar is replaced with a 30-degree scope through the existing sheath.

An 18-gauge spinal needle is then inserted into the knee joint under direct visualization to determine placement of a third incision. This incision creates an opposite portal for the insertion of the probe and operative instruments. The location of this incision depends on the results of the EUA or other preoperative diagnostic exams.

Through the scope, the surgeon begins viewing the knee joint and surrounding surfaces, including the synovium.

The surgeon checks for the presence of loose bodies or pathology.

OPERATIVE ARTHROSCOPY

Arthroscopic resection and repair of a meniscal tear is a very common procedure. A diagnostic arthroscopy is performed before any corrective procedures are started.

The menisci are structures in the knee that distribute load across the joint and produce capsular stability. A tear in the meniscus is the most common knee injury. The medial meniscus is injured more often than the lateral meniscus. The treatment of meniscal tears is aimed at preserving the structure. Meniscectomy may be partial or complete. Complete meniscectomy leaves the medial rim of the structure to share load bearing and stabilize the knee.

When the meniscus is in view, the surgeon locates the tear using the probe. The tear is removed with a hook knife, a sharp grasping instrument, or a motorized shaver. Meniscal tears that occur outside the outer vascular zone (the outer 10%) do not heal well and cannot be sutured.

ARTHROSCOPIC ANTERIOR CRUCIATE LIGAMENT REPAIR

Surgical Goal

The surgical goal of this procedure is to reconstruct the ACL in active individuals who have an unstable knee that interferes with their activity.

Pathology

The ACL is the knee ligament torn most often. Injury usually results from stepping and twisting the knee at the same time. ACL repair most often includes replacement of the ligament with a substitute, such as autograft, allograft, or synthetic ligament. Autografts are currently the substitute of choice, particularly the patellar tendon attached to the patellar and tibial bone blocks.

Instrumentation for arthroscopic ACL repair includes all the diagnostic arthroscopy equipment and the ACL reconstruction system. In addition, the procedure requires some type of fixation device (e.g., screws, staples, spiked washers, interference screws) and bone plugs. Power equipment includes drills, a microsagittal saw, and a motorized arthroscopy shaver. Figure 27-31 illustrates and describes arthroscopic ACL repair.

Technique

1. The diagnostic arthroscopy is preformed.
2. Any meniscal tears or injuries are treated.
3. The remaining ACL is debrided with an arthroscopic full-radius shaver.
4. A notch plasty is performed with a 4.5-mm arthroplasty bur, rasp, osteotomes, or curettes.
5. A small incision is made at the distal lateral aspect of the femur. A femoral aiming device is positioned, and a guide pin is inserted (Figure 27-31, A).
6. Another small incision is made below the knee.

7. When the isometric positioning has been determined, a longitudinal skin incision is made medial to the midline near the patellar tendon so that graft can be harvested.
8. The graft is sized. Heavy sutures are placed through drill holes made at the ends of the graft in the bone (Figure 27-31, B).
9. The guide pins are then reinserted and over-drilled with cannulas that are close in width to the prepared graft.
10. Both ends of the graft are fixed with an interference screw (staple, bone screw, or ligament button) as the surgeon desires (Figure 27-31, C).
11. The joint is irrigated and closed.
12. A pressure dressing is applied, and a hinged knee brace is placed before the patient emerges from anesthesia.

Discussion

The patient is prepped and draped for a diagnostic arthroscopy. The arthroscopy is performed and the torn ACL is visualized. Any meniscal tears or injuries are treated.

The remaining ACL is debrided with an arthroscopic full-radius shaver. A notch plasty is performed with a 4.5-mm arthroplasty bur, rasp, osteotomes, or curettes. The notch plasty facilitates visualization during the procedure and protects the graft from wear and from amputation postoperatively.

A small incision is made at the distal lateral aspect of the femur. A femoral aiming device is positioned, and a guide pin is inserted (Figure 27-31, A), allowing reconstruction of the ACL to begin.

Another small incision is made below the knee. The tibial aiming device is positioned, and a guide pin is inserted from the anterior tibial incision to the intercondylar notch. The pins are replaced with heavy suture that passes through the femoral and tibial pin sites. The guide pins are checked for isometric positioning with a tensioning device that is attached with a heavy suture. The surgeon puts the knee through several range-of-motion (ROM) exercises to determine the correct measurement.

When the isometric positioning has been determined, a longitudinal skin incision is made medial to the midline near the patellar tendon so that graft can be harvested. The graft is sized and heavy sutures are placed through drill holes made at the ends of the graft in the bone (Figure 27-31, B).

The guide pins are then reinserted and over-drilled with cannulas that are close in width to the prepared graft. Over-drilling the holes establishes tunnels so that the drilled holes are in the center of the previous insertion sites of the ACL.

Both ends of the graft are fixed with an interference screw (staple, bone screw, or ligament button) of the surgeon's choice (Figure 27-31, C).

The joint is irrigated, and typically a closed drainage system is inserted at closure of the wound. The tourniquet is released, and a pressure dressing is applied, followed by a hinged knee brace. The knee brace must be placed before the

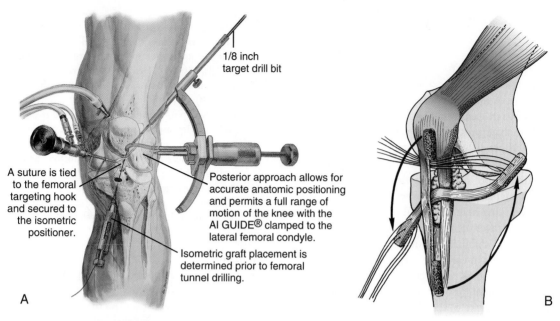

A

B

A suture is tied to the femoral targeting hook and secured to the isometric positioner.

1/8 inch target drill bit

Posterior approach allows for accurate anatomic positioning and permits a full range of motion of the knee with the AI GUIDE® clamped to the lateral femoral condyle.

Isometric graft placement is determined prior to femoral tunnel drilling.

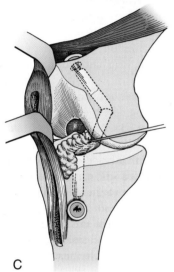

C

FIGURE 27-31
A, Femoral aiming device in position during ACL reconstruction. **B,** The patellar tendon is taken, and drill holes placed in each end of the bone graft. Heavy sutures are placed in the holes to help "pull" the graft through the notch and up through the tunnels. **C,** Both ends of the graft are fixed, in this case with ligament buttons. (**A** courtesy Johnson & Johnson. **B** from Laurin CA et al: *Atlas of orthopedic surgery,* vol 3, 1992, Masson. **C** from Rothrock JC: *Alexander's care of the patient in surgery,* ed 12, St Louis, 2003, Mosby.)

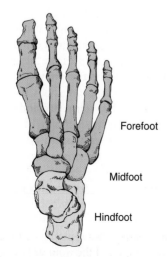

Forefoot

Midfoot

Hindfoot

FIGURE 27-32
Anatomical regions of the foot. (Modified from Wiesel SW and Delahay JN: *Essentials of orthopaedic surgery,* ed 2, Philadelphia, 1997, Saunders.)

patient emerges from anesthesia to protect the new graft from being torn before the bone graft heals.

ANKLE ARTHROSCOPY
Surgical Goal
Ankle arthroscopy is used to visualize the ankle joint.
Pathology
The ankle itself is generally divided for descriptive purposes into three anatomical regions: the midfoot, the hindfoot, and the forefoot (Figure 27-32). The talus is indeed the "keystone" of the foot-ankle relationship, helping to create a "hinge" joint. The ankle also is unique in that about 65% of its surface is covered with articular cartilage and that it has *no* musculotendinous attachments.

Arthroscopy is used to identify abnormalities that have not been identified by radiographic studies or to identify the causes of other symptoms the patient may have, such as pain, swelling, and instability of the ankle (Figure 27-33).

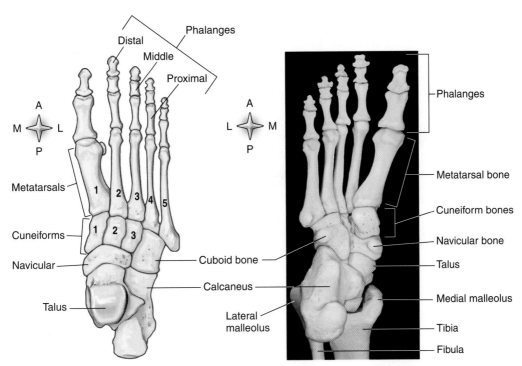

FIGURE 27-33
Radiologic photographs and bony anatomy of the normal foot and ankle. (From Thibodeau GA and Patton KT: *Anthony's textbook of anatomy and physiology,* ed 17, St Louis, 2003, Mosby; photo from Vidic B, Suarez FR: *Photographic atlas of the human body,* St Louis, 1984, Mosby.)

Technique

1. An anteromedial incision is made with a #15 blade.
2. A cannula is inserted.
3. A syringe is used to infuse the joint with saline.
4. An 18-gauge needle is inserted into the ankle and visualized through the scope.
5. The needle is removed, and a #15 blade is used to make an anterolateral incision.
6. A port is inserted into the ankle.
7. A mini shaver or a regular shaver may be used to clear any tissue.
8. The joint is irrigated and closed.
9. A dressing is applied.

Discussion

The patient is placed in the supine position. The unaffected leg is placed in a leg holder. The patient may have a spinal block, general anesthesia, or an ankle block as anesthetic; a primary consideration is that the surgeon needs adequate relaxation to distract the ankle. An ankle distractor is illustrated in Figure 27-34.

A tourniquet is applied to the upper thigh, following all the precautions for using a tourniquet. Often the bleeding can be controlled by the irrigation, and the tourniquet may not be needed. The patient is then prepped from the knee to the toes. The patient is draped with a towel and then an extremity drape. The foot is wrapped with an Esmarch bandage or Ace wrap to exsanguinate the foot.

The anteromedial incision is made with a #15 blade, and a cannula is inserted. A syringe is used to infuse the joint with saline. This port is used for the initial arthroscopy, and later is used for insertion of instrumentation.

When the joint has been distended with saline and can be seen through the arthroscope, an 18-gauge needle is inserted into the ankle. This needle marks the location of the anterolateral portal. The needle then is removed, and an incision is made with a #15 blade. A hemostat may be used to bluntly dissect the capsule.

The scope is inserted into the anteromedial port. Through this port, the surgeon then can view the deltoid ligament, medial malleolus, medial gutter in the medial talomalleolar joint, and any osteochondral lesions. A mini shaver as well a regular shaver may be used to clear any synovitis or other diseased tissue. The joint is then irrigated and closed with 4-0 nylon, and a compression dressing is applied.

SHOULDER ARTHROSCOPY

Surgical Goal

In shoulder arthroscopy, the shoulder joint is visualized with the use of an arthroscope.

Pathology

With an arthroscope, a surgeon can perform extensive visualization to help manage disorders of the shoulder joint, rotator cuff, subacromial bursa, biceps tendon, glenoid, humeral head, and subscapularis tendon. Some pathology may be identified and repaired through the scope. Figure

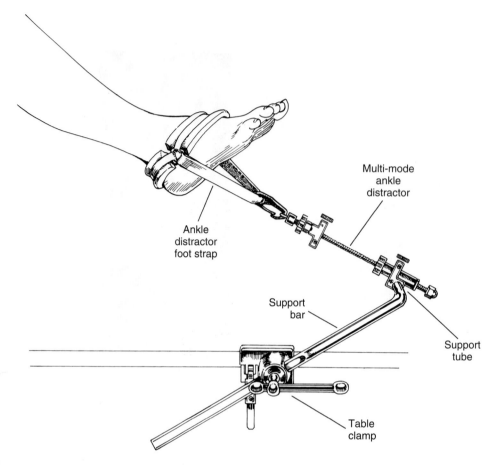

FIGURE 27-34
Noninvasive ankle distractor. (From Rothrock J: *Alexander's care of the patient in surgery,* ed 12, St Louis, 2003, Mosby; courtesy McConnell Orthopaedic Manufacturing Company, Greenville, Tex.)

27-35 illustrates the normal acromioclavicular (AC) joint, and Figure 27-36 illustrates common AC separations.

If the surgeon cannot repair the defect through the scope, he or she may have to open the shoulder. Operating rooms staff members should be prepared to convert the case to open repair.

Indications for a shoulder arthroscopy may include:

▶ Impingement syndrome
▶ Osteophytes of the AC joint
▶ Thickening of the rotator cuff
▶ Bursitis
▶ Frozen shoulder
▶ Rupture of the biceps tendon
▶ Superior labrum anterior-posterior (SLAP) lesion
▶ Removal of loose bodies

Technique

1. The surgeon infiltrates the glenohumeral joint space with 60 ml of saline through an 18-gauge spinal needle.
2. A small puncture is made with a #11 blade.
3. The inflow cannula is inserted, and the joint is distended.
4. A stab incision is made with a #11 blade.
5. The scope sleeve is inserted into the joint.
6. A 30-degree scope is inserted into the sleeve.
7. The anatomy of the shoulder is visualized.
8. An 18-gauge spinal needle is inserted through the skin.
9. A third incision is made.
10. A hook is used to check the stability of the labrum and the rotator cuff.
11. A 4.5 mm full-radius shaver is used to shave any diseased tissue and correct any defects.
12. The joint is irrigated and closed.
13. The dressing is applied, and an arm sling or immobilizer is used as indicated.

Discussion
The patient is placed in a modified Fowler's position, in a lateral decubitus position, or in a beach-chair position. The arm is extended, wrapped, and suspended from a shoulder tower (shoulder traction device).

Depending on the size of the patient, proper weight is added to the tower to distract the shoulder joint. The patient is prepped, beginning at the anterior aspect of the shoulder, extending from the neck to the inferior costal margin, and extending down the back of the shoulder, forearm, hand,

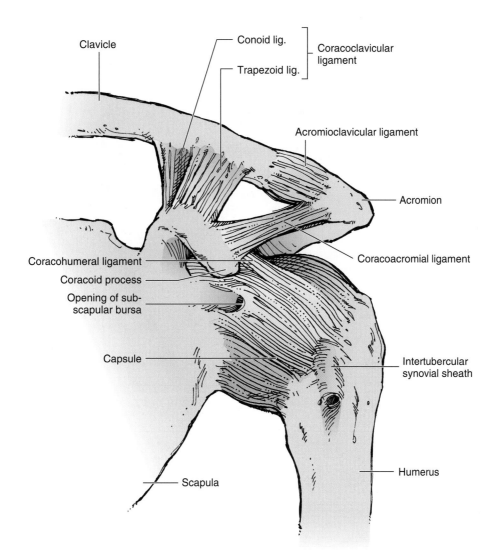

Clavicle

Conoid lig.

Trapezoid lig.

Coracoclavicular ligament

Acromioclavicular ligament

Acromion

Coracoacromial ligament

Coracohumeral ligament

Coracoid process

Opening of sub-scapular bursa

Capsule

Intertubercular synovial sheath

Humerus

Scapula

FIGURE 27-35
Normal AC joint surrounded by ligament and capsule. (Redrawn from Wiesel SW and Delahay JN: *Essentials of orthopaedic surgery,* ed 2, Philadelphia, 1997, Saunders.)

and fingers. The patient is then draped according to the surgeon's preference.

A marking pen is then used to identify the bony landmarks. The surgeon uses an 18-gauge spinal needle and 60 ml of saline with or without epinephrine to infiltrate and expand the joint space. This distracts the joint space, giving the surgeon easier entry into the joint. A small puncture is then made with a #11 blade, and the inflow cannula is inserted.

Irrigation is then connected, and the tubing is unclamped. While the joint is being infiltrated, a third incision is made. The scope sleeve and the 30-degree scope are inserted, and the biceps tendon is identified. Figure 27-37 illustrates the placement of the operative scopes and instruments during a routine shoulder arthroscopy.

The patient's arm is rotated and moved as needed to allow the surgeon to visualize the various structures in and around the joint. Instruments that may be needed to complete the procedure endoscopically are a blunt hook for

checking the rotator cuff and exploring the surrounding tissue and the microbur to smooth bone.

The shoulder is irrigated, incisions are closed with 4-0 nylon, 4 × 4 dressings are applied, and either a shoulder immobilizer or an arm sling is applied.

ARTHROSCOPIC ROTATOR CUFF REPAIR
Surgical Goal
The goal of rotator cuff repair (endoscopic and open) is to restore stability to the shoulder joint, alleviate pain, and allow the patient to return to normal activities.
Pathology
The rotator cuff comprises the supraspinatus muscle, the subscapularis, the infraspinatus, and the teres minor. Most rotator cuff tears occur through the insertion of the tendinous fibers of the supraspinatus muscle that attaches onto the greater tuberosity of the proximal humerus. Rotator cuff tears and impingement syndrome affect middle-aged people

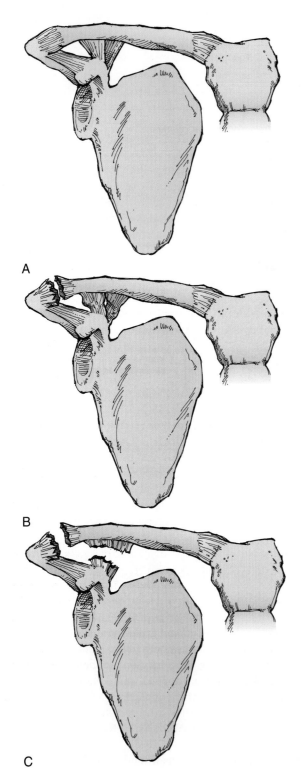

FIGURE 27-36
AC separations. **A,** Grade I: the AC joint is sprained.
B, Grade II: the AC joint is disrupted (coracoclavicular
sprain). **C,** Grade III: disruption of the AC joint and the coracoclavicular ligament. (Modified from Wiesel SW and Delahay JN: *Essentials of orthopaedic surgery,* ed 2, Philadelphia, 1997, Saunders.)

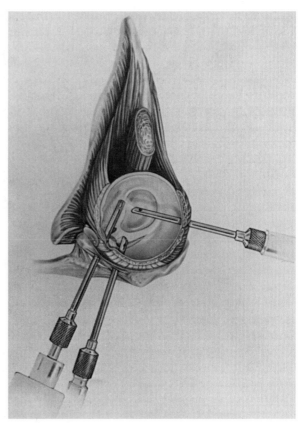

FIGURE 27-37
Placement of the operative instruments during an arthroscopic
repair of the rotator cuff. (From Rothrock J: *Alexander's care
of the patient in surgery,* ed 12, St Louis, 2003, Mosby;
courtesy Smith & Nephew, Andover, Mass.)

most often, and the cause is degenerative. Other causes are
sports injury and accidental injury in younger patients.

Patients with rotator cuff tears may not be able to initiate
abduction of the shoulder because the stabilizing forces of
the ruptured tendons on the humeral head are lost. Methods
of repair depend on the size and shape of the tear.

Technique

1. Entry is the same as a diagnostic shoulder arthroscopy. A
   complete diagnostic arthroscopy is performed.
2. When the tear has been identified, the subacromial space
   is examined.
3. The bursa is removed with an arthroscopic shaver.
4. A bur is used to shave the tissue from the undersurface of
   the acromion (acromioplasty), creating a smooth, flat undersurface.
5. The cuff is then shaved to remove any loose or frayed tissue.
6. A punch and tap are used to create a hole for the anchors.
7. The anchors are impacted.
8. With a suture grasper, the surgeon moves the suture into
   the proper position.
9. With a suture punch, the surgeon threads the suture to the
   tendon from the bone.
10. Suture is then placed, tied down, and cut.
11. The joint is irrigated and closed.
12. The dressing is applied.

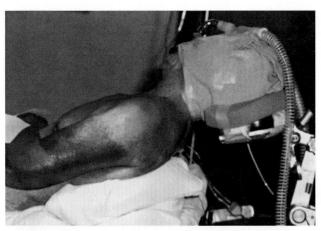

FIGURE 27-38
A patient in the beach-chair position. (From Browner BD, Jupiter JB, Levine AM, et al: *Skeletal trauma: basic science, management, and reconstruction,* ed 3, Philadelphia, 2003, Saunders.)

Discussion

The patient is placed in the beach-chair position (Figure 27-38) and prepped and draped in the usual fashion for an arthroscopy. A complete diagnostic arthroscopy and inspection of the bursa is performed.

The biceps tendon, labrum, glenoid, humeral head, and tendons all are inspected. If there is any pathology, it is addressed after initial inspection.

When the tear has been identified, a subacromial space is examined. If the bursa is inflamed, it may be removed for better visualization with the 4.5 mm full-radius shaver. When the bursa has been removed, the subacromial decompression then is performed. A tissue ablator then is used to cauterize and remove the coracoacromial ligament and tissue. The acromion and the AC joint should be checked for overhangs and spurs.

When the tissue has been removed, a bur is used to smooth the undersurface of the acromion, creating a smooth, flat inferior surface. The cuff is shaved to remove any loose flaps or tissue, as these can create a source of impingement. The surgeon then selects the spot for the anchors. A punch and tap then are used to create a hole for the anchor. The anchor is then impacted into the articular surface. The sutures are separated from each other and identified. The sutures are passed through the tendon and pulled out of the cannula. This is performed with a suture punch, which takes the suture and captures the edge of the tendon. The surgeon then pulls the suture up through the cannula, making sure not to pull it completely out. This step is performed a few times, depending on the number of anchors needed.

When the anchor has been placed, it is then tied down and cut. A hook may be used to check for stability. When all the anchors have been placed and tied, the shoulder is then rotated and checked for stability. The shoulder is irrigated, and the incision site is closed with 4-0 nylon.

Shoulder Procedures
ANTERIOR GLENOHUMERAL DISLOCATION
Surgical Goal
The surgical goal of this procedure is to put the glenohumeral head back into anatomical position.
Pathology
Although some dislocations may remain stable, some shoulders dislocate repeatedly, resulting in soft-tissue trauma. Often the surgery crew will be called on an emergent basis to relocate a dislocated shoulder. The procedure is not emergent, but if the soft tissue swells around the dislocation, the shoulder may be very difficult to relocate.
Technique
The patient is put under general anesthesia. The muscles must be relaxed to allow reduction. The techniques for reducing an anterior dislocation is illustrated in Figure 27-39.

If the shoulder becomes unstable or the dislocations become frequent, the patient may need a Bankart procedure.

BANKART PROCEDURE
Surgical Goal
A Bankart procedure is used to correct a recurrent anterior dislocation of the shoulder.
Pathology
Of all the joints in the body, the glenohumeral joint is the one most often dislocated. The skeletal construction of the shoulder favors mobility at the expense of stability. The rather flat glenoid fossa, which articulates with the large humeral head, makes for a basically unstable, shallow, ball-and-socket design. The stability of the joint depends on the surrounding soft tissue. Injury to the capsular envelope of the joint leads to subluxation or dislocation.

Recurrent anterior glenohumeral dislocation usually is produced by a force on the outstretched hand with the shoulder in abduction, external rotation, and elevation, a position that causes anterior levering of the humeral head and secondary stretching of the anterior and inferior capsular tissues. This injury can happen when one swims the backstroke or reaches into the back seat from the front seat of a car. Figure 27-40 illustrates the separation between the anterior glenoid rim and the detached anterior capsule. This separation illustrates a "Bankart lesion," which is responsible for recurrent anterior shoulder dislocations.

Technique
1. The patient is positioned, prepped, and draped according to procedure.
2. The surgeon makes an incision using a #10 blade.
3. The surgeon deepens the incision using sharp dissection with Metzenbaum scissors and Ferris Smith forceps.
4. If the coracoid process is to be removed to produce better operative exposure, this step is performed with an oscillating saw.
5. The wound is irrigated.

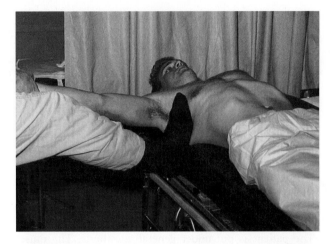

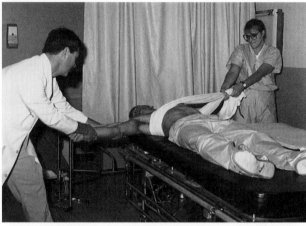

FIGURE 27-39
Traction, countertraction technique of reduction of anterior glenohumeral dislocation. (From Green NE and Swiont-kowski MF: *Skeletal trauma in children*, ed 3, Philadelphia, 2003, Saunders.)

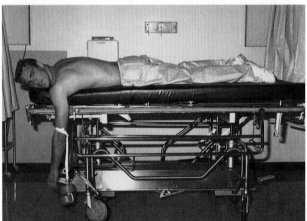

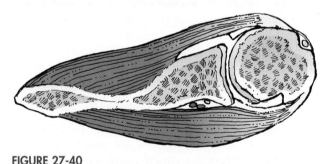

FIGURE 27-40
The pathology of the Bankart lesion. The anterior capsule has been detached from the anterior glenoid rim. (Modified from Wiesel SW and Delahay JN: *Essentials of orthopaedic surgery*, ed 2, Philadelphia, 1997, Saunders.)

6. The attenuated anterior capsule is reattached to the rim of the glenoid fossa with heavy sutures.
7. The glenoid fossa rim is decorticated with a curette, a rasp, or a bur.
8. The capsule is attached with bone anchors, staples, or heavy sutures.
9. The wound is irrigated and closed.
10. The shoulder is immobilized in an arm sling or a shoulder immobilizer.

Discussion

The patient is placed in a semi-sitting or beach-chair position. Unlike other shoulder procedures, in this procedure the scapula is *not* elevated with a sandbag. The shoulder is prepped and draped according to procedure, leaving the arm draped free and allowing the surgeon to manipulate the shoulder by moving the arm throughout the procedure.

The surgeon makes an anterior curved or longitudinal incision in the anterior axillary fold over the shoulder joint. The surgeon deepens the incision using sharp dissection with Metzenbaum scissors and Ferris Smith forceps until the capsule is opened. If the surgeon plans to remove the coracoid process to obtain better operative exposure, this step is performed with an oscillating saw. The wound is irrigated to remove any "bone dust" or debris, and the extended anterior capsule is reattached to the rim of the glenoid fossa with heavy sutures, such as 2-0 Ethibond sutures.

The glenoid fossa rim is decorticated with a curette, a rasp, or a bur to produce a raw surface on the bone to which the capsule will be attached. The capsule is attached with special bone anchors, staples, or heavy sutures (Figure 27-41). The wound is irrigated and closed. The shoulder is immobilized in an arm sling or a shoulder immobilizer.

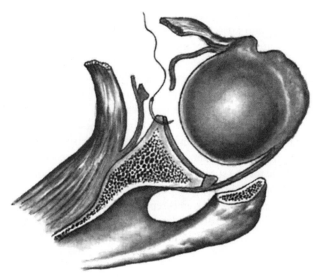

FIGURE 27-41
The Bankart repair: Holes are made in the rim of the glenoid (with an awl or a micro bur), and the free lateral margin of the capsule is sutured to the rim of the glenoid. (From Gregory B: *Orthopaedic surgery,* St Louis, 1994, Mosby.)

BRISTOW PROCEDURE

Surgical goal
This surgical procedure is used to repair recurrent dislocations of the anterior glenohumeral joint.

Pathology
Surgical stabilization of the glenohumeral joint is considered in traumatic instability if the condition repeatedly compromises shoulder comfort or function despite a reasonable trial of internal and external rotator strengthening and coordination exercises.

Technique

1. The operation begins as would a Bankart procedure.
2. When the capsule is open, the surgeon dissects the tip of the coracoid process from the scapula just distal to the insertion of the pectoralis minor muscle.
3. A vertical slit is made in the subscapularis tendon.
4. The joint is exposed.
5. The anterior surface of the neck of the scapula is scraped, leaving bone exposed.
6. The coracoid process with its attached tendons is then passed through the slit in the subscapularis.

Discussion
The operation begins as would a Bankart procedure.

In this procedure, the surgeon dissects the tip of the coracoid process from the scapula just distal to the insertion of the pectoralis minor muscle, leaving the conjoined tendons (i.e., the short head of the biceps and the coracobrachialis) attached.

Through a vertical slit in the subscapularis tendon, the joint is exposed and the anterior surface of the neck of the scapula is scraped with rasps or a micro bur. This leaves "bare bone" to facilitate the healing process. The surgeon then passes the coracoid process with its attached tendons through the slit in the subscapularis and keeps it in contact with the raw area on the scapula by suturing the conjoined tendon to the cut edges of the subscapularis tendon. In effect, a subscapularis tenodesis is performed.

Closure and dressings are the same as for a Bankart procedure.

PUTTY-PLATT PROCEDURE

Surgical Goal
A Putty-Platt procedure is used to correct a recurrent anterior dislocation of the shoulder.

Pathology
The pathology of Putty-Platt is the same as for a Bankart repair.

Technique

1. Prep, drape, and incision are the same as for a Bankart procedure.
2. The joint capsule is sutured (or anchored) to the glenoid rim.
3. The subscapularis muscle is advanced laterally.
4. The surgeon inspects the glenoid and humeral head, using palpation to access osteochondral changes.
5. The lateral portion of the subscapularis is sutured to the anterior glenoid rim.
6. The medial portion of the subscapularis is sutured to the rotator cuff at the greater tuberosity.
7. The layers of the joint are overlapped.
8. The incision is closed and dressed, and the shoulder is immobilized.

Discussion
In the Putty-Platt procedure, the joint capsule is sutured (or anchored) to the glenoid rim. The surgeon advances the subscapularis muscle laterally. This protects the shoulder from future dislocation by placing a physical barrier, the muscle. The subscapularis tendon is divided $2\frac{1}{2}$ cm medial to its insertion. The glenoid and humeral heads are inspected with palpation to identify osteochondral changes. The lateral portion of the subscapularis is sutured to the anterior glenoid rim. The medial portion of the subscapularis is sutured to the rotator cuff at the greater tuberosity. The layers of the joint are overlapped, a technique used often in soft-tissue reconstruction. The incision is closed, dressed, and the shoulder immobilized.

The procedure is rarely useful when the anterior capsular is of poor quality preoperatively.

OPEN ROTATOR CUFF REPAIR

Surgical goal
The goal of rotator cuff repair is to correct the disruption in the rotator cuff, thereby reducing pain and shoulder dysfunction.

Pathology

The shoulder is uniquely designed to produce power and precision through a nearly limitless ROM. The price of such mobility is instability, one of the most common problems affecting the shoulder joint. For normal function, the shoulder requires power and strength, which are derived from the coordinated interaction of at least 26 muscles.

Although the shoulder is not subjected to the same type and magnitude of load as the knee and the hip and has been described as a non–weight-bearing joint, it is load bearing. The rotator cuff and deltoid each provide approximately 50% of the power needed for overhead lifting and 90% of the power needed for external rotation. Disruption of the rotator cuff can result in pain and shoulder dysfunction.

The rotator cuff comprises the following muscles:

▶ Supraspinatus
▶ Subscapularis
▶ Infraspinatus
▶ Teres minor

Most rotator cuff repairs are performed through the insertion of the tendon fibers of the supraspinatus muscle that attaches onto the proximal humerus. Any of the four structures making up the rotator cuff can be involved in the tear. Supraspinatus syndrome also is called *impingement syndrome*. The approach to diagnosis and treatment is similar for both.

Technique

1. The patient is positioned, prepped, and draped as for a Bankart procedure.
2. A 10-cm to 12-cm incision is made in the anterior-superior deltoid.
3. After soft tissue has been explored, a subacromioplasty is performed.
4. The tear is identified and sutured.
5. Closure is per the surgeon's preference.
6. Dressings are applied, and the shoulder is immobilized in an arm sling.

Discussion

The patient is placed in a modified beach-chair position with a "bump" placed under the patent's scapula on the affected side. The affected arm is then elevated, and the fingers are placed in finger traps. The shoulder is prepped and draped as per a Bankart procedure.

The surgeon then makes a 10-cm to 12-cm skin incision in the anterior-superior aspect of the shoulder. The incision extends just inside the acromion lateral to the coracoid. Soft tissue is exposed with the ESU, Metzenbaum scissors, and retractors such as Gelpi retractors.

The AC joint and the acromion should be identified. An incision is made through the deltoid muscle, extending just anterior to the AC joint to the lateral edge of the acromion. The deltoid is then split with the needle-tip ESU.

The bursa is opened, and the coracoacromial ligament is identified and dissected off the acromion. Special shoulder retractors and instrumentation may be employed at this time, depending on the type of repair being performed (Figure 27-42). The acromion is removed with either an osteotome or a sagittal saw. A rongeur and a rasp then are used to smooth the surface of the bone. The tear then may be identified.

Stay sutures are placed in the edges of the torn tendon. A bur is used to create a small trench in the articular surface. When this step has been completed, a drill bit is used to create a hole for the suture. A suture, such as a 2-0 Ethibond suture, is passed through the bone and the tendon and is held with a hemostat. This step is repeated until the tear is closed. Only after all the sutures are in place does the surgeon tie them down in place. The patient's arm should be elevated, keeping the tension off the soft tissue and the new suture line.

The incision is irrigated, checked for bleeders, and cleaned of debris. The incision is closed with 2-0 and 3-0 absorbable suture. The subcutaneous tissue is closed with staples or a 4-0 absorbable suture and Steri-Strips. The incision is covered with 4 × 4 gauze and a bulky dressing and is immobilized with a sling or a shoulder immobilizer.

HUMERAL FRACTURES

Surgical Goal

Fractures of the humerus can be distal, proximal, or in the shaft of the bone. Treatment of each type of fracture differs. In general, proximal humeral fractures are managed by closed techniques. The need for reduction is determined by the extent of displacement of the bone. Nondisplaced fractures are treated with a sling-and-swath immobilization method.

Displaced proximal humeral fractures may be treated by placement of percutaneous pinning (Figure 27-43). This

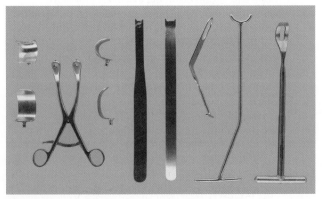

FIGURE 27-42
Shoulder retractors: *Left to right,* glenoid self-retaining retractor with four blades, two short and two long (front view and side view); glenoid retractor, narrow; glenoid retractor (Batman), medium; shoulder retractor, angled, short; Bankart retractor; shoulder retractor, angled, long. (From Tighe S: *Instrumentation for the operating room,* ed 6, St Louis, 2003, Mosby.)

type of pinning requires the use of specialized instrumentation and the C-arm radiograph intraoperatively. It is not unusual to see a rotator cuff tear with a proximal humerus fracture that is displaced.

Mid-shaft humeral fractures are treated with long plates and screws or with IM rods. The IM procedure and instrumentation will be discussed as a femoral fracture. The technique is roughly the same, but the instruments are smaller. A mid-shaft fracture that was reduced with a plate and screws is illustrated in a radiograph in Figure 27-44.

Distal humeral fractures can greatly compromise the function of the elbow, and special care must be taken in the treatment of these fractures. These fractures result most often from a fall on an outstretched arm or hand that produces hyperextension of the elbow (Figure 27-45). The fracture is common in pediatric patients and is reduced with the patient under general anesthesia. Using C-arm radiography, the surgeon pins the fracture with the arm hyperflexed (Figure 27-46), and the pin placement is confirmed in the anteroposterior (AP) and lateral planes (Figure 27-47).

Hand Procedures

METACARPOPHALANGEAL JOINT ARTHROPLASTY
Surgical Goal
The surgical goal of MCP joint arthroplasty is to eliminate pain and align the joints, producing joint stability.

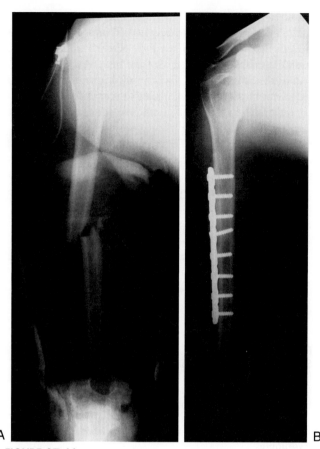

A   B

FIGURE 27-44
A, A displaced mid-shaft humeral fracture. **B,** Open reduction internal fixation (ORIF) with a limited-contact dynamic compression plate. (From Browner BD, Jupiter JB, Levine AM, et al: *Skeletal trauma: basic science, management, and reconstruction,* ed 3, Philadelphia, 2003, Saunders.)

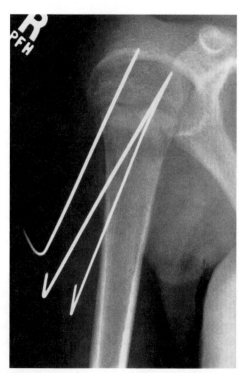

FIGURE 27-43
Placement of percutaneous pins in a proximal humeral fracture. (From Green NE and Swiontkowski MF: *Skeletal trauma in children,* ed 3, Philadelphia, 2003, Saunders.)

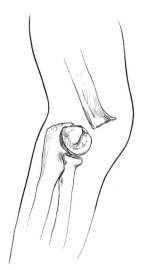

FIGURE 27-45
Supracondylar humerus fracture. (From Herring JA: *Tachdjian's pediatric orthopaedics from the Texas Scottish Rite Hospital for Children,* ed 3, Philadelphia, 2002, Saunders.)

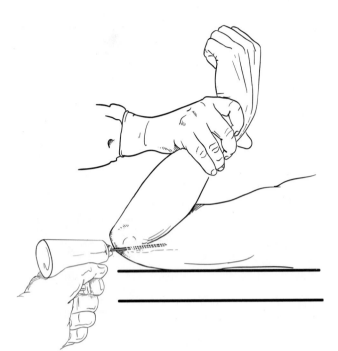

FIGURE 27-46
Supracondylar fractures are pinned with the arm hyper-flexed. (From Herring JA: *Tachdjian's pediatric orthopaedics from the Texas Scottish Rite Hospital for Children*, ed 3, Philadelphia, 2002, Saunders.)

Pathology

Older patients tend to develop loose, unstable joints with loss of MCP flexion and ulnar drifting. The cause of the MCP joint disease in adults is longstanding rheumatic arthritis (Figure 27-48) The treatment of choice for adults is MCP joint arthroplasty.

Children with juvenile arthritis have just the opposite of the typical adult deformity. In juvenile arthritis, the joints are left stiff, not loose. The MCP joint is stiff in extension, and radial deviation is seen. The treatment of choice for children is MCP arthrodesis, and implant arthroplasty of the fingers of children is generally avoided.

Technique

1. Incisions are made on the dorsal side of the appropriate fingers.
2. The proximal and distal portions of the joints are excised, and the IM canals are reamed.
3. The trial prosthesis is employed to help in choosing the size of the final prosthesis.
4. If necessary, the tendons and ligaments may be repaired.
5. The implants are inserted (Figure 27-49).
6. The incision is irrigated and closed.
7. The dressing and posterior splint are applied.

Discussion

The patient is positioned supine with the affected arm extended on an arm table. A tourniquet then is applied. The patient's arm is prepped from the fingertips to the elbow.

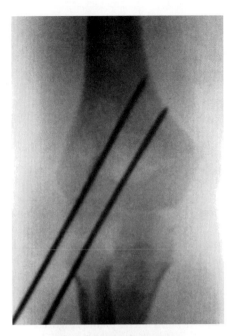

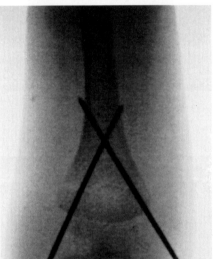

FIGURE 27-47
Radiograph of a reduced supracondylar fracture. (From Herring JA: *Tachdjian's pediatric orthopaedics from the Texas Scottish Rite Hospital for Children*, ed 3, Philadelphia, 2002, Saunders.)

The arm is then draped with an extremity drape. A small bone set, the implant instruments, and a micro bur are needed.

A transverse incision is made over the dorsum of the metacarpals, exposing the tendon. Tenotomy scissors and a #15 blade are used to release the extensor tendon. The joint capsule and collateral ligaments are then elevated on both sides of the metacarpal and on the proximal phalanx. A micro saw is used to resect the metacarpal head. Two small (Hohmann) retractors should be placed under the bone to protect the underlying tissue when the saw is used. A small diamond rasp then is used to smooth the ends of the bones, creating a smooth surface.

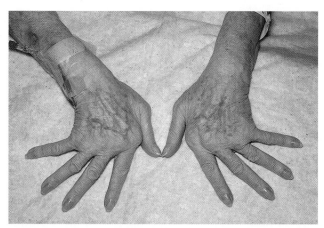

FIGURE 27-48
Arthritic hands. (From Swartz MH: *Textbook of physical diagnosis,* ed 3, Philadelphia, 1998, WB Saunders.)

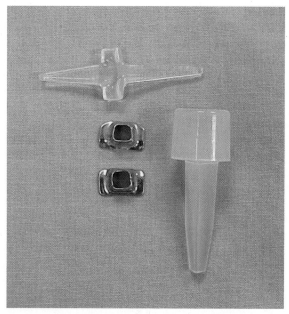

FIGURE 27-49
Swanson Silastic finger joint implant with grommets and a trapezium implant on the right. (Picture courtesy of the College of Southern Idaho, Twin Falls, Idaho.)

The surgeon holds the proximal phalanx with one hand while using a micro bur to enter the medullary canal. This bur is used to widen the canal for the implant. (If broaches are used, the broaching starts with the smallest and progresses to the largest until the prosthesis trial fits.)

When the intramedullary canal is open, the trials are used to measure implant size, and the site is irrigated. The implants are inserted, the joint is irrigated, and the skin is closed.

The dressings are applied, and the hand is placed in a posterior splint with the finger or fingers held in extension.

DE QUERVAIN'S CONTRACTURE RELEASE

Surgical Goal

The surgical goal of this procedure is to release the tendon affected by De Quervain's contracture and thereby eliminate pain and numbness in the fingers.

Pathology

De Quervain's stenosing tenosynovitis presents with painful wrist and thumb motion. Grasping the thumb and abruptly deviating the wrist toward the ulna causes pain over the radial styloid and first extensor compartment housing the abductor pollicis longus and extensor pollicis brevis tendons.

Initial treatment of the affliction should include splinting or administration of nonsteroidal antiinflammatory drugs (NSAIDs). If this treatment is unsuccessful, then De Quervain's release is needed.

Trigger finger is a form of stenosing tenosynovitis. An enlargement of the flexor tendon or inflammation of the sheath can lead to a discrepancy in the size of the tendon and the pulley, particularly the first annular pulley over the volar plate of the MCP joint. Difficulty flexing the digit and a painful "snap" are experienced when trying to extend the digit.

This condition is not congenital, but it is fairly common in infants and young children. The condition of *trigger finger* or *trigger thumb* is a mechanical problem, and the most effective treatment is trigger finger or trigger thumb release.

Technique	TRIGGER THUMB OR TRIGGER FINGER RELEASE

1. A small incision is made across the affected pulley.
2. Complete release of the offending proximal pulley is performed.
3. The inflamed tissue and the surrounding tissue are removed from the tendon sheath by careful dissection with a Steven's tenotomy scissors or other small scissors.
4. The incision is irrigated and closed.
5. A bulky dressing is applied.

Discussion

The patient is placed in the supine position with the operative arm on an arm board. Anesthesia appropriate for the age of the patient is given. If the surgeon prefers a tourniquet, one may be applied to the upper arm to control bleeding. Appropriate prepping and draping techniques are employed.

The surgeon uses a #15 blade (or a Beaver blade if the patient is a child) to make an incision across the affected pulley. Steven's tenotomy scissors and toothed Adson forceps are used to carefully dissect the tissue to expose the tendons.

When the tendons have been exposed and the fingers can be moved without impingement, the tourniquet is released, hemostasis is achieved, and the wound is irrigated. The skin then is closed, and the wound is dressed with a bulky dressing.

DUPUYTREN'S CONTRACTURE RELEASE

Surgical Goal

The goal of Dupuytren's contracture release is to return the hand and fingers to normal anatomical position and function.

Pathology

Dupuytren's contracture is a common condition, affecting primarily older men, in which the fascia of the palm and/or fingers contracts. The affliction begins as a nodule that may be tender at onset and progresses unpredictably but somewhat inevitably to fibrous bands that cause the contractures in the fingers. The ring and little finger are those affected most often.

There is a strong familial component, particularly when the onset is in younger men and the deformity progresses rapidly. The contractures are seldom painful, but they cause restriction of extension but not of flexion because they do not involve the flexor tendons (Figure 27-50). Treatment is surgical.

Technique

1. The surgeon makes an incision with a #15 blade on the ulnar side of the palmar fascia.
2. Steven's tenotomy scissors and toothed Adson forceps are used to dissect the tissue and expose tendons.
3. The palmar fascia is removed entirely, freeing up the contractures.
4. The incision is irrigated and closed.
5. A dressing is applied.

Discussion

The patient is placed in the supine position with the operative arm on an arm board. A Bier block or general anesthetic may be given to produce anesthesia. A tourniquet may be applied to the upper arm to control bleeding. Prepping and draping are appropriate for a hand procedure.

The surgeon uses a #15 blade to make the incision on the ulnar side of the palmar fascia as well as the apex of the fascia. Tenotomy scissors and light forceps are used to carefully dissect the tissue and expose the tendons. After the tendons have been freed and the fingers can be moved without impingement, the tourniquet is released and the wound is checked for hemostasis and irrigated. The skin is closed and dressed based on the surgeon's preference.

Foot Procedures
BUNIONECTOMY
Surgical Goal

Severe pain and the inability to fit shoes generally mandate surgical treatment for bunions. The goal of the treatment then is to relieve pain and return the foot to a normal anatomical position.

Pathology

Three classic abnormalities are found in bunions:

▶ *The exostosis* itself is a red, tender, and painful bursa overlying the bony exostosis.
▶ In *hallux valgus*, a big toe deviates in a lateral direction. It also often rotates or pronates.
▶ In *metatarsus primus varus*, the first metatarsal is deviated medially.

Figure 27-51 illustrates hallux valgus and exostosis. These three abnormalities can occur together or individually.

Bunions have a female preponderance, with up to 88% of adolescent patients being girls. There is usually a strong family history, with most patients inheriting the condition from their mothers.

Many different types of bunion repair are performed, as illustrated in Figure 27-52.

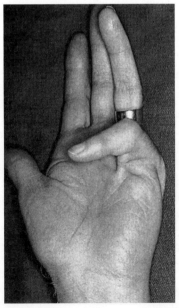

FIGURE 27-50
Dupuytren's contracture. (From Mercier LR: *Practical orthopedics*, ed 4, St Louis, 1995, Mosby.)

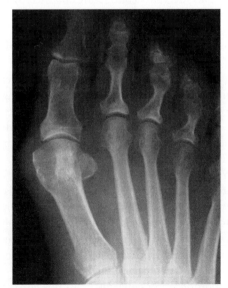

FIGURE 27-51
Classic abnormalities in a bunion hallux valgus and bunion exostosis. (From Brier SR: *Primary care orthopedics*, St Louis, 1999, Mosby.)

Technique KELLER BUNIONECTOMY

1. The surgeon makes an incision at the great toe (Figure 27-53).
2. Sharp dissection is extended to the joint capsule.
3. A flap is made to expose the underlying hypertrophic bone.
4. All soft-tissue attachments are removed from the base of the phalanx.
5. The proximal third of the proximal phalanx is resected with a micro-oscillating saw.
6. Proper alignment of the toe is maintained by one or two K-wires placed in the center of the medullary canal and then driven into the metatarsal head, neck, and shaft.
7. The wound is irrigated, the capsule closed, and the skin is closed.
8. The wound is dressed, and the foot placed in a bunion shoe.

Discussion

The patient is placed in the supine position. The patient may have an ankle block before the foot is prepped. After the toe has been anesthetized, the foot is prepped from the mid-calf to the toes. The draping is performed in the usual fashion.

The surgeon makes a longitudinal skin incision. The subcutaneous tissue and bursa are then elevated. The metatarsal head is made visible by sharp dissection with either a #15 blade or tenotomy scissors. When the bone is exposed, a micro-sagittal saw is used to remove about 40% of the bone. Proper alignment of the toe is maintained by one or two .062

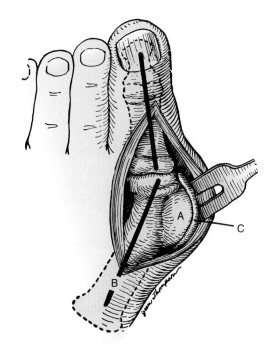

FIGURE 27-53
Incision for a Keller bunionectomy. (From Richards V: *Surgery for general practice*, St Louis, 1956, Mosby.)

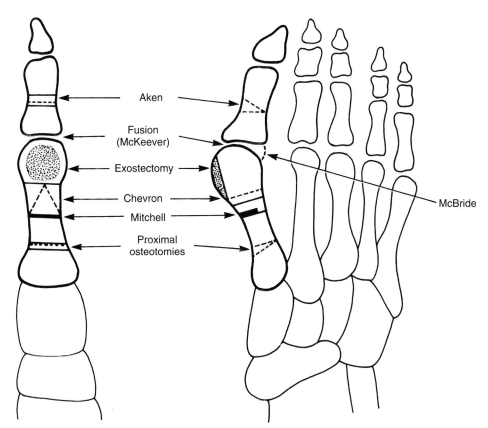

FIGURE 27-52
Types of bunionectomies. (From Rothrock J: *Alexander's care of the patient in surgery*, ed 12, St Louis, 2003, Mosby.)

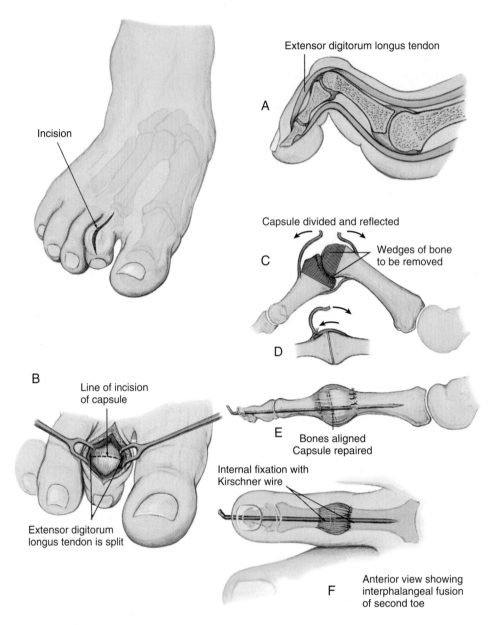

FIGURE 27-54
Hammer toe repair. (From Herring JA: *Tachdjian's pediatric orthopaedics from the Texas Scottish Rite Hospital for Children,* ed 3, Philadelphia, 2002, Saunders.)

K-wires placed in the center of the medullary canal. A radiograph is taken (or C-arm is used) to confirm the placement of the pins.

The incision is irrigated, and the capsule is closed. A dressing is applied, holding the toe in abduction to release any tension on the repair, and a postoperative bunion shoe is fitted to the foot.

HAMMERTOE CORRECTION

A hammertoe is a condition in which a toe has contracted at the proximal interphalangeal (PIP) joint (middle joint in the toe), potentially leading to severe pressure and pain. Ligaments and tendons that have tightened cause the toe's joints to curl downward. Hammertoes may occur in any toe except the big toe. There is often discomfort at the top part of the toe caused by rubbing against the shoe.

To correct a hammertoe deformity, the cartilaginous articulating surfaces are resected. After the joint is removed, the raw edges are "fused" with a small K-wire. The wire is driven through the end of the toe and both joint edges to hold the toe straight until the bone is healed (Figure 27-54). Hammertoes often are associated with bunions.

ACHILLES TENDON REPAIR
Surgical Goal
The goal of Achilles tendon repair is to reapproximate the proximal and distal ends of the ruptured Achilles tendon.

Immediately after the tendon repair, the assistant or the surgical technologist takes the responsibility of keeping the foot in a plantar flexed position (toes down) to keep stress off the new suture line in the tendon. When the assistant has assumed the responsibility of keeping the foot flexed, the foot must stay in this position until the anterior cast or short leg cast is in place and the cast has cured.

PERCUTANEOUS REPAIR OF THE ACHILLES TENDON
Percutaneous repair of an Achilles tendon is an option for patients who live in an area where the procedure is performed. Benefits of this technique include:

▶ A smaller incision is used.
▶ Scar formation is smaller.
▶ The tendon sheath holds the blood clot that is formed at the time of rupture, permitting rapid healing of the tendon.
▶ No general anesthetic is given.
▶ The rehabilitation program is accelerated.
▶ Full return to sports is expected.

The technique for this abbreviated procedure begins with patient sedation followed by local infiltration into the incision area. The proximal portion of the tendon, as identified by palpation and MRI, is sutured with a heavy nonabsorbable suture placed transversely through the skin and the tendon and out the opposite side.

This suture then is intersected through the tendon, through the gap at the rupture site, and finally through the distal portion of the tendon just above the calcaneus and through the skin punctures. A second stitch is placed after the first one and is tied with the foot in plantar flexion. Surgical dressings and a cast are applied as for an open procedure.

TENORRHAPHY
A tenorrhaphy is the surgical repair of a torn tendon. If the tendon is completely torn, the edges must first be approximated so that healing may begin. There are several ways to repair a tendon. The Z-plasty described above in the Achilles tendon repair is one method, and a U incision is another (Figure 27-56).

After a repair, the patient may be placed in a splint to protect the tendon from movement.

TRIPLE ARTHRODESIS
Surgical Goal
The surgical goal is to reduce the pain of an unstable ankle resulting from rheumatoid arthritis.
Pathology
A triple arthrodesis involves fusion of the talocalcaneal, talonavicular, and calcaneocuboid joints. These joints become painful or unstable in clubfoot, poliomyelitis, and rheumatoid arthritis.

This surgery uses fusion to prevent full range of motion in the ankle. After the procedure, movement of the foot and ankle is limited to plantar flexion and dorsal flexion.

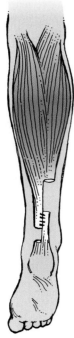

FIGURE 27-55
Achilles tendon repair. (From Herring JA: *Tachdjian's pediatric orthopaedics from the Texas Scottish Rite Hospital for Children*, ed 3, Philadelphia, 2002, Saunders.)

Pathology
Although the patient rarely gives a history of trauma, the Achilles tendon is often the site of small, low-grade collagen disruptions. The Achilles tendon rupture presents with inability to plantar flex the foot. After the diagnosis has been established, surgical repair is a treatment of choice.

Technique
1. The surgeon makes a posteromedial skin incision.
2. The skin and subcutaneous tissue are retracted with rakes or a self-retaining Gelpi retractor.
3. The ends of the tendon are pulled into the incision site, and the edge is cut to make a clean edge.
4. The tendon is reanastomosed with a tendon-suturing technique.
5. The wound is irrigated and closed.
6. The foot is placed in an anterior splint or a short leg cast.

Discussion
A posteromedial skin incision is made. The surgeon avoids making a midline incision to prevent future problems with the shoe wearing on the incision site. When the tendon edges have been identified, they are pulled into the incision with a heavy suture. The surgeon checks the remaining length of the tendon remnants to see where the suture line will be. The tendon may be debrided of any tendon threads and then attached via a Z-plasty technique using 0 or 2-0 Ethibond or other nonabsorbable suture (Figure 27-55).

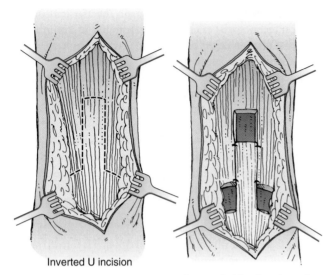

Inverted U incision

Underlying soleus
muscle left intact

Sutures holding lengthened
tendo Achilles in place

FIGURE 27-56
U-plasty versus Z-plasty technique in Achilles tendon repair.
(From Herring JA: *Tachdjian's pediatric orthopaedics from the Texas Scottish Rite Hospital for Children,* ed 3, Philadelphia, 2002, Saunders.)

Technique

1. The surgeon makes the incision.
2. The joints are exposed.
3. Cartilage and joint capsules are dissected and removed.
4. The articular surfaces of the calcaneocuboid joint, the subtalar joint, and the talonavicular joint all are removed.
5. The removed bone is prepared for grafting.
6. A Steinmann pin, staples, or screws are used for internal fixation.
7. A drain is inserted.
8. The wound is closed.
9. A short leg cast or splint is applied over the surgical dressing.

Discussion
The patient is placed in a supine position. The leg is prepped and draped per standard procedure.

An anterior or anterolateral incision is made. This type of approach avoids injury to the superficial peroneal nerves. The cartilage and soft tissue are dissected and removed from the joints with a rongeur, #15 blade, and tissue forceps. The capsules of the talonavicular, calcaneocuboid, and subtalar joints are incised circumferentially to obtain as much mobility as possible. The foot should be placed in as normal a position as possible.

The articular surfaces of the calcaneocuboid joint, the subtalar joint, and the talonavicular joint are removed with an osteotome, a power saw, or a rasp. All of the bone removed is a potential bone graft and should be preserved on the back table.

When the bone has been removed, one processes it by cutting it into small pieces. If there is not enough bone for

the graft, bone can be harvested from the anterior ilium. Most of the bone graft should be placed at the talonavicular joint. Smooth Steinmann pins, staples, or screws are used for internal fixation.

A closed drainage system such as a Hemovac drain is inserted, the wound is closed, and a surgical dressing is placed. A short leg cast or splint is applied.

Knee Procedures
ANTERIOR CRUCIATE LIGAMENT REPAIR
Surgical Goal
The goal of ACL repair is the same as for an arthroscopic ACL repair.
Pathology
The pathology of ACL repair is the same as for an arthroscopic ACL repair.

Technique

1. A midline incision is made across the knee joint with a #10 blade.
2. The soft tissue is retracted with knee retractors or rakes.
3. The ESU is used for soft-tissue dissection.
4. When the knee has been opened, the patellar tendon is harvested.
5. When the graft has been removed, it is prepped for placement in the patient and then protected from drying until needed.
6. If any repairs are needed (e.g., meniscectomy) they are performed at this time.
7. When the ACL has been identified, any remnants of the ACL tissue are removed.
8. A large drill bit is used to make a notch plasty.
9. After the notch plasty has been performed, a tibial aiming guide is inserted into the joint space.
10. A guide then is drilled through the tibia until the tip exits the center proximal tibia.
11. The surgeon then slowly reverses the drill, pulling the pin and the graft through the tibia and the femur.
12. The drill and pin are removed, and the surgeon pulls the suture tight to make sure there is a secure fit.
13. The patient receives passive ROM.
14. An interference screw is placed into the bone.
15. The knee is then irrigated.
16. The incision is closed and dressed.
17. The knee is placed in a knee immobilizer.

Discussion
The patient is placed in the supine position and prepped and draped as for a knee arthroscopy. The leg then is exsanguinated, and the tourniquet is inflated.

A midline incision is made across the knee joint with a #10 blade. The soft tissue is retracted with knee retractors or rakes, and the ESU is used for soft-tissue dissection. When the knee has been opened, the patellar tendon is harvested.

The tendon is identified, and a hemostat or a joker elevator is inserted under the patellar tendon and is moved proximally and distally to mobilize the tendon. The surgeon then uses a sterile skin marker and ruler to mark the length of the incision in the tendon well as the bone. The tendon is split with a scalpel and tissue forceps. When the tendon is free, an oscillating saw is used to remove a 1-inch patellar and tibial bone plug and the attached tendon between them.

After the graft is removed, it is taken to the back table, where the assistant cleans the graft, sizes the graft, and drills holes at both ends of the bone plug (refer to Figure 27-32, B). After the holes have been drilled, a large Ethibond suture is placed through all the drill holes. The graft should be kept damp with a lap sponge until needed.

If any repairs are needed (e.g., meniscectomy) they are performed at this time. After the ACL has been identified, any remnants of the ACL tissue are removed.

A large drill bit is used to make a notch plasty to create a wider intracondylar space. This wide space keeps the new graft from "rubbing" and causing future abrasions that would weaken the graft. After the notch plasty has been performed, a tibial aiming guide is inserted into the joint space. The guide is placed at the entry of the old ACL on the tibia. With the guide in place, a hole is drilled through the tibia until the tip exits the center proximal tibia.

The surgeon then slowly reverses the drill, pulling the pin and the graft through the tibia and the femur. The drill and pin are removed, and the surgeon pulls the suture tight to make sure there is a secure fit.

The surgeon checks the stability of the knee as well as the strength of the graft by putting the patient through passive ROM while the knee incision is still open. If the knee is found to be stable, an interference screw is placed into the graft and screwed down to secure the graft. The knee then is irrigated. The incision is closed and dressed. The knee is placed in a knee immobilizer.

Procedures of the Femur
FEMORAL RODDING
Surgical Goal
Femoral "rodding" or **nailing** is used to stabilize closed or open femoral fractures.
Pathology
Femoral fractures occur in trauma cases, such as multivehicle accidents (MVAs), in slips and falls, and in pathological fractures resulting from neoplasms. The technique described here is the same as for a humeral fracture, with only mild variations.

Technique

1. The patient is placed on a fracture table.
2. A C-arm is used to x-ray the femur.
3. The surgeon performs a closed reduction.
4. The surgeon makes an incision across the greater trochanter.
5. The fascia is dissected.
6. The trochanteric fossa is viewed.
7. A curved awl is inserted.
8. A ball-tip guide is introduced down the medullary canal.

9. The cannulated reamer is passed over the guide and drilled to the proper depth.
10. The nail is inserted into the femoral canal.
11. The lag screw is drilled and placed.
12. The proximal and distal screws are placed.
13. Final x-rays are taken.
14. The incision is irrigated and closed, and the dressing is applied.

Discussion
The patient is given a spinal or general anesthetic and then placed on the fracture table in the supine position with the affected leg placed in an ankle brace (see the fracture table in Figure 27-16). The unaffected leg is then placed into a cradle.

Preoperative C-arm radiographs are taken, the fracture is reduced, and the patient is prepped and draped as appropriate or as directed by the surgeon.

The surgeon then makes an incision from the proximal tip of the greater trochanter and continues medially for about 5 cm. The fascia is then dissected with a ¾-inch Key elevator. A curved awl is inserted in line with the femoral shaft to create an opening into the femur.

A ball-tipped guide then is introduced through the opening and advanced down the medullary canal past the fracture site. AP and lateral x-rays then are taken to follow the guide rod down the femoral shaft and across the fracture to the distal femur.

A cannulated reamer then is introduced over the guide wire, and the medullary canal is reamed to the appropriate width. The nail is then assembled onto the inserter with either a 130-degree or a 135-degree target vise for the lag screw. The surgeon then inserts the nail into the femoral canal to the fracture site, keeping the correct reduction while impacting the nail.

X-rays are taken to confirm that the nail is in position. After the nail is set, the guide sleeve is passed through the target guide and into the lag screw.

The wire is left in place, and the depth gauge is used to determine the length of the screw. The drill is passed over the guide wire, and the correct lag screw is placed.

The distal screw is sited with the C-arm and a distal targeting device. When the hole has been centered, a small stab incision is made and the pin is impacted through to the implant. A drill guide is then placed over the pin, and the pin is removed. Using the procedure for placement of screws, both screws are placed, and a final x-ray is taken. The incision is irrigated and closed, and a dressing is applied.

OPEN REDUCTION INTERNAL FIXATION
Surgical Goal
ORIF is performed to internally reduce a fracture under direct visualization of the fracture site.

Pathology

Intertrochanteric fractures, subtrochanteric fractures, and basilar neck fractures all are good candidates for ORIF. Each of these fracture types is approached differently and can be corrected with different fixation devices. The technique for performing ORIF of a fracture of a femoral head using a dynamic compression nail and a four-hole side plate is described here.

Technique

1. The patient is placed on the fracture table.
2. A C-arm is used for imaging.
3. If possible, a closed reduction is performed.
4. A lateral incision is made down the femur.
5. Rakes are used to retract subcutaneous tissue.
6. A periosteal elevator is used to dissect the tissue from fascia.
7. Bennett retractors are placed.
8. A 2.5-mm pin is used with a 135-degree guide and drilled through the femoral head.
9. The reamer is set to the correct depth and drilled over the pin.
10. The screw hole is tapped.
11. The plate must be placed under the compression screw before the screw is placed.
12. The screw and plate are placed over the pin and screwed down.
13. A 3.2-mm drill bit is used.
14. Screws then are placed through the plate.
15. The compression screw is applied.
16. The incision is irrigated and closed, and a pressure dressing is applied.

Discussion

The patient is administered general or spinal anesthesia and then is placed on a fracture table in the supine position. The affected leg is placed into a leg holder and stabilized with an ankle cuff (see Figure 27-16 for patient positioning on the fracture table). The unaffected leg then is placed up and over, and into a leg holder. A C-arm is brought into the OR to x-ray the fracture site, and a closed reduction will be performed.

The patient is prepped and draped per standard procedure and the surgeon's preference. A straight lateral incision then is made down the length of the femur. Curved Mayo scissors, Ferris Smith forceps, and the ESU are used to dissect the soft tissue, and Israel rakes are used to retract the subcutaneous tissue during this task. The periosteum is dissected from the femur with a ½-inch Key periosteal or Cobb elevator. When the bone is exposed, the Bennett retractors are positioned under the bone to retract the soft tissue from the bone.

Surgical technologists must be familiar with this instrumentation set. This is often an emergent case, and the instruments are sterilized unassembled (which is the case with many orthopedic specialty instruments).

A 2.5-mm graduated pin is inserted, with the C-arm for guidance, and the pin is placed through the center of the femoral head with a 135-degree angle guide. Lateral and AP x-rays are used to confirm the correct placement of the pin. The pin is measured to confirm the size of hip screw that is needed. The pin is graduated to facilitate measuring.

The reamer then is set to the correct depth (using the measurement just taken) and is slid over the pin until it contacts the bone. The surgeon then reams the femoral head, leaving the Steinmann pin in place. The bone is tapped and made ready to accept a screw. Using all the principles for proper placement of a screw, the surgeon taps the bone with a T-handle tap. The plate and the screw are placed simultaneously. The screw fits into the plate, and although the plate is not anchored at the same time, it must be placed at the same time as the lag screw.

When the long lag screw is in place, the surgeon uses the procedure for placement of screws to fill the four-hole plate with the proper length of screw. Figure 27-57 illustrates the final position of the dynamic compression screw and side plate. Note the fracture site and the action of the plate and partially threaded screw in "pulling" the bone in toward the fracture (i.e., compressing it).

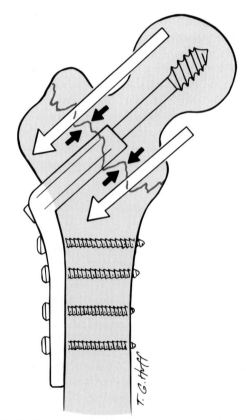

FIGURE 27-57
Dynamic compression sliding hip screw. Functional loading of a sliding hip screw causes dynamic compression at the fracture site. With functional loading, the screw slides through the barrel of the side plate, allowing the fracture to impact or compress. Note the placement of the cannulated screw in the inferior third of the femoral neck. (From Browner BD, Jupiter JB, Levine AM, et al: *Skeletal trauma: basic science, management, and reconstruction,* ed 3, Philadelphia, 2003, Saunders.)

Finally, the surgeon may place a compression screw that has been threaded into the back of the lag screw with a large fragment screwdriver. A final set of AP and lateral x-rays are taken. The surgical site is irrigated and checked for hemostasis. The incision is closed, and a pressure dressing is applied.

A Note About Pressure Dressings

Dynamic compression screws and side plates typically are used in elderly patients who have fallen and broken the femoral head. Because of their advancing age, they have a high risk for skin problems, and the pressure dressing used as a dressing may cause more harm than good. Care must be taken to individualize this dressing to each patient. Many types of tape used in pressure dressings have stretch, and the pull on the fragile elderly skin may cause blisters or actually tear the skin. Remember that intact skin is the first line of defense against infection, and care must be exercised with this specialty dressing that is used in many orthopedic procedures.

ORIF OF PELVIC FRACTURE

Surgical Goal

The surgical goal is to reduce a displaced or unstable pelvic fracture.

Pathology

Pelvic fractures can be life threatening. Complications of pelvic fractures include injury not only to the major vessels and nerves, but also to the major visceral organs, such as the intestines, the bladder, and the urethra.

Pelvic fractures are classified as stable (type A), rotationally unstable (type B), and vertically stable but rotationally and vertically unstable (type C). Treatment is based on the classification and may include closed manipulation and reduction of the fracture, closed reduction external fixation, and ORIF. Type-A fractures (stable) usually are nonsurgical. External fixation is the most widely recommended treatment for type-B fractures. Type-C fractures may treated with ORIF, with external fixation devices, or with a combination of both.

Technique

The technique for application of an external fixation device follows the same principle as the technique for application of external fixation to a forearm.
1. The pelvis is reduced manually.
2. Reduction is confirmed with a C-arm radiograph.
3. K-wires are inserted percutaneously, and the skin is tented.
4. Parallel rows of pins are placed in the anterior iliac crest.
5. Three universal frames are placed over the pins.
6. Optimal reduction of the fracture is achieved and confirmed with radiographs.
7. The cross bar is attached, and the joints of the frame are tightened.
8. The pin sites are dressed.

Discussion

The pelvis is reduced manually. The reduction is confirmed with C-arm radiography. K-wires are inserted percuta-

neously, and the skin is tented (a small slit is made in the skin to reduce the postoperative tension on the skin). Parallel rows of pins are placed in the anterior iliac crest. Three universal frames are placed over the pins, and optimal reduction of the fracture is achieved. The reduction is confirmed again with radiography. The cross bar is attached, and the joints of the frame are tightened. The pin sites are dressed with iodine or antibiotic ointment and gauze.

TOTAL HIP ARTHROPLASTY

Surgical Goal

The surgical goals of total hip arthroplasty are to return the hip to proper anatomical position and relieve the patient of hip pain.

Pathology

Indications for an arthroplasty are degenerative joint disease, rheumatoid arthritis, severe hip fracture, and osteoarthritis.

Technique

1. An incision is made at the anterosuperior iliac spine, extending to the greater trochanter.
2. Retractors are placed.
3. The capsule is opened.
4. The hip is dislocated.
5. Hohmann retractors are placed under the femoral neck.
6. The femoral trial is used to mark the cut of the neck.
7. An oscillating saw is used to amputate the femoral head.
8. The acetabulum is checked for osteophytes, and tissue is removed.
9. Acetabular reamers are used.
10. The trial is used and checked for size.
11. The permanent acetabular implant is opened onto the sterile field and then impacted.
12. The trial liner then is applied.
13. A box osteotome is used to create an opening in the femur.
14. Straight reamers and then flexible reamers are passed sequentially through the canal.
15. Trial broaches then are impacted.
16. The head and neck are then assembled on the trial broach.
17. The hip is reduced and put through ROM tests.
18. The hip is dislocated.
19. The trials are removed, and the canal and wound are irrigated.
20. The cement is mixed.
21. Final implants are inserted, and the hip is reduced.
22. The incision is irrigated.
23. A drain such as a Hemovac drain is inserted.
24. The incision is closed.
25. Surgical dressing is applied.
26. An abduction splint is applied before the patient is moved or awakened from anesthesia.

Discussion

The patient is given an appropriate anesthetic and placed in a lateral position using either a bean bag or a hip-positioning device. The leg is raised in a leg holder for an appropriate prep.

The draping is performed according to the surgeon's preference. The leg then is placed in a 60-degree flexion, and the landmarks are drawn out. The skin incision begins proximally at the anterosuperior iliac spine parallel to the posterior edge of the greater trochanter; the incision is extended along the femoral shaft about 1 cm distal from the greater trochanter.

The subcutaneous tissues are then dissected from the fascia with a ¾-inch elevator. A #10 blade is used to cut the fascia just 1 or 2 cm, curved Mayo scissors are used to extend the fascial incision, and muscles are split proximally with an ESU. After the muscle and fascia have been dissected, a Charnley retractor and other hand-held retractors are used for further exposure.

The capsule is then opened, and the femoral head is exposed. The hip is then dislocated. The surgeon places a bone hook around the femoral neck to assist with the dislocation of the hip from the acetabulum. With the hip subluxed, blunt Hohmann retractors are placed above and beneath the femoral neck. The knee must remain flexed to keep the hip in place. Soft tissue is removed from the neck and from the medial side of the greater trochanter. A femoral trial is used to mark the level of the proposed osteotomy of the femoral neck.

The oscillating saw then is used to cut the femoral head from the femur. The femoral head then is removed with a corkscrew or with a sharp bone clamp. The femoral head is then measured with a caliper.

A self-retaining retractor or blunt Hohmann retractors are used to retract tissue from the acetabulum opening. A long, heavy hip curette is used to scrape the acetabulum.

The femur is retracted anteriorly to allow the acetabular reamers to pass. The bone shavings from the deep acetabular reaming should be saved for bone graft. The final reamer size is determined by complete contact between the reamer and the acetabular rim. A trial-size shell then is inserted and impacted with the correct amount of anteversion. If the fit is not proper, the next size of trial is used. When the final cup size has been established and impacted, the antebellum liner is inserted. The trial liner then is snapped or screwed into the cup.

The patient's foot is then lowered toward the floor, with the hip internally rotated to expose the proximal end of the femur. Retractors are placed, and the femur is then inspected for any remaining soft tissue. A box osteotome then is used to create a straight entry in the femoral canal. The IM reamer is inserted to expose the canal's opening. A series of flexible reamers are used next; the size of the reamer is determined by the width of the canal. Reaming should stop when the cortex is felt (or heard). Surgeons describe this contact as "chatter."

With the canal opened, the smallest femoral rasp is inserted and is used to enlarge the back of the trochanter. The rasps are used to enlarge the femoral canal to facilitate entry of the femoral component.

The calcar is used to clean any excess bone around the implant. A head-and-neck trial is assembled and placed into the femoral canal. The hip then is reduced and brought into flexion and extension, adduction, and internal and external rotation. The length of the leg is checked bilaterally.

When the size of the femoral implant has been determined, the hip is dislocated. The trial acetabulum and femoral components are removed, and the wound is irrigated. If cement is to be used, a cement restrictor is placed into the distal femoral canal to prevent cement from traveling further down the canal than desired.

The acetabular components are implanted first, and the femoral components are impacted last. The components can be used with bone glue or without glue. If glue is used, after the glue has cured, the hip is reduced slowly so that the greater trochanter does not fracture.

ROM and stability are tested. The wound then is irrigated and checked for hemostasis, a Hemovac or Surtran closed drainage system is inserted, the hip is closed and dressed, and a hip adduction pillow is placed between the patient's legs.

TOTAL KNEE ARTHROPLASTY

Surgical Goal
Total knee arthroplasty is performed to replace the worn surfaces of the knee joint.

Pathology
Indications for an arthroplasty are degenerative joint disease, rheumatoid arthritis, severe hip fractures, and osteoarthritis. There are many types of knee replacement systems, and the technique listed here gives only guidelines for a total knee replacement. Surgical technologists should be familiar with the type and brand of total joint system being used. Total knee replacements may be:

▶ Unicompartmental, replacing only one side of the knee
▶ Bicompartmental, replacing the femoral and tibial components
▶ Tricompartmental, replacing the femoral, tibial, and patellar components

Technique

1. A tourniquet is placed for this procedure.
2. An incision is made from the distal end of the femur to the medial tibial tuberosity.
3. Retractors are placed.
4. The femoral and tibial cartilage ends are removed with various jigs from specialized instrumentation.
5. Trial tibial components and trial femoral components are placed.
6. The skin of the knee is closed with towel clips, and the knee is put through ROM to check for length and function.
7. The articulating surface of the patella is removed, and a patellar button is sized.
8. The knee is irrigated.
9. Cement is mixed.
10. The implants are placed.
11. Excess cement is removed from around the implant.

12. The site is irrigated.
13. A Hemovac or Surtran closed drainage system is inserted.
14. The incision is closed.
15. The surgical dressing is applied.

Discussion

The patient is placed under appropriate anesthesia. The patient is placed in the supine position on the table with a bump under the affected hip. A tourniquet may be placed at the patient's thigh.

The knee is prepped and draped according to the surgeon's preference. The surgeon exposes the knee using a midline incision across the knee. With the knee joint exposed, retractors are placed, the knee is flexed to 90 degrees, and the patella is turned with the soft tissue. The surgeon may release any soft-tissue attachments if needed. Specialty jigs and cutting guides may be used throughout the procedure. Specialty jigs and cutting guides are available for each type of replacement knee.

The distal cutting alignment guide is positioned extramedullary to the proximal tibial spines, and the osteotomy saw is used to resect the proximal portion of the tibia. The tibia is then sized with the templates.

The surgeon reduces the knee joint and checks to see whether the knee can come back into proper alignment before proceeding. The AP cutting guide then is used to size the femur. With the AP cutting guide in place, the anterior and posterior portions of the femur are resected. Using appropriate jigs, the surgeon flexes the knee and resects the distal portion of the femur.

The appropriate spacer is inserted. The knee is placed in flexion, and the femoral notch and chamfer guide are centered between the epicondyles and impacted until fully seated. The anterior and posterior chamfers are cut with the oscillating saw. The femoral trial then is positioned. The tibial size is reassessed with the tibial templates.

A trial reduction is performed. If the reduction proves satisfactory, the permanent components are placed. The trials can be placed with or without glue.

Drains are placed, the wound is closed, and surgical dressings are placed. The surgeon may order a passive ROM machine starting in the postanesthesia care unit (PACU) for the patient.

TOTAL SHOULDER ARTHROPLASTY

Surgical Goal

The goals of the total shoulder arthroplasty are to alleviate the patient's pain from an arthritic joint and/or return the shoulder joint to normal range of motion.

Pathology

Some of the indications for a total shoulder arthroplasty are excessive external rotation, restrictive external rotation, and end-stage degenerative joint disease (DJD). Osteoarthritic changes may be a factor in the indications for surgery. X-rays

and other tests may show more pathological problems, such as:

- Rotator cuff tear
- Severe arthritis and osteophytes
- Biceps tendon rupture/tear
- SLAP lesion

Technique

1. An incision is made, beginning at the AC joint and continuing over the coracoid process.
2. Soft tissue is dissected to the point of the joint capsule.
3. The joint capsule is opened, and the humeral head is visualized.
4. Osteophytes are trimmed away from the humeral head.
5. The humeral head is removed.
6. The IM canal finder is inserted into the humerus.
7. Reamers and broaches are used to open the humeral IM canal.
8. The trial head is attached to the trial stem, and the arm is reduced and tested for stability.
9. The humerus is dislocated, and trials are removed.
10. If bone cement is to be used, it is mixed.
11. The wound is irrigated.
12. Bone graft is placed to fill any gaps.
13. The humeral stem and head then are impacted.
14. The arm is reduced and irrigated.
15. The incision is closed.
16. The surgical dressing is applied.
17. The arm is placed in an arm sling.

Discussion

The patient is placed in a beach-chair position. Positioning for this case is very important; an improper position may interfere with access to the humerus, which may cause a humeral fracture.

With the patient in position, the surgeon performs an EUA. The patient then is prepped and draped per standard procedure and the surgeon's preference.

The surgeon makes the incision, beginning at the AC joint and continuing over the coracoid process. The soft tissues are dissected with the ESU, Mayo scissors, forceps, and shoulder retractors. When the joint capsule is reached, it is opened, allowing the humeral head to be visualized. The humeral head is dislocated, and a blunt Hohmann retractor then is placed behind the head to maintain the position.

The arm is extended, adducted, and externally rotated to maximize the exposure of the humeral head. Osteophytes are trimmed away from the humeral head with a rongeur or wide osteotome. This creates normal anatomy of the neck of the humeral head.

A saw is used to remove the head of the humerus. This cut should be almost identical to the anatomical neck of the humerus. Saline irrigation should be dripped onto the saw blade to cool the blade if necessary to keep the saw from burning the bone. This is typically very hard bone, so excessive heat is not uncommon.

A starting IM canal finder is inserted into the humerus and is used to break up any cancellous bone and widen the canal for the implant. Reamers are introduced into the humerus, beginning with a small-diameter reamer and working up to larger ones. With the IM canal opened, the broaches then are impacted until the prosthesis fits snugly into the canal. The trial head then is attached to the trial broach. The arm then is reduced. Stability tests are performed. Traction, rotation, and extension are tested.

When using the trials, one should take care so that the humeral head is not left "proud." Leaving the head "proud" will excessively tighten the capsule, which will limit the elevation during the reduction.

When the surgeon is satisfied with the fit of the trials, the humerus is dislocated, the trials are removed, and the joint is irrigated with saline or antibiotics. Two different types of humeral stem implants are available—the cemented prosthesis and the press fit prosthesis. The surgeon will have chosen the type of prosthesis previously.

If bone graft is to be used, it is placed along the transected edge of the proximal humeral shaft and any other gaps. The implant is chosen and then either cemented or press fitted. The humeral head is then impacted on the humeral stem and slowly reduced. ROM tests are then repeated. The wound is closed, and a dressing and arm sling or immobilizer are applied before the patient is aroused from the anesthetic.

TOTAL ELBOW ARTHROPLASTY
Surgical Goal
Total elbow arthroplasty is performed to treat excessive bone loss resulting from arthritis or DJD. Such bone loss causes a loss of normal function and rotation and pain to the patient.
Pathology
The joint may become unstable, causing pain and discomfort resulting from stiffness and joint fusion. Other indications are major cysts at the olecranon-coronoid junction and loss of extension beyond 60 degrees. The pathology also may have been the direct result of a traumatic fracture that is unhealed or has considerable bone deficit.

Technique

1. A posterior incision is made at the elbow.
2. The ulnar nerve is identified.
3. Triceps are elevated, and the tip of the olecranon is removed.
4. The MCL is released to improve exposure.
5. A portion of the trochlea is removed.
6. The IM canal finder is inserted.
7. A portion of the distal humerus is removed.
8. The drill and rasps are used to enter the medullary canal of the ulna.
9. Trial implants are inserted.
10. Cement is mixed.
11. The wound is irrigated.
12. Bone graft is used to fill any open spaces and to treat any rotational displacement.
13. Cement is applied, and the final implant is impacted.
14. The incision is closed.
15. The surgical dressing. a posterior splint, and an arm sling are applied.

Discussion
The patient is placed in the supine position with the arm over the chest. The tourniquet is then applied. The arm is then prepped and draped following standard procedure and the surgeon's preference.

The surgeon makes a posteromedial incision at the elbow. The ulnar nerve is identified and protected. The medial half of the triceps is elevated, and the tip of the olecranon is removed. The MCL is released to improve exposure. The forearm is then rotated in the lateral position to produce exposure of the distal humerus. An oscillating saw is used to remove a portion of the trochlea. Access to the medullary canal of the humerus is then complete. An IM canal finder is inserted and exchanged for an alignment stem with an attached cutting block. The surgeon uses the oscillating saw and removes the distal humerus.

The surgeon enters the medullary canal of the ulna using a high-speed drill or bur. Additional bone is then removed from the tip of the olecranon to make room for the reamers. After the reaming, a rasp is impacted down the ulna carefully to avoid a proximal ulnar fracture or other complication.

After the humerus and ulna have been prepared, the surgeon inserts the trials. When the trials are in place, ROM, including flexion and extension, is tested. The trials then are removed, and the surgical site is irrigated.

Following the guidelines for mixing bone cement, one mixes the cement and places it in a cement gun for injection into the humeral and ulnar canals. Bone graft is placed into any open spaces and behind the humeral implant. The bone graft helps the humerus resist posterior and rotational displacement. The humeral implant is then impacted, and the ulnar implant is inserted.

When the bone cement has cured, the tourniquet is deflated and hemostasis is obtained with the ESU. The surgical site then is irrigated with antibiotic irrigant. The incision then is closed, dressing is applied, and the elbow is placed in neutral position with a posterior splint and an arm sling.

TOTAL ANKLE ARTHROPLASTY
Surgical Goal
The goals of this procedure are to restore normal range of motion to the ankle joint and allow the patient to move without arthritic pain.

Pathology

The pathology in patients undergoing total ankle arthroplasty is a chronic progression. The ankle may have been treated initially with steroids, NSAIDs, or splinting. If this treatment has failed, ankle arthrodesis may have been attempted unsuccessfully, leading to total ankle arthroplasty.

Indications for total ankle arthroplasty may include a failed talectomy resulting in avascular necrosis, or revision of a previous arthroplasty.

Technique

1. An anterior incision is made over the ankle joint.
2. The tibiotalar joint and talus dome are exposed.
3. A sizing template is used to mark the tibia.
4. Anchoring holes are made in the tibia, and the template is positioned while the foot is distracted.
5. The talus is marked, and a groove is made to accommodate the talar component.
6. The trial talar component is inserted, and the ankle is put through ROM exercises.
7. When the trial reduction is complete, the talar and tibial components are cemented.
8. The ankle joint is irrigated.
9. A drain may be used.
10. Surgical dressings are placed.
11. A posterior splint is placed.

Discussion

An anterior incision is made over the ankle joint. The tibiotalar joint and talus dome are exposed, and soft tissue is retracted with small, self-retaining retractors. When the center of the talus has been identified and marked with a marking pen, a sizing template is used to mark the tibia. A small defect is made with the 1-inch drill, and anchoring holes are made in the tibia. The template is positioned while the foot is distracted.

The talus is marked, and a groove is made to accommodate the talar component. The groove is made with a small osteotome or a small oscillating saw. The trial talar component is inserted, and the ankle is put through ROM exercises to check the fit. When the trial reduction is complete, the talar and tibial components are cemented. The ankle joint is irrigated, and if a drain is needed, it may be inserted at this time. A small drain, such as a Jackson-Pratt drain, may be used for this procedure.

Surgical dressings are placed, and a posterior splint is placed to help immobilize the ankle for a few days.

LOWER EXTREMITY AMPUTATION (BELOW-THE-KNEE AMPUTATION)

Surgical goal

Specialty orthopedic amputations are performed for trauma, malignancy, and infection. The goal of the orthopedic surgeon is to retain or repair the function of the limb, and BKA usually is performed only as the final option.

Pathology

Amputations are necessary because of trauma, malignancy, infection, or ischemia.

Technique

1. The level of amputation is determined, and the incision line is marked.
2. The incision is made.
3. Muscle and soft tissue are divided.
4. The periosteum is raised.
5. The bone is cut and beveled.
6. The wound is irrigated.
7. A drain is inserted.
8. The fascia is closed with interrupted sutures.
9. The skin is approximated.
10. An immediate postoperative stump dressing and splints may be applied.

Discussion

The level of amputation is determined, and the incision line is marked to create a long posterior flap. The incision is made. Muscle and soft tissue are divided, and the periosteum is raised with a Cobb or Key elevator. The bone is cut with an oscillating saw, reciprocating saw, or Gigli saw. The bone is beveled at the anterior aspect and smoothed with a rongeur and a rasp. The wound is irrigated, a Penrose or Hemovac drain is inserted, and the fascia is closed with heavy Vicryl sutures or other absorbable sutures. The skin is closed with staples or interrupted nonabsorbable suture such as nylon. An immediate postoperative stump dressing and splints may be applied, depending on the surgeon's preference.

LIMB REATTACHMENT

Surgical Goal

In this procedure, a severed limb is reattached to the body through bone-to-bone contact and by treatment of the surrounding area so that all soft tissues (blood vessels, muscles, tendons, and nerves) are regenerated.

Pathology

Indications for reattachment of hand, wrist, forearm, or leg include amputated limb or finger in children, multiple fingers involved in trauma, amputated thumb, and clean amputation. Several presurgical factors may increase or decrease the likelihood of successful replantation surgery.

The severity of the injury can determine the parts of the hand or fingers that can be saved.

Cooling the amputated part can substantially increase the time that can elapse between injury and surgery. When preparing patients for transfer to a replantation center, emergency medical personnel package the amputated limb or digits on ice to optimize the chance for successful replantation.

A key factor in improving the success of patients with finger and hand amputations is the emergency hospital network. This includes rapid transportation by ambulance or air. Emergency technicians arrange for transportation and ensure that bandages, x-rays, antibiotics, intravenous fluids, and tetanus shots are provided rapidly.

Technique

1. The patient's injuries are cleaned very carefully to avoid deep infection.
2. Any fractured bones first are stabilized.
3. The tendons are repaired.
4. Delicate nerves, arteries, and veins are repaired in the last stage of the procedure.
5. In severe injuries, vein or skin grafts are taken from another site, such as the forearm, foot, or thigh.
6. Skin grafts are necessary when the injury or swelling prevents the skin edges from closing.
7. Wounds are considered dirty and generally are not closed.
8. The wound and the anastomosis site are surgically dressed and protected from injury with a posterior splint.

Discussion

The amputated digits should be kept cool before surgery. One does this by wrapping the digits in gauze moistened with saline or a salt solution. The digits and gauze are placed inside a bag and set on ice to keep them cool. This helps to preserve the amputated parts. For best results, the replantation should be performed within 4 to 6 hours of the injury.

The bone ends of the affected finger or toe are shortened to reduce tension on the repaired arteries, veins, and nerves. K-wires may be used in hands and feet to stabilize bones. Bones of arms or legs are stabilized with long plates and screws. The tendons are then repaired. Because they are so small, the nerves and vessels are repaired under a microscope. When the repair is completed, the hand or foot is wrapped in a sterile surgical dressing. A posterior splint may be applied after surgery to protect the replanted digit and allow for swelling.

Remarkable advances in microsurgery have made it possible to reattach amputated limbs. Special microsutures and microscopes have been developed that allow a microvascular surgeon to repair the blood supply to the reattached limb. Microvascular surgeons have developed new techniques for repairing these very small blood vessels.

Complications

The success rate for replantation surgery averages about 80%, but complications do arise. Complications from replantation include death of the replanted tissue, reduced nerve function, reduced motor function, and cosmetic deformity. Risk factors for failed limb reattachment include amputation through the proximal phalanx (especially of the index and small fingers), tobacco abuse, and a crushed or significantly contaminated wound.

REFERENCES

Anderson KN: *Mosby's medical, nursing, and allied health dictionary,* ed 6, 2002, Saunders.
Avioli LV: *The osteoporotic syndrome: detection, prevention, and treatment,* ed 4, 2000, Academic Press.
Bowden B, Bowden J: *An illustrated atlas of the skeletal muscles,* 2002, Morton.
Browner BD, Jupiter JB, Levine AM et al: *Skeletal trauma in children, ed 3,* Philadelphia, 2003, Saunders.
Core curriculum for surgical technology, ed 5, 2002, Association of Surgical Technologists.
Green NE and Swiontkowski MF: *Skeletal trauma in children,* vol 3, ed 3, Philadelphia, 2003, Saunders.
Gregory B: *Orthopaedic surgery,* St Louis, 1994, Mosby.
Herring JA: *Tachdjian's pediatric orthopaedics from the Texas Scottish Rite Hospital for Children,* vol 1-3, ed 3, 2002, Saunders.
Phillips N: *Berry and Kohn's operating room technique,* ed 10, 2004, St. Louis, Mosby.
Rothrock JC: *Alexander's care of the patient in surgery,* ed 12, St Louis, 2003, Mosby.
Shier, Butler, and Lewis: *Hole's essentials of human anatomy and physiology,* ed 7, Boston, 1996, McGraw-Hill.
Tighe SM: *Instrumentation for the operating room: a photographic manual,* ed 6, St Louis, 2003, Mosby.
Weisel SW and Delahay JN: *Essentials of orthopaedic surgery,* ed 2, Philadelphia, 1997, Saunders.

Chapter 28

Peripheral Vascular Surgery

Behavioral Objectives

After studying this chapter the reader will be able to:

- Identify the anatomical structure and functions of arteries and veins
- Identify common obstructions of vessels
- Describe the scheme for performing bypass grafts
- Identify the goal of peripheral vascular surgery
- Identify various grafts used for peripheral vascular surgery

Terminology

Angioplasty—A process of remodeling the lumen of a blood vessel. This term usually refers to the removal of plaque or the release of a stricture in the vessel wall.

Arteriosclerosis—Disease characterized by thickening, hardening, and loss of elasticity of the walls of arteries.

Arteriotomy—An incision made in the artery, usually to perform an anastomosis with a graft or another vessel, or to remove plaque or a thrombus from inside the artery.

Arteriovenous fistula—Also called an AV fistula; a naturally occurring or surgically created connection between an artery and a vein. In surgery, an AV fistula is created surgically to prepare a vessel for hemodialysis.

Atherosclerosis—The most common form of arteriosclerosis. The formation of thick, yellowish plaque (containing cholesterol and lipoid materials, and lipophages) that infiltrates and deposits in the inner layer of the arterial wall. This plaque causes stricture and loss of arterial blood flow to a part of the body.

Bifurcation—A Y shape in an artery or graft.

Diastolic pressure—The lowest pressure exerted on the arterial wall during the resting phase of the cardiac cycle.

Doppler duplex ultrasonography—Doppler ultrasonography amplifies sounds that pass through tissue. Doppler duplex technology uses this technology plus ultrasound to produce a visual image of blood flow through a vessel.

Electroencephalogram (EEG)—A diagnostic tool that measures the electrical activity of the brain. During vascular surgery, EEG may be used to determine the patient's neurophysiologic response.

Embolus—A clot of blood, air, or organic material that moves freely in the vascular system. An embolus travels from larger to smaller vessels until it cannot pass through a vessel. At that level it interrupts the flow of blood and may result in severe disease or death.

Endarterectomy—The surgical removal of atherosclerotic plaque from inside an artery.

Etiology—The origin or cause of a disease.

Extracorporeal—Outside the body. In extracorporeal hemodialysis, the blood is shunted outside the body for filtering and cleansing.

Hemodialysis—A process in which blood is shunted out of the body and through a complex set of filters. It is performed on patients with end-stage renal disease to remove extra electrolytes and waste products from the body.

Terminology

Infarction—A blockage in an artery leading to ischemia and tissue death.

In situ—In the natural position or normal place, without disturbing or invading surrounding tissues.

Intravascular ultrasound—A diagnostic tool in which a transducer is introduced into an artery and ultrasound used to translate the physical characteristics of the lumen into a visible image.

Ischemia—Lack of blood and therefore oxygen in tissue.

Lumen—The inside of a hollow structure such as a blood vessel.

Percutaneous—Literally means "through the skin." In a percutaneous approach in surgery, an incision is not made, but a catheter or other device is introduced through a puncture site.

Stent—A tubular device placed inside an artery to hold it open to treat and prevent stricture.

Systolic pressure—The greatest amount of pressure exerted on the arterial wall during the pumping action of the heart.

Thrombus—Any organic or nonorganic material blocking an artery. Generally refers to a blood clot or atherosclerotic plaque. However, infected tissue or a large bacterial colony that separates from its origin (e.g., from a heart valve) also may become a thrombus.

Tunica adventitia—The outermost covering of an artery.

INTRODUCTION TO PERIPHERAL VASCULAR SURGERY

Peripheral vascular surgery encompasses procedures of the arteries and veins, excluding those in or near the heart, brain, or cranial vessels. Many surgical procedures of the vascular system are performed to treat arteriosclerosis, **atherosclerosis,** or thromboembolic disease. These procedures often must be performed quickly and efficiently while one or more major vessels are clamped.

Vascular surgery requires focused concentration and preparation for surgical emergency. Operations on blood vessels present a risk of sudden uncontrolled hemorrhage, which can lead to irreversible hypovolemia or hypotension. The scrub must acquire thorough knowledge of instruments and equipment. He or she also must have excellent organizational skills and the ability to remain alert for long periods of time. Many vascular surgeries are performed as emergency procedures. "Routine" vascular surgery can quickly develop into a critical emergency.

ANATOMY OF THE PERIPHERAL VASCULAR SYSTEM

The peripheral vascular system is a complex network of vessels whose function is to carry blood to all parts of the body. When the heart beats, it sends blood to all parts of the body. The blood then returns to the heart, which sends it to the lungs for reoxygenation. This system is called the *peripheral vascular system.* The organs of this system are the arteries, veins, and capillary networks. The technologist preparing to scrub on any peripheral vascular case should be familiar with the vascular anatomy as well as regional structures. The system must be considered as a whole rather than a snapshot appearing through a fenestration of the drape. Changes that occur during surgery affect the whole body. This is because the vascular system provides active, ongoing transport of nutrients and oxygen necessary for survival. Interruption or changes in the cycle quickly affect anatomical regions beyond the operative site.

The peripheral vascular system encompasses two parallel vascular systems: the pulmonary and systemic vascular systems (Figure 28-1). The *pulmonary system* begins at the heart. Deoxygenated blood is pumped through the pulmonary arteries into the lungs, which oxygenate the blood. The oxygenated blood then returns to the heart via the pulmonary veins (Figure 28-2).

The *systemic vascular* system begins with the great arteries that arise from the heart. The arterial and venous vascular system is illustrated in Figure 28-3. These vessels carry blood away from the heart (all arteries except the pulmonary arteries carry oxygenated blood) to increasingly smaller branches. The smallest artery is called an *arteriole.* Finally, the arterioles join into a meshed network called the *capillary bed* or *capillary network* (Figure 28-4). Oxygen and other cellular nutrients are delivered at the capillary beds inside tissues. At the point of exchange, the arterioles become *venules,* the smallest veins of the body. Blood returns to the heart via the venules, veins, and finally the vena cava, the largest vein in the body. Blood enters the heart through the inferior and superior vena cava, and the cycle begins again.

Structure of the Vessels

Blood vessels are complex organs with multiple tissue layers, each having separate functions (Figure 28-5). Except at the capillary level, all blood vessels have three layers: the **tunica adventitia,** or outside layer, the middle *tunica media,* and the inner *tunica intima.* The intima layer is made of squamous epithelium, which prevents blood cells from sticking to the vessel walls. When the intima is disrupted or damaged by disease, this layer can no longer serve this function. Clots form easily, and the vessel can become narrowed.

The *media* is smooth muscle. It provides elasticity to the vessel, allowing it to expand and contract with changing blood pressure and volume. This layer is thicker in the artery than in the vein. Some vasodilating drugs act on this muscle layer to relax it and prevent constriction or spasm.

The *adventitia* is the protective connective-tissue layer of the vessel. It attaches to the surrounding tissue. When a ves-

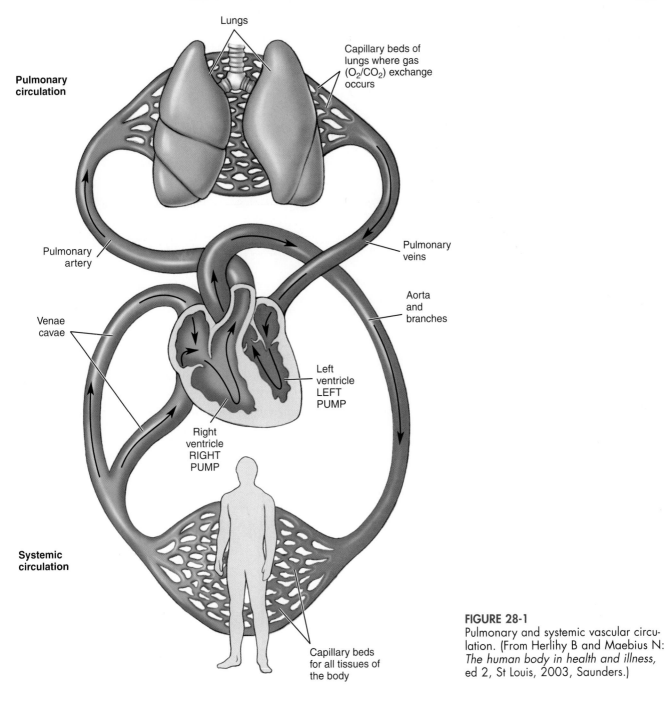

Pulmonary circulation

Lungs

Capillary beds of lungs where gas (O_2/CO_2) exchange occurs

Pulmonary artery

Pulmonary veins

Venae cavae

Aorta and branches

Left ventricle LEFT PUMP

Right ventricle RIGHT PUMP

Systemic circulation

Capillary beds for all tissues of the body

FIGURE 28-1
Pulmonary and systemic vascular circulation. (From Herlihy B and Maebius N: *The human body in health and illness,* ed 2, St Louis, 2003, Saunders.)

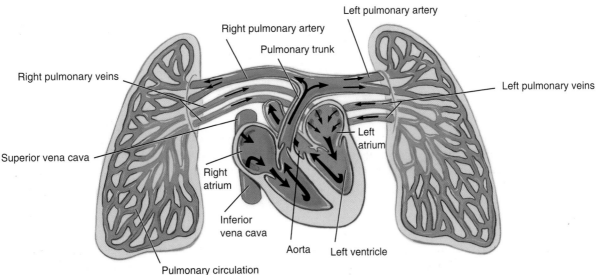

Right pulmonary artery

Left pulmonary artery

Pulmonary trunk

Right pulmonary veins

Left pulmonary veins

Superior vena cava

Left atrium

Right atrium

Inferior vena cava

Aorta

Left ventricle

Pulmonary circulation

FIGURE 28-2
Pulmonary circulation. (From Applegate E: *The anatomy and physiology learning system,* ed 2, St Louis, 2000, Saunders.)

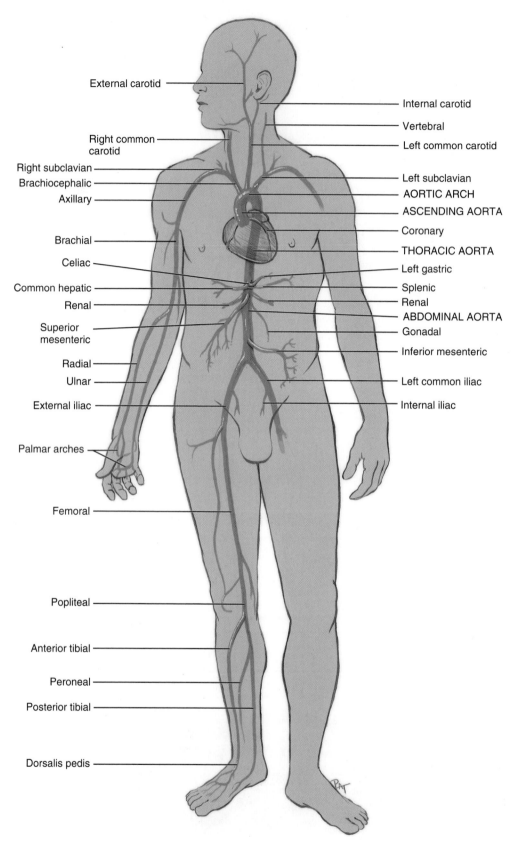

External carotid

Internal carotid

Vertebral

Right common carotid

Left common carotid

Right subclavian

Left subclavian

Brachiocephalic

AORTIC ARCH

Axillary

ASCENDING AORTA

Coronary

Brachial

THORACIC AORTA

Celiac

Left gastric

Common hepatic

Splenic

Renal

Renal

ABDOMINAL AORTA

Superior mesenteric

Gonadal

Inferior mesenteric

Radial

Ulnar

Left common iliac

External iliac

Internal iliac

Palmar arches

Femoral

Popliteal

Anterior tibial

Peroneal

Posterior tibial

Dorsalis pedis

FIGURE 28-3
A, Major systemic arteries.

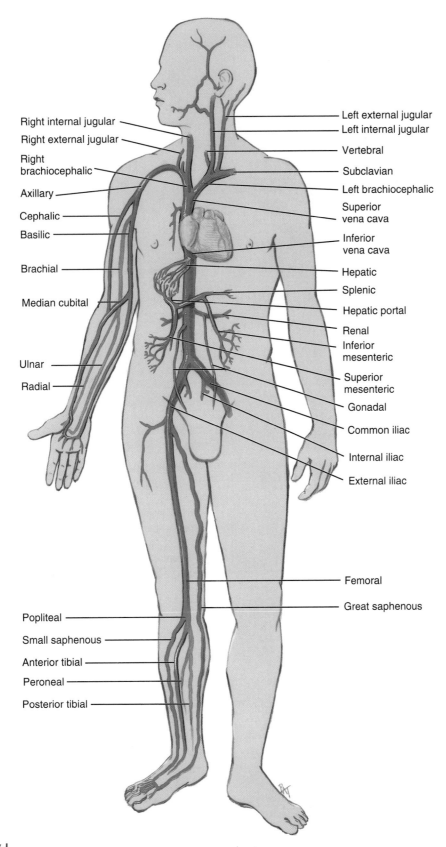

FIGURE 28-3, cont'd
B, Major systemic veins (From Applegate E: *The anatomy and physiology learning system,* ed 2, St Louis, 2000, Saunders.)

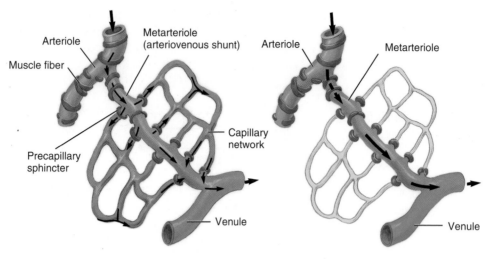

FIGURE 28-4
Organization of a capillary network (From Applegate E: *The anatomy and physiology learning system,* ed 2, St Louis, 2000, Saunders.)

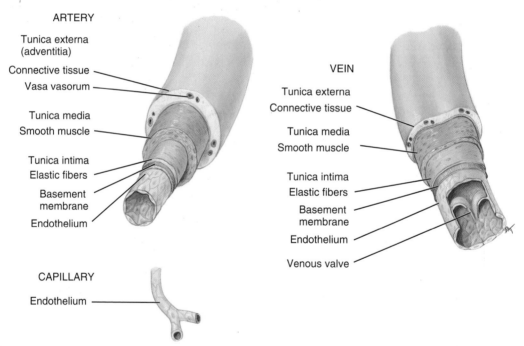

FIGURE 28-5
Structure of blood vessels. (From Applegate E: *The anatomy and physiology learning system,* ed 2, St Louis, 2000, Saunders.)

sel is *mobilized* or freed, it is this layer that is separated from the bed of tissue surrounding the artery or vein. Veins have a thicker adventitia than arteries.

Differences between Arteries and Veins

Structural differences between veins and arteries reflect their function. An *artery* is a vessel that carries blood away from the heart. The arteries carry oxygenated blood to the rest of the body (except for the pulmonary arteries, which carry deoxygenated blood to the lungs). Arteries are under considerable internal pressure from the pumping of the heart and therefore are much thicker than their corresponding vessels, the veins.

An artery is more elastic than a vein. This is because it must withstand changing pressures and recoil easily. When the artery loses its ability to recoil, as in atherosclerotic disease, it cannot convey arterial blood efficiently. As mentioned above, arteries contain an important inner layer, the intima. Atherosclerosis (see below) destroys this layer by infiltrating it with lipids. The plaque seen on the inside of the artery does not merely lay over the intima, but invades it in advanced disease. As more and more plaque covers the intima, the vessel loses its ability to respond to pressure. Lipids stick more readily to the plaque, and the vessel finally becomes occluded. This causes ischemia (loss of blood to the tissue), pain, and eventual tissue death.

Veins are vessels that carry blood toward the heart. Veins carry deoxygenated blood from body tissues back to the heart (except for pulmonary veins, which carry oxygenated blood to the heart). Veins move blood back to the heart by the pumping action of the skeletal muscles and changes in the thoracic pressure when the lungs inflate. Within each vein, small valves open as the blood is pumped through the vein. When the pressure beyond the valve exceeds the pumping pressure, the valve closes. Venous blood pressure is lower than arterial pressure because the venous pumping mechanism is weaker than the heart.

Blood Pressure

Blood pressure is the force that is exerted on the arterial wall by the pumping action of the heart. The **systolic pressure** is the highest pressure that occurs when the heart beats (called *systole*). The lowest pressure is the **diastolic pressure,** and this is the pressure that occurs during the relaxation phase of the cardiac cycle, called *diastole.*

EQUIPMENT AND INSTRUMENTS

Instruments

Vascular surgery requires both vascular and general surgical sets. The exact instruments needed depend on the operative site. For superficial surgery, short, delicate instruments are required. Large vessels, such as the descending aorta, require longer, heavier instruments.

Vascular instruments include vascular clamps, fine-tipped needle holders, atraumatic forceps such as Cushing or DeBakey forceps, sharp dissecting scissors, right-angle clamps, and retractors. Right-angle clamps are used throughout the procedure to reach under and around vessels without causing trauma. Suction is critical during all vascular procedures.

Dissection in vascular surgery requires delicate, *sharp* scissors. Both blunt and sharp dissection is required to gain access to blood vessels. The risk of traumatizing nearby structures is minimized when instruments are maintained properly. Common vascular instruments are illustrated in Figure 28-6.

Suture

MATERIALS AND DESIGN

Vascular suture materials include polypropylene, expanded polytetrafluoroethylene (PTFE, Gore-Tex), Ethibond (polyester), and silk. Sizes range from 3-0 to 8-0. Laser-drilled swaged sutures are superior because the diameter of the suture matches the needle head and creates less trauma. Round, tapered, or beveled needles in sizes $\frac{1}{2}$ inch to $\frac{3}{8}$ inch usually are used. Double-armed sutures commonly are used to create a circumferential anastomosis.

HANDLING OF SUTURE MATERIAL IN THE FIELD

One must take special care when handling vascular suture materials in the sterile field. Fine polypropylene sutures must be carefully removed from the packet and delicately stretched. The needle holder must be the appropriate size for the needle so it does not damage the needle body. Gore-Tex suture is not pliable and must not be pulled or stretched as it is removed from the needle package. A rule of thumb for the scrub in peripheral vascular surgery is to always stay one suture ahead, so when the scrub hands the surgeon the last 5-0 Prolene suture on the field, the scrub should request another from the circulator so the scrub is prepared with a suture in case of bleeding or hemorrhage.

The surgeon may want the double-armed sutures loaded on both ends with needle holders, or one needle loaded with a needle holder and the other needle with a rubber-shod mosquito hemostat. The scrub should not remove any rubber shods or needle drivers from the operative field; the scrub should let the surgeon pass them back. The sutures are double armed and attached to shods and needle drivers, so retrieving instruments from the field could potentially rip apart an anastomosis of a vessel or graft and cause hemorrhage.

Vascular Grafts
MATERIALS AND DESIGN

Vascular grafts are used to replace a blood vessel or to make a patch. Synthetic grafts are made of Dacron, polyester, or Gore-Tex. Sources of natural materials are banked human umbilical cord, bovine grafts, and autografts. Grafts may be straight or **bifurcated** (Y-shaped). The length is measured in centimeters, and the diameter reflects *outside* diameter (OD).

ON-SITE PREPARATION

Vascular grafts are extremely expensive. They must not be opened until the surgeon is ready to insert them and has verbally requested the size required.

Synthetic grafts require no preinsertion preparation except trimming.

Patch grafts are cut into elliptical sections and sutured into place with a double-armed suture as shown in Figure 28-7. Bovine grafts are packaged in preservative, which must be thoroughly rinsed from the graft before insertion.

All commercially prepared grafts are intended for use as directed by the manufacturer, and specific protocol is necessary for safe implantation. Each graft has an identification number, which must be recorded on the patient's operative record.

GRAFT TUNNELING

Vascular grafts often must be tunneled through subcutaneous tissue to connect one vessel to another. Two techniques are used. The surgeon may use his fingers to separate the tissue digitally, or a graft tunneler can be used (see above). This is a long metal shaft with bunt tips that is manually pushed through the tissue. The subcutaneous tissue has scant blood supply, so the risk of hemorrhage is small. As the tunneler is advanced, it leaves a tubular space through which the graft can be threaded. This surgeon usually performs this step by inserting a long clamp such as a Péan into the tunnel and grasping the graft from the entry site. If the tunnel is short, the surgeon can pass it easily. Longer grafts may require an intermediate incision in the skin and subcutaneous tissue.

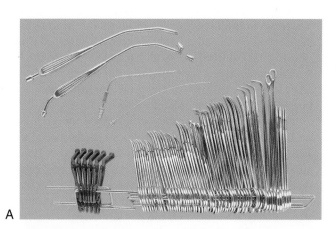
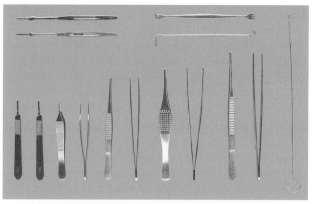
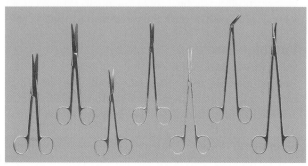
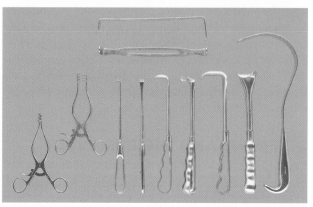

FIGURE 28-6
Peripheral vascular set. **A,** *Top to bottom,* 2 Yankauer suction tubes with tips; 1 Frazier suction tube with stylet. *Bottom, left to right,* 6 paper drape clips; 10 Halsted mosquito hemostatic forceps, curved; 6 Crile hemostatic forceps, 5½ inch, curved; 6 Providence hemostatic forceps (delicate tip), 5½ inch, curved; 4 Crile hemostatic forceps, 6½ inch, curved; 4 Allis tissue forceps; 4 Westphal hemostatic forceps; 6 tonsil hemostatic forceps; 2 Mayo-Péan hemostatic forceps, long, curved; 2 Carmalt hemostatic forceps, long; 2 Adson hemostatic forceps, long; 2 Mixter hemostatic forceps, long, fine and heavy tips; 2 Foerster sponge forceps; 2 Crile-Wood needle holders, 7 inch; 2 Ayer needle holders, 7 inch, fine tips. **B,** *Top, left to right,* 2 Bard-Parker knife handles, no. 7; 2 Miller-Senn retractors. *Bottom, left to right,* 2 Bard-Parker knife handles, no. 3; 2 Adson tissue forceps with teeth (1 × 2), side view and front view; 2 DeBakey vascualr Atraugrip tissue forceps, short, side view and front view; 2 Ferris-Smith tissue forceps, side view and front view; 2 DeBakey vascular Atraugrip tissue forceps, medium, side view and front view; 1 eyed obturator (stylet) for Rumel tourniquet. **C,** *Left to right,* 1 Mayo dissecting scissors, straight; 1 Mayo dissecting scissors, curved; 1 Metzenbaum scissors, 5 inch; 1 Metzenbaum scissors, 7 inch; 1 Lincoln Metzenbaum scissors; 1 Potts-Smith cardiovascular scissors, 45-degree angle; 1 Strully scissors, probe tip. **D,** *Top,* 2 Army-Navy retractors, side view and front view. *Bottom, left to right,* 2 Weitlaner retractors, sharp, medium; 2 vein retractors, side view and front view; 2 Richardson retractors, small, side view and front view; 2 Richardson retractors, medium, side view and front view; 1 Deaver retractor, small, side view. (From Tighe S: *Instrumentation for the operating room,* ed 6, St Louis, 2003, Mosby.)

Intravascular Ultrasound

Intravascular ultrasound is used in both peripheral and coronary surgery to map the **lumen** of a vessel. A rotating flexible catheter carrying a transducer is introduced into the vessel. Ultrasonic energy is generated and interpreted by the transducer. The lumen of the vessel, including density, accumulation of atherosclerotic plaque, and thickness of the wall, then can be mapped and a visual image can be produced. Because of its ability to rotate, intravascular ultrasound produces a 360-degree image.

Doppler Scanning

Doppler scanning intensifies the sounds made by blood flowing through a vessel. The pitch, rhythm, and quality of the sound reflect pressure, volume, and flow rate. The tip of the Doppler probe is placed over a pulse point or other area that requires evaluation. The probe gathers the sound generated by the body structure and transmits the sound to the Doppler unit. When the sensing probe is placed over an artery, high-frequency sound saves generated by the probe are reflected back from the blood cells. Specific pitches, generated by the blood flowing through the artery, are associated with velocity, and these are interpreted by the surgeon. The surgeon may assess blood flow before, during, and after surgery. A nonsterile Doppler probe may be used preoperatively and postoperatively, and a sterile probe should be available for intraoperative use.

Doppler Duplex Ultrasonography

Doppler duplex ultrasonography combines Doppler scanning, which intensifies the sound (or lack of it) of blood

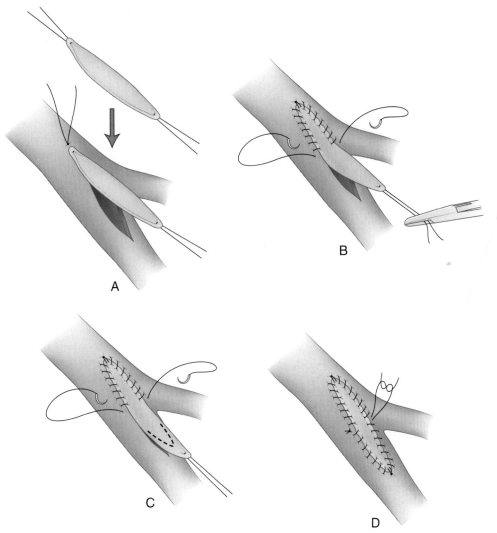

FIGURE 28-7
Patch angioplasty. **A,** Mattress sutures are placed at each end of the graft. **B,** Suturing begins at one corner of the arteriotomy towards the middle. **C,** The graft may be trimmed (along dotted lines to fit the arteriotomy). **D,** The closure is continued from the opposite end toward the midline, where the sutures are tied together. (From Rutherford R: *Atlas of vascular surgery: basic techniques and exposures,* Philadelphia, 1993, Saunders.)

flowing through a vessel, with ultrasound, which produces visual images of the vessel. It measures strictures, **thrombi,** venous insufficiency, and other abnormalities that can be measured by their density. Gray-scale and color images are produced. A data recorder produces a permanent record of the information.

Pulse Volume Recording (Arterial Plethysmography)

The pulse volume recorder is used to measure the waveform of the arterial pulse during systole. To perform this test, one places three blood pressure cuffs around the leg and inflates them to 65 mm Hg. Each cuff reading produces a waveform, which is compared with the others. A reduced wave in one area can indicate reduced blood flow at that point.

OPERATIVE TECHNIQUES

Endarterectomy

Atherosclerosis is a disease of the arterial vascular system. In this condition, a fatty fibrotic plaque develops in the intima layer of the arteries. As plaque builds and invades the intima layer of the vessel, the endothelium is damaged. This causes hardening and loss of elasticity (Figure 28-8).

Plaque is found in large and medium-size arteries. The coronary arteries are often affected, leading to heart disease. Other common sites are the **bifurcations** of the femoral, iliac, and carotid arteries. Atherosclerosis is associated with smoking, hyperlipidemia, and advancing age. Atherosclerosis is a major health problem in the United States. Coronary artery disease is the leading cause of death in the United States.

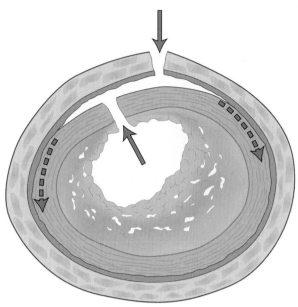

FIGURE 28-8
Cross section of a diseased artery showing incision to the correct level (cleavage plane in outer media), which is then continued circumferentially. (From Rutherford R: *Atlas of vascular surgery: basic techniques and exposures*, Philadelphia, 1993, Saunders.)

Many vascular procedures require removal of atherosclerotic plaque from the inside of the artery. Plaque is a rubbery substance that adheres to the intima (innermost) layer of the blood vessel, causing occlusion. When the surgeon removes plaque, there is a risk of breaking it apart and causing an **embolus.** This procedure requires meticulous technique and fine instruments. Plaque can be removed in one piece, as shown in Figure 28-9. The surgeon may use a Penfield or Freer elevator to separate the plaque from the intima while applying gentle traction. In another method, the blood vessel is opened at its bifurcation (**Y** split) and the plaque is removed circumferentially.

Retraction
Retraction of the vessel is maintained with a long, flat strip of cotton (called an umbilical tape), flexible Silastic vessel loops, or a small Penrose drain. These vessel retractors are used to manipulate the vessels without causing trauma. To place a vessel loop around a blood vessel, the scrub mounts it on a right-angle clamp that can be passed underneath the vessel and looped around the vessel. The two ends of the vessel loop are clamped with a hemostat. One can achieve a tourniquet effect by sliding a short length of flexible tubing called a **Rumel** tourniquet along the free ends of the vessel loop, as shown in Figure 28-10.

Closure and Anastomosis
Longitudinal incisions in the blood vessel are closed with a double-armed suture. Traction sutures may be placed at one or both ends of the incision (Figure 28-11). Circumferential incisions (in an anastomosis) are closed with a double-armed suture, as shown in Figure 28-12.

Hemostasis
A dry surgical site is critical in vascular surgery, and suction must be available at all times. Because vascular suction tips clog easily, the technologist should keep one on the field and another in reserve. This allows the clogged tip to be flushed or cleared with a metal stylet while one remains in use.

Large vessels such as the abdominal aorta require larger suction tips. A Poole or Yankauer suction tip is used in retroperitoneal surgery. Two suctions may be necessary to maintain a dry field. In general, suction is used more often than sponges to maintain a dry operative field.

Hemostasis is maintained at anastomosis sites with collagen or fibrin products such as microfibrillar collagen hemostat (Gelfoam, Avitene) and topical thrombin. Small (1-cm) squares of Gelfoam often are soaked in topical thrombin and used to control bleeding at anastomosis sites. Surgicel also may be placed on the site of the anastomosis.

Anticoagulation
During vascular surgery the operative area must be irrigated with heparinized saline solution. This prevents the formation of thrombi at the surgical site and reduces the risk of embolus. Systemic heparin is administered before the blood vessels are exposed and is infused into the operative vessel after it has been opened. The scrub prepares heparin irrigation by attaching a vascular irrigation tip, such as an Abrahms or Stoney needle tip, to a 20-ml or 30-ml syringe.

Because both thrombin and heparin are distributed to the scrub, there is a risk that the wrong drug may be offered to the surgeon. It is critically important that all medications on the field be clearly marked. Intravenous administration of thrombin can cause a fatal embolus.

After the administration of heparin, local coagulation time is longer than normal, which is desired. Additional sutures, topical thrombin, or vascular clamps may be required after vessel closure. Systemic heparin is reversed with protamine sulfate, which is administered by the anesthesia care provider. Protamine sulfate is the only medication that reduces the effects of heparin.

Vasospasm
Vasospasm is spasm of an artery or vein. This can occur when the vessel is handled and can cause damage to the structure. Lidocaine or papaverine is injected into the vessel to prevent vasospasm during surgery. The lidocaine should be clearly labeled and available on the Mayo stand before the initial incision is made.

SURGICAL PROCEDURES
Intraoperative Angiography
SURGICAL GOAL
Preoperative angiography is the injection of contrast media into a selected artery and its branches to determine the exact location of strictures, occlusion, or malformation. During surgery, *intraoperative* angiography is used in conjunction

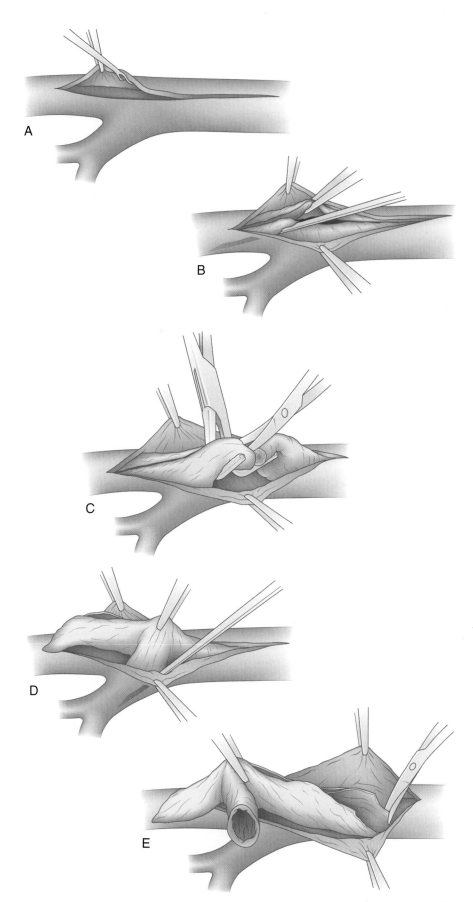

FIGURE 28-9

Open endarterectomy. **A,** The correct cleavage plane is developed. **B,** The plaque is freed up circumferentially. **C,** The plaque is divided over a right-angle clamp. **D,** The plaque is freed up distally into the major outflow branches. **E,** The proximal end of the plaque is trimmed off. (From Rutherford R: *Atlas of vascular surgery: basic techniques and exposures,* Philadelphia, 1993, Saunders.)

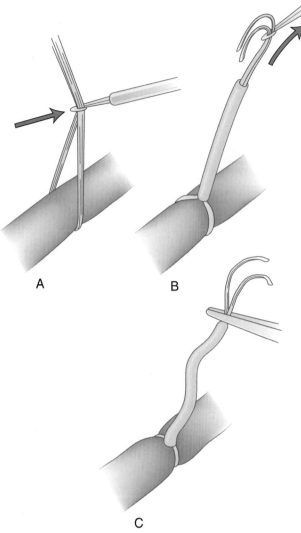

FIGURE 28-10
Application of a Rumel tourniquet. **A,** The two ends of the umbilical tape are hooked. **B,** The tape is pulled through the rubber catheter. **C,** The tourniquet is cinched down and secured with a hemostat. (From Rutherford R: *Atlas of vascular surgery: basic techniques and exposures,* Philadelphia, 1993, Saunders.)

with **angioplasty,** especially stent placement and embolectomy, to allow the surgeon to see the position of the stricture and place the catheter in the correct location.

DISCUSSION

Intraoperative angiography is performed with intravascular ultrasound and other imaging techniques because it allows the surgeon to see obstructions or emboli distal and proximal to the operative area.

Technique

1. All team members don a lead shield before surgery.
2. The circulator distributes contrast media to the scrub.
3. The scrub prepares the contrast media and sterile saline.

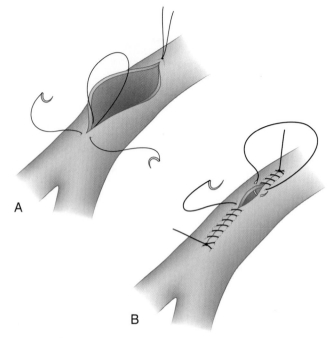

FIGURE 28-11
Longitudinal arteriotomy. **A,** Suture placed at each end. **B,** A continuous suture is run from each end toward the middle. (From Rutherford R: *Atlas of vascular surgery: basic techniques and exposures,* Philadelphia, 1993, Saunders.)

4. The operative site is prepared for x-ray or C-arm fluoroscopy.
5. Metal instruments are removed from the field, and the operative site is covered with a sterile drape.
6. The surgeon injects the artery with contrast media, and images are recorded during injection.
7. The contrast media is flushed from the artery with sterile saline.

In this procedure, contrast media is injected directly into the operative artery and its branches. Contrast media does not allow penetration of x-rays and is seen on radiograph or fluoroscopy as a white tract. The outline and interior configuration of the vessel are observed on x-ray or fluoroscopy. The media is flushed through the vessel with sterile saline at the completion of the procedure. Repeat injections and data recording may be required to clarify an image.

Whenever angiography is planned, all personnel must wear a lead shield over their scrub attire. This includes scrubbed personnel.

Equipment needed for intraoperative angiography includes:

▶ Two or more 30-ml or 50-ml syringes
▶ Contrast media as specified by the surgeon
▶ An arterial needle
▶ One or two vinyl catheters with a stopcock attached
▶ An intravenous catheter for injection of dye intraluminally
▶ Sterile intravenous saline

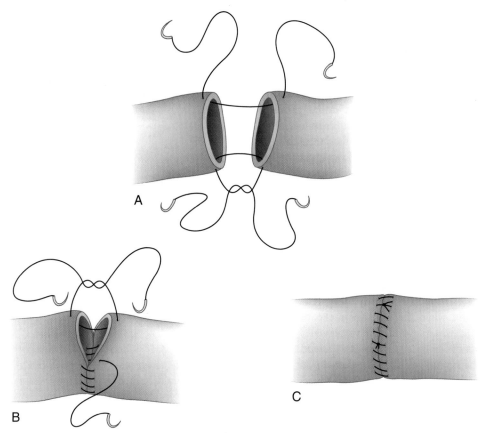

FIGURE 28-12
Closure of a circumferential incision. **A,** Placement of two double-arm sutures 180 degrees apart. **B,** The sutures are run continuous and toward each other. **C,** Completion of closure. (From Rutherford R: *Atlas of vascular surgery: basic techniques and exposures*, Philadelphia, 1993, Saunders.)

The circulator distributes contrast media to the scrub, who draws it up into two syringes. A solution of 60% Renografin usually is used. A third syringe of *intravenous* saline also is prepared to flush the media from the arteries when x-rays have been completed. The scrub attaches the angiogram needle to a short length of vinyl tubing and attaches the other end to one syringe of dye. All air bubbles must be removed from the tubing to ensure that air is not introduced into the artery. A Kelly or Mayo hemostat placed across the tubing prevents air from backing into it. If a stopcock is used, air bubbles are flushed out and the stopcock is secured in the closed position.

The surgeon may choose one of several techniques to inject the dye:

▶ If the **arteriotomy** (incision in the artery) has already been sutured closed, an angiography needle attached to the vinyl tubing and syringe is inserted between the sutures.
▶ A catheter can be inserted into the vessel and snugged down with a Rumel tourniquet.
▶ The arterial needle can be secured inside the cut end of the vessel with silk suture.

If standard x-rays are to be taken, the technologist uses sterile technique to receive the cassette in a cassette pouch. The technologist folds the outer edge of the cover, making a wide sterile cuff. After the cassette has been dropped inside, the edges of the pouch are turned up and secured. The cassette is then placed under the limb, the x-ray machine is placed in position, and films are taken. The cassette is removed from the field. If C-arm fluoroscopy is used, the C-arm is draped and a still series of pictures is taken during injection. The artery and branches are immediately flushed with saline. Additional pictures may be required.

Angioplasty
SURGICAL GOAL

Angioplasty is a general term that describes various methods of remodeling the inner surface of an artery that has narrowed because of stricture or atherosclerosis. The surgical goal is to reestablish patency and circulation of arterial blood. Peripheral angioplasty is often performed on the femoral, iliac, and carotid arteries. *Interventional angioplasty* is commonly performed in the outpatient setting. Intraoperative angioplasty may follow surgical **endarterectomy**.

PATHOLOGY

Angioplasty is performed to treat atherosclerosis or stricture of the blood vessel.

DISCUSSION

Angioplasty is performed *during angiography,* with C-arm fluoroscopy. Contrast media is injected to verify the correct placement of the stent, embolectomy catheter, or intravascular shaving device.

Stent

A vascular **stent** is a small metal implant designed to fit against the wall of an artery. Many different types of stents are available. They are made of stainless steel, titanium, or metal alloy called Nitinol. The common principle among all types is that they are a meshed tube that adheres to the lumen of the vessel. The tube produces continuous vessel patency so that blood can flow freely. Atherosclerotic plaque is pushed against the vessel wall and prevented from entering the lumen by the stent that covers it.

Most stents are implanted permanently. Two types of stents are commonly used. These are the *balloon expandable stent* and the *self-expanding stent.* The balloon expandable stent is a fine catheter with a balloon tip. The stent is fixed over the balloon, and when the balloon is expanded, the stent is pushed into position against the vessel wall.

For implantation of the balloon expandable stent, the patient is placed in the supine position and a large-bore needle is inserted into the vessel distal to the stenting site. A flexible guide wire is passed over the needle, which is then withdrawn, and the angioplasty balloon catheter is inserted. A tuberculin syringe is used to expand the balloon. The stent is discharged, and the catheter is removed. A common type of balloon expandable stent is the *Palmaz stent* (Figure 28-13, *A*).

The self-expanding stent is placed in the same manner except that the stent is preloaded into a delivery system that is passed over the guide wire. When the stent is discharged, it opens and adheres to the lumen wall. The *Wallstent* is a commonly used self-expanding stent (Figure 28-13, *B*).

Balloon Angioplasty

In this procedure, a stricture in the artery is expanded with a balloon catheter that has been inserted to the level of the plaque. When the balloon is inflated, it pushes the plaque against the vessel wall and releases the stricture. Angioplasty balloons are available in graduated lengths and widths.

Before the balloon angioplasty is performed, contrast media is injected into the artery, and the area of stricture is marked on films produced by the data recorder. The balloon catheter is inserted into the artery to the level of the stricture. The catheter is left in place at a specific pressure and specific length of time. The balloon catheter is filled with contrast media, and both the vessel walls and catheter balloon are observed on fluoroscopy. The catheter is withdrawn, and final angiography films are taken.

Thrombectomy (Open Procedure)
SURGICAL GOAL

A thrombus is a stationary blood clot in the arterial or venous system that blocks blood supply distal to it. The surgical goal of thrombectomy is to surgically remove the clot while it is stationary. This restores circulation and prevents

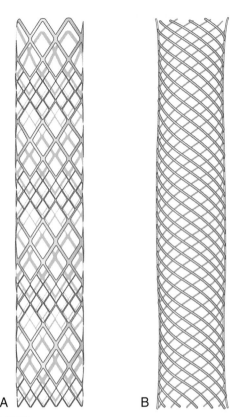

FIGURE 28-13
A, Balloon balloon expandable stent. **B,** Self-expanding stent.

the clot from moving. Thrombectomy is commonly performed with an embolectomy catheter.

PATHOLOGY

Many different conditions can result in a thrombus. When a thrombus breaks away from a blood vessel wall and travels through the vascular system, it is called an embolus (a free moving thrombus).

An embolus can consist of any material, including atherosclerotic plaque, necrotic tissue from an infected heart valve, or a blood clot. As an embolus travels through increasingly smaller vessels of the vascular system, it can lodge in the heart, brain, kidney, mesentery, or other vital organ. This causes an **infarction** or area whose blood supply is *blocked.* An infarction leads to ischemia, an area of tissue devoid of the oxygen and other nutrients that the blood normally supplies. Without blood, the tissue dies. Thrombectomy therefore can be a life-saving procedure.

This discussion focuses on the **etiology** (origin or cause of a disease condition) of a blood thrombus. Common causes of thrombi are:

▶ Trauma, especially surgery, when large blood vessels are exposed to air and clots form at the surgical site
▶ Obesity
▶ Childbirth
▶ Genetic predisposition

▶ **Pulmonary emboli** (those which lodge in the lung) usually originate from the venous system of the lower extremities. These are caused by venous system disease resulting in stasis.

In addition to surgical interventions, the patient receives anticoagulation therapy to prevent further formation of clots. This does not dissolve existing clots but aids in the prevention of new ones.

Technique

1. The surgeon exposes and mobilizes the target vessel.
2. Vessel loops are placed around the artery.
3. The vessel is clamped.
4. An incision is made into the artery (arteriotomy).
5. The embolectomy catheter is threaded into the arteriotomy and past the thrombus.
6. The balloon is inflated and slowly retracted, pulling the thrombus through the arteriotomy.
7. Intraoperative Doppler duplex ultrasonography may be performed.
8. The arteriotomy is closed.
9. The wound is closed.

DISCUSSION

The most common method of removing thrombi is with a Fogarty-type **embolectomy catheter.** This is a narrow, flexible catheter with a firm tip and an inflatable balloon at the tip. The length of the catheter varies widely, as the entry site may be close to or far from the thrombus itself. Balloons are round or elliptical, and catheters are available in sizes ranging from 1 Fr to 6 Fr. The balloon is filled with air or saline, according to the manufacturer's recommendations. A tuberculin syringe is used to fill the balloons, which have a volume of 0.2 ml or more. The balloon must be tested before use and never overinflated. To set up the catheter for use, one attaches the proximal end to a length of vinyl tubing with or without an intervening three-way stopcock. The tuberculin syringe is placed at the proximal end of the tubing. All connections must be tight.

Patient preparation depends on the location of the thrombus as determined by angiograms, duplex Doppler ultrasonography, and magnetic resonance imaging (MRI). Thrombi from the lower extremities often are removed from the groin. Mesenteric thrombi require an abdominal approach (laparotomy). In the following description of thrombectomy, the techniques are described beginning with the isolation of the vessel and actual use of the embolectomy catheter. Surgical incisions and closures are found in chapters associated with a particular anatomical area.

The patient is placed in supine position for abdominal, lower-extremity, and upper-extremity surgery. A general or regional anesthetic is used. The surgical site is prepped in normal fashion.

The scrub should have heparinized saline, vessel irrigation tips, vascular sutures, ties, and hemostatic agents avail-

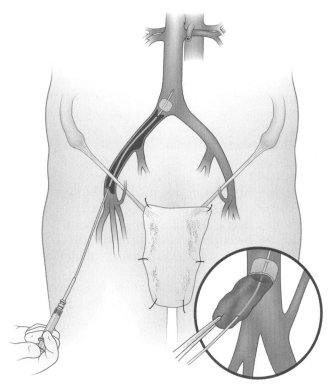

FIGURE 28-14
A thrombectomy catheter is introduced through a femoral venotomy to extrude the thrombosis. (From Ouriel K and Rutherford R: *Atlas of vascular surgery: operative procedures,* Philadelphia, 1998, Saunders.)

able. A variety of vascular clamps matched to the size of the vessel (or surgeon's preference) also should be available on the instrument table. Small-bore suction and larger atraumatic suction tips are needed. Vascular forceps are used throughout the procedure. Catheters should not be opened until the surgeon requests the size and type needed.

After surgical exposure of the target vessel, the surgeon places several vessel loops around the vessel and its nearby tributaries. This allows manipulation of the vessel and traction as needed.

To perform the embolectomy, the surgeon clamps the vessel distal to the thrombus. A vascular clamp is selected to fit the configuration of the vessel and its position in the wound. An arteriotomy then is made with a #11 scalpel blade. Suction is applied at the arteriotomy site.

The prepared embolectomy catheter then is carefully threaded into the vessel past the site of the thrombus. The balloon is inflated, and the catheter is withdrawn (Figure 28-14). This pulls the thrombus ahead of the catheter and out of the vessel. The catheter may require reinsertion if a false passage was entered. Angioscopy and angiography are performed to ensure that the procedure was successful. The thrombus that is removed should be retained or preserved as a specimen.

The arteriotomy or venous incision is closed with size 7-0 nonabsorbable vascular suture. The wound is closed in layers according to the incision site.

Vascular Access for Renal Hemodialysis
SURGICAL GOAL
Patients with end-stage renal disease require frequent **hemodialysis.** This treatment requires long-term access to the patient's vascular system. An anastomosis between the arterial and venous systems is created surgically to produce this access. Two techniques usually are used to create vascular access. These are described below.

PATHOLOGY
End-stage renal disease results in serious electrolyte imbalance and severe uremia (nitrogenous wastes in the blood). When the kidney's filtering ability drops below 5%, hemodialysis is necessary for survival. During dialysis, the patient's blood is shunted **extracorporeally** (outside the body) through an artery. The blood is pumped through a series of filters to remove the waste products and excess electrolytes that normally would be filtered by the kidney. The blood is then returned to the body through a vein.

DISCUSSION
Arteriovenous Shunt: Arm
The patient is placed in the supine position with the arm extended on a large arm board. The arm is prepped and draped free. A local anesthetic is used.

A skin incision is made over the cephalic vein and carried through the fascial layer with a curved hemostat and tenotomy or other plastic surgery scissors. Two small vessel loops are placed around the vein, and the ends are clamped with mosquito hemostats. A small *bulldog* or similar vascular clamp is placed over the proximal end of the vessel. The distal end is divided and ligated with silk or polypropylene suture. This technique is repeated on the artery. A graft tunneler may be used to bring the graft in close approximation to both vessels. The graft is sutured in place with 6-0 or 7-0 polypropylene (Figure 28-15, *A*). The incisions then are closed in layers and dressed with dry gauze.
Arteriovenous Fistula
An **arteriovenous fistula** is a direct anastomosis between an artery and a vein. The site is selected for patency and accessibility. After a routine prep and draping of the area, an incision is made over the vessels. The vessels are mobilized with sharp dissection and anastomosed as for an arteriovenous shunt (Figure 28-15, *B*). The wound is closed in layers.

Insertion of Vena Cava Filter
SURGICAL GOAL
The vena cava filter is a metal umbrella-shaped filter inserted into the inferior vena cava to prevent emboli from entering the pulmonary system. The filter can be temporary or permanent.

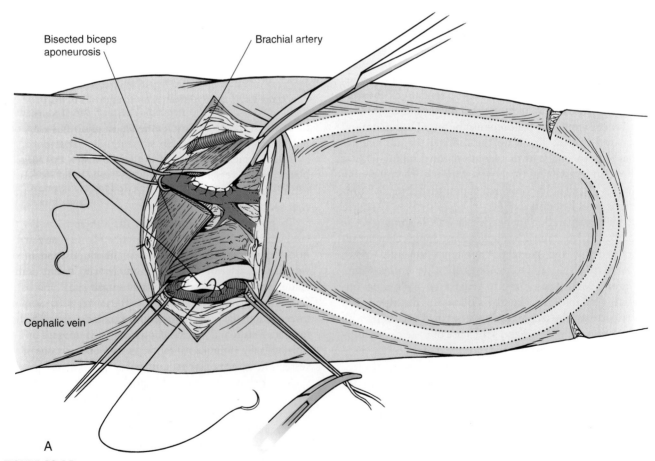

FIGURE 28-15
A, Anastomoses of the loop forearm graft.

PATHOLOGY

Pulmonary emboli occur when one or more thrombi move from the venous system into the pulmonary vascular system (**pulmonary emboli**). The vena cava filter is a method of capturing and preventing further movement of emboli. Candidates for the surgery include the following:

▶ Patients who have venous thromboemboli but cannot tolerate anticoagulant therapy. These include patients who have had recent surgery or have suffered a hemorrhagic stroke.

▶ Patients who have had a massive pulmonary embolism and survived but for whom a subsequent embolism would be fatal.

▶ The patient who has had chronic or venous thromboemboli in spite of anticoagulant therapy.

Technique

1. A large-bore needle is inserted into the femoral artery.
2. A guide wire is threaded through the needle, and the needle is withdrawn.
3. The filter and introducer are inserted over the guide wire under fluoroscopy.
4. The filter is deployed from the introducer, and the introducer is then withdrawn.
5. The position of the filter is verified.
6. A pressure dressing is applied to the insertion site.

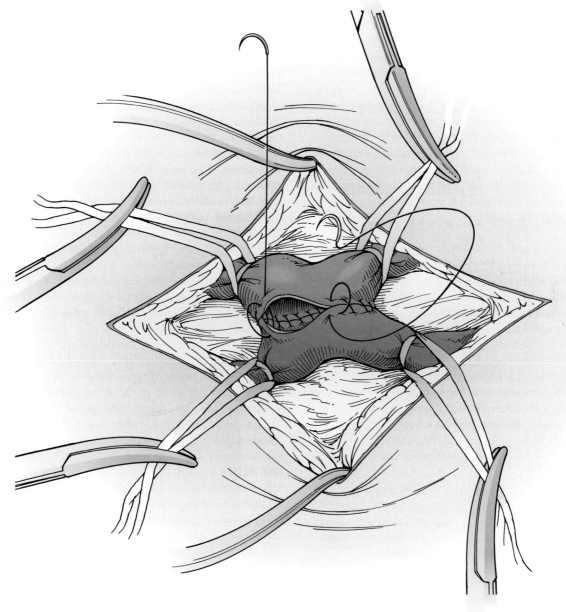

B

FIGURE 28-15, cont'd
B, Continuous suture placement over the anterior wall of the anastomosis. (From Moody F: *Atlas of ambulatory surgery,* Philadelphia, 1999, Saunders.)

DISCUSSION

Insertion of a vena cava filter is commonly performed in the radiology department under fluoroscopy. New filter devices can be inserted at the patient's bedside in the ICU.

The vena cava filter device is inserted via needle insertion. This is called a **percutaneous** (through the skin) approach. The procedure requires a guide wire and filter introducer. The guide wire is a fine, flexible wire coated with a chemical such as PTFE that resists platelet aggregation and allows the wire to slide easily through the vessel. The filter itself, which resembles an umbrella without fabric, is made of titanium, stainless steel, or Nitinol. When the filter is deployed, it opens out to the edges of the vessel.

All personnel working in interventional radiology wear lead aprons over their scrub attire.

The patient is placed in the supine position on the fluoroscopy or radiology table. The groin is prepped with Betadine solution, and the area is draped in the usual manner. Regional anesthesia with or without sedation is administered.

The surgeon or radiologist begins the procedure by inserting a large-bore needle into the femoral artery. A guide wire is inserted through the needle, and the needle is withdrawn. With the aid of fluoroscopy, the introducer is passed over the guide wire, and the filter is ejected from the tip. The introducer and guide wire are withdrawn, and pressure is applied to the puncture site for 10 to 15 minutes. A pressure dressing is placed over the site. The patient must remain in flat supine position for at least 4 hours after the procedure to prevent stress on the artery.

Carotid Endarterectomy
SURGICAL GOAL

Carotid endarterectomy is the surgical removal of atherosclerotic plaque from the carotid artery. Plaque is removed through an open incision in the artery. This reestablishes the flow of oxygenated blood to the brain.

PATHOLOGY

Obstruction of the carotid artery commonly forms at the birfucation of the common carotid artery with the internal and external carotid branches. The occlusion causes restricted arterial blood flow to the brain and neurologic symptoms.

Technique

1. An incision is made along the anterior border of the sternocleidomastoid muscle and carried to deep tissue.
2. The common, external, and internal carotid arteries are mobilized and controlled with vessel loops and Rumel tourniquets. Loops ends are clamped together.
3. Lidocaine may be injected into the arteries to prevent spasm.
4. The internal, common, and external carotid arteries are clamped.
5. The electroencephalogram is monitored.
6. An arteriotomy is made into the common carotid artery and extended upward.

7. An intraluminal shunt may be put in place to provide continuous cerebral blood flow.
8. Atherosclerotic plaque is dissected from the vessel wall.
9. A patch graft may be sutured over the arteriotomy, or the incision may be closed by primary intention.
10. If a shunt has been used, it is removed just before the incision is closed.
11. After the clamps are removed, the graft is checked for leaks, and extra sutures are placed if needed.
12. All bleeders are controlled with the electrosurgical unit (ESU).
13. The wound is closed in layers.

DISCUSSION

During carotid endarterectomy, the surgeon may need to temporarily occlude the carotid arteries while removing plaque. This is a critical phase in the procedure because blood flow to the brain is interrupted. It is therefore important that the scrub clarify the steps of the procedure with the surgeon before surgery. The instrument and Mayo table must be kept neat and organized to ensure maximum efficiency during the procedure. All essential instruments, catheters, and vascular clamps must be prepared and in view. Attention to the surgical wound is important throughout the procedure.

Carotid endarterectomy may be performed under general or regional anesthetic. When performed under regional anesthetic, the patient may respond to simple neurologic tests such as hand strength tests or speaking. **Electroencephalogram (EEG)** is commonly used to measure the brain's electrical activity during the procedure. Electrical activity is affected by oxygen supply to the tissue, a critical component of carotid surgery.

The patient is placed in the supine position, and the head is turned away from the affected side. A small pad may be placed under the shoulders to hyperextend the neck. If EEG monitoring will be used, electrodes are placed. The scrub prep extends from the face to the axillary line. Draping is similar to that of thyroidectomy.

The surgeon begins the procedure by incising the neck along the anterior border of the sternocleidomastoid muscle. The incision is carried deeper with the vascular forceps, ESU, Metzenbaum scissors, and sponge dissectors to the level of the common, internal, and external carotid arteries. The scrub should have a variety of retractors available, including two dull Weitlaners, dull rakes, and Army-Navy retractors. The rake retractors should have *dull* rather than sharp teeth to avoid trauma to the large vessels that lie in close proximity.

The common, external, and internal carotid arteries are mobilized with fine vascular tissue forceps and Metzenbaum scissors. The bifurcation itself is not mobilized fully. Vessel loops are then placed around each of the three arteries. Small hemostats are used to clamps the ends of the loops. Small sections of tubing or Rumel tourniquets also may be placed around the loops for control.

Before the surgeon makes the arterial incision, the anesthesia care provider administers intravenous heparin to the patient. This prevents clotting and reduces the risk of emboli. The artery may be injected with 1% lidocaine to prevent spasm during the procedure.

Before the actual endarterectomy, the scrub should have the following instruments ready: a #11 scalpel blade, Potts and DeMartel scissors, neurosurgical elevators (Penfield or similar), a Freer elevator, and straight hemostats. Wide-tip atraumatic suction also is needed. The surgeon indicates which vascular clamps he or she prefers.

To begin the endarterectomy, the surgeon clamps the internal, common, and external carotid arteries. He or she notifies the anesthesia care provider and circulator that the arteries have been clamped. The period of time the artery is occluded is timed. The EEG is closely monitored until clamps are released.

The surgeon then makes a small incision into the common carotid artery with a #11 scalpel blade. The incision is extended with Potts or DeMartel scissors. Arterial plaque is identified as thick, yellow, rubbery material adhering to the lumen (intima layer) of the artery.

Internal Shunt Device

To provide continuous blood flow to the cerebrum while plaque is being removed, the surgeon may insert a flexible internal shunt (also called a *Javid shunt*) into the internal and common carotid arteries. The scrub must flush the shunt with heparinized saline before passing it to the surgeon.

If a shunt is to be used, it is inserted at this point. A shunt *ring clamp* (called a *Javid clamp*) and vessel tourniquets are used to maneuver and hold the shunt in place. Clamps may be released when the shunt is in place.

The surgeon grasps the edge of the plaque with vascular forceps or a straight hemostat and lifts it gently from the intima. Penfield or Freer elevators are used to create a dissection plane between the plaque and the inner lumen. The arterial plaque and lumen of the artery are flushed with heparinized saline during this portion of the procedure.

After dissection, the plaque is passed to the scrub as a specimen. The arterial lumen is then flushed with heparinized saline solution.

The arterial incision is closed with size 5-0 or 6-0 cardiovascular sutures, or a patch graft may be put in place at this time. The patch graft is cut to size from a sheet of PTFE or other grafting material.

Before the arteriotomy is closed, the external, common, and internal carotid artery clamps are *opened and closed, in that order.* This allows any debris to flow out and restores blood flow. At this point the arteries are clamped.

NOTE: If a shunt has been placed, it is removed just before the arterial incision is completely closed. The ring clamp holding the shunt is released from the internal carotid artery, and the shunt is removed. The artery is then partially reclamped.

When the incision has been closed, the surgeon removes the clamps from the external, common, and finally the internal carotid arteries.

The suture line is observed for leaks, which are repaired with additional sutures and controlled with topical hemostatic agents.

Angiograms may be taken at this time to check patency of the vessel superior to the surgical site. Doppler and intravascular ultrasound also may be used. All bleeders are controlled with the ESU, and the neck incision is irrigated with warm saline. The deep layers of the arterial incision are closed with synthetic absorbable sutures, size 3-0. Skin is closed with nylon or other synthetic nonabsorbable material in size 4-0. A gauze dressing is used to cover the wound. See Figure 28-16 for illustrations of carotid endarterectomy.

Saphenous Vein Harvesting

SURGICAL GOAL

The greater saphenous vein is surgically removed to provide an autograft for peripheral or coronary artery bypass. The surgical goal is to remove the vein while retaining its structural and physiological soundness.

PATHOLOGY

The autograft is an ideal graft for arterial bypass. The greater saphenous vein has been more successful for the small-diameter arterial bypass than other materials. It is readily accessible, and its connective tissue layer thickens with increased pressure. This makes it strong and able to withstand high arterial pressure.

Technique

1. The surgeon incises the groin and inner aspect of the leg over the saphenous vein.
2. The distal vein is exposed, the branches are divided, and the vein is excised.
3. Branches of the vein are clamped, ligated, and divided.
4. The vein is injected with papaverine or lidocaine to prevent spasm.
5. The vein is mobilized and then removed.
6. The surgeon attaches an irrigation syringe to one end of the vein to check for leaks.
7. All tributaries are clamped and tied.
8. The leg wound is closed.
9. The graft is protected in moist saline.

DISCUSSION

A general anesthetic usually is administered because the procedure is performed in conjunction with a peripheral or cardiac bypass surgery. The patient is placed in the supine position, and the selected leg is prepped from the groin to the foot. Drapes expose the leg and groin, with the foot occluded.

A common problem experienced during vein harvesting results from the practice that one surgeon harvests the vein while the rest of the team prepares the implant site, such as during coronary artery bypass. In this case, the two overhead operating lights are dedicated to the top of the surgical field, leaving no direct light for the saphenous vein harvest. A third light or headlight should be available to provide lighting on the leg.

The knee is flexed to gain access to the medial aspect of the leg. To begin the surgery, the surgeon makes a long incision directly over the saphenous vein from the groin to the point of removal, usually below the knee.

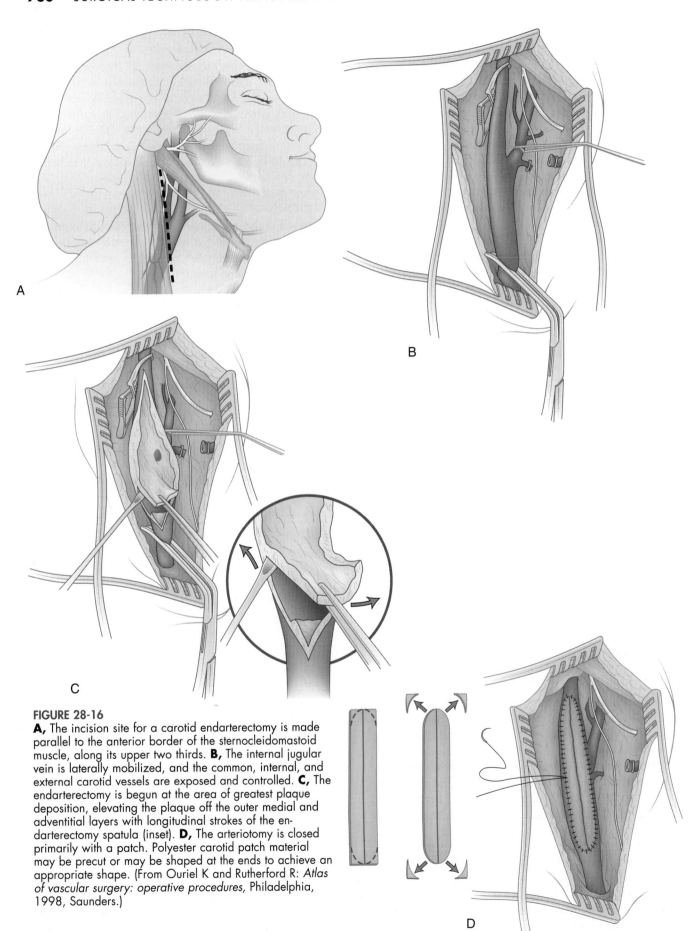

FIGURE 28-16
A, The incision site for a carotid endarterectomy is made parallel to the anterior border of the sternocleidomastoid muscle, along its upper two thirds. **B,** The internal jugular vein is laterally mobilized, and the common, internal, and external carotid vessels are exposed and controlled. **C,** The endarterectomy is begun at the area of greatest plaque deposition, elevating the plaque off the outer medial and adventitial layers with longitudinal strokes of the endarterectomy spatula (inset). **D,** The arteriotomy is closed primarily with a patch. Polyester carotid patch material may be precut or may be shaped at the ends to achieve an appropriate shape. (From Ouriel K and Rutherford R: *Atlas of vascular surgery: operative procedures,* Philadelphia, 1998, Saunders.)

The groin incision is made parallel to the upper thigh crease, directly over the saphenous vein. Bleeders are coagulated with the ESU or ligated with silk suture, size 3-0. A *dull* Weitlaner retractor may be placed in the wound. Branches of the vein are clamped and ligated with silk or clipped and divided. The vein is ligated with heavy silk sutures and divided with scissors.

The surgeon performs the distal excision by first clamping tributaries and ligating them. The surgeon then carefully dissects the vein along its length to avoid creating wide tissue flaps on each side. The surgeon locates the tributaries, clips or ligates them with silk, and divides them.

The scrub or assistant must keep the vein and incision moist during the surgery. Frequent irrigation with saline solution is necessary. An Asepto syringe can be used for irrigation. Some surgeons inject papaverine or lidocaine into the subcutaneous tissue to prevent vein spasm.

The surgeon places Silastic vessel loops around the vein for retraction rather than using forceps, which can damage the vessel. When all tributaries have been divided, the vein is removed and placed in a kidney basin.

The vein then must be prepared for use. The scrub attaches a blunt-tip irrigation needle to a 30-ml syringe. The needle is inserted into the tip of the vein and secured with a heavy silk tie. Saline is used to irrigate the vein during the repair. If ordered, heparinized papaverine may be used. The surgeon injects solution into the vein and occludes the branches with silk ties. The vein must be kept moist at all times.

After preparation, the graft is maintained in a moist saline environment until needed. The vein also may be placed in a basin with heparinized papaverine and normal saline solution. This is often called a "vein bath." The vein must be carefully monitored and protected at all times.

The leg incision is closed with interrupted sutures of synthetic nonabsorbable material. Skin is closed with staples or monofilament synthetic suture. This procedure is illustrated in Figure 28-17.

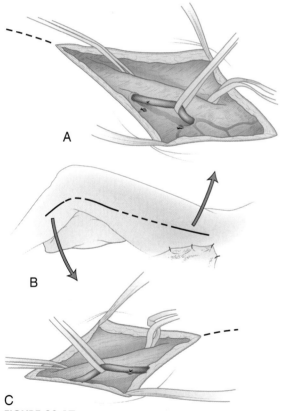

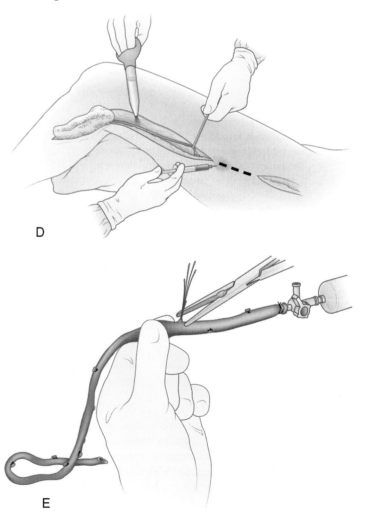

FIGURE 28-17
Harvesting of the saphenous vein. **A,** Exposure of the saphenous vein and femoral artery in the groin. **B,** The hip is rotated externally, and the knee is flexed to facilitate venous harvest without a skin flap. **C,** The vein is exposed below the knee level. The popliteal artery is surrounded with an umbilical tape proximally and a vessel loop distally. **D,** Harvest of the greater saphenous vein. The exposed vein is kept from desiccation using moist packs and saline irrigation. **E,** The vein is gently irrigated with heparinized papaverine solution. Open branches are grasped with fine forceps, and the stump is ligated with fine silk suture. (From Ouriel K and Rutherford R: *Atlas of vascular surgery: operative procedures,* Philadelphia, 1998, Saunders.)

Axillofemoral Bypass
SURGICAL GOAL

The axillofemoral bypass creates circulation between the femoral arteries and the axillary artery to restore circulation to the lower extremity or in emergency bypass for an infected aortic graft or aneurysm.

PATHOLOGY

Circulation to the lower extremities is derived from the descending aorta and the iliac and femoral arteries. Atherosclerotic disease of the aortoiliac region results in obstruction to the lower extremities. One achieves bypass by shunting the blood directly from the femoral arteries through a femorofemoral bypass to the axillary artery (axillofemoral bypass).

An important indication for axillofemoral bypass is an infected aortic graft. Perfusion (blood flow and oxygen exchange in the tissues) of the leg can be restored after excision of the graft. Axillofemoral bypass offers an alternative. It avoids the risks of major aortic surgery, but long-term patency of the graft is possible only if outflow from the axillary artery is brisk.

Technique

1. A 45-degree incision is made in the subclavicular area on the affected side.
2. The pectoralis major muscle is bluntly divided, and the deep fascia is incised.
3. The pectoralis minor muscle tendon is divided.
4. The axillary artery is mobilized and clamped.
5. A synthetic graft is tunneled through the subcutaneous tissue from the axillary incision to the femorofemoral graft.
6. The axillary artery and tributaries are clamped.
7. The axillary artery is incised, and the proximal end of the graft is anastomosed to the artery.
8. The groin is entered, and the femoral graft is mobilized and controlled.
9. The distal graft is anastomosed to the femorofemoral graft.
10. The incisions are checked for leakage.
11. Angiograms are performed.
12. The wounds are closed in layers and dressed.

DISCUSSION

The patient is placed in the supine position. The skin prep includes the affected arm, shoulder, clavicular and neck areas, abdomen, and groin. The arm is placed on a wide arm board and draped as for an upper-arm procedure (excluding the hand). The groin is occluded with towels and an adhesive drape. Separate drapes are used to expose the operative area, and both legs may be draped with split sheets or U drapes. A body sheet or procedure drape then is placed on top of the drapes.

Two surgeons may work simultaneously, one at the subclavicular incision and the other at the groin. To begin the procedure, the surgeon makes a 45-degree incision in the subclavicular region. The subcutaneous layer is entered with the ESU, and a rake or retractors are placed at the incision edges. The pectoralis major muscle is divided manually, and the deep fascia is incised. However, the tendon attachment of the pectoralis minor must be severed with the ESU. A deep self-retaining retractor or small Richardson retractors replace the rakes.

The surgeon then mobilizes the axillary artery and places vessel loops around it and nearby tributaries. Small branches are clamped with small bulldog or spring clamps, divided, and ligated.

A tunnel is then made in the subcutaneous incision between the upper incision and the groin with a graft tunneler. If the patient is very tall, an intermediary incision may be necessary.

The groin is entered as previously described, and the femoral artery graft and bifurcation are mobilized. Vessel loops are placed around the graft and controlled with Rumel tourniquets.

The patient is given intravenous heparin, and the axillary artery is clamped. The artery is incised with a #11 scalpel blade, and the anastomosis is performed with 5-0 or 6-0 polypropylene suture.

The distal end of the graft is brought into contact with the femoral graft. The distal tip of the graft is beveled with scissors and anastomosed with size 6-0 Gore-Tex sutures. A double-arm suture is commonly used.

Suture lines are checked for leaks, and heparin is reversed with protamine. An angiogram may be performed to ensure patency of the graft. Both wounds are irrigated and closed in layers. Highlights of the procedure are illustrated in Figure 28-18.

Femoral Popliteal Bypass
SURGICAL GOAL

In this procedure, a synthetic graft or autograft is implanted between the femoral and popliteal arteries. **In situ** grafting uses the greater saphenous vein as a shunt.

PATHOLOGY

Femoral popliteal bypass is indicated for atherosclerosis of the femoral artery. (See the section on atherosclerosis.)

Technique

1. The surgeon makes an incision on the medial side of the thigh and carries it to deep tissues using sharp and blunt dissection.
2. The femoral artery is mobilized, and vessel loops are placed around it.
3. The distal incision is made on the medial side of the knee inferior to the patella.
4. The popliteal artery is located and mobilized.
5. Angiograms are performed.
6. A synthetic graft is tunneled through the subcutaneous tissue, connecting the two wound sites.
7. Heparin is administered to the patient.

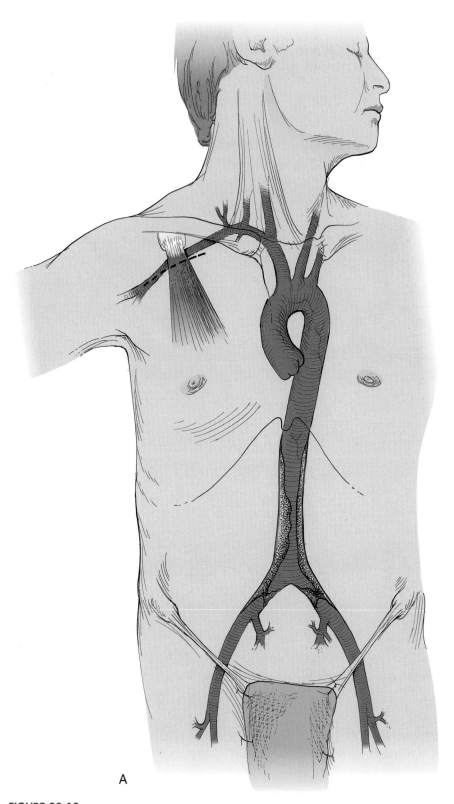

A

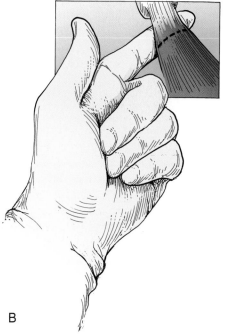

B

FIGURE 28-18
A, The axillary artery is exposed through an oblique incision placed over the pectoralis minor muscle. **B,** The pectoralis minor muscle will then be divided with the ESU.

FIGURE 28-18, cont'd
C, The axillary artery and its large branches are clamped. **D,** Placement of graft, which runs parallel to the axillary artery. (From Ouriel K and Rutherford R: *Atlas of vascular surgery: operative procedures,* Philadelphia, 1998, Saunders.)

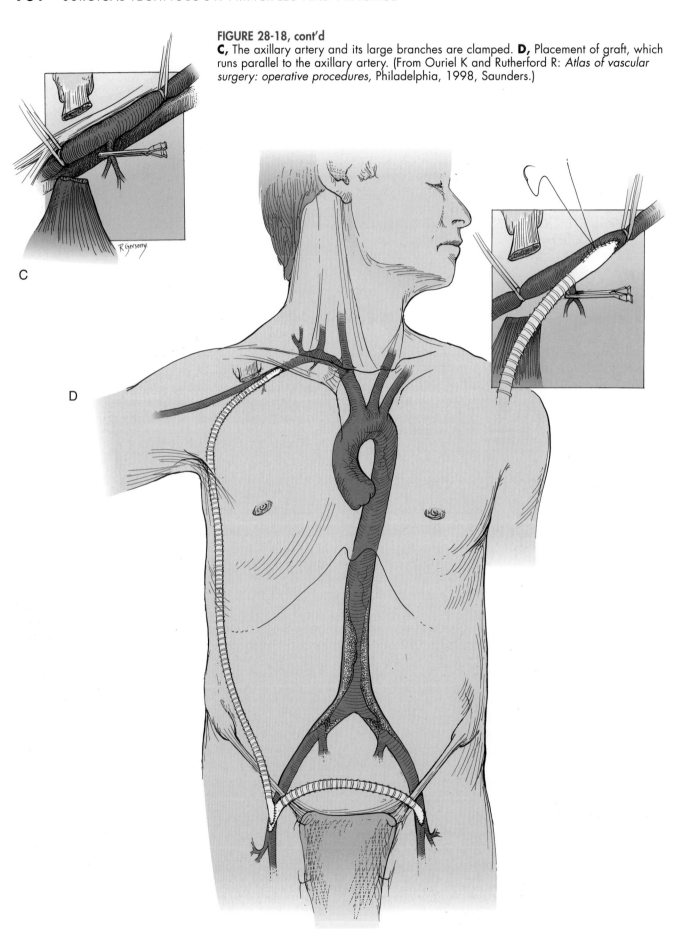

C

D

8. The femoral artery is clamped, and an arteriotomy is performed.
9. The proximal limb of the graft is anastomosed to the femoral artery.
10. The popliteal anastomosis is performed.
11. Angiograms are taken, and pulses are verified.
12. The wounds are closed after all bleeding has been controlled.

DISCUSSION

The patient is placed in the supine position, prepped, and draped with the affected leg and groin exposed. The surgeon makes an incision on the medial side of the thigh, below the groin. Dissection is performed with the scalpel, Metzenbaum scissors, sponge dissectors, and the ESU. A Weitlaner or Gelpi retractor is used for superficial retraction. For deeper retraction, Army-Navy retractors or small Richardson retractors may be used.

The surgeon mobilizes the femoral artery with careful dissection. One or more vessel loops are placed around the artery for retraction and manipulation.

A second vertical incision is made on the medial side of the knee below the patella. The surgeon dissects the subcutaneous, fascial, and muscle layers using both sharp and blunt dissection. A self-retaining retractor is used to expose the popliteal space. The popliteal artery then is mobilized with sponge dissectors and scissors. A vessel loop is placed around the artery. Angiography may be performed at this time to verify that the popliteal artery is patent.

The surgeon chooses an appropriate-size graft. The greater saphenous vein may be used in place of a synthetic graft. This technique is explained below in the section on in situ saphenous femoropopliteal bypass.

The surgeon makes a tunnel in the subcutaneous tissue and carries the graft from the upper to the lower wound. The graft then can be drawn back easily into the popliteal space.

To perform the anastomosis, the surgeon first places a vascular clamp across the femoral artery. A small incision is made in the artery with a #11 scalpel blade or vascular scissors. Using running sutures of size 5-0 or 6-0 polypropylene, the surgeon creates the anastomosis between the femoral artery and graft.

The popliteal anastomosis is created in the same manner as the femoral anastomosis. During both anastomoses, the scrub should have heparinized saline solution available for irrigation of the arterial sites. Hemostatic agents are used to check bleeding at the anastomosis and additional sutures are placed if needed.

Angiograms are taken at this time, and the patency of the arterial system is monitored with the Doppler or intravascular ultrasound. The wound is then irrigated and closed in layers. The popliteal space is closed with interrupted sutures of absorbable synthetic, size 2-0 or 3-0. Skin is commonly closed with staples or nylon sutures. The groin incision is closed in layers and dressed with gauze squares.

This procedure is illustrated in Figure 28-19.

In Situ Saphenous Femoropopliteal Bypass
SURGICAL GOAL

In situ saphenous vein bypass is a surgical alternative to using a synthetic graft to bypass a diseased femoral artery. The saphenous vein is not removed but is left in anatomical position. In the technique described here, a continuous incision is made along the entire saphenous vein. This is the safest method and allows complete ligation of tributaries. The distal or narrow end of the vein is anastomosed to the popliteal artery, and the proximal vein is anastomosed to the large end of the femoral artery. The goal is to produce vascular continuity with an autograft.

Technique

1. One single incision or multiple incisions are made on the medial thigh, following the path of the saphenous vein.
2. The surgeon ligates and divides the branches of the vein.
3. The proximal and distal ends of the vein are clamped and divided.
4. Internal valves are obliterated with microvascular valve scissors, a valvulotome and angioscope, or a valvulotome alone.
5. The saphenous vein is anastomosed to the femoral and popliteal arteries.

DISCUSSION

The patient is prepped and draped with the operative leg and thigh exposed. The medial aspect of the thigh is incised from above the ankle to the groin, following the saphenous vein. The incision is carried deeper with dissecting scissors and the ESU. This exposes the saphenous vein, which is partly or completely mobilized. Vessel loops are placed along its length for manipulation.

The branches of the vein then are clamped with mosquito hemostats or clipped. Each is divided from the vein. Fine silk sutures also may be used to ligate the tributaries. The distal and proximal ends of the saphenous vein are clamped and divided.

Before the anastomoses are performed between the saphenous vein and the femoral and popliteal arteries, the valves must be incised so that arterial blood can flow through the valves easily. Several techniques are used. The angioscope is passed through the lumen of the vein, and a system is used to both sever the valves and remove tributaries. This avoids extensive dissection of the vein. An alternative method is to incise the first two valves under direct vision with valve scissors, and then use a valvulotome with or without the angioscope to release the others.

The surgeon then performs the anastomoses between the saphenous vein and femoral artery. The vein is trimmed to a bevel, and a small incision is made in the femoral artery with Potts scissors or a #11 scalpel blade. An end-to-side anastomosis is formed with 6-0 or 7-0 nonabsorbable sutures with a double-arm or single-arm needle. The profunda femoris also can be used for anastomosis. The distal anastomosis is made with the same technique.

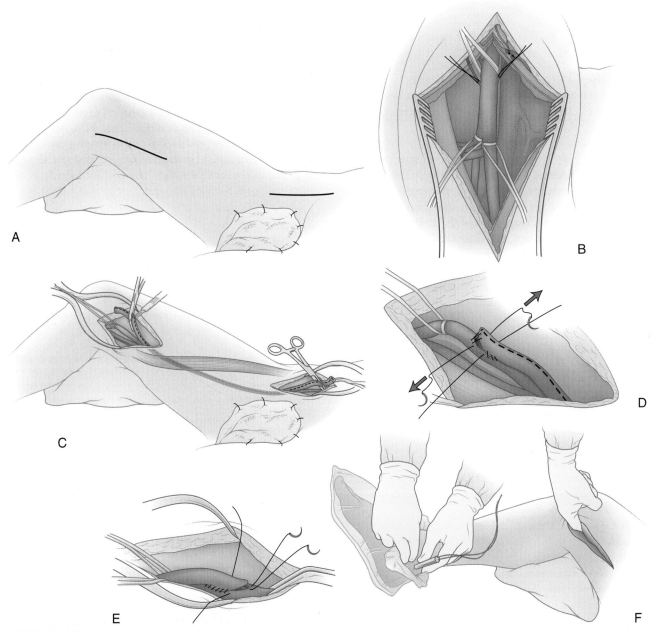

FIGURE 28-19
Femoral popliteal bypass. **A,** The femoral incision is placed at the level of the inguinal ligament, and the popliteal incision runs from the medial condyle of the femur to a point overlying the adductor hiatus. **B,** The common femoral, superficial femoral, and profunda femoris arteries are exposed in the groin. **C,** The graft is beveled for the anastomoses using a curved hemostat and the knife blade. **D,** Completion of the popliteal anastomosis is achieved using a two-suture technique. **E,** The proximal anastomosis is completed with a two-suture technique. **F,** Intraoperative assessment of the hemodynamic result is performed intraoperatively with evaluation of the Doppler signal at the ankle and palpation of the pulse in the popliteal artery beyond the anastomosis. (From Ouriel K and Rutherford R: *Atlas of vascular surgery: operative procedures,* Philadelphia, 1998, Saunders.)

The small tributaries that branch from the saphenous vein next must be occluded. These are located with the Doppler unless the vein is completely exposed. The surgeon applies digital pressure over the vein while observing the Doppler wave. Increased flow indicates an area of arteriovenous fistula (vascular connection between the arterial circulation and the venous flow). These areas are exposed, and each individual tributary is clipped or ligated and incised.

Angiography is performed at this time to check for patency. The wounds are irrigated and closed in layers, with absorbable synthetic sutures used for subcutaneous and fascial tissue. Skin is closed with clips or nonabsorbable suture.

The wounds are dressed with nonadherent dressing followed by gauze squares and roller gauze.

Femorofemoral Bypass
SURGICAL GOAL
Femorofemoral bypass is implantation of a prosthetic graft connecting the femoral artery on the affected side to the opposite femoral artery. This is performed to bypass unilateral atherosclerotic disease in the iliac artery.

PATHOLOGY
Refer to the section on atherosclerosis. This approach is performed only when the iliac system on the donor side is free of disease. Iliac disease is usually bilateral. In this case, stenting or balloon angioplasty of the donor iliac system may be necessary. Perfusion to the recipient iliac system can result in a drop in pressure at the donor site. This can result in worsening symptoms and disease in the donor arterial system. The femorofemoral bypass is not effective if the superficial femoral artery is diseased. This technique prevents retrograde ejaculation and impotence in the male patient. These complications sometimes arise from dissection of the aorta when there is damage to the parasympathetic system.

Technique
1. The surgeon makes bilateral groin incisions and isolates the common femoral arteries.
2. The surgeon uses his or her fingers and a tunneling instrument to separate the tissues and create a subcutaneous tunnel between the groin incisions.
3. A synthetic graft is pulled through the tunnel and anastomosed to each femoral artery.
4. The wounds are closed.

DISCUSSION
The patient is prepped and draped for bilateral groin incisions. A Foley catheter may be inserted during the prep. The genitalia are excluded from the prep with towels and an occlusive drape. A general or regional anesthetic may be used.

The procedure begins with groin incisions. These incisions are made with the scalpel and carried to the deeper layers with sponge dissectors, Metzenbaum scissors, and the ESU. Large bleeders may be clamped and ligated with silk suture of size 3-0. The scrub should have right-angle clamps and two or more self-retaining retractors available for the dissection. Army-Navy retractors and small Richardson retractors also may be needed. The groin incision is carried to the level of the common femoral artery, which is isolated with Silastic loops. The iliac artery also may be looped for manipulation. The procedure is then repeated on the opposite side.

The surgeon then creates a subcutaneous tunnel in the skin between the two incisions using his or her fingers. An aortic clamp is used to puncture the fascial attachments at the midline. The surgeon grasps one end of the graft with the curved aortic clamp and pulls it through the tunnel. The graft must be pulled through the tunnel without kinks or twists.

An end-to-side anastomosis is performed between the graft and the profunda femoris on each side. Running sutures of 5-0 or 6-0 polypropylene are commonly used to perform the anastomosis. Air is pushed out of the graft, and the vascular clamps are removed. Hemostatic agents are applied to the suture lines, and protamine sulfate is given intravenously to reverse the effects of heparin. When the wound is dry and the suture lines are secured, the wound is closed in layers. The femorofemoral bypass is illustrated in Figure 28-20.

Varicose Vein Excision
SURGICAL GOAL
In this procedure, dilated and tortuous (varicose) veins and their tributaries are surgically removed to prevent symptoms and to improve cosmetic appearance.

PATHOLOGY
Blood returns to the heart from the lower extremities through the pumping action of muscles and the changes in abdominal and intrathoracic pressure. The intraluminal valves of the veins prevent blood from returning by gravity to the extremities. Failure of the pumping action or valve incompetency results in the return of blood into the veins. The thin-walled veins bulge out, causing pain, swelling, and venous **stasis** (pooling of blood in the vessels). This also can lead to venous insufficiency. In primary varicose veins, the superficial saphenous veins are affected. Secondary varicose veins originate from the deep saphenous vein. Surgical treatment is removal of the deep saphenous vein, superficial saphenous veins, or both. Tributaries of the veins that are visible through the skin are removed separately.

Technique
1. The surgeon exposes the greater saphenous vein at the medial malleolus.
2. The vein is ligated to the stripper and divided.
3. A vein stripper is passed through the vein to the groin.
4. The groin is incised to expose the proximal end of the vein.
5. The proximal end is ligated, and all tributaries are divided and ligated.
6. The surgeon removes the vein by extracting the vein stripper.
7. Superficial veins are removed by excision.

DISCUSSION
Before surgery the paths of the superficial veins are marked with indelible ink. The patient is placed in the supine position, prepped, and draped with the affected leg and groin exposed. A general or regional anesthetic is administered.

The surgeon makes an incision anterior to the medial malleolus. The incision is carried deeper with a curved hemostat and Metzenbaum scissors. A small Weitlaner retractor or Senn retractors may be placed in the wound.

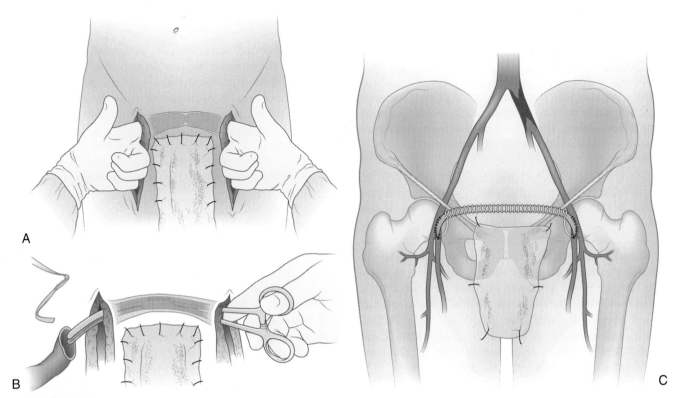

FIGURE 28-20
Femorofemoral bypass. **A,** The suprapubic tunnel is created digitally. **B,** The midline fascia is pierced with a long clamp, grasping a Penrose drain or an umbilical tape to facilitate delivery of the graft without kinks or twists. **C,** Bilateral end-to-side anastomoses are constructed, each anastomosis being run onto the profunda femoris artery if the superficial femoral arteries are occluded. (From Ouriel K and Rutherford R: *Atlas of vascular surgery: operative procedures,* Philadelphia, 1998, Saunders.)

When the distal saphenous vein is located, it is dissected free. The severed distal end is ligated with 2-0 silk. The surgeon then threads a disposable vein stripper through the lumen until resistance is felt. Small tributaries (*perforators*) that connect the deep saphenous vein to the superficial vein may impede passage of the stripper. A small incision is made over the tributary, which is clamped, divided, and ligated. The stripper is advanced to the terminal end at the femoral junction.

The groin is incised with the scalpel, and bleeders are coagulated with the ESU. A rake, Army-Navy, or Weitlaner retractor is placed in the wound. The proximal end of the saphenous vein is isolated with a vessel loop. The branches then are double clamped, divided, and ligated with silk suture of size 3-0.

When all branches have been secured, the vein stripper is pulled out at the groin incision while the assistant applies pressure over the calf and thigh using folded towels.

To remove small superficial tributaries, the surgeon makes an incision directly over them and mobilizes them with a curved hemostat and dissecting scissors. The vessels are then double clamped, divided, and ligated with silk ties.

The leg is dressed with nonadherent gauze strips and rolled gauze followed by an elastic compression bandage. Varicose vein stripping is illustrated in Figure 28-21.

Abdominal Aortic Aneurysmectomy with Graft Insertion

SURGICAL GOAL
Abdominal aortic aneurysm is a condition in which a section of the abdominal aorta bulges because of atherosclerotic plaque and progressive weakening of the aortic wall. The surgical goal is to remove the aneurysm and implant a graft extending from the aorta to both iliac arteries. This restores circulation to the lower extremities and pelvis.

PATHOLOGY
Aortic aneurysms can occur at any location in the artery. They usually occur just below the renal arteries and extend to the bifurcation of the common iliac arteries or just above it. If the disease remains undiagnosed, the walls of the aorta become increasingly stretched and finally rupture. This usually results in death. A **dissecting aneurysm** is one in which blood seeps between the layers of the vessel, causing it to tear and split. Atherosclerosis and degeneration of the muscular layer of the vessel are the most common causes of aortic aneurysm. Although the aneurysm may not extend into the iliac arteries, a bifurcated graft often is used in repair.

Technique

1. A surgeon performs a laparotomy through a long midline incision.
2. The retroperitoneal space is entered.
3. The abdominal aorta is partially dissected.
4. The renal veins may be ligated and divided.
5. The aorta is cross-clamped.
6. The aneurysm is incised and opened.
7. Blood clots and plaque are removed from the aneurysm sac.
8. A graft is implanted in the aorta above the proximal end of the aneurysm, extending to the bifurcation of the iliac arteries.
9. Angiograms are taken.
10. The retroperitoneal space is closed.
11. The abdomen is closed as a single layer with polydioxanone surgical (PDS) suture or in multiple tissue layers.

DISCUSSION

An aortic aneurysm may be scheduled (elective) or an emergency procedure. If the procedure is an emergency, recall that the most important stages of the surgery are exposure of or access to the target tissue, adequate visualization of the trauma site, immediate control of hemorrhage, and rapid repair or restoration of circulation.

The scrub should have long instruments immediately available because the target site is anterior to the posterior body wall or retroperitoneum. Right-angle clamps, the surgeon's choice of vascular clamps, abdominal suction tips, and an ESU are needed. A long Penrose drain and vascular loops also should be available for vessel retraction. Because of the depth of the wound, deep hand-held retractors, such as a Deaver retractor, or a self-retaining retractor, such as a Thompson or Bookwalter retractor, with multiple attachments may be required. Grafts should be available but not opened until the surgeon has prepared the vessels. A blood-recovery system, such as the Cell Saver or Haemonetics system, usually is used in emergency surgery.

The patient is placed in the supine position, prepped, and draped for a midline incision extending from the xiphoid to the pubis. A Foley catheter is inserted before the skin prep.

The surgeon enters the abdomen through a long midline incision. Many moist laparotomy sponges are used to prevent the bowel from drying out during the procedure. If the intestines must be brought out of the abdominal cavity, a plastic pouch may be used to keep them moist. Long vessel loops should be prepared at this time. Each should be tagged with a hemostat. Right-angle clamps are used to pass the loop under the vessels.

Retractors are placed, and the retroperitoneum is incised with a #10 blade mounted on a long scalpel handle. Using blunt and sharp dissection with long Metzenbaum scissors and vascular forceps, the surgeon exposes the aorta and places a vessel loop around it.

If the aneurysm extends to or above the renal veins, they are clamped, ligated, and divided. Using finger dissection

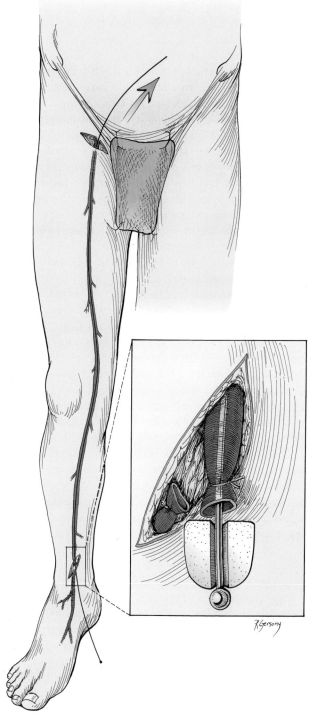

FIGURE 28-21
The traditional method of varicose vein stripping. The vein is tied over the rod, and the bullet is attached to extract the vein. (From Ouriel K and Rutherford R: *Atlas of vascular surgery: operative procedures*, Philadelphia, 1998, Saunders.)

and sponge dissectors, the surgeon frees the upper end of the aorta. There is a risk of damaging the vena cava at this stage. If damage occurs, it is repaired immediately with size 4-0 or 5-0 vascular suture. The inferior mesenteric arteries are clamped, ligated, and divided.

Dissection continues until the aorta is freed from the vertebral column. If excessive bleeding occurs, pressure is applied with laparotomy sponges. A Crafoord coarctation forcep, Satinsky clamp, or Cooley clamp is placed across the aorta to occlude it. Heparinized saline is injected into the upper aorta above the clamp.

The aneurysm next is prepared for opening. If there is a risk of excessive bleeding in spite of cross-clamps on the aorta, a Foley catheter with a 30-ml balloon may be prepared for use as an intraluminal tamponade in the aorta. In any event, the scrub should be prepared for excessive bleeding when the aneurysm is opened. Extra aortic clamps, suction, and mounted sutures should be prepared. A basin is used to collect large clots and debris.

The surgeon uses a #15 blade or ESU to make a midline incision into the aneurysm sac, leaving the *anterior* surface of the aorta and aneurysm intact. He or she then scoops out any blood clots. The plaque is grasped with vascular forceps and gently separated from the wall of the aorta. The scrub should keep the basin on the field to collect the specimens. The lumbar arteries, which enter the aorta from the poster side, may be occluded with size 4-0 or 5-0 polypropylene. A graft is selected, and the straight portion is anastomosed to the aorta with a double-arm polypropylene suture.

The iliac arteries then are prepared for anastomosis. The arteries are mobilized carefully by blunt dissection, and the common iliac artery is clamped with a right-angle DeBakey clamp. Heparinized saline is injected above the clamp. This technique is repeated on the opposite side.

Each artery is opened, and the proximal ends are irrigated with heparinized saline. The graft is trimmed and anastomosed with size 5-0 or 6-0 polypropylene suture. The surgeon checks the graft for leaks by slowly releasing the clamps. Additional sutures may be required. Hemostatic agents may be applied to the suture lines until all bleeding has been controlled. Angiograms and ultrasound are used to verify patency of the vessels. Pedal pulses also are monitored.

The wound is irrigated with saline solution. The retroperitoneum is closed with a running suture of 2-0 or 3-0 absorbable suture. The abdominal contents are replaced, and the abdominal wound is irrigated before closure. A single-layer closure of PDS suture may be used, or the abdomen can be closed in layers. See Figure 28-22 for illustrations of this procedure.

Aortofemoral Bypass
SURGICAL GOAL
Aortofemoral bypass is performed to treat aortoiliac occlusive disease. A graft is implanted between the aorta and femoral arteries, and the graft bypasses the iliac arteries and produces free circulation.

PATHOLOGY
The iliac artery is a common site of atherosclerosis. The aortofemoral bypass is performed in place of endarterectomy or aortoiliac bypass because it produces increased patency and can be performed in patients with extensive calcification of the arteries.

Technique
1. The surgeon makes bilateral groin incisions to expose the femoral arteries.
2. The surgeon performs a laparotomy through a long midline incision and exposes the aorta.
3. The patient is heparinized, and the aorta is clamped below or at the renal arteries.
4. The distal portion of the aorta is oversewn with heavy vascular sutures.
5. The proximal end of a bifurcated graft is anastomosed to distal aorta.
6. Bilateral subcutaneous tunnels are made in the retroperitoneal tissue to accommodate the two limbs of the graft, which are then pulled through the tunnels.
7. Bilateral arteriotomies are made in the femoral arteries, and the graft limbs are anastomosed to each artery.
8. Angiography and ultrasound are used to verify patency.
9. The wound is checked for bleeders and closed in the routine manner.

DISCUSSION
The prep area extends from the axillary line to the midthighs. Both legs are draped circumferentially, and the genitalia are covered with a towel and barrier drape. A Foley catheter is inserted before the skin prep. The patient is placed in the supine position.

The procedure begins with bilateral groin incisions, which are carried deeper to expose the femoral arteries. Dissection is performed with Metzenbaum scissors, sponge dissectors, and the ESU. Weitlaner or Gelpi self-retaining retractors are used superficially, and Richardson retractors are used for deeper hand retraction. After the femoral vessels have been exposed, the incisions may be covered with sterile towels during laparotomy.

A midline abdominal incision is made and carried to the aorta, as described in the previous procedure. The proximal portion of the aorta is dissected to the renal veins.

Heparin is administered to the patient, and the femoral arteries are clamped with right-angle vascular clamps. The inferior mesenteric artery is clamped to prevent an embolus from entering it when the aortic clamp is applied.

The aorta then is mobilized with blunt dissection. The surgeon then can clamp the aorta below the level of the renal arteries. The aorta then is severed, and the distal end is oversewn with polypropylene sutures, size 2-0 or 3-0. The proximal end of a bifurcated graft is trimmed to fit and anastomosed to the distal aorta. Size 3-0 polypropylene is used.

The surgeon then creates retroperitoneal tunnels in the loose connective tissue of the groin to accommodate the graft limbs. The surgeon separates the tissue using his finger.

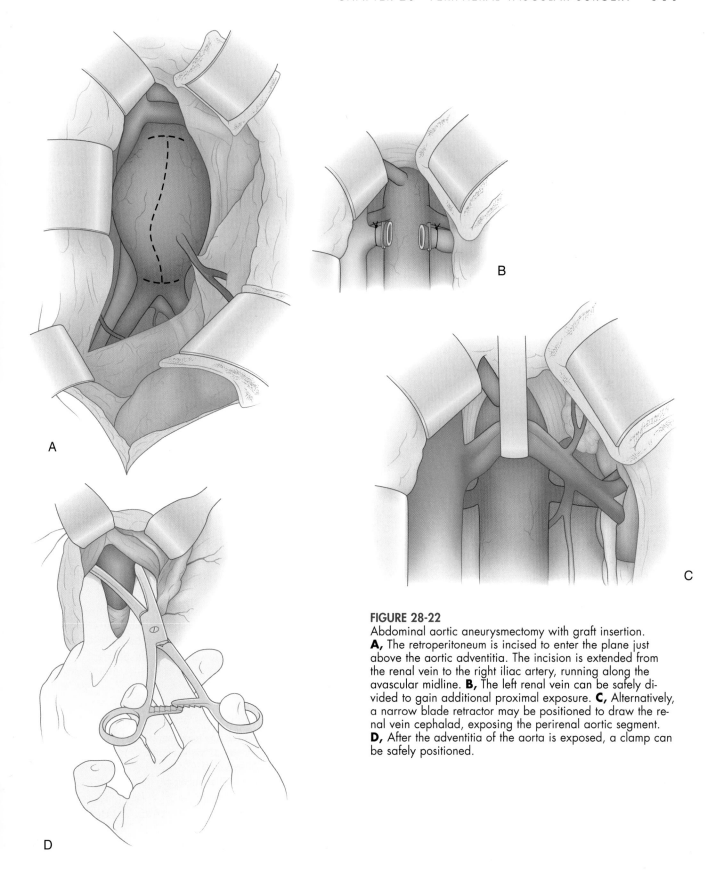

FIGURE 28-22
Abdominal aortic aneurysmectomy with graft insertion.
A, The retroperitoneum is incised to enter the plane just
above the aortic adventitia. The incision is extended from
the renal vein to the right iliac artery, running along the
avascular midline. **B,** The left renal vein can be safely divided to gain additional proximal exposure. **C,** Alternatively,
a narrow blade retractor may be positioned to draw the renal vein cephalad, exposing the perirenal aortic segment.
D, After the adventitia of the aorta is exposed, a clamp can
be safely positioned.

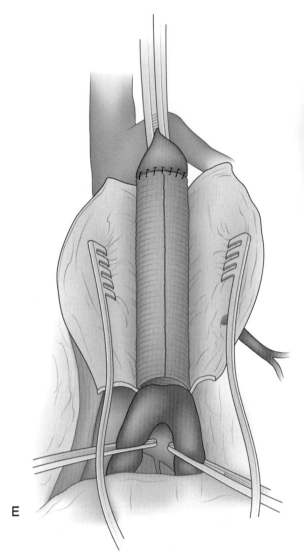

E

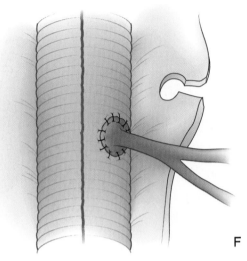

F

FIGURE 28-22, cont'd
E, Graft placement with proximal anastomosis is completed. **F,** A large inferior mesenteric artery with minimal back bleeding is reimplanted onto the body of the graft. (From Ouriel K and Rutherford R: *Atlas of vascular surgery: operative procedures,* Philadelphia, 1998, Saunders.)

A graft tunneler can cause life-threatening injury to the veins. The two limbs of the graft then are pulled through the tunnels and into the femoral wounds. A vascular clamp may be placed across the graft limb to prevent it from twisting.

Using suture scissors, the surgeon trims the ends of the graft to a 45-degree angle, rounding the tips. Each limb of the graft then is sutured into the femoral artery through an arteriotomy. Size 4-0 double-armed polypropylene is commonly used.

After the anastomoses, the femoral clamps are slowly released. Angiograms and ultrasound are performed to verify the patency of the grafts. The wound is irrigated and closed as described in the previous procedure.

Above-Knee Amputation
SURGICAL GOAL
This procedure is the surgical removal of the leg.

PATHOLOGY
Although amputation may not be considered strictly a vascular procedure, the operation is usually performed when vascular insufficiency caused by arteriosclerotic or thromboembolic disease causes the lower limb to necrose. Above-knee rather than below-knee amputation is chosen when the vascular supply in the lower limb is insufficient for proper healing at the amputation site. The procedures closely resemble each other.

Technique
1. The surgeon incises the leg circumferentially.
2. The incision is carried to the femur.
3. The femur is severed.
4. The popliteal vessels are ligated.
5. The sciatic nerve is ligated.
6. The wound is closed.

DISCUSSION
The patient is placed in the supine position, and the affected leg is prepped. Many surgeons prefer to place the gangrenous foot in a plastic bag to protect the wound site from possible contamination. The foot is then excluded from the scrub prep.

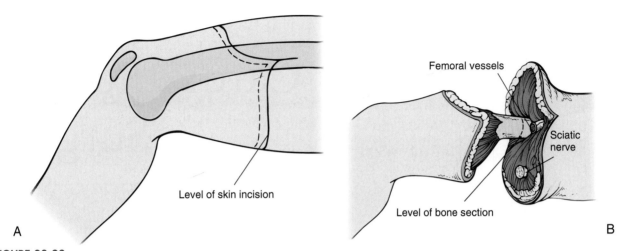

FIGURE 28-23
Above-knee leg amputation. **A,** Skin incision site at middle third of thigh. **B,** Level of bone resection. (From Rothrock J: *Alexander's care of the patient in surgery,* ed 12, St Louis, 2003, Mosby.)

To begin the procedure, the surgeon incises the leg. The incision is carried through the subcutaneous, muscle, and fascial layers with the deep knife, heavy scissors, or electrocautery pencil. Large rake retractors such as Israel rake retractors often are useful in drawing the wound edges back to expose the femur. The surgeon may sever the femur with the Gigli saw or with an amputation saw, such as the Satterlee saw.

When the femur has been severed, the surgeon completes the amputation by severing the soft tissues that lie on the posterior side of the femur. The scrub removes the limb from the field and may pass it directly to the circulator. The surgeon ligates the popliteal artery and vein and grasps the sciatic nerve with a Kocher or other heavy clamp. The end of the nerve is crushed with the clamp to prevent the formation

of a neuroma (tumor at the end of a nerve). It is then ligated with a suture ligature, size 0 or 2-0. The end of the nerve is cut with the scalpel or scissors and allowed to retract back into the femoral stump.

The stump is closed in layers with Dexon or other absorbable sutures, size 0 or 2-0. The skin is sutured with the surgeon's choice of material and dressed with bulky gauze and an Ace wrap.

Highlights of this procedure are illustrated in Figure 28-23.

REFERENCES

Moody F: *Ambulatory surgery,* Philadelphia, 1999, Saunders.

Ouriel K and Rutherford R: *Atlas of vascular surgery: operative procedures,* Philadelphia, 1998, Saunders.

Rutherford R: *Atlas of vascular surgery: basic techniques and exposures,* Philadelphia, 1997, Saunders.

Chapter 29

Cardiothoracic Surgery

By Patricia C. Seifert

Learning Objectives

After studying this chapter the reader will be able to:

- Identify the instrumentation and equipment used in cardiac and pulmonary surgery
- Explain endoscopic procedures of the lungs and mediastinum
- Describe the proper method of handling specimens in cardiopulmonary surgery
- Explain the use of a water-seal chest drainage system
- Describe common cardiac and pulmonary procedures

Terminology

Alveoli—Small air sacs found in the lungs, through which oxygen and carbon dioxide are exchanged during respiration.

Aneurysm—A bulging in an artery caused by a weakening in the arterial wall. The weakening may be a congenital defect or the result of atherosclerosis, arteriosclerosis, infection, trauma, or degenerative disease.

Apex—(1) The lower left tip of the left ventricle of the heart; (2) the rounded upper portion of each lung.

Arrhythmia—An abnormal heartbeat (also called dysrhythmia).

Asystole—The absence of a heartbeat; cardiac standstill.

Atria—The two upper chambers of the heart.

Atrial appendage—A small, muscular, ear-shaped portion of the atrium.

Bicuspid valve—A valve with two leaflets. Commonly refers to the valve between the left atrium and the left ventricle (the mitral valve). Also may refer to an anomalous aortic valve containing two (rather than the normal three) leaflets.

Bolster—A small tube made from soft vinyl or plastic. A bolster is threaded over the ends of an umbilical tape or suture tie that is placed around a vessel. A Rumel tourniquet is a type of bolster.

Bradycardia—A slow heart rate; usually a heart rate of less than 60 beats per minute.

Bucking—A patient's involuntary reaction to stimulation of the larynx. It occurs when the patient is sedated. The patient recoils and arches the neck in a bucking motion.

Cardioplegia—The intentional stopping of the heart during cardiac surgery. It is performed with cardioplegia solution, which often contains a mixture of potassium chloride, lidocaine, dextrose, insulin, albumin, tromethamine, and Plasmanate.

Coarctation—A congenital narrowing or stricture in the descending thoracic aorta.

Commissurotomy—A surgical incision into a commissure, a band of tissue that connects two anatomical structures. In the heart, the valves may be banded together by scar tissue. In this case, a commissurotomy is a surgical incision made into this scar tissue to separate the valve leaflets.

Congenital—A condition present at birth.

Cross-clamp—To place a clamp across a structure (usually a blood vessel) to occlude it. The term often is used to describe the clamping of the aorta and other large blood vessels.

Dysrhythmia—A disturbance in the heartbeat (also called an arrhythmia).

Epinephrine—A medication that stimulates the heart muscle and produces vasoconstriction.

Fibrillation—A cardiac dysrhythmia in which the heart ceases to pump and instead quivers and undulates. This results in cardiac standstill and stasis of blood in the heart.

Terminology—cont'd

Fusiform aneurysm—A type of aneurysm that involves the entire circumference of a blood vessel.

Heparin—An anticoagulant medication.

Infarction—Necrosis and death of tissue after the cessation of blood supply. A myocardial infarction occurs when a blood vessel to a portion of the heart is blocked and the tissue distal to the blood vessel receives no oxygen and nutrients carried by blood.

Ischemia—A condition of reduced blood supply in a localized area, often caused by a narrowing of the blood vessel supplying the tissue.

Lidocaine—Medication used to reduce ventricular arrhythmias. Also known as Xylocaine.

Lobectomy—The surgical removal of one or more lobes of the lung.

Mediastinum—An enclosed cavity in the chest containing the heart, large vessels, trachea, esophagus, and lymph nodes.

Off-pump procedure—Procedure performed without a cardiopulmonary bypass (i.e., "the pump").

Pacemaker—A device that generates electrical impulses that stimulate the heart muscle to contract at a predetermined rate.

Pericardial fluid—Fluid lying between the visceral and parietal membranes that provides lubrication to the tissues, thereby reducing friction to the tissues.

Pleural cavities—Right and left enclosed cavities in the chest that contain, respectively, the right and left lungs.

Pneumonectomy—The surgical removal of one lung.

Preclotting—Process of soaking a graft or patch of synthetic graft material in the patient's blood or plasma before insertion. Most grafts no longer need preclotting.

Protamine sulfate—Medication that reverses the anticoagulation effects of heparin.

Regurgitant valve—A heart valve that is unable to close tightly, thereby allowing regurgitation (leaking) of blood into the heart chamber from which it came.

Saccular aneurysm—A type of aneurysm in which a saclike formation with a narrow neck projects from the side of the artery.

Shunt—This term is used in various contexts in cardiovascular surgery. To shunt blood or fluids means to carry blood from one location to another (e.g., in cardiopulmonary bypass, blood is shunted from the body to the bypass equipment). A shunt can be a blood vessel or tube that carries the blood. In shunting procedures, the existing route of blood is changed or a vessel is removed and a synthetic graft shunt is implanted.

Stenosis—The narrowing of a cardiac valve or lumen of a blood vessel.

Sternotomy—An incision made into the sternum (breast bone).

Syncope—A temporary loss of consciousness caused by an interruption or decrease in the flow of blood to the brain.

Tachycardia—A fast heart rate, usually over 120 beats per minute.

Tag—A hemostat (or other clamp) placed on the ends of traction suture, umbilical tape, or vessel loop to hold the ends together.

Tamponade—Accumulation of blood within the pericardium that compresses the outer walls of the heart and prevents adequate intraventricular filling of the heart. A chest tube must be inserted, or the chest opened, for the blood surrounding the heart to be drained.

Thoracostomy—Incision in the chest wall for the purpose of drainage

Thoracotomy—An incision made into the thoracic cavity.

Tricuspid valve—The heart valve found between the right atrium and the right ventricle.

Vasoconstriction—Narrowing of blood vessels, caused by hormones, drugs, or some other source.

Ventricles—The lower right and left chambers of the heart.

Wedge resection—The surgical removal of a section of a lobe of the lung.

Xylocaine—Medication used to reduce ventricular arrhythmias. Also known as lidocaine.

INTRODUCTION TO CARDIOTHORACIC SURGERY

The goals of cardiothoracic surgery are to repair, replace, or correct **congenital** (present at birth) or **acquired** anatomical abnormalities and to improve the function of the cardiac, pulmonary, and vascular systems. Both traditional "open" techniques and video-assisted, minimally invasive endoscopic procedures are employed. A thorough knowledge of the anatomy and instrumentation, and the surgeon's technical requirements is required for optimal care of the patient. Before surgery, the patient undergoes diagnostic imaging studies to identify pathological changes or anomalies to be surgically treated. Box 29-1 lists common tests used to diagnose patient problems. The choice of diagnostic tests is determined by the anticipated underlying pathology. The tests are used to confirm or deny pathology. Of particular interest are the results of the cardiac catheterization, listed in Table 29-1.

Laboratory tests also are performed to identify abnormalities of the blood, urine, or other body fluids affecting the patient's status. Table 29-2 lists normal and abnormal values of common laboratory tests.

ANATOMY OF THE THORACIC CAVITY

The thoracic cavity is separated from the abdominal cavity by the diaphragm and contains the heart and its great vessel, the lungs and their associated respiratory structures, the mediastinum, and a portion of the esophagus.

Diagnostic Tests Usually Performed for Cardiovascular Disorders

Noninvasive*

▶ Resting ECG
▶ Exercise ECG (stress test)
▶ Chest radiography
▶ Echocardiogram
▶ Resting MUGA
▶ Exercise thallium
▶ Exercise MUGA
▶ CT scan
▶ PET scan with stress test
▶ MRI, MRA

Invasive

▶ Aortography
▶ Electrophysiology
▶ Cardiac catheterization
▶ Endomyocardial biopsy

*When dye is injected into the vascular system, the test is considered semi-invasive.
ECG, electrocardiogram; *MUGA*, multiple uptake gated acquisition; *CT*, computed tomography; *PET*, positron emission tomography; *MRI*, magnetic resonance imaging; *MRA*, magnetic resonance angiography.
Modified from Beller GA: Relative merits of cardiovascular diagnostic techniques. In Braunwald E, Zipes DP, Libby P, editors: *Heart disease: a textbook of cardiovascular medicine,* ed 6, Philadelphia, 2001, Saunders.

The Heart

The heart is a muscular organ that consists of four hollow spaces or *chambers*. The two upper chambers are called the right and left atria; the two lower chambers are called the right and left ventricles (Figure 29-1). The heart lies between the two lungs, posterior to the sternum and anterior to the vertebrae and esophagus. It is contained within a closed cavity called the *mediastinum.* Most of the heart lies to the left of the midline.

Enclosing the heart is a double-layered membrane called the *pericardium* (Figure 29-2). Between the inner layer of the pericardium (the visceral pericardium) and the outer layer (the parietal pericardium) is the pericardial fluid, which lubricates the two tissue layers and prevents friction.

The walls of the heart contain three layers. The outer layer is called the *epicardium,* the muscular middle layer is the *myocardium,* and the inner layer is the *endocardium.*

The heart's four chambers are divided by a wall (the *septum*) (Figure 29-3). The *right ventricle* receives deoxygenated blood from the *right atrium.* From there, the blood is pumped through the pulmonary artery to the lungs, where it is oxygenated. The *left ventricle* receives oxygenated blood from the *left atrium.* From there, the blood is pumped into the aorta and the systemic circulation.

The heart's own blood supply is delivered by the *coronary artery circulation* (Figure 29-4).

HEART VALVES

The valves of the heart maintain unidirectional blood flow. The atria are separated from the ventricles by the atrioventricular (AV) valves. The *tricuspid* valve lies on the right side, while the *bicuspid* (mitral) valve lies on the left side. The leaflets of the valves open as blood is pumped and close when the pressure on the other side of the valve exceeds the entry pressure. The AV valve leaflets are attached to the papillary muscle of the ventricles by connective tissue called *chordae tendineae.* The valves are illustrated in Figure 29-5. The large vessels of the heart also contain valves. The *semilunar* valves connect the ventricles to the large vessels. The *pulmonary valve* connects the right ventricle with the pulmonary artery. The *aortic valve* on the left connects the left ventricle to the aorta.

THE CARDIAC CYCLE

The cardiac cycle consists of two parallel pumps. The right ventricle pumps blood through the pulmonary valve to the lungs; the left ventricle pumps blood through the aortic valve into the systemic circulation (Figure 29-6). Congenital defects produce abnormal blood flow.

THE CONDUCTION SYSTEM

The conduction system of the heart causes the heart to beat (Figure 29-7). The myocardial cells have an intrinsic ability to generate a beat (contraction). The conduction system is a complex network of special cardiac cells that are capable of generating electrical activity through special conduction pathways. These cells are located in specific areas of the heart and relay electrical stimulation that produces the heart's pumping action.

The *sinoatrial* or *SA node,* located at the junction of the superior vena cava and the right atrium, is the pacemaker of the heart. Electrical impulses begin here. From here, the impulse travels to the *AV* node in the interatrial septum. Impulses are further relayed to the *bundle of His* at the AV junction. Conduction continues through the right and left bundle branches and out to the ventricular muscle walls and *Purkinje fibers.* Disease or interference in the conduction system results in uncoordinated electrical activity or electrical activity that results in abnormal pumping action of the heart.

The Lower Respiratory System

The pulmonary system begins with the trachea, located on the midline of the neck at the inferior larynx. The lower respiratory system includes the lungs and bronchi.

LUNGS

The lungs are paired organs that are separated in the thoracic cavity by the *mediastinum.* This space contains the heart, large vessels, bronchi, trachea, and esophagus (Figure 29-8, *A*). Each of the lungs is enclosed in a *pleural cavity.* The *hilum* of each lung is located on its medial side. Large blood vessels and primary bronchi enter the lung here. The *apex* of

Text continued on p 802

Table 29-1 CARDIAC CATHETERIZATION DATA

Hemodynamic Data	Normal Values		
Flow			
Cardiac output (CO)	4.0-8.0 L/min		
Cardiac index (CI)	2.5-4.0 L/min/m^2		
Ejection fraction (EF)	60%-70%		
Left ventricular end-diastolic volume (LVEDV)	90-180 ml		
Stroke volume (SV)	60-130 ml/beat		
Stroke volume index (SVI)	35-70 ml/beat/m^2		
Resistances	Systolic	Diastolic	Mean
Systemic vascular resistance (SVR)	<20 Wood units		
Total pulmonary resistance	<3.5 Wood units		
Pulmonary vascular resistance (PVR)	<2.0 Wood units		
Shunts (Q$_P$/Q$_S$)			
Pulmonary flow/systemic flow		1:1	
Oxygen Saturations			
Venae cavae		70%	
Right atrium		70%	
Right ventricle		70%	
Pulmonary artery		70%	
Pulmonary veins		97%	
Left atrium		97%	
Left ventricle		97%	
Aorta		97%	
Valve Orifices (Adult)			
Aortic	2-4 cm^2		
Mitral	4-6 cm^2		
Tricuspid	10 cm^2		
Pressures (mm hg)			
Venae cavae			0-5
Right atrium (RA)			2-6
Right ventricle (RV)	20-30	0-5	
Pulmonary artery (PA)	20-30	10-20	10-15
Pulmonary artery wedge pressure (PAWP)			4-12
Left atrium (LA)			4-12
Left ventricle (LV)	120	0-5	
Left ventricular end-diastolic pressure (LVEDP)			5-12
Aorta	120-140	60-80	70-90
Brachial artery	120	70	
Femoral artery	125	75	

ANGIOGRAPHIC DATA	Findings
Coronary arteries	Anatomy/function of coronary vascular bed; distal coronary flow; AV fistula; atherosclerosis; anomalous origin of coronary arteries
Ventriculography	Anatomy/function of ventricles and associated structures; LV aneurysm; congenital abnormalities; valvular stenosis/regurgitation; shunts
Valvular angiography	Intact mitral/tricuspid complex; valvular incompetence/stenosis/regurgitation
Pulmonary angiography	Pulmonary embolism; congenital abnormalities
Aortography	Patency of aortic branches; normal mobility, competence, and anatomy of aortic valve; aneurysms: saccular, fusiform; origin of aortic dissection; shunts or anomalous connections; congenital defects or obstructions

Modified from Pagana KD and Pagana TJ: *Mosby's diagnostic and laboratory test reference,* ed 5, St Louis, 2001, Mosby.
AV, atrioventricular; *LV,* left ventricular.

Table 29-2 LABORATORY DATA

Test	Conventional Values
Arterial Blood Gases	
pH	7.38-7.44
PO_2	95-100 mm Hg
PCO_2	35-40 mm Hg
Blood Chemistry	
Glucose (fasting)	70-110 mg/dl
Protein (total)	6.8-8.5 g/dl
Blood urea nitrogen (BUN)	8.0-25 mg/dl
Uric acid	3.0-7.0 mg/dl
Cardiac Enzymes	
Creatine kinase (CK)	5-75 mU/ml
CK-MB (isoenzyme)	0%
Troponin T	<0.2 μg/L
Troponin I	<0.35 μg/L
Coagulation Profile	
Platelet count	150,000-400,000/μl
Prothrombin time (PT)	Depends on thromboplastin reagent used; typically 9.5-12.0 sec
Thrombin time	Depends on concentration of thrombin reagent used; typically 20-29 sec
Partial thromboplastin time (PTT)	Depends on phospholipid reagent used; typically 60-85 sec
Activated PTT (aPTT)	Depends on activator and phospholipid reagents used; typically 20-35 sec
Fibrinogen	200-400 mg/dl
Fibrinogen split products	10 mg/dl
Complete Blood Cell Count	
Hemoglobin (Hgb)	
1-3 days old	14.5-22.5 g/dl
2 mo old	9.0-14.0 g/dl
6-12 yr old	11.5-15.5 g/dl
Adult	
Male	13.5-18.0 g/dl
Female	12.0-16.0 g/dl
Hematocrit (Hct)	
2 days old	48%-75%
2 mo old	28%-42%
Adult	
Male	42%-52%
Female	35%-47%
Red blood cells (RBCs)	
1 week old	$3.9\text{-}6.3 \times 10^6/\mu l$
3-6 months old	$3.1\text{-}4.5 \times 10^6/\mu l$
2-6 years old	$3.9\text{-}5.3 \times 10^6/\mu l$
Adult	
Male	$4.6\text{-}6.2 \times 10^6/\mu l$
Female	$4.2\text{-}5.4 \times 10^6/\mu l$

Table 29-2 LABORATORY DATA—CONT'D

Test	Conventional Values
Complete Blood Cell Count—cont'd	
White blood cells (WBCs)	
1 day old	$9.4\text{-}34.0 \times 10^3/\mu l$
1 mo old	$5.0\text{-}19.5 \times 10^3/\mu l$
Adult	$4.5\text{-}11.0 \times 10^3/\mu l$
Creatinine (Urine, 24-hr)	
Male	20-26 mg/kg/24 hr
Female	14-22 mg/kg/24 hr
Electrolytes	
Potassium (K^+)	3.8-5.0 mEq/L
Sodium (Na^+)	136-142 mEq/L
Chloride (Cl^-)	95-103 mEq/L
Magnesium (Mg^{++})	1.5-2.0 mEq/L
Lipids	
Cholesterol	<200 mg/dl
Triglycerides	10-190 mg/dl
Phospholipids	150-380 mg/dl
Free fatty acids	9.0-15.0 mM/L
Liver Function	
Albumin (serum)	3.5-50 g/dl
Alkaline phosphatase	20-90 IU/L
Globulin (serum)	2.3-3.5 g/dl
Serum bilirubin (total)	0.2-1.4 mg/dl
Pulmonary Function	Normal values vary depending on the patient's age, gender, weight, and race. The following are generally calculated: Residual volume (RV), Tidal volume (TV), Expiratory reserve volume (ERV), Inspiratory reserve volume (IRV), Total lung capacity (TLC), Vital capacity (VC)
Urinalysis	
Color	Amber, yellow
Clarity	Clear
pH	4.6-8.0
Specific gravity (SG)	1.002-1.035
Protein	0.0-8.0 mg/dl
Sugar, ketones, RBCs, WBCs, casts	Negative

Modified from Malarkey LM and McMorrow ME: *Nurse's manual of laboratory tests and diagnostic procedures,* ed 2, St Louis, 2000, Saunders.

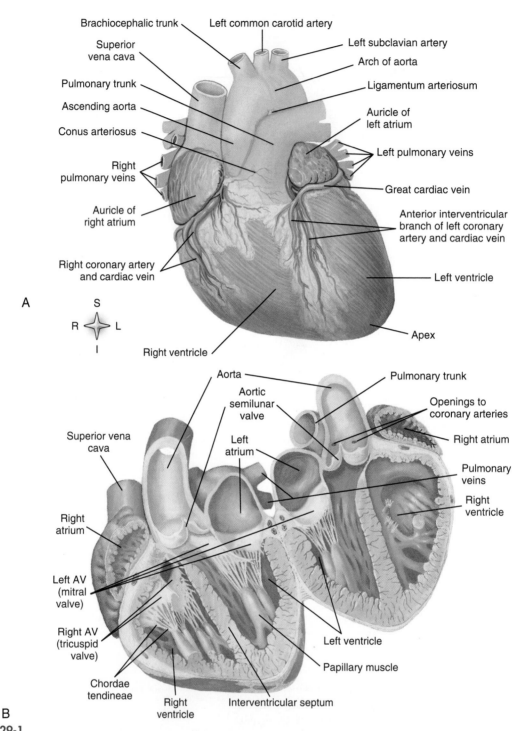

FIGURE 29-1
A, Anterior view of the exterior of the heart. **B,** Interior of the heart. (From Thibodeau GA and Patton KT: *Anatomy and physiology,* ed 5, St Louis, 2003, Mosby.)

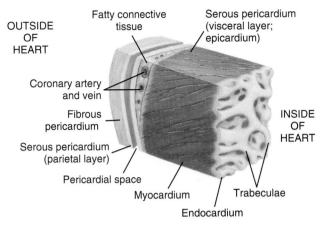

FIGURE 29-2
The pericardium. (From Thibodeau GA and Patton KT: *Anatomy and physiology*, ed 5, St Louis, 2003, Mosby.)

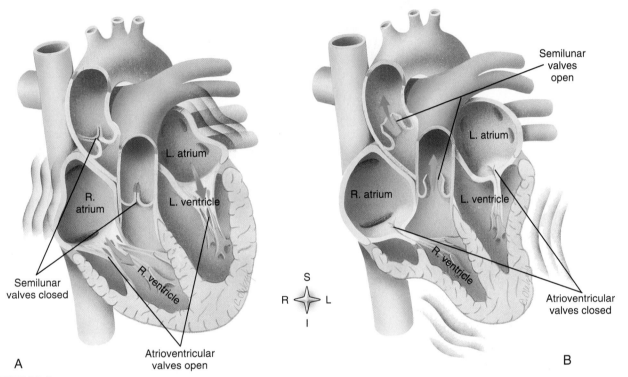

A

B

FIGURE 29-3
The heart's chambers and valves. **A** illustrates the action of heart chambers and valves when the atria contract. **B** illustrates the action of heart chambers and valves when the ventricles contract. (From Thibodeau GA and Patton KT: *Anatomy and physiology*, ed 5, St Louis, 2003, Mosby.)

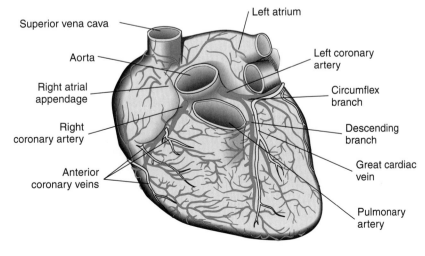

ANTERIOR VIEW

FIGURE 29-4
Coronary artery circulation. (Modified from Berne RM and Levy MN: *Cardiovascular physiology*, ed 8, St Louis, 2001, Mosby.)

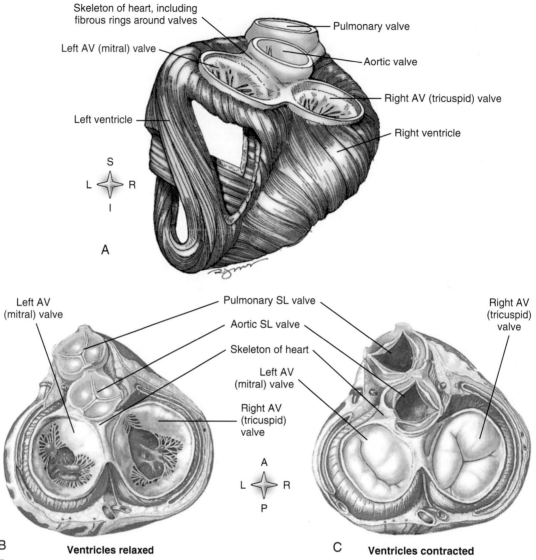

FIGURE 29-5
Structure of the heart valves. **A,** Posterior view. **B,** View from above with ventricles relaxed. **C,** View from above with ventricles contracted. (From Thibodeau GA and Patton KT: *Anatomy and physiology,* ed 5, St Louis, 2003, Mosby.)

the lung is located at the upper portion and extends just above the clavicle.

Each lung is composed of segments called bronchopulmonary segments. The right lung has three lobes, and the left lung has two lobes. The pleura is a two-layered membrane that surrounds each lung (Figure 29-8, *B*). Pleural fluid fills the space between the two layers. The outside layer adheres to the thoracic cavity. The potential space between the two layers of the pleura creates negative pressure. It is this negative pressure that causes the lungs to expand.

BRONCHI
The bronchi are derived from the trachea. The two main branches are the *right* and *left primary bronchi.* As they enter the segments of the lungs, the bronchi branch into smaller

and smaller branches or bronchioles, forming a tree-like structure of airways. At the end of the bronchioles are the *alveolar* ducts, sacs, and finally the *alveoli.* The alveolus is the structure that exchanges oxygen and carbon dioxide in the blood during respiration.

BREATHING
The act of breathing or inspiration is caused by the contraction of the diaphragm and intercostal muscles. As the diaphragm contracts, it elongates the thoracic cavity and causes the pressure within the lungs to decrease. This pulls air into the lungs. Expiration occurs when the diaphragm and intercostal muscles relax. The alveoli contract and air escapes passively out of the lungs. This allows the pressure between the outside atmosphere of the body and the lungs to equalize.

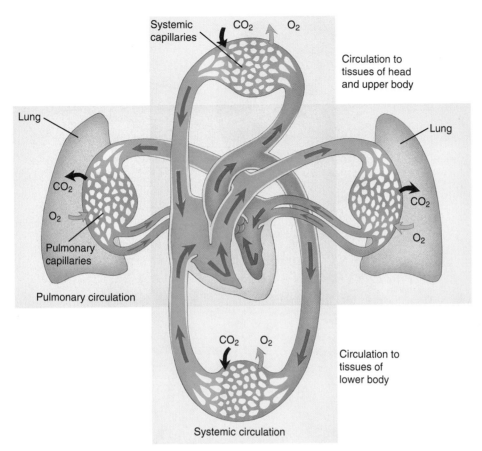

FIGURE 29-6
Blood flow through the circulatory system. (From Thibodeau GA and Patton KT: *Anatomy and physiology,* ed 5, St Louis, 2003, Mosby.)

INSTRUMENTS

In addition to general surgery instruments, three major sets of instruments are used in cardiothoracic procedures: general thoracic instruments (including stapling devices), cardiac instruments, and lung instruments. The exact nature of the procedure determines which sets are needed. Specific instruments for coronary artery, valve, and aneurysm surgery may be added (Figure 29-9).

Coronary Artery Instruments

The coronary artery instruments include fine instruments, particularly scissors and needle holders that are used when operating on very small vessels such as the coronary arteries.

For minimally invasive coronary procedures, performed through small thoracic incisions, longer instruments are required. In off-pump coronary anastomosis, a flexible, suction-tip coronary stabilizing device can be positioned on either side of the coronary artery to minimize cardiac movement. Figure 29-10 shows the stabilizer attached to a sternal retractor.

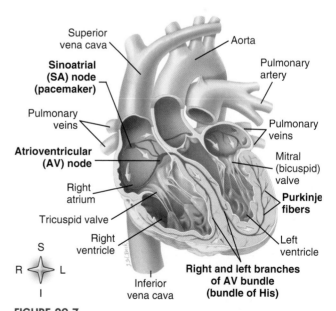

FIGURE 29-7
Conduction system of the heart. (From Thibodeau GA and Patton KT: *Anatomy and physiology,* ed 5, St Louis, 2003, Mosby.)

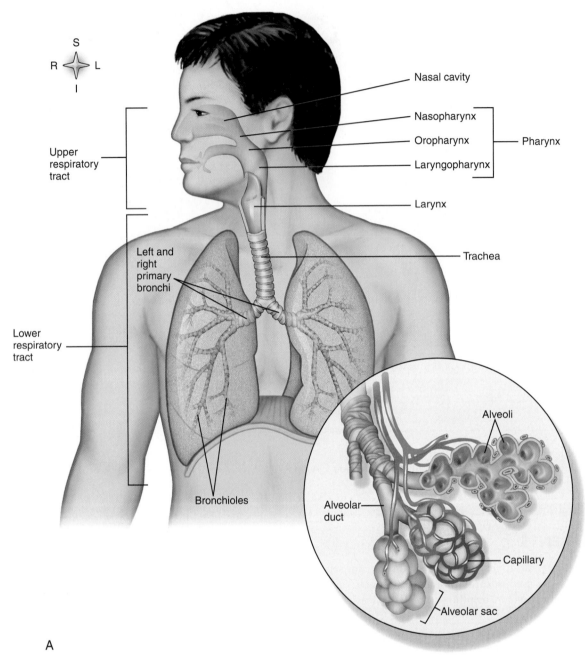

A

FIGURE 29-8
A, Location of the lungs in the respiratory system.

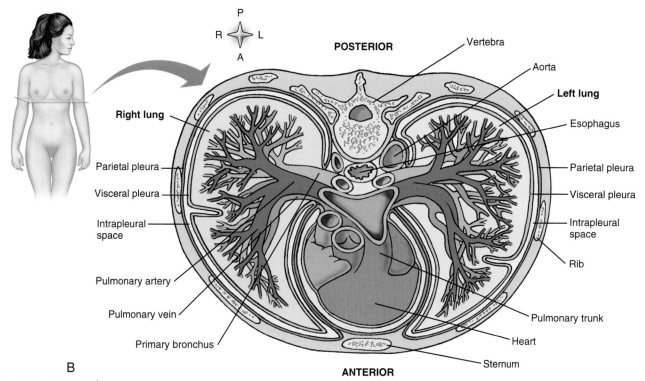

POSTERIOR

Vertebra

Aorta

Left lung

Esophagus

Parietal pleura

Visceral pleura

Intrapleural space

Rib

Pulmonary trunk

Heart

Sternum

Right lung

Parietal pleura

Visceral pleura

Intrapleural space

Pulmonary artery

Pulmonary vein

Primary bronchus

B

ANTERIOR

FIGURE 29-8, cont'd
B, Transverse section of the lungs and pleura. (From Thibodeau GA and Patton KT: *Anatomy and physiology,* ed 5, St Louis, 2003, Mosby; **B** courtesy Barbara Cousins.)

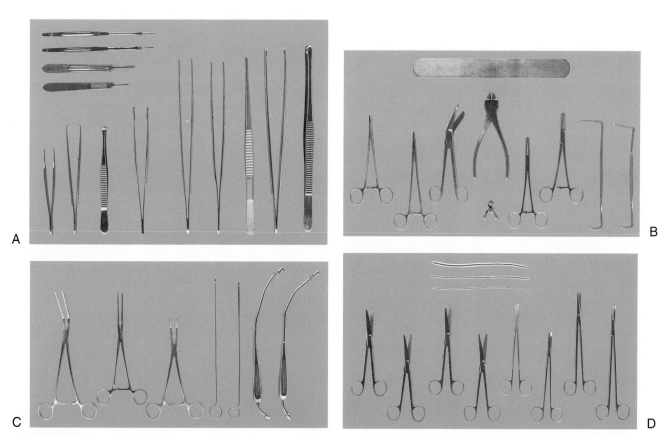

A B C D

FIGURE 29-9
Cardiac instruments. **A,** *Top left,* 2 Bard-Parker knife handles, no. 7; 1 Bard-Parker knife handle, no. 4; 1 Bard-Parker knife handle, no. 3. *Bottom, left to right,* 1 Adson tissue forceps with teeth (1 × 2); 2 Hayes Martin tissue forceps with multiteeth, front view and side view; 1 Ferris-Smith tissue forceps; 3 DeBakey vascular Atraugrip tissue forceps with post, long, 2 front views and 1 side view; 2 Russian tissue forceps, long, front view and side view. **B,** *Top,* 1 Ochsner malleable retractor, medium. *Bottom, left to right,* 1 Jarit sternal needle holder, 7 inch; 1 Jarit sternal needle holder, 8 inch; 1 bandage scissors, heavy; 1 wire cutter, heavy; 1 bed cord–holding clip; 2 Jarit (Vorse) tubing occluding clamps; 2 Army-Navy retractors. **C,** *Left to right,* 1 DeBakey multipurpose vascular clamp, obtuse angle, 60 degrees, jaw length 4 cm, overall length 9 inches; 1 Glover patent ductus clamp, straight; 1 Beck aorta clamp; 2 eyed obturators (stylets) for Rumel tourniquet; 2 Yankauer suction tubes with tips. **D,** *Top,* 3 Hegar dilators: 7 and 8, 5 and 6, 3 and 4. *Bottom, left to right,* 1 Mayo dissecting scissors, curved; 3 Mayo dissecting scissors, straight; 2 Metzenbaum scissors, 7 inch; 1 Metzenbaum scissors, 8 inch; 1 Strully scissors with probe tip. *Continued*

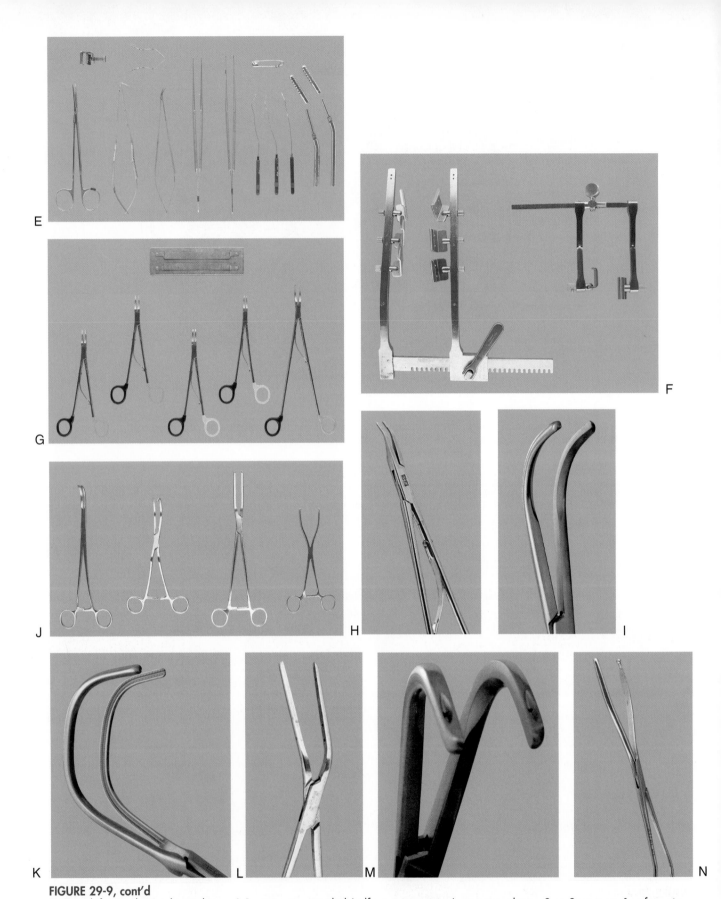

FIGURE 29-9, cont'd

E, *Top, left to right,* 1 tubing clamp; 1 Parsonnet epicardial (self-retaining spring) retractor, sharp, 3 × 3 prongs; 1 safety pin with rings. *Bottom, left to right,* 1 Snowden Pencer scissors, straight; 1 Yasargil scissors, bayonet handle, 125-degree angle; 1 You-Potts scissors, fine, thin 10-mm blades, 45-degree angle; 2 Snowden-Pencer dressing forceps, 8 inch; 3 Garrett dilators: 2.0 mm, 1.0 mm, and 1.5 mm; 2 metal coronary suction tubes with tips. **F,** *Left to right,* 1 Ankeney sternal retractor; 1 Himelstein sternal retractor. **G,** *Top,* 1 hemoclip cartridge base. *Bottom, left to right,* 5 Weck EZ Load hemoclip appliers: 2 medium, 7.75 inch; 2 small, 7.75 inch; 1 large, 10.75 inch and tip. **H,** Close-up of Weck hemoclip applier. **I,** Semb ligature-carrying forceps, 9 inch; **J,** *Left to right,* 1 Semb ligature-carrying forceps, 9 inch; 1 Lambert-Kay aorta clamp; 1 Fogarty clamp-applying forceps, angled; 1 bulldog clamp applier. **K,** Lambert-Kay aorta clamp. **L,** Fogarty clamp-applying forceps, angled. **M,** Semb ligature-carrying forceps, close-up of tip; **N,** Bulldog clamp applier. (From Tighe SM: *Instrumentation for the operating room,* ed 6, St Louis, 2003, Mosby.)

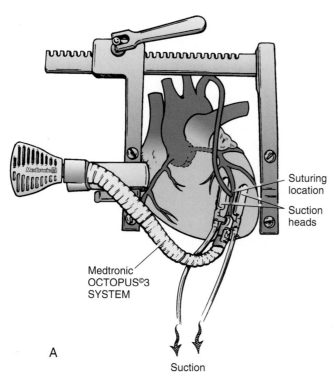

A

Medtronic
OCTOPUS©3
SYSTEM

Suturing
location

Suction
heads

Suction

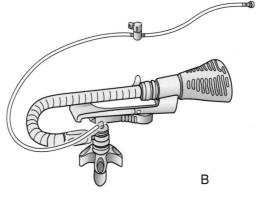

B

FIGURE 29-10
A, The Octopus 3 coronary stabilizer attaches to
the sternal retractor proximally and immobilizes
the coronary artery. The device uses suction pads
to minimize tissue motion at the anastomotic site.
B, The Starfish left ventricular suction device holds
the left ventricle apex and allows it to be retracted
for access to lateral and posterior coronary arteries. (From Seifert PC: *Cardiac surgery: perioperative patient care*, St Louis, 2002, Mosby; courtesy
Medtronic, Inc., Minneapolis, Minn.)

Valve Instruments
Valve instruments include special retractors to expose the
valve, suture holders, and accessories to the valve prosthesis
of choice.

Aneurysm Instruments
These include an array of vascular clamps in addition to the
dissecting instruments.

PROSTHETIC GRAFTS

Tube and Patch Grafts
Prosthetic grafts are used to replace abnormal, diseased, or
injured segments of an artery or vein. Many types of grafts
are available in assorted sizes (Figure 29-11). The technologist should be familiar with those used by the surgeons in
their health facility. The two most common types of grafts
are knitted and woven grafts. Knitted grafts are more porous
and softer and allow the suture needle to pass through more
easily. They are preferred for small artery anastomosis or
when an artery is very fragile. Woven grafts are used for large
artery replacement because their tight weave prevents loss of
blood through the graft.

Preclotting is seldom required because most woven and
knitted grafts are impregnated with collagen to reduce
bleeding through the graft. Rarely, some synthetic grafts require preclotting with the patient's blood. To do this, the surgeon aspirates 30 to 50 ml of blood from the patient before
heparinization. The surgeon or technologist then flushes the
graft with the blood. The graft is then placed in a small basin

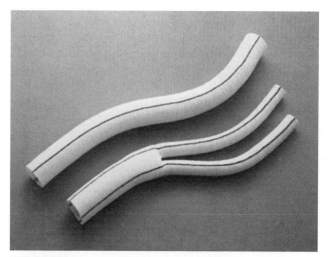

FIGURE 29-11
Straight and bifurcated arterial tube grafts. (From Rothrock
JC: *Alexander's care of the patient in surgery*, ed 12, St
Louis, 2003, Mosby; courtesy Meadox Medicals, a division
of Boston Scientific Company, Natic, Mass.)

until the surgeon needs it. The blood clots and seals the
spaces between the fibers of the graft.

Grafts are available as straight or bifurcated tubes made
of Teflon, Dacron, or polytetrafluoroethylene (PTFE). To
avoid waste and expense, only the appropriate size graft, as
specified by the surgeon using graft sizers, should be opened
for a procedure. The size, type, and serial number of the
graft are checked and then recorded on the patient's operative record by the circulator.

Patch grafts, also made of Teflon or PTFE, are used to strengthen a suture line or close a defect (abnormal opening in the tissue). Patches are cut to size as needed. Teflon felt material in the form of small pledgets is used on the suture or along the suture line to reinforce the anastomosis. The scrub should place a mosquito clamp in the middle of the pledget so that the surgeon can pass the suture through each end of the pledget.

Prosthetic Valves

A full set of prosthetic heart valves, their sizers, handles, and holders are required when valve replacement is to be performed. The technologist should be familiar with the different type of valves and accessory equipment (Figure 29-12). Valves are extremely expensive and should be handled as little as possible. The scrub and the circulator must verify the type, size, and identification number of the valve. The circulator then records the information on the patient's operative record. Two valves commonly used are the St. Jude Medical (mechanical) and the Hancock porcine (biological) valves.

SPECIAL EQUIPMENT

Rumel Tourniquet

The Rumel tourniquet is commonly used in cardiovascular surgery. This is a short length of rubber tubing either commercially prepared or cut from a Robinson urinary catheter. The tourniquet is threaded over cannulation sutures to help hold the cannulae in place. The Rumel tourniquet also is used when large vessels are occluded or isolated with a vessel loop or umbilical tape (length of cotton passed under a vessel for retraction). A stylet such as that from a Rumel tourniquet is used to snare the strands of suture or tape and bring

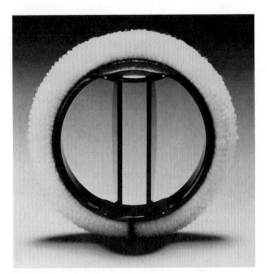

FIGURE 29-12
St. Jude Medical bileaflet valve prosthesis. (From Rothrock JC: *Alexander's care of the patient in surgery*, ed 12, St Louis, 2003, Mosby; courtesy St. Jude Medical, Inc., St. Paul, Minn. Copyright 2005.)

them through the lumen of the tubing. One then tightens the tubing against the cannula or vessel by pulling on the strands. The tubing is held securely by a hemostat placed across its upper end.

Pacemaker

A pacemaker is a device that produces electrical impulses that stimulate the heart muscle. This process is called *pacing* the heart. Pacing batteries may be temporary (external) or permanent (internal). Temporary electrodes are implanted on the surface of the heart at the time of cardiac surgery. Permanent electrodes are of two types: endocardial (transvenous) and epicardial. The endocardial electrode is inserted into a vein and advanced into the right ventricle under fluoroscopy (Figure 29-13). The epicardial electrode is sutured directly to the heart, on the atrium, ventricle, or both. Endocardial transvenous insertion is more common. The electrode(s) are connected to a generator.

The technologist should have a basic understanding of the purpose of pacemakers and should be able to identify their components. An alligator cable is used to connect the electrode(s) to the external battery for temporary pacing of the heart. This cable also may be used as a fibrillator when it is connected to the fibrillator power source. The heart is fibrillated (causing it to quiver) when there is a risk that air may be drawn into it and ejected into circulation by its normal beating action. Fibrillation also may be used during the repair of a leaking anastomosis.

Defibrillator

The defibrillator paddles are required to convert **fibrillation** (ineffectual quivering of the heart) into a normal rhythm (Figure 29-14). The two paddles are kept readily available on the sterile field. When needed, such as during heart arrhythmia, the surgeon places a paddle on each side of the heart and instructs the circulator to set the charge on the defibrillator. The application of electricity to the heart shocks the cells, converting the rhythm back to normal. When the defibrillator is in use, all personnel must stand clear of the patient to avoid receiving an electric shock.

DRUGS

Heparin

Heparin sodium is an anticoagulant. It prevents fibrinogen from converting to fibrin, an essential phase of the body's clotting mechanism. The drug does not dissolve blood clots but only prevents them from forming. It is administered through a large vein or the right atrium before cannulation for cardiopulmonary bypass. It prevents clot formation in the bypass circuit while the patient is on the heart-lung machine. The drug dosage is calculated according to body weight. Heparin also may be distributed to the technologist for local use on the field.

Protamine Sulfate

Protamine sulfate is a medication that, when combined with heparin, reverses the anticoagulant effects of heparin. Intravenous protamine is administered after bypass has been completed and the cannulae have been removed. Some patients have a reaction to protamine, and the surgeon may elect to allow heparin reversal to proceed without it.

Lidocaine

Lidocaine (Xylocaine) 1% is commonly used in the treatment of ventricular arrhythmias. This drug controls particular rhythmic patterns, including *premature ventricular contractions* and *ventricular tachycardia*. These arrhythmias can develop into ventricular fibrillation in which the heart ceases to beat but instead quivers without coordination, effectively stopping circulation.

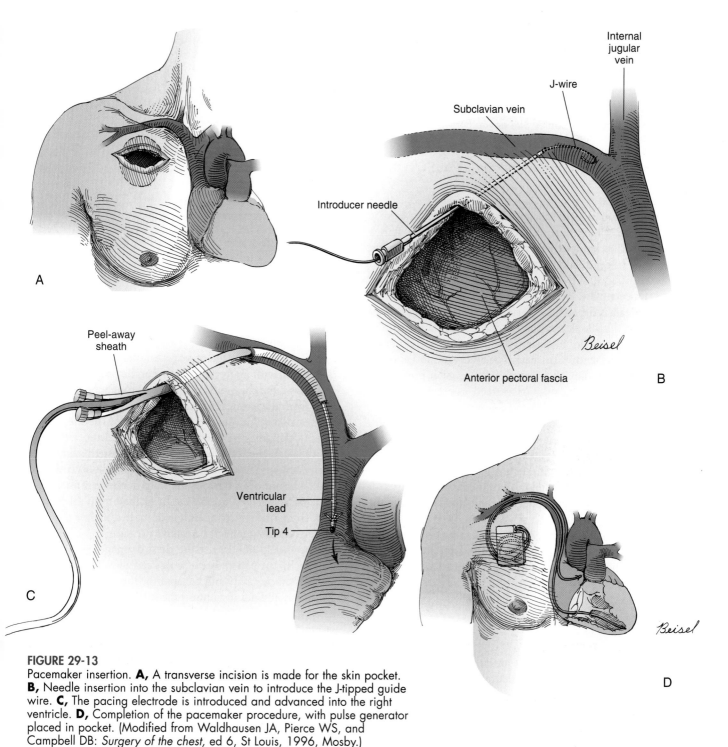

FIGURE 29-13
Pacemaker insertion. **A,** A transverse incision is made for the skin pocket. **B,** Needle insertion into the subclavian vein to introduce the J-tipped guide wire. **C,** The pacing electrode is introduced and advanced into the right ventricle. **D,** Completion of the pacemaker procedure, with pulse generator placed in pocket. (Modified from Waldhausen JA, Pierce WS, and Campbell DB: *Surgery of the chest,* ed 6, St Louis, 1996, Mosby.)

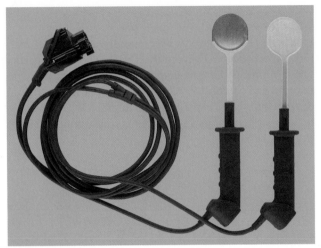

FIGURE 29-14
Internal defibrillator paddles with power cord. (From Tighe SM: *Instrumentation for the operating room*, ed 6, St Louis, 2003, Mosby.)

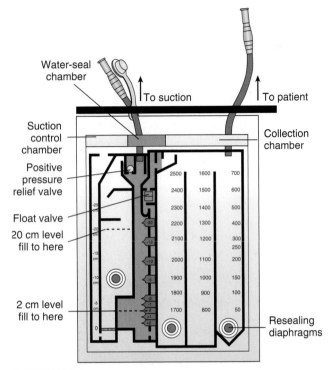

FIGURE 29-15
Chest drainage system. (From Lewis SM, Heitkemper MM, and Dirksen SR: *Medical surgical nursing*, ed 6, St Louis, 2004, Mosby.)

Epinephrine

Epinephrine has many different actions, including cardiac stimulation. Under normal circumstances it cannot start a heart that has stopped beating (called **asystole**) but rather stimulates the adrenergic receptors in the heart.

Cardioplegia

Cardioplegia is the purposeful stopping of the heart's pumping action. Cardioplegic solution may contain a mixture of potassium chloride, lidocaine, dextrose, insulin, albumin, tromethamine, and Plasmanate. The exact type and amount of the drugs in the solution vary with surgeon preference. The solution may be cooled or warmed, as required, for administration.

Cardioplegic solution is administered with two methods. In *antegrade* cardioplegia (after the aortic cross-clamp has been applied), a needle is placed in the aorta (proximal to the aortic clamp) where it exits the left ventricle (the aortic "root"). Cardioplegic solution is infused into the aorta. It then flows into the right and left coronary ostia and into the coronary circulation.

In *retrograde* cardioplegic infusion, a catheter is placed in the coronary sinus of the right atrium and into the coronary sinus. Cardioplegic solution is then infused into the coronary venous system.

SURGICAL PROCEDURES

Thoracostomy

After spontaneous or traumatic air leak, or a surgical procedure in which the right or left pleural cavity is opened, negative pressure must be restored to allow the lungs to expand. The surgeon achieves this by making an opening into the affected pleural cavity via a small thoracic incision. Through this thoracostomy, one or more chest tubes are inserted and connected to a water-seal chest drainage system to remove air, blood, and other fluids from the thoracic or pericardial cavity. Suction is applied.

Chest tubes are made of heavy Silastic or polyvinyl chloride tubing with many perforations at the proximal end. After surgery, the chest tube is inserted through a stab incision away from the surgical incision. Chest tubes may be placed in one or more locations. If two are required (in one or both pleura), they may be joined with a Y connector. The tubes are then attached to a closed drainage system with three compartments (Figure 29-15). Two compartments contain a small amount of water, and the third is reserved for collection. Suction is used to pull the air or fluid from the thorax. Each compartment of the unit is connected to the other by a tube, which maintains the negative pressure.

One should never raise the chest drainage system above the level of the patient because this can allow fluid to return to the thoracic cavity and collapse the lungs.

One should not disconnect the suction until immediately before patient transport because the blood may accumulate inside the pericardium and produce cardiac tamponade.

Video-Assisted Thoracoscopic Surgery

Video-assisted thoracoscopic surgery (VATS) is a minimally invasive method of performing many surgical procedures of the thoracic cavity. Preparation of the patient, equipment, and instruments are discussed in this section. Selected procedures are described in more detail throughout the chapter.

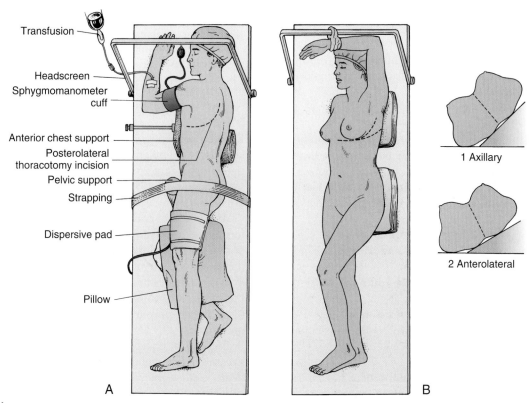

FIGURE 29-16
Positions for thoracotomy incisions. **A,** Lateral position for posterolateral incision. **B,** Semilateral position for axillary or antero-lateral position. (From Rothrock JC: *Alexander's care of the patient in surgery,* ed 12, St Louis, 2003, Mosby; courtesy Zimmer Inc., Warsaw, Ind.)

SURGICAL GOAL

The goal of endoscopic surgery is to achieve the desired surgical effect with less tissue trauma, less postoperative pain, and a shorter recovery time than usually associated with thoracic procedures.

PATIENT PREPARATION

The thoracoscopy patient is placed in the lateral position with the operative side up (Figure 29-16). Recall that the right or left lateral decubitus position describes which side is *down.* Thus the right lateral decubitus position means that the right side of the patient is in contact with the operating table. Review this position in Chapter 10, Transporting, Transferring, and Positioning, before proceeding. A critical safety point in lateral decubitus positioning is the position of padding under the patient's thorax.

An *axillary roll* is positioned to *avoid* pressure on the axillary nerves and blood vessels; if the roll is not properly positioned, severe nerve damage may result.

A general anesthetic is administered through a double-lumen endotracheal tube. The double lumen allows the lung on the affected side to collapse while anesthetic and oxygen are administered to the other lung.

The patient is prepped from the lower neck to the level of the iliac crest from bedside to bedside. The exposed shoulder

and arm also may be prepped and the arm placed on an overhead arm board or the upper arm placed at a 90-degree angle over the upper chest with padding to prevent pressure on the ulnar nerve and decubital tunnel.

TROCAR AND CANNULA SITES

Locations of ports depend on the procedure. However, the telescope port is placed farthest from and most inferior to the target tissue. The anterior port often is placed in the midclavicular line in the fourth interspace. Three or four ports usually are required. A combination *mini thoracotomy* (small thoracotomy incision) and thoracoscopy may be performed for some surgeries.

EQUIPMENT

Thoracoscopy in the adult requires 10-mm lenses in sizes 0 degrees and 30 degrees. The scope, camera, and light source are connected in the usual manner (see Chapter 18, Endoscopic Surgery and Robotics).

Instruments used in thoracic endoscopic procedures include general surgery, cardiovascular, and lung instruments. Instruments with curved shanks often are used in the thoracic cavity because they permit better access to structures. Endoscopic stapling devices are used for biopsy and resection procedures (see the section on instruments above).

Bronchoscopy
SURGICAL GOAL
Bronchoscopy is the insertion of a fiberoptic or rigid telescope into the trachea and bronchi to make a diagnosis or for surgical intervention.

PATHOLOGY
Diseases of the bronchi often are visible with the aid of endoscopy. Although lung disease may not be visible through the endoscope, the encroachment of tumor sometimes can affect the shape and inner structure of the bronchial tree. Some common indications for bronchoscopy include:

▶ Controlling hemorrhage from a tumor or mass
▶ Obtaining bronchial secretions and washings from the lower respiratory tract
▶ Finding the cause of blood in the sputum, wheezing, or persistent cough
▶ Assessing the patency of the bronchial tree
▶ Determining the extent of burn injury from toxic inhalation or smoke inhalation
▶ Performing laser ablation
▶ Removing foreign bodies that the patient has aspirated (food or objects, especially in the pediatric patient)
▶ Assessing lesions seen on chest x-rays
▶ Assessing traumatic injury

Technique　　**RIGID BRONCHOSCOPY**

1. The surgeon inserts the bronchoscope into the trachea and advances it.
2. The respiratory structures are examined.

3. Interventional procedures, such as removal of tissue or extraction of a foreign body, may be performed.
4. Bronchial washings, cytological biopsy, or sputum samples may be taken.
5. The bronchoscope is gently withdrawn.

DISCUSSION
Rigid bronchoscopy is generally reserved for the removal of large tissue or foreign bodies. This is because the lumen of the rigid scope is larger than the lumen of the flexible bronchoscope (Figure 29-17). A general anesthetic is used for rigid bronchoscopy. Side channels deliver oxygen or anesthetic gas.

An important complication of rigid bronchoscopy is injury to the tracheobronchial structures if the patient moves during the procedure. The autonomic gag reflex may cause the patient to arch and cough even during heavy sedation or light general anesthesia. This is called **bucking**. A local anesthetic is sprayed into the trachea before the endoscope is inserted to help prevent bucking and serious injury during the procedure.

The patient is placed in the supine position with the neck hyperextended slightly. A body drape is applied. The patient's eyes may be protected with pads.

Before the procedure begins, the scrub should make sure that all light cables and fittings are in good working order. An eyepiece adapter should be placed over the scope to protect the surgeon from contamination by the patient's body fluids. A tooth guard is placed in the patient's mouth to protect the teeth.

The surgeon inserts the rigid scope into the trachea. Side channels on the bronchoscope allow for insertion of irriga-

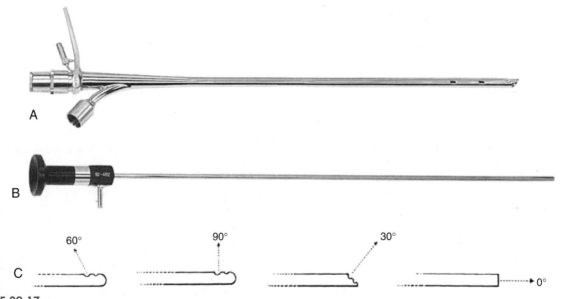

FIGURE 29-17
Instruments for bronchoscopy. **A,** Holinger ventilating fiberoptic bronchoscope. **B,** Fiberoptic light carrier. **C,** Fiberoptic bronchoscopic telescopes: left to right, forward oblique 60 degree; lateral 90 degree; right angle 30 degree; forward 0 degree. (From Rothrock JC: *Alexander's care of the patient in surgery,* ed 12, St Louis, 2003, Mosby; courtesy Pilling Co., Fort Washington, Penn.)

tion, suction, and other instruments. The scrub should assist by guiding the instruments into the side channels.

If sputum or fluid samples are to be taken, suction tubing adapted with a Lukens trap is attached to the endoscope. The surgeon injects fixative solution into the scope with a syringe. Cells are washed free from the bronchus and retrieved with the suction cannula attached to a Lukens trap. This is a small vial that collects solutions as they are suctioned. The trap must be held upright to avoid losing the specimen. The surgeon performs bronchial lavage by injecting saline into the side channel.

Cytology brushing is performed with a small brush inserted into the scope. When the brush is retrieved, the scrub dips it into the specimen container with a small amount of saline, or transfers the specimen according to the surgeon's directions.

Biopsy tissue is removed with cup forceps. The scrub is responsible for removing the tissue from the forceps. A hypodermic needle may be used to remove the tissue; the tissue then is placed on a moistened Telfa pad to prevent its loss. One should be sure when removing the tissue from the forceps not to crush the specimen, as that may distort the pathology of the tissue.

Foreign bodies are retrieved with a basket similar to that used to remove kidney stones. The basket instrument is threaded into the side channel. Grasping forceps also may be used to retrieve a foreign body.

At the close of the procedure, before the scope is withdrawn, the surgeon suctions the patient free of all secretions. The scope is then withdrawn.

Technique FLEXIBLE BRONCHOSCOPY

1. The fiberoptic tube is inserted through the patient's mouth or nose.
2. The surgeon examines the tracheobronchial tree.
3. Cytology or biopsy specimens are taken.
4. The bronchial tree is suctioned.
5. Video data are recorded.

DISCUSSION

Flexible bronchoscopy is used to examine the lower respiratory tract and to obtain biopsy specimens. Interventional procedures through the flexible scope are more limited than with the rigid scope because of the small diameter of the tip (Figure 29-18). Like all endoscopes, the fiberoptic bronchoscope has video capability, and the images gathered through the scope are projected onto the video screen.

The advantage of fiberoptic bronchoscopy is the ability to reach deeply into the bronchial tree, and the ability of the tip to rotate. This allows a more complete view of the anatomy. Accessory instruments used with the flexible bronchoscope are smaller than those used with the rigid scope. Simultaneous imaging studies (e.g., x-ray film) may be performed during the procedure. The patient with a neck injury is a candidate for flexible bronchoscopy because hyperextension of the neck is unnecessary for insertion.

The patient is placed in semi-Fowler's position. A local anesthetic is sprayed into the throat, and the patient usually is sedated. The flexible fiberoptic tube is passed through the patient's mouth or nose. Unlike rigid bronchoscopy, which allows the patient to be ventilated through the tube, the patient must breathe *around* the flexible endoscope.

The surgeon inserts the fiberoptic scope and advances it through the trachea and bronchial tree. He or she then examines the tissues and uses the video data recorder to see and make a permanent record of the images.

The surgeon obtains cytology samples by inserting a small brush through the operating channel. The technologist must be sure that the instrument is long enough to extend outside the tip of the scope. When the brush has been removed, the scrub dips the brush in a specimen container holding a small amount of saline. This process may be repeated several times.

Biopsy forceps may be used to take small tissue samples. These must be carefully handled, because they are very small and easily lost. After the forceps has been withdrawn from the scope, one should immediately place the specimen in a specimen container or on a Telfa pad.

A suction cannula is used to remove secretions. These are trapped in the Lukens specimen trap just as in rigid bronchoscopy.

Mediastinoscopy
SURGICAL GOAL

The mediastinoscope is inserted to examine the area for masses or lymph tissue.

Technique

1. The surgeon makes an incision in the suprasternal notch.
2. The surgeon incises the fascia and uses his or her fingers to create a tunnel into the mediastinum.
3. The surgeon inserts the mediastinoscope through the tunnel along the trachea.
4. The trachea, bronchial tree, aortic arch, and lymph nodes are examined for evidence of disease.
5. Lymph node tissue may be aspirated.
6. The mediastinoscope is withdrawn.
7. The wound is closed.

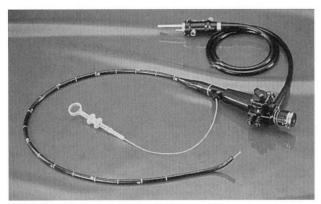

FIGURE 29-18
Flexible bronchoscope. (Courtesy Olympus, New Hyde Park, NY.)

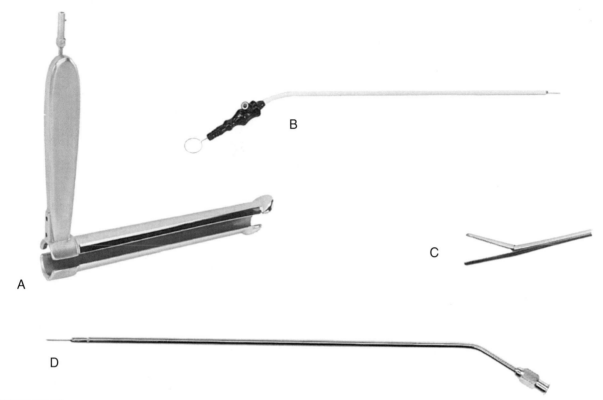

FIGURE 29-19
Instruments for mediastinoscopy. **A,** Carlens mediastinoscope. **B,** Insulated suction tube. **C,** Jackson laryngeal forceps. **D,** Aspirating needle. (From Rothrock JC: *Alexander's care of the patient in surgery,* ed 12, St Louis, 2003, Mosby; courtesy Pilling Co., Fort Washington, Penn.)

DISCUSSION

The mediastinoscope is a lighted endoscope (Figure 29-19). Video-assisted endoscopy is available and allows the scope's field of vision to be projected on a video screen.

The patient is placed in the supine position with the neck hyperextended. He or she is prepped and draped for an upper thoracic incision. The procedure is performed under general anesthesia. The surgeon may stand at the patient's head or side.

A small incision is made over the suprasternal notch with a #10 knife blade. The incision is carried through the subcutaneous and muscle layers, commonly with Metzenbaum scissors and tissue forceps. The fascial layer on the anterior surface of the trachea is identified. The surgeon clamps small veins with mosquito hemostats and ligates them with fine silk ties. The electrosurgical unit (ESU) is used for smaller bleeders.

The surgeon uses blunt finger dissection to make a plane between the tissues into the superior mediastinum. The scope is then inserted into this plane.

Major arteries and veins of the thoracic cavity lie close to the area being visualized and can be injured inadvertently. Good lighting and suction are critical to preventing trauma to the tissues. The technologist must exercise care when handing instruments to the surgeon to avoid jarring the patient or surgeon.

When the scope is in proper position, the surgeon performs further dissection with small sponges mounted on grasping forceps. He or she identifies the nodes or tissue to be biopsied. To differentiate between lymph-node tissue and the wall of the pulmonary artery, a special needle has been designed that is attached to a metal stylet and used to pierce the tissue. The technologist attaches a syringe to the stylet before handing it to the surgeon, who then aspirates the contents of the tissue. If there is no evidence of blood return from the tissue, the surgeon uses cup biopsy forceps to obtain a pathology specimen. The technologist removes the tissue from the forceps and places it in a specimen container or Telfa pad moistened with saline.

After specimens have been obtained, the surgeon dries the wound and checks for bleeding. The ESU and hemostatic agents such as *Gelfoam* and *Surgicel* may be used to control bleeding. The surgeon then withdraws the scope and closes the incision with synthetic absorbable sutures and skin staples or suture.

Scalene Node Biopsy
SURGICAL GOAL

Scalene node biopsy is performed on patients with palpable nodes in the area of the scalene fat pads. The biopsy is performed to diagnose and stage malignant and nonmalignant thoracic diseases (Figure 29-20).

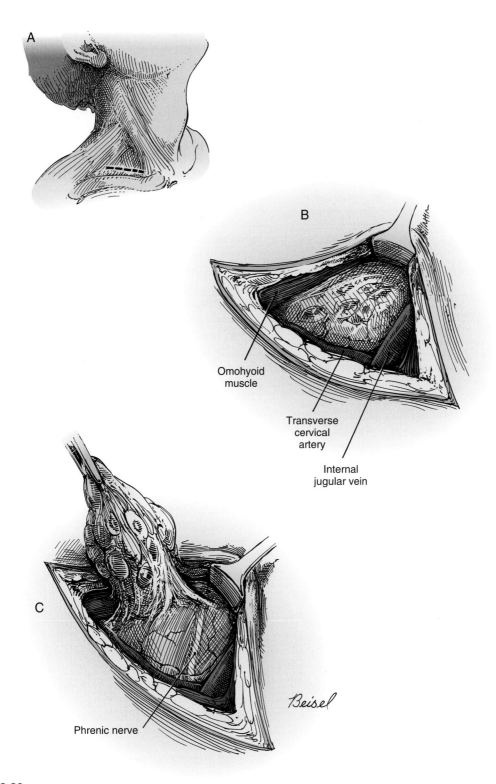

FIGURE 29-20
Scalene node biopsy. **A,** Location of transverse incision. **B,** A triangular incision is made at the boundaries of the fat pad.
C, The scalene fat pad is removed; the anterior scalene muscle lies behind the fat pad at the lateral aspect. (Modified from
Waldhausen JA, Pierce WS, and Campbell DB: *Surgery of the chest,* ed 6, St Louis, 1996, Mosby.)

PATHOLOGY

Lung cancer spreads through the intrathoracic and mediastinal lymphatics to the supraclavicular nodes (the last nodes in the drainage chain). The excision and biopsy of the scalene fat pad should be performed before thoracotomy is performed.

Technique

1. The patient's head is turned away from the operative site.
2. The surgeon makes a transverse incision, 5 cm to 7 cm long, approximately 2 cm above the clavicle. The medial end of the incision is located at the posterior border of the sternocleidomastoid muscle.
3. The incision continues through the platysma muscle; retractors are inserted.
4. The scalene fat pad is bounded inferiorly by the subclavian vein and the transverse cervical artery; medially by the internal jugular vein and the sternocleidomastoid muscle; and laterally by the omohyoid muscle.
5. The scalene fat pad is removed, exposing the phrenic nerve and the anterior scalene muscle.
6. The wound is closed.

DISCUSSION

Scalene node biopsy is one of the ancillary procedures often performed in conjunction with bronchoscopy and is used to identify patients most likely to benefit from thoracotomy for malignant disease. If the biopsy findings demonstrate "positive" nodes, thoracotomy usually is not advised because a resection is unlikely to be curative.

The patient is placed in the supine position with the head turned away from the surgical site. He or she is prepped and draped for an upper thoracic incision. The procedure is performed under general anesthesia. The surgeon stands on the operative side.

Thoracotomy
SURGICAL GOAL

A thoracotomy is an incision made in the thoracic cavity to allow surgery on the cardiothoracic structures (see Table 29-3 for a list or thoracic incisions). The thoracotomy incision is used to provide wide exposure of the surgical site; it may be required when the endoscopic approach is contraindicated (e.g., because of severe adhesions).

Technique

Opening
1. The surgeon incises the skin.
2. The subcutaneous tissue and muscle layers are divided.
3. The ribs are divided.
4. The surgeon enters the intercostal space.
5. The surgeon enters the thoracic cavity.

Closing
1. Sutures are placed around the divided ribs.
2. The ribs are brought together with a *rib approximator.*
3. The muscle, subcutaneous tissue, and skin are closed in layers.

DISCUSSION
Opening
The patient is placed in the lateral position, prepped, and draped for a lateral thoracotomy. The surgeon makes the incision, following the curve of the rib. Subcutaneous and muscle layers then are divided with the knife or ESU. Bleeders are coagulated or clamped and ligated with silk ties.

The surgeon inserts a scapular retractor beneath the shoulder muscles and elevates the scapula. An intercostal incision is made with the knife or ESU. If a rib is to be removed, the surgeon incises the periosteum along its anterior surface. A periosteal elevator or rib raspatory is used to strip periosteum from the rib. The surgeon cuts the rib free from its attachment at the spine and sternum using Bethune rib shears. The entire rib is removed. The surgeon then trims the sharp edges of the remaining rib end using Sauerbruch rib shears. This prevents possible trauma to surrounding tissue and the surgeon's gloves during the procedure.

The surgeon covers the edges of the wound with laparotomy sponges to protect the wound edges from bruising. He or she then places a self-retaining retractor in the wound and opens it slowly to prevent rib fracture or tissue trauma.

The steps of this procedure are illustrated in Figure 29-21.
Closing
After chest tubes have been inserted and instruments have been removed, the surgeon places pericostal sutures such as #2 or #1 absorbable suture around the two ribs and tags the suture ends with a hemostat. Four to six sutures usually are required. A rib approximator (such as the *Bailey approximator*) is used to bring the ribs together. The pericostal sutures then are tied securely while the approximator is in place.

A continuous absorbable suture of size 0 may be used to approximate the periosteum between the two ribs. The surgeon then closes the muscles with a size-0 continuous or interrupted nonabsorbable suture. Subcutaneous tissue is closed with size 3-0 nonabsorbable synthetic sutures. Skin is closed with staples or the surgeon's preferred suture material. Chest tubes are connected to the water-chest drainage system, and the wound is dressed with absorbent pads and tape.

The steps of this procedure are illustrated in Figure 29-22.

Median Sternotomy
SURGICAL GOAL

Median sternotomy is a midline incision used for surgical procedures of the anterior thoracic cavity.

Technique

Opening
1. The surgeon makes a midline thoracic incision.
2. The xiphoid is divided.
3. The sternum is divided.

Closing
1. Wires are placed through the sternum.
2. The sternal edges are approximated.
3. The fascia and periosteum are reapproximated.
4. The subcutaneous tissue and skin are closed.

Table 29-3 THORACIC INCISIONS

Incision	Position	Indications	Special Patient Needs
Median sternotomy: Incision down center of sternum	Supine	Most adult cardiac procedures except those on branch pulmonary arteries, distal transverse aortic arch, and descending thoracic aorta	Padding for hands, elbows, feet, back of head, dependent bony prominences
Mini-sternotomy: Partial upper or lower sternal incision starting either from sternal notch or xiphoid process and extending to midportion of sternum; lower-end sternal splitting (LESS)	Supine	MAS, on-CPB or off-CPB procedures	Same as median sternotomy
Parasternotomy: Resection of right or left costal cartilages (from second to fifth cartilage, depending on surgical target)	Supine; small roll may be placed under affected side	Left: MAS CABG Right: MAS CABG, valve procedures	Same as median sternotomy; risk of postoperative chest-wall instability
Anterolateral thoracotomy: Curvilinear incision along subpectoral groove to axillary line	Supine with pad or pillow under operative site; arm supported in sling or overarm board; arm on unaffected side may be tucked along side	MAS, MIDCAB, trauma to anterior pericardium and left ventricle; repeat sternotomy	Padding for extremities; pillow or other device to elevate affected side; armboard or sling for arm on affected side
Left anterior small thoracotomy (LAST), right anterior mini-thoracotomy: Curvilinear incision along subpectoral groove, right or left side	Supine with small roll under affected side	Left: MAS, MIDCAB Right: MAS valve procedures or CABG	Same as anterolateral thoracotomy
Lateral thoracotomy: Curvilinear incision along costochondral junction anteriorly to posterior border of scapula	Placed on side with arms extended and axilla and head supported; knees and legs protected	Lung biopsies; first-rib resection; lobectomy	Armboard, overarm board, axillary roll, padding for extremities, pillow between legs; sandbags, straps, wide tape, or other devices to support torso
Posterolateral thoracotomy: Curvilinear incision from subpectoral crease below nipple, extended laterally and posteriorly along ribs almost to posterior midline below scapula (location of intercostal incision depends on surgical site); used less often with availability of VATS techniques	Lateral with arms extended and axilla and head supported; knees and legs protected	First-rib resection; lobectomy	Similar to needs for lateral thoracotomy
Transsternal bilateral anterior thoracotomy (clamshell): Submammary incision extending from one anterior axillary line to the other across sternum at fourth interspace	Supine	Lung transplant; emergency access to heart when sternal saw not available	Same as median sternotomy; requires transection of left and right IMA
Subxiphoid incision: Vertical midline incision from over xiphoid process to about 10 cm inferiorly (may divide lower portion of sternum to improve exposure)	Supine	Pericardial drainage, pericardial biopsy, attachment of pacemaker electrodes, MAS	Same as median sternotomy

Continued

Table 29-3   THORACIC INCISIONS—CONT'D

Incision	Position	Indications	Special Patient Needs
Thoracoabdominal incision: Low curvilinear incision on left side, extended to anterior midline, continued vertically down abdomen	Anterior thoracotomy with chest at 45-degree angle to table; abdomen supine	Thoracoabdominal aneurysm	Same as anterolateral thoracotomy

CPB, cardiopulmonary bypass; *CABG,* coronary artery bypass grafting; *MAS,* minimal access surgery; *MIDCAB,* minimal access direct coronary artery bypass; *IMA,* internal mammary artery; *VATS,* video-assisted thoracoscopic surgery.

Modified from Rusch VW and Ginsberg RJ: Chest wall, pleura, lung, and mediastinum. In Schwartz SI, ed: *Principles of surgery,* ed 7, New York, 1999, McGraw-Hill; Waldhausen JA, Pierce WS, and Campbell DB: *Surgery of the chest,* ed 6, St Louis, 1996, Mosby; Arom KV and Emery RW: Ministernotomy for coronary artery bypass surgery. In Yim APC et al: *Minimal access cardiothoracic surgery,* Philadelphia, 2000, WB Saunders; Arom KV and Emery RW: Alternative incisions for cardiac surgery. In Yim APC et al: *Minimal access cardiothoracic surgery,* Philadelphia, 2000, WB Saunders.

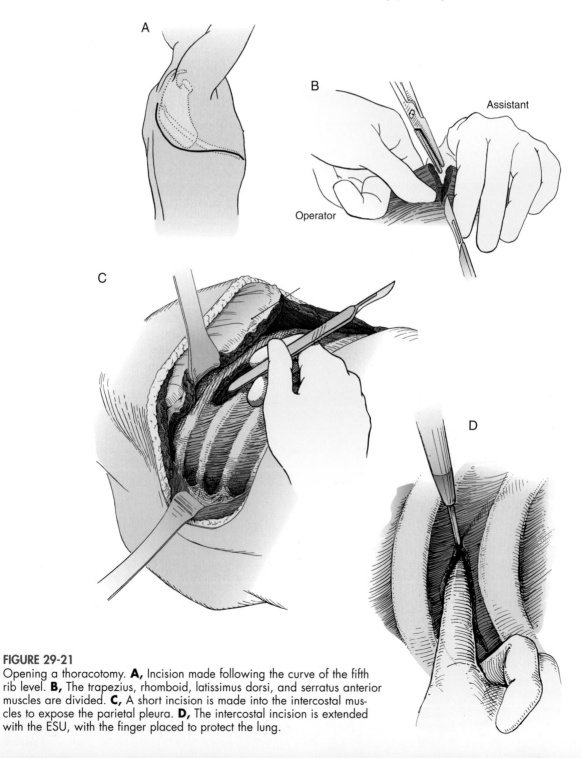

FIGURE 29-21

Opening a thoracotomy. **A,** Incision made following the curve of the fifth rib level. **B,** The trapezius, rhomboid, latissimus dorsi, and serratus anterior muscles are divided. **C,** A short incision is made into the intercostal muscles to expose the parietal pleura. **D,** The intercostal incision is extended with the ESU, with the finger placed to protect the lung.

E

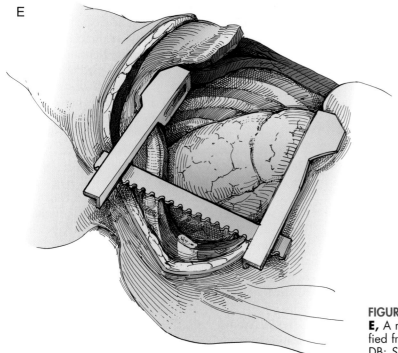

FIGURE 29-21, cont'd
E, A rib retractor is inserted to expose the lung. (Modified from Waldhausen JA, Pierce WS, and Campbell DB: *Surgery of the chest,* ed 6, St Louis, 1996, Mosby.)

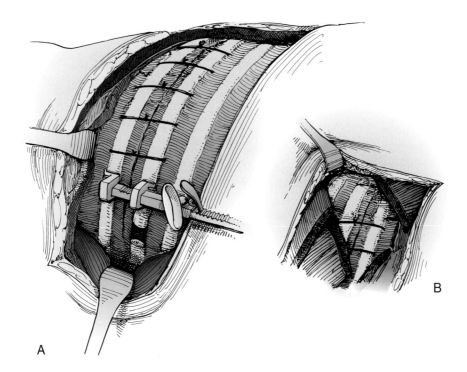

A

B

FIGURE 29-22
Closing a thoracotomy. **A,** Use of a rib approximator, and placement of pericostal sutures. **B,** Completion of pericostal closure. (Modified from Waldhausen JA, Pierce WS, and Campbell DB: *Surgery of the chest,* ed 6, St Louis, 1996, Mosby.)

DISCUSSION

Opening

The patient is placed in the supine position, prepped, and draped for a midline thoracic incision. The surgeon makes a midline incision from the sternal notch to 2 to 3 inches below the xiphoid. The subcutaneous tissue and linea alba (fascial layer distal to the xiphoid) are divided with the knife or ESU. The surgeon separates the underlying tissue from the sternal notch and xiphoid using finger dissection. He or she then divides the xiphoid on the midline with heavy curved scissors. A sternal saw then is placed in the center of the xiphoid, and the bone is divided.

The assistant elevates the cut edges of the sternum using hand-held retractors (such as Army-Navy retractors) while the surgeon coagulates bleeders using the ESU. A small amount of bone wax may be applied to the cut edges.

Before placing a self-retaining retractor, the surgeon protects the edges of the bone with moist laparotomy sponges. The retractor then is opened slowly. This exposes the pericardium, which is incised with the ESU or scissors.

The surgeon grasps the pericardium with vascular forceps or a clamp to elevate it and prevent injury to the heart. The pericardium is incised to expose the heart and ascending aorta. Lateral incisions are made as needed.

If the procedure requires bypass, silk traction sutures are placed through the edges of the pericardium and sewn to the periosteum. An umbilical tape may be used to encircle and retract the aorta. The heart and aorta are then cannulated for cardiopulmonary bypass. If an **off-pump** procedure (cardiopulmonary bypass is not needed) is to be performed, cannulation is not required.

This procedure is illustrated in Figure 29-23.

Closing

After the surgical procedure, temporary pacing wires are placed on the epicardial surface of the heart. The surgeon places six to eight #5 wire sutures through each sternal edge. The scrub holds the free ends of the wire while passing the sutures to control the end. The surgeon tightens the wires and twists each one until it is snug against the sternum to bring the sternal edges together. The surgeon uses a wire twister to make a final twist, burying the ends in the periosteum.

When Wolvek sternal-approximation fixation instruments are used, the ends of the wires are threaded through

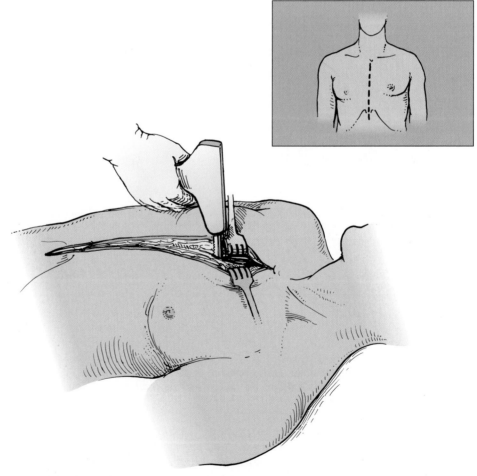

FIGURE 29-23
Opening a median sternotomy with an oscillating saw. (Modified from Waldhausen JA, Pierce WS, and Campbell DB: *Surgery of the chest*, ed 6, St Louis, 1996, Mosby.)

small metal plates. The surgeon then tightens the ends and locks the wire into position by crimping the plate. The excess wire is cut with wire cutters, and sharp tips are buried in the periosteum with the wire twister. Other approximation systems also are available.

The surgeon approximates the fascia and periosteum with interrupted sutures, such as size-0 polyester sutures.

This procedure is illustrated in Figure 29-24.

Repair of Pectus Excavatum
SURGICAL GOAL
Pectus excavatum (also known as "funnel chest") is the most common congenital deformity of the sternum (Figure 29-25). Deformity of the costal cartilages causes a concave deformity of the sternum. Although surgery may be performed for pulmonary or cardiac dysfunction, cosmetic considerations are the most common indication for surgery. The procedure often is performed between the ages of 10 and 16, when undressing in front of one's peers becomes embarrassing, although it may be performed earlier in life.

Technique

1. The surgeon makes a midline sternotomy or transverse submammary incision between the nipples.
2. The pectoralis muscles are elevated from the thoracic wall.
3. The perichondrium of each deformed cartilage is elevated (but not excised).
4. The cartilage may be removed in two pieces from the costochondral junction to the sternum.

5. The sternum is fractured through the anterior sternal table.
6. A K-wire or metal strut often is inserted to stabilize the sternum's new position.
7. Pectoralis muscles are reattached to the sternum and periosteum.
8. A mediastinal drain is placed. Pleural chest tubes are inserted if the pleural cavity has been entered.
9. The incision is closed.

DISCUSSION
The patient is placed in the supine position and is prepped and draped for an anterior thoracic (sternal) incision. The procedure is performed under general anesthesia. In addition to thoracic instruments, the surgeon may use osteotomes or chisels, bone hooks, bone-holding forceps, periosteal elevators, and a Gigli saw and handles. A roll may be placed under the upper chest to elevate the sternum.

Pectus carinatum ("pigeon breast") is another sternal deformity, wherein the sternum protrudes rather than being depressed. Repair usually is performed after the child's growth spurt when the defect becomes readily apparent. Excess bone is removed with a knife or osteotomes.

Cervical Rib Resection for Thoracic Outlet Syndrome
SURGICAL GOAL
Thoracic outlet syndrome refers to the compression of the subclavian vessels and the brachial plexus at the apex of the

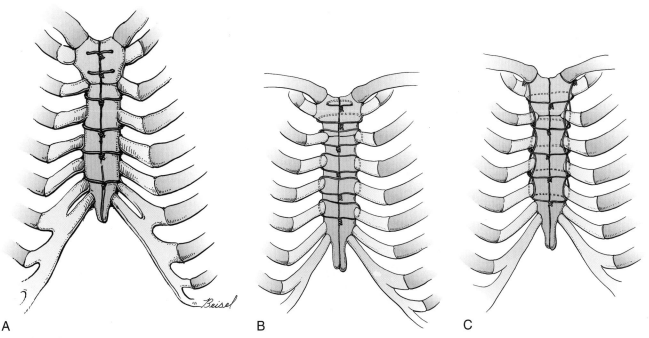

A   B   C

FIGURE 29-24
Closure techniques for median sternotomy. **A,** Normal closure of the sternal incision with heavy wire sutures. **B,** Box wiring technique used for brittle, thin, or fragile bone. **C,** Robicsek technique, used when the two halves of the sternum have been fractured in the case of sternal revision for nonunion, with placement of cerclage wires to allow firm impaction of the two sides. (Modified from Waldhausen JA, Pierce WS, and Campbell DB: *Surgery of the chest,* ed 6, St Louis, 1996, Mosby.)

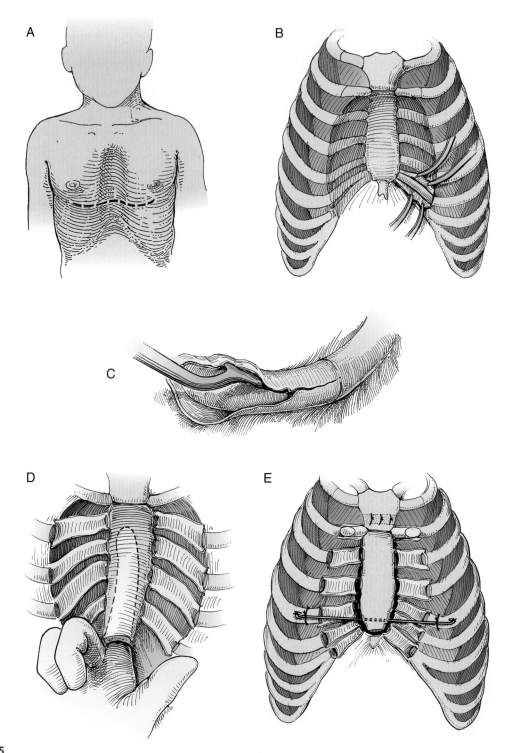

FIGURE 29-25
Repair of pectus excavatum or pectus carinatum. **A,** Location of transverse submammary incision. **B,** The pectoralis muscles are elevated from the thoracic wall. **C,** The perichondrium of each deformed cartilage is elevated, and the cartilage is removed. **D,** The sternum is fractured through the anterior table, to be mobilized anteriorly. **E,** K-wires or a metal strut is inserted to stabilize the new position of the sternum. (Modified from Waldhausen JA, Pierce WS, and Campbell DB: *Surgery of the chest*, ed 6, St Louis, 1996, Mosby.)

thorax. This syndrome also has been called *cervical rib syndrome, first thoracic rib syndrome, costoclavicular syndrome,* and *hyperabduction syndrome.* The various names given to thoracic outlet syndrome generally refer to the compression of the neurovascular structures to the upper extremities. The surgical goal is to release the compression of the neurovascular tissue and restore neurovascular function to the affected upper extremity, neck, or shoulder.

Technique

1. The patient is placed in the lateral position with the arm abducted 90 degrees and attached to an ether screen or an IV pole; occasionally an assistant holds the arm.
2. The patient's arm, neck, and upper chest are prepped.
3. The surgeon makes a transaxillary incision between the pectoralis muscle and the latissimus dorsi muscle on the affected side.
4. Dissection is carried out to the level of the cervical rib (if present) or the first rib.
5. The mid-portion of the rib is removed with a periosteal elevator, followed by removal of the anterior and posterior sections of the rib.
6. A drain is placed.
7. The incision is closed.

DISCUSSION

The orifice of the thoracic outlet is formed by the first ribs, the spine, and the sternum. Thoracic outlet syndrome occurs when the brachial plexus and the subclavian vein or artery are compressed as they pass from the neck into the upper extremity (in the region between the thoracic outlet and the insertion of the pectoralis minor muscle).

Compressing structures may include the first rib and the clavicle, the pectoralis minor tendon, and, less often, the cervical rib. Cervical ribs are rare anatomically, occurring in approximately 1% of the population (Harding and Silver, 1991); they usually are bilateral. When present, they are removed during the procedure, which often includes removal of the first rib.

Complete rib resection is necessary to prevent recurrent symptoms. Soft-tissue dissection instruments as well as rib cutters, elevators, and rongeurs are added to the instruments.

Thoracoscopy: Lung Biopsy (Video-Assisted Thoracoscopic Surgery)
SURGICAL GOAL

In this procedure, a small portion of lung tissue is removed for pathological examination.

PATHOLOGY

Lung biopsy is performed most often when other diagnostic tests such as CT scan, bronchoscopy, and x-ray do not reveal the cause of lung disease or when a lesion indicates the possibility of cancer, tuberculosis, sarcoidosis, or pulmonary fibrosis.

Technique

1. The surgeon makes a 2-mm intercostal incision between the ribs.

2. A 10-mm or 12-mm trocar is inserted.
3. A 0-degree telescope is inserted.
4. One or more additional trocar sites are incised for instrumentation.
5. A small section of lung is removed.
6. The edges of the divided lung tissue are checked for hemostasis and the absence of an air leak.
7. A chest tube is inserted through one puncture site.
8. The wounds are closed.

DISCUSSION

The patient is placed in the lateral position, prepped, and draped for a thoracostomy. A 2-mm skin incision is made, and a 12-mm port is created. A 10-mm thoracic telescope is introduced, and two additional trocars are introduced through incisions. The sites are based on CT scan and x-ray findings.

A small sponge forceps is inserted through one of the instrument ports, and a 30-mm endoscopic linear stapler is introduced through the other port. The instruments can interfere with each other if they overlap (called "fencing"). The biopsy specimen is removed with a surgical cutting and stapling device. An additional specimen may be removed.

A **wedge resection** is a large tissue biopsy or the removal of a small peripheral lesion. These are commonly removed with the linear surgical stapler during thoracoscopy.

The surgeon carefully inspects the suture line for air leaks by filling the chest cavity with warm saline solution. The anesthesia care provider than inflates the lung and observes the suture line for bubbles. The surgeon or assistant suctions the solution, and more sutures are placed as needed.

The instruments are withdrawn, and a chest tube is inserted into the lower incision. The wounds are sutured with synthetic absorbable suture and skin staples.

This procedure is illustrated in Figure 29-26.

NOTE: If a small open incision is necessary for biopsy, the procedure is performed as described, with the linear stapler. A chest tube is inserted, and the wound is closed with synthetic absorbable sutures and skin staples.

Lobectomy
SURGICAL GOAL

In this procedure, a lobe is surgically removed to prevent the spread of metastatic cancer or to treat a benign tumor.

PATHOLOGY

A lobectomy may be performed to treat many types of lung disease, including resectable tumor, benign tumor, and sarcoidosis, or to remove tissue that has been traumatized.

Technique

1. A thoracotomy is performed.
2. The hilum of the lobe is identified, and individual arteries and veins are divided.
3. The bronchus is mobilized and separated from the hilum.
4. The lobe is removed.

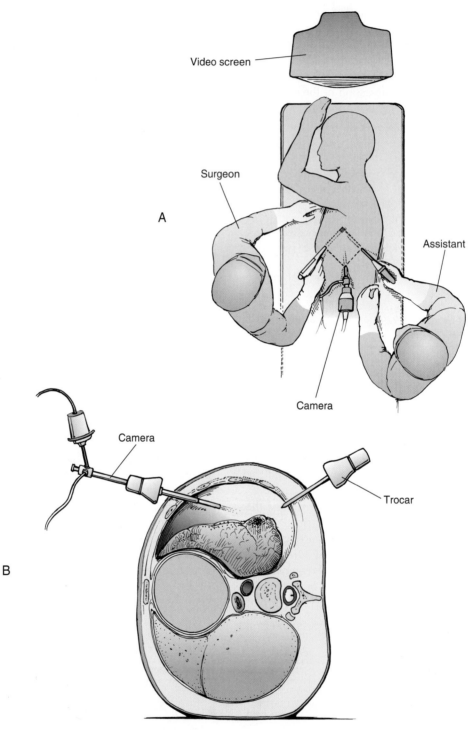

FIGURE 29-26
Thoracoscopy: lung biopsy (video-assisted thoracoscopic surgery; VATS). **A,** Diamond for trocar placement. **B,** The thoracoscope is inserted, and the pleural space is inspected.

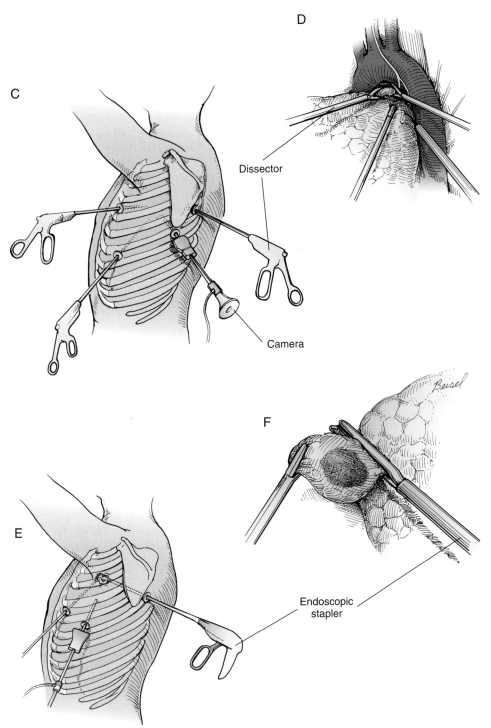

FIGURE 29-26, cont'd
Thoracoscopy: lung biopsy (video-assisted thoracoscopic surgery; VATS). **C,** Insertion sites for endoscopic dissectors, forceps, and scissors. **D,** Location and isolation of tissue for biopsy. **E,** Insertion of an endoscopic stapler for wedge resection or lung biopsy. **F,** Removal of lesion with the endoscopic linear stapler. (Modified from Waldhausen JA, Pierce WS, and Campbell DB: *Surgery of the chest,* ed 6, St Louis, 1996, Mosby.)

5. The suture line is tested for leaks, and extra sutures are placed as needed.
6. The bronchial stump is covered with pleura.
7. Chest tubes are inserted and the incision(s) are closed.

DISCUSSION

Lobectomy may be performed as a VATS procedure or an open procedure. The principles and anatomical divisions are the same for open and closed procedures. If a thoracoscopy is planned, instruments for converting to an open procedure must be available.

The patient is placed in the lateral position and prepped and draped for a thoracotomy incision.

A posterolateral thoracotomy is performed. The surgeon examines the entire lung and mediastinum closely to make certain that there is no evidence of disease beyond that previously diagnosed. The lobe is then retracted with lung-grasping forceps, and the peritoneal covering over the hilum is incised. The pulmonary artery and vein are dissected free at the hilum. Sponge dissectors are used to aid in separating the vessels from the connective tissue around the hilum.

The vessels and bronchus may be encircled with a vascular loop for retraction. Individual vessels are mobilized with scissors and clamped with right-angle clamps. Silk ties of size 2-0 are used for ligation.

The surgeon uses a bronchus clamp to occlude the bronchus. Suction is very important while the bronchus is open to prevent blood or fluid from draining into the opposite lung. The scrub may be needed to manage the suction while the surgeons transect and suture the bronchus. Interrupted sutures of 3-0 silk, 4-0 synthetic absorbable suture, or a linear stapler are used to occlude the proximal bronchus, which is then divided with the knife.

When all vessels and the bronchus have been occluded, the lobe can be removed. The surgeon covers the bronchial stump with the pleura, using interrupted sutures of size 3-0 polyethylene. The wound is irrigated, and the lung is inflated to check for leaks. A chest tube is inserted, and the wound is closed in layers.

Lobectomy is illustrated in Figure 29-27.

Thoracoplasty

Classic thoracoplasty for inflammatory pulmonary disease (notably tuberculosis) no longer is considered appropriate treatment since the development of effective medical treatment with antituberculosis medications. Thoracoplasty includes the removal of usually three to four ribs from the chest wall; in the past the procedure often led to serious complications, such as the formation of scoliosis, limited shoulder motion, and paradoxical motion of the lung.

A more recent form of thoracoplasty involves the transfer of one or more bulky chest-wall muscles to repair the pleural defect after lobectomy or to fill the space left after sternectomy for mediastinitis. The muscular tissue flaps may include the pectoralis major, the rectus abdominis, or the latissimus dorsi muscles.

Pneumonectomy
SURGICAL GOAL

Pneumonectomy is the removal of an entire lung to debulk (reduce the size) of a malignant tumor and slow the spread of cancer. Extensive abscess or bronchiectasis also may be treated by pneumonectomy.

PATHOLOGY

Removal of a lung reduces the size of a tumor and slows the spread of the disease. Extensive or chronic abscess may result in extensive pulmonary damage requiring drainage and lobectomy. Bronchiectasis is chronic dilation of the bronchi as a result of infection, pulmonary obstruction, tuberculosis, or chronic bronchitis.

Technique

1. The surgeon performs a thoracotomy.
2. The mediastinal pleura is incised.
3. The major vessels (bronchus, pulmonary artery, and superior and inferior pulmonary veins) are divided.
4. The vagus, phrenic, and recurrent laryngeal nerves are identified.
5. Regional lymph nodes are dissected.
6. The bronchus is divided and closed.
7. The lung is removed, and the wound is closed.

DISCUSSION

The patient is placed in the lateral position, and a thoracotomy is performed. The entire lung and surrounding tissues are examined closely to evaluate the extent of the disease. The lung is retracted with nonmalleable or malleable retractors or Duval lung forceps to expose the mediastinal pleura. The surgeon incises the mediastinal pleura using scissors and smooth tissue forceps. Blunt dissection is carried out with a sponge dissector along the edge of the parietal pleura.

Dissection is carried to the hilum of the diseased lobe. The surgeon isolates the major structures connected to the lung. These include the bronchus, pulmonary artery, and pulmonary vein. The pulmonary artery and vein are carefully separated, clamped with right-angle vascular clamps, and divided. Heavy silk sutures are used to ligate the vessels. The vagus, recurrent laryngeal (left side only), and phrenic nerves pass close to these vessels. To protect these nerves from injury, they are isolated with vessel loops or moist umbilical tapes. The assistant then may retract them. The pulmonary artery is then clamped, divided, and ligated. The surgeon may oversew the cut edges of the artery with a fine suture such as 4-0 or 5-0 silk or polypropylene. The superior and inferior veins are ligated and divided in similar fashion. Ligation clips may be used for smaller vessels.

The bronchus is commonly occluded with a Sarot clamp and divided with the knife. The lung is then removed from

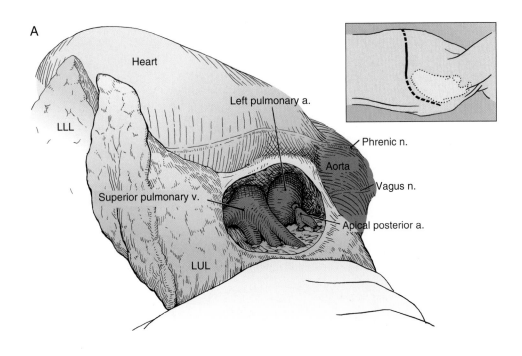

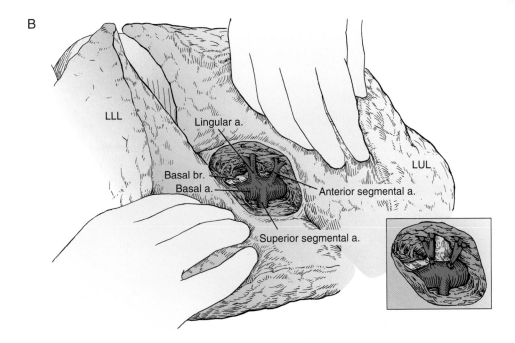

FIGURE 29-27

Lobectomy. **A,** The left main pulmonary artery is identified and followed distally to the first upper lobe branch. **B,** The fissure is divided between the upper and lower lobes and is opened to allow division of the arteries to the anterior and lingular segments.

Continued

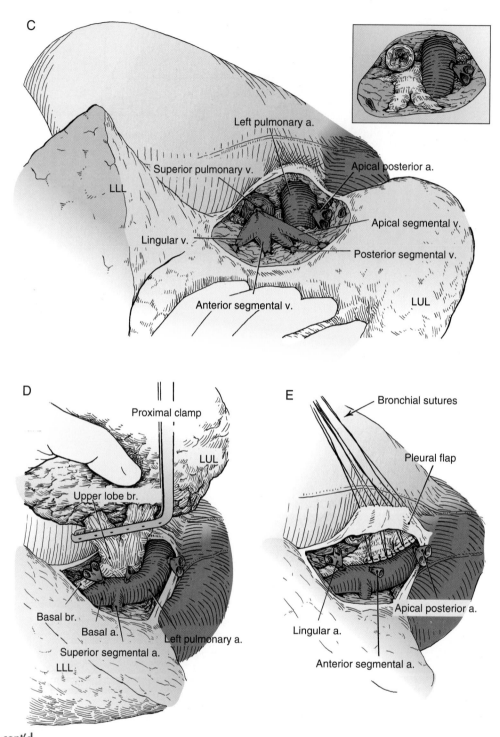

FIGURE 29-27, cont'd
Lobectomy. **C,** Dissection of the superior pulmonary vein. **D,** Placement of the proximal bronchus clamp 1.5 to 2 cm from main bronchial trunk. **E,** Closure of the upper lobe bronchus with fine synthetic absorbable sutures. (Modified from Waldhausen JA, Pierce WS, and Campbell DB: *Surgery of the chest,* ed 6, St Louis, 1996, Mosby.)

the wound. The surgeon closes the open end of the bronchus using interrupted sutures, such as size 3-0 polypropylene sutures, or the stapler. The scrub may manage the suction while the bronchus is being closed. The bronchus is then divided, and the lung is removed from the wound.

The wound is irrigated with warm saline, and any leaks are identified and repaired. The pleura is sutured over the bronchus. Bleeders are coagulated with the ESU. Often two chest tubes are inserted and brought out through stab wounds adjacent to the incision. These are secured with heavy silk sutures. The upper mediastinal pleura is

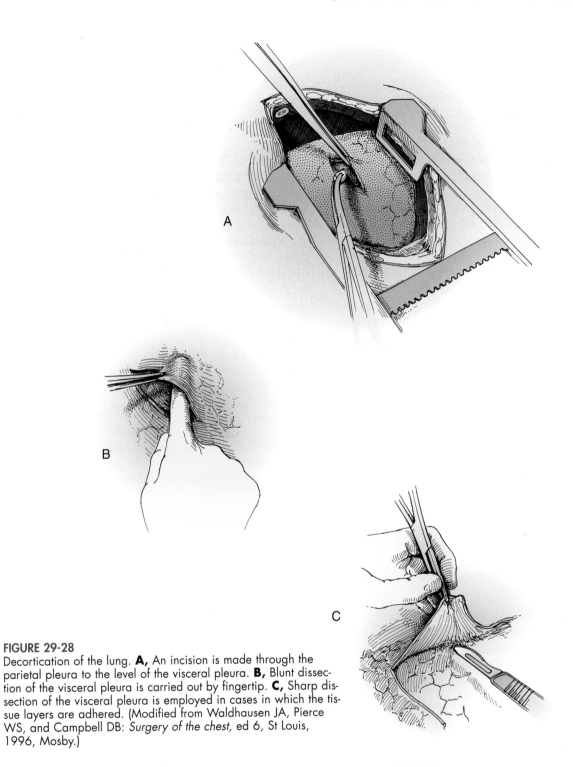

FIGURE 29-28
Decortication of the lung. **A,** An incision is made through the parietal pleura to the level of the visceral pleura. **B,** Blunt dissection of the visceral pleura is carried out by fingertip. **C,** Sharp dissection of the visceral pleura is employed in cases in which the tissue layers are adhered. (Modified from Waldhausen JA, Pierce WS, and Campbell DB: *Surgery of the chest,* ed 6, St Louis, 1996, Mosby.)

closed with absorbable suture, and the wound is closed in layers.

Decortication of the Lung
SURGICAL GOAL
Decortication of the lung is the surgical removal of the fibrin layer of the lung, which covers the visceral and parietal pleura, and that is preventing complete expansion of the lung (Figure 29-28).

Technique

1. The patient usually is placed in a posterolateral thoracotomy position.
2. An incision is made in the fifth intercostal space.
3. Clotted blood is removed.
4. Adhesions below the parietal and visceral pleura are sharply divided.
5. When the visceral pleura is reached, the dissection is continued alternately with a gauze pledget ("sponge stick") or

the fingertip until the fibrotic covering is removed sufficiently to allow full expansion of the lung.

6. Drainage tubes are inserted.
7. The incision is closed.

DISCUSSION

The fibrinous exudates that form over the visceral pleura can result from pus in the pleural cavity (a complication of pneumonia), trauma, lung abscesses, foreign bodies in the bronchial tree, or other factors that lead to chronic inflammation and the subsequent development of scar tissue.

Thoracic instrumentation is used. Culture tubes often are required for tissue samples. After the thoracic incision has been made, the skin, subcutaneous tissue, and muscle are dissected with scissors and electrocautery. A rib spreader is inserted to expose the affected portion of the lung(s). A portion of the fifth or sixth rib may be resected with rib shears. Both sharp and blunt dissection are performed. Empyema or other fluid is drained and cultured. The anesthesia provider expands the lung intermittently to demonstrate areas requiring additional decortication. After sufficient dissection and removal of the scar tissue, drainage tubes are inserted, and the incision is closed.

Lung Volume Reduction
SURGICAL GOAL

Patients with chronic pulmonary emphysema may benefit from resection of portions of a lung in which air is trapped in emphysematous lung tissue. Lung function, exercise capacity, and respiratory muscle strength are improved postoperatively.

Technique

1. The surgeon makes a transverse anterior thoracotomy, sternotomy, or lateral thoracotomy incision; a sternal saw is used to split the sternum.
2. Adhesions are sharply dissected.
3. The lungs are deflated to identify areas of trapped air.
4. The surgeon uses lung clamps to grasp the portion of the lung to be excised and applies surgical stapling devices lined with bovine pericardium to each side of the lung tissue to be excised.
5. The lung is inspected to identify residual air leaks; these are closed.
6. Chest tubes are placed in each pleural space.
7. The ribs and sternum are closed with wire.
8. The remaining incision is closed in layers.

DISCUSSION

Lung volume reduction surgery (LVRS) is useful for patients with chronic pulmonary emphysema who have targeted areas of severity (versus global air entrapment). Depending on the location of the areas to be resected and reduced, the surgeon will select the appropriate position for the patient.

To inspect the lung, the surgeon has the anesthesia provider inflate and deflate areas of the pulmonary tissue.

Stapling devices are commonly used. Placing a strip of bovine pericardium on each side of the lung tissue to be stapled and resected minimizes residual air leaks (and the need for multiple staples to seal the leak). Bovine pericardium must be rinsed to remove the preservative solution, so basins and sterile normal saline to rinse the bovine tissue must be available.

Lung Transplantation
SURGICAL GOAL

Lung transplantation of one or both lungs is performed to remove a diseased, poorly functioning lung (or lungs) and replace it with an optimally functioning lung procured from an organ donor. In part because of the severe shortage of donor organs, single-lung transplantation is increasingly employed as a way to maximize the allocation of donor lung organs. In patients whose right and left lungs both are diseased (with cystic fibrosis or chronic infection), bilateral transplantation is indicated.

Technique   LUNG PROCUREMENT

1. The donor is prepped from chin to knees. (The donor can be living or deceased.)
2. A median sternotomy is performed; occasionally a thoracotomy is performed.
3. A sternal (or rib) retractor is inserted.
4. The pleura are opened longitudinally, and the pericardium is divided.
5. Umbilical tapes are placed around the aorta and the superior and inferior venae cavae.
6. Pleural adhesions are divided, and the proximal pulmonary arteries are dissected.
7. Heparin is given.
8. The superior vena cava is ligated with heavy silk ties.
9. The aortic arch is dissected free, and the ligamentum arteriosum (the remnant ductus arteriosus) is divided.
10. The pulmonary artery is encircled with an umbilical tape and separated from the ascending aorta.
11. Cardioplegia solution is infused through the proximal aorta into the heart via the coronary arteries; pulmoplegia solution is infused into the pulmonary organs.
12. Cardiac veins and arteries are separated, and the heart is removed and placed in a cold preservative solution.
13. The pulmonary arteries are separated from the mediastinum.
14. The trachea is dissected free.
15. The lungs are inflated and then stapled and removed.
16. The lungs are placed in a cold preservative solution.

DISCUSSION

Both single-lung and double-lung transplantation are indicated for patients with restrictive lung disease, emphysema, pulmonary hypertension, and other noninfectious end-stage pulmonary diseases. Single-lung transplantation has increased the availability of donor organs and is widely used.

The donor patient is placed supine because this position allows the best exposure of the various organs to be excised. The procurement of lung tissue (and other organs) is a very precise procedure that requires knowledge of protocols and procedures, and problem-solving abilities. Procurement teams generally must be self-sufficient and not assume that the facility that will host the procurement has all the supplies that the procurement team needs. Thus the team must have a sternal saw (battery-powered saws are recommended), the basic thoracic and/or cardiac instruments, and the supplies (such as cold preservative solutions and sterile containers for the organs).

Speed is usually important because many organs have a limited period of viability. If the technologist has any questions (as either a member of the procurement team coming from the recipient hospital, or as a member of the team from the donor hospital), he or she should not hesitate to ask for clarification. Organ transplantation is a team effort, and all members of the staff play a role in a successful transplantation outcome.

Technique   SINGLE-LUNG IMPLANTATION

1. The patient is placed laterally with the lung-procedure side up and prepped from chin to knees.
2. A thoracotomy incision is made, and a retractor is inserted.
3. If the recipient's right lung is to be removed, the pulmonary vein, pulmonary artery, and azygous vein are isolated and divided.
4. If the recipient's left lung is to be removed, the ligamentum arteriosum is divided.
5. The lung to be removed is collapsed, and the proximal pulmonary artery is occluded. If there is hemodynamic instability, femoral-femoral bypass may be instituted.
6. The lung is removed.
7. The pulmonary veins are divided, and branches of the pulmonary artery are separated.
8. The bronchus is divided, and the diseased lung is removed.
9. The bronchus-to-bronchus anastomosis is performed with a 3-0 absorbable suture.
10. The pulmonary-artery-to-pulmonary-artery anastomosis is performed with a running 4-0 polypropylene suture.
11. The recipient pulmonary veins are attached to the donor atrial cuff with a running 4-0 polypropylene suture.
12. The new lung is inflated and inspected.
13. Chest tubes are inserted, and hemostasis achieved.
14. The chest is closed.
15. Bronchoscopy may be employed to suction secretions and confirm an intact anastomosis.

DISCUSSION

The recipient patient for single-lung transplantation is placed laterally with the affected side up. A double-lumen endotracheal tube is inserted to inflate either lung selectively. Generally the groin is prepped and exposed in case a femoral-femoral bypass is required. With single-lung transplantation, thoracotomy instruments are used; cardiopulmonary bypass instruments and supplies should be available in the operating room in case bypass is required. The choice of suture materials varies with each surgeon;

the description above may be different in other institutions.

The incidence of bronchial anastomotic complications has been reduced through a variety of techniques. These techniques may be used during the procedure and include shortening the donor bronchial stump, wrapping the anastomosis with omentum or an intercostal muscle pedicle, or employing an intussuscepting (e.g., telescoping) bronchial anastomosis technique.

Technique   DOUBLE-LUNG TRANSPLANTATION

1. The patient is placed in the supine position and prepped from chin to knees. The arms are placed above the head and supported with an ether screen or similar device.
2. The surgeon makes a bilateral anterior thoracotomy ("clam shell") incision.
3. If bilateral sequential transplantation is to be performed, the first lung is inserted as described above; the process is repeated on the opposite side for the second lung. This often avoids the need for cardiopulmonary bypass.
4. If a bilateral en-bloc procedure is to be performed (both donor lungs are removed and implanted as one unit), cardiopulmonary bypass usually is required.
5. Bibronchial, pulmonary artery, and atrial anastomoses are performed as described for single-lung procedures.
6. The procedure is completed as described above.

DISCUSSION

Bilateral lung procedures often require cardiopulmonary support. Bypass may be avoided with the bilateral sequential technique, in which the more diseased native lung is removed first and the other lung is capable of maintaining adequate oxygenation. Femoral cannulation supplies should be readily available.

Diaphragmatic Hernia
SURGICAL GOAL

A congenital diaphragmatic hernia is a weakness in the diaphragm that allows abdominal organs (such as the small and large intestines, stomach, spleen, and liver) to enter the thoracic cavity. Surgery is performed to return the abdominal contents to their appropriate location in the abdomen and to reduce the respiratory impairment that accompanies diaphragmatic hernias.

Technique

1. Extracorporeal cardiopulmonary support may be required if conventional ventilation cannot prevent respiratory failure.
2. The surgeon makes an abdominal incision. In some cases, a subcostal incision (or low thoracotomy) is made.
3. The retroperitoneal posterior rim of the diaphragm is mobilized from the periosteal attachments.
4. The abdominal contents that have moved into the thorax are returned to the abdominal cavity.

5. The anterior and posterior rims of the diaphragmatic tissue are approximated with nonabsorbable mattress sutures. Reinforcing pledgets may be used; a prosthetic patch may be used for large defects.
6. A chest tube may be inserted for drainage.
7. The incision is closed.

DISCUSSION

The diaphragm is the primary muscle of inspiration and separates the thoracic organs from the abdominal organs. Weaknesses in the diaphragmatic muscle allow abdominal organs to protrude into the thoracic cavity, with subsequent respiratory and cardiac impairments. The most common location of a diaphragmatic hernia is in the posterolateral foramen of Bochdalek.

If cardiopulmonary support is required to support respiratory function, the surgeon may institute **extracorporeal membrane oxygenation (ECMO)** support a few days before the repair of the surgical hernia. A cannula is inserted into the right internal jugular vein. Venous blood returning to the heart is diverted into this cannula and enters the oxygenator, where gas exchange occurs (e.g., carbon dioxide is removed and oxygen is added to the blood). The freshly oxygenated blood then is pumped back into the systemic circulation through a cannula inserted into the right or left internal carotid artery.

The procedure is performed under general anesthesia. The patient is placed in the supine position, and the anterior chest and abdomen are prepped and draped. The decision to make an abdominal or a thoracic incision is based on the location of the hernia and the position of the affected organs. The diaphragm is dissected from its attachments, and the organs are identified. The abdominal organs are identified, inspected, and gently returned to the abdominal cavity. The surgeon looks for a hernia sac (rarely found); if a hernia sac is found, it is excised. The diaphragmatic muscle is repaired with 2-0 or 3-0 nonabsorbable mattress sutures to prevent future migration of abdominal tissue into the chest cavity. If there is too much abdominal tissue to fit into the abdominal cavity, the muscle may be left open and the skin closed over the organs (to create a ventral hernia). The ventral hernia is repaired after the patient spends a few days on ECMO support.

This procedure is illustrated in Figure 29-29.

Thymectomy
SURGICAL GOAL

Excision of the thymus is commonly performed for malignant tumors and occasionally for myasthenia gravis.

Technique

1. The surgeon makes a median sternotomy to expose the thymus.
2. A sternal retractor is inserted.
3. The thymus is separated from the pericardium and the mediastinal pleura by blunt and sharp dissection.

4. The phrenic nerves are identified and preserved.
5. Hemostasis is achieved.
6. A closed suction drain is inserted.
7. The incision is closed.

DISCUSSION

The thymus is a bilobed structure that is joined in the midline. The thymus receives its blood supply from branches of the internal thoracic artery; venous blood drains into the innominate vein (Figure 29-30).

The patient is placed in the supine position, and the anterior chest is prepped and draped. Median sternotomy is performed with a sternal saw; a sternal retractor is inserted. Thymal blood vessels are clamped, divided, and ligated. The gland is removed, and hemostasis is achieved. Frozen-section studies may be performed on suspected malignant tissue to ensure that adequate clean (nonmalignant) margins have been attained. A mediastinal drain is inserted, and the sternum is reapproximated with sternal wire in the adult. Heavy nonabsorbable sutures may be used in young patients.

Closure of Patent Ductus Arteriosus
SURGICAL GOAL

Surgical closure of a patent ductus arteriosus is performed to prevent arterial blood from recirculating through the lungs. The ductus may be approached via an open incision or via the endoscopic route.

Nonsurgical closure of the ductus increasingly is achieved in the neonatal intensive care unit with the use of indomethacin (Indocin), a medication that constricts ductal tissue. Ductal occluder devices also may be used; these are inserted in the cardiac catheterization suite.

PATHOLOGY

A patent ductus arteriosus is a persistent fetal communication between the pulmonary artery and the descending thoracic aorta. During fetal development, blood is pumped from the right ventricle into the systemic circulation by way of the ductus. The lungs are largely bypassed and remain unexpanded. At birth, the lungs expand and the ductus closes spontaneously within a relatively short time. If the ductus fails to close, arterial blood returns to the lungs, causing an added burden on the lungs and heart. The heart becomes enlarged and may fail. The ductus is surgically closed to correct this defect, most often while the patient is in infancy.

Technique

1. The surgeon performs a left thoracotomy.
2. The mediastinal pleura is incised.
3. The ductus is isolated.
4. The ductus is closed.
5. A chest tube is inserted, and the chest is closed.

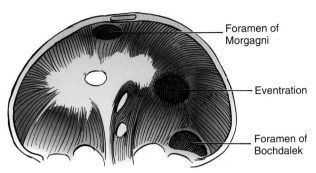

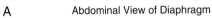

A   Abdominal View of Diaphragm

FIGURE 29-29
Sites of congenital diaphragmatic hernias. **A,** Abdominal view of the diaphragm. The most common congenital hernia is a defect in the posterolateral foramen of Bochdalek. **B,** Extracorporeal membrane oxygenation (ECMO) support is instituted before repair of the diaphragmatic defect. **C,** Location of incision site. **D,** The intraabdominal organs are reduced out of the chest. (Modified from Waldhausen JA, Pierce WS, and Campbell DB: *Surgery of the chest,* ed 6, St Louis, 1996, Mosby.)

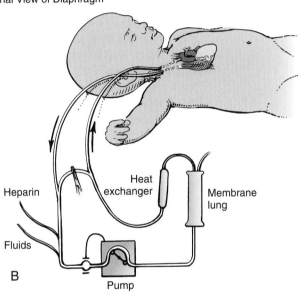

B

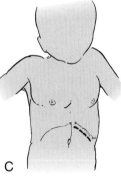

C

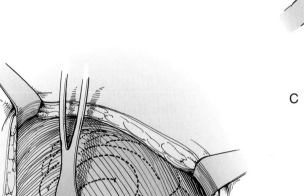

D

A

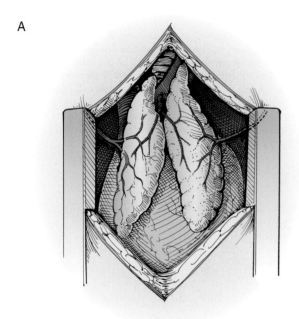

B

Short vein
from thymus

Thymic
tissue

Innominate
vein

FIGURE 29-30
Thymectomy. **A,** Anterior thymectomy. The thymus is separated from the pericardium and mediastinal pleura, preserving the phrenic veins. **B,** Cervical thymectomy. The thymus is removed through a transverse suprasternal incision. (Modified from Waldhausen JA, Pierce WS, and Campbell DB: *Surgery of the chest,* ed 6, St Louis, 1996, Mosby.)

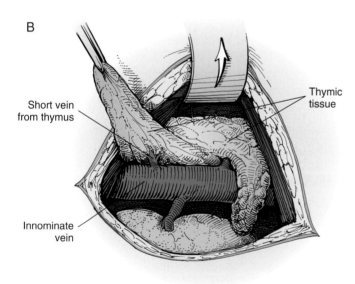

DISCUSSION

The patient is placed in the supine position, prepped, and draped for a thoracotomy. This procedure increasingly is performed endoscopically.

A thoracotomy is performed as previously described. To begin the repair, the surgeon places a traction suture through the edges of the pleura. Size 3-0 silk usually is used. The ends are tagged with a hemostat. The assistant retracts the pleura with the suture. The surgeon then carefully dissects the aorta and pulmonary artery with fine dissecting

scissors to expose the ductus. The surgeon is careful to distinguish between the aorta and the ductus (which may be as large as or larger than the aorta). A heavy silk suture may be passed around the ductus.

The surgeon continues the dissection until the ductus is fully isolated. The surgeon differentiates between the ductus and the aorta. In some cases, the ductus can be larger than the aorta. Straight or slightly angled vascular clamps are placed across the ductus, one close to the aorta and the other close to the pulmonary artery. In the newborn or small infant, the surgeon may simply tie the ductus with size 0 silk because the ductus is small and may not allow placement of the vascular clamps. Vascular clips also may be used.

In other situations, the surgeon may divide and oversew the cut edges. The surgeon cuts halfway through the ductus using Potts scissors or a knife. A size 5-0 or 6-0 polypropylene suture is used to begin the closure of the ductus on the aortic side. The surgeon continues to incise the ductus and continues the suture to close the defect on the aortic side. The vascular clamp then is slowly released. Additional sutures are placed if needed. The end of the ductus closest to the pulmonary artery is sutured in the same manner. Vascular clips may be used instead of sutures. Hemostasis at the suture line may be maintained with a topical hemostatic agent.

The mediastinal pleura is closed with a continuous suture of size 3-0 or 4-0 silk or chromic gut. An appropriate size chest tube is inserted, and the wound is closed in layers. Some surgeons remove the chest tube after the skin incision is closed.

Highlights of this procedure are illustrated in Figure 29-31.

Correction of Coarctation of the Thoracic Aorta
SURGICAL GOAL
Correction of a coarctation is performed to restore blood flow to the lower body and reduce stress on the heart.

PATHOLOGY
Coarctation of the thoracic aorta is a congenital **stenosis** (narrowing), usually occurring near the junction of the fetal ductus arteriosus and the aorta. Severe narrowing obstructs the normal flow of blood through the thoracic aorta and to the lower body. The heart becomes enlarged because of the burden of pumping blood through a stricture. The lower body may be underdeveloped as a result of the defect.

Technique
1. A thoracotomy is performed.
2. The mediastinal pleura is incised.
3. The ligamentum arteriosum is ligated and divided.
4. The aorta is occluded proximal and distal to the coarctation.
5. The aorta is transected and reanastomosed, or a prosthetic graft is inserted.
6. The aorta is unclamped.
7. The wound is closed.

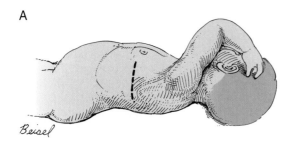

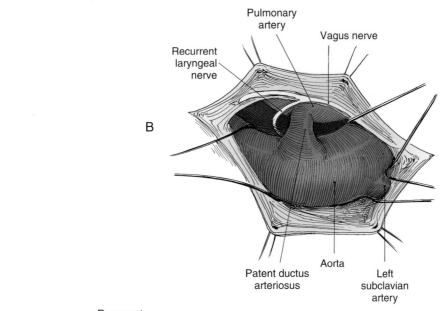

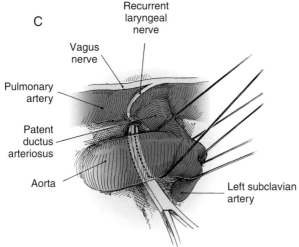

FIGURE 29-31

Closure of patent ductus arteriosus. **A,** Incision site at the fourth intercostal space. **B,** Dissection is carried to the patent ductus arteriosus, then across the ductus toward the pulmonary artery. **C,** Dissection of the posterior wall of the ductus is performed.

Continued

DISCUSSION

The patient is commonly placed in the lateral position, prepped, and draped for a thoracotomy. The thoracic cavity is entered through a posterolateral thoracotomy. A moist laparotomy sponge is placed over the lung, which is retracted by the assistant. The surgeon incises the mediastinal pleura and places traction sutures of size 3-0 or 4-0 silk in the edges.

This exposes the aorta. A moist umbilical tape is placed around the aorta for mobilization and retraction.

The intercostal arteries are mobilized. Fine dissecting scissors are used to dissect the aorta in the area of the coarctation.

The surgeon ligates and divides the ductus (a ductus that has closed naturally is called the *ligamentum arteriosum*) to

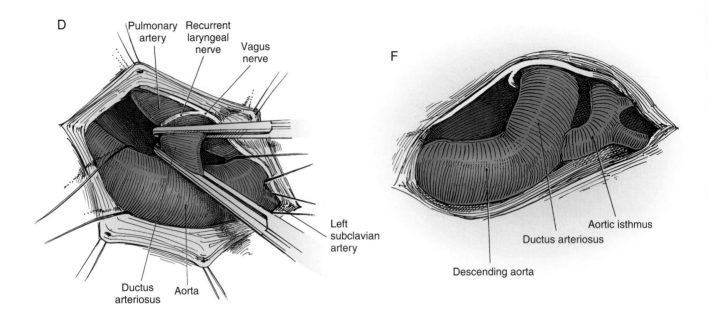

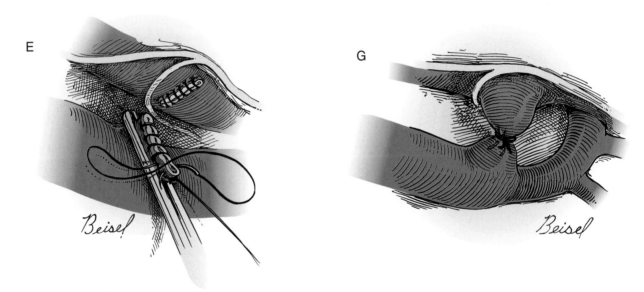

FIGURE 29-31, cont'd
Closure of patent ductus arteriosus. **D,** Ductus clamps are applied, and the ductus is divided. **E,** Each end of the ductus is closed with a running mattress suture followed by an over-and-over suture of 6-0 Prolene. **F,** Ligation technique in the newborn. Enlargement of the ductus to the size of the descending aorta, whereas the aortic isthmus is smaller. **G,** Placement of a no. 1 silk ligature around the ductus to occlude the lumen. (Modified from Waldhausen JA, Pierce WS, and Campbell DB: *Surgery of the chest,* ed 6, St Louis, 1996, Mosby.)

free the aorta and prevent bleeding from the ductus or ligamentum if it is still patent. Additional sutures of size 4-0 silk are placed in the ductus if needed.

The surgeon occludes the aorta proximal and distal to the coarctation with straight or angled vascular clamps. The arteries that supply the coarctated segment also are ligated, and bulldog clamps may be placed on other vessels that lie between the coarctated segment and the cross-clamps of the aorta. The aorta is then transected, and the stricture is removed.

The two ends of the aorta then are anastomosed with a continuous suture of size 5-0 or 6-0 for the pediatric patient.

Interrupted sutures often are used in the pediatric patient to allow growth. In adults, a size 3-0 or 4-0 polypropylene suture is used. If the two limbs of the aorta cannot be brought together easily (often the case in adults), a synthetic tube graft may be inserted or a proximal portion of the left subclavian artery may be used to form a patch. In this technique, a part of the artery wall is swung around and anastomosed to the resected coarctation. The distal artery then is ligated.

The surgeon removes all clamps from the aorta and intercostal arteries. Blood flow to the lower body is restored. The surgeon inspects all suture lines for hemostasis, and ad-

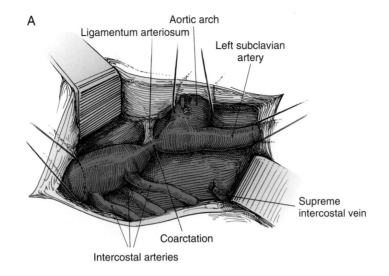

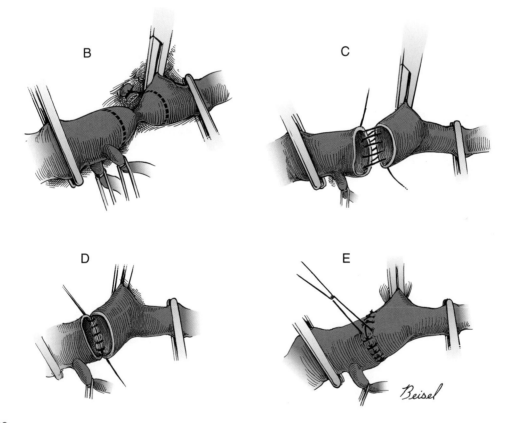

FIGURE 29-32
Correction of coarctation of the thoracic aorta. **A,** Dissection of tissue exposes the location of the coarctation. **B,** Arterial clamps are applied above and below the constriction. **C** and **D,** A continuous suture of absorbable monofilament is used. **E,** Closure of the anterior wall is completed with interrupted simple sutures or continuation of the continuous suture.

Continued

ditional sutures are placed as needed. Topical hemostatic agents may be applied to control bleeding.

The surgeon closes the mediastinal pleura with size 3-0 or 4-0 silk or chromic gut. A chest tube is inserted, and the wound is closed in layers.

Refer to Figure 29-32 for illustrations of this procedure.

Pericardiectomy
SURGICAL GOAL

Chronic inflammation of the pericardium can produce a fibrotic (and often calcified) coating over the heart that constricts the ventricles. Removal of the adherent scar tissue improves cardiac function.

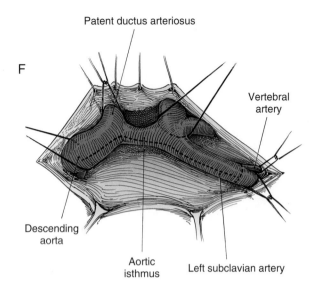

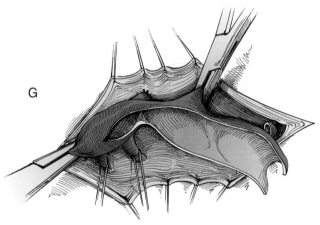

FIGURE 29-32, cont'd
Correction of coarctation of the thoracic aorta. **F,** Subclavian flap technique. The patent ductus arteriosus is ligated with a heavy silk ligature. The subclavian artery is ligated at the origin of the vertebral artery, which is also ligated. **G,** An incision is made in the aorta distal to the area of narrowing, and the incision is carried on the lateral side through the area of coarctation into the isthmus and the left subclavian artery. (Modified from Waldhausen JA, Pierce WS, and Campbell DB: *Surgery of the chest*, ed 6, St Louis, 1996, Mosby.)

Technique

1. Median sternotomy is commonly performed, although bilateral thoracotomy with a transverse sternotomy may produce better exposure in cases with extensive scarring.
2. Removal of the fibrous tissue usually begins over the left ventricle between the parietal pericardium and the epicardium (visceral pericardium).
3. Both ventricles, atria, and venae cavae are decorticated until hemodynamic pressure demonstrates improved filling of

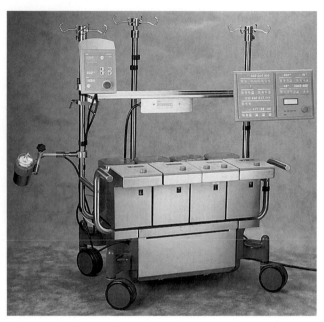

FIGURE 29-33
Cardiopulmonary bypass pump: Stöckert S III modular HLM with integrated centrifugal pump driver. (Courtesy Stöckert Instrumente, Gmbh, Munich; photo courtesy of US distributor: COBE CV, division of Sorin Biomedica, Arvada, Colo.)

the right and left ventricles and increased blood pressures.
4. Hemostasis is achieved.
5. Chest drainage tubes are inserted.
6. The sternum is reapproximated with wire.
7. The incision is closed.

DISCUSSION

Constrictive pericarditis may develop as a result of viral infection, tuberculosis, or chronic pericarditis. The heart becomes encased within an adherent layer of scar tissue.

The patient is placed in the supine position, and the anterior chest is prepped and draped. External defibrillator pads should be applied in anticipation of ventricular fibrillation resulting from manipulation of the heart during dissection. Median sternotomy is performed with a sternal saw. Dissection of the dense adhesions can cause increased bleeding; suture ligatures of 4-0 or 5-0 polypropylene or silk, on pledgets if desired, may be used. Cardiopulmonary bypass (below) often is available on a stand-by basis.

Basic sternotomy instruments are used in addition to lung retractors. An ultrasound debridement system occasionally is used for very dense calcification. Portions of adherent scar may be left in place if the risk of injury to underlying structures is great. Common examples are areas of the right and left coronary artery. Bilateral dissection is performed to the phrenic nerves (which are identified and preserved).

Cardiopulmonary Bypass
SURGICAL GOAL

Cardiopulmonary bypass is a method of perfusion and oxygenation of blood by temporarily diverting blood away from

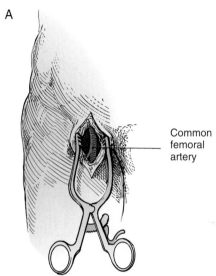

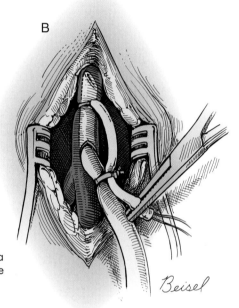

Common
femoral
artery

FIGURE 29-34
Femoral vein–femoral artery bypass. **A,** A Weitlaner retractor is used to expose the femoral vein and femoral artery. **B,** The cannula is inserted into the artery and secured with a tourniquet tied to the cannula; the process is repeated for the femoral vein. (Modified from Waldhausen JA, Pierce WS, and Campbell DB: *Surgery of the chest,* ed 6, St Louis, 1996, Mosby.)

the heart and lungs during surgery of the heart and major vessels through a pump oxygenator, allowing the surgeon to stop the heart and perform surgical procedures on it.

CONSIDERATIONS

Although an increasing number of cardiac procedures are performed without the use of cardiopulmonary bypass, many types of surgery, such as valve replacement and aneurysm repair, do require bypass.

To perform cardiopulmonary bypass, a special heart-lung pump is used to collect the blood, remove excess carbon dioxide, oxygenate the blood, and return it to the body (Figure 29-33). The pump tubing is connected to cannulae that are inserted into the venae cavae and ascending aorta through a median sternotomy incision. The femoral artery and femoral vein occasionally are used when the great vessels are not accessible because of disease.

Cardiopulmonary bypass may be total or partial. The surgeon performs total bypass by tightening umbilical tapes around the venae cavae and cannulae. This forces all blood returning to the right side of the heart into the cannula and thus to the pump. It also prevents air from entering the venous line and obstructing the flow of blood to the pump when the right side of the heart is opened, such as during repair of the tricuspid valve. Total bypass also is used for procedures such as mitral valve replacement, repair of septal defects, and resection of left ventricular aneurysm. In partial bypass, blood can escape around the cannula and enter the heart. Partial bypass often is used during aortic valve replacement. It also is used to support a patient in emergency situations such as cardiac arrest or ruptured aneurysm.

Figure 29-34 illustrates femoral vein–femoral artery bypass, and Figure 29-35 illustrates caval-aortic bypass.

HEART-LUNG MACHINE

The tubing and oxygenator for the heart-lung machine are assembled and primed by a perfusionist (pump technician).

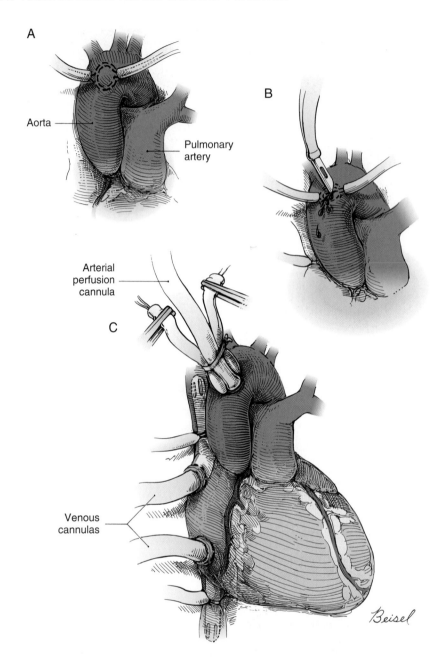

FIGURE 29-35
Caval-aortic bypass. **A,** Insertion site location is high into the ascending aorta. **B,** A purse-string suture is placed around the adventitia, and a stab wound is placed for insertion of the aortic cannula. **C,** The purse-string sutures are tightened to secure the aortic cannula with rubber keepers, which are held to the cannula with a heavy ligature. Venous cannulae are inserted through purse-string sutures into the upper and lower portions of the right atrium. (Modified from Waldhausen JA, Pierce WS, and Campbell DB: *Surgery of the chest,* ed 6, St Louis, 1996, Mosby.)

Before cannulation is performed, the surgical technologist should be familiar with the basic function and operation of the pump, the size of the pump lines, and how the lines connect to and from the patient.

The scrub must know which lines infuse blood and which lines remove blood because the introduction of air or particulate material into the infusing line can cause a stroke (cerebral infarction).

The scrub also should be familiar with the various types of cannulae and catheters, and know where they are used in the body. The cannulae and catheters discussed here are shown in Figure 29-36:

▶ *Venous* cannulae are straight ended with multiple holes in the distal tip and are used to drain the blood from the body. The two-stage venous cannula also contains openings in the mid-portion of the catheter.

▶ The *aortic* cannula may have a straight or an angled tip to direct the blood toward the descending thoracic aorta. This cannula carries oxygenated (arterial) blood.

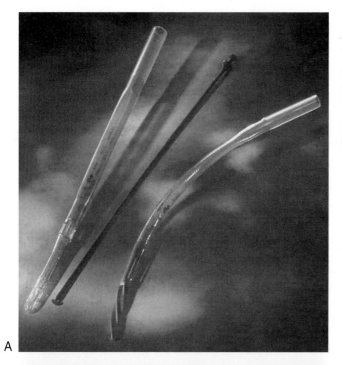

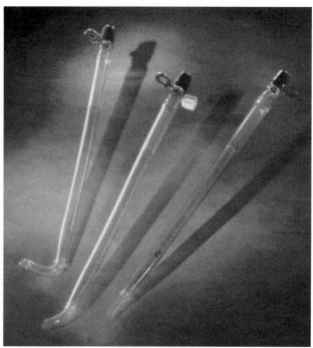

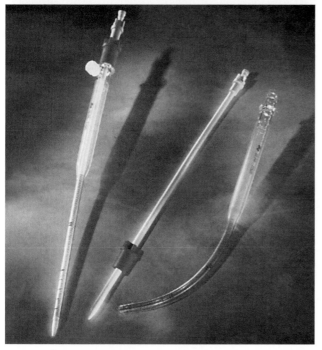

FIGURE 29-36
A, Venous cannulae. **B,** Aortic cannulae. **C,** Elongated arterial cannulae. (From Seifert PC: *Cardiac surgery: perioperative patient care,* St Louis, 2002, Mosby; courtesy Medtronic, Inc., Minneapolis, Minn.)

▶ The *femoral* cannula, which also carries oxygenated (arterial) blood, is tapered to match the size of the artery and has a beveled end to allow easier insertion.
▶ The *coronary perfusion* cannula has a cuff near its tip to prevent the cannula from being inserted too far into the coronary arteries, thus occluding or injuring the lumen of the artery. It is used to infuse cardioplegic solution directly into the heart.
▶ The *left ventricular sump (vent) catheter* drains air and blood within the heart, and prevents blood accumula-

tion, which can cause distension of the ventricle and injure the heart muscle.
▶ A *right superior pulmonary vent catheter* also is used to decompress the left ventricle.

In both types of bypass, blood returns to the pump through the cannula by gravity drainage and is pumped back into the circulation by the roller head (or a centrifugal pump) on the bypass machine. When the right side of the heart is opened and the patient is on bypass, there is a risk of air entering the venous line. This can cause an "air lock" (a large amount of air in the venous line). This can obstruct the flow of blood to the pump.

The vacuum created by the pump draws the air away from the heart and down into the pump.

The technologist must always watch for the presence of air in the heart or pump lines and alert the surgeon immediately if air is noticed.

Air must be removed immediately to prevent an air embolus. The technologist should have a needle and syringe readily available for this purpose. A 10-ml syringe with a 19-gauge needle can be used for both adult and pediatric patients.

Technique   CANNULATION OF THE AORTA

1. The surgeon places a purse-string suture on the anterior portion of the aorta and snares its ends through a tube tourniquet.
2. The aorta is incised.
3. The cannula is inserted and positioned.
4. The suture is tightened.
5. The cannula and tubing are tied together with heavy silk suture and sewn to the drape.
6. The cannula is allowed to fill to remove all air.
7. A tube-occluding clamp is placed across the cannula.
8. The cannula is connected to the arterial perfusion line from the pump, ensuring that there is no air in either the cannula or the arterial line.

DISCUSSION

A purse-string suture is placed on the anterior portion of the ascending aorta, and its ends are snared through a Rumel tourniquet. A stab incision is made into the aorta, and the incision is dilated with an aortic dilator or clamp. The surgeon controls bleeding by holding one finger over the hole as the cannula is inserted. The assistant controls the top end of the cannula, which is occluded by a tube-occluding clamp. The surgeon positions the cannula, and the assistant tightens the suture to form a tourniquet. The tourniquet then is tied to the cannula with heavy silk suture. The surgeon momentarily clamps and unclamps the cannula to allow it to fill with blood and remove the air. The cannula then is connected to the arterial perfusion line from the pump.

Technique   CANNULATION OF THE SUPERIOR AND INFERIOR VENAE CAVAE

1. A portion of the right atrial wall is clamped with a partial occlusion clamp.
2. A purse-string suture is placed in the occluded portion, and the ends are snared through a Rumel tourniquet.
3. The atrium is opened, and its walls are retracted.
4. As the clamp is opened, the cannula is inserted and the clamp is fully removed.
5. The cannula is introduced into the vena cava.
6. The purse-string is tightened around the cannula, and the suture ends are drawn tightly through the tubing, thus forming a tourniquet.

7. The cannula and tubing are tied together with a heavy silk suture.
8. The cannula is allowed to fill with blood and is then occluded with a *tube-occluding* clamp.
9. A second venous cannula is introduced in the same manner.
10. The cannulae are connected to a Y connector attached to the venous return line going to the pump.

DISCUSSION

Before cannulation, heparin is administered to the patient by the anesthesia care provider. If two cannulae are to be inserted, the surgeon uses vascular forceps to grasp the right atrial appendage (a small muscular pouch attached to the atrium) and places a curved partial-occlusion vascular clamp (*Beck* or *Glover*) across it. A purse-string suture of size 2-0 polyester or polypropylene is placed through the occluded portion of the appendage. The assistant snares the ends of the suture through a piece of tubing and tags the ends with a hemostat.

The surgeon then excises the tip of the appendage with scissors and applies clamps or forceps to the two edges of the atrial wall. The assistant controls the vascular clamp and retracts the atrial wall. The surgeon retracts the atrial wall and inserts the cannula. The technologist should control the end of the cannula during this procedure. The assistant removes the vascular clamp and controls the suture to prevent bleeding from the atrium.

The surgeon introduces the cannula into the superior vena cava. The assistant forms a tourniquet around the suture as previously described. The surgeon ties the cannula and tourniquet together with a heavy silk tie and then allows blood to fill the cannula by gravity or by lung inflation. The assistant places a tube-occluding clamp across the cannula. Caution is needed to avoid clamping the wire-reinforced portion of the cannula.

The inferior vena cava is cannulated through a similar technique. The major difference is that the cannula is inserted through the atrial wall instead of through the appendage. A knife blade and scissors may be used to open the atrium. The cannulae are connected to the venous return line from the pump.

Venous Cannulation with a Two-Stage Cannula

This procedure is similar to that used for bicaval cannulation except that only one cannula is used. The cannula has holes both in the distal end (which is inserted into the inferior vena cava to drain the lower body) and in the mid portion of the cannula (which lies in the atrium to drain blood from the superior vena cava) (Figure 29-37).

Technique   CANNULATION OF THE FEMORAL ARTERY AND VEIN

1. The surgeon makes an incision in the groin over the area of the femoral artery.
2. The tissue layers are divided, and a self-retaining retractor is inserted.

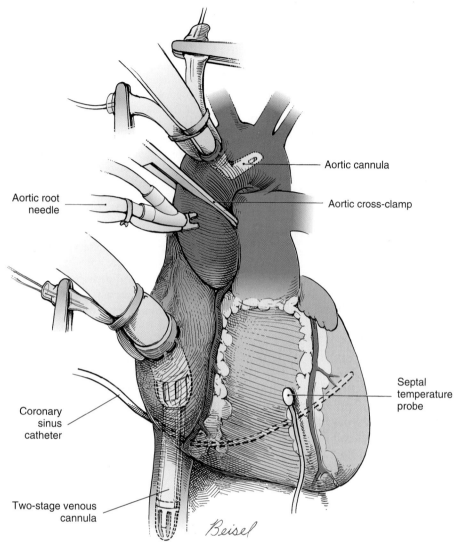

Aortic cannula

Aortic cross-clamp

Aortic root needle

Septal temperature probe

Coronary sinus catheter

Two-stage venous cannula

Beisel

FIGURE 29-37
Venous cannulation with a two-stage cannula. (Modified from Waldhausen JA, Pierce WS, and Campbell DB: *Surgery of the chest,* ed 6, St Louis, 1996, Mosby.)

3. The common femoral artery is isolated and encircled with umbilical tapes, whose ends are placed through a tube tourniquet.
4. The femoral vein is isolated through the above technique.
5. The artery is occluded with vascular clamps, and an arteriotomy is performed in the common femoral artery.
6. The cannula is inserted as the upper clamp is removed.
7. The cannula is allowed to fill with blood to evacuate all air, and a tube-occluding clamp is applied across the cannula.
8. The cannula is connected to the perfusion line from the pump.
9. The femoral vein is cannulated with the same technique.

DISCUSSION

Cannulation of the femoral artery and vein is performed when partial bypass is needed to support the patient's circulation in an emergency or during surgical resection of the descending thoracic aorta and ascending aorta. The femoral artery also is cannulated whenever the ascending aorta cannot be cannulated, and in some minimally invasive cardiac procedures.

After heparin has been given, the surgeon makes an incision in the groin over the femoral vessels with the knife. The subcutaneous tissue and fascial layers are divided with scissors. A self-retaining retractor is placed in the incision. The surgeon then isolates the common femoral artery with Metzenbaum scissors. The vessel is encircled with umbilical tape and secured in the jaw of a right-angle clamp. The assistant places a tube tourniquet over the ends of the tapes. The femoral vein is isolated with the same technique.

The surgeon occludes the femoral artery with small angled vascular clamps, such as a Glover or Cooley clamp. An arteriotomy is performed in the occluded segment with a #11 knife, and the incision is extended with Potts scissors. The opening may be dilated with a clamp. The surgeon inserts the cannula as the assistant removes the superior vascular clamp. The assistant tightens the umbilical tape to hold the cannula in place. The surgeon ties a heavy silk suture around the cannula and the tape, and releases the tube-occluding clamp to allow blood to fill the cannula and evacuate air. The cannula is then connected to the arterial perfusion line.

In patients with pulmonary emboli, partial cardiopulmonary bypass using the femoral vein and the femoral artery can be employed (Figure 29-38, *A*). Left heart bypass may be used to perfuse the lower body when the descending aorta is cross-clamped (Figure 29-38, *B*).

Technique | INSERTION OF A SUMP CATHETER INTO THE APEX OF THE LEFT VENTRICLE

1. The apex is elevated, and a purse-string suture is placed through it.
2. The ends of the suture are brought through a tube tourniquet.
3. The surgeon makes a stab incision in the ventricle and dilates the incision.
4. The catheter is inserted into the ventricle and secured with the tube tourniquet.
5. The catheter is tied to the tubing with heavy silk suture.
6. The apex of the ventricle is lowered to its normal position.

DISCUSSION

As soon as bypass is initiated, the surgeon elevates the apex of the left ventricle with a laparotomy sponge. A purse-string suture is placed in the apex and snared through a tube tourniquet. The technologist connects the sump catheter to the pump line.

The surgeon makes a stab incision in the apex with a #11 knife blade and dilates the opening with a Schnidt clamp, or similar clamp. He or she inserts the catheter, which is secured with the tourniquet. The surgeon ties the catheter and tourniquet together with heavy silk suture and lowers the apex into normal position.

Technique | INSERTION OF A SUMP CATHETER INTO THE RIGHT SUPERIOR PULMONARY VEIN

1. The surgeon retracts the right atrium to the left to expose the right superior pulmonary vein.
2. A purse-string suture is placed in the vein.
3. A stab incision is made in the vein, and the incision is dilated.
4. The catheter is inserted and manipulated into the left atrium across the mitral valve and then into the left ventricle.
5. A tube-occluding clamp is placed across the cannula.
6. The tubing is tightened against the catheter and secured.
7. The catheter is connected to the pump line.

DISCUSSION

A right superior pulmonary vein catheter is used more often than a left ventricular apical catheter, which can cause injury to the ventricular muscle.

The assistant retracts the right atrium to expose the right superior pulmonary vein while the surgeon places a purse-string suture. A tourniquet is placed over the suture ends. The surgeon makes a stab incision in the vein with a #11 knife blade, dilates the incision with a clamp, and inserts the catheter into the vein. He or she then manipulates the catheter into the left atrium, across the mitral valve, and into the left ventricle. The tourniquet is then snugged down, and a tube-occluding clamp is put in place across the catheter. The surgeon ties the catheter to the tourniquet with heavy silk suture and connects it to the pump suction line.

Technique | DECANNULATION OF THE VENTRICLE, VENAE CAVAE, AND AORTA

1. A tube-occluding clamp is placed across the catheter or cannula.

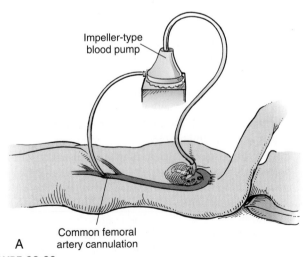
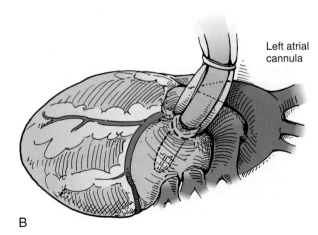

FIGURE 29-38
Left heart bypass. **A,** Preparation of the common femoral artery for cannulation. **B,** Insertion of the arterial cannula into the left atrium through a stab incision in two purse-string sutures. (Modified from Waldhausen JA, Pierce WS, and Campbell DB: *Surgery of the chest,* ed 6, St Louis, 1996, Mosby.)

2. Suture ties are removed from the catheter.
3. The catheter is withdrawn, and the suture is tied.

DISCUSSION

The left ventricular catheter usually is removed from the ventricle before bypass is discontinued. The catheter is occluded with a tube-occluding clamp, and the silk suture and tourniquet are removed. The catheter is withdrawn, and the suture is tied securely to occlude the cannulation site. Additional sutures (often on pledgets) may be used for hemostasis. Decannulation of the venae cavae and aorta uses the same technique after bypass has been discontinued.

Technique	DECANNULATION OF THE FEMORAL ARTERY AND FEMORAL VEIN

1. The cannula is occluded.
2. The umbilical tape is released.
3. The cannula is withdrawn, and the vein is occluded with a vascular clamp.
4. The venotomy is closed, and all clamps and tapes are removed.
5. The artery is decannulated with the same technique.

DISCUSSION

At the conclusion of bypass, the surgeon occludes the femoral vein cannula. The assistant releases the cannula from the drapes and other attachments on the field. The surgeon then withdraws the cannula and occludes the vein with a vascular clamp. The venotomy is closed with a continuous suture of 5-0 or 6-0 polypropylene. All clamps are removed, and the artery is decannulated with the same technique.

Cardioplegia Infusion
SURGICAL GOAL

Cardioplegia solution is used to stop the heart, thereby reducing the energy required by the cardiac muscle by eliminating the energy requirements of contraction. The process of infusing cardioplegic solution into the coronary arteries protects the cardiac muscle from damage while the aorta is occluded and the blood supply is interrupted. The solution may be infused directly into the coronary artery or transatrially into the coronary sinus. Cardioplegia solution can be infused indirectly into the aortic root just above the aortic valve.

Technique	DIRECT CORONARY ARTERY INFUSION (ANTEGRADE)

1. The ascending aorta is occluded and opened below the clamp.
2. The surgeon identifies and cannulates the ostia (openings) of the coronary arteries.
3. Solution is infused, and the cannulae are removed immediately after each infusion.
4. The aorta is closed when the surgery has been completed.

DISCUSSION

The surgeon occludes the ascending aorta and opens it below the clamp. The coronary ostia are located, and the correct sizes of cannulae are determined. The technologist connects the appropriate-size cannulae to the tubing. The surgeon then gently inserts the cannulae into the ostia of the coronary arteries and holds them in position until the pump perfusionist or anesthesia care provider completes the infusion. Solution is infused until the heart ceases to beat (Figure 29-39). The technologist should keep the cannulae and tubing secure in a towel until they are needed for subsequent infusions. The surgeon closes the aorta at the completion of surgery.

Technique	INDIRECT CORONARY ARTERY INFUSION (ANTEGRADE)

1. The surgeon occludes the ascending aorta.
2. An indwelling catheter is inserted into the aortic root above the valve.
3. The catheter is connected to the tubing and filled with cardioplegic solution.
4. The solution is infused.
5. The indwelling catheter is removed immediately before the aorta is unclamped.
6. The defect made by the catheter is repaired with suture.

DISCUSSION

This technique and the transatrial retrograde method (below) are the methods most commonly used. The surgeon places a polypropylene purse-string suture in the aorta below the site of the cross-clamp. He or she then occludes the ascending aorta and inserts an indwelling catheter, such as a 14-gauge Angiocath, into the aorta below the clamp. The assistant connects the tubing from the cardioplegic solution to the catheter. A Y connector can be inserted into the cardioplegia tubing and a suction line inserted to vent air from the aorta. Each line from the Y (cardioplegia and vent) can be occluded. When cardioplegic solution is being infused, the suction line is occluded; when the suction line is opened, the cardioplegia line is occluded.

Cardioplegic solution is infused as often as necessary during the procedure. The surgeon withdraws the indwelling catheter and removes the clamp from the aorta. Air in the aorta is suctioned through the vent line. When the catheter has been removed, the surgeon closes the defect with size 5-0 polypropylene suture.

Technique	TRANSATRIAL CARDIOPLEGIA VIA THE CORONARY SINUS (RETROGRADE)

1. A small purse-string suture is placed in the atrial wall, and an incision is made in the center.
2. A retrograde cardioplegia catheter is passed through the atrial stab wound, inserted into the opening of the coronary sinus, and positioned in the coronary vein.

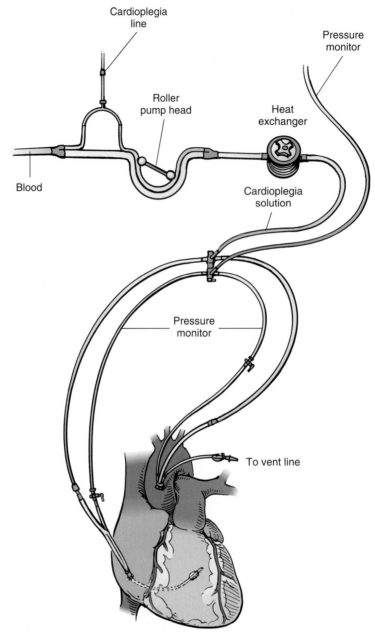

FIGURE 29-39
Cardioplegia infusion. (Modified from Waldhausen JA, Pierce WS, and Campbell DB: *Surgery of the chest,* ed 6, St Louis, 1996, Mosby.)

3. The proximal end of the catheter is connected to a line leading to the cardioplegia source.
4. Cardioplegia solution is infused to stop the heart.
5. When cardioplegia is no longer needed, the catheter is removed and the purse-string is tied to close the wound.

DISCUSSION

Cardioplegia solution often is infused through the retrograde route (into the coronary venous system) rather than through the arterial antegrade route. The cardioplegia solution flows from the coronary veins through the capillaries and into the coronary arteries, stopping the heart.

After placing a 5-0 polypropylene purse-string suture in the atrial wall, the surgeon incises the atrium with a #15 or #11 blade. The retrograde cardioplegia catheter is inserted into the atrium and guided at the entrance of the coronary sinus. Palpating the outer atrial wall, the surgeon positions the catheter in the sinus opening and advances it into the vein. The catheter is attached to tubing connected to the cardioplegia source in the bypass circuit.

When it is no longer needed, the catheter is removed and the atrial incision is closed.

Resection of Aneurysms of the Descending Thoracic Aorta

SURGICAL GOAL

The goal of surgical repair of an aneurysm is to prevent rupture and life-threatening hemorrhage.

PATHOLOGY

An aneurysm is a widening or dilation of the walls of the artery that may be caused by atherosclerosis, arteriosclerosis, infection, syphilis, trauma, or congenital abnormality. Aneurysms obstruct the normal flow of blood, leading to ischemia and tissue necrosis.

Two classifications of aneurysms are saccular and fusiform. A **saccular aneurysm** is a ballooning out of a localized area in the artery. A **fusiform aneurysm** involves the entire circumference of the artery, causing it to become spindle shaped. **Dissection** occurs when a tear occurs in the intima, allowing blood to flow between the layers of the vessel wall. Dissections of the descending aorta are surgically repaired most often when there is impending rupture of the lesion.

Technique

1. The surgeon performs a thoracotomy.
2. The mediastinal pleura is incised.
3. The aneurysm or dissection is mobilized from the surrounding tissue.
4. Vascular occluding clamps are applied to the aorta, and the aneurysm or dissection is resected.
5. The intercostal arteries are ligated.
6. A prosthetic graft is implanted.
7. The occluding clamps are removed from the aorta.
8. The graft may be enclosed by the remaining vascular wall.
9. The mediastinal pleura is closed.
10. Chest tubes are inserted, and the wound is closed.

DISCUSSION

The patient usually is placed in the lateral position, prepped, and draped for a thoracotomy.

A thoracotomy is performed as described above. When the chest has been opened and the retractors placed, the surgeon retracts the edges of the pleura with size 2-0 silk sutures.

The surgeon begins to free the aneurysm from the surrounding tissue. Femoral vein–femoral artery cardiopulmonary bypass may be employed to perfuse the kidneys and the rest of the lower body. If bypass is not employed, speed is essential at this time because there is no flow to the lower body. The technologist must be very alert and avoid unnecessary movements and loss of time while handling instruments.

The surgeon occludes the aorta proximal and distal to the aneurysm. The surgeon then makes a longitudinal incision

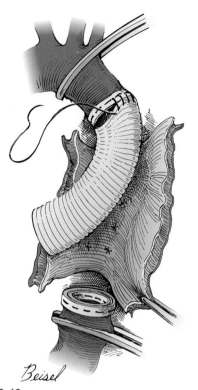

FIGURE 29-40
Resection for descending thoracic aortic aneurysm. (Modified from Waldhausen JA, Pierce WS, and Campbell DB: *Surgery of the chest*, ed 6, St Louis, 1996, Mosby.)

into the aneurysm with the knife and extends the incision with scissors. The outer layer of the aneurysm is preserved and retracted with sutures of size 2-0 or 3-0 silk. These flaps will be used later in the procedure to cover the grafts and prevent them from adhering to the lung.

The surgeon removes all debris and blood clots inside the aneurysm using suction and tissue forceps. The technologist should have a small basin to receive loose debris and blood clots and a moist sponge to wipe debris from the surgeon's instruments. The surgeon ligates the intercostal vessels along the posterior wall of the aneurysm with polyester sutures. Identifying the origin of these vessels may be difficult. To aid in identification, the surgeon may irrigate the area with warm saline solution and look for bleeding points, indicating an open vessel. When hemostasis is secured, the graft is anastomosed to the aorta.

The surgeon transects the aorta immediately above and below the aneurysm and removes the middle segment. A graft is then implanted to replace the diseased segment.

Resection of an aneurysm is show in Figure 29-40.

Anastomosing the Graft

The surgeon performs the proximal anastomosis with a continuous suture of polypropylene or polyester suture of size 3-0 or 4-0. A straight vascular clamp may be placed across the graft while the surgeon momentarily releases the proximal aortic clamp to check for leaks. The surgeon reapplies the aortic clamp, removes the graft clamp, and places any additional sutures needed to control leakage. Teflon pledgets may be used to bolster the sutures.

After the surgeon completes the proximal anastomosis, he or she trims the graft to the appropriate length and performs the distal anastomosis. Before the surgeon ties the suture, the graft is flushed to clear it of clots and debris. The suture is then tied, and all clamps are removed, restoring blood flow to the lower body.

If cardiopulmonary bypass has been used, it is discontinued at this stage, and the cannulae are removed. To complete the procedure, the surgeon covers the graft with remaining aneurysm tissue (if it has not been excised) using an absorbable continuous or interrupted suture material of size 2-0 or 3-0. The mediastinal pleura is closed, chest tubes are inserted, and the wound is closed in layers.

Implantation of a Pacemaker
SURGICAL GOAL
A pacemaker is implanted to provide electrical simulation to the heart to increase a slow heart rate (**bradycardia;** heart rate of less than 40 to 60 beats per minute). Bradycardia is one type of dysrhythmia. Pacemakers currently are often implanted in the cardiac catheterization suite. When concomitant cardiac surgery is performed, the pacemaker electrodes and generator may be inserted during surgery, or they may be inserted postoperatively via the transvenous route (a temporary pacer is employed until it is replaced by a permanent pacing system).

PATHOLOGY
Cardiac **arrhythmia** is an abnormal pattern of conductivity in the heart. Some healthy individuals may have arrhythmias. When the heart's conduction mechanism is affected by disease, however, certain arrhythmias can be life threatening. Arrhythmias are named by type and origin (e.g., atrial flutter). Some common arrhythmias include the following:

▶ **Ventricular tachycardia:** heart rate over 100 beats per minute
▶ **Atrial flutter:** heart rate of 240 to 450 beats per minute
▶ **Ventricular fibrillation:** chaotic, disorganized stimulation of the ventricle(s) that does not pump the blood
▶ **Atrial fibrillation:** chaotic, disorganized stimulation of the atrium (atria) that prevents atrial contraction (which normally helps to fill the ventricle with blood)
▶ **Bradycardia:** abnormally slow electrical impulses and heart beat below 40 to 60 beats per minute

Conduction problems in the heart can arise from many different disease conditions, including ischemic heart disease resulting from blocked coronary arteries or congenital defects. The cardiac pacemaker provides electrical stimulation to the heart to increase the heart rate.

Pacemaker implantation (see Figure 29-13) may be performed on a temporary basis such as during cardiac procedures, or the implantation may be permanent. Three approaches are used for permanent implantation: transvenous,

epicardial, and subxiphoid. The transvenous and subxiphoid procedures, which do not require a thoracotomy, are commonly performed with the patient under local anesthesia with monitored anesthesia care. When the transvenous approach is used, the electrodes are placed with the aid of fluoroscopy.

A right or left subclavian venotomy is performed, and the electrode is advanced into the right atrium, through the tricuspid valve, and into the right ventricle, where it is placed in the right ventricular apex. The pulse generator is then placed within the superficial tissues of the chest wall. An atrial electrode also may be placed in the atrial appendage for dual-chamber (atrial and ventricular) pacing.

The implantation of both permanent and temporary pacemakers through a thoracotomy is less common than placement through the transvenous approach; the procedures are discussed below.

Technique   TEMPORARY PACEMAKER

1. An electrode is sutured to the right atrium and/or the right ventricle.
2. The free end of the electrode is brought through the skin and secured with a suture.
3. The electrode is connected to an alligator cable attached to a temporary, external pacemaker generator.

DISCUSSION
Temporary pacemaker leads are implanted before cardiopulmonary bypass is discontinued because the field is more accessible with the lungs deflated (as occurs on bypass). Another reason the leads are implanted before bypass is discontinued is that if the touching of the heart during lead attachment causes an arrhythmia, perfusion to the body is not compromised. The surgeon sutures the metal wire electrode to the heart with size 5-0 silk. Only the tip of the electrode is exposed wire; the remaining section is insulated. The technologist should have the electrode open and loaded on a needle holder before or after bypass is discontinued. The assistant cuts the needle off the electrode after the surgeon places it through the myocardium. The surgeon then secures the electrode with sutures of size 5-0 silk. The surgeon brings the opposite end of the electrode through the skin and secures it with 2-0 silk sutures. The electrode then is connected to an alligator cable and pacemaker generator. The anesthesiologist or circulator then can pace the heart as necessary.

Technique   PERMANENT PACEMAKER (EPICARDIAL INSERTION)

1. The chest is opened to expose the right ventricle.
2. The coiled metal tip of the electrode, placed in a Silastic casing, is positioned in the ventricular epicardium.
3. The surgeon places the sutures to secure the electrode.
4. The electrodes are tested with the alligator cables and then connected to the permanent generator and tested.
5. The generator is implanted in the chest wall.
6. The wound is closed.

DISCUSSION

Although permanent epicardial pacemakers are inserted less often than transvenous pacers, there are times when the intravenous route is not feasible, such as in the presence of subclavian vein stenosis. A sternotomy for cardiac surgery is not necessarily an indication for epicardial lead attachment because leads may be inserted transvenously after sternotomy when temporary pacing is sufficient to maintain an acceptable heart rate.

The techniques for implanting the permanent pacemaker through a thoracotomy or short transverse incision are similar. The surgeon makes a short transverse incision below the xiphoid and across the diaphragm using the skin knife. The subcutaneous, fascial, and muscle layers are divided with the scalpel or ESU. A self-retaining retractor, such as a small Finochietto retractor or a large Weitlaner retractor, is placed in the wound.

The surgeon exposes the right ventricle by opening the pericardium with the knife or dissecting scissors. Size 2-0 silk sutures are placed on the edges of the pericardium so that the assistant can offer traction on the tissue. The surgeon then places several sutures of size 4-0 silk or polyester through the ventricle and into the electrode Silastic casing. The coiled metal tip of the electrode is placed into the myocardium, and the sutures are tied. Additional sutures may be needed to secure the electrode. In addition to the coiled (pig-tail) lead, a harpoon-like lead also is available (Figure 29-41).

To test the electrode, the surgeon connects it to an alligator cable attached to the temporary external pacemaker generator. The circulator or anesthesia care provider activates the battery. If the electrode functions normally, it is then connected to the permanent battery. The surgeon makes a pocket for the battery beneath the fascia of the chest, or less often, the abdomen. The surgeon inserts the battery into the pocket and closes the pocket with interrupted size 0 or 2-0 nonabsorbable sutures. Size 0 or 2-0 absorbable sutures are used to approximate the subcutaneous tissue, and the skin is closed with the surgeon's suture of choice.

Replacement of Pacemaker Battery
SURGICAL GOAL

In this procedure, a malfunctioning pacemaker generator is replaced to produce continuous pacing.

Technique

1. The surgeon incises the skin over the generator.
2. The tissue layers are divided to expose the generator and electrode(s).
3. The generator is removed from the tissue pocket.
4. The electrode is connected to an alligator cable and tested.
5. The electrode is inserted into the new generator.
6. The new generator is inserted into the tissue pocket, and the wound is closed.

DISCUSSION

The surgeon incises the skin over the generator. The underlying tissue layers are divided with sharp dissection to expose the electrodes and generator. The generator is removed from the tissue pocket, and the electrodes are disconnected. The surgeon immediately connects the electrodes to the alligator cable of an external pacer generator so that the heart can be continually paced during the exchange of generators. The electrodes are then connected to the new generator. The surgeon places the new generator into the tissue pocket. Interrupted sutures of size 3-0 absorbable suture are used to approximate the tissues over the generator. The skin is then closed with the surgeon's suture of choice.

Implantable Cardioverter Defibrillator
The implantable cardioverter defibrillator (ICD) is an electronic cardiac defibrillating and monitoring device used in patients susceptible to ventricular fibrillation or ventricular tachycardia. Most ICDs also have pacing functions to treat bradycardia that may occur after an episode of defibrillation. The device consists of a generator, sensing electrodes, and defibrillation/pacing electrodes. Newer ICDs have largely replaced the older models that used epicardial patch electrodes applied during open procedures.

The ICD may be implanted through a thoracotomy, subxiphoid, or median sternotomy incision, although most are inserted transvenously. The sensing leads are commonly placed in the right ventricle through a transvenous approach. The ventricular defibrillation leads are inserted into the heart transvenously, and the generator is placed within the superficial tissue of the chest or abdominal wall. A subcutaneous thoracic patch occasionally is used to optimize defibrillation.

Insertion of an ICD is shown in Figure 29-42.

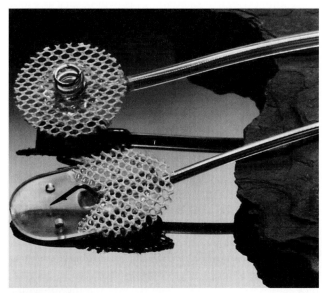

FIGURE 29-41
Permanent epicardial screw-in (top) and stab (bottom) pacemaker leads. (From Seifert PC: *Cardiac surgery: perioperative patient care*, St Louis, 2002, Mosby; courtesy Medtronic, Inc., Minneapolis, Minn.)

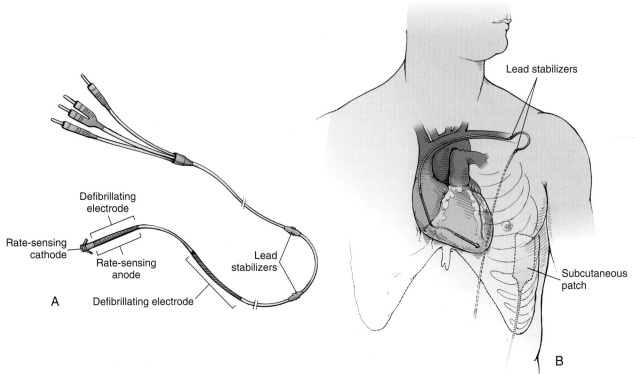

FIGURE 29-42
Insertion of an ICD. **A,** Lead system composed of sensing and defibrillating electrodes combined in one unit. **B,** Placement of electrodes in patient. (Modified from Rothrock JC: *Alexander's care of the patient in surgery,* ed 12, St Louis, 2003, Mosby.)

Coronary Artery Bypass

SURGICAL GOAL

Coronary artery bypass of a narrow segment of one or more coronary arteries is performed to improve circulation to the heart. An autograft (tissue from the patient's own body) usually is used as the bypass graft.

PATHOLOGY

Arteriosclerosis and atherosclerosis commonly cause narrowing of the coronary arteries.

Technique

1. The surgeon makes a median sternotomy incision.
2. A segment of the saphenous vein is removed. The internal mammary artery (IMA) is dissected from its retrosternal bed.
3. The heart is cannulated for cardiopulmonary bypass unless an off-pump procedure is planned.
4. The aorta is occluded, and cardioplegic solution is administered into the aortic root.
5. The coronary artery is incised, and the vein, IMA, or other graft conduit is anastomosed to the coronary arteriotomy.
6. The aorta is unclamped.
7. Venous and other free grafts are anastomosed to the ascending aorta. These may be anastomosed while the cross-clamp is applied.
8. Cardiopulmonary bypass is discontinued, and decannulation is performed.
9. Pacing wires and chest tubes are inserted, and the wound is closed.

DISCUSSION

The surgeon performs a median sternotomy and cannulates for cardiopulmonary bypass. However, an increasing number of coronary bypass procedures are performed without the use of cardiopulmonary bypass. Proponents of off-pump procedures prefer to avoid the risks of bypass, such as stroke and systemic inflammation. In patients with very complex, multi-vessel disease, bypass often is required. The assistant removes the greater saphenous vein from the leg, or the left or right radial artery may be harvested for use as a free graft (Figure 29-43). The right gastroepiploic artery occasionally is used as a pedicle graft (Figure 29-44). Video-assisted endoscopic vein harvesting may be performed.

Preparation of Internal Mammary Artery
The IMA is dissected free from its retrosternal bed (Figure 29-45). The sternal edge may be elevated with a self-retaining retractor attached to the side from which the IMA is dissected. The left IMA is commonly used; the right also may be employed.

Coronary Artery Bypass
After cardiopulmonary bypass has been instituted (if used), the surgeon identifies the segment of coronary artery to which the bypass graft will be anastomosed. The surgeon removes excess epicardial fat from the arteriotomy site with a #64 Beaver blade or a #15 blade. The surgeon then occludes the ascending aorta and inserts the indwelling catheter for infusion of cardioplegic solution and venting of air.

Next, the surgeon opens the coronary artery with a #11 knife blade (or Beaver blade) and extends the incision with

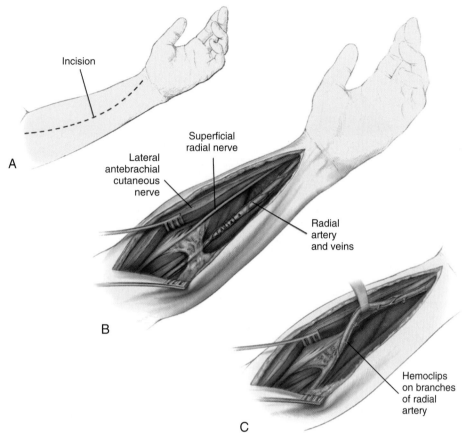

FIGURE 29-43
Dissection of radial artery. **A,** Incision line. **B,** Deep forearm dissection exposes the radial artery and vein pedicle. **C,** Radial artery pedicle is mobilized, and the multiple side branches are clipped. The artery is removed and may be irrigated with a vasodilator. A continuous intravenous infusion of diltiazem helps to prevent vasoconstriction of the artery. (Modified from Doty DB: *Cardiac surgery: operative technique,* St Louis, 1997, Mosby.)

Diethrich or fine Potts coronary scissors. A Garrett dilator may be inserted into the lumen of the artery to assess its size. The technologist places the vein in a small basin with heparinized blood solution to keep the graft moist. The surgeon bevels the free end of the vein with Potts scissors. The vein is then sutured to the coronary artery with continuous or interrupted sutures, such as size 6-0 or 7-0 polypropylene. When the anastomosis is complete, the assistant inflates the vein with physiological solution to test for leaks and to determine the diameter of the graft when it is filled.

The surgeon performs all other anastomoses using the same technique (8-0 polypropylene may be used for the IMA). The aorta is then unclamped, and the indwelling catheter is removed. A portion of the aorta is occluded with a vascular clamp such as the Lambert-Kay clamp. A #11 knife blade and aortic punch are used to create a hole in the occluded portion.

The surgeon inflates the vein to make certain it is not twisted and does not have any leaks, and to determine the length needed to reach the aorta. He or she then cuts the vein to the appropriate length and bevels the end with Potts scissors. The anastomosis is performed between the vein and the hole in the aorta. The surgeon completes each of the anastomoses and removes the clamp from the aorta. When the procedures are performed off-pump, a small horseshoe retractor is positioned over the coronary arteriotomy to minimize cardiac movement during the distal anastomosis. The proximal aortic anastomosis is performed with partial occlusion of the aorta.

Air is evacuated from the vein grafts with a 25-gauge or 27-gauge needle. The surgeon inspects each anastomosis for possible leaks; these are repaired before bypass is discontinued. The cannulae are removed, and a pacemaker electrode may be sutured to the heart. Metal rings or radiopaque material may be placed around each vein graft on the aorta. These mark the veins in the event cardiac catheterization is performed in the postoperative period.

A coronary artery bypass is illustrated in Figure 29-46.

Minimally Invasive Direct Coronary Artery Bypass

Minimally invasive direct coronary artery bypass (MIDCAB) is an off-pump procedure that employs a left anterior thoracotomy incision placed over the area of the left anterior descending (LAD) coronary artery. The procedure is performed infrequently because of the considerable postoperative pain from the thoracic incision, the fact that access is limited to the LAD artery (and occasionally the diagonal coronary artery), and the technical ability required to perform the anastomosis in a small exposed area on a beating heart.

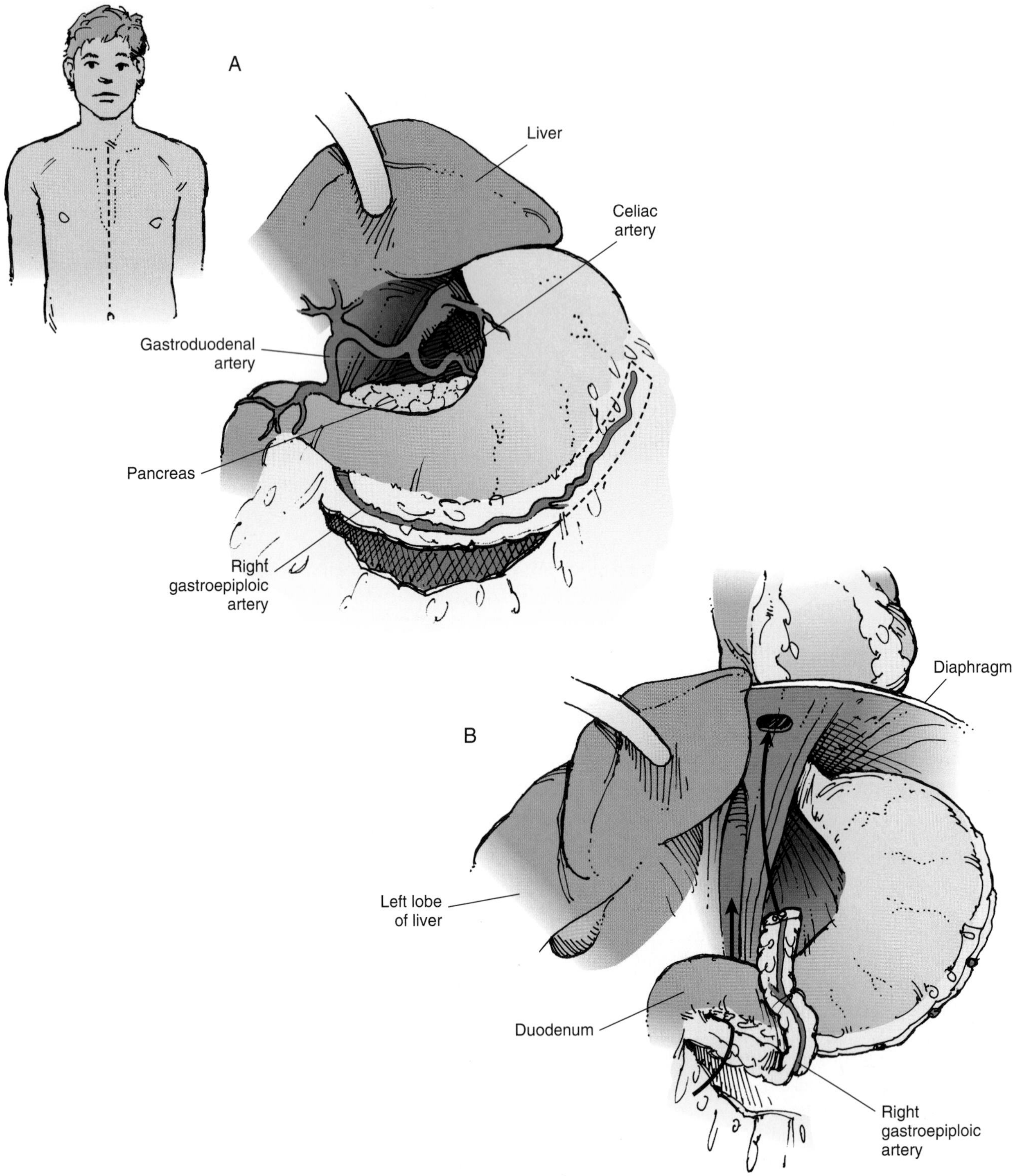

FIGURE 29-44
Right gastroepiploic artery mobilization. **A,** Exposure of the upper abdomen through a median sternotomy incision; the liver is retracted superiorly and to the right. **B,** The right gastroepiploic arterial pedicle may be taken superiorly or anteriorly and passed through an opening created in the diaphragm and into the pericardial sac.

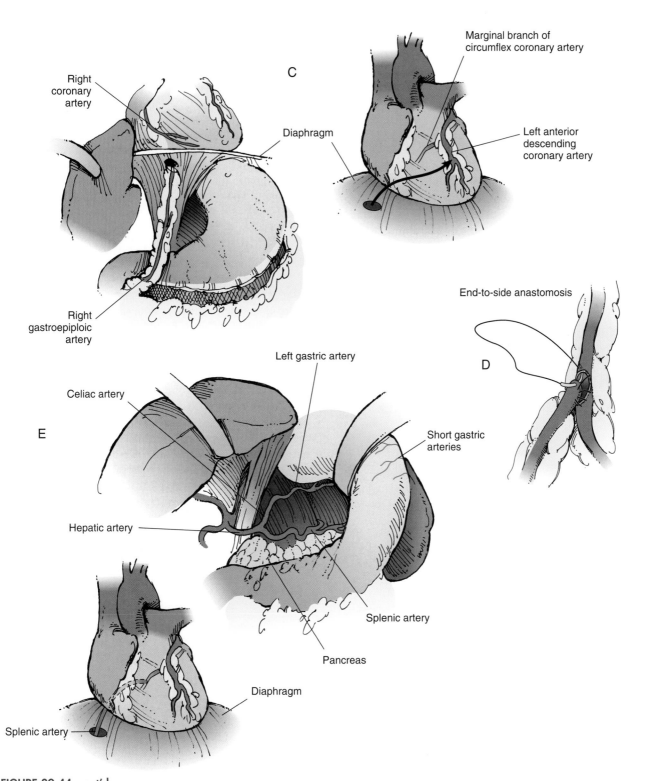

FIGURE 29-44, cont'd
Right gastroepiploic artery mobilization. **C,** The right gastroepiploic artery may be used to revascularize nearly any artery on the surface of the heart. **D,** End-to-side technique to anastomose the right gastroepiploic artery to the coronary artery. **E,** In unusual situations, the splenic artery may be used as a bypass conduit. (Modified from Doty DB: *Cardiac surgery: operative technique,* St Louis, 1997, Mosby.)

A special rib retractor with endoscope is used to harvest the left IMA. The rib retractor is exchanged for another small thoracotomy retractor positioned to expose the anastomotic site of the LAD. A stabilizing device is used to minimize cardiac movement during suturing. The anastomosis is performed in the traditional manner.

Transmyocardial Revascularization
SURGICAL GOAL

Transmyocardial revascularization (TMR) is a procedure in which a series of small-bore, transmural channels are created with a laser (carbon dioxide laser or holmium:yttrium-aluminum-garnet [YAG] laser) to allow oxygenated blood from the left ventricle to perfuse the myocardium. The goal

is to increase blood flow to the heart in patients with coronary disease that is not amenable to coronary artery bypass (CAB) or to medical management. TMR may be used in conjunction with standard CAB.

Technique

1. In patients not undergoing CAB, a mini-thoracotomy is made on the side of the affected coronary artery.
2. The surgeon opens the pericardium to expose the heart.
3. The sterile laser probe is given to the surgeon, who places the probe tip on the epicardium and makes channels into the heart muscle.
4. Hemostasis is achieved.
5. A chest tube may be inserted.
6. The incision is closed.

DISCUSSION

Laser precautions are instituted: protective eyewear for the entire operative team, moist sponges over the patient's eyes, and "Do not enter" signs posted on all entry doors. The surgical team must be properly trained in the use of the laser.

If TMR is performed in conjunction with CAB, only laser-specific instruments and supplies should be added to the set-up. If TMR is to be performed through a thoracotomy, chest instruments as well as the laser supplies and equipment are used. External defibrillator patches are applied to all patients; pediatric internal defibrillator paddles also may be requested.

The surgeon uses a sterile laser probe to make the myocardial channels from the epicardium to the endocardium. The technologist must ensure that the sterility of the laser probe is maintained between channel formations. Both the

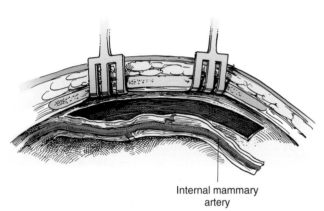

FIGURE 29-45
Dissection of internal mammary artery (IMA). (Modified from Waldhausen JA, Pierce WS, and Campbell DB: *Surgery of the chest*, ed 6, St Louis, 1996, Mosby.)

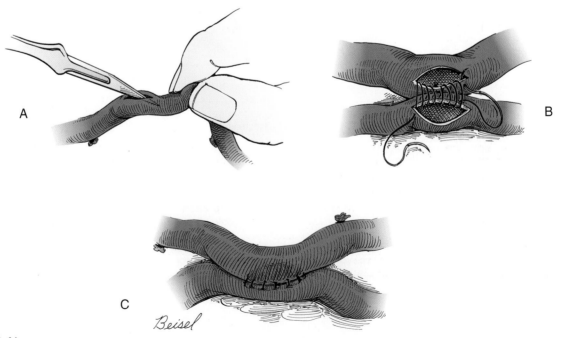

FIGURE 29-46
A coronary artery bypass. **A,** The proximal anastomosis of the bypass graft. Aortotomy made with a punch in the ascending aorta. **B,** F-1 parallel anastomosis technique. **C,** F-2 diamond-shaped anastomosis. (From Waldhausen JA, Pierce WS, Campbell DB: *Surgery of the chest*, ed 6, St Louis, 1996, Mosby.)

scrub and the circulating personnel keep a running count of the number of channels formed.

A percutaneous transvenous method of lasering can be performed. The channels are made from the endocardium to the epicardium.

Coronary Artery Angioplasty and Stent Insertion
This procedure is performed to relieve stricture in a coronary artery or to restore circulation in patients who are not candidates for coronary bypass. The procedure for stenting is described in Chapter 30. The femoral artery is commonly used for the insertion of the catheter carrying the stent and other angioplasty devices. The brachial artery occasionally is used as the catheter insertion site.

Batista Procedure
SURGICAL GOAL
The Batista procedure was introduced to treat end-stage heart disease not amenable to conventional therapy (such as insertion of a ventricular assist device or cardiac transplantation). It is infrequently performed in the United States.

Introduced by a Brazilian surgeon, the Batista procedure is an attempt to remodel the anatomy of the heart. By excising a portion of the dysfunctional, dilated left ventricular myocardium, the surgeon improves ventricular function by creating a smaller, more effective pumping chamber.

Technique

1. The surgeon makes a median sternotomy to expose the heart.
2. The myocardium is inspected.
3. A triangular portion of dilated left ventricular myocardium is excised.
4. The myocardial edges are reapproximated with bolstered, heavy nonabsorbable sutures.
5. Chest drains are inserted.
6. The sternum is closed with wire.
7. The incision is closed.

DISCUSSION
The lack of modern technological devices and techniques in some countries has promoted the use of innovative procedures to treat end-stage heart disease. The Batista procedure is one such attempt to improve ventricular function in situations in which cardiac support technology may not be available.

Another technique with similar indications is the **Dor technique,** also called the *endoventricular circular patch plasty* procedure. A portion of scarred myocardium is excised, and the remaining defect is repaired with a Dacron patch. Both the **Batista** procedure and the **Dor** procedure are similar to the repair of a left ventricular aneurysm by excision and plication or by endoaneurysmorrhaphy (described later in this chapter).

Aortic Valve Replacement
SURGICAL GOAL
The aortic valve maintains one-way blood flow from the left ventricle to the aorta. In this procedure, a diseased valve is replaced to restore valve function.

PATHOLOGY
Common causes of valve insufficiency are rheumatic fever, endocarditis, and congenital anomalies. A **regurgitant** (leaky) valve loses its ability to close tightly and thus allows blood to leak back into the left ventricle instead of going through the aorta (aortic valve regurgitation is also known as aortic insufficiency). The left ventricle eventually fails because of the added strain of trying to eject the excess blood out into the aorta.

The valve leaflets also may become **stenotic** (stiff) because of calcification or other thickening. This can reduce the opening of the valve to a small slit. The ventricle must work harder to pump a sufficient amount of blood through the narrowed orifice of the stenotic valve. This can lead to ventricular failure and insufficient blood flow to the brain, coronary arteries, and other organs. **Syncope,** a form of temporary unconsciousness caused by a lack of oxygen to the brain, heart failure, and sudden death may occur when stenosis is severe.

Technique

1. The surgeon performs a median sternotomy.
2. Cannulation for cardiopulmonary bypass usually is performed with a two-stage venous cannula.
3. The ascending aorta is occluded, and cardioplegic solution is infused through the aortic root or through the coronary sinus and into the coronary circulation.
4. A transverse incision is made in the anterior aortic wall.
5. A prosthetic valve is selected and sutured in place.
6. The aortotomy is closed, and the aorta is unclamped.
7. Cardiopulmonary bypass is discontinued and cannulae are removed.
8. Pacing wires and chest tubes are inserted, and the wound is closed.

DISCUSSION
The surgeon performs a median sternotomy and cannulates for cardiopulmonary bypass. A retrograde cardioplegia catheter is inserted into the coronary sinus. The ascending aorta is occluded, and cardioplegia solution is infused (Figure 29-47). The route through which cardioplegia solution is delivered depends on the valve pathology. If there is aortic stenosis, the cardioplegia solution initially is infused through the aortic root. After the aorta has been opened, subsequent cardioplegia infusions are given through the retrograde catheter. If there is aortic insufficiency, cardioplegia solution infused into the aortic root will preferentially flow into the left ventricle. Fluid in the ventricular chamber will distend and injure the ventricular wall. In these situations, retrograde cardioplegia solution is infused. Direct coronary perfusion rarely is required.

The surgeon opens the aorta with a transverse incision or, occasionally a vertical incision. He or she incises the valve cusps with forceps and scissors or a long knife. If there is extensive calcification of the valve leaflets, the surgeon may debride the calcium with rongeurs. The technologist should intermittently clean the instruments with a wet laparotomy sponge to prevent calcium particles and other materials

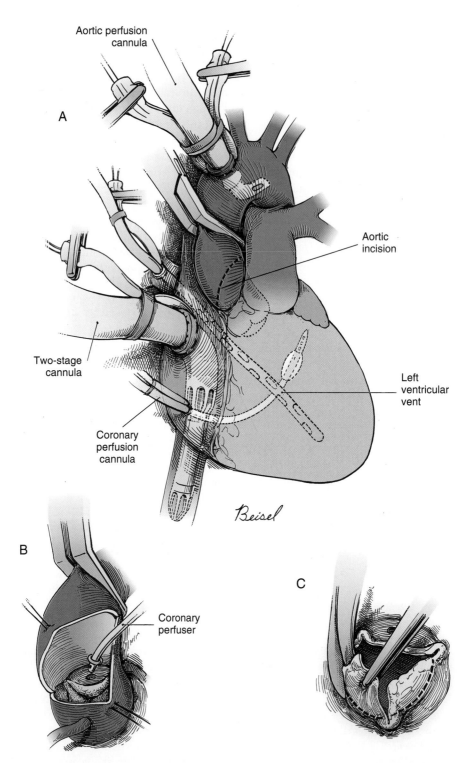

FIGURE 29-47
Aortic valve replacement. **A,** Incision and placement sites for aortic valve procedures. Cannulation, retrograde cardioplegia, and vent sites. **B,** An alternative technique if retrograde cardioplegia is not used; hand-held coronary ostial catheters are used to deliver cardioplegic solution. **C,** Excision of the diseased valve.

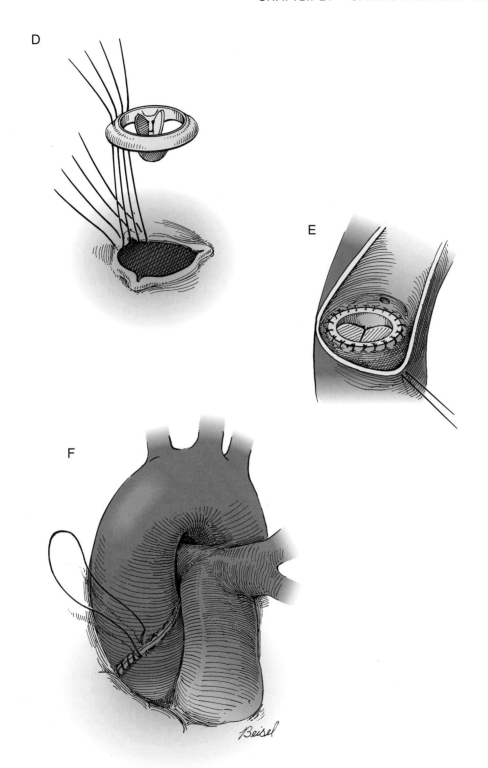

FIGURE 29-47, cont'd
Aortic valve replacement. **D,** Sutures are placed in the prosthetic sewing ring and the valve. **E,** Completion of valve replacement. **F,** The aortic suture line is closed. (Modified from Waldhausen JA, Pierce WS, and Campbell DB: *Surgery of the chest,* ed 6, St Louis, 1996, Mosby.)

from dropping back into the wound where they might cause an embolism.

The annulus is measured with obturators. Different types of valve prostheses have their own unique sizing obturators. The scrub obtains the correct size of prosthesis from the circulating nurse. The surgeon places interrupted sutures through the annulus of the prosthetic sewing ring. Some surgeons prefer to use a continuous suture of 2-0 or 3-0 polypropylene. Interrupted sutures in the aortic valve may be inserted in three series, corresponding to the three cusps of the valve. The distal suture ends are tagged with mosquito clamps or placed in a suture holder. When biological valves are used, they must be kept moist with saline because if the leaflets become dry, the prosthesis can be injured and may not function properly.

The surgeon seats the valve in position and ties all sutures. The aortotomy is closed with two 2-0 or 3-0 polypropylene sutures. One suture begins on the left side, and the other suture begins on the right side. The sutures are tied in the middle portion of the aortotomy. Before tying the sutures, the surgeon allows air to escape from the suture line. He or she then ties the sutures securely. The aortic clamp is removed, and the aortic vent line is turned on to aspirate air. The surgeon also may elevate the left ventricular apex and insert a 19-gauge needle into the chamber to allow air to escape.

Bypass is discontinued, and cannulae are removed. Temporary pacemaker electrodes may be sutured to the heart. Chest tubes are inserted, and the wound is closed in layers.

Mitral Valve Replacement and Repair
SURGICAL GOAL
In this procedure, a diseased mitral valve is replaced to prevent blood from regurgitating into the left atrium or to open a stenotic valve. If the valve is severely damaged, the valve is replaced. When possible, the valve is repaired with an annuloplasty (or other reparative techniques) rather than replaced.

PATHOLOGY
The mitral valve is situated between the left atrium and left ventricle. Over time, a stenotic valve causes the left atrium to become dilated and can lead to arrhythmias such as atrial fibrillation. Mitral valve disease is commonly caused by rheumatic heart disease.

Technique
1. The surgeon performs a midline sternotomy.
2. Cannulation of the superior and inferior venae cavae is performed for total cardiopulmonary bypass.
3. The ascending aorta is occluded, and cardioplegic solution is infused through the aortic root and into the coronary arteries.
4. A left atriotomy is performed, and the mitral valve is excised.

5. A prosthetic valve is sutured in place.
6. The atriotomy is closed, and the aorta is unclamped.
7. Cardiopulmonary bypass is discontinued, and the cannulae are removed.
8. Chest tubes and pacing wires are inserted, and the wound is closed.

DISCUSSION
Mitral Valve Replacement
The surgeon performs a median sternotomy and cannulates both venae cavae for total cardiopulmonary bypass. The ascending aorta is occluded, and cardioplegic solution is infused through the aortic root and into the coronary arteries.

The surgeon opens the left atrium with the long knife, extends the incision with scissors, and inserts an atrial retractor, which the assistant uses to expose the valve. The surgeon grasps the valve with a valve hook or long Allis clamp and excises the cusps with valve scissors or the knife. The chordae tendineae and papillary muscles of the anterior leaflet are cut; the posterior leaflet chordae often are left intact.

The annulus is then measured so that the technologist can obtain the correct size of prosthetic valve from the circulator. The surgeon places the sutures through the annulus and the prosthetic sewing ring using the same technique as described for aortic valve replacement. The valve is then seated in position, and sutures are tied. The atriotomy is closed with continuous suture of size 3-0 polypropylene. Before tying the sutures, the surgeon temporarily releases the vena cava tourniquets and allows the heart to fill with blood. The blood is allowed to spill out of the heart to remove air bubbles. The surgeon then ties the sutures securely. The aortic clamp is removed, and the aorta is aspirated with a vent catheter to ensure that no air remains in the heart.

Cardiopulmonary bypass is discontinued, and the cannulae are removed. A temporary pacemaker electrode may be sutured to the heart. Chest tubes are inserted, and the wound is closed.

Mitral valve replacement is illustrated in Figure 29-48.
Mitral Commissurotomy
Occasionally a mitral **commissurotomy** (opening of the commissures that bring the cusps of the valve together) is performed rather than valve replacement (Figure 29-49). This technique can be used to relieve a stenosis when the valve leaflets are sufficiently flexible to allow it. The procedure is performed during bypass. The surgeon incises the commissures with a knife or breaks them apart with a mitral valve dilator such as the Gerbode or Tubbs dilator to separate the cusps. The atrium then is closed as described for mitral valve replacement.
Mitral Ring Annuloplasty
A dilated mitral valve annulus can be repaired by placement of an annuloplasty ring in the annulus to allow the valve leaflets to come together more efficiently (Figure 29-50). Sutures are placed in the annulus and the annuloplasty ring

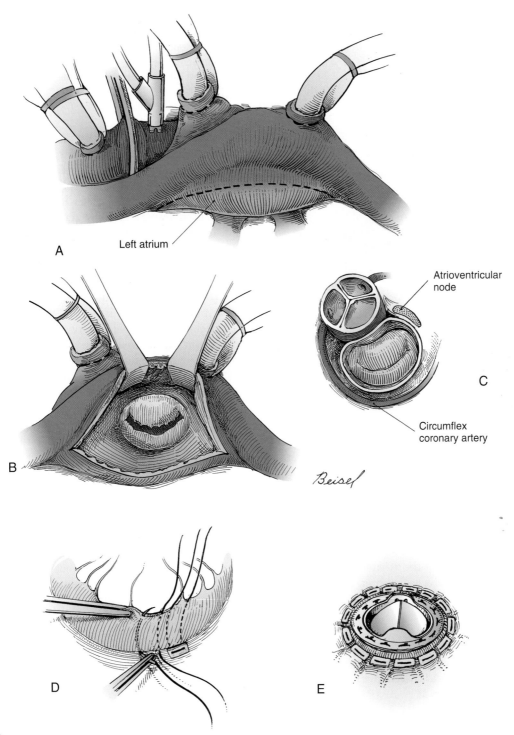

Left atrium

Atrioventricular node

Circumflex coronary artery

Beisel

A

B

C

D

E

FIGURE 29-48
Mitral valve replacement. **A,** Location of incision and cannulation sites for bypass. **B,** Exposure of the valve. **C,** Anatomical re-
lationship between the mitral and aortic valves. **D,** Pledgets are placed with double-armed sutures in native valve annulus.
E, The completed valve replacement illustrating a bi-leaflet prosthesis with pledgets surrounding the prosthetic sewing ring.
(Modified from Waldhausen JA, Pierce WS, and Campbell DB: *Surgery of the chest*, ed 6, St Louis, 1996, Mosby.)

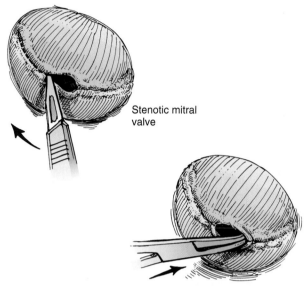

Stenotic mitral valve

FIGURE 29-49
Mitral commissurotomy. (Modified from Rothrock JC: *Alexander's care of the patient in surgery*, ed 12, St Louis, 2003, Mosby.)

and are tied. This procedure reduces the annular orifice, thereby allowing the valve leaflets to close properly.

Tricuspid Valve Replacement or Repair

In replacement procedures, the tricuspid valve is excised and replaced with a prosthetic valve through a right atriotomy. Total cardiopulmonary bypass is required. Tricuspid ring annuloplasty (similar to mitral annuloplasty) is often preferred over replacement.

Resection of Aneurysm of the Ascending Aorta

SURGICAL GOAL

An aneurysm or dissection of the ascending aorta can rupture or prevent the aortic valve leaflets from closing properly. The goal of this procedure is to repair the aneurysm and restore function to the valve.

PATHOLOGY

Arteriosclerosis and atherosclerosis contribute to an aneurysm of the ascending aorta. Aortic dissection results from pathological changes in the aortic wall.

Technique

1. The surgeon performs a median sternotomy.
2. The femoral artery is isolated and cannulated.
3. The venae cavae are cannulated.
4. Total cardiopulmonary bypass is initiated, and a vent catheter of the right superior pulmonary vein is inserted.
5. The aorta is occluded distal to the aneurysm or dissection, and the aortic wall is opened.
6. Retrograde cardioplegia solution is infused; the coronary arteries rarely are directly perfused.

7. A prosthetic graft is anastomosed to the proximal and distal aorta, and the aorta is unclamped.
8. Cardiopulmonary bypass is discontinued, and the cannulae are removed.
9. Chest tubes are inserted, and the wound is closed.

DISCUSSION

A median sternotomy may be performed after the femoral artery and vein have been isolated for cannulation if there is a risk of the aorta rupturing upon the opening of the chest. After cannulation has been completed and the right superior pulmonary vein sump catheter has been inserted, the surgeon occludes the aorta distal to the aneurysm. The aneurysm is opened with scissors, and all clots and debris are removed. If the aorta is dissected, the location of the aortic tear is identified (Figure 29-51, *A*).

Retrograde cardioplegic solution is administered through the coronary sinus. The surgeon examines the aortic valve to determine the extent of injury and to replace it, if necessary. The technologist should have valve instruments available on the set-up tray to avoid delay. Valve suture should be ready for immediate opening if needed.

The surgeon obtains the appropriate-size graft from the technologist and performs the distal anastomosis with a continuous suture of size 3-0 polypropylene (Figure 29-51, *B*). When the anastomosis is complete, the surgeon occludes the graft with a vascular clamp and temporarily releases the aortic clamp to test the suture line. Additional sutures are placed as needed. Teflon felt pledgets are used to reinforce the suture line. If the aneurysm extends into the aortic arch, the arch vessels must be anastomosed to the graft (Figure 29-52).

The surgeon cuts the graft to an appropriate length and performs the proximal anastomosis. Before tying the suture, the surgeon temporarily releases the aortic clamp to fill the graft and flush out air and clots.

The surgeon removes the right superior pulmonary vein sump catheter. After cardiopulmonary bypass has been discontinued, the cannulae are removed. The surgeon may cover the graft with aneurysm tissue. The assistant closes the groin incision while the surgeon inserts chest tubes and closes the sternotomy.

The surgeon occasionally must replace both the aorta and the aortic valve. Special composite graft-valve prostheses are available for these procedures (Figure 29-53).

Resection of Left Ventricular Aneurysm

SURGICAL GOAL

In this procedure, an aneurysm of the left ventricle is resected to reduce the risk of embolization of clots from the aneurysm and to prevent the rupture of the aneurysm.

PATHOLOGY

Aneurysm of the left ventricle is most commonly caused by a reduced blood supply from an infarcted coronary artery.

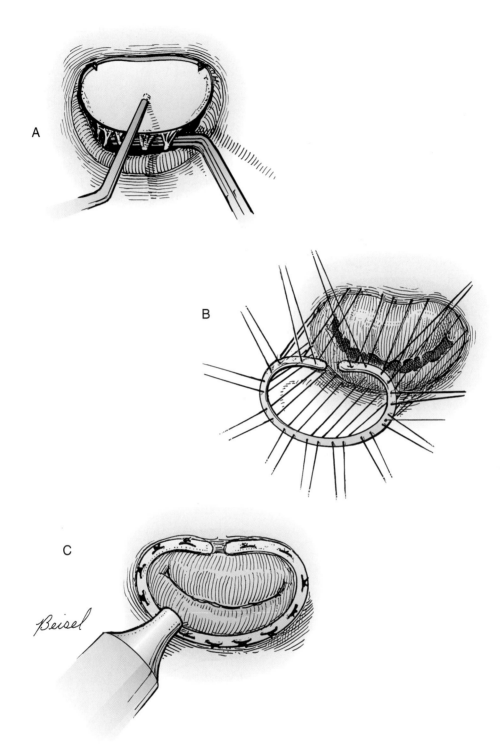

FIGURE 29-50
Mitral valve annuloplasty. **A,** An obturator is used to determine the appropriate size of ring. **B,** Interrupted sutures are placed around the circumference of the annulus and then into the ring. **C,** Ring placement is completed and repaired valve competency is tested with saline-filled bulb syringe. (Modified from Waldhausen JA, Pierce WS, and Campbell DB: *Surgery of the chest,* ed 6, St Louis, 1996, Mosby.)

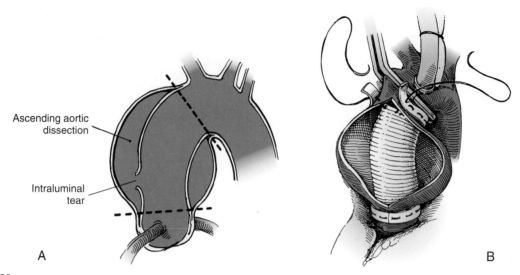

FIGURE 29-51
A, Aortic dissection. **B,** Resection and graft repair of ascending aortic aneurysm. (Modified from Waldhausen JA, Pierce WS, and Campbell DB: *Surgery of the chest,* ed 6, St Louis, 1996, Mosby.)

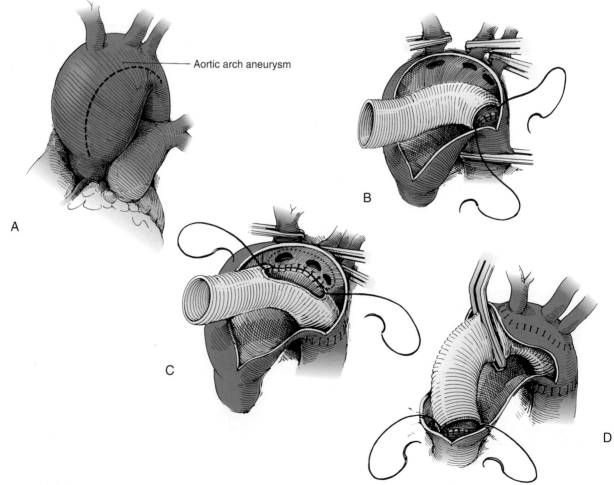

FIGURE 29-52
Repair of aortic arch aneurysm. **A,** Incision. **B,** Distal anastomosis. **C,** Anastomosis of graft to common origin of arch vessels. **D,** Proximal anastomosis. (Modified from Waldhausen JA, Pierce WS, and Campbell DB: *Surgery of the chest,* ed 6, St Louis, 1996, Mosby.)

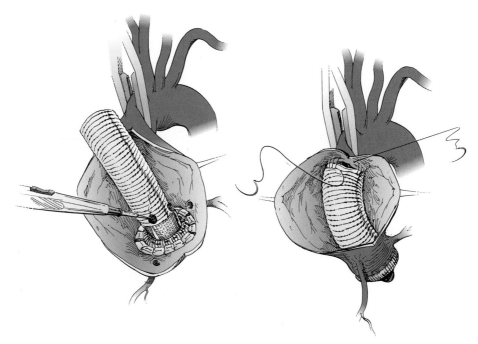

FIGURE 29-53
A composite graft-valve is used in the Bentall-DeBono procedure. (Modified from Townsend CM: *Sabiston textbook of surgery,* ed 16, Philadelphia, 2001, Saunders.)

The surrounding tissue becomes necrotic, softens, and then dilates.

Technique

1. The surgeon performs a median sternotomy.
2. Cannulation and total cardiopulmonary bypass is initiated.
3. A left ventriculotomy is performed, and the aneurysm is resected.
4. The ventricle is closed.
5. The cannulae are removed.
6. Pacer electrodes are sutured to the heart, chest tubes are inserted, and the wound is closed.

DISCUSSION

After a median sternotomy has been performed and bypass has been initiated, the surgeon cross-clamps the ascending aorta and places a laparotomy sponge beneath the heart to elevate the left ventricle. The ventricle is then incised with the long knife, and the incision is extended with curved Mayo scissors. Allis clamps may be applied to the edges of the aneurysm for traction.

The surgeon assesses the mitral valve and removes any clots with forceps or suction. The technologist should keep the instruments clean to prevent clots from entering the bloodstream.

The surgeon then excises the aneurysm tissue with curved Mayo scissors and inserts a Dacron patch to repair the ventricle. An alternate technique is to resect the aneurysm tissue and then bring together the edges of the ventricle with a suture of size 0 polypropylene or polyester. Strips of Teflon felt or pledgets then are incorporated with the suture. A second or third row of sutures is placed through the ventricular edges for a more secure closure. The surgeon decompresses the ventricle using the sump catheter from the heart-lung machine to prevent distension as blood accumulates in the ventricle. The catheter is removed before the final suture is placed. The suture then is tied. The apex of the ventricle may be aspirated with a 19-gauge needle. The wound then is prepared for closure as previously described, and the incision is closed.

Resection of left ventricular aneurysm is illustrated in Figure 29-54.

Pulmonary Valvulotomy
SURGICAL GOAL

Valvulotomy is performed to release fused valve leaflets and restore circulation from the right ventricle to the lungs.

PATHOLOGY

Pulmonary valve stenosis usually is a congenital anomaly in which the right ventricle must work harder to pump blood through the narrowed valve into the pulmonary circulation.

Technique

1. The surgeon performs a median sternotomy and opens the pericardium.
2. Cardiopulmonary bypass is initiated.
3. The venae cavae are encircled with umbilical tapes.
4. The pulmonary artery is opened, and the fused leaflets are separated.
5. The pulmonary artery is closed.

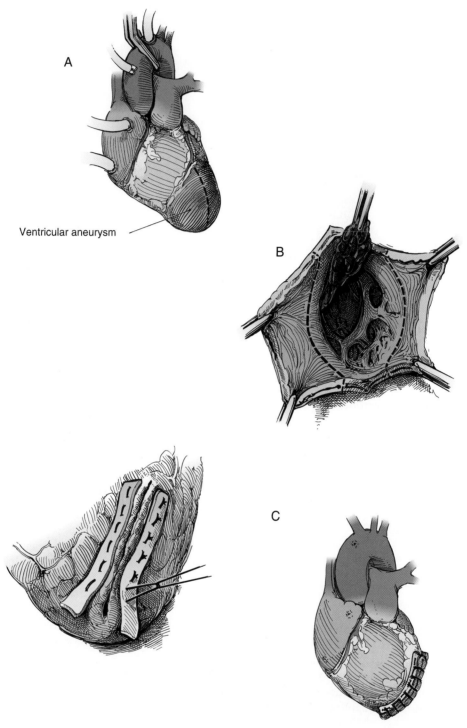

Ventricular aneurysm

FIGURE 29-54
Resection of left ventricular aneurysm. **A,** Placement of the arterial cannula in the ascending aorta, double venous cannulae, and antegrade cardioplegia solution. **B,** The incision is made into the central portion of the aneurysm, and the mural clot is removed. **C,** Linear closure technique of the defect with a side strip of felt on each side of the aneurysm sutured in place, and the two edges brought together and oversewn to complete the repair.

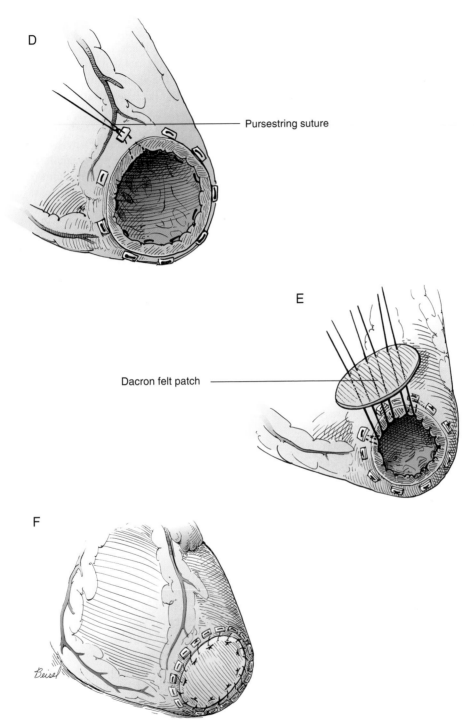

D

Pursestring suture

E

Dacron felt patch

F

Beisel

FIGURE 29-54, cont'd
Resection of left ventricular aneurysm. **D,** Dacron felt patch technique to repair the defect. Placement of purse-string suture with felt pledgets through the thickened rim of the scar. **E,** A patch of woven Dacron polyester is secured with interrupted mattress sutures. **F,** The edge is reinforced with a running polypropylene suture, and the repair is complete. (Modified from Waldhausen JA, Pierce WS, and Campbell DB: *Surgery of the chest,* ed 6, St Louis, 1996, Mosby.)

6. Cardiopulmonary bypass is discontinued, and the wound is prepared for closure.
7. The wound is closed.

DISCUSSION

The surgeon enters the chest through a median sternotomy. The pericardial sac is incised with scissors, and the incision is extended downward to the diaphragm and upward to the innominate vein. Cannulae of the correct size are obtained, and bypass is initiated.

An umbilical tape is placed on the aorta, and a purse-string suture of size 4-0 polypropylene or polyester is placed. The assistant brings the ends of the suture through a **bolster** (short vinyl or Silastic tube used to hold suture ends together) and holds the suture with a hemostat.

Heparin is administered to the patient. Bicaval venous cannulation and aortic cannulation are performed as described above. Cardiopulmonary bypass is begun.

To begin the repair, the surgeon isolates the vena cava with umbilical tapes, and a tourniquet is placed as previously described. The surgeon opens the pulmonary artery above the valve with scissors. The aorta may be temporarily occluded to create a drier field. The fused leaflets are separated with a knife, Metzenbaum scissors, or Potts scissors. The surgeon closes the pulmonary artery with continuous suture (often of size 5-0). If the pulmonary artery is stenotic, a piece of prosthetic graft may be inserted to enlarge the artery.

Refer to Figure 29-55 for illustrations of this procedure.

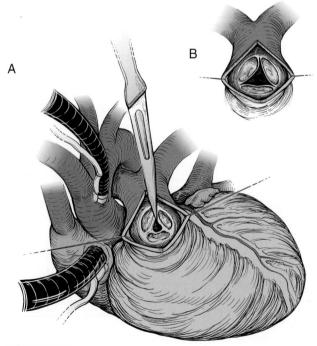

FIGURE 29-55
Pulmonary valvulotomy. **A,** Fused leaflet commissures are incised to the pulmonary artery wall. **B,** Completed valvulotomy. (Modified from Mavroudis C and Backer CL: *Pediatric cardiac surgery,* ed 3, St Louis, 2003, Mosby.)

Closure of Atrial Septal Defect
SURGICAL GOAL

Atrial septal defect is a congenital anomaly in which a hole in the interatrial septum allows blood from the left atrium to flow to the right atrium. The goal of surgery is to close the defect and reduce excessive blood flow to the lungs.

PATHOLOGY

Blood normally flows from the left atrium to the left ventricle before entering the systemic circulation. An atrial septal defect causes the blood to shunt from the left atrium to the right atrium. This creates increased pressure on the right ventricle and lungs, causing the heart to enlarge and eventually fail. Atrial septal defect usually is closed surgically during childhood. However, some patients reach adulthood before developing symptoms that require surgical repair.

Technique

1. The surgeon performs a median sternotomy.
2. Total cardiopulmonary bypass is initiated.
3. The aorta is occluded.
4. A right atriotomy is performed, the defect is closed, and the atriotomy is closed.
5. Cardiopulmonary bypass is discontinued, and the wound is prepared for closure.
6. The wound is closed.

DISCUSSION

The patient is prepped and draped for a median sternotomy. The sternotomy is performed, and bypass is initiated. The surgeon may fibrillate the heart and occlude the aorta before performing a right atriotomy. A Cooley (adults) or Richardson (pediatric) retractor is placed in the wound, and the surgeon examines the defect. Additional supplies may be needed depending on this assessment.

The surgeon may repair the defect with a primary closure (infants) or by inserting a patch or pericardial graft (older children, adults) (Figure 29-56). Large defects require a patch graft, which is cut to size and sutured in place with polypropylene or nylon sutures. Air is removed from the left side of the heart before final sutures are placed and tied.

Bypass is discontinued, and the wound is prepared for closure. The incision then is closed in layers.

Closure of Ventricular Septal Defect
SURGICAL GOAL

A ventricular septal defect causes increased pulmonary pressure by allowing blood from the left ventricle to flow into the right ventricle and to the lungs, leading to congestive heart failure. The septal defect is repaired to restore normal cardiac circulation.

PATHOLOGY

A ventricular septal defect is a hole in the intraventricular septum and can occur in a variety of locations (Figure

29-57). The higher pressure in the left ventricle causes blood to flow through the defect into the area of lower pressure, the right ventricle. The increased volume of blood in the right ventricle creates a volume overload in the lungs and can cause congestive heart failure. Surgical closure of the defect is performed most often in the pediatric patient although post–myocardial infarction ventricular septal defects can occur in the adult patient.

Technique

1. The surgeon performs a median sternotomy.
2. Cannulation for total cardiopulmonary bypass is performed.
3. The aorta is occluded, and cardioplegic solution is infused into the coronary arteries.
4. A ventriculotomy is performed, and the defect is closed.
5. The aorta is unclamped, and the ventricle is closed.
6. Bypass is discontinued, and the cannulae are removed.
7. A temporary pacemaker electrode is sutured to the heart.
8. Chest tubes are inserted, and the wound is closed.

DISCUSSION

The surgeon performs a median sternotomy and cannulates for total cardiopulmonary bypass for the pediatric patient as described above.

The surgeon occludes the aorta with a pediatric vascular clamp and infuses retrograde cardioplegia solution through the coronary sinus. A right ventriculotomy is performed with the knife or Mayo scissors. The surgeon may place sutures through the edges of the ventricle for traction.

The defect is assessed, and a patch graft is sutured into place. Teflon pledgets may be used to reinforce the suture line. Air is removed from the left ventricle before final closure.

After removing the aortic clamp, the surgeon closes the ventricle with continuous suture. Bypass is discontinued,

and the cannulae are removed. A temporary pacemaker lead may be sutured to the right ventricle and right atrium. Chest tubes are inserted, and the wound is closed.

Total Correction of Tetralogy of Fallot
SURGICAL GOAL

Tetralogy of Fallot is a combination of congenital defects that include pulmonary stenosis, ventricular septal defect, right ventricular hypertrophy, and dextraposition (displacement) of the aorta. The surgical repair is performed to correct cyanosis and restore normal blood flow.

PATHOLOGY

Tetralogy of Fallot causes cyanosis as a result of reduced pulmonary blood flow and the right-to-left shunting (from the right ventricle to the left ventricle) of blood. This shunting results in the mixing of deoxygenated blood with oxygenated blood; this mixed blood then is pumped into the systemic circulation. The right ventricle becomes **hypertrophied** (enlarged) because of the work needed to pump the blood through the obstructed pulmonary system. Patients are cyanotic, and any increase in oxygen demand results in reduced pulmonary blood flow. It is best to correct the defects early in infancy. If delayed repair is necessary, a systemic-pulmonary shunt may be performed to increase blood flow

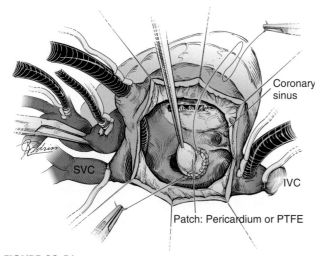

FIGURE 29-56
Closure of atrial septal defect. (Modified from Mavroudis C and Backer CL: *Pediatric cardiac surgery,* ed 3, St Louis, 2003, Mosby.)

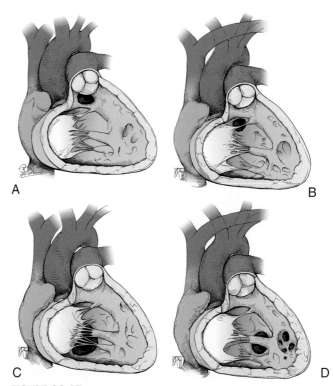

FIGURE 29-57
Types of ventricular septal defects. **A,** Type I (conal, supracristal, infundibular, subarterial). **B,** Type II or paramembranous. **C,** Type III (atrioventricular canal type or inlet septum type). **D,** Type IV (single or multiple), also called muscular. (Modified from Mavroudis C and Backer CL: *Pediatric cardiac surgery,* ed 3, St Louis, 2003, Mosby.)

to the lungs. This shunt improves oxygenation and allows the baby to grow to a stage at which total correction is possible.

Technique

1. The surgeon performs a median sternotomy.
2. Bypass is initiated.
3. Cardioplegia is performed.
4. A right ventriculotomy is performed, the infundibular muscle is resected, and a pulmonary valvulotomy is performed.
5. The ventricular septal defect is closed, and the right ventricle is closed with a patch.
6. Bypass is discontinued.
7. A temporary pacemaker lead is inserted.
8. Chest tubes are inserted, and the wound is closed.

DISCUSSION

The incision used for this procedure depends on whether a palliative shunt previously was performed. Total correction in the absence of a previous shunt is performed through a median sternotomy. After the chest has been opened, bypass is initiated. Cardioplegia then is performed as previously described.

The surgeon performs the right ventriculotomy using a knife and curved Mayo scissors. Retractors are inserted, and a portion of the infundibular muscle is excised. The technologist should wipe all instruments clean after use to prevent emboli from forming.

A pulmonary vavulotomy then is performed, and the ventricular septal defect is closed as previously described. After air is evacuated from the left ventricle, the clamp is removed from the aorta.

The surgeon closes the ventricle with a continuous suture of polypropylene of size 4-0. A patch of woven Dacron or Teflon is used to enlarge the right ventricular outflow tract (area beneath the pulmonary valve). The pulmonary artery also may be enlarged with a patch, using a suture of a smaller size.

Pulmonary artery pressure and right ventricular pressure are measured to determine whether the surgery was successful. If the results indicate that additional surgery is required, additional surgical supplies are needed.

After successful surgery, bypass is discontinued and the wound is prepared for closure as described previously. Chest tubes are inserted, and the wound is closed.

Highlights of this procedure are illustrated in Figure 29-58.

Insertion and Removal of Intraaortic Balloon Catheter

SURGICAL GOAL

The intraaortic balloon catheter reduces the workload of the heart after myocardial infarction or in patients who cannot be taken off of bypass.

PATHOLOGY

The intraaortic balloon catheter is inserted retrogradely via the femoral artery into the descending thoracic aorta. The distal tip of the catheter should be positioned just below the

left subclavian artery. The balloon increases the supply of oxygen to the heart by increasing coronary blood flow during diastole and improves distal perfusion of the body's organs. When the ventricle contracts, the balloon deflates, creating a vacuum that lowers the pressure in the aorta. When the ventricle relaxes, the balloon inflates, increasing the volume of blood into the coronary arteries and distal organs (Figure 29-59). This produces additional blood flow to the brain, kidneys, and other organs. The size of the balloon is determined by the size of the femoral artery.

Technique

Insertion

1. The femoral artery is exposed and isolated through a groin incision.
2. The surgeon ties a heavy silk suture around the proximal end of the balloon catheter to mark the level of insertion.
3. The femoral artery and branches are occluded, and the artery is incised.
4. The catheter is inserted into the femoral artery and advanced into the descending thoracic aorta up almost to the left subclavian artery.

Removal

1. The groin is reopened, and the femoral artery is isolated.
2. The balloon catheter is withdrawn, and the artery is occluded.
3. The femoral artery is unclamped, and the wound is closed.

DISCUSSION

Insertion

The patient is placed in the supine position, prepped, and draped for a bilateral femoral incision. This is a precaution in case the first attempt to insert the balloon percutaneously is not possible because of aortoiliac stenosis. The procedure is performed under local anesthesia or during cardiac surgery if the heart requires support.

The groin is incised, and the incision is carried to the femoral artery and branches with sharp and blunt dissection. A small self-retaining retractor is placed in the wound. The common femoral artery and branches are mobilized with dissecting scissors, and umbilical tapes or vessel loops are placed around the vessels for traction. Bolsters may be inserted over the loops and the ends tagged.

The surgeon measures the catheter against the distance between the patient's subclavian artery and the femoral artery. He or she then marks this level by tying a suture around the proximal end of the catheter. The catheter is deflated with a syringe before insertion.

The femoral arteries then are occluded with vascular clamps such as Glover or DeBakey peripheral vascular clamps, or the umbilical tapes are used as tourniquets. The surgeon makes an incision in the common femoral artery with a #11 blade. Potts scissors are used to extend the incision as needed.

The scrub moistens the balloon with saline solution. The proximal clamp is removed from the artery, and the

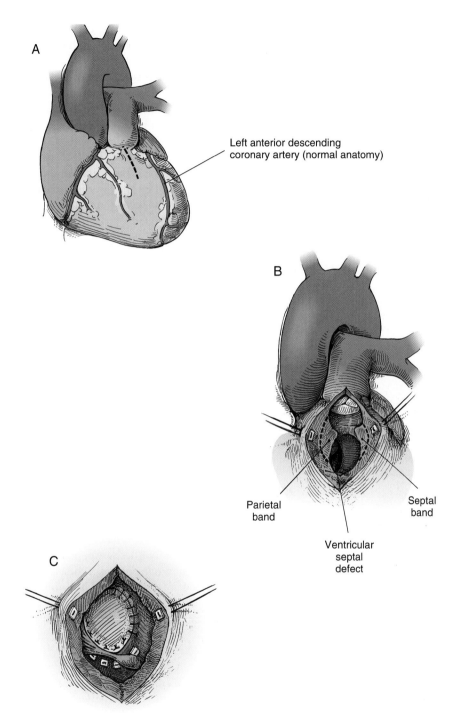

FIGURE 29-58
Total correction of tetralogy of Fallot. **A,** Location of incision for exposure of the ventricular septal defect. **B,** Incision into the ventricular septal defect, with excision of the hypertrophied parietal and septal bands. **C,** Closure of the ventricular septal defect with mattress sutures.   *Continued*

surgeon inserts the catheter into the arteriotomy. The catheter then is advanced to the level of the suture mark. The assistant controls bleeding while holding tension on the umbilical tape.

The pump technician evacuates the atmospheric air from the catheter with a 50-ml syringe, and the pump is activated.

The surgeon secures the catheter to the patient's leg with size 2-0 silk suture. The wound may be irrigated with antibiotic solution.

The wound is closed in layers with absorbable and non-absorbable sutures. A pressure dressing is applied to prevent hematoma.

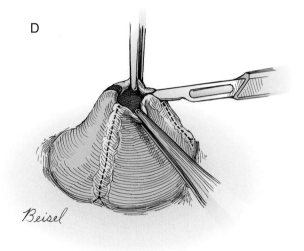

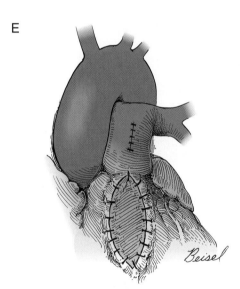

FIGURE 29-58, cont'd
Total correction of tetralogy of Fallot. **D,** The dome-shaped pulmonary valve is inverted, and the fused commissures are incised. **E,** The outflow tract is closed with a pericardial patch. (Modified from Waldhausen JA, Pierce WS, and Campbell DB: *Surgery of the chest,* ed 6, St Louis, 1996, Mosby.)

Removal

The previous wound is reopened, and the femoral artery is isolated. The balloon is deflated, and the catheter is slowly withdrawn. The femoral artery is occluded, and the incision is oversewn with continuous suture of polypropylene in size 5-0. Two sutures may be used. One suture is started at one side of the incision, and the other suture is started on the opposite side; the two sutures are tied in the center of the femoral artery incision.

Ventricular Assist Device
SURGICAL GOAL

A ventricular assist device (VAD) is used to wean patients from the cardiopulmonary bypass when other means are ineffective. Patients awaiting a heart transplant also may be candidates for VAD, which may consist of a polyurethane blood sac, flexible diaphragm, and pump assembly. The VAD maintains perfusion through cannulae that are placed into the chambers of the heart and the great vessels according to the patient's need. Power is provided by pneumatic, electric, or battery-powered pumps.

DISCUSSION

During *left ventricular assistance,* blood is directed from the left ventricle through the inflow cannula and into the assist device, and returned to the ascending aorta through the outflow cannula (Figure 29-60). Inflow and outflow are distinguished by the direction of the blood flow relative to the VAD pump. Some VAD pumps can be implanted in the chest cavity. Drivelines from the pump exit through incisions in the chest.

During *right ventricular assistance,* blood is directed from the right atrium into the pump and into the pulmonary artery. The outflow cannula is sutured to the pulmonary artery. During *biventricular assistance,* both left ventricular and right ventricular devices support both ventricles simultaneously.

An extracorporeal VAD is used for temporary, short-term assistance. The pump is connected to inflow and outflow cannulae that are passed into the thoracic cavity through the chest wall. The pump itself is secured to the outer chest wall and covered with an occlusive dressing. An implantable VAD is used for long-term support and utilizes a pump that is implanted into the patient's chest or abdomen. If a battery pack is used, it is external and its cannulae are passed through the abdomen. VADs may be used as a bridge to transplant, as an investigational tool, or as end-stage therapy.

Heart Transplantation
SURGICAL GOAL

Excision of the native heart and replacement with a donor heart is indicated for patients with end-stage cardiac disease. Other surgical modalities (such as VAD support) often are employed before transplantation.

Technique	HEART PROCUREMENT

1. The donor is prepped from chin to knees.
2. The surgeon performs a median sternotomy.
3. A sternal retractor is inserted.
4. The pericardium is divided.
5. Umbilical tapes are placed around the aorta and the superior and inferior venae cavae.
6. Heparin is given.

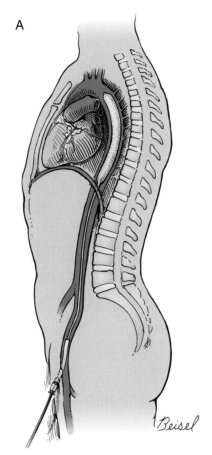

A

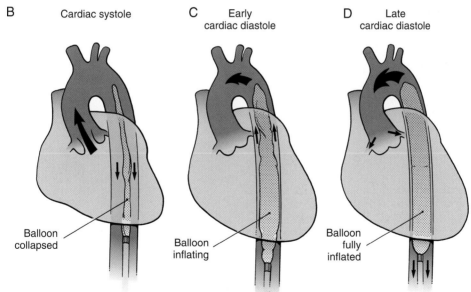

B   Cardiac systole

Balloon
collapsed

C   Early
cardiac diastole

Balloon
inflating

D   Late
cardiac diastole

Balloon
fully
inflated

FIGURE 29-59
Phases of balloon pumping. **A,** Placement of balloon in descending aorta. **B,** Deflation of balloon. **C,** Early inflation of balloon.
D, Completed inflation of balloon. (Modified from Waldhausen JA, Pierce WS, and Campbell DB: *Surgery of the chest,* ed 6,
St Louis, 1996, Mosby.)

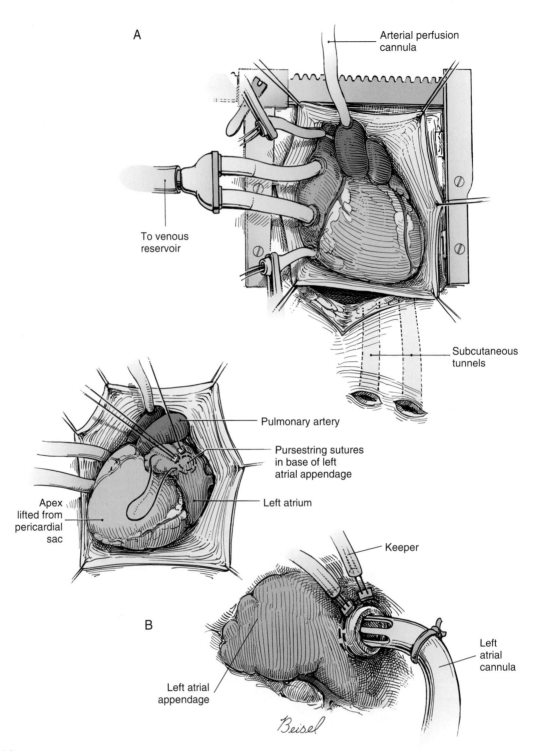

FIGURE 29-60
Left ventricular assistance. **A,** Tunnels are developed from the pericardial space to the skin in preparation for placement of the arterial and atrial cannulas. **B,** Two purse-string sutures are placed at the neck of the left atrial appendage, the atrium is incised, and the atrial cannula is inserted.

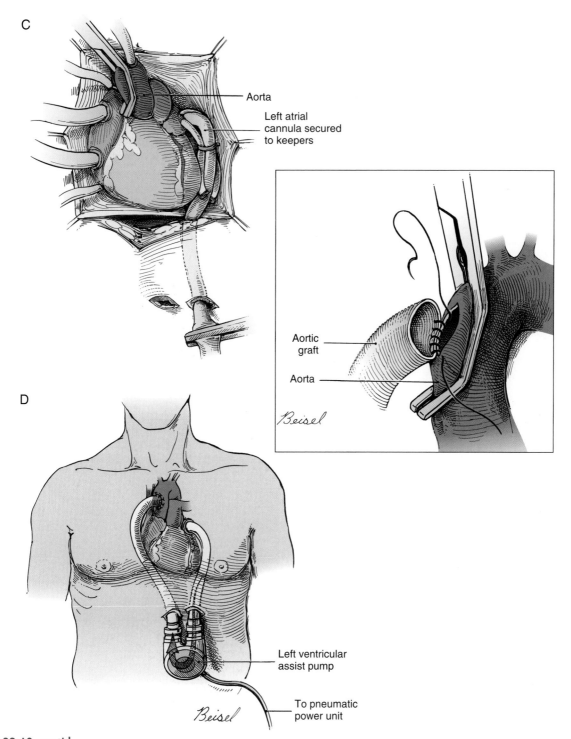

C

Aorta

Left atrial
cannula secured
to keepers

Aortic
graft

Aorta

Beisel

D

Left ventricular
assist pump

To pneumatic
power unit

Beisel

FIGURE 29-60, cont'd
Left ventricular assistance. **C,** The Dacron graft portion of the composite arterial cannula is anastomosed to the side of the ascending aorta. The cannula is clamped and passed through the medial subcostal tunnel. **D,** Attachment of the pump. (Modified from Waldhausen JA, Pierce WS, and Campbell DB: *Surgery of the chest,* ed 6, St Louis, 1996, Mosby.)

7. The aorta, the superior and inferior venae cava, and the main pulmonary artery are dissected.

8. The superior vena cava is ligated with heavy silk ties.

9. Cardioplegia solution is infused through the proximal aorta into the heart via the coronary arteries.

10. The venae cavae and the aorta are divided; the heart is lifted to expose the pulmonary veins. The veins are divided.

11. The pulmonary artery is divided just distal to the bifurcation.

12. The heart is removed and placed in a sterile bag containing cold preservative solution.

DISCUSSION

Two types of cardiac transplantation can be performed. *Orthotopic* transplantation is performed more often and is the replacement of one heart with another (Figure 29-61). *Heterotopic* ("piggy back") transplantation is the insertion of a second (donor) heart into the recipient patient's right pleural cavity (Figure 29-62). The donor heart works in tandem with the recipient's native heart. This procedure occasionally is performed when there is a significant size mismatch between a small donor and a large recipient. Combined heart-lung procedures also may be performed.

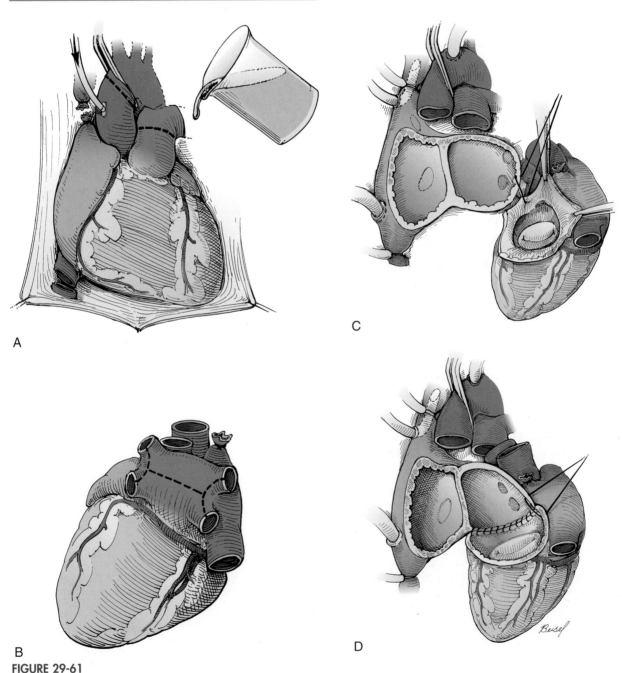

FIGURE 29-61
Orthotopic heart transplantation. **A,** Incision lines in the donor heart. **B,** Posterior portion of heart incision lines connecting pulmonary veins. **C** and **D,** Left atrial anastomosis.

As with other transplantation procedures, it is important to minimize any delay in removing the donor heart and transporting it to the recipient.

NATIVE HEART EXCISION

1. The recipient patient is placed in the supine position and prepped from chin to knees.
2. A median sternotomy incision is made to expose the heart and great vessels.
3. Heparin is given.
4. Bicaval cannulation for cardiopulmonary bypass is performed.
5. Caval tapes are placed around each vena cava.
6. The patient is cooled, the aorta is cross-clamped, and the caval tapes are tightened around the venae cavae.
7. The pulmonary trunk and aorta are divided.
8. The atria are incised to leave intact the posterior portions of the right and left atrial walls and the interatrial septum.
9. The recipient's native heart is excised.

DISCUSSION

The native (recipient) heart is not removed until the donor procurement team has confirmed that the donor heart is acceptable. Unexpected problems occasionally may appear with the donor heart that preclude its use as a donor organ. Tissue-matching protocols must be scrupulously followed to avoid donor-recipient mismatch.

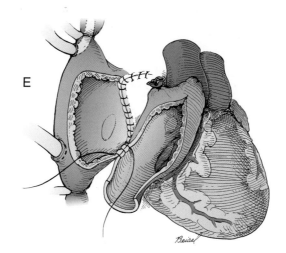

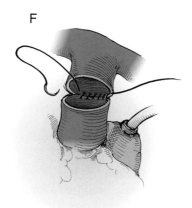

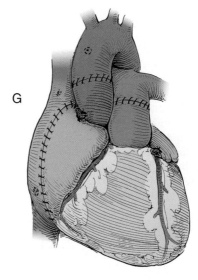

FIGURE 29-61, cont'd
Orthotopic heart transplantation. **E,** Right atrial anastomosis. **F,** Pulmonary artery anastomosis. **G,** Completed transplant. (Modified from Waldhausen JA, Pierce WS, and Campbell DB: *Surgery of the chest,* ed 6, St Louis, 1996, Mosby.)

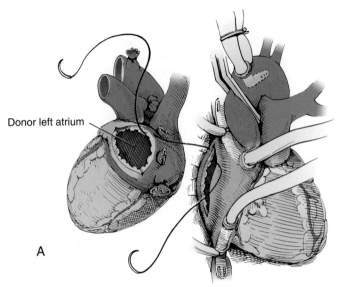

Donor left atrium

A

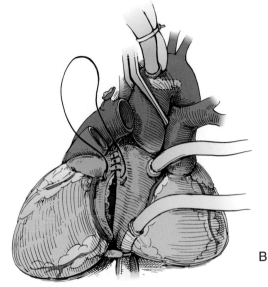

B

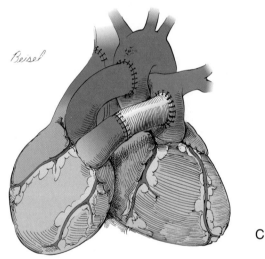

C

FIGURE 29-62
Heterotopic heart transplantation. **A** and **B,** Left atrial anastomoses. **C,** Aortic and pulmonary artery anastomoses. (Modified from Waldhausen JA, Pierce WS, and Campbell DB: *Surgery of the chest,* ed 6, St Louis, 1996, Mosby.)

Technique   DONOR HEART IMPLANTATION

1. The donor heart is removed from the transport container and placed in a basin on the back table.
2. The surgeon inspects the heart and trims the atrial walls and great vessels in preparation for the anastomoses.
3. The donor heart is placed in the pericardial cavity and aligned with the remnant interatrial septum and the right and left atrial wall remnants of the recipient's heart.
4. The donor left atrial wall is anastomosed with a running 3-0 polypropylene suture (suture size and type may vary according to surgeon preference).
5. The right atrial wall is anastomosed with a running 3-0 polypropylene suture, followed by the pulmonary artery anastomosis with a 4-0 polypropylene suture.
6. The aorta is anastomosed with a 3-0 running polypropylene suture.
7. Air is removed from the heart.
8. Chest drainage tubes and epicardial pacing wires are inserted.
9. The chest incision is closed.

DISCUSSION

A pulmonary pressure monitoring line may be inserted before the patient leaves the operating room. Postoperatively, the patient is placed on life-long immunosuppression medication therapy to prevent rejection of the donor heart. Endomyocardial biopsies are taken regularly to monitor for rejection.

A modification of the orthotopic implantation technique has been developed that reduces some of the cardiac rhythm problems that have occurred after transplantation. End-to-end anastomoses between the superior vena cava and the inferior vena cava are performed rather than the traditional

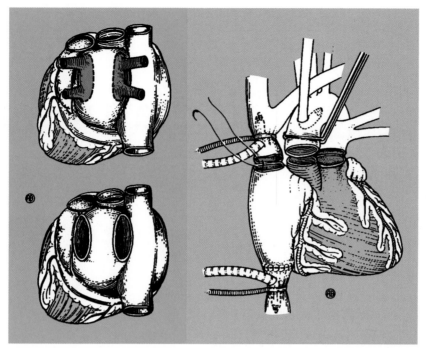

FIGURE 29-63
Modified heart transplantation technique with caval anastomoses and pulmonary venous anastomoses. (From Braunwald E, Zipes DP, and Libby P, eds: *Heart disease: a textbook of cardiovascular medicine,* ed 6, Philadelphia, 2001, Saunders.)

atrial-to-atrial anastomoses (Figure 29-63). A cuff of the recipient left atrium is sewn to the donor left atrium; pulmonary artery and aorta anastomoses are performed in the usual manner.

REFERENCES

Altman L: Brazil surgeon develops a bold, promising operation for patients with heart failure, *New York Times* June 14, 1996, p A16.

Berne RM, Levy MN: *Cardiovascular physiology,* ed 8, St Louis, 2001, Mosby.

Braunwald E, Zipes DP, and Libby P: *Heart disease: a textbook of cardiovascular medicine,* ed 6, Philadelphia, 2001, WB Saunders.

Cameron A, Davis KB, Green G, et al: Coronary bypass surgery with internal-thoracic-artery grafts—effects on survival over a 15-year period, *N Engl J Med* 334 (4):216-219, 1996.

Carpentier A: Cardiac valve surgery: the French correction, *J Thorac Cardiovasc Surg* 86:323, 1983.

Chapek PE: A review of minimally invasive cardiac surgery, *Semin Periop Nurs* 6 (3):165-169, 1997.

Cooley DA, Frazier OH, Kadipasaoglu KA, et al: Transmyocardial laser revascularization: clinical experience with twelve-month follow-up, *J Thorac Cardiovasc Surg* 111 (4):791-799, 1996.

Coulson AS, Quarnstrom JA, Holmes K, et al: Right thoracotomy approach to mitral valve surgical procedures, *AORN J* 65 (2):347-364, 1997.

Crawford ES: The diagnosis and management of aortic dissection, *J Am Med Assoc* 264 (9):2537, 1990.

David TE, Feindel CM, Armstrong S, et al: Reconstruction of the mitral annulus: a ten-year experience. *J Thorac Cardiovasc Surg* 110:1323-1332, 1995.

Dickstein ML, Spotnitz HM, Rose EA, et al: Heart reduction surgery: an analysis of the impact on cardiac function, *J Thorac Cardiovasc Surg* 113:1032-1040, 1997.

Doty DB: *Cardiac surgery: operative technique,* St Louis, 1997, Mosby.

Fremes SE, Christakis GT, Del Rizzo DF, et al: The technique of radial artery bypass grafting and early clinical results, *J Cardiac Surg* 10:537-544, 1995.

Harding A and Silver D: Thoracic outlet syndrome. In Sabiston DC, ed: *Textbook of surgery,* ed 14, Philadelphia, 1991, WB Saunders, pp 1757-1761.

Julian DG and Wenger NK: *Women and heart disease,* St Louis, 1997, Mosby.

Kouchoukos NT, Blackstone EH, Doty DB, et al: *Cardiac surgery,* ed 3, Philadelphia, 2003, Churchill Livingstone.

Mavroudis C and Backer CL: *Pediatric cardiac surgery,* ed 3, St Louis, 2003, Mosby.

Moghissi K, Thorpe JAC, and Cuilli F, eds: *Moghissi's essentials of thoracic and cardiac surgery,* ed 2, New York, 2003, Elsevier.

Phippen ML and Wells MP: *Perioperative nursing practice,* Philadelphia, 1994, WB Saunders.

Piwnica A and Westaby S, eds: *Surgery for acquired aortic valve disease,* Oxford, 1997, Isis Medical Media.

Seifert PC: *Cardiac surgery,* St Louis, 2002, Mosby.

Seifert PC: Cardiac surgery. In Rothrock JC, ed: *Alexander's care of the patient in surgery,* ed 12, St Louis, 2003, Mosby.

Vongpatanasin W, Hillis LD, and Lange RA: Prosthetic heart valves, *N Engl J Med* 335 (6):407-416, 1996.

Waldhausen JA, Pierce WS, and Campbell DB: *Johnson's surgery of the chest,* ed 6, St Louis, 1996, Mosby.

Wieczorek P, Riegel MB, Quattro L, et al: Marfan's syndrome and surgical repair of ascending aortic aneurysms, *AORN J* 64 (6):895-913, 1997.

Wisniowski C and Stephen L: Minimally invasive treatment for coronary artery disease, *AORN J* 66 (6):1002-1009, 1997.

Zenati M, Domit TM, Saul M, et al: Resource utilization for minimally invasive direct and standard coronary artery bypass grafting, *Ann Thorac Surg* 63:S84-S87, 1997.

Chapter 30

Pediatric Surgery

By Margaret Mulcrone

Learning Objectives

After studying this chapter the reader will be able to:

- Understand the difference between pediatric and adult patient physiology
- Assist in setting up for pediatric surgical procedures
- Assist in pediatric surgical procedures reviewed in this chapter
- Recognize instruments commonly used in pediatric surgery
- Recognize the supplies and equipment commonly needed for any pediatric surgery
- Understand the importance of hemostasis in pediatric surgery

Terminology

Aganglionic—Without nerve tissue.

Atresia—A congenital absence or closure of a normal body opening or tubular structure.

Atrioventricular—Pertaining to both the atrium and ventricle.

Branchial cleft cyst—A cavity that is a remnant from embryologic development, present at birth in one side of the neck just in front of, and on either side of, the large angulated muscle (the sternocleidomastoid muscle).

Choanal—The communicating passageways between the nasal fossae and pharynx.

Coarctation—Narrowing of the passageway of a blood vessel, such as coarctation of the aorta, a congenital condition.

Ductus arteriosus—A normal fetal structure, allowing blood to bypass circulation to the lungs. If this structure re-

mains open after birth, it is called a patent ductus arteriosus.

Endocardial cushion—Areas of the fibrous skeleton forming between the atrium and ventricle.

Exstrophy—The eversion or turning out of any organ.

Gastroschisis—The herniation of abdominal contents through the abdominal wall without involvement of the umbilical cord.

Intussusception—The telescoping of one portion of the intestine into another.

Midgut—The middle part of the alimentary canal from the stomach, or entrance of the bile duct, to, or including, the large intestine.

Nephroblastoma—Wilms' tumor.

Omphalocele—A protrusion of abdominal contents through an opening at the navel, especially occurring as a congenital defect.

Pyloric stenosis—A narrowing of the part of the stomach (pylorus) that leads to the small intestines.

Sternocleidomastoid—One of two muscles located on the front of the neck that serve to turn the head from side to side.

Syndactyly—A congenital condition present at birth in which fingers or toes are fused.

Thermogenesis—The production of body heat.

Thyroglossal duct—A transitory endodermal tube in the embryo, carrying thyroid-forming tissue at its caudal end. The duct normally disappears after the thyroid has moved to its ultimate location in the neck; its point of origin is regularly marked on the base of the adult tongue by the foramen cecum.

INTRODUCTION TO PEDIATRIC SURGERY

The care of the pediatric patient is a distinctive and separate specialty. Pediatric patients range from newborns, infants, and children through adolescents. In addition, pediatric patients differ from each other according to age, body weight, and physiological development. Pediatric patients do not act like adults in their physiological and psychological responses and so should not be treated as such.

Pediatric patients typically are grouped according to the following biological age groups:

Neonate	Birth to 1 month
Infant	up to 18 months
Toddler	19 months to 3 years
Preschooler	4 to 6 years
School-age child	7 to 12 years
Adolescent	13 to 16 years

Pediatric surgery involves all surgical specialties and usually is classified into three major surgical groups of defects or diseases: (1) congenital anomalies, (2) systemic and specific organ infections or disease, malignant tumors, or benign lesions, and (3) trauma or accidental injuries.

PHYSIOLOGICAL NEEDS

Airway and Pulmonary Management

Airway management is a priority because of the smaller diameter of the trachea in children. The development of cartilage before the growth of muscle also makes the airway more prone to collapse than in the adult. In the lungs, alveolar maturation is not complete in the child until 8 to 10 years of age. Thus, to satisfy increased oxygen demand, alveolar ventilation in children is twice that of adults. Consequently, if cold stress, hypoglycemia, hypovolemia, or sepsis occurs, the young child is prone to respiratory arrest.

Cardiovascular

The heart rate differs widely among infants, toddlers, and preschoolers and varies with activity versus rest. The infant younger than 1 year of age tolerates a heart rate of 200 to 250 beats per minute without hemodynamic consequence. Disturbance in heart rhythm is uncommon unless a cardiac anomaly is present. Cardiac complications occur with respiratory conditions more often than with cardiac dysfunction.

Temperature Regulation

It is not easy to maintain the body temperature of the young pediatric patient. The pediatric patient, especially the neonate, tends to become hypothermic during anesthesia and the surgical procedure. Heat regulation is difficult because the young child suffers heat loss through a variety of factors. Young children have a larger surface area in relation to body size. They have only a thin layer of subcutaneous fat. Their ability to produce heat is much less because they do not have the ability to shiver and do not have chemical thermogenesis in brown adipose tissue.

Metabolism

The resting metabolic rate of an infant is two to three times that of an adult. This increased metabolic rate in infants and toddlers often consumes their already meager energy source. Glycogen, the energy source, usually is stored immediately before birth. Glycogen stores can be lower in children who are small for gestational age and those with malnutrition and hypoxia. In the young child, cold stress, sepsis, and hypoxia add to the metabolic and energy requirements. In surgery, complications increase proportionately with the increased time of fluid restriction because infants and toddlers are prone to hypovolemia and dehydration. Procedures on infants and toddlers should have priority on the surgical schedule so that these pediatric patients may return to a normal feeding and fluid regimen.

Fluid and Electrolyte Balance

The maintenance of proper fluid balance in the child is a serious physiological need. Infants have a comparatively larger ratio of body-surface area to body mass than adults. In addition, increased evaporative water losses result from the greater surface area and thin epidermis of the child. When children become dehydrated, which can occur rapidly, body functions become disturbed, as does the acid–base balance. Fluid and electrolyte replacement is necessary. Children have a larger percentage of their body weight in extracellular water than do adults. Infants can have 70% to 90% of their body weight in water. The child's higher metabolic rate also makes the need for fluids greater than in adults. In addition, children have a limited renal function because the glomerular filtration rate is 25% of that of an adult. Thus the kidneys of children are immature and have a lesser ability to concentrate urine.

PSYCHOLOGICAL NEEDS

Children differ from adults in their psychological responses and reactions to procedures and the environment. Children often experience some common fears in responding to hospitalization and surgery. The immediate fear is separation from loved ones and things. Other fears common to the pediatric surgical patient are feelings of abandonment, thoughts of punishment, and fear of rejection. The real and fantasy fears of pain and injury, including all the apprehensions about surgical procedures, injections, anesthesia, and surgery, are great psychological concerns of the pediatric patient.

GENERAL CONSIDERATIONS

Because of the unique qualities of the pediatric patient, the surgical technologist must be aware of several factors that affect the outcome of the surgical event. These factors include, but are not limited to, metabolism, fluid and electrolyte balance, temperature regulation, cardiovascular and pulmonary responses, infection safety, and pain management. Following are some recommendations for providing care to the pediatric patient:

▶ Maintain the child's body temperature.
▶ Transport neonates and infants in a heated isolette.
▶ Regulate the OR temperature at least 10 minutes before the start of the procedure. The room temperature should be kept at 85° F (29.4° C).
▶ For the premature or critically ill patient, the room temperature should be kept at 85° F (29.4° C).
▶ Use thermal blankets, head covering, wrapping of the extremities, a radiant heat lamp, or a combination of these to help preserve body heat.
▶ Warm the IV, irrigation, and skin-prep solutions before administering or using them.
▶ Monitor external and/or internal body temperature throughout the surgical procedure.
▶ Monitor fluids and electrolytes.
▶ Accurately measure all irrigation solutions used.
▶ Weigh sponges.
▶ Report all fluid and blood loss to anesthesia provider for prompt intervention.
▶ Effectively use suture material and the electrosurgical pencil to achieve hemostasis and to identify and clamp bleeding vessels.
▶ Be prepared to use hemostatic agents.
▶ Ensure safety measures and proper positioning of the patient.
▶ Never leave a child unattended on the operating table.
▶ For small infants and neonates, drop the foot and/or head of the operating bed to produce easier access to the patient.
▶ Avoid hyperextension and/or hyperflexion of the joint areas.
▶ Prevent cardiovascular compromise or respiratory embarrassment while the patient is restrained.
▶ Adhere to skin-care precautions to avoid chemical burns and skin breakdown.
▶ Do not allow solutions to pool under the patient.
▶ Avoid direct application of adhesive tape whenever possible.
▶ Pad pressure points.

SPECIAL EQUIPMENT AND SUPPLIES

Instruments

Very small and delicate instruments must be used to protect and preserve anatomical structures. Lightweight instruments should be used to avoid inhibiting or restricting the pediatric patient's bodily functions (e.g., breathing, circulation, nervous system). In addition, instruments should never be laid on top of the patient when not in use, because they could restrict circulation to the area or cause bruising. Needle holders have fine-pointed jaws to hold small, delicate needles. When the pediatric patient is an adolescent, the instruments used in the surgical procedure may need to be adult size.

Draping

Disposable drape sheets without a fenestration often are preferred. The surgeon can create the opening to fit the proposed surgical approach, especially for neonates and small infants. Towels with small towel clips and a pediatric drape sheet may be used for most surgical procedures involving children, while adult drape sheets usually are preferred for adolescents.

Sponges

Raytec sponges often are used with small lap sponges (4 × 8) in place of the large laparotomy sponges. Dissector sponges (Kitners) often are used for blunt dissection, preserving surrounding structures.

Electrosurgery

The electrosurgical unit (ESU) may be replaced by a hand-held battery-operated cautery unit for neonatal and infant surgery, or a fine-tipped bipolar cautery may be used. If the surgeon prefers the ESU, a pediatric grounding pad is chosen based on the size of the patient.

Sutures

Sutures ranging from size 0-0-0 to 5-0 are used most often for delicate, fragile tissue. The material can be either absorbable or nonabsorbable, depending on the wound need, and is swaged to a ½-inch or ⅜-inch circle needle. A subcuticular closure usually is performed, with small Steri-Strips used to help approximate the skin edges.

Catheters

When needed for the pediatric patient, catheters as small as 8 Fr are available. For urinary retention, a Foley catheter with a 3-ml balloon is preferred. If a stomach tube is needed, a plain or whistle-tipped catheter may be used, depending on the surgeon's preference.

Dressings

Because adhesive tape often is abrasive to young, tender skin, a topical skin adhesive, or collodion, often is used with Steri-Strips over a small incision (especially when a subcuticular closure has been used).

Medication and IV Fluids

In the treatment of the pediatric patient, most dosages of medications and intravenous fluids are based on the child's body weight.

SURGICAL PROCEDURES

Choanal Atresia
SURGICAL GOAL

Surgical repair of choanal atresia is performed to restore the normal nasal passage and prevent damage to growing structures that are important in facial development.

PATHOLOGY

Choanal atresia is a congenital anomaly of the anterior skull base characterized by closure of one or both posterior nasal cavities. It causes a narrowing or blockage of the nasal airway by membranous or bony tissue (Figure 30-1). This condition occurs in 1 out of every 7000 to 8000 live births. Unilateral atresia with a right-side predominance appears in 60% of reported cases. The newborn may be known as an "obligate nose breather," meaning he or she must breathe through the nose because the oral airway has not yet developed sufficiently to allow for frequent mouth breathing. Choanal atresia generally is recognized shortly after birth while the infant is still in the hospital.

Choanal atresia that blocks both sides (bilateral) of the nose causes acute breathing problems with cyanosis and breathing failure. Bilateral choanal atresia causes respiratory distress at birth. Most newborns with the condition require early intubation. Bilateral choanal atresia should be repaired shortly after birth.

Most unilateral cases are isolated anomalies. Blockage on only one side causes less severe problems. A unilateral case may go undiagnosed until the child presents with persistent unilateral nasal drainage. Repairs of unilateral choanal atresia are performed at about 2 to 3 years of age.

Surgical procedures to correct choanal atresia can be broadly classified into transnasal and transpalatal approaches. The choice of approach is based on the surgeon's assessment of the choanal anatomy. The transpalatal approach is described here.

Technique

1. Under general anesthesia, the patient is positioned, prepped, and draped.
2. The nasopharynx is exposed through a U-shaped incision in the mucosa of the hard palate.

3. The mucosal flap is elevated to the posterior edge of the hard palate, and the soft palate muscular layer is incised where it inserts into the posterior edge of the hard palate.
4. The surgeon uses a drill to remove the bone along the posterior edge of the hard palate, vomer, and pterygoid region.
5. Nasal mucosal flaps are elevated and preserved.
6. Stents then are positioned through the new choanal opening and secured with the anterior ends of the stent just within the nasal vestibule.
7. The nasal stents usually are removed under general anesthesia 6 to 10 weeks after repair.

DISCUSSION

The transnasal approach requires less operative time and causes slightly less morbidity related to the incision. The transnasal procedure is best for thin membranous atresias in older children. It does not allow sufficient exposure for extensive bone removal. The transnasal puncture, with or without a microscope, has become unpopular because of the high rate of failure requiring revision resulting from the insufficient exposure of the choanal area. In the transseptal technique, a window is made in the septum anterior to the atretic plate. The transpalatal approach produces better exposure and more accurate bone removal. The palatal incision increases operative time and blood loss.

The transpalatal approach possibly reduces the risk of major vascular injury, intracranial complications, and restenosis. The transpalatal approach is best for thick bony atresia, for bilateral atresias in neonates, and in cases in which there are anomalies affecting the anterior nasal cavities or nasopharynx. Transpalatal repair is a technique that produces excellent exposure and has a high success rate but requires more operative time. Increased blood loss and risk of palatal fistula, palatal dysfunction, and maxillofacial growth disturbance are drawbacks of this procedure.

Endoscopic technique (nasal or retropalatal), with or without powered instrumentation, offers excellent visualization with great ease in the removal of the bony choanae. This technique has excellent long-term results.

Branchial Cleft Cyst
SURGICAL GOAL

In this procedure, the branchial cleft cyst is surgically excised.

PATHOLOGY

A branchial cleft cyst is an embryonic developmental defect that develops from the primitive branchial apparatus (branchial arch, cleft, and pouches). These abnormalities usually result from the incomplete closure of the branchial plate between the cleft and pouch (Figure 30-2). These anomalies typically are lined with stratified squamous epithelium and contain other dermal structures such as hair follicles, sweat glands, and sebaceous glands.

Branchial cysts, sinuses, and fistulas can become apparent at any age but are seen more often in childhood or young adulthood. The cyst is not more common in either gender,

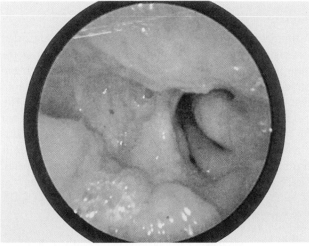

FIGURE 30-1
Nasopharyngoscopic view of an infant with unilateral choanal atresia. The left choana is clearly patent, but the right is atretic. (From Zitelli BJ, Davis HW: *Atlas of pediatric physical diagnosis,* ed 4, St Louis, 2002, Mosby.)

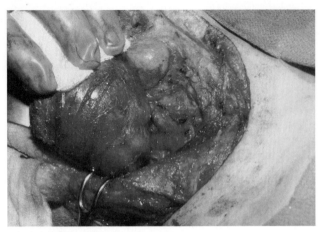

FIGURE 30-2
Intraoperative photograph of a branchial cleft cyst in an infant. (From Townsend CM, Beauchamp D, Evers BM et al: *Sabiston textbook of surgery*, ed 17, Philadelphia, 2004, Saunders.)

and only rare familial occurrence has been noted; 2% to 3% of cases are bilateral.

Branchial cleft cysts, sinuses, and fistulas are classified into first, second, third, or fourth branchial abnormalities.

First branchial abnormalities are located near or in contact with the external auditory canal and are divided into two types by their location. These cysts account for 8% of branchial abnormalities.

Second branchial cleft cysts make up the majority of branchial abnormalities. The external opening or cyst is found along the anterior border of the sternocleidomastoid muscle. The tract passes superior and lateral to the carotid artery, cranial nerve (CN) IX, and CN XII. Superior to CN IX, the path turns medial between the internal and external branches of the carotid artery. The tract may end near the middle constrictor muscle or may open into the oropharynx in the area of the tonsillar fossa.

Third branchial cleft cysts are rare. These abnormalities also are found along the anterior border of the sternocleidomastoid muscle and are lateral and superior to the common carotid. The tract of these abnormalities travels lateral and superior to CN XII before traveling posterior and medial to the internal carotid artery. It continues to track medial to the thyrohyoid membrane and opens into the piriform sinus.

Fourth branchial cleft cysts are extremely rare. A left-side abnormality would start from its opening in the apex of the piriform sinus, travel inferiorly into the mediastinum, loop posteriorly around the aortic arch, track superiorly into the neck of the carotid artery, pass superior to CN XII, again descend in the neck, and exit in the skin anterior to the lower portion of the sternocleidomastoid muscle. On the right, the tract would loop around the right subclavian artery before ascending in the neck.

Technique

1. Before incision, the cyst is filled with methylene blue to facilitate dissection. A Fogarty catheter sometimes is used to facilitate dissection.

2. The surgeon creates a stepladder incision for removal of the benign lesion (cyst).
3. An elliptical incision is made around the external opening of the sinus tract or fistula.
4. An adequate amount of supporting connective tissue around the tract is excised in a cephalad (head) direction up to the point at which the second parallel stepladder incision is made.
5. If suspected recurrent neck abscesses have resulted from an infected branchial pouch sinus, tonsillectomy from the internal tract may be performed.
6. With the first branchial anomaly operation, a superficial parotidectomy and facial nerve dissection may be performed.

DISCUSSION

General anesthesia usually is recommended because of the complexity of the dissection. The patient is positioned supine with a shoulder roll for hyperextension of the neck to better expose the surgical site. Depending on the surgeon's preference, the area from the chin to the nipples may be prepped.

Every effort is made to minimize the scar because it is a benign lesion, but adequate surgical exposure is needed to remove the cyst. The stepladder incision technique is used to help minimize the scar. Careful dissection is vital to preserve the nerves and arteries of the region.

Complications of operations for branchial anomalies include secondary infection and damage to nearby anatomical structures, including facial, recurrent laryngeal, hypoglossal, spinal accessory, and glossopharyngeal nerves.

Thyroglossal Duct Cyst
SURGICAL GOAL

In this procedure, the thyroglossal duct cyst, as well as the thyroglossal tract up to the base of the tongue, is excised.

PATHOLOGY

A thyroglossal duct cyst is a freely movable cystic mass that lies high in the neck at the midline and is attached to the base of the tongue. The cyst usually is located near the hyoid bone. It is the most common malformation of the thyroid that requires surgical intervention. A few are present at birth, but most present in early childhood. Most children present for medical evaluation because of a mass in the neck that is identified by its elevation in the neck when the tongue is protruded. Males are affected more often than females. Nearly one third of these lesions contain thyroid tissue.

Technique

1. The surgeon makes a skin incision in the center of the neck along the natural skin crease near the cyst.
2. A superior and inferior flap is created to expose the cyst. The superior flap is elevated to the level of the hyoid bone, and the inferior flap is elevated until the inferior portion of the cyst is identified.

3. The strap muscles are separated, and the cyst is dissected from the surrounding structures until it is attached only to the hyoid bone superiorly.
4. Muscle is removed from around the body of the hyoid bone and then transected on each side of the pedicle.
5. A curved retractor is placed orally, which facilitates excision of the tract up to the base of the tongue with the addition of a 5-mm to 10-mm core of muscle.
6. The incision is closed with a Penrose drain in place, and the neck is wrapped with a pressure dressing at the end of the operation.

DISCUSSION

The primary management technique for thyroglossal duct cysts is surgical excision. The procedure of choice is the Sistrunk procedure. The Sistrunk procedure includes excision of the cyst in continuity with the mid portion of the body of the hyoid bone and a small block of muscle around the foramen cecum (base of the tongue).

The procedure is performed under general anesthesia. The patient is placed in the supine position with a shoulder roll in place.

If the infection is secondary to abscess formation, the patient will need to return to surgery for incision and drainage, or repeated aspiration in combination with antibiotic treatment may be required.

Coarctation of the Aorta
SURGICAL GOAL

In this procedure, the narrow section of the aorta is removed, and the two severed ends of the aorta are sewn together or joined with a graft

PATHOLOGY

Coarctation of the aorta is a birth defect in which the aorta is narrowed somewhere along its length, most often just past the point where the aorta and the subclavian artery meet. The aorta is the main artery that sends oxygen-rich blood from the heart to the body. Coarctation of the aorta is a constriction of a segment of the aorta, obstructing the flow of blood to the body (Figure 30-3). As a result, the left ventricle must pump harder because the resistance is greater. If not treated, this increased workload may contribute to enlargement of the heart. Coarctations typically occur as isolated defects but also may occur with a ventricular septal defect, subaortic stenosis, or complex congenital heart defect.

Coarctation usually occurs in a short segment of the aorta just beyond the point at which the arteries to the head and arms branch off, as the aorta arches inferiorly toward the abdomen and legs. Coarctation occurs in the "juxtaductal" part of the aorta, the part near the point at which the ductus arteriosus attaches.

Coarctation forces the left ventricle to work harder. It must generate higher pressure than normal to force blood through the narrow segment of the aorta to the lower part of the body.

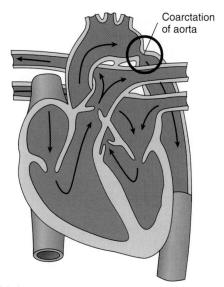

FIGURE 30-3
Coarctation of the aorta. (From Wong DL: *Nursing care of infants and children,* ed 7, St Louis, 2003, Mosby.)

In approximately 50% of cases of isolated coarctation, the problem is severe enough to cause symptoms in the first day of life coinciding with the time the ductus arteriosus closes. If the coarctation is not detected in the newborn, it may go unrecognized for many years in some cases. Aortic coarctation occurs in approximately 1 out of 10,000 people. It usually is diagnosed in children or adults under 40. Early surgical intervention (before 10 years of age) usually is advised. Today, coarctation typically is diagnosed and surgically repaired during infancy.

A surgeon may repair the area of coarctation in several ways:

▶ The narrowed area of the aorta may be removed and the two ends reconnected (end-to-end anastomosis).
▶ A patch may be added to the aorta to enlarge it (patch augmentation).
▶ A bypass-like graft may be placed in the area of narrowing (jump graft).
▶ The area of coarctation may be removed and replaced (tube graft).
▶ Rarely, an ascending-to-descending aortic bypass graft may be used to bypass an area of narrowing in the aorta. This can be performed from a different approach and allows the surgeon to perform valve replacement simultaneously.

The resection and end-to-end anastomosis is the preferred surgical method and is described here.

Technique

1. Under anesthesia, the patient is placed in the right lateral position, prepped, and draped.
2. An incision is made on the left side of the chest, between the ribs and below the armpit.

3. The left chest is entered through an incision between the ribs. The ribs are gently spread, the pleura is incised, and the lung is gently moved aside.
4. The surgeon continues careful dissection with fine vascular forceps to visualize and mobilize the aorta. The laryngeal nerve is identified and protected. The ductus arteriosus is ligated and divided between ductus clamps.
5. The aorta is cross-clamped above and below the obstruction, and the narrow segment is resected.
6. The two ends of the aorta are reanastomosed with a continuous, everting mattress technique for the posterior wall and interrupted, everting mattress sutures for the anterior wall. Clamps are removed slowly, and flow through the aorta is reestablished.
7. If the segment with the coarctation is short or if a longer segment must be removed, a Dacron (a synthetic material) graft is used to fill the gap.
8. A small chest tube then is placed for drainage, and the chest incision is closed. Dressing is applied.

DISCUSSION

Repair of aortic coarctation usually is performed via a left thoracotomy without cardiopulmonary bypass. Thoracotomies sometimes require the use of a heart-lung cardiac bypass machine that delivers oxygen to the body while the heart is stopped for repair of the coarctation. It may be possible to perform the surgery without the use of cardiac bypass, depending on the severity of the coarctation and the repair.

A number of techniques are available for repair of the coarctation. With resection and end-to-end anastomosis, still the preferred surgical method, the aorta is isolated and the aortic isthmus and ductal tissue are resected. The distal aortic arch is incised along its inferior side, the lower aorta is incised along its lateral side, and the two are sewn together. The advantages of end-to-end technique are that the subclavian artery is not sacrificed, and complete relief of obstruction is easily obtained.

During the minimally invasive procedure, which takes approximately 4 hours, the patient is sedated and a small, thin, flexible tube (catheter) is inserted into a blood vessel in the groin and guided to the area of the coarctation. When the catheter is in position, a balloon at the tip of the catheter is inflated. The balloon pushes open and stretches the narrow segment, improving blood flow. The balloon then is deflated, and the catheter with balloon is guided back out of the body. In some patients, a stent also is placed in the dilated area to hold it open.

Tracheoesophageal Fistula
SURGICAL GOAL

In this procedure, congenital defects of the airway and the digestive tract, esophageal atresia and tracheoesophageal fistula (TEF) respectively, are repaired.

PATHOLOGY

TEF is an abnormal opening between the trachea and esophagus. Esophageal atresia often is associated with TEF.

Esophageal atresia is characterized by incomplete formation of the esophagus or a pouch. There are many anatomical variations of esophageal atresia with TEF. The most common fistula occurs at the upper segment of the esophagus, ending in a blind pouch with the lower segment of the esophagus connected by a fistula to the trachea. This congenital anomaly is thought to occur in 1 in 1500 to 3000 infants. Associated congenital anomalies of the heart, gastrointestinal tract, and nervous system are common.

The neonate with TEF (with esophageal atresia) experiences episodes of rattling respirations, coughing, choking, and cyanosis. The episodes may be exaggerated during feeding. Abdominal distension develops as air builds up in the stomach. Prompt surgical intervention may prevent respiratory and eating difficulties.

Technique

1. The surgeon may need to perform a gastrostomy first to decompress the air-distended stomach.
2. If a transpleural approach is used, a right posterolateral incision is made over the fifth rib and the pleura is entered via the fourth intercostal space.
3. The mediastinal pleura is incised, and the lower esophagus is exposed and mobilized.
4. The surgeon transects, closes, and tests the TEF for air leaks by filling the chest with a small amount of saline.
5. Depending on the diameter and thickness of the upper and lower muscular wall segments, esophageal continuity is established by one of several one-layer or two-layer techniques.
6. A small gastrostomy feeding tube may be passed transnasally into the esophagus, across the anastomotic site, and into the stomach for postoperative feeding.
7. A chest tube is positioned, and the incision is closed.
8. If the chest is entered retropleurally, a chest tube is not necessary, but a small Penrose drain may be inserted close to the anastomosis and brought out through the lateral corner of the wound.

DISCUSSION

The patient is placed on his or her left side with the right arm extended above the head. The patient is prepped with iodophor-povidone solution and draped.

A colon interposition may be necessary if the distance between anomalies is too great.

Wilms' Tumor
SURGICAL GOAL

In this procedure, an entire intraabdominal tumor and involved surrounding tissue are excised.

PATHOLOGY

Wilms' tumor, also known as nephroblastoma, is the most common intraabdominal childhood tumor. It presents as a painless mass whose enlargement may laterally distend the abdomen. Often, the pediatrician on routine exam or a parent while playing with the child will notice a large, firm mass

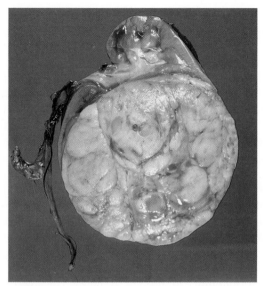

FIGURE 30-4
Pediatric adenosarcoma, called Wilms' tumor, pictured here in the lower pole of the kidney. Note the tumor's tan to gray color and its confined margins. (From Kumar V, Cotran R, Robbins S: *Basic pathology,* ed 7, Philadelphia, 2002, Saunders.)

below the rib cage on either the right or left side of the abdomen (Figure 30-4).

The tumor may spread from the abdomen to the lungs, which is the most common site of distant spread. Most of these tumors can be initially resected, particularly if they are on one side only. If the tumor extends from the kidney to the vena cava, preoperative chemotherapy is preferred to shrink the tumor and reduce the risk to the patient. Of these patients, 5% to 7% may have bilateral tumors. If the tumor involves only one kidney and does not extend into the vena cava, the treatment of choice is to remove the kidney and connecting lymph nodes. Bilateral tumors are biopsied, and chemotherapy is instituted before partial or total resection of the kidney.

Technique

1. The transabdominal approach, which may be extended to a combined transabdominal-transthoracic approach, is used to inspect abdominal contents and clamp the vessels of the renal pedicle before tumor dissection.
2. All suspicious lymph nodes are removed, placed into separate containers, and labeled. If no suspicious nodes are present, biopsy specimens are obtained of nodes in adjacent areas.
3. The opposite kidney is explored before dissection of the tumor.
4. The extent of the tumor can be marked with hemostatic clips to facilitate radiation therapy.
5. The entire primary tumor is removed if doing so does not place the patient in jeopardy.
6. Any residual tumor is marked with clips.

7. Because of its proximity to the kidney, the adrenal gland usually is removed.
8. The abdominal cavity and viscera are thoroughly inspected for evidence of tumor extension or metastases. Extensive surgery may include partial colectomy or partial resection of the diaphragm.
9. After hemostasis is secure and the abdomen has been thoroughly explored, closure is performed without drainage.

DISCUSSION

The child is positioned supine with a roll under the affected side. Both chest and abdomen are prepped and draped. Infrequently the tumor extends into the inferior vena cava as well as the atrium, and in such cases cardiopulmonary bypass should be available. Because of the possible need to clamp the vena cava, lines are placed into the arm and neck. Clean gloves and instruments should be available for inspection of the contralateral kidney. Careful attention should be given when handling tumor and lymph nodes to avoid spillage.

Pyloromyotomy
SURGICAL GOAL

A pyloromyotomy is the incision and suturing of the muscles of the pylorus to treat congenital hypertrophy of the pyloric sphincter (pyloric stenosis), which can cause pyloric and/or gastric obstruction. The Ramstedt-Fredet pyloromyotomy is the procedure of choice to correct the defect surgically.

PATHOLOGY

Pyloric stenosis is seen most often in infants 2 to 4 weeks of age. There is a strong familial association. Males are affected four times as often as females, with a high incidence of the disorder occurring in first-born males.

Signs and symptoms of high gastrointestinal obstruction usually appear at about 2 to 6 weeks of age, with the first symptoms being projectile vomiting that is free of bile. The vomitus usually does not contain bile because the obstruction occurs proximal to the ampulla of Vater. The hypertrophied muscle usually can be palpated as a firm, movable mass in the right upper quadrant. Other associated symptoms include dehydration, weight loss, and general failure to thrive. Peristalsis often can be identified by involuntary wavelike movement of the alimentary canal. On barium swallow examination, diagnosis is made from evidence of active peristalsis with delayed or absent emptying.

In the Ramstedt procedure, the muscle of the hypertrophic pylorus is split, leaving the mucosa intact.

Technique

1. A right upper (subcostal) transverse incision is made through subcutaneous tissue; through external oblique, internal oblique, and transversus abdominis muscles; and through the peritoneum.
2. The liver edge is retracted superiorly to expose the greater curvature of the stomach (near the pylorus), which is

grasped with a noncrushing clamp and brought out through the incision.

3. A damp gauze sponge is used to grasp the stomach, and with traction inferiorly and laterally, the pylorus can be delivered through the incision.

4. The surgeon then makes the incision through the muscle of the anterior pylorus from the junction of the pylorus and duodenum to the antrum of the stomach.

5. A blunt instrument (often curved jaws of the hemostat or a pyloric spreader) is used to split the muscle fibers, with care taken to avoid perforation of the mucosa. Air can be placed in the stomach per nasogastric tube to check for perforation.

6. The pylorus is returned to the abdominal cavity and, after verification of hemostasis, the incision is closed with running absorbable suture.

7. The skin is closed with subcuticular suture.

8. Adhesive strips and possibly a small dressing are applied.

DISCUSSION

General anesthesia is given via an endotracheal tube. Before induction of anesthesia, the stomach is aspirated. The patient is positioned supine. The chest and abdomen are prepped with an iodophor-povidone solution and then draped.

The surgeon makes a right upper quadrant transverse incision of approximately 2.5 to 3 cm over the right rectus muscle just superior to the liver edge. The fascial layers are divided transversely, but the rectus muscle is either retracted laterally or split in the middle. The liver edge is retracted superiorly, exposing the greater curvature of the stomach (near the pylorus), which is grasped with a noncrushing clamp and brought out through the incision. A damp gauze sponge is used to grasp the stomach, and with traction inferiorly and laterally, the pylorus is delivered through the incision. Grasping the duodenum or pylorus directly with a forceps may result in injury or perforation and therefore is to be avoided.

The serosa on the anterior wall of the hypertrophied pylorus is incised with a scalpel from just proximal to the pyloric vein to the antrum just proximal to the area of hypertrophied muscle down to the level of the submucosa. A careful check for a leak in the stomach or duodenum is performed before the pylorus is returned to the peritoneal cavity.

For better cosmetic appearance, some surgeons make a supraumbilical, curvilinear incision. This incision, however, is associated with a higher incidence of wound-related complications.

With improvements in technical equipment and surgical skills in minimally invasive techniques, laparoscopic techniques are increasingly becoming available for use with children and infants. Although operating times initially may be longer and complications may occur, operating times and results for laparoscopic pyloromyotomy are improving with experience, and the patients enjoy the benefits of minimally invasive surgery: reduced surgical stress, improved patient recovery, shortened hospital stay, and superior cosmetic results.

Gastroschisis
SURGICAL GOAL

In this procedure, the abdominal contents are returned into the abdominal cavity. A Silastic pouch may be placed over the abdominal contents to contain the bowel and aid in the reduction until surgical closure.

PATHOLOGY

Gastroschisis is an abdominal wall defect caused by the failure of the abdominal wall to develop just to the right of the umbilical ring (the most common site). All abdominal wall layers are missing, including the peritoneum. The bowel is herniated outside the abdomen without a covering (Figure 30-5). The abdominal cavity is underdeveloped because of the extraabdominal location of the bowel. The bowel has no peritoneal or skin coverage to protect it from the amniotic fluid, which causes chemical irritation and inflammation of the peritoneum, which may cause peritonitis. Bowel malrotation and other anomalies may occur.

Technique

1. The patient is placed in the supine position. The chest and abdomen are prepped and draped.

2. The surgeon makes the incision.

3. The surgeon carefully inspects the intestines.

4. The bowel lying outside the abdomen and not covered by peritoneum may be debrided because of chemical peritonitis. But if debridement cannot be performed, a bowel resection may be performed.

5. The abdominal contents are inspected for any other abnormalities. Any intestinal atresia detected is resected, and primary anastomosis is completed.

6. The bowel is returned to the abdominal cavity, and primary closure is attempted.

7. The fascia is approximated with interrupted nonabsorbable monofilament (or delayed absorbing sutures).

8. The skin is closed with absorbable subcuticular suture to produce optimal cosmetic results. An umbilicoplasty may be performed at the time of skin closure.

9. If the abdominal wall is too tight to allow primary closure, a "silo" of material such as Silastic sheeting may be constructed, which is sutured (with monofilament suture) to the abdominal wall (rectus fascia) at the margins of the defect.

10. After the silo is constructed, it is wrapped with sterile gauze soaked in povidone-iodine for support. Thick gauze is applied to protect the silo and prevent evaporation and contamination.

DISCUSSION

Surgery is performed with the patient under general endotracheal anesthesia with muscle relaxation. An orogastric tube is placed for decompression of the gastrointestinal tract.

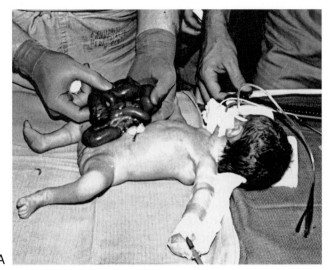

A

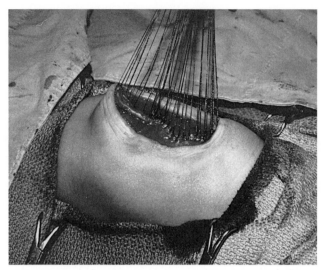

B

FIGURE 30-5
A, An infant with gastroschisis. **B,** Closure of the fascia in an infant with gastroschisis. (From Ashcraft KW, Holcomb GW, Murphy JP: *Pediatric surgery,* ed 4, Philadelphia, 2005, Saunders.)

After the intestines have been inspected, the diaphragm is carefully examined because a diaphragmatic hernia may not be apparent until the intestine is returned to the abdominal cavity. The loops of intestine are carefully returned to the abdominal cavity, with care taken to orient the mesentery correctly to avoid twisting and vascular compromise of the intestines. If the liver is herniated, the surgeon must be careful not to kink or injure the hepatic veins, obstruct the stomach, or compress the inferior vena cava.

If staged prosthetic closure is chosen for treatment, Dacron-reinforced Silastic sheeting is used to construct the silo. As much intestine as possible is returned to the abdominal cavity. The Silastic sheeting is sutured to the abdominal wall. All skin is saved and not sutured to the Silastic sheeting. The surgeon then constructs a closed silo around the remaining exposed intestine by stapling or suturing the sheet to itself. The silo is placed perpendicular to the defect, and the upper end of the silo, tied with an umbilical tape, is kept parallel to avoid a constriction at the base of the silo where the prosthesis joins the abdominal wall. The silo is compressed daily, forcing the abdominal contents to gradually enter the abdominal cavity until primary closure is obtained.

In some cases a skin expander is placed into the peritoneal cavity for several days. After the expander progressively enlarges a sufficient volume of skin, the expander is removed and the abdomen is closed.

Omphalocele
SURGICAL GOAL
In this procedure, the abdominal contents are returned through the abdominal wall and the abdomen is surgically closed.

PATHOLOGY
An omphalocele is a congenital malformation in which variable amounts of abdominal contents protrude into the base

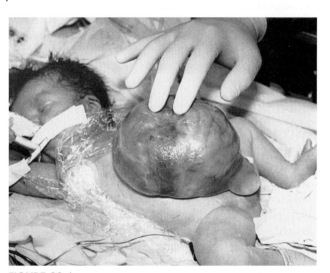

FIGURE 30-6
A newborn with a giant omphalocele that contains both liver and intestine. (From Ashcraft KW, Holcomb GW, Murphy JP: *Pediatric surgery,* ed 4, Philadelphia, 2005, Saunders.)

of the umbilical cord. The omphalocele is covered by a clear sac or membrane. The size and extent of the omphalocele can vary from one containing the greater portion of the abdominal viscera, including the spleen and liver, to one containing only a small loop of bowel or intestines. The condition results from a herniation through a midline defect in the abdominal wall around the area of the umbilicus (Figure 30-6).

Usually there is no skin covering the defect, which greatly increases the incidence of a life-threatening infection for the already compromised infant. Additional congenital anomalies usually are present in these pediatric patients, and depending on the capability of the abdominal cavity to contain the contents of the omphalocele, a one-stage or two-stage procedure may be performed.

Technique

Single-stage repair (small omphalocele)

1. The omphalocele is covered with a warm saline laparotomy sponge.
2. The surgeon makes an incision separating the skin from the peripheral borders of the sac.
3. The hernia sac is separated from the sac contents.
4. Bowel contents are returned to the abdominal cavity after they are inspected for abnormalities.
5. The base of the hernia sac is ligated, and excess sac is removed.
6. The umbilical vessels are ligated, and the sac and rim of the defect are excised.
7. The abdominal contents are reduced within the abdomen, and the abdomen is closed routinely.

Two-stage repair (large omphalocele)

1. When the defect cannot be closed and/or the abdominal cavity cannot safely accommodate the contents of the omphalocele, an attempt is made to mobilize the surrounding skin to cover the protruding viscera.
2. If this is impossible, the surgeon uses a synthetic material (e.g., Silastic or silicon mesh) to cover the defect by suturing it around and over the viscera.
3. As growth permits (age 6 to 24 months) an initial repair procedure may be performed, requiring one or two additional procedures.

DISCUSSION

Close attention must be paid to maintaining the body temperature of the massive exposed surface area from which the body can lose heat. The use of nitrous oxide as an anesthetic agent is avoided during the procedure because it causes increased gas in the intestines, which in turn makes the reduction of abdominal contents into the peritoneal cavity more difficult.

Surgery is performed with the patient under general endotracheal anesthesia with muscle relaxation. The infant is positioned supine; the abdomen, umbilical cord, and sac are gently prepped with a povidone-iodine prep solution and rinsed with warm, sterile saline to reduce any bacterial contamination. Rectal irrigation with warm, sterile saline helps to evacuate any meconium from the intestines and reduce intestinal mass. The skin is prepped, and the infant is draped for the surgical procedure. A Foley catheter is inserted after the sterile field has been established.

When only small defects have been treated, primary closure is attempted after abdominal contents have been gently returned to the peritoneal cavity. The abdominal cavity is closed with 3-0 nonabsorbable suture.

When the defect is of medium or large size, a staged procedure is performed with prosthetic to reduce the defect. During the first stage:

▶ Gastrostomy may be performed. In this procedure, an artificial opening into the stomach is created with insertion of a gastrostomy tube or catheter, permitting the drainage of stomach contents during the healing process.

▶ The sac is excised, and the umbilical vein and arteries are ligated.
▶ A silo is created with Silastic mesh and secured though all layers of the edge of the defect with a continuous locking suture of 2-0 nonabsorbable suture. The open end of the silo is closed; thus a cylinder of mesh is created extending upward from the abdomen.
▶ The open end of the silo is tied closed with umbilical tape. A roller clamp is attached to the end of the silo to aid in gently reinserting the abdominal contents back into the abdomen.
▶ The mesh suture line is wrapped with Kling (rolled gauze) dipped in iodophor solution to prevent infection. Plastic wrap is placed on the silo to prevent heat loss.
▶ In the neonatal intensive care unit, the daily reduction of abdominal contents is performed by the addition of a lower tie of umbilical tape or adjustment of the roller clamp.

During the second stage:

▶ In 5 to 10 days, the abdominal viscera are completely reduced and the infant is returned to the operating room.
▶ The silo is removed, and the fascia is closed with interrupted 2-0 or 3-0 nonabsorbable suture.
▶ The skin is closed with interrupted 4-0 nonabsorbable suture. The surgeon attempts to create an umbilicus by using a purse-string suture in closing the inferior 2 cm of incision.

Resection and Pull-Through for Hirschsprung's Disease (Aganglionic Megacolon)

SURGICAL GOAL

In this procedure, the entire aganglionic segment of the colon and rectum is removed, and the proximal normal colon is anastomosed to the distal rectum or anus.

PATHOLOGY

Hirschsprung's disease is characterized by a congenital absence of ganglion cells in the distal colon, resulting in a functional obstruction. A segment of the colon or rectum lacks the necessary ganglion cells, resulting in reduced tone and reduced or absent peristalsis proximally. Because the colon contents cannot pass normally through the involved segment, the colon becomes distended, causing increased abdominal distension. Although the distal colon is involved more often, the disease may encompass the entire colon.

Nearly one half of all infants with Hirschsprung's disease have a history of delayed first passage of meconium (beyond age 36 hours). Older infants and children typically present with chronic constipation. Children with Hirschsprung's disease usually are diagnosed by age 2 years. On barium enema, one sees proximal distension of the colon and then a transition zone where the bowel appears funnel shaped, followed by the distal aganglionic segment, which is narrowed.

The definitive diagnosis of Hirschsprung's disease is confirmed by rectal biopsy (i.e., findings that indicate an absence of ganglion cells).

The problem may be recognized soon after birth or in later infancy, and may develop into necrotizing enterocolitis, which often is fatal in the neonate if not treated promptly.

Technique

1. A left paramedian incision is made, and if a colostomy is present, it is excised.
2. The sigmoid colon is mobilized, and the superior hemorrhoidal vessels are divided.
3. Frozen section specimens may be taken to determine the presence of ganglia.
4. The pelvis is entered, the lateral rectal ligaments are cut, and the rectum is further mobilized, staying close to the bowel.
5. A long clamp (Babcock or ring forceps) is inserted transanally, and a segment of the dissected colon is seized from within. Using counter pressure from the pelvis, the colon is everted and "pulled through" the anus.
6. Should the portion be too large, it may need to be excised abdominally before the proximal portion of the intestine is pulled through the anus.
7. The layers of the everted bowel are circumferentially incised, and absorbable suture is used to anchor the rim of the retained portion of the colon to the anal canal, in either a single or double layer.
8. The specimen is amputated, and the anastomosis is performed with absorbable suture or internal staples.
9. At the completion of this portion of the procedure, gowns, gloves, and set-up should be changed in preparation for the abdominal portion of the procedure.
10. The proximal edge of the muscular cuff is approximated to the seromuscular layer of the colon, completing the abdominal anastomosis.
11. The abdomen is irrigated and closed routinely, usually without the insertion of drains.

DISCUSSION

Before definitive surgery is performed, a colostomy may be created to relieve the obstruction and allow for normal bowel function.

The *Swenson pull-through* procedure is used most often, but several other procedures can be used to relieve this condition, usually depending on the extent of the disease and the surgeon's preference. The procedure may use the perineal approach, the abdominal approach, or a combination similar to the abdominal-perineal resection. The infant is prepped and draped from the nipples down to and including the buttocks, genitals, perineal area, and upper thighs to permit positioning of the perineal stage without redraping. An indwelling catheter is inserted to keep the bladder empty during the procedure.

Intussusception
SURGICAL GOAL

Intussusception, a telescoping of one portion of the intestine into another, is relieved either by reduction via hydrostatic

pressure (usually barium enema) or by a laparotomy with manual manipulation If the intussusception does not reduce spontaneously, by hydrostatic pressure, or by prompt surgical intervention, gangrene ultimately will result.

PATHOLOGY

Intussusception is the most common cause of intestinal obstruction in the age group of those 3 months to 6 years old, and thus one of the most common surgical emergencies in this age group. The most common site of intussusception is around the ileocecal valve, wherein the terminal ileum becomes invaginated into the cecum. Invagination, a broader term, is the insertion of one part of a structure into another part of the same structure.

Intussusception causes an obstruction to the passage of intestinal contents beyond the problem. In addition, the two walls of the intestines can compress against each other, causing inflammation, edema, and swelling, and eventually reducing blood flow. If this process continues, necrosis could result, causing internal bleeding, perforation, and peritonitis. This condition calls for immediate treatment.

Technique

1. A transverse or low right paramedian incision is made, and the peritoneum is entered.
2. The entire bowel is carefully inspected to determine whether the bowel wall at the intussusception is viable.
3. Manual manipulation is attempted to reduce the intussusception.
4. The bowel may require fixation after reduction to prevent recurrence.
5. Alternatively, if the viability of the bowel is in question, a resection is performed in an approach similar to that of an adult bowel resection, with a bowel anastomosis or with the ends of the bowel brought out as a stoma through separate incisions.
6. With the latter, the anastomosis is performed as a secondary procedure.
7. The abdomen is closed routinely.

DISCUSSION

Surgery is performed under general anesthesia with monitoring in a warmed operating room. The intussusception must be reduced quickly either nonoperatively or operatively because the bowel wall will lose its blood supply, become gangrenous, and perforate. A barium enema often will show the obstruction and may correct the problem. The force of the flow of the barium enema may be enough to force the bowel to move back into place. An air enema also may be used to correct this problem.

The chance of nonoperative reduction (e.g., via barium enema) is 50% if the reduction is performed within 24 to 48 hours. However, surgery may be needed if the barium enema does not work. Surgery uses an abdominal incision through which the surgeon pushes the telescoping part of the intestine back into place and through which the surgeon may remove any part of the bowel that is not functioning. An appendectomy may be performed at the same time.

Reduction of Volvulus
SURGICAL GOAL
Reduction of a volvulus is performed to relieve intestinal obstruction by untwisting (counterclockwise detorsion of) the affected bowel, removing any structural causes, and depending on viability of the affected bowel, resecting a bowel with anastomosis; or an ileostomy or colostomy may need to be created.

PATHOLOGY
Volvulus is a clockwise rotation or twisting of a loop of intestine around itself, affecting its own blood supply. This can lead to strangulation of the blood vessels and ultimately death or gangrene of the affected portion of bowel (Figure 30-7). Volvulus is rare and affects babies or children most often, but it can occur at any age. The birth abnormality that causes volvulus in babies or children is a developmental weakness called malrotation. The central part of the intestine normally rotates into its final position in about the tenth week of pregnancy. Occasionally this part of the intestine does not rotate fully, leaving the bowel predisposed to later twisting.

When the volvulus involves the entire small bowel, it is referred to as midgut volvulus. Most patients with acute midgut volvulus present in the first month of life. Chronic midgut volvulus is detected more often in children older than 2 years.

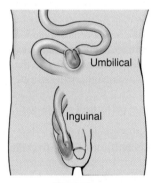
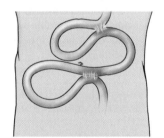
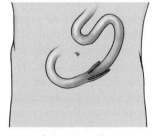
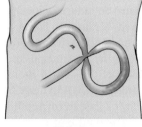

FIGURE 30-7
Four common intestinal obstructions in pediatric patients are herniation, adhesions, intussusception, and volvulus. (From Cotran RS, Kumar V, Collins T: *Robbins pathologic basis of disease*, ed 6, Philadelphia, 1999, Saunders.)

Emergency surgery to repair the volvulus is necessary. Early recognition of the volvulus and prompt treatment generally result in a good outcome. A second-look laparotomy may be performed 36 hours after the initial surgery to ensure viability of the remaining bowel.

Technique
1. The patient is placed in the supine position, and the abdomen is prepped and draped.
2. The surgeon makes a supraumbilical right transverse incision extending from the midline laterally. The incision must be long enough to permit adequate inspection of the entire midgut.
3. The bowels are inspected, and the volvulus is reduced. This means that the bowels are untwisted, checked for damage, and allowed to regain pink coloration indicating that the blood supply has been restored.
4. After reduction of the volvulus, any duodenal (Ladd's) bands causing obstruction are identified; the bands are then dissected (Ladd's procedure).
5. If a small segment of bowel is necrotic (dead from lack of blood flow), the bowel is resected. The ends of the bowels are reanastomosed or used to form a colostomy or ileostomy.
6. The appendix is removed to prevent future diagnostic problems.

DISCUSSION
The incision is made long enough to permit adequate inspection of the entire midgut. The entire bowel is removed from the abdomen so that its orientation and improper fixation may be examined completely.

With midgut volvulus, the colon is not apparent as the abdomen is opened because it lies posteriorly. In addition, the small bowel may appear congested and blue, with dilated mesenteric veins.

The entire mass of small and large intestine is delivered from the peritoneal cavity, avoiding traction on the mesentery. With this maneuver, the twist of the base of the mesentery may be visualized. The surgeon cradles the bowel between his or her hands and untwists the volvulus in a counterclockwise direction. The bowel is reduced in steps of 180-degree turns until the transverse colon and cecum are brought into view anterior to the mesenteric pedicle. The color of the intestine usually improves after the reduction unless the bowel already has been compromised. In general, two to three full rotations of the bowel are required to completely reduce the volvulus.

Imperforate Anus
SURGICAL GOAL
In this procedure, colorectal continuity is established to correct the absence of an anal orifice, and/or to close a fistula, if present.

PATHOLOGY
Imperforate anus is the absence of a normal anal opening (Figure 30-8). The diagnosis is made shortly after birth by a

routine exam. The imperforate anus can be a high or low lesion.

There are four classes of imperforate anus.

I: Stenosis at the anus or distal rectum; treated by dilation and/or incision.

II: Membranous barrier at the anal opening; treated with incision and dilation.

III: Rectum ends in a blind pouch above the perineum, usually associated with various fistulas; correction depends on the pathology present.

IV: Anal canal and distal rectum end in a blind pouch proximally. The more proximal rectum ends in a blind pouch above the distal segment.

Type IV is rare and usually treated by preliminary colostomy, with a second-stage repair several months later. Type III also may be treated initially with a colostomy, with definitive repair occurring at about 3 months of age, depending on the child's general health.

Technique TYPE III IMPERFORATE ANUS

1. The tract is identified via a small clamp inserted into the fistula.
2. The surgeon makes a perineal incision in the midline of the tract and carries dissection through the skin and subcutaneous tissue.
3. The fistula is identified and divided; the exterior end is left open to allow postoperative drainage.
4. The rectum is freed on all sides, and the rectoanal repair is started with absorbable suture.
5. The rectum is opened, and the bowel wall is trimmed back. Traction sutures are placed through the skin and the full thickness of the bowel.
6. Repeated dilation may be necessary as the opening may shrink in the succeeding few months.

DISCUSSION

The type of surgery performed depends on the severity of the condition. A low imperforate anus can be repaired in the

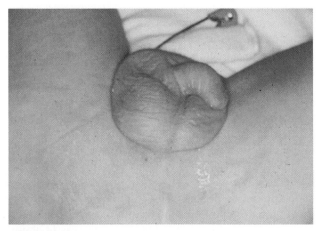

FIGURE 30-8
An infant with imperforate anus. Note that there is no visible external opening. (From Ashcraft KW, Holcomb GW, Murphy JP: *Pediatric surgery,* ed 3, Philadelphia, 2005, Saunders.)

newborn period through a procedure called a perineal anoplasty. For a high imperforate anus, a colostomy usually is performed. The infant with a high lesion therefore is given time to grow until a definitive repair can be performed with a pull-through operation.

Bladder Exstrophy
SURGICAL GOAL

In this procedure, the bladder and pelvis are surgically closed; a cosmetically pleasing and functioning penis in the male or external genitalia in the female are constructed; and urinary continence is achieved while kidney function is preserved.

PATHOLOGY

Bladder exstrophy is a congenital birth defect of malformation of the bladder and urethra in which the bladder is turned "inside out." The bladder does not form into its normal round shape but instead is flattened and exposed outside the body. The lower portion of the bladder, a funnel-shaped bladder neck, made up of muscles that open and close the bladder, fails to form correctly. The urethra and genitalia are not formed completely, and the anus and vagina appear anteriorly displaced. In addition, the pelvic bones are widely separated.

Exstrophy is rare, occurring in about 1 out of 40,000 births. Of these, bladder exstrophy is one of the most common congenital bladder abnormalities. It occurs more often in boys.

Exstrophy can involve the rectum and large bowel and coexist with hernias. Thus the obvious bladder exstrophy seen at birth will prompt immediate action and a search for other anomalies. The surgery to repair the defect usually is performed within 48 hours of birth.

Bladder exstrophy requires surgical repair, usually a staged "reconstruction." The primary goals of reconstruction are closure of the bladder and urethra, closure of the abdominal wall, preservation of kidney and sexual function, improved appearance of genitalia, and urinary continence. Reconstruction usually is performed in three stages (varying with each child and with the surgical strategy chosen by the surgeon):

First stage: Closure of bladder and abdomen (24 to 48 hours of life)

Second stage: Epispadias repair (2 to 3 years old)

Third stage: Achieve urinary continence (4 to 5 years old)

The repair of the exstrophic bladder in the male is described here.

Technique

1. Under anesthesia, the patient is placed in the supine position, a wide area is prepped, including the entire body anteriorly and posteriorly below the level of the nipple so that turning is possible, and the area is draped.

2. Traction suture of 5-0 Prolene is placed in the glans penis, and ureteral catheters are secured in each ureteral orifice.
3. The surgeon incises and completely dissects around the periphery of the bladder and urethral plate.
4. The incision is then extended distally to the verumontanum, the area where the ejaculatory ducts join the urethra, on both sides of the urethra.
5. The umbilical cord is excised, and an umbilicoplasty is performed during or after the initial procedure.
6. A paraexstrophy flap may be created if there is any question about the urethral length.
7. The bladder is completely mobilized with preservation of its blood supply.
8. The surgeon performs inversion of the bladder plate and approximation of the corpora as a first stage in epispadias repair.
9. The corpora are then approximated carefully in the midline to promote penile elongation.
10. The surgeon performs further closure of the skin over the skin inferiorly with approximation to the urethral plate.
11. The urethral plate is made tubular, and ureteral catheters are placed bilaterally and brought out on each side of the bladder.
12. After two-layer closure of the bladder and urethral plate, the bladder is reduced into the pelvis and fixed with suture.
13. Sutures are placed to encourage approximation of the pubic halves. The drainage tubes then are brought out superiorly, and fascia, subcutaneous tissue, and skin are approximated.

DISCUSSION

The technique for initial closure in the female with bladder exstrophy is similar. An exception with this technique is that a traction suture is placed above the vagina, and the vagina then is brought downward to assume a caudal angle of entry.

The female patient usually presents with a normal uterus, fallopian tubes, and ovaries. The vagina may be slightly higher in placement and somewhat narrowed. The clitoris is separated into two parts, and the labia and mons pubis (hair-bearing skin) are spread apart. Reconstructive surgery is performed to bring the clitoris, mons pubis, and labia (if necessary) together. This surgery produces functional and cosmetically acceptable genitalia.

The male patient may have a short, curved penis that may appear somewhat flat at the top. The urethral opening is epispadial (on the upper surface of the penis). There is usually a space between the base of the penis and the scrotum. The patient may have bilateral inguinal hernias. The testes may be undescended (not in the scrotum) or retractile (capable of being drawn back into the scrotum). If hernias are present, they are repaired. Reconstructive surgery is performed to repair the penis. This surgery results in functional and cosmetically acceptable genitalia.

Orchiopexy
SURGICAL GOAL
Orchiopexy is surgical correction of an undescended testicle. The goal of surgery is to bring the testicle into the scrotum

and attach it to the scrotal wall. The procedure is performed before the child reaches school age.

PATHOLOGY
During normal fetal life, the testicles are retained within the abdomen. Just before birth, the testicles should descend into the scrotum. Occasionally one or both testicles fail to descend into the scrotum. Undescended status can cause sterility as a result of the increased temperature in the abdominal cavity.

Technique

1. The surgeon enters and explores the inguinal region.
2. The testicle is identified.
3. The spermatic cord is dissected free.
4. The testicle is mobilized by sharp and blunt dissection.
5. A tunnel is made through the inguinal canal into the scrotum.
6. The testicle is brought through the tunnel and secured with sutures.
7. The inguinal layers are closed.

DISCUSSION
The patient is placed in the supine position, prepped, and draped with the inguinal and groin areas on the affected side exposed. The surgeon makes an incision over the external ring as for a hernia repair. The incision is carried into the deep inguinal tissues with sharp dissection.

Small bleeders are coagulated with the ESU or clamped with mosquito hemostats and ligated with fine absorbable sutures. The spermatic cord then is identified and dissected with blunt and sharp dissection. The cord is dissected high in the internal ring to create sufficient slack to bring the testicle into the scrotum.

To create a tunnel for the testicle, the surgeon uses his or her finger or a blunt clamp such as a Mayo or sponge forceps. The surgeon advances the clamp through the external oblique fascia and manually separates the tissue, forming a pocket in the scrotum.

The testicle then is brought through the tunnel, and the scrotum is incised to expose the scrotal septum. Several sutures of size 3-0 or 4-0 absorbable material are placed through the septum and testicle, securing the testicle in place.

Otoplasty
SURGICAL GOAL
Otoplasty is performed to correct the shape of the ear.

PATHOLOGY
Otoplasty can be performed in children or adults. In children, it usually is performed to repair a congenital deformity (commonly called lop ears) that causes the ear to abnormally protrude from the side of the head. This condition usually is due to the absence or insufficiency of the antihelical fold of the external ear. This condition can be either unilateral or bilateral. The repairs usually are performed before

the patient starts school. In adults, otoplasty usually is required after an injury such as a burn or trauma.

1. The surgeon creates the antihelical fold by bending the external ear backward. The surgeon marks the position by placing methylene blue on 22-gauge needles and placing them through the ear (anterior to posterior).
2. The posterior ear is injected with local medication containing epinephrine, and an ellipse of skin is excised.
3. Cartilage near the antihelical fold is incised, and the anterior surface is scored.
4. Suture is placed in the cartilage.
5. The skin is closed.
6. Dressings are applied.

DISCUSSION

The patient is placed in the supine position with the affected ear up and the unaffected ear heavily padded to cushion pressure. The arms are tucked to give the surgeon full access to the head. The patient is prepped and draped, including the use of a head drape, to allow exposure of the affected ear. If both ears are affected, a Mayfield headrest may be useful in the positioning of the head. This headrest allows access to both ears.

The surgeon marks the antihelical fold by placing 22-gauge needles that have been dipped in methylene blue. The surgeon performs this step by bending the external ear backward and then inserting and withdrawing the needles from anterior to posterior. The scrub must have a calipers available to give the surgeon a precise method of measuring when marking. The surgeon then injects the posterior ear with epinephrine with or without local anesthetic and excises an ellipse of skin using a #15 blade and Adson toothed forceps or Brown-Adson forceps. Double-prong skin hooks are used to retract the skin flaps, and the underlying tissue is elevated with a Freer elevator.

The surgeon then addresses the cartilage of the antihelical fold. This can be done in several ways. The cartilage can be scored with a #15 blade, thus making it more pliable, and then sutured into place. The cartilage can be excised in a fashion that allows the antihelical fold to be created. The cartilage also can be thinned with a drill to allow it to be molded. A 4-0 permanent suture, such as a Mersilene, clear nylon, or polydioxanone surgical (PDS) suture, may be used to hold the cartilage in place. The skin incision then is closed with a 3-0 absorbable suture of the surgeon's choosing. A bulky "mastoid"-style dressing consisting of Telfa, Kerlix fluffs, and Kerlix rolls is applied to the ear. This gives the newly formed ear adequate support and protection.

Syndactylism
SURGICAL GOAL

In this procedure, syndactylism, a condition characterized by fusion of the fingers or toes, is surgically corrected.

PATHOLOGY

Syndactyly (or syndactylism) is a congenital condition in which the digits of the hand or feet are joined from birth. The most common form of syndactyly is symmetric webbing in two otherwise normal hands (Figure 30-9). It may be associated with other abnormalities in the hand, such as extra fingers (polydactyly) or bony abnormalities. In syndactyly with otherwise normal digits, a web of skin joins adjacent fingers; each finger, however, has its own tendons, vessels, nerves, and bony phalanges. Surgical correction of syndactyly, separation of the fused digits, is performed at any time after 12 months of age.

Toe syndactyly is treated surgically less often than finger syndactyly because proper functioning of the foot does not require fine movements of individual toes. The setup and process of repairing finger syndactyly also can be applied to the correction of toe syndactyly. The goal in treating syn-

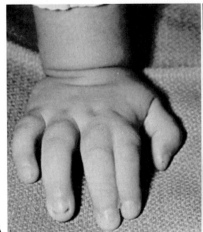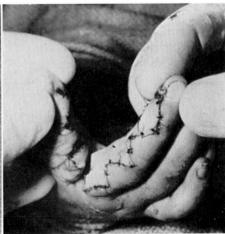

FIGURE 30-9
A, Syndactyly involving index and long fingers. **B,** Surgical repair of syndactyly; the skin web has been separated, and triangular flaps and skin grafts have been placed along the sides of both the involved fingers. (From Rothrock JC: *Alexander's care of the patient in surgery,* ed 12, St Louis, 2003, Mosby.)

dactyly is to allow the proper function of the digits and to produce a cosmetically acceptable appearance.

Technique

1. The patient is positioned supine with the affected arm prepped, draped, and placed on an arm/hand table.
2. The sites of skin incisions are marked, and the tourniquet is inflated.
3. The skin is incised, and small flaps at the sides of fingers and in the web are elevated.
4. After these flaps have been sutured into position, the surgeon makes patterns of areas of absent skin on the sides of fingers and transfers the patterns to the skin-graft donor site.
5. The skin graft is taken. If a full-thickness skin graft is used, it must be defatted before the graft is sutured into place.
6. The donor-site wound is dressed appropriately.
7. Stent dressings are placed over the skin grafts. The entire hand is immobilized in a bulky dressing or a long-arm plaster cast.

DISCUSSION

Although the skin web may appear loose, a skin deficiency always appears when surgical separation is undertaken. Preparations for taking a skin graft (usually full thickness) always should be made.

A plastic local instrument set is required, along with a marking pen, unexposed x-ray film, a pediatric pneumatic tourniquet, and an Esmarch bandage.

Under general anesthesia, the patient is placed in the supine position on the OR bed with the affected arm extended on an arm table. The affected hand is prepped and draped, and both inguinal areas (donor for full-thickness skin grafts) are prepped and draped. Some surgeons prefer to use the wrist and forearm as donor sites. The surgery creates flaps of skin to best cover the fingers after they have been separated. Skin grafts always are needed because of the geometry of the digits. Full-thickness grafts usually are taken from the groin crease because this approach leaves minimal scarring.

Other Pediatric Procedures

Throughout this text, many pediatric procedures are featured in various chapters that focus on surgical specialties. For your convenience, the following pediatric procedures can be found in other chapters that focus on surgical specialties:

Technique

Chapter 23, Genitourinary Surgery
Repair of hypospadias
Repair of epispadias

Chapter 24, Ophthalmic Surgery
Dacryocystorhinostomy
Lacrimal duct probing

Chapter 25, Otorhinolaryngological, Oral, and Maxillofacial Surgery
Myringotomy
Tonsillectomy
Adenoidectomy
Cochlear implant

Chapter 26, Plastic and Reconstructive Surgery
Repair of cleft lip
Repair of cleft palate
Repair of microtia

Chapter 29, Cardiac Surgery
Repair of pectus excavatum
Closure of patent ductus arteriosus
Closure of atrial septal defect
Closure of ventricular septal defect
Total correction of tetralogy of Fallot
Repair of diaphragmatic hernia

Chapter 31, Neurosurgery
In vitro shunting procedures
Myelomeningocele repair
Craniostenosis

REFERENCES

Atkinson LJ and Fortunato N: *Berry & Kohn's operating room techniques*, ed 8, St Louis, 1996, Mosby.

Brock JW III and O'Neill JA Jr: Bladder exstrophy. In: *Pediatric surgery*, vol 2, ed 5, St Louis, 1998, Mosby.

Cartwright CC, Jimenez DF, Barone CM, et al: Endoscopic strip craniectomy: a minimally invasive treatment for early correction of craniosynostosis, *J Neurosci Nurs* 35:3, 2003.

Cilley RE and Krummel TM: Disorders of the umbilicus. In: *Pediatric surgery*, vol 2, ed 5, St Louis, 1998, Mosby.

Fairchild SS: *Perioperative nursing: principles and practices*, Boston and London, 1993, Jones and Bartlett Publishers.

Meeker MH and Rothrock JC: *Alexander's care of the patient in surgery*, ed 11, St Louis, 1999, Mosby.

O'Neill JA, Rowe MI, Grosfeld JL, et al: *Pediatric surgery*, ed 5, vol 1, St Louis, 1998, Mosby.

O'Neill JA, Rowe MI, Grosfeld JL, et al: *Pediatric surgery*, ed 5, vol 2, St Louis, 1998, Mosby.

Phippen ML and Papanier Wells M: *Patient care during operative and invasive procedures*, Philadelphia, 2000, WB Saunders.

Schwartz MZ: Hypertrophic stenosis. In: *Pediatric surgery*, ed 5, vol 2, St Louis, 1998, Mosby.

Swoveland B, Medrick C, Kirsh M, et al: The Nuss procedure for pectus excavatum correction, *AORN J* 74:6, 2001.

Touloukian RJ and Smith EI: Disorders of rotation and fixation. In: *Pediatric surgery*, ed 5, vol 2, St Louis, 1998, Mosby.

Young DG: Disorders of the umbilicus. In: *Pediatric surgery*, ed 5, vol 2, St Louis, 1998, Mosby.

Chapter 31

Neurosurgery

By Christina L. Baumer
and Janet Anne Milligan

Learning Objectives

After studying this chapter the reader will be able to:

- Assess the anatomy, physiology, and pathology of the brain and the central nervous system
- Analyze the diagnostic and surgical interventions for a patient undergoing neurological procedures
- Plan the intraoperative course for a patient undergoing neurological procedures
- Identify and select proper instrumentation and equipment for neurological procedures
- Identify how to safely position the patient for neurological procedures
- Describe the proper care of specimens from neurological procedures
- Discuss the postoperative considerations for a patient undergoing neurological procedures
- Analyze and describe the sequence of procedural steps in many neurological procedures

Terminology

Acoustic neuroma—A benign tumor of the eighth cranial nerve.

Arachnoid—The middle layer of the meninges, which is a very delicate serous membrane that resembles a spider's web.

AV malformation—Arteriovenous malformation. An abnormal communication between the arteries and veins (called a fistula).

Berry aneurysm—A small saclike bulge of a cerebral artery, usually found in the circle of Willis.

Bur—Drill tip designed to make holes in bone; also spelled burr.

Central nervous system—Part of the nervous system containing the brain and spinal cord.

Cerebellum—Gray matter lying in the posterior cranial fossa that is divided into fissures. The cerebellum is responsible for coordination and movement.

Cerebral aqueduct—A narrow pathway for the cerebrospinal fluid to flow to the fourth ventricle and then to the brain stem and spine.

Cerebral cortex—The outer tissue layer of the cerebrum, composed of gray matter and divided into lobes.

Cerebral peduncle—A bundle of nerves found in the anterior portion of the midbrain that carries impulses to and from the cerebrum.

Cerebrospinal fluid—A nourishing fluid that circulates around the brain and spinal cord, acting like a watery cushion to prevent injury.

Cerebrum—The main portion of the brain, divided into two hemispheres. The cerebrum controls motor activities and sensory impulses. Its forebrain is responsible for memory, intelligence, and reason. The cerebrum is the largest portion of the brain.

Corpora quadrigemina—Four rounded masses found in the midbrain responsible for auditory and visual impulses.

Cryosurgery—The use of subfreezing temperature to destroy tissue.

Dura mater—The very fibrous outer layer of the meninges.

Endoneurium—A protective sheath that surrounds the fascicles.

Epineurium—The outer protective covering of a peripheral nerve.

Fascicles—Small bundles of nerve fibers.

Fissure—A narrow cleft in the brain tissue between the folds of the gyri.

Foramen magnum—The large opening in the occipital bone between the cranial cavity and the spinal canal.

Frontal lobe—The lobe of the brain containing the forehead; the anterior portion of the cerebrum.

Galea—A tough fibrous tissue sheet resembling a helmet that protects the brain.

Gray commissure—Portion of the spinal cord that includes the spinal canal and that covers the spinal cord.

Gray matter—Areas of the nervous system where fibers are unmyelinated. Gray matter contains the bodies of nerve cells.

Gyri—The folds or convolutions of the brain tissue.

Terminology—cont'd

Hypothermia—Having a body temperature below normal.

Interventricular foramen—A passage from the third to the lateral ventricle of the brain.

In vitro—Done in a laboratory; usually describing a test involving isolated tissue, organs, or cells.

Ligamentum flavum—A ligament that connects one spinous process of a vertebra to another.

Medulla oblongata—Gray matter that serves as a continuous connection between the spinal cord and the pons. The impulses that pass to and from the spinal cord pass through here. The medulla is responsible for the body's vital functions, such as heart rate, respiration, and control of the circulatory system.

Meninges—The three layers of membranes that cover the brain and spinal cord.

Midbrain—Portion of the brain located between the forebrain and hind brain. The corpora quadrigemina and cerebral aqueduct are located here.

Occipital lobe—The most posterior portion of the cerebrum.

Parietal lobe—The upper central portion of gray matter of the cerebrum lying between the frontal, occipital, and temporal lobes. Coordination and sensory integration take place here.

Pericranium—Periosteum of the skull.

Perineurium—Fibers of connective tissue that bind nerve fibers together.

Peripheral nervous system—Part of the nervous system containing the cranial and spinal nerves and branches.

Pia mater—The vascular meningeal membrane lying closest to the brain.

Pons—A structure of white matter lying between the midbrain and medulla, serving as a relay between the medulla and cerebral peduncles. The fifth, sixth, seventh, and eighth cranial nerves originate here.

Rami—A forked division of a spinal nerve.

Scalp—Multilayered skin of the skull usually covered by hair.

Skull—The bone covering the head.

Spinal cord—The section of the central nervous system found in the spinal canal that contains both white and gray matter extending from the foramen magnum to the upper lumbar region.

Stereotactic—The use of complex mechanisms (specifically algebraic equations) to locate and destroy target structures in the brain.

Subarachnoid space—The space between the pia mater and the arachnoid.

Sulcus—A groove, furrow, or linear depression in the cerebral tissue.

Suture—Joints or small membranes of the skull that are flexible at birth and close and harden with age.

Temporal lobe—A lobe of cerebrum found at the lower lateral portion of each hemisphere.

Trephination—The process of cutting out a piece of bone with a trephine.

Trephine—A cylindrical saw used for cutting a circular piece of bone out of the skull.

Ventricle—A small chamber of the brain containing cerebrospinal fluid.

Vertebra—A bony segment of the spinal column.

Vertebral lamina—A pair of broad plates of bone flaring out from the vertebral body to form an arch that provides a base for the spinous process of the vertebrae.

White matter—Nervous tissue covered by a myelin sheath. This is the conductive tissue of the brain and spinal cord.

INTRODUCTION TO NEUROSURGERY

Neurosurgical procedures are performed to remove pathological lesions, relieve pressure on the brain caused by disease or injury, relieve pain, and repair injured or diseased peripheral nerves. Neurosurgery is a highly specialized area of surgery, and many hospitals reserve a special team to assist the neurosurgeon. In some craniotomy procedures, two circulators may be needed.

ANATOMY OF THE NERVOUS SYSTEM

The nervous system is divided into two parts: the **central nervous system**, which includes the brain and **spinal cord**, and the **peripheral nervous system**, which includes the cranial and spinal nerves and their branches.

Central Nervous System
SKULL
The **skull** is the protective housing of the brain. It is composed of 24 bones, each connected by a thin membrane called a **suture**. The skull is covered by the multilayered **scalp**, which contains the skin and the extremely vascular subcutaneous tissues. Directly superficial to the skull is the **pericranium**, the periosteum of the skull bones. This is followed by the occipitofrontalis muscle and the **galea**, which is a tough fibrous tissue sheet. Directly over the galea lies the subcutaneous tissue, which contains a highly vascular layer that bleeds profusely when cut. The *skin* of the scalp is very thick and covered with hair.

MENINGES
Directly beneath the skull lie the three protective coverings of the brain, the **meninges.** The outermost layer, the **dura mater**, is composed of very dense fibrous tissue. The middle layer is the **arachnoid**. This is a very delicate serous membrane that has the appearance of a spider web. Beneath the arachnoid is the **subarachnoid space,** which is filled with **cerebrospinal fluid.** The **pia mater** is the layer closest to the brain. This is a vascular membrane that contains portions of areolar connective tissue. This membrane dips down into the various crevices and convolutions of the brain. The lay-

ers of the scalp, superficial brain, and associated structures are illustrated in Figure 31-1.

VENTRICLES

The **ventricles** are the spaces of the brain. These spaces lie between the various sections of the brain and are filled with cerebrospinal fluid, which bathes and nourishes it. Four ventricles lie within the brain. Two *lateral ventricles* occupy the two halves of the **cerebrum.** These are connected to each other by the **interventricular foramen,** which leads to the *third ventricle.* This ventricle opens into a narrow path called the **cerebral aqueduct,** which leads directly into the *fourth ventricle,* lying near the base of the brain. The fluid leaves the fourth ventricle through three openings, where it then circulates around the brain stem and cord. The ventricles are illustrated in Figure 31-2.

BRAIN

The brain itself is divided into three main sections, and these sections are further divided into subdivisions as follows:

▶ Forebrain
   Cerebrum
▶ Midbrain
   Corpora quadrigemina
   Cerebral peduncles
▶ Hindbrain
   Cerebellum
   Pons
   Medulla oblongata

Forebrain

The *cerebrum* governs all motor activities and sensory impulses. This section of the forebrain is also responsible for memory, intelligence, and reason. The cerebrum is the largest portion of the brain, occupying seven eighths of the total weight of the organ. The surface of the cerebrum is convoluted, with small bulges that occur throughout its surface. These bulges are called **gyri** (singular, *gyrus*). Between the bulges are shallow indentations called **sulci** (singular, *sulcus*). Larger, deeper furrows in this area are known as **fissures.**

The cerebrum is divided into two distinct halves, which are separated by the *longitudinal fissure.* Each half is called a *cerebral hemisphere.*

The outer tissue layer of the cerebrum is known as the **cerebral cortex.** This layer is composed of gray matter and is divided into lobes, which receive their names from the bones that lie over them. The lobes include the **frontal lobe, parietal lobe, temporal lobe,** and **occipital lobe.** The lobes and functional areas of the cerebrum are illustrated in Figure 31-3.

Midbrain

The **midbrain** is situated between the forebrain and the hindbrain. The cerebral aqueduct, which was previously mentioned, courses through the middle of the midbrain. On the ventral side of this portion of the brain are two masses of **white matter** called the **cerebral peduncles.** These peduncles carry impulses to and from the cerebrum. On the dorsal side are four rounded tissue masses called the **corpora quadrigemina.** This section is responsible for relaying auditory and visual impulses.

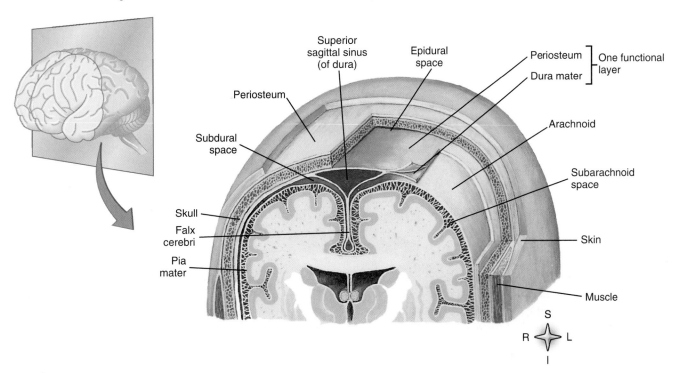

FIGURE 31-1
Surgical layers of the scalp, galea, meninges, and brain. (From Thibodeau GA and Patton KT: *Anthony's textbook of anatomy and physiology,* ed 17, St Louis, 2003, Mosby.)

Hindbrain

The **cerebellum** lies in the posterior cranial fossa and closely resembles the cerebrum in structure (Figure 31-4). Like the cerebrum, it is covered by a cortex composed of **gray matter** and is divided into lobes by fissures. The cerebellar lobes include the anterior, posterior, and flocculonodular. The first two, the anterior and posterior lobes, help control coordination and movement. The flocculonodular lobe helps control equilibrium.

The **pons** lies between the midbrain and the medulla, in front of the cerebellum (see Figure 31-4). It consists mainly of white matter and serves as a relay between the medulla and the cerebral peduncles. The fifth, sixth, seventh, and eighth cranial nerves have their origin in this portion of the hindbrain.

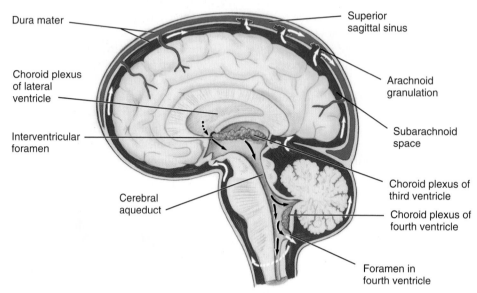

FIGURE 31-2
The ventricles of the brain. (From Applegate E: *The anatomy and physiology learning system,* ed 2, St Louis, 2000, Saunders.)

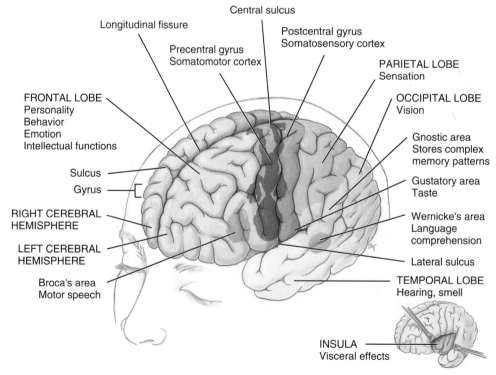

FIGURE 31-3
Lobes and functional areas of the cerebrum. (From Applegate E: *The anatomy and physiology learning system,* ed 2, St Louis, 2000, Saunders.)

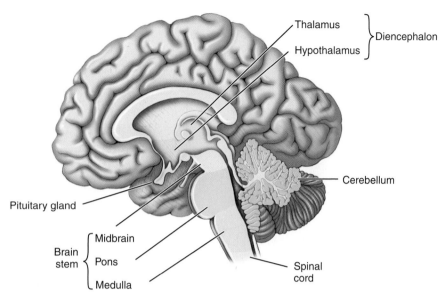

FIGURE 31-4
Diencephalon, brain stem, and cerebellum. (From Herlihy B and Maebius N: *The human body in health and illness,* ed 2, St Louis, 2003, Saunders.)

The **medulla oblongata** is a continuous connection between the spinal cord and the pons (see Figure 31-4). It is made up primarily of gray matter and closely resembles the spinal cord in internal structure except that it is much thicker. Lines of white matter are interspersed within the gray matter, and all impulses into and out of the spinal cord are located here. The medulla is responsible for vital functions such as control of the circulatory system, respiration, and heart rate.

Spinal Cord

The spinal cord is located within the vertebral canal and is continuous with the medulla oblongata of the hindbrain. The cord begins at the **foramen magnum,** a large foramen at the base of the skull, and terminates at the first and second lumbar **vertebrae** (Figure 31-5, *A*). Structurally, the spinal cord is somewhat flat on the dorsoventral side and contains an outer layer of white matter and an inner body of gray matter. A cross section of the cord reveals that the gray matter forms a rough "H" shape. The two dorsal portions of the "H" are called the *dorsal horns,* and the two ventral portions are called the *ventral horns.* The cross portion of the "H" is called the **gray commissure,** and this portion encompasses a canal that traverses the length of the cord (Figure 31-5, *B*). The cord is surrounded by the meninges down to the level of the second or third sacral vertebra.

Peripheral Nervous System
CRANIAL NERVES

The cranial nerves are 12 pairs of nerves that originate in the brain and are responsible for sensory and motor functions of the body. Each of the 12 pairs has a separate name and function:

   I. *Olfactory:* Responsible for the sense of smell.
  II. *Optic:* Conveys impulses for sight.

  III. *Oculomotor:* Controls muscles that move the eye and iris.
  IV. *Trochlear:* Controls the oblique muscle of the eye.
  V. *Trigeminal:* Sensory nerve controlling the sensations of the face, forehead, mouth, nose, and top of the head.
  VI. *Abducens:* Controls lateral movement of the eye.
  VII. *Facial:* A motor nerve responsible for the muscles in the face and scalp; also controls tears and salivation.
  VIII. *Acoustic:* Controls hearing and equilibrium.
  IX. *Glossopharyngeal:* Serves the sense of taste and pharyngeal movement. This nerve also controls the parotid gland and salivation.
  X. *Vagus:* Innervates the pharyngeal and laryngeal muscles, heart, pancreas, lungs, and digestive systems. This nerve also controls the sensory paths of the abdominal viscera, the pleura, and the thoracic viscera.
  XI. *Accessory:* Contains two parts: a cranial and a spinal portion. The cranial portion joins the vagus nerve to help control the pharyngeal and laryngeal muscles. The spinal portion controls the trapezius and sternocleidomastoid muscles.
  XII. *Hypoglossal:* Innervates the muscles of the tongue.

The cranial nerves and their origins, exit points, and functions are listed in Table 31-1 and illustrated in Figure 31-6.

SPINAL NERVES

There are 31 pairs of spinal nerves that originate from the cord and are attached at various points along the length of the entire cord. These nerves exit the spinal column through the *vertebral foramina.* Each nerve is composed of small bundles of nerve fibers called **fascicles,** which are surrounded by a sheath called the **endoneurium.** The **peri-**

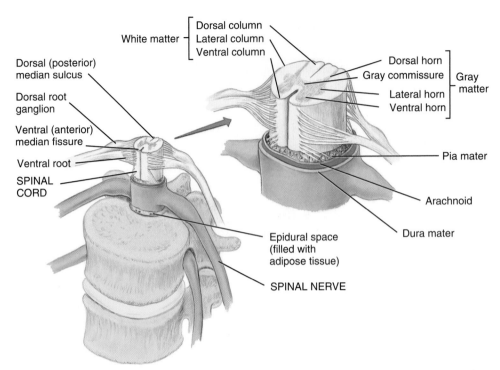

FIGURE 31-5
Cross section of the spinal cord. (From Applegate E: *The anatomy and physiology learning system,* ed 2, St Louis, 2000, Saunders.)

Table 31-1	CRANIAL NERVES		
Number	Name	Origin	Action
I	Olfactory	Telencephalon	Smell
II	Optic	Diencephalon	Vision
III	Oculomotor	Mesencephalon	Somatic motor for eyeballs, iris, and ciliary body
IV	Trochlear	Mesencephalon	Somatic motor for eyeballs
V	Trigeminal	Metencephalon	Motor and sensory
VI	Abducens	Myelencephalon	Somatic motor
VII	Facial	Myelencephalon	Motor and sensory
VIII	Vestibulocochlear	Myelencephalon	Hearing and balance
IX	Glossopharyngeal	Myelencephalon	Visceral motor and sensory, general sensory
X	Vagus	Myelencephalon	Visceral motor and sensory, general sensory
XI	Spinal accessory	Myelencephalon	Visceral motor
XII	Hypoglossal	Myelencephalon	Somatic motor

From Phillips N: *Berry & Kohn's operating room technique* ed 10, St Louis, 2004, Mosby.

neurium, fibers of connective tissue, extends within the spaces between the nerve fibers and binds them together. The nerve unit is then bound together by the **epineurium.**

The 31 pairs of spinal nerves correspond to the same number of *spinal segments,* each segment containing one pair of nerves (Figure 31-7). There are 8 cervical pairs, 12 thoracic, 5 lumbar, 5 sacral, and 1 coccygeal. Each spinal nerve has two roots: one dorsal and one ventral. The dorsal root contains an area of enlargement called the *dorsal root ganglion.* Each spinal nerve forms two branches; these are called **rami.**

POSITIONING, PREPPING, AND DRAPING

The patient may be placed in one of several positions, depending on the procedure. In most cases, the neurosurgeon is available to direct and assist in positioning of the patient.

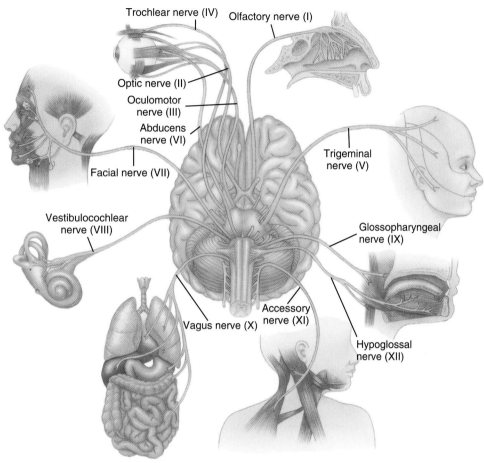

FIGURE 31-6
Ventral surface of the brain showing attachment of the cranial nerves. (From Thibodeau GA and Patton KT: *Anthony's textbook of anatomy and physiology*, ed 17, St Louis, 2003, Mosby.)

The supine position may be used for many craniotomy and anterior cervical spine procedures and for the repair of peripheral nerves. A modified Fowler position may be used for selected craniotomy procedures and for posterior cervical spine operations. Laminectomy procedures are performed with the patient in the laminectomy position, with or without the use of a special laminectomy brace that elevates the thorax. A complete description of these positions and related safety precautions can be found in Chapter 10, Transporting, Transferring, and Positioning.

When the patient is to be prepped for a craniotomy procedure, the hair is first shaved with electric clippers (this should be done outside the operating room suite) and then with a razor, as described in Chapter 11, Surgical Preparation and Draping. The patient's hair must be saved and returned to the patient as personal property. In preparation for cervical spine procedures, the surgeon may order the patient's nape to be shaved to the level of the ears. If the patient's hair is long, it should be secured to the top of the head with an elastic band.

Because most surgeries involving the brain require complex draping routines, the surgeons may direct and complete the draping themselves. Drapes may be sewn directly to the scalp with silk sutures, adhesive drapes may be used, or surgical skin staples may be used. In any case involving the head, it is wise to have extra drapes available to secure a large sterile field. (See Chapter 11, Surgical Preparation and Draping, for a complete discussion of draping techniques.)

SPECIAL EQUIPMENT

In neurosurgical procedures involving the brain, special equipment should be available according to the surgeon's preference or specific need.

The *microscope* is often used when microsurgical techniques are employed (see Chapter 24, Ophthalmic Surgery). It may be needed for cranial, spinal, or peripheral nerve procedures. When less magnification is needed, the surgeon may choose to wear *surgical loupes* and a *headlight*.

The *electrosurgical unit* and *bipolar unit* are used often during cranial procedures. When the skull flap has been created and the brain is exposed, the *cutting* selection on the electrosurgical unit should be turned off to avoid inadvertent injury to the delicate brain tissue.

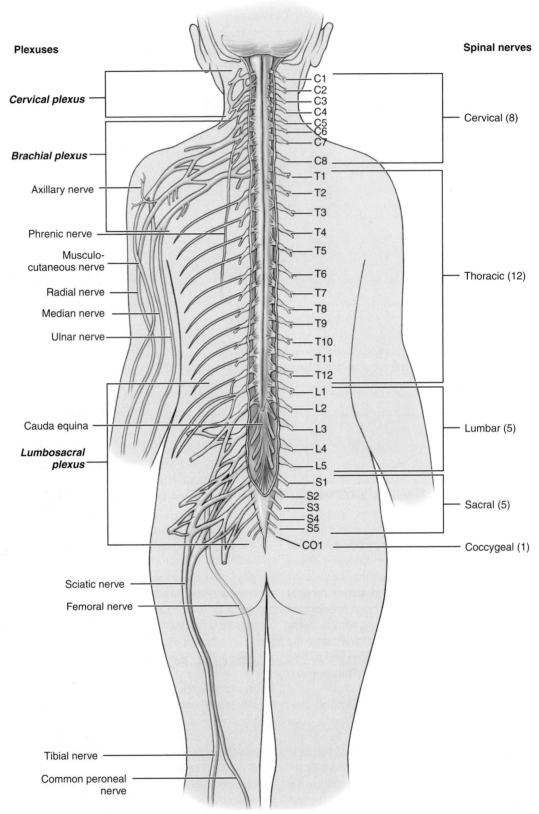

FIGURE 31-7
Spinal nerves. (From Herlihy B and Maebius N: *The human body in health and illness*, ed 2, St Louis, 2003, Saunders.)

A special overhead table (Mayfield table) is used in place of the Mayo stand during craniotomy procedures (Figure 31-8). With the surgeon standing at the patient's head, the table can be positioned, raised, or lowered into the optimum location from which instruments and supplies can be passed. The table offers the scrub ample working area on which to arrange the many supplies and solutions needed during a craniotomy procedure. In many cases, the Mayfield table is draped continuously with the patient to produce one large sterile field.

Drills and perforators (powered instruments used to penetrate the skull) are used for all brain procedures. These specialized instruments vary according to the manufacturer, and the scrub and circulator should become familiar with those used in his or her operating room.

The patient's head is maintained in a fixed position during craniotomy or cervical spine procedures by a *headrest* that attaches to the operating table. Many different types of headrests are available, some designed with detachable pins that can be sterilized and then placed into the patient's skull. The patient is positioned with the headrest in place, and then the pins are reattached to the headrest to immobilize the head completely. Three common types of headrests are the Light-Veley, the Mayfield, and the three-pin suspension (Figure 31-9).

The Cavitron Ultrasonic Surgical Aspirator (CUSA) is a system that removes body tissue through fragmentation, irrigation, and suction, and that includes a console and a hand-held device (Figure 31-10). The CUSA is used in the removal of certain brain tumors. The sterile hand-piece held by the surgeon contains an electrical device that causes the tip to vibrate in and out 23,000 times per second. The vibrating tip fragments tissue that it touches, and an irrigation solution flowing from a source near the tip

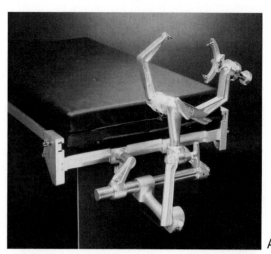

A

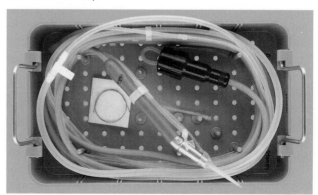

B

FIGURE 31-9
A, Three-pin suspension skull clamps. **B,** Mayfield headrest. (From Rothrock J: *Alexander's care of the patient in surgery,* ed 12, St Louis, 2003, Mosby; courtesy Omi Surgical Products, a division of Ohio Medical Instrument Company, Cincinnati, Ohio.)

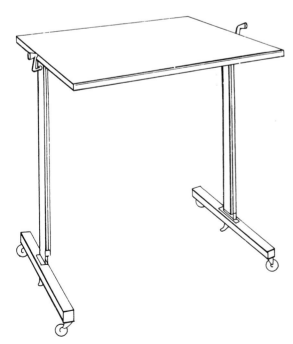

FIGURE 31-8
Mayfield instrument table. (From Rothrock J: *Alexander's care of the patient in surgery,* ed 12, St Louis, 2003, Mosby.)

FIGURE 31-10
CUSA handpiece and attachments. (From Tighe S: *Instrumentation for the operating room,* ed 6, St Louis, 2003, Mosby.)

suspends the fragmented tissue so it can be aspirated through the tip and transported to a reservoir in the console unit.

At least one surgical technologist or nurse from each hospital in which the unit is used is required to attend an in-service program given by the system's manufacturer. This program ensures that the system is set up and operated properly.

The CUSA system must be stored in an area that is free of dirt, blood, and water. It must be drained before storage, and the hand-piece should be stored in its case.

Cryosurgery, the use of subfreezing temperature to destroy tissue, is becoming more popular in neurosurgical procedures. Cryosurgery is used to destroy the ganglion of nerve cells in the thalamus for treatment of Parkinson's disease. Cryosurgery is effectively used to destroy the pituitary gland to stop the progress of many types of metastatic cancer and in many types of brain tumors. During the procedure, the coolant is circulated through a metal probe that has been chilled to as low as –160° C (–320° F) depending on the chemical used. The moist tissue adheres to the cold metal and freezes. Cells become dehydrated, and the membranes burst.

Suction and irrigation are essential in every craniotomy procedure. Because the skull does not expand to accommodate an increase in tissue fluid or blood, the wound must be kept free of bleeding vessels. Otherwise, increased intracranial pressure (ICP) caused by the accumulation of blood or fluid may damage the delicate nerve tissue and cause irreparable damage. Two separate suction tubes and tips should be available on the sterile field at all times. Frazier suction tips are commonly used. A suction tip equipped with a fiberoptic light at the end, if available, also is useful. In addition to removing fluid, the suction tip also may be used to evacuate tumor material, aid in dissection, or aspirate necrotic tissue, pus, or cystic matter.

Irrigation solutions that help the surgeon identify bleeding and clear the wound of debris should be available at all times. Lactated Ringer's solution and physiological saline solution are commonly used. The scrub should have two bulb syringes filled with the surgeon's preferred solution at all times and readily available to the surgeon. Irrigation solutions are kept at 105° F to 115° F at all times. Fluid that exceeds 120° F causes cell damage to the cortex and must never be used. In addition, fluid that drops below 105° F can cool the patient's core body temperature to below normal ranges, causing **hypothermia**.

Special *neurosurgical sponges* are used during cranial and spinal procedures (see Chapter 15, Surgical Technique). These may be in the form of flattened radiopaque squares of feltlike material or cotton balls to which a string is attached. They are offered to the surgeon on a flat metal plate (or ribbon retractor, if a plate is not available) and should be moistened with saline solution before use. The scrub should account for all sponges according to the hospital's policy and procedures. Routine 4-inch × 4-inch Raytec sponges are used *only* when the brain is not exposed, because their rough texture can damage delicate brain tissues.

DRUGS

Drugs used specifically during cranial procedures may be classified as hemostatics, diuretics, and antibiotics. As discussed previously, hemostasis is one of the critical concerns during any cranial procedure. Agents commonly used are bone wax (applied to the skull), Gelfoam, Surgicel, topical thrombin, Avitene (microfibrillar collagen), and hydrogen peroxide. The scrub should cut the Gelfoam into several different sizes before use, unless otherwise directed by the surgeon (Figure 31-11). These pieces may or may not be soaked in topical thrombin, according to the surgeon's preference. Surgicel and Avitene are both delivered to the surgeon in their *dry* state. Avitene should be offered to the surgeon with a *dry* thumb forceps for placement in the wound; otherwise, the Avitene could stick to the forceps. Thrombin always should be delivered to the patient topically.

Intravenous diuretics are administered to the patient before, during, and after any cranial procedure to prevent the brain from swelling as the result of surgery. This practice reduces the likelihood of increased ICP and resulting tissue damage. Mannitol is a commonly used diuretic.

Most neurosurgeons use an antibiotic solution as a final wound irrigant in cranial procedures and in some peripheral nerve repairs. The choice of antibiotic varies according to the surgeon's preference.

Anesthesia

Brain tissue itself is insensitive to pain. Only the scalp, extracranial arteries, and portions of the dura mater are sensitive to pain. Local anesthetic injected into the incisional area of the scalp aids in hemostasis of this highly vascular area. When the procedure is performed under a general anesthetic, the level of anesthesia can be much lighter and therefore safer for the patient.

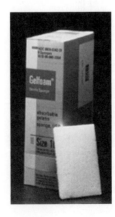

FIGURE 31-11
Gelfoam. (From Snyder K and Keegan C: *Pharmacology for the surgical technologist*, Philadelphia, 1999, Saunders.)

DIAGNOSTIC PROCEDURES

There are many neurological diagnostic procedures that may or may not involve surgical personnel, but the technologist and nurse should be familiar with these (see Chapter 19, Diagnostic Procedures, for a complete discussion). If any of the procedures have been performed before surgery, the results should be readily available during surgery.

Angiography

During angiography, a contrast medium such as diatrizoate compound is injected into the vessels of the cranium to reveal aneurysms, certain tumors, or other vascular lesions. After the dye is injected, radiographs are taken in rapid succession.

Myelography

Myelography, a procedure similar to angiography, employs a contrast medium that is injected into the subarachnoid space of the spinal canal. Radiographs may reveal lesions such as a herniated disk, spinal cord tumor, or other anomaly. Fluoroscopy is employed to visualize affected areas. The radiologist then takes spot films, which become a permanent record of the patient's condition.

Pneumoencephalography

During pneumoencephalography, a lumbar puncture needle is introduced into the subarachnoid space and air is injected. Radiographs then are taken to determine the outline of the ventricular system and subarachnoid cisterns.

Ventriculography

During ventriculography, air or contrast medium is substituted for cerebrospinal fluid. This study is particularly useful in diagnosing tumors. The procedure is performed when there is an obstruction between the ventricular system and the spinal canal. The ventricular fluid is aspirated, air is introduced through small **bur** holes, and radiographs then are taken.

Echoencephalography

This study uses ultrasonic waves in identifying brain abscesses, tumors, and hematomas. The procedure is used most often in emergencies.

Computed Tomography

Computed tomography (CT) produces radiographs of the brain (or other areas of the body) represented in cross-section. The pictorial radiographs outline the ventricles of the brain, nerves, blood vessels, tumors, or other structures. The tissues are depicted according to their relative absorption coefficient (density of tissue) and photographed onto radiographs, allowing the radiologist to determine the exact location and pathological consideration of the tissues.

SURGICAL PROCEDURES

Peripheral Nerve Repair (Neurorrhaphy)
SURGICAL GOAL

In this procedure, a severed nerve, usually in the hand or forearm, is anastomosed to restore function.

PATHOLOGY

Peripheral nerve injuries may be caused by an industrial accident or other type of accident. Successful repair depends on the age of the patient, extent of injury to adjacent tissue, and type of injury to the nerve. Two types of injuries are the clean cut, such as that caused by glass, and an injury that causes the nerve to shatter. If the nerve is severely damaged, it may be replaced by a nerve graft taken from another location in the body, usually the leg (sural nerve).

Technique

1. The extent of the injury is evaluated.
2. The nerve is trimmed if necessary.
3. The surgeon anastomoses the nerve.
4. The wound is closed and dressed with supportive material.

DISCUSSION

The operation to repair a severed peripheral nerve usually is performed as an emergency procedure. If nerve repair is delayed, the possibility of full recovery is reduced. Two common methods of peripheral nerve repair are used—the *funicular* suture technique and the *epineural* suture technique. In the funicular technique, the funiculi (fibers that make up the nerve) are joined together individually. In the epineural technique, the epineurium (component of connective tissue that surrounds the nerve) is anastomosed, and the individual funiculi are not sutured together.

In preparation for peripheral nerve repair, the scrub should have microinstruments or eye instruments available. In addition, the microscope or surgical loupes, bipolar coagulation unit, physiological saline solution such as that used in eye surgery, and a pneumatic tourniquet should be available. Fine sutures of sizes 10-0, 7-0, and 6-0 swaged to small cutting needles also are needed. The choice of suture material and size depends on the surgeon's preference, but monofilament nylon usually is used.

The patient should lie in the supine position with the affected arm or hand resting on an arm board or hand table, such as the one described in Chapter 27, Orthopedic Surgery. If there has been extensive damage to the limb, the surgeon may want to debride (excise any devitalized or ragged tissue) before beginning the nerve repair. The debridement usually takes place in conjunction with the skin prep or immediately after it. If the surgeon wishes to perform the skin prep and debridement, the scrub or circulator should supply the surgeon with copious amounts of sterile saline solution, sponges, antiseptic soap, a fine scalpel, tissue forceps, and dissecting scissors.

When debridement has been completed, the limb is draped in routine fashion. Some surgeons drape the limb first and then perform the debridement. The first step of the actual procedure is the mobilization of the injured nerve. The surgeon gently frees the severed nerve from its surrounding tissue using fine dissecting scissors and thumb forceps.

Before the anastomosis begins, the jagged ends of the nerve must be severed. Two fine traction sutures are placed through each end of the nerve and are used to bring the nerve ends into approximation. To sever the nerve ends, the surgeon may use a scalpel or a razor blade breaker (commonly called a "breaker blade"). A moistened wooden tongue blade may be used as a firm surface on which to place the nerve. The scrub should have one or two new razor blades available. The surgeon then breaks a corner from the blade and uses the fragment to sever the nerve ends. The nerve ends are cut serially in 1-mm slices until the ends appear satisfactory for anastomosis.

In the epineural technique, the surgeon places several sutures of size 6-0 or 7-0 nylon, one through each quadrant of the nerve (Figure 31-12). For funicular repair, each individual funiculus is joined with interrupted sutures of size 10-0 nylon. During the anastomosis, the scrub should irrigate the nerve frequently with balanced saline solution, such as that used in eye surgery, to prevent the nerve from drying out.

After the repair, the tissue layers are approximated with fine interrupted sutures. A dressing of cotton gauze and plaster of Paris or other casting material is used to immobilize the limb until healing is complete.

Sympathectomy
SURGICAL GOAL
In this procedure, the sympathetic nerve fibers and ganglia of the autonomic nervous system are interrupted.

PATHOLOGY
The lumbar sympathectomy is commonly performed to relieve arterial spasm caused by vascular disease. A sympathectomy may be performed in other locations along the spinal column to treat intractable pain caused by advanced carcinoma or to increase vascular circulation. A *lumbar sympathectomy* is described below.

Technique

1. The surgeon enters the retroperitoneal space.
2. The nerves are grasped and divided, and clips are applied.
3. The wound is closed.

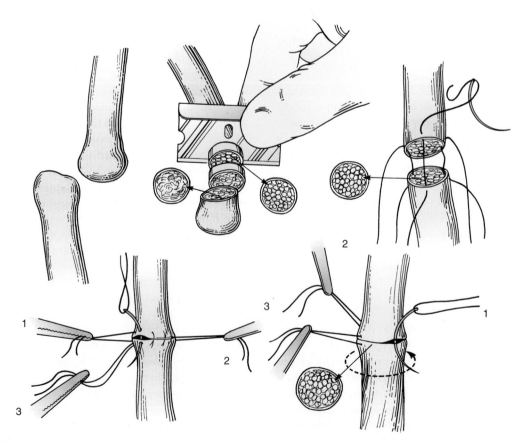

FIGURE 31-12
The nerve-repair anastomosis is made with multiple fine sutures placed through the nerve sheath or epineurium. (From Sachs E: *Diagnosis and treatment of brain tumors and the care of the neurological patient,* ed 2, St Louis, 1949, Mosby.)

DISCUSSION

The patient may be placed in the Sims or supine position, depending on the approach the surgeon wishes to take. The surgeon may reach the sympathetic chain through a flank incision or transperitoneally through a paramedian incision. The flank incision is used more often. The surgeon enters the retroperitoneal space through this incision. The scrub should have deep hand-held retractors available, such as a Harrington, wide Deaver, or wide ribbon retractor. The assistant places these in the wound along with several moist lap sponges to help expose the sympathetic chain and associated ganglia.

When the chain has been exposed, the surgeon elevates it using a long nerve hook (Smithwick hook). The scrub should have two long ligating clip appliers available at this time. The surgeon clips the chain in several places and divides it using long Metzenbaum scissors. The wound is then closed in layers.

RELATED PROCEDURES

▶ Rhizotomy
▶ Cordotomy
▶ Thoracic sympathectomy
▶ Cervical sympathectomy

Lumbar Laminectomy
SURGICAL GOAL

In this procedure, an opening is created in the **vertebral lamina** to expose the spinal cord and/or disk.

PATHOLOGY

There are four common indications for a laminectomy. These are to remove a herniated disk, spinal cord tumor, or aneurysm; or to repair the spinal cord injured by trauma, such as a bullet wound. See Figure 31-13 for different locations of possible disk herniations. The operating microscope is used for aneurysms or tumors or whenever fine dissection is required. The microscope is brought into the surgical field when the surgeon reaches the spinal cord dura, and microsurgical instruments are used to repair the defect. A lumbar laminectomy for the removal of a herniated disk is described here.

Technique
1. The back is incised over the affected disk.
2. A cavity in the lamina is created.
3. The disk is removed piece by piece.
4. The wound is closed.

DISCUSSION

The patient is placed in the laminectomy position and turned onto a laminectomy brace *after* induction. Alternatively, the patient may be placed on sandbags and rolled bath blankets to elevate the chest. (A complete description of proper padding and positioning is presented in Chapter 10.) The back is then prepped in routine fashion.

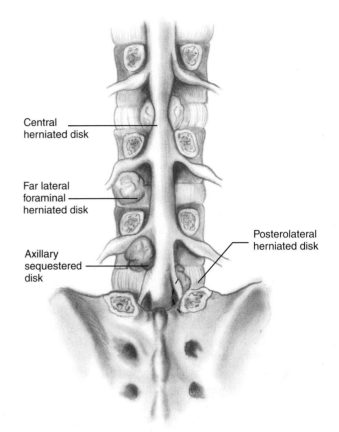

FIGURE 31-13
Locations of possible disk herniations. (From Vaccaro AR, Betz RR, and Zeidman SM: *Principles and practice of spine surgery,* St Louis, 2003, Mosby.)

To begin the procedure, the surgeon may inject the incisional site with a small amount of local anesthetic with epinephrine added to aid in hemostasis. The surgeon makes a midline vertical incision over the spine using a #20 knife blade. The surgeon deepens the wound with the knife or cautery pencil to the level of the fascia and incises the fascia with toothed forceps and the cautery pencil. Two angled Weitlaner retractors are inserted into the wound for better exposure.

The scrub should have a large number of unfolded Raytec sponges available at this time. The surgeon packs the sponges along the vertebra with periosteal elevators. This is done both to aid in hemostasis and to expose the vertebrae by retracting the larger back muscles. Because the wound is now deep, the surgeon may replace the Weitlaner retractors with Beckman-Adson retractors, or Taylor retractors may be used. If Taylor retractors are used, the scrub should supply the surgeon with roller gauze. The surgeon wraps the gauze around the tail of the retractor and drops the opposite end to the circulator, who secures it to the table frame or a sandbag to keep the retractors in place.

The surgeon uses a large rongeur to bite off the protruding bony spinous process and expose the lamina. Up-biting and down-biting Kerrison rongeurs then are used to excise the lamina and create access to the disk. It is the scrub's responsibility to clean the end of the rongeur as the surgeon makes each small bite into the bone. This is best done with a moist Raytec sponge. These bits of bone must be retained as specimens. After the lamina has been reduced, cottonoid sponges are used instead of Raytec sponges. To prevent the dura from tearing, the surgeon uses a dental probe or Freer-type elevator to loosen any dura attached to the lamina. At this time the scrub may offer the surgeon bone wax on the end of a Penfield elevator or on the edge of a small medicine glass to aid in hemostasis.

The surgeon then identifies the yellowish **ligamentum flavum** (ligament that connects each vertebra to the next) and incises it with a #15 knife blade mounted on a #7 handle. Down-biting Kerrison rongeurs are used to remove any ligament that obstructs the surgeon's view of the disk. The disk is now approachable.

The assistant retracts the vertebral nerve using a Love retractor or similar nerve-root retractor as the surgeon snips off pieces of the bulging disk with a Takahashi or pituitary rongeur. As the disk is removed, the surgeon may use a curette for further evacuation. The scrub must clean the tips of the instrument with each bite, as when the bits of lamina were removed, and retain the bits of disk as specimens. These specimens should be kept separate from the bone fragments previously retrieved. The scrub must remain alert during this maneuver, because the surgeon cannot turn his or her head away from the wound (because the risk of spinal-cord damage is great).

When the herniated disk has been removed, the surgeon closes the wound. The fascial layer usually is closed with absorbable synthetic sutures mounted or swaged to a large cutting needle. Size-0 suture usually is used. Before closing the muscle layer, the surgeon may inject a local anesthetic to help alleviate postoperative pain. The muscle and subcutaneous layers are closed with size 2-0 synthetic absorbable sutures. The skin is closed according to the surgeon's preference (a variety of materials may be used), and the wound is dressed in routine fashion.

This procedure is illustrated in Figure 31-14.

Microdecompression Endoscopic Spinal Diskectomy

In microdecompression endoscopic spinal diskectomy, the surgical goal and the pathology are the same as in a lumbar laminectomy.

SURGICAL GOAL

In this procedure, a microscopic opening is created in the **vertebral lamina** to expose the spinal cord and/or disk.

PATHOLOGY

This procedure is less invasive than the traditional open procedure and requires less postoperative recovery time for the patient. Several different surgical approaches currently are used, with the lateral approach considered to have a distinct

advantage. The surgeon chooses the surgical incision that will work best with each patient.

With the help of x-rays, fluoroscopy, and video endoscopy for magnification and guidance, the surgeon inserts a small tube with special tiny surgical instruments. With the use of a diskotome, the surgeon removes enough of the disk to decompress the nerve root before applying the laser probe. After the surgeon inserts the laser probe into the disk space, the remaining disk is removed, tightened, burned, or shrunk by the laser (thermodiskoplasty).

This procedure uses no traumatic muscle dissection, bone removal, or bone fusion. The procedure usually takes about 40 minutes, and x-ray exposure is minimal. The incision is small enough to close with a small bandage.

Microdecompression endoscopic spinal diskectomy is specifically designed for patients with uncomplicated herniated disks; however *endoscopic spinal fusion* also is being performed with the use of C-arm fluoroscopy and specialized instrumentation.

Cervical Diskectomy (Discectomy)
SURGICAL GOAL

The surgical goal of a cervical diskectomy is the same as that of lumbar laminectomy: to create an opening in the lamina to expose the spinal cord and/or cervical disk. The cervical lamina is much less prominent than the lumbar or thoracic spine, and the scrub needs instrumentation of a slightly smaller diameter for this procedure.

PATHOLOGY

The first of seven cervical vertebrae, the atlas, supports the skull. The second, the axis, is easily identified by its vertical projection extending onto the foramen of the atlas. Ligaments hold the first two cervical vertebrae together while allowing for substantial rotational movement.

The remaining five cervical vertebrae are structurally more like the thoracic and lumbar spine. Each has a body and an elastic cushion, called an intervertebral disk, that separates the bodies from one another. A median section through the lumbar vertebrae shows that the intervertebral disk is similar in location and structure to the cervical spine. The facet joints between the vertebrae and the elastic intervertebral disks work together to allow for movement of the spine.

The most common neurosurgical problem of the intervertebral disk is herniation. This results from weakness or rupture of the circular ligament (annulus fibrosus), which normally confines the soft center of the disk (nucleus pulposus), much like the soft pillow inside a starched pillowcase. Herniation of the disk causes pain in the shoulders and numbness and/or weakness in the arms and/or hands. The pain results from nerve-root compression and can be bilateral or unilateral. Surgical excision of the disk decompresses the nerve roots and relieves the patient's pain.

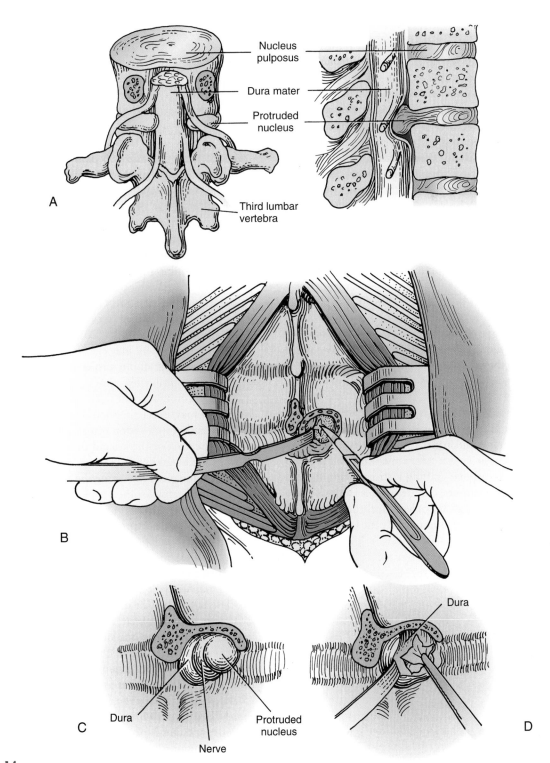

FIGURE 31-14
A, Normal and herniated disk. **B,** A window has been made in the lamina, and ligament has been incised to expose the underlying dura mater and nerve root. **C,** Normal anatomy of the dura mater, nerve root, and herniated disk. **D,** Nerve root retractor is in place and the disk is removed. (From Carini E, Owens G: *Neurological and neurosurgical nursing,* ed 6, St Louis, 1974, Mosby.)

TECHNIQUE

The surgical technique for cervical diskectomy is the same as for lumbar laminectomy and diskectomy.

DISCUSSION

The patient is positioned prone with his or her head in a Gardner or Mayfield headrest or in a sitting position with skull clamps to keep the head and neck stable for the procedure. If the patient is sitting, anesthesia requires additional patient-monitoring devices because of the increased risk of air emboli. This is always a risk when the surgical incision is higher than the patient's heart.

The scrub must understand that the smaller stature of the cervical vertebrae requires the instruments (e.g., Kerrison rongeurs, nerve retractors, and pituitary rongeurs) to be much smaller than those used in lumbar laminectomy.

Anterior Cervical Fusion
SURGICAL GOAL

In this procedure, one or more herniated cervical intervertebral disks are excised, and bone grafts are placed between the vertebrae to fuse them together (Figure 31-15).

PATHOLOGY

The patient with a herniated cervical disk experiences pain in the shoulders or arms accompanied by numbness and weakness in the hands and arms.

In addition to basic laminectomy instruments, the scrub should have Cloward bone-grafting instruments, a bipolar coagulation unit, osteotomes, curettes, and a Hudson brace available. The surgeon also may elect to use the operating microscope or surgical loupes to magnify the operative site.

Iliac crest graft

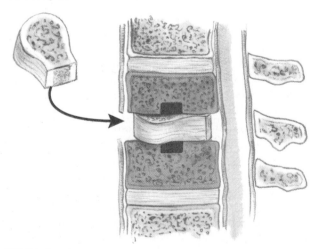

FIGURE 31-15
Anterior cervical diskectomy and fusion. The interspace is distracted, and the disk is removed. The graft then is placed in the empty interspace. (From Vaccaro AR, Betz RR, and Zeidman SM: *Principles and practice of spine surgery,* St Louis, 2003, Mosby.)

Technique

1. The surgeon incises the neck.
2. The cervical vertebra is exposed.
3. The herniated disk is removed.
4. A bone graft is taken from the iliac crest and placed in the intervertebral space.
5. The wounds are closed.

DISCUSSION

Two approaches are used to treat diseased cervical vertebrae: anterior and posterior. The approach to be used depends on the location of the diseased disk. When the posterior approach is used, the patient is placed in Fowler's position. For an anterior approach, the patient is placed in the supine position with the head turned to the left and the right hip elevated on a sandbag or rolled bath blanket. This facilitates exposure to the iliac crest, from which the bone graft is taken

Both operative sites are prepped and draped in routine fashion. The exposed iliac crest can be covered with a sterile towel after draping until the surgeon is ready to take the bone graft. The patient may elect to use a cadaver bone plug instead of an allograft plug from the iliac crest. If this is the case, the prep of the iliac crest is unnecessary.

The surgeon may mark the cervical incision with a knife blade and may inject the incisional site with a local anesthetic. A transverse incision is made in the skin crease of the neck at the level of the cricoid cartilage. The surgeon then deepens the wound with the deep knife, Metzenbaum scissors, or cautery pencil, severing the platysma muscle. A small self-retaining retractor then is placed in the wound. Hemostasis is maintained with the cautery unit or with fine ligatures of absorbable suture.

The surgeon identifies the carotid artery digitally and incises the muscle fibers lying medially to expose the vertebrae. A layer of fascia lying over the vertebra is incised with a #15 knife blade mounted on a #7 handle. A U.S. Army-Navy or small Deaver retractor may be needed to help expose the vertebra.

The surgeon then incises and removes the anterior longitudinal ligament. With the disk then clearly visible, the surgeon may put a hypodermic needle into it and request that radiographs be taken of the disk. This determines the level of the disk to ensure that it is indeed the diseased one.

The bone graft may be taken at this time or after the surgeons have removed the diseased disk. A Cloward self-retaining retractor is placed in the wound. The surgeon then incises the disk with a #15 knife blade. To remove the disk, the surgeon uses pituitary rongeurs and fine curettes. The disk is removed piece by piece, as in a laminectomy, and the scrub must retrieve the bits of disk from the rongeur or curette in the same manner as for a laminectomy. The surgeon may use a Cloward intervertebral spreader to further expose the disk. A small drill bit or bur may be used to expose the dura within the interspace. The dura then is elevated with a sharp nerve hook or dura hook and incised with a #15 knife blade. When the interspace has been adequately enlarged and all traces of disk have been removed, the bone graft is taken (if it has not been taken before the disk removal). While the graft is excised, the neck wound should be covered with a saline-soaked Raytec sponge to prevent tissue drying and with a sterile towel to protect it from contamination.

Two methods are used to take the bone graft. The Cloward method uses a special dowel cutter that creates a "plug" of bone from the iliac crest. Alternatively, an osteotome and mallet can be used to shear the surface of the iliac crest and create short slivers of bone for the graft. Regardless of the method, the surgeon incises the iliac crest and deepens the incision with the cautery pencil. When the bone has been exposed, a self-retaining retractor is placed in the wound. The surgeon then uses a periosteal elevator to strip the crest of periosteum.

The graft then is taken by one of the methods previously discussed. The scrub may be required to trim the bone graft with a rongeur. The graft is then placed in a basin; it may be moistened with saline solution or left dry (some surgeons believe that the saline solution destroys some of the bone cells). Bleeding vessels on the surface of the iliac crest are controlled with bone wax, and the surface is smoothed with a rasp or rongeur.

The surgeon examines the graft and cuts it to the appropriate size to fit in the intervertebral space. Any extra bits of bone from the graft must be saved because they may be used later to fill the interspace. The surgeon places the graft in the interspace and taps it so that it fits snugly between the vertebrae. If the Cloward dowel cutter has been used, the Cloward impactor is used to place the graft.

The wound then is irrigated. Bleeding vessels are controlled with the cautery pencil or a topical hemostatic agent. The iliac wound and neck wound can be closed simultaneously, by the surgeon and the surgeon's assistant. The iliac wound is closed with heavy absorbable suture, such as Dexon or Vicryl, mounted on cutting needles. The cervical incision is closed in layers with fine absorbable sutures, such as Dexon or silk. Both wounds are dressed in routine fashion.

When the patient is moved from the operating table to the stretcher, particular care is taken to keep the head in alignment with the body to prevent the graft from dislodging.

Spinal Fixation
SURGICAL GOAL
Spinal fixation devices provide stability and restore anatomical alignment to the spine.

PATHOLOGY
Spinal fixation procedures are performed to treat fractures, degenerative disease, infection, and tumors and to correct congenital deformities such as those seen in scoliosis. Bone-grafting material often is used to promote fusion and to replace bone after resection. Internal spinal fixation is performed to maintain position and alignment and to prevent motion as the spine fuses. This procedure is illustrated in Figure 31-16.

Technique
1. The surgeon makes an incision along the border of the iliac crest.
2. The muscles on the outer table of the ilium are stripped, elevated, and retracted.
3. Strips of the iliac crest can be removed with an osteotome or curved gouges.
4. A cortical window also may be made in the outer table, and the cancellous bone chips may be obtained with curettes or gouges.
5. The deep superficial layers may be drained to prevent formation of a hematoma.
6. The wound is closed in layers, and a pressure dressing is applied.
7. The scrub must do a sponge and sharps count at closure of the hip.

DISCUSSION
Depending on the extent of the injury or degeneration, an anterior or posterior approach may be used to place the bone graft and fixation hardware. If an anterior approach is used, fusion instrumentation, neurological instruments, and a general surgical laparotomy set must be used. A full instrument count is needed if the anterior approach is used.

If the posterior approach is used, the patient prep and position will be the same as for lumbar laminectomy. The prep includes the area of the iliac crest for the taking of a graft.

The surgeon makes a midline incision above the unstable vertebra and incises the muscle and periosteum as for a lumbar laminectomy. The surgeon places the spinal fixation system, following the manufacturer's instructions. The surgeon chooses a system most appropriate for the patient and the type of instability involved. Many types and makes of instrumentation are available, but they all have similar components.

A spinal fixation system may include a connector, a spinal rod, a spinal fixation component, and a fastener. The spinal fixation component preferably includes a fixation device, such as a hook or screw, for securing the spinal rod to vertebrae of the thoracic or lumbar spine. Tightening the fastener draws the connector through the tapered cavity, which compresses the receiving end about the spinal rod to connect the spinal rod and the spinal fixation component.

Before placing the hardware, the surgeon takes a **graft from the iliac crest.** A cancellous bone graft consists of spongy bone usually taken from the anterior or posterior crest of the ilium.

A cortical bone graft consisting of hard, dense bone is removed from the crest of the ilium or the tibia. The location of the crest of the ilium is subcutaneous, allowing exposure without difficulty.

After the insertion of hardware, the surgeon places the bone graft across and around the remaining lamina. A Hemovac or Jackson-Pratt drain may be placed before closure of the back wound. The closure is the same as for a lumbar laminectomy.

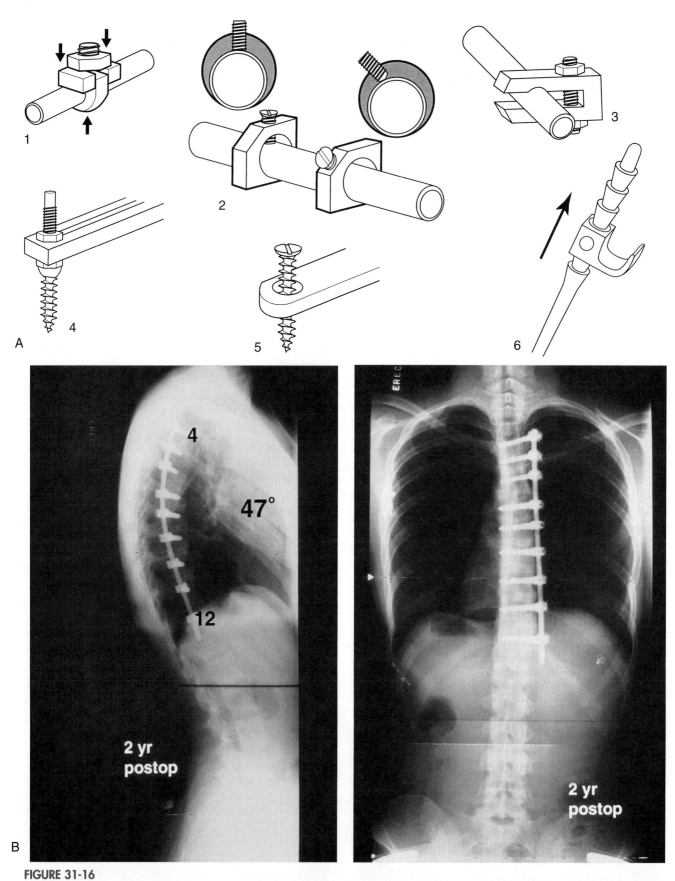

FIGURE 31-16

A, Spinal fixation system: (1) three-point shear clamps; (2) lock screw connectors, end-on *(left)* or tangential *(right)* application; (3) circumferential grip connector; (4) constrained bolt-plate connector; (5) semiconstrained screw-plate connector; (6) semiconstrained component-rod connector with an exaggerated depiction of allowed toggle. **B,** A postoperative x-ray of a patient with Scheuermann's disease. The patient had a spinal fusion. Note the placement of the hardware in the x-ray. (From Vaccaro AR, Betz RR, and Zeidman SM: *Principles and practice of spine surgery,* St Louis, 2003, Mosby.)

The scrub must be aware that the instrument sets can be very large. The Texas Scottish Rite Hospital (TSRH) implant and insertion trays include 10 separate trays full of instruments, trials, and prostheses. Two separate sterile back tables may be needed for this procedure.

Bioabsorbable Implants in Spinal Fusion and Spinal Fixation Procedures

The use of bioabsorbable implants in spine surgery is growing rapidly. These implants mimic the function of traditional metallic devices. The implants are similar in that they maintain stability, act as carriers for grafting substances, and promote the biological mechanisms of fusion.

The implants currently in use are made of alpha-polyesters. The two products most widely used are polylactide and polyglycolide. The breakdown products of these two materials are glycolic acid and lactic acid, which occur in the physiological function of the human body and are easily absorbed over time.

Craniotomy
SURGICAL GOAL

In this procedure, an opening is made in the skull to expose the brain and intracranial structures, usually a diseased or injured portion of the brain (Figure 31-17).

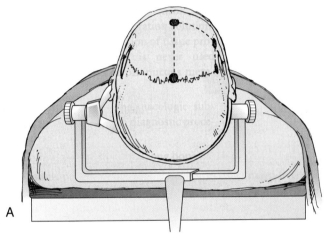

A

FIGURE 31-17
A, Bur holes. **B,** Leroy-Raney scalp clips, clip applier, and clip holder. (**A** from Meyer F: *Atlas of neurosurgery: basic approaches to cranial and vascular procedures,* Philadelphia, 1999, Churchill Livingstone. **B** from Rothrock J: *Alexander's care of the patient in surgery,* ed 12, St Louis, 2003, Mosby; courtesy Codman and Shurtleff, Inc., Raynham, Mass.)

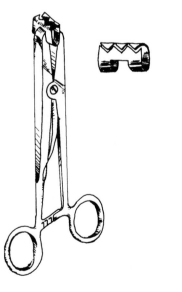

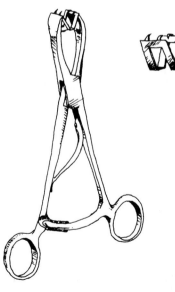

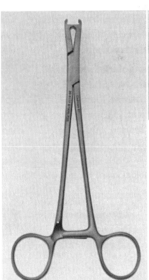

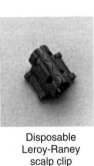

Disposable
Leroy-Raney
scalp clip

Applier for
Leroy-Raney clip

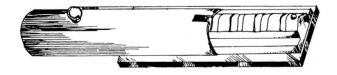

B

PATHOLOGY

Craniotomies are classified according to their location, such as anterior, middle, or posterior fossa; a craniotomy also may be classified as frontal, parietal, temporal, or occipital, depending on the planned location of the incision. In performing a craniotomy, the surgeon creates a bone flap. When a bone flap is created, the bone may be left attached to muscle and turned back with the soft tissue to which it is attached, or it may be removed as a free bone flap. If the surgeon removes bone instead of creating a flap, the procedure is called a *craniectomy*. In the event of intracranial hemorrhage, bur holes are drilled into the skull to relieve the pressure of blood against the brain.

Technique

1. The surgeon makes an incision in the scalp.
2. A bone flap is created.
3. The diseased or injured portion of the brain is exposed.
4. The pathological condition is removed or repaired.
5. The bone flap is reattached, and the incision is closed.

DISCUSSION

Depending on the location and size of the diseased portion of brain, the surgeon may request a microscope. If the pathology is superficial, however, the surgeon may choose to wear magnifying loupes only. The scrub or circulator would be wise to check with the surgeon on this point before the procedure begins.

The patient is positioned on the operating table with the head stabilized on a headrest. The surgeon usually assists in the positioning of the patient so as to ensure that the position creates maximum exposure of the lesion. The skull is prepped and draped in routine fashion. Before beginning the procedure, the surgeon may mark the incision site with a needle, scalpel blade, or marking pen, particularly if the incision is to be long, because this aids in proper approximation of skin at the close of the procedure.

To aid in hemostasis, the surgeon may inject the scalp with local anesthetic combined with epinephrine. The incision is made with a #20 knife blade. When the initial incision has been made, the surgeon uses many Raytec sponges and digital pressure to maintain hemostasis. Hemostatic scalp clips such as Raney or Leroy-Raney scalp clips are then applied to the tissue edges. These remain in place throughout the procedure. The galea (tough fibrous layer of tissue around the skull) and pericranium are incised with the electrocautery pencil, thus exposing the skull itself.

A small, angled Weitlaner retractor is placed at each end of the incision, and the assistant may use a Cushing retractor or similar retractor to aid in holding back the skin flap. The surgeon then uses a periosteal elevator to strip the pericranium farther from the skull so that it can be drilled. Two or more bur holes are made in the skull with the perforator and extended with the craniotome. After each bur hole is made, the surgeon removes the bone debris and dust with a curette and enlarges the holes. Kerrison rongeurs may be used to excise more bone, if necessary. The scrub should have bone wax available at this time to aid in hemostasis.

The surgeon then uses a Penfield #3 or Sachs dura separator to loosen the dura from the skull. A Gigli saw guide and wire or Hall Neurairtome is used to cut the skull between the bur holes, thus creating the skull flap. The surgeon then wedges two periosteal elevators under the flap to lift it from the dura. If any dura remains attached to the skull flap, a joker elevator may be used to release it. To retract and protect the flap, the surgeon may wrap it in wet Raytec sponges, turn it back, and suture it to the scalp. The Weitlaner retractors are removed and replaced with Gelpi retractors. Gelfoam and cottonoid sponges then may be placed at the periphery of the open dura.

In preparation for entry into the brain tissue, the scrub should have a bipolar cautery unit and a #6 Frazier suction tip available. The surgeon may request the microscope at this time, as previously discussed. The surgeon uses a dura hook to lift the dura away from the brain and incises it with a #15 knife blade mounted on a #7 handle. The incision is lengthened with Frazier dura scissors or Lahey-Metzenbaum scissors and toothed Adson or Cushing tissue forceps. The scrub should have prepared traction sutures of size 4-0 Ethibond or silk, swaged to a fine needle or threaded in French-eye needles. These sutures are used to retract and tack the dura away from the wound. The brain then is exposed.

In the event of tumor or other pathological lesion, the surgeon uses brain spoons, curettes, delicate rongeurs, or the CUSA to remove the diseased tissue. The scrub should have irrigation available at all times during the procedure. A 30-ml or 50-ml syringe or an ear syringe is used to hold the irrigation fluid. A variety of cottonoid sponges and topical hemostatic materials also should be readily available to surgeons throughout the dissection of the brain tissue.

After the removal of the lesion, the surgeon irrigates the wound with antibiotic solution. The dura then is closed with fine Ethibond or silk sutures, although some surgeons prefer to leave the dura open. The surgeon then uses the craniotome to drill small holes in the bone flap and edges of the skull through which short lengths of #28 steel wire are passed, thereby reattaching the flap to the skull. A wire twister is used to snug the ends of the wire against the bone. With a pediatric patient, the surgeon may elect to attach the bone with a 2-0 Vicryl suture instead of the wire. Bur hole covers made of silicone, rubber, or metal then are applied over the previously made bur holes. The surgeon attaches the loose pericranium and galea over the bur holes and bone flap using 2-0 Vicryl or silk sutures. The scalp clips then are removed, and the muscle and subcutaneous layers are approximated with size 3-0 Vicryl, Dexon, or silk sutures. The skin is closed with size 4-0 synthetic suture (Ethiflex, silk, or other Dacron suture) mounted on a cutting needle.

Highlights of a craniotomy are illustrated in Figure 31-18.

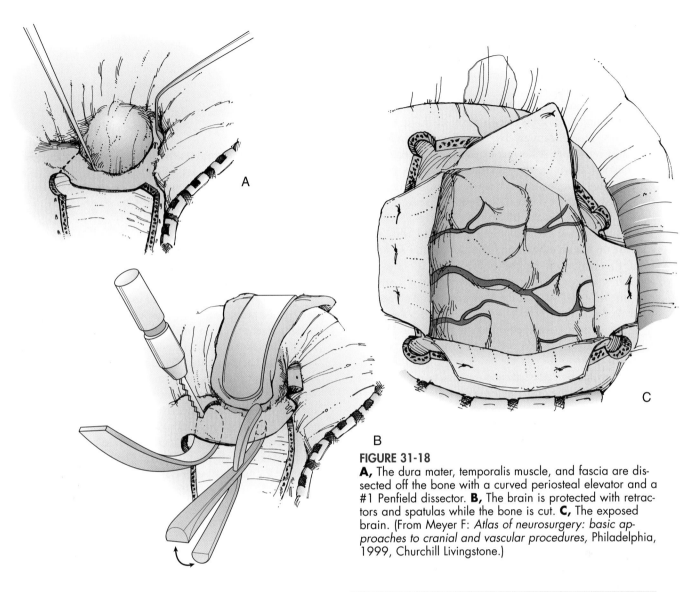

A

B

C

FIGURE 31-18
A, The dura mater, temporalis muscle, and fascia are dissected off the bone with a curved periosteal elevator and a #1 Penfield dissector. **B,** The brain is protected with retractors and spatulas while the bone is cut. **C,** The exposed brain. (From Meyer F: *Atlas of neurosurgery: basic approaches to cranial and vascular procedures,* Philadelphia, 1999, Churchill Livingstone.)

Posterior Fossa Craniectomy
SURGICAL GOAL
In this procedure, the posterior occipital bone is perforated and removed and the foramen magnum is exposed to remove a lesion in the posterior fossa.

PATHOLOGY
This procedure is performed to remove a lesion or to repair damage caused by trauma. The procedure varies depending on the size and type of the lesion being removed. The operation may use a unilateral or bilateral incision and may include the removal of the arch of the atlas. The posterior approach gives the surgeon access to the fourth ventricle.

Technique

1. The patient is placed in a sitting position.
2. A bur hole must be made before the initial incision is made.
3. The incision is made from mastoid tip to mastoid tip in an upward curve.
4. Bleeding is controlled, and the skin flap is retracted.
5. The muscles are freed with a Key elevator.
6. Bur holes are made in the occipital bone and then extended.
7. The dura mater is stripped from the underside of the bone.
8. Bleeding is controlled.
9. The dura mater is opened.
10. The brain is explored for tumor or other pathology and resected if necessary.
11. Hemostasis is achieved.
12. The dura mater is closed.
13. The wound is closed per the surgeon's preference.
14. The patient is returned to the supine position, and the skull clamps are removed before the patient emerges from anesthesia.

DISCUSSION
The patient is prepped and placed in a sitting or beach-chair position. Care is taken to stabilize the patient's head at the forehead with a headrest such as the Mayfield or the Gardner skull clamp.

Before the surgeon makes the initial incision over the occipital bone, a **trephine** (bur hole) must be made to allow placement of a ventricular catheter. If this step was not taken before the exploration, the bur hole can be made concurrently with the procedure.

The incision is made bilaterally between the mastoid tips. Scalp bleeding is controlled with the electrocautery, hemostats, and suture ligatures. The skin flap is retracted with Weitlaner retractors. A Key periosteal elevator is used to free the muscles, which are then divided with an electrocautery cutting blade. The incision is deepened until the laminae of the first two or three cervical vertebrae are exposed.

One or more holes are drilled into the occipital bone with a Trephinator, and the osteotomy is widened with a large rongeur or a craniotome bur. The dura mater is stripped from the underside of the bone, and a double-action rongeur, such as a Kerrison or Leksell rongeur, is used to enlarge the hole and smooth the bone edges. Bone bleeding is controlled with bone wax.

The dura mater is opened with a dura hook and a #7 knife handle with a #15 blade. A cottonoid strip may be placed on the brain tissue to protect the brain as the dural incision is widened with a pair of Metzenbaum scissors.

The extent of the posterior fossa exploration depends on the nature of the disease. The exploration may include opening of the cisterna magna, draining of the spinal fluid, and inspection of the cerebellar hemispheres.

When the brain has been exposed, brain retractors are placed over cottonoid strips to increase exposure. The scrub must keep the handles of the hand-held retractors dry to prevent them from slipping in the surgeon's hand; however, the inserted edge should be kept wet to prevent damage to the brain. During the procedure, cranial nerves may be identified with a nerve stimulator.

After the lesion has been removed, the surgeon must check for adequate hemostasis because of the increased venous pressure in the patient's head. The dura mater may be partially or fully closed, and the muscle, fascia, and skin are closed as for a craniotomy. The patient must remain anesthetized until returned to a supine position and the prongs of the headrest are removed.

Steps of this procedure are illustrated in Figure 31-19.

Stereotactic Procedure
SURGICAL GOAL
These stereotactic neurosurgical procedures use three-dimensional coordinates to destroy target structures in the brain with heat, cold, x-rays, and ultrasound.

PATHOLOGY
Common conditions and/or parts of the body for which use of the stereotactic approach is indicated include tumors, basal ganglia, the thalamus, hypophysis, aneurysms, and anterolateral spinal tracts. Target areas undergo biopsy, are destroyed by chemical or mechanical means, or are electrically stimulated to control intractable pain.

Technique
1. The patient's head is placed in the stereotactic frame, and the patient is sent to magnetic resonance imaging (MRI) or CT.
2. The target lesion is located, and the computer coordinates are determined.
3. The patient is transferred to the operating room.
4. The stereotactic procedure is performed using precise coordinates.
5. Instruments are introduced into the brain tissue and lesion through a bur hole.
6. Closure is performed according to the placement of the bur hole and the surgeon's preference.

DISCUSSION
The patient is sedated and placed in a sitting position, and the surgeon uses local infiltration to place Mayfield pins and an apparatus that fits on the head to help locate structures in the brain by means of x-ray and algebraic coordinates. The patient is sent to CT or MRI, where predetermined anatomical landmarks are used as guides and the coordinates are determined. The computer determines target trajectory. The use of stereotaxis allows the surgeon to plan the best line of sight with the least amount of tissue damage to the patient for many surgical approaches.

The patient is transferred to the operating room. The patient is placed under general anesthesia if the procedure will be extensive. The surgeon places bur holes. After making the bur holes, the surgeon uses hollow cannulae, coagulating electrodes, cryosurgical probes, wire loops, and other biopsy instruments to destroy target areas in the brain. Stereotaxy also may be used on the spinal cord.

This is a relatively new procedure, and advancements in technology will allow laser and endoscopy to be used with the stereotactic equipment.

Refer to Figure 31-20 for illustrations of this procedure.

Craniostenosis
SURGICAL GOAL
Craniectomy is performed to correct the premature closure of an infant's cranial suture lines by separating the two involved bones and treating the bones to prevent resealing until the brain has completed most of its growth.

PATHOLOGY
Craniostenosis is a congenital deformity of the skull that results from premature closure of one or more of the cranial sutures of the skull. Fusion of each of the major cranial vault sutures can have different types of effects on the skull (Figure 31-21, *A*).

Technique
1. The surgeon makes the scalp incision over the appropriate suture line.
2. The periosteum is lifted from the outside surface of the bone.
3. The dura mater is stripped from the underside of the skull.

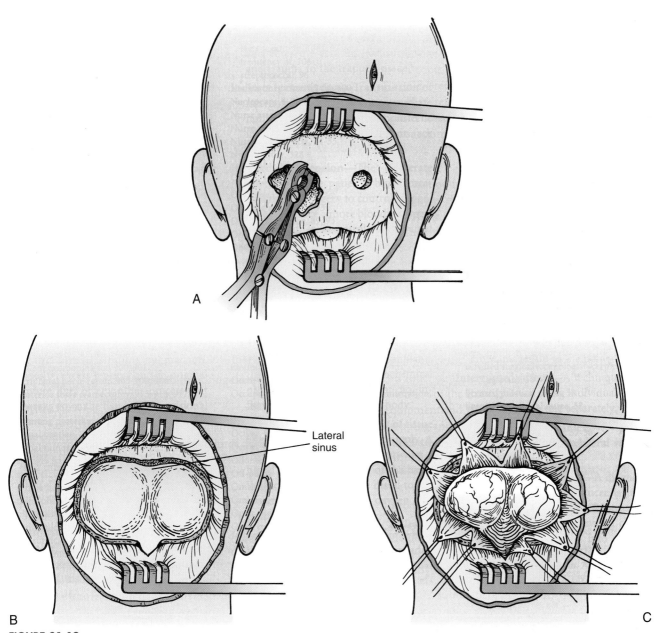

A

B

Lateral
sinus

C

FIGURE 31-19
Suboccipital craniectomy. **A,** Craniectomy. **B,** The dura is exposed. **C,** The dura is incised, and the cerebellum is exposed.
(From Sachs E: *Diagnosis and treatment of brain tumors and the care of the neurological patient,* ed 2, St Louis 1949, Mosby.)

4. A surgeon then removes a generous strip of the bone edges that have formed the premature closure.
5. The bone edges are waxed.
6. Silastic sheeting may be placed to prevent the bone edges from separating.
7. The wound edges are closed.

DISCUSSION

The scalp is incised over the area at which the premature closure of the infant's suture line has caused a deformity. The periosteum is lifted from the bone with a small Key elevator. A small hole is made in the bone with a rongeur. The dura mater is then stripped from the underside of the skull with blunt dissection with a nerve hook. A generous strip of bone then is removed with a heavy scissors, craniotome, or small Kerrison rongeur. The ostectomy should follow the skull's normal suture lines (Figure 31-21, *B* and *C*). The bone edges are then waxed, and preformed Silastic sheeting can be inserted over the bone edges bordering the craniectomy and sutured into place.

Intracranial Aneurysm

An intracranial aneurysm is the bulging of an artery whose origin is the internal carotid or mid cerebral artery. The so-called **berry aneurysm** is located near the base of the brain

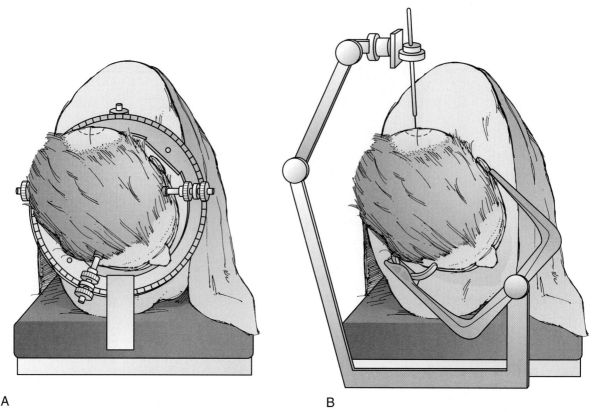

A   B

FIGURE 31-20
A, Framed stereotaxy. **B,** Frameless stereotaxy. Both techniques allow the surgeon to plan many surgical approaches with the least amount of cortical disruption and brain retraction. (From Meyer F: *Atlas of neurosurgery: basic approaches to cranial and vascular procedures,* Philadelphia, 1999, Churchill Livingstone.)

at the circle of Willis, the most common site of an intracranial aneurysm.

Aneurysms are caused by a weakening of the arterial wall, usually resulting from a congenital defect. These aneurysms can range from the size of a pea to the size of a baseball (Figure 31-22). As blood flows past the weakened area, it pushes on the vessel wall and causes subsequent thinning of the area. Sudden rupture and hemorrhage are the life-threatening results.

The aneurysm is approached through a standard suboccipital or subfrontal craniotomy, as previously described. The operating microscope often is used to locate the area of the aneurysm and to complete the procedure. When the arachnoid tissues have been freed with delicate sharp dissection, the base of the aneurysm and often its "parent" or subbranches are occluded.

Occlusion is achieved with the use of aneurysm clips or by suture ligation (Figure 31-23). In some cases, methyl methacrylate or similar epoxy is used to wrap the aneurytic area.

Intracranial Microneurosurgery

Advanced technology in lighting and magnification, afforded by the operating microscope, allows the neurosurgeon to perform intracranial microneurosurgery. A number of microprocedures have been developed.

EXCISION OF AN ACOUSTIC NEUROMA

Although removal of an **acoustic neuroma** (a lesion on the eighth cranial nerve) through the middle fossa or labyrinth of the ear is performed by the otologist, the neurosurgeon can resect an acoustic neuroma that extends into the posterior fossa of the cranial cavity (Figure 31-24).

DECOMPRESSION OF CRANIAL NERVES

Microvascular decompression (release of pressure) of cranial nerves is performed to treat trigeminal neuralgia, glossopharyngeal neuralgia, and acoustic nerve dysfunction. In these conditions, an artery or small tumor may cause extreme pain or dysfunction.

During decompression surgery, a retromastoid (behind the mastoid bone) incision is used. The artery or vein that is the cause of some types of compression is freed from the nerve, or a small piece of Silastic sponge can be placed between the nerve and artery. If no decompression is found, the nerve may be removed to relieve pain.

CEREBRAL REVASCULARIZATION

This is the anastomosis of an extracranial artery to an intracranial artery to bypass a stricture or blockage below the bifurcation of the common carotid artery. This bypass es-

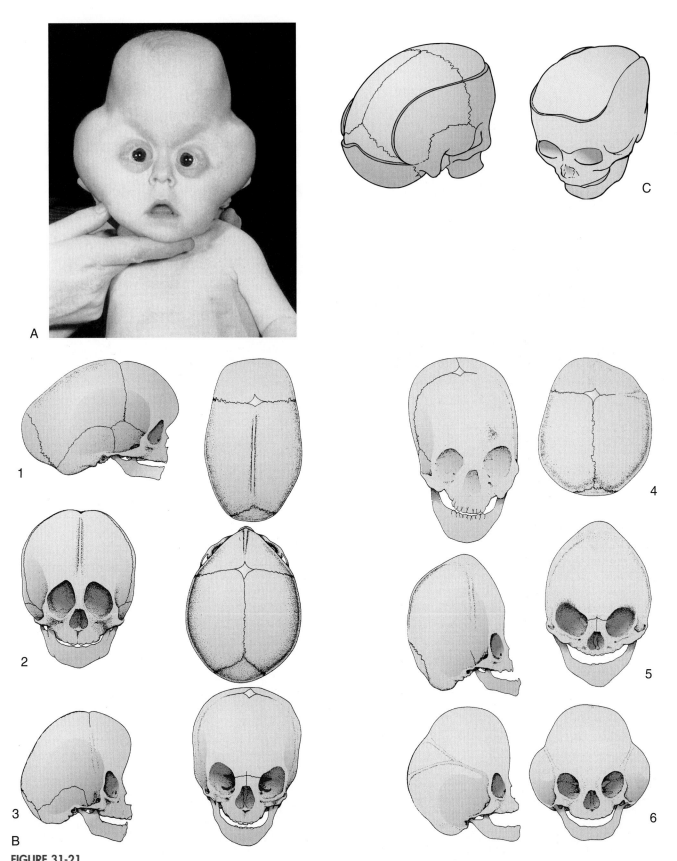

FIGURE 31-21
A, A severe cloverleaf skull deformity. **B,** Effects on the skull from fusion of each of the major cranial vault sutures. (1) Sagittal sutures, (2) metopic suture, (3) coronal suture, (4) single coronal suture, (5) coronal sutures, (6) cloverleaf suture. **C,** Wide vertex craniectomy for treatment of scaphocephaly involving the sagittal suture line. (From Choux M, DiRocco C, Hockley A, et al: *Pediatric neurosurgery,* London, 1999, Churchill Livingstone.)

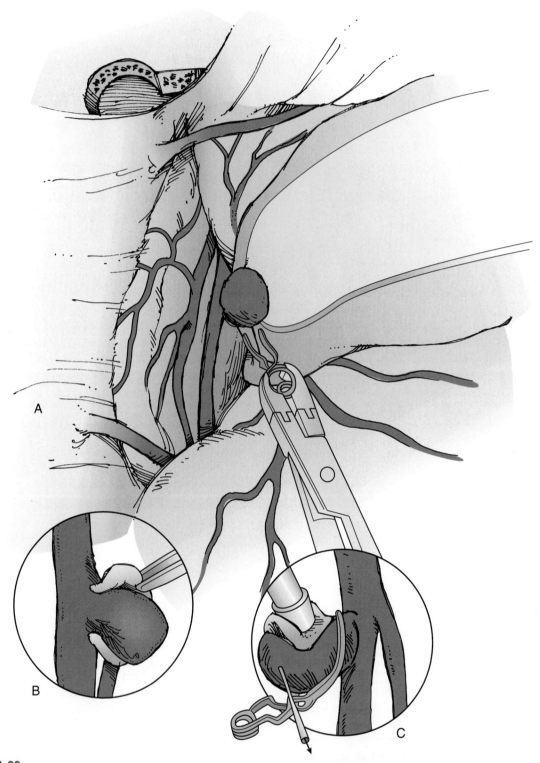

FIGURE 31-22
Sequential steps in aneurysm clipping. Note the placement of the aneurysm clips. **A,** The right hemisphere is retracted, and the proximal parent artery is identified. **B,** A small piece of Gelfoam is placed around the neck of the aneurysm to facilitate placement of the clip. **C,** Once the clip is placed, the aneurysm contents are aspirated. (From Meyer F: *Atlas of neurosurgery: basic approaches to cranial and vascular procedures,* ed 1, Philadelphia, 1999, Churchill Livingstone.)

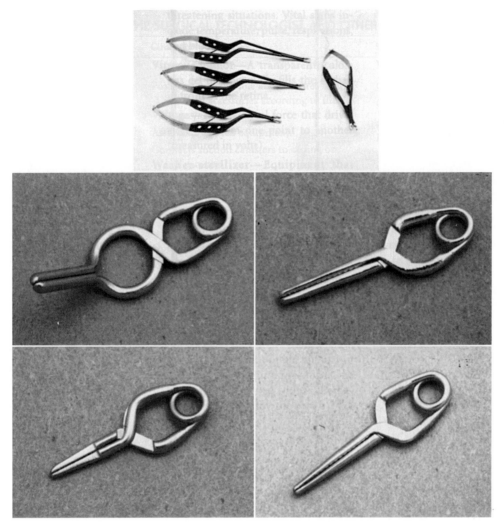

FIGURE 31-23
Standard aneurysm clips and appliers. (From Rothrock J: *Alexander's care of the patient in surgery,* ed 12, St Louis, 2003, Mosby; courtesy Aesculap, Burlingame, Calif.)

tablishes increased blood flow to the cerebral circulation. An artery in the scalp is anastomosed to a branch of the middle cerebral artery. This procedure prevents a major stroke. If the diseased artery is blocked with plaque, the surgeon can remove the material from the cerebral artery rather than bypassing the artery altogether.

EXCISION OF ARTERIOVENOUS MALFORMATION
An **arteriovenous malformation** (AV malformation) is an abnormal communication between the arteries and veins (called a fistula). As the connection becomes larger under pressure, blood is diverted from surrounding brain tissue. When this occurs, multiple hemorrhages from the dilated blood vessels can cause seizures and subarachnoid hemorrhage. The goal of surgery is to resect the fistulas by coagulation or by application of ligation clips.

Bur Holes
The creation of bur holes (**trephination**) is one of the steps performed during a craniotomy but can be a separate oper-

ative procedure. This procedure includes an incision of the scalp and underlying tissue and the creation of one or more holes in the skull, with possible entry into the tissues that lie directly beneath it.

The bur hole procedure is performed most often to treat brain abscess or subdural hematoma. Because the brain is encased in a rigid housing (the skull), any pressure exerted from within can potentially damage the brain itself. After traumatic head injury, one or more ruptured blood vessels may cause a hematoma to form under the dura. The goal of bur hole surgery, then, is to locate the hematoma, remove it, and thereby relieve the pressure.

The procedure is carried out as for a craniotomy to the level of the dura. If a hematoma is suspected, the scrub should have suction available and ample irrigation fluid to help clear the traumatized area of blood and tissue debris so that the bleeding area can be located and controlled. A typical subdural hematoma near the temporal lobe is illustrated in Figure 31-25.

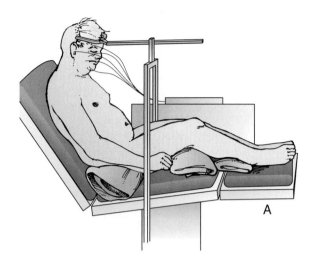

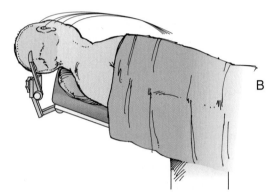

FIGURE 31-24
Two patient positions used for resecting acoustic neuromas. Note the placement of the pins in the headrest. **A,** The patient is in the sitting position. **B,** The patient is in the supine position. (From Meyer F: *Atlas of neurosurgery: basic approaches to cranial and vascular procedures,* Philadelphia, 1999, Churchill Livingstone.)

Cranioplasty

SURGICAL GOAL
In this procedure, an area of bone in the skull is replaced with a methyl methacrylate plate, autograft, or metal prosthesis.

PATHOLOGY
Deformities in the skull resulting from trauma or disease may leave a portion of the brain and dura mater exposed. In trauma cases in which an emergency craniectomy has been performed, the patient often returns to surgery for a cranioplasty when he or she is more stable. The patient's own bone might be saved and used in the cranioplasty in these cases. In other circumstances, a prosthesis is used to cover the exposed area, protect it from injury, and improve the appearance. The use of methyl methacrylate is described below.

Technique

1. The surgeon incises the scalp.
2. If present, bone fragments are trimmed away.

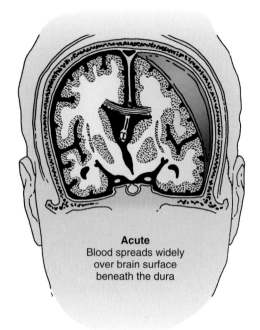

Acute
Blood spreads widely over brain surface beneath the dura

FIGURE 31-25
A subdural hematoma. (From Rothrock J: *Alexander's care of the patient in surgery,* ed 12, St Louis, 2003, Mosby.)

3. A plate of methyl methacrylate is formed.
4. The plate is drilled and wired in place.
5. The wound is closed.

DISCUSSION
The patient is positioned, prepped, and draped for access to a particular area of the skull. The scalp is incised over the defect, as for a craniotomy. Depending on the nature of the previous injury or disease, there may or may not be remnants of bone in the affected area. If bone fragments are present, the surgeon may use a rongeur to trim away the fragments. If the affected area is completely devoid of bone, the surgeon trims the periphery of the area with rongeurs to form a saucerlike ledge. This prevents the prosthesis from slipping below the level of the skull and aids in seating it in place. The scrub should retain all the bits of bone that are trimmed as specimen. When the surgeon has completed this procedure, the wound is irrigated with warm saline solution. An antibiotic irrigant also may be used at this time.

The scrub prepares the methyl methacrylate. While the cement is still doughy, the surgeon may place the mass of cement in a plastic bag. The mass is flattened and molded over the cranial defect until it fits. The surgeon then removes the molded cement from the defect to allow the cement to harden. While the cement is drying and hardening, the scrub should prepare a dental or similar drill and fine drill point.

When the cement plate has hardened, the surgeon drills several holes in its edge. Similar holes are drilled at the periphery of the skull defect. Any rough spots in the cement plate are smoothed with the use of a large bur attached to a power drill or craniotome. The surgeon then fits the cement plate into the defect and secures it by passing fine stainless steel wires through the holes. The wound is then irrigated and closed in routine fashion.

Shunting Procedures

SURGICAL GOAL

This is the diversion of cerebrospinal fluid away from the ventricles of the brain to another location in the body.

PATHOLOGY

The condition of *hydrocephalus* is a congenital anomaly that results in an increased amount of cerebrospinal fluid in the ventricles (Figure 31-26). This may be the result of overproduction of the fluid, or it may be the result of a condition that interferes with the normal absorption of fluid. In selected cases, surgical intervention is aimed toward removing the excess fluid to relieve pressure on the brain.

DISCUSSION

Many different techniques are employed in shunting procedures. The distal shunt may be placed in the atrium of the heart (ventriculoatrial shunt) or in the peritoneal cavity (ventriculoperitoneal shunt). The shunt may or may not contain a reservoir or flushing valve. Because of the many different types of shunts available from manufacturers and thus the different techniques associated with their use, it is best to read the manufacturer's specifications before the actual procedure is performed. As with all Silastic or other implant materials, the shunt should be handled carefully and protected from contamination by lint, dust, or glove powder.

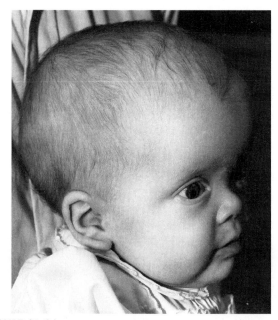

FIGURE 31-26
A 3-month-old baby with hydrocephalus. (From McCullough DC: *Pediatric neurosurgery,* Philadelphia, 1989, WB Saunders.)

Specific guidelines on handling implant materials are presented in Chapter 29. In addition, the scrub must be aware of the size of the patient and adjust the instruments and sutures accordingly. These shunting procedures may be performed on adults, adolescents, children, and newborns; and most recently this procedure has been performed as an **in vitro** procedure.

Ventriculoatrial Shunt

During ventriculoatrial shunting, the proximal end of the shunt is positioned in the ventricle through a frontal bur hole (trephine). A second incision is made in the postauricular area, and the shunt is guided to the internal jugular vein. The shunt is then threaded into the vein through a small incision and advanced to the atrium under fluoroscopy (the shunt is radiopaque).

Ventriculoperitoneal Shunt

During ventriculoperitoneal shunting, the proximal end of the shunt is placed in the peritoneal cavity, usually near the liver, through a tunnel made in the subcutaneous tissue (Figure 31-27). The tunnel may be made with uterine packing forceps or a tunneler, such as the one used during vascular surgery. All types of shunts may be altered as the patient grows and may require additional repair because of obstruction or mechanical failure.

In Vitro Shunting Procedures

Shunting procedures as well as procedures to correct myelomeningocele currently are being performed successfully as in vitro interventions. The scrub must be aware of the patient's small size and may need to prepare small instrument sets to accompany the neurological instruments. The fetus often weighs only 1 or 2 pounds. These procedures require an incision into the uterus of a woman who is 22 to 25 weeks pregnant to access the fetus with the anomaly. A multidisciplinary team will be involved in an in vitro neurological procedure, including a neurosurgeon, an OB/GYN surgeon, a pediatrician, and a pediatric monitoring nurse.

Ventriculoscopy

SURGICAL GOAL

In this procedure, the surgeon examines the ventricles of the brain with an endoscope. A prerequisite for safe endoscopic procedures is clear visualization of the anatomy.

PATHOLOGY

Preformed cavities filled with crystal-clear cerebrospinal fluid, such as the ventricular system, provide optimum conditions for the application of endoscopes. Conditions such as hydrocephalus, intraventricular lesions, or cysts are ideal for the use of the endoscopic approach.

Technique

1. The patient is placed under general anesthesia and placed in the supine position with head stabilization.

2. The scalp incision is made and followed by placement of a bur hole.
3. The surgeon opens the dura and inserts the operating sheath.
4. Retractors are placed.
5. The surgeon performs the procedure of choice.
6. The bur hole is closed as per protocol.

DISCUSSION

After induction of general anesthesia, the patient is placed in the supine position with the head stabilized in a horse-shoe headrest or pin fixation. A 3-mm straight scalp incision and a 10-mm bur hole are made. After the dura has been opened, the operating sheath with trocar is inserted free-hand or under navigational guidance in the lateral ventricle and fixed with two Leyla retractor arms (Figure 31-28). The trocar then is replaced with the endoscope. The surgeon identifies the target area through common landmarks such as the choroid plexus, fornix, and veins. The procedure is performed as needed. Hydrocephalus currently remains the most common intracranial disease treated endoscopically.

Neuroendoscopy is still in its infancy. Like microsurgery, it has a steep learning curve. With proper selection of patients and improvement in the technical equipment, the results will certainly improve, endoscopic techniques will be used more often, and the indications for their use will expand.

Lumbar Diskoscopy

SURGICAL GOAL

Diskoscopy is a minimally invasive endoscopic approach for the treatment of various spinal disorders.

PATHOLOGY

Lumbar diskoscopy aided by fluoroscopy is used to diagnose, treat, and repair herniated lumbar disks or disk fragments, or to stabilize unstable spinal segments. Diskoscopy is a cost-effective approach to the visualization of the spinal

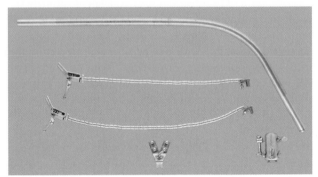

FIGURE 31-28
Leyla retractor: 1 fixation base for the 2 flexible arms, 2 flexible arms, square block, table brace. (From Tighe S: *Instrumentation for the operating room,* ed 6, St Louis, 2003, Mosby.)

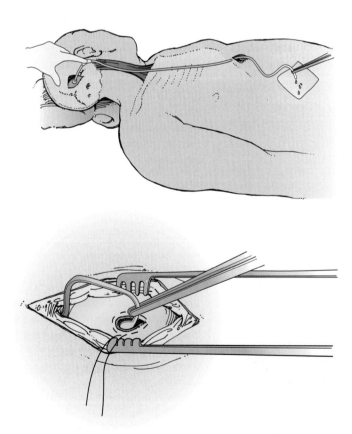

FIGURE 31-27
Ventriculoperitoneal shunt placement. (From Meyer F: *Atlas of neurosurgery: basic approaches to cranial and vascular procedures,* Philadelphia, 1999, Churchill Livingstone.)

canal and results in reduced hospital stays and shorter patient recovery time.

Diskoscopy is contraindicated in patients who have a known coagulopathy, renal insufficiency, chronic liver disease, a history of an adverse reaction to local anesthetics or anti-inflammatory medications, or a history of gastrointestinal ulcers, or who are pregnant.

Diskoscopy has been explored as alternative to major spinal surgery for more than 60 years. As technology improves, the imaging and instrumentation used in this specialty surgery continue to improve the overall result of the procedure for the patient.

Technique

1. The surgeon incises the epidural space at the caudal region.
2. A 17-gauge needle is inserted into the sacral canal and advanced.
3. Placement of the needle is confirmed with fluoroscopy.
4. A guide wire is placed.
5. A dilator and sheath are introduced.
6. The fiberoptic cable is passed.
7. Arthroscopic instrumentation may be introduced through a second portal.
8. The herniated disk, disk fragment, or spinal segment is stabilized.
9. The wound is closed.

DISCUSSION

The patient must be placed in the prone position on a radiolucent table. A pillow should be placed under the abdomen to allow for ample expansion of the chest and abdomen as well as to adequately support the anterosuperior iliac spine. To widen the height of the intervertebral disks, the table may be flexed. The C-arm fluoroscope must be sterilely draped and placed in a position to provide lateral visualization during the procedure.

Aided by C-arm fluoroscopy, the surgeon confirms a midline position of the incision while advancing a 17-gauge needle into the sacral canal. Contrast (preferably nonionic) is injected to confirm placement and anatomy of the nerve roots, fat, and adhesions.

A guide wire is placed through the needle under fluoroscopy, and the insertion needle is removed. The canal passage then may be widened with a #11 knife to allow for the easier insertion of the introducer sheath and dilator. The dilator and sheath are passed over the guide wire, and the surgeon again confirms the position via fluoroscopy. When the sheath is in place, the guide wire and dilator are removed.

A flexible fiberoptic cable is passed through the introducer. Approximately 10 to 15 ml of normal saline is used to distend the epidural space at this time. The surgeon views the anatomy. The surgeon may use fluoroscopy and direct guidance to place a second port for arthroscopic instrumentation.

Before the closing of the incision, a postoperative film is taken. The surgeon may elect to inject Depo-Medrol and lidocaine to prevent the formation of adhesions and aid in postoperative pain control. The incision may be closed with skin suture and covered with a bandage or dressing.

Cordotomy is the division of the anterolateral tracts of the spinal cord for treatment of intractable pain. This procedure can be performed unilaterally or bilaterally as needed. The patient is prepped and draped as for a laminectomy, and the surgeon makes a midline incision over the affected branches. The laminae are left intact, and only the spinal-cord tracts are transected. As technology improves, the laser is being used in the procedure, and the procedure is performed percutaneously in the radiology department.

Rhizotomy is performed through an exposure similar to that of cordotomy. When the spinal cord and roots have been exposed and the posterior root has been identified, the posterior root is resected.

Open Carpal Tunnel Release
SURGICAL GOAL

The goal of the surgical carpal tunnel release is to free an entrapped median volar nerve and restore function of the wrist.

PATHOLOGY

The median nerve lies on the wrist's volar surface. Repetitive hand movements, rheumatoid synovitis, a malaligned Colles' fracture, and obesity, can result in entrapment of this nerve within the carpal tunnel. As a result of pressure or entrapment of the median nerve, patients often report symptoms of pain, numbness, tingling of the fingers, and loss of motor control of the thumb. A physical exam and electrical studies to measure nerve function often are performed to diagnose carpal tunnel syndrome.

Technique

1. The surgeon makes a curvilinear or longitudinal incision on the palmar surface of the wrist.
2. The deep transverse carpal ligament is retracted and divided.
3. A tenosynovectomy may be performed.
4. The wound is irrigated.
5. The skin is closed.
6. A compression bandage and splint are applied.

DISCUSSION

The patient is positioned supine on the operating room (OR) bed with the affected arm resting on an arm table. A tourniquet is placed on the upper operative arm. Before the tourniquet is insufflated, an Esmarch bandage is applied and used to exsanguinate the operative site. The surgeon may mark the palmar surface of the wrist with a marking pen to guide the skin incision.

The surgeon uses a #15 blade to create a longitudinal or curvilinear incision in the skin. The fascia is retracted with tiny Weitlaner retractors, skin hooks, or sharp Senn retractors. The flexor tendon is exposed and retracted. The surgeon identifies both the flexor tendon and the neurovascular bundle that lies close to the tendon. The carpal ligament then is well visualized, and the mid section is cut with either scissors or a knife blade to release the carpal ligament. The incision is irrigated with sterile saline. The fascia and skin are closed, and a compression dressing with splint is applied.

Endoscopic Carpal Tunnel Release
SURGICAL GOAL
See the section on open carpal tunnel release.

PATHOLOGY
See the section on open carpal tunnel release.

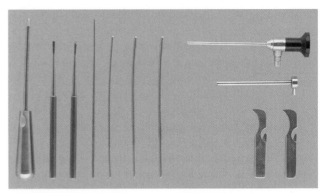

FIGURE 31-29
Carpal tunnel instruments. *Left to right,* ridged obturator, straight blunt dissector, curved blunt dissector, right-angle probe, Hegar dilators. *Right, top to bottom,* carpal tunnel video endoscope, slotted cannula, gold handles for disposable carpal tunnel blades. (From Tighe S: *Instrumentation for the operating room,* ed 6, St Louis, 2003, Mosby.)

Technique

1. The surgeon makes one or two small incisions over the palm of the hand.
2. The endoscope is inserted into one of the incisions.
3. The carpal ligament is incised longitudinally, releasing the pressure on the nerve.
4. The surgeon visualizes the nerve.
5. The subcutaneous tissue over the carpal tunnel is closed.
6. A posterior wrist splint and a pressure dressing are applied.

DISCUSSION
Endoscopic carpal tunnel release uses one or two small incisions over the palm of the hand. The surgery can be performed endoscopically with a small camera attached to a monitor. Most endoscopic carpal tunnel instrumentation sets include all the instruments needed for the procedure (Figure 31-29). The carpal ligament is directly below the incisions, in the distal area of the palm just below the wrist. The carpal ligament is cut longitudinally. This releases the pressure on the nerve as it passes through the ligament. The surgeon then closes only the subcutaneous tissues over the carpal ligament, leaving the carpal tunnel uncovered. The wrist is immobilized with a posterior splint and a heavy bandage for about 7 days.

Myelomeningocele Repair
SURGICAL GOAL
The surgical goal of a myelomeningocele repair is to preserve the neural tissue and close the dural and cutaneous defect. Immediate surgical repair is essential if the defect is leaking cerebrospinal fluid.

PATHOLOGY
Myelomeningocele is a congenital defect in which the neural tube fails to close while the fetus is developing. It is the most common major birth defect, seen at a rate of approximately 4.4 to 4.6 per 10,000 births. The level of the neural tube lesion determines the neurological defects the child will experience.

When a myelomeningocele occurs, many other congenital abnormalities often are found in the infant. These abnormalities include cleft lips and palates, hydrocephalus, heart malformations, and genitourinary anomalies. In addition,

the lesion may be infected, which may initially delay the closure of the lesion.

Early detection of a myelomeningocele can be obtained through various screening methods during pregnancy. One method is the drawing of maternal blood for assessment of alpha-fetoprotein (AFP) level. The higher the level is, the greater is the risk of the fetus having a myelomeningocele. A second test usually performed after a high blood level of AFP is discovered is an amniocentesis. This study of the amniotic fluid surrounding the developing fetus indicates the presence of acetylcholinesterase, an enzyme that appears with this congenital abnormality. Ultrasonography is another valuable study for detecting a defect in the neural tube of the fetus.

When a myelomeningocele is detected, a cesarean section is performed to eliminate the risk of further damage to the neural tissue that occurs as the fetus passes through the birth canal. Corrective surgery usually is performed within 24 to 48 hours after birth but can be delayed for several days or weeks if the infant requires stabilization. If the condition is left untreated, the infant likely will die within the first year of life.

Technique

1. The surgeon dissects and frees the neural tube deficit.
2. Shunting for hydrocephalus may be needed.
3. The surgeon closes the dura.
4. The muscular defect is closed.
5. The fascia and skin are closed.

DISCUSSION
Specialty equipment such as headlights, loupes, and a surgical microscope may be required during this procedure and should be readily available. The patient is placed prone on an OR table with rolls placed under the hips and chest. The patient is prepped and draped according to the surgeon's preference.

The surgeon makes a vertical midline incision. The laminae are identified and removed if necessary. The dura is opened, and the cord is inspected and released if tethered. The dura is tightly closed and reapproximated with either a running suture or a dural patch. The lateral fascial flaps are elevated to aid in closure. The fascia and skin are closed. See Figure 31-30 for an example of the sequential steps in the primary closure of a myelomeningocele.

Almost 75% of infants who undergo surgery for repair become ambulatory as they grow and mature. More than 75% of children born with myelomeningoceles develop an IQ of 80 or higher. Most of these children will require clean intermittent catheterizations throughout their lives.

This operation currently is being performed as an in vitro procedure, increasing the chance of the child becoming ambulatory at an early age.

Spinal Tumor Excision
SURGICAL GOAL
The goals of surgical removal of a spinal tumor are removal of the lesion, restoration of circulation of spinal fluid, restoration of mobility, and lessening or eradication of pain.

PATHOLOGY
Spinal tumors are classified according to their location; they are either extradural (outside the dura mater) or intradural (inside the dura mater). Intradural tumors can be further identified by their proximity to the spinal cord. Intramedullary tumors are found within the spinal cord, and extradural tumors are found inside of the dura mater but outside the spinal cord.

Extradural tumors, those outside the dura mater, include sarcomas, carcinomas from a metastasis, lipomas, neurofibromas, chondromas, angiomas, granulomas, and abscesses. Intradural extramedullary tumors, those inside the dura mater but outside the spinal cord, usually are benign tumors that originate from either the dura mater or the arachnoid space around the spinal cord. Gliomas are the most common intramedullary tumors inside the spinal cord; they have a very poor prognosis because of their ability to infiltrate the cord, making them hard to remove.

Spinal tumors can be diagnosed in several ways. Most patients complain of radicular pain and motor and sensory deficits below the level of involvement. Diagnostic studies used to confirm spinal tumors include the MRI and myelogram.

Technique

1. The surgeon makes an incision over the site of the spinal tumor.
2. The surgeon removes the postvertebral arches.
3. The surgeon exposes the dura.
4. The dura is incised and retracted with sutures.
5. The surgeon excises the tumor.
6. The dura is closed tightly.
7. The operative area is irrigated.
8. The incision is closed.

DISCUSSION
Spinal tumor excision procedures involve the dissection and manipulation of fine tissues and structures. The surgeon may require the use of a headlight, loupes, or a microscope. These items should be noted on the preference card and should be made available for the surgeon's use.

The patient is placed prone on the operating table with the aid of a positioning device. The frame used to position the patient is determined by tumor location, surgeon preference, and patient safety issues. After the prepping and draping of the patient, the surgeon makes a midline fascial incision. The spinous processes are dissected out, and the paraspinous muscles are released bilaterally. A retractor such as a Beckman or Scoville retractor is placed within the incision to aid in the visualization of the surgical site. The surgeon then performs a midline laminectomy using a bone cutter, while the laminae are removed with various rongeurs. The flaval ligament is removed with scissors, a scalpel, or Kerrison or Cloward rongeurs. The epidural fat is removed, and the dura mater is exposed. The dura mater is elevated with a nerve hook, and the surgeon uses a #15 blade to nick

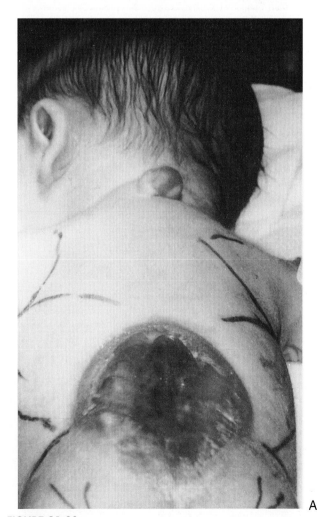

A

FIGURE 31-30
A, A neonate with two separate myelomeningocele lesions, cervical and lumbar.

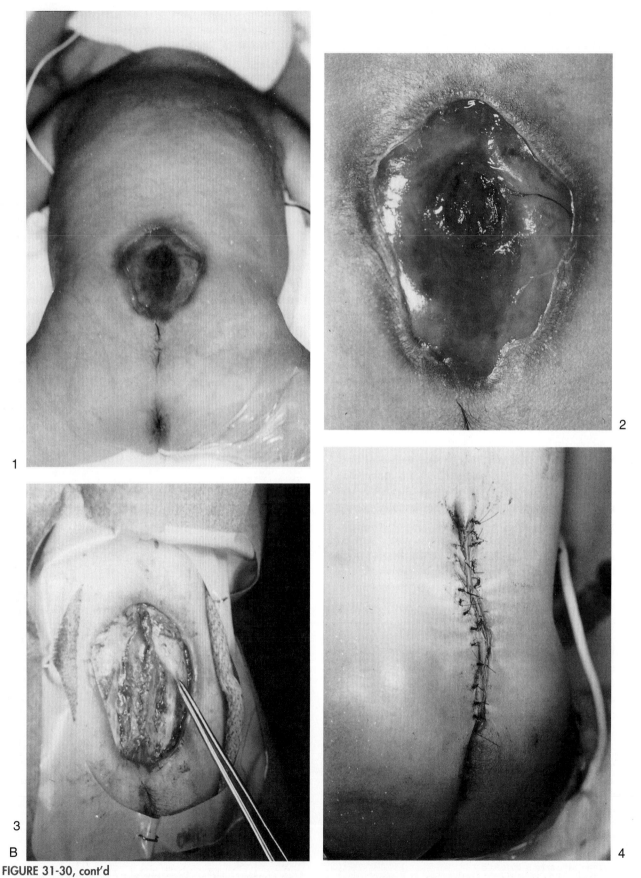

FIGURE 31-30, cont'd
B, The final and sequential steps in the primary closure of a myelomeningocele. (1) The myelomeningocele. (2) A close-up of the defect. (3) The skin is undermined surrounding the defect and approximated in two layers. (4) The final skin closure. (From Vaccaro AR, Betz RR, and Zeidman SM: *Principles and practice of spine surgery*, ed 1, St Louis, 2003, Mosby.)

it. Using a groove director, the surgeon extends the dural incision. The dural edges are retracted with 4-0 silk and dural needles. The cord then is exposed.

When the tumor has been identified, it is gently dissected free and removed. Dissection can be performed with suction, electrosurgical forceps, pituitary scoops, curettes, rongeurs, or an ultrasonic aspirator. Bleeding is controlled with cottonoids, hemostatic clips, Gelfoam, and topical hemostatic agents. The wound is irrigated, and the dura is tightly closed. The paraspinous muscles are reapproximated, and the incision is closed.

Not all spinal tumors can be completely dissected and removed through the surgical approach. Some tumors may require surgical reduction with follow-up radiation therapy.

Ulnar Nerve Transposition
SURGICAL GOAL
The surgical goal of an ulnar nerve transposition is to free the ulnar nerve from a groove on the medial epicondyle, thereby restoring function and eliminating desensitization of the affected arm.

PATHOLOGY
The ulnar nerve is a peripheral nerve that travels through the groove of the medial epicondyle from the upper to lower arms. The ulnar nerve can be injured by trauma, elbow fractures and dislocations, and the repeated bending of the elbow as part of one's occupation or activities. Symptoms generally include reduced sensation in the affected arm, hand atrophies, or, in severe cases, a claw-hand deformity. Surgery is indicated when lifestyle and activity modifications and antiinflammatory medications fail.

Technique
1. The surgeon makes an incision on the lateral elbow.
2. The fascia and carpi ulnaris muscle are divided.
3. The surgeon frees the ulnar nerve.
4. The ulnar nerve is transposed anteriorly and placed deep into the origin of the brachialis flexor muscle.
5. The wound is irrigated.
6. The incision is closed.
7. A splint or cast is applied.

DISCUSSION
The patient is placed supine on the OR bed. The operative arm is placed on an arm table, suspended over the patient, or laid across the patient's body, depending on the surgeon's preference. A tourniquet is applied to the upper operative arm, and the limb is exsanguinated with an Esmarch bandage before the incision is made.

The surgeon makes the skin incision. The longer the incision is, the better is the visualization of the delicate structures. The ulnar nerve is identified in the medial epicondylar groove, and the bands exerting pressure on the nerve are released. The nerve is transposed from the groove at the back of the medial epicondyle of the humerus to the front of the

epicondyle. The ulnar nerve is placed and secured deep within the origin of the brachialis flexor muscle. The pronator muscles may be lifted from the bone to lengthen them to reduce compression on the nerve's new position. The wound is irrigated with sterile saline or an antibiotic solution and closed. A splint or cast is applied to prevent the patient from flexing and extending the elbow until inflammation decreases and healing occurs.

Transsphenoidal Hypophysectomy
SURGICAL GOAL
The goal of hypophysectomy is to remove all or a portion of the pituitary gland. This procedure may be performed to slow the growth and spread of endocrine-dependent malignant tumors or to excise a pituitary tumor. The gland is removed only if other treatment fails to destroy all pituitary tissue.

PATHOLOGY
The complete extracapsular enucleation of the pituitary gland in cases of hypophysectomy and possible complete removal of small pituitary tumors, with the remaining normal portion of the pituitary gland left intact, can be obtained by transsphenoidal hypophysectomy. In this approach, the sella turcica is accessed through the sphenoid sinus.

This procedure is performed to treat endocrine pituitary disorders, hypopituitarism, advanced metastatic carcinoma of the breast and prostate, diabetic retinopathy, and uncontrollable severe diabetes.

Technique
1. The patient is placed in a semi-Fowler's position.
2. The head is slightly flexed and tilted to allow for maximum exposure.
3. The C-arm fluoroscope is positioned lateral to the patient's head, with the monitor placed so that the surgeon can see the screen during the procedure.
4. The surgeon makes the incision under the upper lip horizontally at the junction of the gingivae and deep into the maxilla.
5. The nasal mucosa is elevated from each side of the nasal septum.
6. Bone and nasal cartilage are resected and preserved.
7. The sphenoid sinus is examined.
8. The sinus is opened until the floor of the sella turcica can be identified.
9. The floor is opened with a pneumatic drill.
10. The microscope is used to visualize the pituitary tumor and other lesions.
11. The lesions are resected.

DISCUSSION
Transsphenoidal hypophysectomy is performed with the use of general anesthesia combined with local anesthetic. The patient is supine in a semi-sitting position with the head slightly flexed. A portable C-arm intensifier is used throughout the procedure and should be placed to allow the surgeon

to see the monitor. The C-arm intensifier is centered on the sella turcica. A subnasal incision with a midline rhinoseptal approach is used and deepened until the sphenoid sinus is opened and the sella turcica can be identified.

The floor of the sinus is opened with a sphenoidal punch, and the dura mater is incised. When the extracapsular cleavage plane has been identified, the superior surface of the pituitary is dissected. The gland or tumor is removed, and the sellar cavity may be packed with a muscle that has been previously resected from the patient's thigh. The muscle graft packed into the sellar cavity prevents the leakage of cerebrospinal fluid.

The excision of a muscle graft is a clean procedure and must be performed before the gingival incision is made. The graft must be kept in a moist, sterile sponge to prevent the muscle graft from drying while the hypophysectomy is being performed. The gingival incision is closed with a 3-0 or 4-0 chromic or plain suture, and nasal packing may be used for several days postoperatively. The patient should be treated postoperatively as a craniectomy patient.

REFERENCES

Gardner E, Gray DJ, and O'Rahilly R: *Anatomy: a regional study of human structure,* ed 4, Philadelphia, 1975, WB Saunders,.

Guyton AC: *Basic human neurophysiology,* ed 3, Philadelphia, 1981, WB Saunders.

Jacob S, Francone C, and Lossow WJ: *Structure and function in man,* ed 5, Philadelphia, 1982, WB Saunders.

McVay C: *Surgical anatomy,* ed 6, Philadelphia, 1984, WB Saunders.

Pleasants D: Managing hydrocephalus with a ventricular shunt, *AORN J* 35 (5):885-892, 1982.

Sabiston DC Jr, ed: *Textbook of surgery,* ed 14, Philadelphia, 1991, WB Saunders, 1991.

Williams RW: *Surgical techniques: microlumbar discectomy,* Randolph, MA, 1976, Codman & Shurtleff.

Youmans J, ed: *Neurological surgery: a comprehensive reference guide to the diagnosis and management of neurosurgical problems,* ed 2, Philadelphia, 1982, WB Saunders.

Glossary

Abandonment—The failure to stay with a patient who is under one's care.

Abdominal peritoneum—Serous membrane lining the walls of the abdominal cavity.

Abduction—(1) Movement of a joint or body part *away* from the body. (2) To take away from; away from midline.

ABHES—Accrediting Bureau of Health Education Schools.

Ablate—To remove or destroy tissue.

Ablation—Removal and destruction of tissue by erosion or vaporization, usually through intense heat.

Absorbable sutures—Suture materials that are rapidly or eventually digested by enzymes in the body after the wound is healed.

Accreditation—The process whereby a hospital is evaluated by the Joint Commission for the Accreditation of Healthcare Organizations, which examines the hospital's practices, records, procedures, and outcomes to ensure that minimum standards for patient and employee safety are met.

Acetabulum—A hollow, cuplike portion of the hip joint; the hip socket.

Acoustic neuroma—A benign tumor of the eighth cranial nerve.

Acquired immunity—Disease immunity established through cellular memory. Specific protein antigens cause the immune system to create protein antibodies. Antibodies initiate a cascade of host-protective mechanisms that destroy disease organisms when encountered at a later time.

ACS—American College of Surgeons. A professional organization that establishes educational standards for surgeons and surgical residency programs.

Active electrode—An instrument or device used in surgery to deliver concentrated electrical current to tissue.

Adduction—To move toward the midline.

Adhesions—Scar tissue that binds internal tissues together. Adhesions present a technical problem during endoscopic surgery because they can cause wide variations in the anatomical locations of organs. Because the initial incisions often are made blindly, adhesions can result in trauma to tissues.

Adipose tissue—Layer of tissue containing fat cells.

Adnexa—A collective term for the ovaries, fallopian tubes, and their connective and vascular attachments.

Advance directive—A document in which one gives instructions about his or her medical care in the event that he or she cannot speak for himself or herself because of serious illness or incapacity. Examples of this are a living will and a medical power of attorney.

Adverse reactions—Unexpected reactions to a drug that are not related to dose.

Aerosol droplet—A droplet of moisture that is small enough to remain suspended in air and can carry microorganisms within it.

Aesthetic—Having a pleasing shape and form.

Aganglionic—Without nerve tissue.

Aggression—A forceful physical, verbal, or symbolic action. It may be appropriate (self-protective, indicating healthy self-assertiveness) or it may be inappropriate.

Aggressive—Behavior that is demanding, loud, sarcastic, or threatening.

Airborne contamination—Incident in which microorganisms carried in the air by moisture droplets or dust particles make contact with a sterile surface.

Airborne transmission precautions—Precautions to prevent the transmission of airborne disease from a known carrier to others in the environment.

Air exchange—The exchange of fresh air for air that has been recirculated in a closed area.

Allograft—Transfer of tissue between two genetically dissimilar individuals of the same species.

Alternate site burn—A patient burn at a site other than the target tissue. Alternate site burns have many causes.

Alveoli—Small air sacs found in the lungs, through which oxygen and carbon dioxide are exchanged during respiration.

Amnesia—Loss of recall of events or sensations. In anesthesia, amnesia is a desirable component produced by specific drugs such as the benzodiazepines. Patient recall of surgery is seen in about 0.2% of all cases performed under general anesthesia.

Ampere—Unit used to measure the strength of electric current.

Amplification system—In laser technology, a series of mirrors that reflect photons or free electrons within the optical resonant chamber. This causes emission of more photons and creation of laser energy.

Amplitude—The height of an energy wave.

Amputation—The surgical removal of a limb or portion of a limb.

Analgesia—The absence of pain, produced by specific drugs.

Anastomosis—A connection created between two vessels, spaces, or organs that normally are separated.

Anatomical resection—In liver surgery, refers to the removal of a segment by locating and ligating the biliary and vascular structures that drain into it.

Anesthesia—Literally, "without sensation." In medicine, anesthetic agents block nerve impulses that conduct sensation; these agents also may produce loss of consciousness.

Anesthesia care provider (ACP)—A professional licensed to administer anesthetic agents and medically manage the patient throughout the period of anesthesia.

Anesthesia machines—Machines that are capable of delivering anesthetic gases or volatile liquids. An anesthesia machine delivers titrated amounts of an agent mixed with oxygen. Positive pressure ventilation can be controlled mechanically with a ventilator or manually with a bag and mask. The device monitors the patient's vital physiological signs, such as heart rate, heart rhythm, oxygen saturation, and carbon dioxide level.

Anesthesiologist—A physician who is a specialist in anesthesia and pain management.

Anesthetic—A drug that produces a lack of sensation. A general anesthetic produces a state of unconsciousness, while a regional anesthetic blocks nerve conduction in a specific area of the body without producing loss of consciousness.

Aneurysm—A bulging in an artery caused by a weakening in the arterial wall. The weakening may be a congenital defect or the result of atherosclerosis, arteriosclerosis, infection, trauma, or degenerative disease.

Angioplasty—A process of remodeling the lumen of a blood vessel. This term usually refers to the removal of plaque or the release of a stricture in the vessel wall.

Ankylosis—The immobility or fusion of a joint caused by injury, disease, or surgical procedure.

Antagonist—A term used to describe a drug that is designed to counteract the effects of another agent.

Anterograde amnesia—In anesthesia, the patient's inability to recall events that occur while under the effects of certain drugs. After the drug is metabolized in the body, normal recall returns.

Antibiotic—A drug that inhibits the growth of or kills microorganisms in living tissue.

Antibiotic resistant—The ability of a microorganism to resist destruction by antimicrobial therapy. Antibiotic-resistant strains of microorganisms arise through genetic mutations induced by the use of antibiotics in animal feed, improper use of antimicrobial drugs, overprescription of antibiotics, and environmental factors.

Antibodies—Complex glycoproteins produced by the immune system, formed in response to antigens. An antibody makes contact with an antigen to destroy or control it.

Anticoagulant—A drug that prolongs blood clotting time.

Antigens—Macromolecules, such as proteins, glycoproteins, lipoproteins, and polysaccharides, on the surface of cells that identify them as part of the organism ("self") or foreign ("nonself"). Antigens can trigger a response by the immune system, which seeks out and destroys the marked cell. Surface antigens in bacteria include the flagellar (H), somatic (O), and capsular (K or Vi) antigens.

Antisepsis—A process that destroys most pathogenic organisms on animate surfaces.

Antiseptics—Chemical agents that are approved for use on the skin that inhibit the growth and reproduction of microorganisms. Antiseptics are used to cleanse and paint the surgical site to reduce the number of microorganisms to an absolute minimum.

Anxiolysis—Reduction in anxiety.

AORN—Association of periOperative Registered Nurses. The professional organization for surgical nurses; originally known as Association of Operating Room Nurses.

Apex—(1) The lower left tip of the left ventricle of the heart; (2) the rounded upper portion of each lung.

Apnea—Cessation of breathing.

Approximate—To bring tissue together by sutures or other means.

Aqueous humor—Clear, watery fluid that fills the anterior and posterior chambers in the front of the eye.

Arachnoid—The middle layer of the meninges, which is a very delicate serous membrane that resembles a spider's web.

ARC-ST—Accreditation Review Committee for Surgical Technologists. The professional agency for accreditation of surgical technology programs.

Areola—The darkened area surrounding the nipple, which contains sebaceous glands. The areola becomes more deeply pigmented under the influence of hormones, especially during pregnancy.

Arrhythmia—An abnormal heartbeat (also called *dysrhythmia*).

Arterial blood gases (ABGs)—A blood test that uses an arterial blood sample to assess oxygenation and adequacy of ventilation.

Arteriosclerosis—Disease characterized by thickening, hardening, and loss of elasticity of the walls of arteries.

Arteriotomy—An incision made in the artery, usually to perform an anastomosis with a graft or another vessel, or to remove plaque or a thrombus from inside the artery.

Arteriovenous fistula—Also called an *AV fistula*; a naturally occurring or surgically created connection between an artery and a vein. In surgery, an AV fistula is created surgically to prepare a vessel for hemodialysis.

Arthritis—Inflammation of a joint.

Arthrocentesis—Puncture of a joint space through use of a needle.

Arthrodesis—The surgical immobilization of a joint.

Arthrogram—Visualization of a joint by radiographic study after injection of a contrast medium into the joint space.

Arthroplasty—The operative procedure of reshaping or reconstructing a diseased joint.

Arthroscopy—An examination of the interior of a joint for therapeutic and diagnostic purposes with a specially designed endoscope.

Arthrotomy—A surgical incision into a joint.

Articular cartilage—Hyaline cartilage covering the articular surfaces of bones.

Articulation—The place of union between two or more bones; a joint.

Asepsis—The absence of pathogenic microorganisms on an animate surface or on body tissue. Literally, asepsis means "without infection." In surgery, asepsis is a state of minimal or zero pathogens. Asepsis is the goal of many surgical practices.

Aseptic technique—Methods or practices in health care that promote and maintain a state of asepsis. Also called *sterile technique.*

Assertiveness—A quality in people with self-esteem; assertive behavior seeks to protect one's own rights while respecting those of others.

AST—The Association of Surgical Technologists. The professional association for surgical technologists.

Asystole—The absence of a heartbeat; cardiac standstill.

Atherosclerosis—The most common form of arteriosclerosis. The formation of thick, yellowish plaque (containing cholesterol and lipoid materials, and lipophages) that infiltrates and deposits in the inner layer of the arterial wall. This plaque causes stricture and loss of arterial blood flow to a part of the body.

Atresia—A congenital absence or closure of a normal body opening or tubular structure.

Atria—The two upper chambers of the heart.

Atrial appendage—A small, muscular, ear-shaped portion of the atrium.

Atrioventricular—Pertaining to both the atrium and ventricle.

Augmentation—An addition or increase in size.

Autograft—Surgical transplantation of any tissue from one part of the body to another location in the same individual.

AV malformation—Arteriovenous malformation. An abnormal communication between the arteries and veins (called a *fistula*).

Back table—A large stainless steel table that is draped with a sterile sheet before surgery. Equipment and instruments are placed on this table in reserve, available for use during surgery.

Bacteria (pl); Bacterium (sing)—Unicellular microorganisms with a rigid cell wall, classified with respect to motility, reaction to staining with particular dyes, and their pathogenicity for other living organisms including man. Bacteria are classified as belonging to one of the three domains: Bacteria, Archaea, and Eukarya. They are one of the two domains that are classified as prokaryotes (cells that lack nuclear membrane). All of the prokaryotes of medical importance are in the domain bacteria. They are categorized according to different staining techniques (Gram's stain or the acid fast stain) and fall into three categories: gram-positive bacteria, gram-negative bacteria, and acid-fast bacteria.

Bactericidal—Able to kill bacteria.

Bacteriostatic—Capable of inhibiting the growth of bacteria but not killing them.

Baker's cyst—Synovial cyst (pouch) arising from the synovial lining of the knee.

Barrier drape—Drape intended to separate a contaminated area from the incision site. For example, a barrier drape is placed across the perineum between the vagina and anus during gynecological procedures. The barrier drape is plastic and may have a sticky surface along one edge. This edge is placed at the site where a barrier is needed.

Berry aneurysm—A small saclike bulge of a cerebral artery, usually found in the circle of Willis.

Bicoronal—An incision made between the frontal bone and the parietal bone on one side of the head and extending to the same location on the other side.

Bicortical screw—A screw that goes through both the inner and outer layers of a bone.

Bicuspid valve—A valve with two leaflets. Commonly refers to the valve between the left atrium and the left ventricle (the mitral valve). Also may refer to an anomalous aortic valve containing two (rather than the normal three) leaflets.

Bier block—Regional anesthesia administered by intravenous injection, used for surgical procedures performed on the arm below the elbow or on the leg below the knee; performed in a bloodless field maintained by a pneumatic tourniquet that also prevents the anesthetic from entering the systemic circulation.

Bifurcation—An anatomical term that describes a single tubular or hollow structure that leads to a Y or split in the same structure.

Bile—The digestive substance that is produced by the liver. Its main function is to emulsify (break into small particles) fats so that the body can digest them. When the diet contains excess cholesterol, the bile becomes supersaturated and releases bile salts that are irritating to the gallbladder and cause stones.

Biliary—Refers to the gallbladder and its ducts and blood vessels.

Billroth I procedure—A gastroduodenostomy or surgical anastomosis of the stomach and the duodenum.

Billroth II procedure—A gastroduodenostomy or surgical anastomosis of the stomach and the jejunum.

Bilobate—Having two lobes.

Bioburden—Contamination of an item from debris or microorganisms.

Biological indicators—A mechanism for measuring sterility assurance that determines the presence of pathogenic bacteria on objects subjected to a sterilization process.

Biopsy—Removal of a sample of tissue for pathological analysis.

Bleeder—A bleeding vessel.

Blepharoplasty—Surgery to restore or repair the eyelid or eyebrow.

Blood-borne pathogens—Pathogenic microorganisms that may be present in and transmitted through human blood and body fluids. Examples are hepatitis B virus and human immunodeficiency virus.

Blunt dissection—The technique of separating tissue layers by teasing them apart with a rough sponge dissector.

Blunt needle—A curved, tapered needle with a blunt point. This type of needle is usually used in highly vascular organs such as the liver. Surgeons are encouraged to use the blunt needle for other tissue types to reduce the risk of needle-stick injury.

Boggy—A characteristic of diseased tissue that makes it soft and doughy.

Bolster(s)—A small tube made from soft vinyl or plastic. A bolster is threaded over the ends of an umbilical tape or suture tie that is placed around a vessel. A Rumel tourniquet is a type of bolster.

Box lock—The hinge point of many surgical instruments.

BPH—Benign prostatic hypertrophy; a condition in which the prostate gland enlarges and impinges on the urethra.

Bradycardia—A slow heart rate; usually a heart rate of less than 60 beats per minute.

Branchial cleft cyst—A cavity that is a remnant from embryologic development, present at birth in one side of the neck just in front of, and on either side of, the large angulated muscle (the sternocleidomastoid muscle).

Bridle suture—A traction suture placed in tissue and used to retract or maintain tension on the tissue.

Bronchospasm—An involuntary smooth muscle spasm of the bronchi. Like laryngospasm, it can occur as a complication of anesthesia. Patients with a difficult airway, anatomical malformation, and bronchiole disease are prone to bronchospasm. Certain anesthetic agents cause bronchospasm and laryngospasm.

Brown and Sharp (B & S) gauge—Sizing standard used to measure the diameter of wire or stainless steel.

Bucking—A patient's involuntary reaction to stimulation of the larynx. It occurs when the patient is sedated. The patient recoils and arches the neck in a bucking motion.

Buckling component—Silicone bolster that encircles the eye.

Bur—Drill tip designed to make holes in bone; also spelled *burr*.

Bursa—A padlike sac or cavity found in connective tissue near the joint.

CAAHEP—Commission on Accreditation of Allied Health Education Programs. It accredits educational programs in allied health professions.

Calculi—Abnormal stones in body tissues resulting from the precipitation of minerals, such as calcium, and other substances.

Canalplasty—A procedure in which the external auditory canal is reconstructed.

Cancellous bone—A latticework structure of spongy or soft bone.

Capillarity—The ability of suture material to soak up fluid along the strand from the immersed wet end into the dry nonimmersed end. Capillarity is high in braided sutures.

Capsulorrhexis—Derived from the Greek word "rhexis," meaning a bursting, a rupture, or a tearing. This is a surgical technique used in cataract extraction when the capsule of the cataract is torn, and a complete capsulotomy is performed.

Cardiac muscle—The muscles of the heart.

Cardioplegia—The intentional stopping of the heart during cardiac surgery. It is performed with cardioplegia solution, which often contains a mixture of potassium chloride, lidocaine, dextrose, insulin, albumin, tromethamine, and Plasmanate.

C-arm—A type of radiograph that produces "real time" fluoroscopic images for the surgeon or radiographer.

Case-cart system—Organizational method of preparing equipment and instruments for a specific surgery. Equipment is prepared by the central services or supply department and sent to the operating room.

Case planning—The process of organizing the tasks and equipment required for a surgical procedure. Case planning requires the ability to prioritize, organizational skills, and knowledge about the procedure.

Cataract—A condition in which the crystalline lens of the eye, its capsule, or both become opaque, with consequent loss of vision.

Cavitation—A process in which air pockets are imploded (burst inward), releasing particles of soil or tissue debris.

Central core—The restricted area of the operating room in which sterile supplies and flash sterilizers are located.

Central nervous system—Part of the nervous system containing the brain and spinal cord.

Cerclage—A procedure in which a suture ligature is placed around the incompetent cervix and tightened to prevent spontaneous abortion.

Cerebellum—Gray matter lying in the posterior cranial fossa that is divided into fissures. The cerebellum is responsible for coordination and movement.

Cerebral aqueduct—A narrow pathway for the cerebrospinal fluid to flow to the fourth ventricle and then to the brainstem and spine.

Cerebral cortex—The outer tissue layer of the cerebrum, composed of gray matter and divided into lobes.

Cerebral peduncle—A bundle of nerves found in the anterior portion of the midbrain that carries impulses to and from the cerebrum.

Cerebrospinal fluid—A nourishing fluid that circulates around the brain and spinal cord, acting like a watery cushion to prevent injury.

Cerebrum—The main portion of the brain, divided into two hemispheres. The cerebrum controls motor activities and sensory impulses. Its forebrain is responsible for memory, intelligence, and reason. The cerebrum is the largest portion of the brain.

Certified registered nurse anesthetist (CRNA)—A registered nurse trained and licensed to administer anesthetic agents.

Cerumen—Substance produced by the cerumen glands of the ear (i.e., ear wax).

Chain of command—A hierarchy of personnel positions that establishes both vertical and horizontal relationships between positions.

Chemical barrier—The barrier formed by the action of an antiseptic that not only reduces the number of microorganisms on a surface but also prevents recolonization (regrowth) for a limited period of time.

Chemical indicators—Methods used to verify that an item has been exposed to a particular sterilization process. Chemical indicators ensure that specific parameters of a sterilization process have been met.

Chemical sterilization—A process that uses chemical agents rather than steam to achieve sterilization.

Chemistry studies—Various tests that evaluate the presence of or levels of certain chemicals within the blood. Chemistry studies are performed to evaluate cardiac enzymes, liver function, kidney function, thyroid function, and basic metabolic function. Cholesterol, or lipid, studies are an example of a chemistry study.

Chisel—An orthopedic instrument used to slice bone; one side is straight and the other is beveled.

Choanal—The communicating passageways between the nasal fossae and pharynx.

Cholecystectomy—Surgical removal of the gallbladder.

Choledochojejunostomy—A surgical anastomosis of the common bile duct and the jejunostomy.

Cholelithiasis—Condition in which calculi or bilestones are present in the bile duct or gallbladder.

Cholesteatoma—An ectopic growth of squamous epithelium (skin) in the ear.

Chondroradionecrosis—Necrosis of cartilage resulting from radiation.

Choroid—The vascular, intermediate tissue layer that provides nourishment to the other parts of the interior eye.

Chromic salt—Chemical used to treat surgical gut so it resists rapid enzymatic absorption by body tissues, reduces irritation of tissue, and increases tensile strength in the suture strand.

Circuit—The closed path through which current flows.

Circulator—The nonsterile surgical team member who assists in gathering additional supplies and equipment needed during the surgical procedure and advocates for the patient.

Circumcision—Removal of all or part of the prepuce (foreskin) of the penis.

Cirrhosis—Disease of the liver in which the tissue becomes hardened and its venous drainage blocked. It is usually caused by chronic alcoholism but also may result from other disease conditions.

Clamp—Instrument that is designed to occlude or hold tissue, objects, or fabric between its jaws.

Cleaning—A process that removes organic or inorganic soil or debris.

Closed gloving—A technique of gloving in which the bare hand does not come in contact with the outside of the glove. The sterile glove is protected from the nonsterile hand by the cuff of a surgical gown.

Coagulation—Clotting of blood.

Coarctation—Narrowing of the passageway of a blood vessel, such as coarctation of the aorta, a congenital condition.

Cobalt 60 radiation—A method of sterilizing prepackaged equipment; ionizing radiation.

Coherent—A characteristic of light in which all the light waves are lined up so that their peaks and troughs are matched. It is a characteristic of laser light.

Colonization—The process of a group of bacteria living together.

Commissurotomy—A surgical incision into a commissure, a band of tissue that connects two anatomical structures. In the heart, the valves may be banded together by scar tissue. In this case, a commissurotomy is a surgical incision made into this scar tissue to separate the valve leaflets.

Comorbid disease—A disease or condition that exists simultaneously with another unrelated disease in the same patient.

Complaint—The legal document that begins a civil lawsuit and designates who is suing whom and why.

Complete blood count (CBC)—A blood test that measures specific components of blood, including hemoglobin, hematocrit, red blood cells, white blood cells and types, platelets, and several red blood cell indices.

Computed tomography (CT)—A test that allows physicians to obtain cross-sectional radiographic views of the patient. The test also is called a *CT scan* or *computed axial tomography (CAT) scan.*

Concentration—A measure of the quantity of a substance per a specific volume or weight.

Condyle—A rounded protuberance at the end of a bone forming an articulation.

Conformer—A device placed in the socket after enucleation or evisceration to preserve the shape of the fornices.

Congenital—A condition present at birth.

Conjunctiva—The mucous membrane that lines the eyelids and covers the front of the eyeball.

Conjunctival sulcus—Depression at the level of the conjunctiva.

Consensus—Agreement among members of a group.

Contaminated—The condition in which instruments, supplies, or items have been exposed to a nonsterile item, particle, or surface through physical or airborne contact.

Contamination—Result of physical contact between a sterile surface and a nonsterile surface in surgery. Contamination also can result from airborne dust, moisture droplets, or fluids that act as a vehicle for transporting contaminants from a nonsterile surface to a sterile one.

Content—Substance or actual information contained in a message.

Contracture—Fibrosis of muscle, fascia, skin, or joint capsule that cannot be mobilized if flexed or extended.

Contrast medium—A radioopaque (not penetrated by x-rays) solution that is introduced into body cavities to outline their inside surface.

Controlled hypothermia—Deliberate lowering of the patient's core body temperature during general anesthesia in selected cases. This reduces the oxygen requirements of tissues. It can be used in cardiac surgery, procedures that require occlusion or blockage of large blood vessels, and organ transplantation.

Controlled substances—Drugs that have the potential for abuse. Controlled substances are rated according to their risk potential. These ratings are called *schedules.*

Control-release—Suture material with swaged needles that are designed to "pop-off" with a twist of the wrist after the suture has been passed through tissues.

Convalescence—The stage of disease in which damaged cells are repaired and the patient recovers from the effects of the illness or operation.

Corpora quadrigemina—Four rounded masses found in the midbrain responsible for auditory and visual impulses.

Count—A systematic method of accounting for all sponges, needles, instruments, and other items that can be retained in the patient. Counts are performed on all cases in which there is a possibility of leaving an item in the surgical wound.

Coupling—Electrosurgical contact between two or more instruments during endoscopic surgery. This can result in serious burns.

Court (or bench) trial—Trial in which a judge determines factual evidence and makes the final judgment.

Cricoid cartilage—A ring of cartilage between the trachea and the larynx. This is the only true complete circle of cartilage of the entire airway.

Cricoid pressure—Direct manual pressure on the patient's cricoid cartilage, which compresses the trachea, helps to prevent aspiration, and can facilitate intubation.

Critical items—In medicine, those items that must be sterilized before use on a patient; items that penetrate body tissues or the vascular system.

Critical thinking—The process of analyzing information about the patient, comparing it with similar previous experience, and responding to the unique needs of the current patient. For example, your pediatric patient is 8 years old and is having surgery. You know that the developmental needs at this age include a need for information about the environment. In this particular case, however, the patient has a severe hearing deficit. You must plan some way other than speech to communicate information to the patient to help him cope with his fears about the operating room environment.

Cross-clamp—To place a clamp across a structure (usually a blood vessel) to occlude it. The term often is used to

describe the clamping of the aorta and other large blood vessels.

Cross-contamination—The transmission of microorganisms from one source to another.

Cryosurgery—The use of subfreezing temperature to destroy tissue.

Cryotherapy—A technique whereby an instrument or cryoprobe is used to freeze tissue such as the sclera, ciliary body (for glaucoma), or retinal layers after detachment. The cryoprobe also can be used to remove an opaque lens during intracapsular cataract removal.

CST—Certified Surgical Technologist. A surgical technologist who has successfully passed the certification examination distributed by the Liaison Council on Certification for the Surgical Technologist.

CST-CFA—Certified Surgical Technologist–Certified First Assistant. A Certified Surgical Technologist First Assistant who has successfully passed the certification examination distributed by the Liaison Council on Certification for the Surgical Technologist.

Culture—A process in which a sample of exudate, pus, or fluid is grown in culture media and analyzed for the presence of infectious microorganisms. When the microorganisms have colonized, they are examined for type and sensitivity to specific antibiotics. This procedure is called a *C and S (culture and sensitivity)*.

Culture and sensitivity (C & S)—A test used to identify the sensitivity of a microorganism to a particular antimicrobial agent. The test is used to identify the causative agent of an infection and identify the antimicrobial best suited to fight the infection.

Curettage—To remove tissue by scraping with a surgical curette.

Current—The flow of electrons (measured in amperes).

Cutting instrument—An instrument with a sharp edge used to cut and dissect tissue. This group includes scissors, scalpels, osteotomes, curettes, chisels, biopsy punches, saws, drills, and needles.

Cystocele—A bulging of the bladder into the vagina. The condition is related to weakness in the anterior vaginal wall.

Damages—Money awarded in a civil lawsuit to compensate the injured party.

Debridement—Process of removing dead skin, debris, or foreign bodies from a wound.

Decompression—A technique or process in which the stomach contents are continually drained into a collection device. Decompression is required after gastric surgery or disease.

Decontamination—A process of disinfection.

Decontamination area—A room or small department in which soiled instruments and equipment are cleaned of gross soil and decontaminated to remove microorganisms.

De-epithelialization—Removal of skin from a tissue flap.

Deepithelialized—State in which epithelial tissue has been removed.

Defamation—A derogatory statement concerning another person's skill, character, or reputation.

Dehiscence—The separation of the layers of the surgical wound; it may be partial and superficial only, or complete, with disruption of all layers.

Delayed union—A fracture that has not healed within an average amount of time.

Delegate—To assign one's duties to another person. In medicine, the person who delegates the duty retains accountability for the action of the person to whom it is delegated.

Delegation—The transfer of responsibility for an activity from a licensed person to a nonlicensed person; the person initiating the transfer retains accountability for the outcome of that activity.

Delirium—A state of confusion and disorientation. Delirium is a stage of anesthesia induction that produces struggling, coughing, gagging, and possible airway obstruction resulting from bronchospasm or laryngospasm. Delirium, on induction, is seldom observed with the use of modern induction drugs that rapidly bypass this stage.

Dentition—Teeth.

Dependent tasks—Tasks that are delegated to another person and require direct supervision by the person delegating the task.

Deposition—Testimony of a witness, under oath, and transcribed by a court reporter during the pretrial phase of a civil lawsuit.

Dermoid cyst—A primitive disorganized mass of cells and tissues that often contains teeth, hair, and skin.

Desiccation—Tissue drying. Alcohol is a desiccating skin preparation solution. It causes the destruction of tissue protein and therefore is never used around the eyes or on mucous membranes.

Diagnostic agent—Pharmacologic substance used to aid in diagnostic procedures.

Diaphysis—The shaft of a long bone.

Diastolic pressure—The lowest pressure exerted on the arterial wall during the resting phase of the cardiac cycle.

Diathermy—Low-power cautery used to mark the sclera over the area of the retinal detachment.

Differential count—Test that identifies the amount of each type of WBC in a specimen of blood; typically part of the CBC.

Dilator—Graduated smooth instrument used to increase the diameter of an anatomical opening in tissue.

Direct care—Care that is usually "hands on." Direct care is often therapeutic or diagnostic.

Direct inguinal hernia—An acquired weakness in the inguinal floor that leads to protrusion of the abdominal contents. The characteristic bulging usually follows activity that produces increased intraabdominal pressure or "bearing down," and it causes pain. The area of weakness can become larger over time, and the contents of the hernia can become trapped or strangulated (see *Strangulated hernia*).

Direct transmission—The transfer of microbes from their source to a new host by direct physical contact, for example, exhalation by one individual of a water droplet containing respiratory virus and its inhalation by another.

Disinfection—A process that destroys most but not all pathogenic microorganisms on inanimate objects.

Dispersive electrode—The grounding pad applied to the patient that directs current flow from the patient back to the power unit.

Doppler duplex ultrasonography—Doppler ultrasonography amplifies sounds that pass through tissue. Doppler duplex technology uses this technology plus ultrasound to produce a visual image of blood flow through a vessel.

Doppler studies—A technique that uses ultrasound energy to measure motion within blood vessels. The test measures blood flow through a particular vessel.

Dosage—The regulated administration of prescribed amounts of a drug. Dosage is usually expressed as a quantity of drug per unit of time.

Dose—The quantity of a drug to be taken at one time or the stated amount of drug per unit of distribution (e.g., 0.5 mg per milliliter of solution).

Double-action instrument—An instrument with two hinges in the middle. This provides greater leverage and cutting strength than a single-action instrument. Usually used to describe an orthopedic rongeur.

Double-armed sutures—Suture-needle combinations containing a needle at each end of the suture. Double-armed sutures are used to approximate tissue in a circumference, as in joining two ends of a blood vessel.

Drape—Sterile materials, including towels and sheets, placed around the prepared surgical incision site to create a sterile field.

Droplet nuclei—Dried remnants of previously moist secretions containing microorganisms. Droplet nuclei are an important source of disease transmission.

Drug—Chemical substance that, when taken into the body, changes one or more of the body's functions.

Drug administration—The actual giving of a drug to a person by any route.

Ductus arteriosus—A normal fetal structure, allowing blood to bypass circulation to the lungs. If this structure remains open after birth, it is called a *patent ductus arteriosus*.

Duodenostomy—A surgical opening of the duodenum leading to the outside of the body via a tube, or from another hollow anatomical structure such as the stomach.

Dura mater—The very fibrous outer layer of the meninges.

Dye—A drug typically administered to allow a surgeon to observe under direct visualization the patency of a tubular structure (e.g., fallopian tube, ureter).

Dysphagia—Difficulty in swallowing.

Dysrhythmia—A disturbance in the heartbeat (also called an *arrhythmia*).

Echocardiography—The use of ultrasound to diagnose conditions of the heart.

Efficiency—The economic use of time and energy to prevent unnecessary expenditure of work, materials, and time.

Effusion—Fluid in the middle ear.

Elasticity—The amount of stretch exhibited by a suture material.

Electrocardiogram (ECG)—A noninvasive test that measures electrical activity of the heart; also abbreviated *EKG*.

Electroencephalogram (EEG)—A diagnostic tool that measures the electrical activity of the brain. During vascular surgery, EEG may be used to determine the patient's neurophysiologic response.

Electrolyte levels—The measurement of levels of various minerals and elements within the blood.

Electrolytic media—Any solution that conducts electricity. During surgeries that require continuous irrigation for distention of a hollow organ, the media used must *not* be electrolytic. The use of electrolytic media would allow the current to travel through the media, causing a burn or an electrical shock.

Electromagnetic spectrum—Wave energy in the universe that is quantitatively measured. The visible waves of the spectrum appear colored to humans.

Electromyogram—A graphic record of the contraction of a muscle as a result of electrical stimulation.

Elevator—A non-hinged sharp or dull tipped instrument. An elevator is used to separate tissues or to bluntly re-model tissue.

Embolism—Obstruction or occlusion of a blood vessel by a blood clot or trapped air that migrates through the systemic circulation. An embolus may lodge in small vessels of the body, including vessels of the lung, brain, or heart, blocking circulation and causing local ischemia and tissue death.

Embolus—A clot of blood, air, or organic material that moves freely in the vascular system. An embolus travels from larger to smaller vessels until it cannot pass through a vessel. At that level it interrupts the flow of blood and may result in severe disease or death.

Emergence—A stage in general anesthesia in which delivery of the anesthetic agents is stopped. The patient emerges from a state of unconsciousness into a state of wakefulness. Emergence can be an unstable period that is similar to induction except that physiological and somatic events occur in reverse order.

En bloc—In one piece; describing a removal.

Endarterectomy—The surgical removal of atherosclerotic plaque from inside an artery.

Endocardial cushion—Areas of the fibrous skeleton forming between the atrium and ventricle.

Endometriosis—Endometrial tissue growth outside of the uterine cavity.

Endoneurium—A protective sheath that surrounds the fascicles.

Endoscope—The optical instrument inserted into a body cavity during endoscopic surgery.

Endoscopy—The use of endoscopic technology to diagnose pathology.

Endospore (spore)—The dormant stage of some bacteria that allows them to survive without reproducing in extreme environmental conditions, including heat, cold, and exposure to many disinfectants. When conditions are favorable for reproduction, the spore again becomes active and produces bacterial colonies.

Endosteum—A fine membrane that lines the medullary cavity of bone.

Endotoxin—Bacterial toxin, associated with the outer membrane of certain gram-negative bacteria. Endotoxins are not secreted but are released when the cells are disrupted or broken down.

Endotracheal tube—A hollow airway inserted into the patient's trachea to maintain patency and allow delivery of oxygen and anesthetic gases.

Enucleation—Surgical removal of the eyeball after the eye muscles and optic nerve have been severed.

Epigastric—Region of the abdomen above the umbilicus, following the upper edge of the stomach.

Epinephrine—A medication that stimulates the heart muscle and produces vasoconstriction.

Epineurium—The outer protective covering of a peripheral nerve.

Epiphysiodesis—Fusion of the growth plates in bones.

Epiphysis—The center for ossification at each extremity of long bone. The growth plate.

Epispadias—Congenital abnormality in which the opening of the urethra is on the dorsum of the penis.

Epistaxis—Bleeding arising from the nasal cavity.

Eschar—(1) Tissue that is burned to the point of carbonization. (2) A scab or dry crust caused by a thermal or chemical burn, infection, or excoriating skin disease.

Esmarch bandage—A roller bandage made of rubber or latex. It is wrapped around a limb starting at the distal end and extending to the proximal end. The bandage pushes blood away from the limb. A pneumatic tourniquet located at the proximal end is then inflated to prevent the return flow of blood into the extremity. See *Bier block.*

Esophageal varices—Varicose veins of the esophagus resulting from advanced liver disease. The portal vein becomes engorged because fibrous tissue in the liver occludes the circulatory system. Blood then backs into esophageal veins, which become grossly distended and may burst, causing extensive hemorrhage.

ESWL—Extracorporeal shockwave lithotripsy; a procedure in which ultrasonic sound waves are used to pulverize kidney or gall bladder stones.

Ethical dilemma—A situation in which ethical choices involve conflicting values.

Ethics—Standards that govern a specific group of people.

Ethylene oxide—Highly flammable, toxic gas that is capable of sterilizing an object.

Etiology—The origin or cause of a disease.

Eustachian tube—A tube lined with mucous membrane that joins the nasopharynx and the middle ear cavity. It allows for equalization of the air pressure in the middle ear.

Event-related sterility—The interference of environmental conditions or events with the integrity of a package; sterilized items are otherwise assumed sterile between uses.

Eversion—A turning outward.

Evert—To turn outward or inside out.

Evisceration—(1) The protrusion of an internal organ through a wound or through a surgical incision; (2) Surgical removal of the contents of the eyeball, with the sclera left intact.

Excisional biopsy—Removal of a tissue mass for pathological examination.

Exenteration—Removal of the entire contents of the orbit.

Exostosis—A benign bony growth that arises from the surface of a bone.

Exotoxin—A toxic substance produced by microorganisms and excreted outside of the bacterial cell. Exotoxins differ in the particular tissues of the host that they may affect. Examples of these would be Pseudomonas and tetanus.

Exploratory laparotomy—A laparotomy performed to examine the abdominal cavity when less invasive measures fail to confirm a diagnosis.

Exsanguination—The process of expressing blood from a part.

Exstrophy—The eversion or turning out of any organ.

Exteriorized—Surgical term describing any organ or object that has been "brought out" of a cavity or organ, or the abdominal wall.

Extracorporeal—Outside the body. In extracorporeal hemodialysis, the blood is shunted outside the body for filtering and cleansing.

Fascia—Fibrous membrane covering, supporting, and separating muscles.

Fascicles—Small bundles of nerve fibers.

Fasciotomy—A surgical incision and division of the fascia.

Feedback—Physical response to a message; a component of effective communication.

Fenestrated drapes—Sterile body sheets with a hole or "window" that exposes the surgical incision site. The fenestrated drape is positioned after other drapes and towels have been placed in keeping with the procedure. Fenestrated drapes are differentiated by type, such as laparotomy, thyroid, kidney, eye, ear, and extremity drapes.

Fiberoptic—Pertaining to a lighting system that uses bundles of flexible reflective fibers to transmit light through a cable. Fiberoptic light is extremely intense. The source may be a xenon or halogen metal vapor arc lamp.

Fibrillation—A cardiac dysrhythmia in which the heart ceases to pump and instead quivers and undulates. This results in cardiac standstill and stasis of blood in the heart.

Fibroid—See *Leiomyoma*.

First-degree burn—Burn that involves only the outer layer of the epidermis.

First intention wound closure—Wound closure in which all layers of the wound are approximated and the collagen scar formation is minimal; sometimes called *primary intention wound closure*.

Fissure—A narrow cleft in the brain tissue between the folds of the gyri.

Flash sterilize—To sterilize instruments and equipment in a high-pressure autoclave. Used only in an emergency, such as when an instrument is contaminated during surgery and must be sterilized immediately.

Fluoroscopy—A technique that uses continuous exposure of x-rays to improve the physician's view of structures or objects.

Fomite—An intermediate, inanimate source in the process of disease transmission. Any object such as a contaminated surgical instrument or medical device can become a fomite in disease transmission.

Foramen magnum—The large opening in the occipital bone between the cranial cavity and the spinal canal.

Fowler position—Sitting position used for cranial, facial, and some reconstructive breast procedures.

Fracture—A break in a bone.

Frequency—In wave science, the number of waves per second measured in hertz.

Friable—Condition in which tissue tears or fragments easily when handled. Some disease states produce friable tissue. The liver and spleen normally are friable.

Frontal lobe—The lobe of the brain containing the forehead; the anterior portion of the cerebrum.

Frozen section—A microscopic slice of frozen anatomic tissue that is evaluated for the presence of abnormal cells. Frozen section analysis is performed during surgery to diagnose malignancy.

Fulcrum—The area on an instrument at which the lever moves.

Fulguration—An electrosurgical technique in which a spray of electrical energy coagulates and removes tissue. Also called *spray coagulation*.

Full-thickness skin graft—Skin graft that consists of the entire epidermis and dermis.

Fungicidal—Able to kill fungi.

Fusiform aneurysm—A type of aneurysm that involves the entire circumference of a blood vessel.

Galea—A tough fibrous tissue sheet resembling a helmet that protects the brain.

Gas—Matter in its least dense state (e.g., air at room temperature is a gas).

Gas scavenging—The capture and safe removal of anesthetic gases that escape from the anesthesia machine and other devices such as a patient face mask. Repeated exposure to anesthetic gases is known to be a risk to surgical personnel. The Occupational Safety and Health Administration and the Joint Commission for the Accreditation of Healthcare Organizations require effective scavenging systems.

Gastroschisis—The herniation of abdominal contents through the abdominal wall without involvement of the umbilical cord.

Gastrostomy—A surgical opening through the stomach wall connecting to the outside of the body or another hollow anatomical structure.

General anesthesia—Anesthesia associated with a state of unconsciousness. General anesthesia is not a fixed state of unconsciousness but ranges along a continuum from semiresponsive to profoundly unresponsive.

Generic name—The formulary name of a drug.

Genetic mutation—Having the ability to cause permanent change in genetic structure.

GERD—Gastroesophageal reflux disease. A condition in which the gastroesophageal sphincter allows gastric contents to reflux into the esophagus, causing irritation and mucosal burning, possibly leading to cancer of the esophagus.

Germicidal—Able to kill germs.

Glaucoma—A localized eye disease characterized by increased sustained intraocular pressure that causes damage to the eye.

Glisson's capsule—A firm connective tissue that covers and protects the liver surface.

Globe—The eyeball.

Glottis—Area of the larynx from the superior surface of the true vocal cords to about 1 cm below the medial extent of the true vocal cords.

Glycine—See *Sorbitol*.

Gossip—The telling and retelling of events about another's personal life, professional life, or physical condition.

Gout—Hereditary metabolic disease that is a form of acute arthritis. Marked by inflammation of the joints, usually starting in the foot or the knee.

Gram stain—A method of differential staining of bacteria that separates them into one of two groups, gram-positive or gram-negative. Each group has common characteristics that identify its members and aid in diagnosis and treatment.

Gravity displacement sterilizer—Type of sterilizer that removes air by gravity.

Gray commissure—Portion of the spinal cord that includes the spinal canal and that covers the spinal cord.

Gray matter—Areas of the nervous system where fibers are unmyelinated. Gray matter contains the bodies of nerve cells.

Groupthink—In sociology and group behavior theory, the conformity of a group to one way of thinking and behaving. Groupthink creates two factions, those who agree (in-group) and those who disagree (out-group). This generates resentment and conflict in the workplace.

Gynecomastia—An abnormal enlargement of the mammary gland in males, resulting in enlargement of one or both breasts.

Gyri—The folds or convolutions of the brain tissue.

Handwashing—A specific technique used to remove debris and dead cells from the hands. Handwashing with an antiseptic also reduces the number of microorganisms on the skin.

Hasson cannula—A type of blunt-tipped trocar-and-cannula assembly used in "open" laparoscopic procedures that is anchored to the body wall with sutures.

Head drape—A turban-style drape created with two surgical towels that covers the patient's head and eyes. Knowing how to prepare and place this drape is a valuable draping skill.

Hematocrit (Hct)—Test that examines the percentage of red blood cells as a part of the blood; part of the CBC or hemogram.

Hematopoiesis—The production and development of blood cells, normally in the bone marrow.

Hematuria—Condition of blood in the urine.

Hemodialysis—A process in which blood is shunted out of the body and through a complex set of filters. It is performed on patients with end-stage renal disease to remove extra electrolytes and waste products from the body.

Hemoglobin (Hb)—Test that identifies the capacity of oxygen-carrying cells within the blood. A gram of hemoglobin (Hb) carries 1.34 ml of oxygen. Part of the CBC or hemogram.

Hemogram—A blood test similar to the CBC that is limited to hemoglobin, hematocrit, RBCs, WBCs, and platelets.

Hemostat—A surgical clamp used most often to occlude a blood vessel.

Heparin—An anticoagulant medication.

Hiatus—An opening in tissue. For example, the esophagus passes through the hiatus of the diaphragm.

High-efficiency particulate air (HEPA) filters—Filters installed in the operating room ventilation system that remove 99.97% of particles equal to or larger than 0.3 micrometers (μm).

High-level disinfection—Disinfection process that destroys many forms of microorganisms, not including bacterial spores.

High vacuum sterilizer—Type of steam sterilizer that removes air in the chamber by vacuum. Also known as a *pre-vacuum sterilizer.*

Histology—Study of the structure of tissue.

History and physical (H & P)—The process of interviewing a patient and conducting a physical examination to assess various anatomical structures and systems.

Homeostasis—A state of balance between the body's environmental and physiological stimuli and its responses. Homeostasis is maintained through the body's intricate feedback systems. For example, when blood volume decreases, the heart rate increases to push available blood more efficiently.

Honed—Sharpened.

Hook wire—A device used to pinpoint the exact location of a nonpalpable mass detected during a mammogram. A fine needle is inserted into the mass during the examination, and the tissue around the needle is removed for pathological examination and definitive diagnosis.

Hospital policy—A set of rules or regulations that hospital employees are required to follow. They are created to protect patients and employees from harm and to ensure the smooth operation of the hospital.

Host—The organism that harbors or nourishes another organism (parasite).

Hydrodressing—Dressings that have been impregnated with water-based gel.

Hydroxyapatite implant—A porous implant made of calcium phosphate and a naturally occurring body substance that is coupled to an artificial eye with a peg.

Hyperextension—Extension of a joint beyond its normal anatomical range.

Hyperflexion—Flexion of a joint beyond its normal anatomical range.

Hyperkeratotic—A condition of thickening of squamous epithelium (i.e., callus).

Hyperplasia—Abnormal overgrowth of tissue anywhere in the body.

Hypertrophy—An enlargement.

Hypogastric—Below the level of the stomach.

Hypopharynx—The digestive track between the oropharynx and the esophagus. This is where the airway departs from the aerodigestive tract to form the larynx.

Hypospadias—Abnormal congenital condition in which the urethra opens inferior to its normal location. Normally seen in males, where the urethra opens on the undersurface of the penis.

Hypothermia—Condition of abnormally low body temperature.

Hysteroscopy—A diagnostic and surgical method of performing intrauterine surgery. The hysteroscope is inserted through the cervix and surgery is conducted through the scope.

Imbricate—To build a surface with overlapping layers of material.

Impervious—Not able to be penetrated.

Implant—A synthetic or metal replacement for an anatomical structure such as a joint or cranial bone.

Inanimate—Nonliving.

Incarcerated hernia—Herniated tissue that is trapped outside its normal location by a defect in the abdominal wall. Incarcerated tissue requires emergency surgery to prevent a tourniquet effect on the incarcerated tissue, leading to necrosis.

Incise drapes—Plastic self-adhesive drapes that are positioned over the incision site after the surgical skin preparation. The drape creates a sterile surface over the skin. The incision is made directly through the incise drape and skin.

Incisional hernia—Occurs along the incision of a previous abdominal surgery. Incisional hernia, also called a *ventral hernia,* is caused by infection, obesity, excess tension on the original suture line, or any other process that breaks down the tissues. The incisional hernia may start as a small break in tissue continuity and progress to the full length of the incision. Evisceration and infection can result if the incision fully ruptures. More often, incarceration and strangulation require emergency surgery.

Incompetent cervix—A cervix that is unable to tolerate the weight of a growing fetus and allows it to be expelled during gestation.

Incomplete abortion—Demise of the embryo or fetus and expulsion of the tissue.

Independent tasks—Tasks that are transferred to another person and do not require direct supervision by the person delegating the task.

Indirect care—Patient care that requires skills and knowledge about the patient, the disease, and the procedure, and an appropriate response to the individual patient's needs. Indirect care does not include patient assessment, intervention, or evaluation.

Indirect inguinal hernia—A hernia that protrudes across the membranous sac of the spermatic cord. The weakness in this sac usually is present at birth and may require surgery early in life. If the defect enlarges, the intraabdom-inal contents can slide through the deep and superficial inguinal rings and enter the scrotum, causing pain and trauma to the trapped tissue.

Indirect transmission—Transmission of microorganisms by an intermediate nonliving source, such as a nonsterile instrument or surgical implant (see *fomite*).

Induced hypotension—The deliberate lowering of the patient's blood pressure during surgery to control hemorrhage, produce a more bloodless operative field, or control intracranial pressure.

Induction—The time from the beginning of administration of an anesthetic agent until the patient reaches the surgical level of loss of consciousness. Sensation is lost, and the patient is unaware of the environment.

Inert—A type of sutures and implants that, because of their biochemical properties, provoke little or no inflammatory reaction by the body.

Infarction—Necrosis and death of tissue after the cessation of blood supply. A myocardial infarction occurs when a blood vessel to a portion of the heart is blocked and the tissue distal to the blood vessel receives no oxygen and nutrients carried by blood.

Infection—State or condition in which the body or body tissues are invaded by pathogenic microorganisms that multiply and produce injurious effects.

Inflammation—The body's nonspecific reaction to injury or infection that causes redness, heat, swelling, and pain.

Informed consent form—A legal document stating the patient's surgical procedure and the risks, consequences, and benefits of that procedure, that must be signed by the patient or the patient's representative before surgery can proceed. Also known as a *patient operative consent form.*

Infrared—The portion of the electromagnetic spectrum just below visible light. All warm objects give off infrared radiation.

Innate immunity—A nonspecific body response to foreign proteins, sub-stances, tissues, viruses, or microorganisms. It includes the process of inflammation and vascular and cellular responses.

Innervation—State in which a body part or organ is supplied with nerves or nervous stimuli.

In situ—In the natural position or normal place, without disturbing or invading surrounding tissues.

Insufflator—The device used to deliver carbon dioxide gas from the tank to the patient to achieve pneumoperitoneum. The insufflator monitors the amount and rate of flow and contains an alarm system to alert to excessive intraabdominal pressure.

Insurance—A contract in which the insurance company agrees to defend the policy holder if he or she is sued for acts covered by the policy and to pay any damages up to the policy limit.

Interrupted suture—A technique of suturing tissues using individual sutures and tying each one separately.

Interventricular foramen—A passage from the third to the lateral ventricle of the brain.

Intravascular ultrasound—A diagnostic tool in which a transducer is introduced into an artery and ultrasound used to translate the physical characteristics of the lumen into a visible image.

Intubation—The process of inserting an endotracheal tube. Insertion requires adequate muscle relaxation to prevent spasms of the larynx and pharynx. Endotracheal intubation is performed after anesthesia induction.

Intussusception—The telescoping of one portion of the intestine into another.

Inversion—To turn inward.

In vitro—Done in a laboratory; usually describing a test involving isolated tissue, organs, or cells.

Ischemia—A condition of reduced blood supply in a localized area, often caused by a narrowing of the blood vessel supplying the tissue. Prolonged ischemia causes tissue death resulting from lack of oxygen to the tissue.

Jackknife or Kraske position—A type of prone position in which the patient lies on his or her abdomen with the hips flexed into an inverted-V position.

JCAHO—Joint Commission for the Accreditation of Healthcare Organizations. The accrediting organization for hospitals and other health-care settings in the United States.

Joint cavity—The saclike structure that encloses the ends of bones in diarthrodial joints, consisting of an outer fibrous layer, an inner synovial layer, and synovial fluid.

Joint mouse—Free bits of cartilage or bone present in the joint space, especially the knee. Also called *loose bodies*.

Jury trial—Trial in which a case is presented to a selected jury and the facts and final judgment are determined by the jury.

Keith needle—A straight cutting needle used on superficial tissue.

Keratin—A substance created by squamous epithelium.

Keratoplasty—Corneal transplant surgery.

Laminar airflow (LAF) system—A ventilation system that moves a contained volume of air in layers at a continuous velocity, with 800 to 900 air exchanges per hour.

Laparotomy—A procedure in which the abdominal cavity is surgically opened. The techniques used for laparotomy are used for all open surgical procedures of the abdomen.

Laryngeal mask airway (LMA)—An airway consisting of a tube and small mask that is fitted internally over the patient's larynx. It has advantages over an endotracheal tube in that it does not require the use of muscle relaxants to facilitate insertion and it can be used in a patient whose anatomy makes endotracheal intubation technically difficult.

Laryngoscope—A lighted instrument consisting of a blade and removable handle or a fiberoptic light. It is used to assist in endotracheal intubation. The lighted end of the laryngoscope allows direct visualization of the airway to facilitate correct positioning of the endotracheal tube. After the endo-

tracheal tube is in place, the laryngoscope is gently withdrawn.

Laryngospasm—Involuntary spasm of the smooth muscles of the larynx. Some drugs cause laryngospasm, and some patients are prone to spasm because of a medical or anatomical condition. Severe laryngospasm can restrict or block the patient's airway. It can occur during intubation, during induction and emergence from deep sedation, or in periods of relatively light anesthesia.

Laser—Light amplification by stimulated emission of radiation.

Laser medium—The gas, liquid, or solid through which light energy is passed to create a laser beam. The medium is contained within the optical resonant chamber.

Laser safety officer—A person who is knowledgeable in laser safety and use and is assigned by the hospital to monitor and maintain safety standards for laser use.

Lateral position—Position in which the patient is positioned on his or her side on the operating table or bed.

Latex—A naturally occurring sap obtained from rubber trees and used in the manufacture of medical devices and other commercial goods.

Latex allergy—Sensitivity to latex, which can cause itching, rhinitis, conjunctivitis, and anaphylactic shock leading to death. Personnel and patients with latex allergy must not come in contact with any articles that contain latex.

Laws—Standards that apply to all people within a given society.

LCC-ST—The Liaison Council on Certification for the Surgical Technologist. The professional body responsible for developing and administering the national certification examination.

Leads and cues—A therapeutic communication skill that urges the patient to continue speaking or communicating needs. An example of a lead is "I see, tell me more." An example of a cue is nodding one's head as the patient speaks.

LEEP—Loop electrode excision procedure. In this technique, an electrosur-

gical loop is used to remove a core of tissue from the cervical canal.

Leiomyoma—A fibrous benign tumor of the uterus that usually arises from the myometrium.

Leukoplakia—A white plaque on mucosa.

Liable—Legally responsible and accountable.

Libel—Defamation in writing.

Lidocaine—Medication used to reduce ventricular arrhythmias. Also known as *Xylocaine*.

Ligament—Strong band of fibrous connective tissue connecting the articular ends of bones and serving to bind the bones together and to facilitate or limit motion.

Ligamentum flavum—A ligament that connects one spinous process of a vertebra to another.

Ligate—To tie or bind with a ligature.

Ligation—The procedure of tying off blood vessels or ducts with suture or wire ligatures. This procedure may be used to stop or prevent bleeding or block the passage.

Ligature—Any suture substance or wire used to tie a vessel or strangulate a duct.

Linea alba—A tendinous median line on the anterior abdominal wall; separates the rectus muscles.

Lithotomy position—Position used for vaginal, perineal, and rectal surgery. The patient's legs are positioned on stirrups that hold them in place.

Lithotripsy—A procedure in which stones are crushed within a body cavity such as the bladder.

Living will—Legal document stating the patient's wishes to refuse or limit care if the patient becomes incompetent. Living wills are utilized mainly for cases of terminal illness.

Lobectomy—The surgical removal of one or more lobes of the lung.

Lobectomy (liver)—The surgical removal of one or more anatomical sections of the liver.

Log roll—A technique for moving the patient in which one rolls the patient onto his or her side using a bed sheet or draw sheet.

Lumen—The inside of a hollow structure or tube, such as a blood vessel.

Lumpectomy—The wide excision of a malignant mass of breast tissue. Also known as a *segmental biopsy* or *tylectomy.*

Magnetic resonance imaging (MRI)—A test that incorporates a magnetic field to identify structures within the body.

Malignant hyperthermia—A rare condition that occurs in conjunction with general anesthesia. The patient experiences extremely high body temperature, muscle rigidity, seizures, and cardiac arrhythmia. The condition is reversible with specific drugs and management of symptoms but can be fatal if left untreated. Patients with a history of muscular disease are particularly at risk for malignant hyperthermia. Most general anesthetic inhalation agents carry a risk of producing malignant hyperthermia.

Malpractice—Negligence committed by a professional. Malpractice also may be committed if a person deliberately acts outside of his or her scope of practice or while impaired.

Malunion fracture—An imperfect union in which the fragments of a fractured bone grow in a faulty position.

Marginal tissue—Tissue that surrounds a tumor. During tumor surgery, it is important to include a wide margin around the tumor to prevent recurrence of the tumor.

Marrow—The soft tissue occupying the medullary cavities of long bones.

Maslow's hierarchy—A model of human achievement and self-actualization developed by psychologist Abraham Maslow. This model is widely accepted in Western medicine and describes human needs on a hierarchical basis starting with the most basic needs first.

Mastectomy (simple)—Procedure that removes breast tissue, including the skin, areola, and nipple. Lymph nodes are not removed.

Mastoidectomy—A procedure in which the air cells of the mastoid bone are removed.

Mattress suture—A technique of suturing in which one passes the suture material through the tissues on one side of wound, across the incision, and through the tissues on the opposite side, and then passes the suture material through the opposite-side tissues and back through the tissues of the original side.

Maxillomandibular fixation—Fixation of the upper and lower dentition.

McBurney incision—An oblique *right* muscle-splitting incision used for exploration and removal of the appendix.

Medialize—To move to the midline.

Mediastinum—An enclosed cavity in the chest containing the heart, large vessels, trachea, esophagus, and lymph nodes.

Medical power of attorney—Legal document signed by a person giving another person the power to make health-care decisions for the first person if he or she becomes incompetent, unconscious, or unable to make decisions for himself or herself.

Medical practice acts—State laws that define the practice of medicine.

Medication—A naturally occurring substance or a chemical compound (drug) that is used to treat a specific condition.

Medulla oblongata—Gray matter that serves as a continuous connection between the spinal cord and the pons. The impulses that pass to and from the spinal cord pass through here. The medulla is responsible for the body's vital functions, such as heart rate, respiration, and control of the circulatory system.

Memory—For suture material, the recoil of the suture after it has been removed from the package. Some suture materials are more resistant to straightening than others (have high memory).

Meninges—The three layers of membranes that cover the brain and spinal cord.

Mesh—Soft, pliable, synthetic material that resembles a screen. Mesh is used in hernia repair to bridge the tissue edges of the hernia. Nontension patching or plugging gives strength to the weak abdominal wall but allows normal activities and mobility after surgery. Many different mesh systems are available, and choices are based on the type of hernia and compatibility with the patient's tissues.

Metastatic—Condition in which cancer spreads from a primary (original) site to other areas of the body.

Microlaryngoscopy—Procedure in which a rigid laryngoscope is placed and suspended from the patient and an operating microscope is used to produce better visualization of the larynx. Also called *microsuspension laryngoscopy* and *microdirect laryngoscopy.*

Midbrain—Portion of the brain located between the forebrain and hind brain. The corpora quadrigemina and cerebral aqueduct are located here.

Midgut—The middle part of the alimentary canal from the stomach, or entrance of the bile duct, to, or including, the large intestine.

Missed abortion—An abortion in which the products of conception are no longer viable but are retained in the uterus.

Mission statement—A written declaration that defines the central goal of the health-care institution and reflects the organization's ethical and moral beliefs in broad terms.

Mixter—A type of hemostat with a straight shank and a right-angle tip.

Mobilize—To surgically free up tissue. Most tissues of the body are attached by serous membranes or connective tissue. Whenever tissue is removed or remodeled, these attachments must be freed up. This often includes dividing and ligating blood vessels that are attached. This is called *tissue mobilization.*

Modified radical mastectomy—Removal of the entire breast, the nipple, and areolar region. The lymph nodes also are usually removed. This is the most common procedure for malignant breast tumor.

Monitor—The screen used to display the camera image during endoscopy.

Monochromatic—Having a single color.

Monocortical screw—A screw that goes through only the outer layer of bone.

Monofilament suture—Suture composed of a single strand of material.

Morbid obesity—A condition in which the patient's body mass index is 40 or greater and weight is at least 100 pounds more than the ideal weight in spite of aggressive attempts to lose weight.

Morcelization—A process in which tissue is fragmented so it can be withdrawn easily through an endoscopic cannula or suction device.

Mucocele—A cyst that is filled with mucus and lined with mucosa.

Multifilament suture—Suture composed of many fine strands of fiber that are twisted or braided together.

Muscle-splitting incision—Incision that separates muscle tissues along the length of their fibers. The muscle is not cut. This results in little or no bleeding and prevents the moderate to severe postoperative pain associated with muscle cutting.

Myringoplasty—Closure of a myringotomy.

Myringotomy—An incision or hole in the tympanic membrane created to allow aspiration or aeration of the middle ear.

Nasal polyp—A polyp of the nasal cavity or paranasal sinuses.

Nasogastric (NG) tube—A flexible tube inserted into the patient's nose and advanced into the stomach. The NG tube is used to decompress the stomach or to create a means of feeding the patient liquid nutrients and oral medication.

Nasolaryngoscope—A flexible scope that is passed through the nose to visualize the larynx.

Nasopharynx—The portion of the pharynx above the palate.

Necrosis—Tissue death.

Needleless system—A system of parenteral access that does not use needles for the collection or withdrawal of body fluids through venous puncture.

Needle localization biopsy—Procedure in which tissue surrounding a hook wire device is removed.

Negligence—"Omission to do something that a reasonable person, guided by those *ordinary* considerations which ordinarily regulate human affairs would *do*, or doing something which a reasonable and prudent person would *not* do."*

Neoplasm—An abnormal growth of cells.

Nephroblastoma—Wilms' tumor.

Neuromuscular blocking agents—Drugs that block conduction of nerves that control striated muscle tissue. Muscle relaxation or paralysis may be needed to allow access to the operative site during general anesthesia.

Neuropathy—Any disease of the nerves, whether permanent or temporary, that results in numbness or loss of function of a part of the body.

Neutral zone (no-hands) technique—A method of transferring sharp instruments on the surgical field without hand-to-hand contact. A neutral zone is identified, and sharps are exchanged in this zone.

Nonabsorbable sutures—Suture materials that resist breakdown in the body.

Nonanatomical resection—Removal of a section without regard to its segmental boundaries. A wedge resection is nonanatomical.

Noncritical item—Items that are not required to be sterile as they do not penetrate intact tissues (e.g., bedpans, blood pressure cuffs).

Nonelectrolytic—Nonconductive; nonelectrolytic solutions must be used for bladder distension or continuous irrigation whenever the electrosurgical unit (ESU) is used.

Nonelectrolytic media—A solution that does not conduct electrical current.

Nonpathogenic—Refers to an organism that does not cause disease in a healthy individual. About 95% to 97% of all bacteria are nonpathogenic.

Nonprofit hospital—A hospital that provides services to the community and that allocates nontaxable profits to the maintenance or improvement of the facility.

Nonsterile personnel—In surgery, team members who remain outside the boundary of the sterile field and do not come into direct contact with sterile equipment, sterile areas, or the surgical wound. The circulator, anesthesia care provider, and x-ray technician are examples of nonsterile team members.

Nonunion fracture—Failure of fragments of a fractured bone to knit together.

Norms—Behaviors that are accepted as part of the environment and culture of a group. Norms are usually established by custom and popular acceptance rather than by law, although the two may not be mutually exclusive.

Nosocomial infection—An infection that is acquired as a result of being in a hospital or other health-care facility.

Nurse practice acts—State laws that define the practice of nursing.

Objective—The distal end of the endoscopic telescope.

Obligate aerobe—A microorganism that requires oxygen to live and grow.

Obligate anaerobe—An organism that must live in the absence of oxygen to survive.

Obturator—A blunt-nosed tube inserted through the sheath of a rigid endoscope or hysteroscope to protect the tissue as the instrument is advanced.

Occipital lobe—The most posterior portion of the cerebrum.

Occupational exposure—Exposure to hazards in the workplace. Examples include exposure to hazardous chemicals or contact with potentially infected blood and body fluids.

Ocular—The proximal end of the endoscopic telescope.

Off-pump procedure—Procedure performed without a cardiopulmonary bypass (i.e., "the pump").

Omphalocele—A protrusion of abdominal contents through an opening at the navel, especially occurring as a congenital defect.

*Creighton H: *Law every nurse should know,* ed 5, Philadelphia, 1986, WB Saunders.

Open a case—To begin work on a surgical case by opening sterile supplies and equipment using sterile technique. Tables and stainless steel furniture are first draped with sterile sheets, and sterile equipment is opened onto the tables without contamination.

Open gloving—A gloving technique in which the bare skin does not touch any part of the outside of the glove. Open gloving is generally used when a health worker does not wear a sterile gown.

Open procedure—A traditional surgical procedure that includes incision and wide access to the target tissue.

Optical resonant cavity—The chamber that holds the laser medium. When light energy enters the chamber, it passes through the laser medium, and the number of photons increases.

Organizational chart—A graphic depiction of an organization's chain of command that shows the lines of vertical (higher and lower) and horizontal (equal) administrative authority.

Oropharynx—Portion of the pharynx between the palate and base of the tongue, separated from the oral cavity by the tonsillar pillars.

OSHA—Occupational Safety and Health Administration. Section of the U.S. Department of Labor that establishes rules and standards to protect the safety of employees in the workplace.

Osteoarthritis—Inflammation of a joint.

Osteoarthrotomy—Excision of a joint end of a bone.

Osteoblast—A cell of mesodermal origin that is concerned with the formation of bone.

Osteogenesis—Formation and development of bone.

Osteomalacia—A disease marked by increasing softness of the bones; the adult form of rickets.

Osteomyelitis—Inflammation of bone, especially the marrow.

Osteonecrosis—Death of generalized bone tissue rather than of isolated areas.

Osteophyte—A bony outgrowth, usually found around a joint; a "joint mouse" if loose in the joint.

Osteosclerosis—The abnormal thickening of bone (*skleros,* hardening).

Osteotomy—Surgical breaking of or incision into bone.

Otitis Media—Inflammation of the middle ear.

Otorrhea—Drainage from the external auditory canal.

Otosclerosis—Abnormal thickening of the bone in the otic capsule (middle and inner ear).

Ototoxic—A substance that is noxious to the sensory organs of the inner ear.

Pacemaker—A device that generates electrical impulses that stimulate the heart muscle to contract at a predetermined rate.

Palpable—A quality of tissue that allows an examiner to describe and differentiate the tissue by feeling it. Palpation applies to any form of physical examination in which the examiner uses his or her hand to locate and describe tissue.

Pancreatojejunostomy—A surgical anastomosis of the pancreas and the jejunum.

Papilloma—A benign epithelial neoplasm characterized by a branching or lobular tumor. Also called *papillary tumor.*

Parallel—Denoting light in which the light waves move in narrow columns. It is a characteristic of laser light.

Paramedian—An incision of the vertical abdominal wall lateral to the midline.

Paranasal sinus—Air cells surrounding or on the periphery of the nasal cavities. These are maxillary, ethmoid, sphenoid, and frontal sinuses.

Parasite—An organism that lives within, upon, or at the expense of another organism, known as the host, without contributing to the survival of the host.*

Parenchyma—Tissue that makes up an organ. For example, the liver parenchyma is the body of the liver itself. Pancreatic parenchyma is pancreatic tissue. This term is used to differentiate organ tissue from its covering or capsule.

Parenterally—Referring to administration of a drug by injection.

Parietal lobe—The upper central portion of gray matter of the cerebrum lying between the frontal, occipital, and temporal lobes. Coordination and sensory integration take place here.

Patella—A lens-shaped sesamoid bone situated in front of the knee in the tendon of the quadriceps femoris muscle. Also called *kneecap.*

Patency—The condition of being wide open; describes an unobstructed passageway.

Patent—Open or unobstructed, in reference to a tubular or hollow structure. It is usually used to describe the patient's airway, a blood vessel, or a duct.

Pathogenic—Having the potential to cause disease.

Pathogens—Disease-causing microorganisms.

Patient—A person who is ill or injured or who is undergoing any type of medical treatment.

Patient-centered care—Therapeutic care, communication, and intervention provided according to the unique needs of the patient. Every patient is treated as an individual, and a care plan is developed to meet specific needs identified in the assessment.

Pedicle flap—A section of tissue that is partially removed from one area of the body and transferred to a nearby location. The purpose is to retain blood supply within the flap so the reconstructed area remains viable.

Peracetic acid—Chemical capable of rendering objects sterile.

Percutaneous—Literally means "through the skin." In a percutaneous approach in surgery, an incision is not made, but a catheter or other device is introduced through a puncture site.

Percutaneous enterostomy gastrostomy tube (PEG)—A tube inserted in the stomach for enteral feedings or gastric decompression.

---

*Venes D and Thomas CL, eds: *Taber's cyclopedia medical dictionary,* ed 19, Philadelphia, 2001, FA Davis.

Perforation—A defect in the tympanic membrane caused by trauma or infection.

Pericardial fluid—Fluid lying between the visceral and parietal membranes that provides lubrication to the tissues, thereby reducing friction to the tissues.

Perichondrium—Tissue overlying the cartilage that provides its vascular and nervous supply.

Pericranium—Periosteum of the skull.

Perineum—Anatomical area between the posterior vestibule and the anus.

Perineurium—Fibers of connective tissue that bind nerve fibers together.

Periosteum—Fibrous membrane that covers bones except at the articular surfaces and provides bone with its vascualr and nervous supply.

Peripheral nervous system—Part of the nervous system containing the cranial and spinal nerves and branches.

Peritonsillar abscess—A collection of purulent fluid that arises from the blockage of a pit (or crypt) of the tonsil.

Perjury—Crime of intentionally lying or falsifying information given during court testimony after being sworn to tell the truth.

Personal protective equipment—Protective clothing or equipment that protects the wearer from direct contact with hazardous chemicals or potentially infectious body fluids.

Pfannenstiel—A transverse incision of the lower abdomen below the umbilicus and just above the pubis in a natural crease or fold.

Phacoemulsification—A process whereby high-frequency waves are used to emulsify tissue, such as a cataract. The dissolved tissue then can be removed by aspiration.

Phagocyte—Any cell capable of ingesting particulate matter and microorganisms.

Pharmacodynamics—The biochemical and physiological effects of drugs and their mechanisms of action in the body.

Pharmacokinetics—The movement of a drug through the tissues and cells of the body, including the processes of absorption, distribution, and localization in tissues, biotransformation, and excretion by mechanical and chemical means.

Pharmacology—The study of drugs and their action on the body.

Pharyngitis—Inflammation of the pharynx.

Philtrum—The vertical groove in the center of the upper lip.

Phonation—Vibration of the vocal cords; speaking.

Photodamage—Damage to the skin caused by the sun.

Photon—Particle of light that has no mass and no electric charge.

Photothermal ablation—Electrosurgical destruction or laser vaporization for removal of tissue.

Physical barrier—In surgery, a barrier that separates a sterile surface from a nonsterile surface. Examples are sterile surgical gloves, gowns, and drapes. A physical barrier, such as a clean surgical cap, also can prevent a bacteria-laden surface, such as the hair, from shedding microorganisms.

Pia mater—The vascular meningeal membrane lying closest to the brain.

PID—Pelvic inflammatory disease. Caused by sexually transmitted disease or other infection source. Causes scarring of the fallopian tubes and adhesions in the abdominal and pelvic cavity. PID is one of the leading causes of infertility in the United States.

Plasma sterilization—Sterilization process that uses the form of matter known as plasma (e.g., hydrogen peroxide plasma) to achieve sterilization of an item.

Pleural cavities—Right and left enclosed cavities in the chest that contain, respectively, the right and left lungs.

Pliability—The flexibility of a suture material.

Plicate—To fold, shorten, or reduce the size of a muscle or hollow organ by taking it in tucks.

Pneumatic tourniquet—A balloon cuff similar to a blood pressure cuff in design. The pneumatic tourniquet is used to produce a bloodless operative site or to prevent blood flow to an extremity for injection with local anesthetic in a procedure called a *Bier block*.

Pneumonectomy—The surgical removal of one lung.

Pneumoperitoneum—Technique in which the peritoneal cavity is inflated with a compressed gas such as carbon dioxide (CO_2) so that endoscopic surgery can be performed with reduced risk of trauma to tissues and organs.

Points—The tips of a surgical instrument.

Pons—A structure of white matter lying between the midbrain and medulla, serving as a relay between the medulla and cerebral peduncles. The fifth, sixth, seventh, and eighth cranial nerves originate here.

Portal—The portal vein, which traverses the liver. Its branches form complex extensions into the liver.

Portal of entry—In microbial transmission, the sites where microorganisms enter the body (e.g., an anatomic passage such as the nose or mouth, or the skin).

Ports—Cannulated incisions made in the body wall. The ports receive and stabilize the endoscopic instruments used to perform endoscopic surgery.

Positron emission tomography (PET)—A nuclear medicine study that involves the use of positron-emitting radionuclides to identify areas of damaged or diseased tissue.

Posterior chamber—The fluid-filled space between the back of the iris and the front of the lens.

Postexposure prophylaxis—Recommended procedures to help prevent the development of blood-borne diseases after an exposure incident.

Potentially infectious materials—(1) The following fluids: blood, semen, vaginal secretions, cerebrospinal fluid, synovial fluid, pleural fluid, pericardial fluid, peritoneal fluid, amniotic fluid, saliva during procedures involving the mouth, any body fluid that is visibly contaminated with blood, any body fluid in a situation in which it is difficult or impossible to differentiate among various body fluids; (2) any unfixed tissue or organ (other than intact skin) from a human (living or dead); and (3) human immunodeficiency virus (HIV)–containing cell or tissue cultures, organ cultures, and HIV-containing or hepatitis B virus–containing culture medium or other solutions.

Power—The rate at which energy is used (measured in watts).

Preclotting—Process of soaking a graft or patch of synthetic graft material in the patient's blood or plasma before insertion. Most grafts no longer need preclotting.

Prep—The use of antiseptic solutions for cleaning, reducing microbial count, and preventing unnecessary contamination of an area for a sterile invasive (skin incision) or sterile noninvasive (urinary catheterization) procedure.

Prescription—A written order for a drug. Only licensed personnel may prescribe drugs.

Pretrichial—The region anterior to the hairline.

Primary tumor—In oncology (the study and treatment of cancer), the original site of a cancer that spreads to other locations called *secondary sites* via metastasis.

Prion—A protein-like microbe that is highly resistant to common sterilization methods. A common example of a prion-based illness is Creutzfeldt-Jakob disease.

Probe—An instrument placed within a natural lumen or fistula to determine its length and direction.

Prodromal—Referring to the period between the first symptoms and the acute phase of a disease in the process of infection. Many diseases have prodromal symptoms specific to that disease, whereas in others the symptoms are more generalized.

Professional license—Governmental permission to perform specified actions.

Prokaryote—Cellular organism lacking a true nucleus or nuclear membrane. The microorganisms included in this classification are bacteria and blue green algae.

Prone position—Lying position with the abdomen downward.

Proprietary hospital—A hospital that is owned by shareholders, who receive and pay taxes on the profits made by the institution. Also called a *for-profit hospital.*

Proprietary school—Private, for-profit school.

Protamine sulfate—Medication that reverses the anticoagulation effects of heparin.

Pterygium—A triangular membrane that arises from the medial canthus and that can extend over the cornea, causing blindness.

Ptosis—An abnormal condition involving one or both upper eyelids in which the eyelid droops because of a congenital or acquired weakness of the levator muscle or paralysis of the third cranial nerve.

Pulsed wave—Single bursts of laser light. Q-switched lasers produce this type of wave.

Pulse oximeter—A device that measures the patient's hemoglobin oxygen saturation through the use of spectrometry.

Purse-string—A suturing technique in which a continuous strand is passed in and out of the circumference of a lumen, and then is pulled tight like a drawstring.

Pyloric stenosis—A narrowing of the part of the stomach (pylorus) that leads to the small intestines.

Radiant exposure—The total effect of laser energy, which depends on the energy density of the laser beam, the diameter of the beam, and the exposure time.

Rami—A forked division of a spinal nerve.

Receiver—The person who receives the message communicated by a sender.

Rectocele—A bulging of intestinal tissue into the posterior vaginal wall.

Red blood cell (RBC) count—A part of the CBC or hemogram that identifies the number of circulating red blood cells, or erythrocytes, in the blood.

Reduce—To replace herniated tissue; the tissue may reduce without manipulation when the patient lies down or ceases to strain or bear down.

Reel—A continuous strand of suture mounted on a spool for ligation purposes.

Reflection—(1) Communication with the patient that helps him or her connect current emotions with events in the environment; (2) A condition of turning or bending back upon its course, for example the peritoneum attached to the body wall covering an organ with a reattachment to the body wall.

Regional block—Anesthesia and analgesia of a specific area of the body. Regional blocks may be produced by interruption of impulses of one major nerve or a group of nerves. Adjunct drugs usually are administered to sedate and provide anxiolysis.

Regression—An abnormal return to a former or earlier state, particularly infantile patterns of thought or behavior. This can result from feelings of helplessness and dependency in a patient with a serious physical illness.

Regurgitant valve—A heart valve that is unable to close tightly, thereby allowing regurgitation (leaking) of blood into the heart chamber from which it came.

Resect—To cut through and repair a body cavity or solid tissue.

Resection—Surgical removal of an organ.

Resectoscope—An instrument that removes tissue by cutting and coagulating small slices.

Reservoir—In epidemiology, a possible source of disease transmission. A reservoir can be a person or an inanimate surface. For example, soil is a reservoir for tetanus bacteria. A health worker who sheds *Staphylococcus aureus* also is a reservoir of transmission.

Resident flora—Microorganisms that are normally present in specific tissues of people. Resident flora is necessary to the regular function of these tissues or structures. Also called *normal flora.*

Resident microorganisms—Also called *normal flora*, these are microorganisms that normally live in certain tissues of the body.

Residual activity—The microbicidal activity that remains after an antiseptic or disinfectant has dried.

Restricted area—Area of the operating room in which only personnel wearing surgical attire, including masks, shoe coverings, and head coverings, are allowed. Doors are kept closed and air pressure is greater than that in areas outside the restricted area.

Retained object—An item that is inadvertently left inside the patient during surgery.

Retention catheter—A urinary catheter with an inflatable balloon that is used to drain the bladder continuously during surgery. Also called an *indwelling* or *Foley catheter,* it is placed in the patient before surgical skin preparation.

Retention suture—Heavy nonabsorbable suture placed behind the skin sutures and through all tissue layers to give added strength to the closure. Also called *secondary suture line.*

Retrograde—A backward movement of fluid or an anatomical approach from back to front.

Retrograde pyelography—X-ray or fluoroscopic studies of the renal pelvis using contrast media; "pyel" refers to renal pelvis.

Retrovirus—A group of viruses whose genetic information is coded in RNA rather than in DNA. Human immunodeficiency virus is a retrovirus.

Reverse cutting needles—Curved surgical needles with three honed edges. One of the edges is on the outside of the curve of the needle.

Reverse Trendelenburg position—Position in which the prone or supine patient is tilted with the feet down.

Rhinorrhea—Drainage from the nose.

Risk—The statistical probability of a given event based on the number of such events that have already occurred in a certain population.

Risk management—The process of tracking, evaluating, and studying accidents and incidents to protect patients and employees. Risk management produces change in policy or enforcement of policy if the risk reaches an unacceptable level.

Rongeur—A hinged instrument with sharp, cup-shaped tips used to extract pieces of bone or other connective tissue.

Running suture—A method of suturing that uses one continuous suture strand for tissue approximation.

Saccular aneurysm—A type of aneurysm in which a saclike formation with a narrow neck projects from the side of the artery.

Sanitation—A process that cleans an object.

Satellite facilities—Community healthcare offices that are administered by a single institution but are located in communities in surrounding urban or rural areas. These facilities offer primary and preventive health-care services in general medicine and other specialties.

Scalp—Multilayered skin of the skull usually covered by hair.

Scrub—Member of the sterile team who handles instruments, supplies, and equipment necessary for the surgical procedure. The surgical hand scrub is the process of prescribed, thorough hand cleaning before the donning of sterile gloves and gown.

Scrubbed personnel—In surgery, members of the surgical team who work within the sterile field. Also called *sterile personnel.*

Second-degree burn—Burn that involves the entire epidermis and part of the dermis.

Second intention wound closure—Wound closure that is accomplished by leaving the wound open to heal by granulation from the inner layer to the outer surface.

Sedatives—Agents that induce a state of sedation. The depth of sedation is controlled by the administration of specific agents. Levels of sedation range from slight calming to unconsciousness in which the patient is unresponsive even to repeated deep, painful stimulation.

Segmental mastectomy—See *Lumpectomy.*

Segmental resection—The anatomical resection of the liver. This procedure removes segments that are divided by specific blood vessels and biliary ducts. Although not visible from the outside of the liver, these segments are differentiated and can be removed separately after the associated structures have been managed.

Semiconductor—A material, such as silicon, that is neither a conductor of electricity nor an insulator. Its electrical properties can be changed by the addition of minute amounts of other elements. Semiconductors are the basis of transistors and computer chips.

Semicritical items—Items that are required to be free of most pathogenic organisms including *Mycobacterium tuberculosis,* as these items contact mucous membranes (e.g., respiratory equipment, endoscopes).

Semi-Fowler position—Semi-sitting position used for surgery on the neck and thyroid.

Semi-occluding clamp—A nontraumatic clamp with jaws that either do not contact each other when closed, or exert very little pressure on tissue when closed.

Semirestricted area—Designated area in which only personnel wearing scrub suits and hair caps that enclose all facial hair are allowed.

Sender—The person who communicates a message to another.

Sensorineural hearing loss—Hearing impairment arising from the cochlea, auditory nerve, or central nervous system.

Sentinel event—"A sentinel event is an unexpected occurrence involving death or serious physical or psychological injury, or risk thereof. Serious injury specifically includes loss of limb or function. The phrase 'or risk thereof' includes any process variation for which a recurrence would carry a significant chance of serious adverse outcome. Such events are called 'sentinel' because they signal the need for immediate investigation and response."*

Sentinel lymph node biopsy—Procedure in which one or more lymph

---

* Association of periOperative Registered Nurses, *AORN position statement on correct site surgery,* Denver, CO.

nodes are removed to determine whether malignancy has spread. Other lymph nodes may be periodically removed to determine whether metastasis has occurred.

Septoplasty—A procedure in which the septum is manipulated to improve airflow through the nasal cavity.

Sequential compression devices—Pneumatic devices that wrap around the patient's legs and deliver pressure sequentially. The devices are worn to prevent embolism that results from lack of blood flow from the legs to the heart.

Serosa—The delicate outer layer of tissue of most organs.

Sesamoid—Resembling a grain of sesame in size or shape.

Sexual harassment—Sexual coercion, sexual innuendoes, or unwanted sexual comments or touch.

Shank—The area of a surgical instrument between the box lock and finger ring.

Sharp dissection—The technique of cutting tissue with sharp or electronic instruments such as a knife, scissors, or electrosurgical unit tip.

Sharps—Any objects that can penetrate the skin and have the potential for causing injury and infection, including, but not limited to, needles, scalpels, broken glass, broken capillary tubes, and exposed ends of dental wires.

Shear injury—Tissue injury or necrosis that results when two tissue planes are forcefully pulled in opposite directions. Shearing usually occurs when the body is pulled or slides by gravity across a high-friction surface such as a bed sheet. Shearing can lead to a decubitus ulcer.

Shelf life—The amount of time a wrapped item will remain sterile after it has been subjected to a sterilization process.

Shirodkar's procedure—See *Cerclage.*

Shunt—This term is used in various contexts in cardiovascular surgery. To shunt blood or fluids means to carry blood from one location to another (e.g., in cardiopulmonary bypass, blood is shunted from the body to the bypass equipment). A shunt can be a

blood vessel or tube that carries the blood. In shunting procedures, the existing route of blood is changed or a vessel is removed and a synthetic graft shunt is implanted.

Side effects—Anticipated effects of a drug other than those intended. Side effects may be uncomfortable for the patient or may have a positive consequence.

Skin flap—A flap created by incising the skin and cutting it away from the underlying tissue to which it is attached. The flap can be increased in size or "raised" as the flap is made larger by dissection.

Skin preparation sponge—A gauze that does not contain a radioopaque marker and that is used to apply solution during skin cleansing. These sponges are available in many different sizes and types, according to size, configuration, and location of the preparation area.

Skull—The bone covering the head.

Slander—Spoken defamation.

Smoke plume—Smoke created during the use of an electrosurgical unit or laser. This smoke contains toxic chemicals, vapors, blood fragments, and viruses.

Smooth muscle—Muscle activated involuntarily, such as the muscle of the digestive tract.

Solid—Matter in a rigid state, not liquid or gaseous.

Solid-state—Using the electrical properties of solid components (such as transistors) instead of vacuum tubes.

Sorbitol—A nonelectrolytic solution used for distension of a hollow cavity during use of any electrosurgical device.

Spatial relations—One's physical relation to sterile and nonsterile areas or surfaces. Concepts considered in spatial relationships include the varying heights of sterile team members, distance between a nonsterile team member and a sterile surface, and movement within a sterile area.

Spinal cord—The section of the central nervous system found in the spinal canal that contains both white and gray matter extending from the foramen magnum to the upper lumbar region.

Split-thickness skin graft—Skin graft that consists of the epidermis and a portion of the papillary dermis.

Sporicidal—Able to kill spores.

Staging—A complex method of determining the severity of a malignant tumor. Lymph node involvement, size of the tumor, location, and type are considered.

Stain—A substance that is applied directly to anatomical surfaces to differentiate normal from abnormal cells.

Standard Precautions—Guidelines recommended by the Centers for Disease Control and Prevention (CDC) to reduce the risk of transmission of blood-borne and other pathogens.

Stapedectomy—A procedure in which the ear is replaced with a prosthesis. This procedure is used as treatment for otosclerosis.

Stenosis—The narrowing of a cardiac valve or lumen of a blood vessel.

Stent—A tubular device placed inside an artery to hold it open to treat and prevent stricture.

Stent dressing—A type of dressing in which a molded pressure dressing is sutured to the wound site.

Stereotactic—The use of complex mechanisms (specifically algebraic equations) to locate and destroy target structures in the brain.

Sterile—Free from living microorganisms.

Sterile field—An area that includes the draped patient, all sterile tables, and sterile equipment in the immediate area of the patient. The patient is considered the center of the sterile field.

Sterile item—Any item that has been subjected to a process that renders it free of all microbial life, including spores.

Sterility—A guarantee of the absence of all microbial life, including spores. Sterility is assured when an item is properly packaged and subjected to a sterilization process. Items are considered sterile unless they have been exposed to air or another event that renders the item unsterile. An item that is properly opened onto a surgical field is then considered *surgically clean* because it is then exposed to the air or to patient tissues. Sterility is considered absolute.

Sterilization—A process by which all types of microorganisms, including spores, are destroyed.

Sternocleidomastoid—One of two muscles located on the front of the neck that serve to turn the head from side to side.

Sternotomy—An incision made into the sternum (breast bone).

Stick tie—Name given to a suture ligature or transfixion suture; a suture needle combination that is passed through a vessel or duct for ligation, commonly used in deeper cavities. Commonly called a "stitch."

Stoma—A surgically created opening between a portion of the GI tract and the outside of the body. A stoma is created when a section of the GI system is removed and the remaining limbs of the tract cannot be rejoined because of disease or anatomical limitations.

Stoma appliance—A two-piece or three-piece medical device used to collect contents of the GI system through a stoma. One part of the appliance is attached to the patient's skin over the stoma, allowing free drainage into a collection device.

Straight catheter—A nonretention catheter used to drain the bladder just before surgery.

Strangulated hernia—Herniated tissue that is strangulated and has a compromised or absent blood supply. This is a surgical emergency, especially if the bowel is involved.

Striated muscle—Muscle that is under voluntary control, such as those used to move an arm or leg.

Strike-through contamination—An event in which water, fluids, or blood act as a vehicle to carry microorganisms from a nonsterile to a sterile surface. It occurs, for example, when the outside wrapper of a sterile instrument becomes wet and the water conveys bacteria to the inside of the wrapper and contaminates the instrument, or on the surgical gown, when the gown becomes saturated with blood or other fluids.

Subarachnoid space—The space between the pia mater and the arachnoid.

Subcostal—Literally "under the rib." Describes an incision or area of the abdominal wall that follows the oblique slope of the tenth costal cartilage.

Subcutaneous mastectomy—Procedure that removes the breast while leaving the skin, nipple, and areola intact.

Subcutaneous tissue—The superficial fascia layer that covers the abdominal wall. Fatty tissue that attaches to this tissue can range from several millimeters to 7 or 8 inches thick.

Subcuticular—Beneath the skin.

Subphrenic—An anatomical description meaning "under or below the liver."

Subpoena—A court order requiring its recipient to appear and testify at a trial or deposition. Medical records also can be the subject of subpoenas.

Sulcus—A groove, furrow, or linear depression in the cerebral tissue.

Summons—A court-issued document that is received by a person being sued, notifying the person that he or she is a defendant in the lawsuit.

Supine position—Lying on the back with the face upward.

Supraglottic—Portion of the larynx above the surface of the true vocal cords.

Supratarsal crease—A horizontal crease above the lash line of the upper eyelid.

Surgical conscience—In surgery, the ethical motivation to practice strict aseptic technique to protect the patient from infection. The team members place the highest emphasis on safe delivery of care for the patient.

Surgical hand scrub—A specific technique for washing the hands before donning surgical gown and gloves before surgery. The scrub is performed with timed or counted strokes using detergent-based antiseptic. The surgical hand scrub is designed to remove dirt, oils, and transient microorganisms, and reduce the number of resident microorganisms.

Surgically clean—An item that was considered sterile but is now in use in the surgical field, has become exposed to air or patient tissues, and is no longer

considered absolutely sterile. For convenience, items in use within a surgical field are usually called *sterile* instead of *surgically clean*.

Surgical site infection (SSI)—Postoperative infection of the surgical wound, most commonly caused by the normal bacteria found on the patient's skin or shed from the skin or hair of surgical team members. The goal of the surgical skin preparation is to prevent postoperative wound infection.

Suture—(1) Material used to sew tissue together while healing takes place and to tie off blood vessels or ducts during surgery. (2) A joint that connects bones of the skull that are flexible at birth and that close and harden at birth.

Swaged needle—The fused connection of the eyeless needle and the suture strand.

Symphysis—A joint whose bones are connected by a disk of cartilage.

Synchondrosis—A type of cartilaginous joint in which the cartilage is usually converted into bone before adulthood.

Syncope—A temporary loss of consciousness caused by an interruption or decrease in the flow of blood to the brain.

Syndactyly—A congenital condition present at birth in which fingers or toes are fused.

Syndesmosis—A fibrous articulation in which two bones are joined by ligaments.

Synergistic—Term used to describe two drugs that, when combined, produce an effect that is greater than the sum of the effects produced by each drug acting separately.

Systolic pressure—The greatest amount of pressure exerted on the arterial wall during the pumping action of the heart.

Table break—Hinged joint between sections of the operating table that can be flexed in any direction.

Tachycardia—A fast heart rate, usually over 120 beats per minute.

Tag—A hemostat (or other clamp) placed on the ends of traction suture, umbilical tape, or vessel loop to hold the ends together.

Tamponade—Accumulation of blood within the pericardium that compresses the outer walls of the heart and prevents adequate intraventricular filling of the heart. A chest tube must be inserted, or the chest opened, for the blood surrounding the heart to be drained; an instrument or other means of placing pressure on tissue.

Temporal lobe—A lobe of cerebrum found at the lower lateral portion of each hemisphere.

Tendon—Fibrous portion of muscle, serving to attach muscles to bones and other parts.

Tensile strength—The amount of force or stress a suture can withstand without breaking. This term also is used to refer to the strength of tissues as they heal.

Therapeutic communication—A purposeful method of communication in which the caregiver responds to explicit or implicit needs of the patient.

Therapeutic response—Communicative response to the patient. The goal is to encourage the patient to express his or her needs and to show caring and empathy.

Thermogenesis—The production of body heat.

Third intention wound closure—A delayed primary wound closure. A wound that is infected or has dehisced may be left open until the infection subsides, the tissue edges heal, and the healthy granulous tissue can be approximated.

Third-degree burn—Burn that causes the destruction of the entire thickness of the skin.

Thoracic outlet syndrome—A group of disorders attributed to compression of the subclavian vessels and nerves. Such compression can cause permanent injury to the arm and shoulder.

Thoracostomy—Incision in the chest wall for the purpose of drainage.

Thoracotomy—An incision made into the thoracic cavity.

Thromboembolus—A blood clot that breaks loose and enters the systemic circulation, causing obstruction or occlusion of a blood vessel. Also referred to as a *thrombus*.

Thrombus—Any organic or nonorganic material blocking an artery. Generally refers to a blood clot or atherosclerotic plaque. However, infected tissue or a large bacterial colony that separates from its origin (e.g., from a heart valve) also may become a thrombus.

Throw—The wrapping of suture ends to form a knot.

Thyroglossal duct—A transitory endodermal tube in the embryo, carrying thyroid-forming tissue at its caudal end. The duct normally disappears after the thyroid has moved to its ultimate location in the neck; its point of origin is regularly marked on the base of the adult tongue by the foramen cecum.

Tie-down—The ability of a suture to lie flat when knotted.

Tie on a passer—A strand of suture material attached to the tip of an instrument (such as a right angle) for ligation of vessels and ducts.

Tissue drag—The quality that produces friction between the suture and the tissue. Tissue drag can cause microtrauma in the wound or suture fraying.

Tone—The expression of emotion or opinion contained in the delivery of a message. It is not explicit but is implied by intonation, emphasis on certain words, or measured delivery of words. Tone also is established by nonverbal communication.

Topical—Referring to application of a drug to the skin or mucous membranes.

Topical antiseptics (antimicrobials)—Agents applied to skin or mucous membrane that temporarily reduce or prevent the growth of microorganisms.

Torsion—Twisting of an organ or structure that may cause local ischemia and necrosis.

Tort—A wrong, independent of contract law violations, perpetrated by one person against another person or person's property. Any act of negligence or fraud compensable by money damages. Torts may be intentional or negligent in nature.

Total extraperitoneal (TEP) approach—A laparoscopic hernia repair approached from the extraperitoneal space. A pneumoperitoneum is un-

necessary, because the peritoneum is not entered. Rather, the inguinal area is insufflated with a balloon dissector, and the defect is repaired from within this space.

Total mastectomy—Also called a simple mastectomy; procedure that removes the breast, including skin and nipple. Lymph-node dissection is not performed.

Trabeculectomy—Surgical removal of a portion of the trabeculum to improve outflow of aqueous in glaucoma patients.

Tracheostomy—An opening through the neck into the trachea through which an indwelling tube may be inserted.

Tracheotomy—An incision made into the trachea through the neck below the larynx to gain access to the airway.

Traction—The process of drawing or pulling.

Traction injury—Nerve injury caused by stretching or compression of the nerve.

Trade name—The name given to a drug by the company that produces and sells it.

Traffic flow—The movement of people and equipment into, out of, and within the operating room.

Transcervically—Literally, "through the cervix."

Transdermal—Referring to administration of a drug through a skin patch impregnated with the drug.

Transect—To surgically divide an organ by sharp dissection.

Transfer board—A thin Plexiglas, fiberglass, or roller board that is placed under the patient to move him or her from the operating table to the stretcher or bed.

Transient flora—Microorganisms that do not normally reside in the tissue of an individual. Transient microorganisms are acquired through skin contact with an animate or inanimate source colonized by microbes. Transient flora may be removed by routine methods of skin cleaning (see *Handwashing* and *Surgical hand scrub*).

Transient microorganisms—Organisms that do not normally live in the host tissue. Transient microorganisms are crowded out by resident flora, washed off, or find their new environment unsuitable for colonization. Infection can occur when the transient microorganism overwhelms the body's defenses.

Transitional area—Area in which surgical personnel or visitors prepare to enter the semirestricted and restricted areas. This area includes the locker and changing rooms.

Transmission—The transfer of microorganisms from one source to another.

Transmission-based precautions—Standards and precautions to prevent the spread of infectious disease by patients *known* to be infected.

Transperitoneal (TAP) approach—A traditional method of laparoscopic hernia repair. A pneumoperitoneum is created, and the inguinal space is entered via the lower abdominal cavity.

Transurethral—Describes a procedure in which access is gained through the urethral opening. The term also may describe an instrument that enters the bladder through the urethral meatus.

Transverse incision—An incision that follows a line perpendicular to the midline of the body.

Trendelenburg position—Position in which the prone or supine patient is tilted with the head down.

Trephination—The process of cutting out a piece of bone with a trephine.

Trephine—A cylindrical saw used for cutting a circular piece of bone out of the skull.

Tricuspid valve—The heart valve found between the right atrium and the right ventricle.

Trisegmentectomy—In hepatic surgery, the removal of the right lobe of the liver and a portion of the left. In practice, it is a multiple segmental resection.

Trocar and cannula—Instrument inserted through incision site with a sharp or blunt tip. The trocar tip is inserted through the lumen of the cannula and introduced into the incision site. The trocar then is removed and the cannula remains in the incision site for introduction of instruments for endoscopic procedures.

Tunica adventitia—The outermost covering of an artery.

Turbinectomy—A procedure in which a portion of the inferior nasal turbinates is removed.

TURBT—Transurethral resection of a bladder tumor.

Turgid—Swollen, hard, and/or congested.

TURP—Transurethral resection of the prostate.

Tylectomy—Procedure of localized removal of a lesion; synonymous with *lumpectomy.*

Tympanoplasty—A procedure in which a perforated tympanic membrane is repaired.

Tympanostomy tube—A tube that is placed into a myringotomy to produce aeration of the middle ear.

Type and cross (T & C)—A test that specifically matches a patient's blood with a particular unit or units of blood in the blood bank. This test, also called *type and cross-match,* is used whenever large amounts of blood loss are expected or when a patient unexpectedly requires a blood transfusion.

Type and screen (T & S)—A test that is used to ensure that units of blood that match the patient's blood type are available if required by the patient. The test is not as sensitive as the T & C and is not used to determine whether a particular unit of blood is suitable for the patient.

Ultrasonic cleaner—Equipment that cleans instruments through cavitation.

Ultrasound—The use of sound waves to create a picture of structures within the patient.

Undermine—To separate tissues layers on a vertical plane using dissecting scissors. The separation of the two layers results in a "pocket" between the two layers.

Unrestricted area—Area that people dressed in street clothes may enter.

Urinalysis (UA)—The study of a urine specimen to diagnose or rule out certain medical conditions.

U.S. Pharmacopeia (USP)—A compendium of standards for drugs approved by the Food and Drug Administration for their labeled use. All approved drugs have been tested for consumer safety, and written information is available about their pharmacological action, use, risks, and dosage.

Uterine manipulator—A probelike instrument that is inserted into the distal cervix and used to reposition the uterus during gynecological endoscopic procedures.

UTI—Urinary tract infection.

Uvulopalatopharyngoplasty—A procedure in which the tonsils, uvula, and a portion of the soft palate are removed to reduce and stiffen the excess oropharyngeal and oral-cavity tissue in patients with obstructive sleep apnea or snoring.

Values—Beliefs, customs, behaviors, and norms that a person defends and upholds.

Vasoconstriction—Narrowing of blood vessels, caused by hormones, drugs, or some other source.

Vector—A living intermediate carrier of microorganisms from one host to another. An example is the transmission of the bubonic plague. The vector is a flea, and the bacterium is transmitted to the human by a bite from an infected flea. Fleas may cause a similar disease in rodents.

Ventilation—Movement of gases into and out of the lungs. Positive pressure ventilation is produced by the anesthesia care provider when deep general anesthesia and neuromuscular blocking agents inhibit the patient's normal breathing mechanisms. The reservoir bag on the anesthesia machine allows the anesthesia care provider to manually force oxygen or gases into the patient's lungs. This is called "bagging" the patient.

Ventral hernia—See *Incisional hernia.*

Ventricle(s)—A small chamber of the brain containing cerebrospinal fluid; the lower right and left chambers of the heart.

Veress needle—A long, slender needle inserted through the abdominal wall to deliver carbon dioxide gas during the creation of pneumoperitoneum.

Vertebra—A bony segment of the spinal column.

Vertebral lamina—A pair of broad plates of bone flaring out from the vertebral body to form an arch that provides a base for the spinous process of the vertebrae.

Virucidal—Able to kill viruses.

Virulence—The degree to which a microorganism is capable of causing disease.

Virus—A genetic element containing either DNA or RNA that replicates in cells but is characterized by having an extracellular state. It is parasitic in that it is entirely dependent on nutrients inside cells for its metabolic and reproductive needs. They differ from other microbes in that they cannot reproduce their genetic material, but must produce within a living host.

Visualization—A surgical term that means to "see directly."

Vital signs—Basic diagnostic indicators that help to immediately assess life-threatening situations. Vital signs include temperature, pulse, respirations, and blood pressure.

Vitreous humor—A transparent, colorless gel that normally fills the eyeball in front of the retina.

Voltage—The electrical force that drives electrons from one point to another (measured in volts).

Washer-sterilizer—Equipment that washes and sterilizes instruments after an operative procedure.

Wavelength—The distance from the peak of one wave to the peak of the next wave.

Wedge resection—The surgical removal of a small, sometimes pie-shaped portion of the liver. Also the surgical removal of a section of a lobe of the lung. See *Nonanatomical resection.*

White blood cell (WBC) count—A test that identifies the absolute number of white blood cells in a specimen. The test may be combined with a differential count to identify the numbers of each specific type of white blood cell present. This may be expressed as WBC w/diff.

White matter—Nervous tissue covered by a myelin sheath. This is the conductive tissue of the brain and spinal cord.

Win-lose—In conflict resolution, a situation in which one party is satisfied but the other finds the solution unsatisfactory.

Win-win—In conflict resolution, a situation in which both parties in a conflict gain by the solution.

X-ray—Any test that uses x-rays to record a picture of structures or objects within the body. A standard x-ray often is called a *flat-plate x-ray* to differentiate it from fluoroscopy, which uses continuous x-ray exposure to generate a picture.

Xylocaine—Medication used to reduce ventricular arrhythmias. Also known as *lidocaine.*

Index